Fritz Schajowicz

Tumors and Tumorlike Lesions of Bone

Pathology, Radiology, and Treatment

With Contributions by
M. Sundaram, S. Gitelis, and D.J. McDonald

Foreword by Jorge O. Galante

2nd edition

With 635 Figures in 1526 Separate Illustrations
Some in Color

Springer-Verlag
Berlin Heidelberg New York
London Paris Tokyo
Hong Kong Barcelona
Budapest

Fritz Schajowicz, M.D.

Head, W.H.O. Collaborating Center for the Histological Definition and Classification of Bone Tumors

Former Professor of Pathology, National University of Buenos Aires and Director of the Latin American Registry of Bone Pathology, Buenos Aires, Argentina

Professor of Pathology, Department of Orthopedic Surgery, St. Louis University Medical Center, St. Louis, Missouri, U.S.A.

Visiting Distinguished Professor, Rush-Presbyterian-St. Luke's Medical Center, Chicago, Illinois, U.S.A.

ISBN 978-3-642-49956-2 ISBN 978-3-642-49954-8 (eBook)
DOI 10.1007/978-3-642-49954-8

Library of Congress Cataloging-in-Publication Data
Schajowicz, Fritz. Tumors and tumorlike lesions of bone: pathology, radiology, and treatment / Fritz Schajowicz, with contributions by M. Sundarum, S. Gitelis, and D.J. McDonald; foreword by Jorge O. Galante. – 2nd ed. p. cm. Rev. ed. of: Tumors and tumor-like lesions of bone and joints. c1981. Includes bibliographical references and index. ISBN 3-540-55366-5 (Berlin: alk. paper). – ISBN (invalid) 0-378-55366-5 (New York: alk. paper) 1. Bones–Tumors. 2. Joints–Tumors. 3. Bones–Diseases. 4. Joints–Diseases. I. Schajowicz, Fritz. Tumors and tumor-like lesions of bone and joints. II. Title. [DNLM: 1. Bone Neoplasms. 2. Connective Tissue Diseases. 3. Joint Diseases. WE 258 S296t] RC280.B6S32 1992 616.99'271–dc20 DNLM/DLC for Library of Congress 92-49404 CIP

Softcover reprint of the hardcover 2nd edition 1994

Typesetting: Best-set Typesetter Ltd., Hong Kong

21/3130-5 4 3 2 1 – Printed on acid-free paper

To the memory of my teacher and mentor, the eminent Viennese Pathologist Professor Jakob Erdheim, and to Professors José Valls and Carlos E. Ottolenghi (Buenos Aires, Argentina).

To my wife, Adela, for her patience and constant encouragement, and to my daughters, Monica and Graciela.

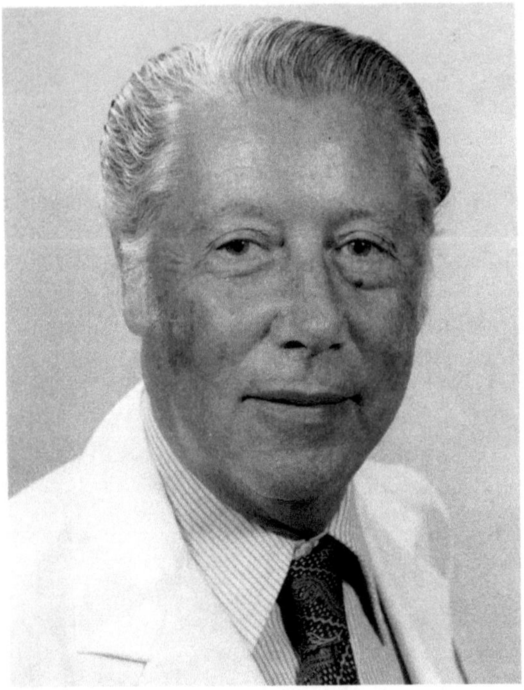

Fritz Schajowicz knew but one goal: ever to deepen our knowledge of bone tumors. To this end he devoted his life and soul, working without haste but without pause and thus coming to excel in diagnosis, treatment, and prognosis. The knowledge so assiduously gained he gladly imparted to "his boys," young doctors from the world over, in lectures delivered with transparent clarity and distinguished by his permanent good humor. With his wisdom and insight he brought hope and inspiration to all who work in this difficult field. His contribution has been unique; his will be an abiding presence.

ADELA M. CASTILLO SCHAJOWICZ

Contents

With contributions by

MURALI SUNDARAM, M.D., F.R.C.R.
Professor of Radiology, St. Louis University
Chief of Diagnostic Radiology, St. Louis University Hospital

STEVEN GITELIS, M.D.
Associate Professor of Orthopaedic Oncology, Rush Medical College
Director, Section of Orthopaedic Oncology,
Rush-Presbyterian-St. Luke's Medical Center,
Chicago, Illinois, U.S.A.

DOUGLAS J. MCDONALD, M.D.
Associate Professor of Orthopedic Surgery, St. Louis University
Head, Section of Orthopedic Oncology,
St. Louis University Medical Center, St. Louis, Missouri, U.S.A.

Foreword to the Second Edition

It was with great pleasure that I accepted the offer to write this foreword to the second edition of *Tumors and Tumorlike Lesions of Bone* by Professor Fritz Schajowicz. Sadly, since this book was completed, the news of Professor Schajowicz's untimely death was received. He lived his life fully and dedicated it without compromise to the advancement of science in the field of musculoskeletal pathology. This book serves as a wonderful tribute to all that Prof. Fritz Schajowicz stood for; he was a unique individual and a close personal friend.

The contributions of Professor Schajowicz to our knowledge of bone and joint pathology are second to none. A native of Vienna, he was a disciple of Professor Jakob Erdheim, a pioneer in the field of musculoskeletal pathology. He trained under him as a student and young doctor until the master's premature death in 1937. In 1938 he moved on to Italy to become the Director of the Pathology Laboratory at the Rizzoli Orthopedic Institute in Bologna, which was then under the direction of another eminent figure, Professor Vittorio Putti. As the drama and tragedy of the Second World War began to unfold, Professor Schajowicz moved to Buenos Aires, Argentina, where he began a distinguished career in 1939. He worked closely there with two orthopedic surgeons of international fame, Professor Jose Valls and Professor Carlos Ottolenghi. He was later appointed Professor of Pathology at the University of Buenos Aires and then became the head of the Pathology Department at the Italian Hospital, a position that he held until 1986. At the Italian Hospital Dr. Schajowicz established a center for bone and joint pathology which served as the nucleus for the Latin American Registry of Bone Pathology, a superb collection which numbered 5274 tumors and 1665 tumorlike lesions of bone by the time he finished his work as head of the Registry at the end of 1985. This unique material, which represents part of Professor Fritz Schajowicz's personal experience in the field, served as the basis for the information and provided all of the statistical data presented in the book.

I met Professor Schajowicz in Gothenberg, Sweden, in 1965, when I had the privilege of collaborating with him and Professor Carl Hirsch in the preparation of a manuscript dealing with degenerative lesions of the cervical spine. That collaboration developed into personal friendship and gave rise to continuing professional contacts. We were fortunate that from 1977 onward, Professor Schajowicz served as a Visiting Professor in our Institution. Through the years he contributed immensely to the education of our residents, fellows, and attending staff and participated in the care of our patients with musculoskeletal lesions. In 1986, Professor Schajowicz retired from his position in Buenos Aires and accepted a post as Professor of Pathology at St. Louis University.

In the course of his professional career, Dr. Schajowicz was the recipient of many honors and distinctions. He was appointed the Director of the International Reference Center for Histopathological

Diagnosis of Bone Tumors and Allied Diseases of the World Health Organization and in that position he had the responsibility for developing, in collaboration with Drs. Ackerman and Sissons, a classification and definition of bone tumors and tumorlike lesions of bone which was published in 1972 under the title *Histological Typing of Bone Tumors*. The classification has recently been updated in collaboration with Dr. L.H. Sobin and it is followed in this most recent edition of his book.

In 1990 Professor Schajowicz returned to his native Vienna to preside over the inauguration of the recently renovated Jakob Erdheim Institute of Pathology. In a special solemn ceremony the government leaders of Vienna also presented Dr. Schajowicz with a golden medal of honor, the highest distinction conferred by Vienna for cultural and scientific merit: in this case for research into and teaching of bone pathology at the international level.

On the occasion of his being in Vienna, the Faculty of Medicine of the University of Vienna granted Dr. Schajowicz a new diploma of Doctor of Medicine, fifty years after his graduation from that institution, as well as a bronze medal given in honor of Professor Rokitansky, first full professor of anatomic pathology at the University of Vienna. These are singular distinctions for outstanding scientific accomplishment by a physician and had a particular emotional and personal value for Professor Schajowicz.

The first edition of this book, which was published in 1981, was written while the author spent a year of sabbatical leave at our Institution. That book received universal acceptance and has served for the last 10 years as the major reference text dealing with tumors and tumorlike lesions of bone. Dr. Rodney Sweetman, reviewing it for the *Journal of Bone and Joint Surgery*, said "I know of no better book on bone tumors," while Dr. Jonathan Cohen called it "the most useful of all available texts on bone tumors." The first edition used the WHO classification and definition of primary bone tumor and tumorlike lesions of bone, and, as mentioned above, this second edition likewise employs the classification, though in its revised form. As in the first edition, the clinical aspects, including diagnosis and treatment of the lesions, are incorporated in the text so that a complete perspective is presented, characteristic of the approach that Professor Schajowicz took in his evaluation of these lesions. The use of new imaging and diagnostic techniques is incorporated, as well as the new concepts involving the staging and treatment of malignant and aggressive bone tumors.

This book will remain the standard text and reference material in the field. It belongs in the library of every orthopedic surgeon and pathologist interested in this particular area of medicine.

I am very grateful for having had the opportunity of writing this foreword. I admired Professor Schajowicz for his unique professional qualifications, for his capacity as a teacher, and for the contributions that he made to this field of medicine. Most of all I admired his enthusiasm, his joy at participating and undertaking new projects and responsibilities, his warmth as an individual and as a personal friend.

JORGE O. GALANTE, M.D.
The William A. Hark, M.D. – Susanne G. Swift Professor and Chairman
Department of Orthopedic Surgery
Rush-Presbyterian-St. Luke's Medical Center

Preface to the Second Edition

More than ten years have elapsed since the publication of the first edition of *Tumors and Tumorlike Lesions of Bone and Joints* in 1981. During this period significant progress has been made in diagnosis, and particularly in staging and treatment of bone tumors. In most centers, limb-sparing surgery has replaced the more radical ablative surgery, with or without preoperative chemotherapy. This became possible due to the introduction and increased application of newer high-quality imaging techniques (CT and MRI) and in particular the use of new cytomorphologic methods of diagnosis, especially immunohistochemistry. These advances in diagnosis and treatment have been reflected by the publication of new editions of several important textbooks, since their authors – pathologists, orthopedic surgeons, and radiologists – felt the necessity of updating their works in recent years. However, in these publications different criteria of classification were adopted. The number of cases compiled at the Latin American Registry of Bone Pathology increased from 4913 primary bone tumors and more than 1100 tumorlike lesions at the time of publication of the first edition of this book, to 5274 bone tumors and 1665 tumorlike lesions by the end of December 1985, when I finished my work as head of the Registry and occupied the positions of Professor of Orthopedic Pathology at St. Louis University Medical Center and Distinguished Visiting Professor at Rush-Presbyterian-St. Luke's Medical Center in Chicago. The material of the Registry has been computerized, and that has permitted me to update the statistical data for use in this new edition.

During recent years the WHO classification and definition of primary bone tumors and tumorlike lesions has been revised by a group of internationally renowned specialized pathologists, headed by this author and a representative of WHO, Dr. L.H. Sobin. The revised classification is now in press with this same publisher (Springer-Verlag) and has been followed in this edition of *Tumors and Tumorlike Lesions of Bone*, as it was in the first edition.

However, some modifications of the original classification were necessary. A limited number of new tumor entities have been included: aggressive (malignant) osteoblastoma, benign and malignant fibrous histiocytoma, primary neuroectodermal tumor, and leiomyosarcoma of bone. Moreover, some existing entities have been subdivided into separate variants because their distinctive histopathologic features are often associated with a different biologic behavior and prognosis, as in the subdivision of osteosarcoma into different surface and central variants. The group of small round-cell tumors has been redefined and discussed at length in the light of the newer classifications, the term "primary reticulum-cell sarcoma of bone" being replaced with "primary malignant lymphoma." The possible neural origin of Ewing sarcoma and its relationship to other tumors with neural features [neuroblastoma and primary neuroectodermal tumor of bone (PNET)] was the object of special interest.

Likewise, to the original group of tumorlike lesions have been added: "intraosseous epidermoid cyst" and "giant-cell (reparative) granuloma" (also called "giant-cell reaction") of short tubular bones of hands and feet.

In general, the framework and concept of the original classification, which was widely accepted, remains essentially the same. It is based on histologic criteria, particularly the type of differentiation shown by the tumor cells and the type of intercellular material they produce. This scheme of nomenclature and classification has proven to be justified because it permits useful prediction of the behavior of the individual cases to which it is applied.

Several illustrations (radiographs and photographs) have been eliminated, and have been replaced by many new figures, often in full color, and particularly illustrating the features shown by the new imaging methods. Only a few electronmicrographs and special immunohistochemical stains, relevant for diagnosis, have been included, because these methods are still of limited value in routine bone tumor diagnosis. A number of the new illustrations correspond to cases observed in St. Louis and Chicago. However, these cases were not included in our statistical data, which are exclusively those of the Latin American Registry of Bone Pathology.

The reference list pertaining to the Introduction is immediately preceded by a list of general references including most well-known textbooks and some comprehensive general articles. Moreover, the reference lists for each chapter have been supplemented by newer articles published since 1980. Besides containing all the references cited in the text, each list includes other important works that may be of interest to the reader.

I am grateful to Dr. Steven Gitelis, Chief of the Division of Oncology in the Department of Orthopedic Surgery at Rush-Presbyterian-St. Luke's Medical Center in Chicago, and Dr. Douglas McDonald, Orthopedic Oncologist of the Department of Orthopedic Surgery at St. Louis University Medical Center in St. Louis, who both generously accepted the difficult task of writing a new chapter updating the principles of staging and treatment of malignant and aggressive bone tumors. I am also deeply indebted to Dr. Murali Sundaram, Chief and Professor of Diagnostic Radiology at St. Louis University Medical Center, who will discuss the indications and diagnostic possibilities of the imaging techniques, at present of fundamental importance for precise staging and correct treatment of bone tumors.

I owe a special debt of gratitude to Professor Robert Burdge, Chairman of the Department of Orthopedic Surgery of St. Louis University Medical Center, for his continuous support and encouragement. He provided me with the necessary financial backing and the opportunity to dedicate a great part of my time to the preparation and completion of this book.

My deep appreciation is given to Bonnie Sabin for her unfailing and skillful assistance in completing the statistical computerized data, and for language editing and word processing the manuscript.

I am greatly indebted to Dr. John Clohisy, Orthopedic Resident of the Department of Orthopedic Surgery at St. Louis University Medical

Center, for his efforts in updating the statistical data that accompany the text.

To the members of the Department of Biomedical Communications, especially Dr. Bill J. Briggs, Chairman, Cliff Pollack, Photography Supervisor, and Kären Engdorf and Kirsten Ellis, Biomedical Photographers, I express my appreciation for the expert preparation of many of the new illustrations.

I wish to thank the following editors and publishers for granting permission to reproduce illustrative material from my own publications, which are acknowledged in the corresponding legends: *The Journal of Bone and Joint Surgery* (British and American editions), J.B. Lippincott Company, *Clinical Orthopedics*, and the American Cancer Society (*Cancer*).

I am also indebted to the staff of my publisher, Springer-Verlag, for the care and efforts taken for the preparation of this edition, especially to William Day, Senior Medical Editor, and Elizabeth Corra, Managing Editor.

Fritz Schajowicz

Foreword to the First Edition

In the past 50 years considerable progress has been made in orthopedics and traumatology. One of the principal reasons for these advances has undoubtedly been the separation of these specialties from general surgery. Alongside this development the number of those devoted to the study and treatment of locomotor disabilities, who could formerly be counted on the fingers of one hand – at least in our country – has multiplied by thousands and even more have subspecialized. This accelerated growth has encouraged the sharpening of diagnostic skills, technical improvement, and the application of advances in other fields of medicine to orthopedics. However, paradoxically enough, one of the most important aspects of orthopedics, bone pathology, has not attracted enough specialists worldwide to handle the complex problems, encountered daily, that only an expert and experienced pathologist is capable of resolving.

Within the modern milieu, the personality and accomplishments of Professor Fritz Schajowicz stand out distinctly. Dr. Schajowicz, of Austrian origin, studied with Professor J. Erdheim of Vienna. Having afterwards been granted a fellowship to extend his knowledge of bone pathology at the Rizzoli Orthopedic Institute of Bologna under the direction of Professor Vittorio Putti, he complemented this work with the study of clinical orthopedics at that prestigious institution. In 1938, Professor Jose Valls visited the Rizzoli Institute and, recognizing the outstanding training of Professor Schajowicz, invited him to move to Argentina where we were in need of an expert pathologist. It has now been 40 years since Dr. Schajowicz joined our team, and his collaboration has been an invaluable aid.

Schajowicz is not only an eminent and expert pathologist and a keen investigator of intricate and complex tissue structures; he is also an excellent clinician, who knows the varying symptoms of lesions – their local, general and humoral reactions – and an expert interpreter of x-rays of lesions of the skeleton as well. It is for these reasons that Dr. Schajowicz does not accept any specimen for study in his Pathology Center that is not accompanied by its corresponding clinical history, laboratory test results, and x-rays, all of which are discussed with the attending surgeon.

Once settled in Buenos Aires, Dr. Schajowicz obtained grants and technical assistance from the World Health Organization and the National Institutes of Health of the United States. With this financial assistance and the aid of volunteers, he was able to set up a Center of Bone and Joint Pathology, the site of the Latin American Register of Bone Pathology, which began its activities in 1962 in the modest locale of the Italian Hospital of Buenos Aires.

So many cases requiring his opinion have come to this center that the collection of radiographs and photographs is enormous, and the

Latin American Register can be considered one of the most complete in the world. The accumulated material has been used not only for research but also for the instruction of many pathologists and orthopedists who want to deepen their knowledge of this difficult field of pathology.

Through the collaboration of Dr. Schajowicz, Professor José Valls and myself, a book was published in 1942 on puncture biopsy in bone lesions, describing a method that became so widely accepted that the number of aspiration biopsies performed and examined by the author of this book totals more than 8000. The most important statistic on aspiration biopsies of the vertebral bodies, now numbering 2200, is maintained at the Center of Bone Pathology. This biopsy technique, which we helped to standardize, is now used routinely throughout the world.

Dr. Schajowicz joined the Department of Pathological Anatomy of the Medical School of the University of Buenos Aires as an Associate Professor and spent three years there as a full professor before he resigned the post because, as a bone pathologist, he did not want to wander from his self-appointed path.

Because his accomplishments have been internationally acclaimed, the World Health Organization named him Head of the International Reference Center for Histo-Pathologic Diagnosis of Bone Tumors and Allied Diseases, collaborating with him an important group of specialists the world over. As they were intrigued by the diversity of opinion with respect to classification of primitive bone tumors, Dr. Schajowicz with Ackerman and Sissons established a classification system published by the World Health Organization, which has been translated into several languages and accepted worldwide.

Dr. Schajowicz has traveled the world, working as a fellow with Hirsch in Sweden on the pathology of the lumbar disc and the cervical spine, working with Trueta in Oxford, England, on osteoarthritis of the hip, teaching courses, lecturing, and above all displaying the abundant material he has collected in order to pass on his knowledge and share his ideas.

Having arrived at such heights in his profession, he has decided to publish this book, in which he summarizes his long, intense life's work. His total dedication to bone and joint pathology has been amply demonstrated by his many articles published in the most prestigious journals of the specialty. We do not hesitate to state that this work will be of fundamental use to pathologists, orthopedists and radiologists and we anticipate its great success.

I would like to give my personal thanks to Dr. Schajowicz for the irreplaceable collaboration that has been such a great help to us in solving the numerous cases sent to us for treatment. With the passing of the years we have established a friendship and mutual regard and it pleases me to recognize them now. Perhaps it is on this account that Dr. Schajowicz has distinguished me with the honor of writing this Foreword to his "masterwork," for which I owe him my gratitude.

Carlos E. Ottolenghi, M.D.
Professor Emeritus, School of Medicine
Department of Orthopedics and Traumatology
National University of Buenos Aires
Full Member, National Academy of Medicine

Preface to the First Edition

Diagnostic pathologists, orthopedic surgeons, and radiologists are often confronted with problems of the diagnosis and treatment of tumors of the locomotor system. It is especially for these groups that I have prepared this work. The experiences of many workers in this field are summarized here, but my personal concepts and experience during more than 40 years of continuous work in osteoarticular pathology are the basis of this book.

During a period of 37 years, 4913 primary bone tumors and over 1100 tumorlike lesions (among 19600 cases of orthopedic pathology) have been studied and documented in our laboratory, which in 1962 became the headquarters of the Latin American Registry of Bone Pathology and in 1965 became the International Reference Center of Bone Tumors of the World Health Organization. In order to limit the size of this volume, metastatic tumors of bone and tumors of jaws of specific odontogenic origin are excluded. On the other hand, I have included a chapter on the controversial group of pseudotumoral and neoplastic processes involving joints.

I have adopted and follow in this volume the World Health Organization classification and definitions of bone tumors, which I published in 1972 with L.V. Ackerman and H.A. Sissons, in collaboration with L.H. Sobin and H. Torloni. This classification, based on histologic criteria, includes benign and malignant neoplasms, primary in bone. Certain tumorlike processes are also included because of their frequent clinical and histologic similarity to bone tumors. Since 1972, only slight modifications of this classification have been necessary, for example, the addition of a few new tumor entities, some of which are still controversial ("malignant osteoblastoma" and "malignant fibrous histiocytoma of bone").

The diagnosis of a bone lesion should be established in every case by combined clinical-radiologic and pathologic investigations. Therefore, clinical, especially radiologic features are described and illustrated extensively here. Preference is given, as far as possible, to the comparative study of the gross pathologic and radiographic appearance of the resection or amputation specimen, preferably of thin slabs of the specimen. The clinical features are complemented by detailed descriptions of the histology and are accompanied by numerous photomicrographs, several in full color, in order to facilitate the task of the practicing pathologist. Only a few electron-micrographs have been included, because electron microscopy as a routine method of bone tumor diagnosis is still of limited value.

For each tumor entity we have briefly commented on the most common and most convenient type of treatment presently in use at our and other specialized centers. The extensive bibliography will guide the interested reader to detailed studies in the literature; however, the rapid increase of original contributions in recent years, especially from the

United States, makes it practically impossible to do full justice to all authors.

Over 90% of the cases included in our statistics came from the various orthopedic departments in Argentina. A limited number of cases referred from other countries are included because of their rarity or special interest, but this does not modify our statistical data greatly. We had also at our disposal the data from the Registry of the Chilean Orthopedic Society, the Committee of Bone Tumors of Uruguay, and from two centers in Brazil dedicated primarily to the study of bone tumors, headed by Dr. Donato de Prospero and Dr. C. Lemos; their kindness and cooperation is gratefully acknowledged. Their figures are very similar to ours and confirm our data on the incidence and relative frequency of the different tumor types.

FRITZ SCHAJOWICZ

Acknowledgments

I wish to express my gratitude to the late professor and chairman of the Department of Orthopedic Surgery of the University of Buenos Aires, Professor José Valls, who gave me the opportunity to equip and organize a laboratory dedicated exclusively to diagnosis and research in orthopedic pathology. After the retirement of Professor Valls, I continued my work under his successor, Professor C.E. Ottolenghi, who during many years of close cooperation contributed his unfailing enthusiasm and friendship to the function of our laboratory, which later became a separate entity, the Center of Osteoarticular Pathology, open to the contribution of all physicians.

I am greatly indebted to my colleagues of the Italian Hospital (Buenos Aires) and to the many orthopedic surgeons in Argentina and other countries, who sent their cases to our Center and granted the use of their material for this and previous publications.

My grateful acknowledgment goes to my colleague and friend, Dr. R.L. Cabrini, for many years of close and fruitful cooperation in orthopedic pathology research, the result of which are the many articles published in this field.

I have a special debt of gratitude to my wife Adela, who since the foundation of the Latin American Registry of Bone Pathology and during more than ten years of indefatigable and enthusiastic cooperation was responsible for its organization and administrative work, thus making the statistical and graphic documentation of this volume possible.

I want to express my appreciation to Dr. E.H. Santini Araujo, who, working under a fellowship of the Argentine Orthopedic Society in my laboratory, has spared no effort in the accumulation of the statistical data that accompany the text.

My thanks to the staff of my laboratory for their unfailing assistance, in particular to the secretary, Mrs. P. Benjuia, the technicians, Mrs. A. Sens and Mrs. S. Turano, and the photographer L. Lobos. I owe a special acknowledgment for the efforts and skillful help of our photographer H.H. Busani, who made the great majority of the excellent gross photographs and reproduced the radiographs and photomicrographs.

The final preparation and publication of this book was made possible by the invaluable encouragement and support of Dr. J. Galante, Chairman of the Department of Orthopedic Surgery of the Presbyterian – St. Lukes Medical Center, and by the financial help of his department and that of the Department of Pathology, directed by Professor R. Wainstein: to both my deep appreciation. Working at this medical center for 14 months as Visiting Professor, I received the efficient collaboration of the medical and technical staff and especially of Dr. D. Petasnick of the Radiology Department.

My debt of gratitude goes to the Technical Administrator of the Department of Orthopedics, Mr. R. Urban, and to the secretaries Mrs. Aerelia Hill and Miss Sue Crow for their careful preparation of a great part of the manuscript. To Mr. Charles Hover of the Medical Illustration Services of the Rush Medical College goes my appreciation for the careful preparation of many of the illustrations.

I warmly acknowledge Dr. H. Torloni, former medical officer of W.H.O.'s Cancer Unit, who participated in every phase of the preparation of the bone tumor classification and the work of our Reference Center, and his successor, Dr. L.H. Sobin, for his encouragement and for obtaining W.H.O.'s permission to use part of the photographic material.

My special thanks go to the following editors and publishers for granting permission to reproduce illustrative material from my own publications which are acknowledged in the corresponding legends: The Journal of Bone and Joint Surgery (British and American editions), American Cancer Society, Inc. (Cancer), Acta Orthopaedica Scandinavica, J.B. Lippincott Company (Clinical Orthopedics), and Butterworths Scientific Publications, London.

I am greatly indebted to my publishers for their careful attention to this volume, especially to Larry Carter and Berta Steiner for their untiring efforts.

FRITZ SCHAJOWICZ

Introduction

Among the wide variety of human tumors, primary bone tumors are comparatively rare, which explains why only a few centers have been able to collect an appreciable number of cases. A major factor in the progress in the study of bone tumors was the establishment in many countries (Holland, Sweden, England, Japan, Latin America, and others) of regional tumor centers or registries, following the American example. Having centralized data collection centers makes it possible to assemble in a relatively short time abundant material that can be used in standardizing terminology and diagnosis, in carrying out research and epidemiologic studies, and above all in teaching and training medical specialists. The latter task is of fundamental importance because the majority of pathologists have little opportunity to acquire sufficient experience with this group of skeletal lesions, the study of which, moreover, requires technical expertise not possessed by all of them.

It is difficult to obtain accurate figures for the overall incidence of bone tumors because most of the available statistical data are compiled from death certificates, which do not specify the type of tumor. From an analysis of the reported cancer deaths in the United States for 1948, Steiner estimated that primary bone tumors constituted about 1% of all fatal malignant tumors. In Great Britain, approximately the same incidence of primary bone tumors was obtained from mortality figures for 1950–1954 (MacKenzie et al. 1961), an incidence of 0.8%–0.9%. A later United States statistic (Miller 1976; Young and Miller 1975) indicated that they account annually for 1.87 deaths per million children under 14 years of age, a figure that rises to 11.96 deaths per million among people between 15 and 19 years of age. More recently the National Cancer Institute of Washington, D.C. (1983–1985) reported an estimated figure of 2100 (1200 males and 900 females) new bone cancer cases among a total of 1 010 600 cancers of all sites. Information on the relative frequencies of different types of primary malignant bone tumors in the various national series may be influenced by an unrepresentative selection of cases and by the way in which the diagnostic definitions are applied (Miller and Dalager 1974). However, a comparison of different series, e.g., from Britain, Holland, the United States (cases treated at the Mayo Clinic, 1909–1977), and Japan (cases from the Bone Tumor Registry, 1966), shows a close similarity between the figures.

Glass and Fraumeni (1970) (United States) examined the death certificates of all children under 15 years of age (n = 1532) who died from these neoplasms between 1960 and 1966 for type of tumor, race, and sex, and found an average annual mortality among white children of 3.04 deaths per million as contrasted with 2.26 among nonwhite children. Among children 15–19 years old during 1965–1966, the corresponding bone tumor mortality rates were 9.93 for whites and 7.84 for nonwhites. This difference in the mortality rates for the two races was due mainly to the extremely low frequency of Ewing sarcoma in nonwhite individuals under 20 years of age. This discrepancy was subsequently demonstrated by others in the United States (Jensen and Drake 1970; Linden and Dunn 1970; Miller and Dalager 1974) and for blacks in Africa, who show a similar near absence of Ewing tumor (Williams 1975). Blacks thus appear to be genetically resistant to this form of bone neoplasia – an important point in differential diagnosis and in tumor etiology.

In general, we are only at the beginning of our research on etiology and pathogenesis. Therefore, the exchange of experience among different groups of investigators is vitally important to progress in this still obscure field. Although experimental and human pathologic evidence is more and more supportive of the hypothesis of the viral etiology of malignant bone tumors, at present a substantial dose of ionizing radiation is the only agent known to be a potential cause of bone cancer in man. It also appears possible that ionizing radiation is able to activate latent tumor viruses.

Despite recent advances, there is still considerable diversity of opinion regarding the histogenesis, nomenclature, classification, and treatment of bone tumors and tumorlike conditions. The close collaboration of research workers with the diagnostic pathologist and the clinician, and the application of modern methods such as histochemical studies, autoradiography, tissue cultures in vitro, genetic studies, fluorescent and electron microscopy, and more recently immunohistochemistry, flow cytometry, and new high-quality imaging techniques are bringing us closer to an understanding and interpretation of the vital processes occurring in skeletal tissue, as also to significant advances in the management of bone tumors.

Diagnosis of Bone Tumors

It is generally agreed that the diagnosis of a bone lesion should be approached from a dynamic standpoint with the pathologist working in close cooperation with the radiologist and orthopedic surgeon.

Although in some cases the diagnosis is readily established without a previous biopsy, there are others which remain a challenge even to the experienced pathologist with full knowledge of the clinicoradiologic features. The surgeon should be aware that there are cases in which the pathologist may find it difficult or is unable to make a definite diagnosis regarding a skeletal lesion.

There are a limited number of aggressive and malignant lesions, some of them recently added to the literature, which present serious, in part still unresolved problems of diagnosis, histogenesis, or classification even to the experienced pathologist.

These problems still persist in spite of the introduction of the newer imaging techniques (computed tomography, magnetic resonance imaging, scintigraphy) and the advances of the new cytomorphologic methods, including immunohistochemistry, study of cellular DNA content by laser-based flow cytometry, and cytogenetic chromosomal investigation.

Radiology is of great importance in the diagnosis of bone tumors. Radiographs should always be available to the pathologist, who should never make a definite diagnosis without knowing the radiologic features. It is also of fundamental importance in providing the pathologist with detailed clinical information (such as duration and type of symptoms, previous trauma or irradiation, pathologic fracture).

Bone reacts to the presence of neoplastic, metabolic, inflammatory, or other processes in two different ways: by new bone formation or by bone resorption. The two processes are often combined, one predominating over the other. The following points should be ascertained from a radiographic examination of a bone lesion:

1. Whether the lesion is monostotic or polyostotic
2. The type of bone affected (tubular or flat)
3. The site of the lesion with reference to the epiphysis, growth plate, metaphysis, or diaphysis, and with reference to its medullary, cortical, or juxtacortical location
4. An estimate of how much of the total length and circumference of the bone is affected
5. The presence or absence of adjoining soft tissue changes with particular mention of fascial planes, tumor tissue, etc.
6. The nature of any bone changes present (destructive or radiolucent of moth-eaten, permeative, or geographic type, proliferative, or mixed)
7. The character of the bony margins of the lesions (sharp, ill-defined, thick, thin, increased or decreased density)
8. The nature of any cortical bone changes, such as the involvement of medullary or periosteal surfaces, cortical invasion, pressure atrophy
9. The density of tumor tissue, with particular regard to the presence of calcification and its roentgenographic characteristics (solid, punctate, smoky)
10. The character of periosteal reaction (laminated or "onion peel," solid, sunburst, or Codman's triangle)

Radiographic techniques may vary in accordance with the nature of bone destruction or proliferation, as well as with the presence or absence of perifocal soft tissue changes.

The different special imaging procedures will be discussed in the following section by Dr. Murali Sundaram.

The Role of Imaging

Murali Sundaram

Since the previous edition of this textbook, magnetic resonance imaging (MRI) has been added to the array of imaging modalities for the evaluation of tumors of bone. This technique either complements, competes with, or replaces preexisting diagnostic modalities that include radiography, conventional tomography, scintigraphy, computed tomography (CT), and arteriography. In order that these imaging modalities are appropriately and judiciously employed, an understanding of their relative strengths, weaknesses, sensitivity, and specificity is required. Diagnosing and staging tumors of bone accurately, expeditiously, and cost-effectively must be the objective and this can be achieved only by applying a consistently logical approach in the evaluation of the tumor or tumorlike lesion of bone. Aside from imaging, it is important to have an appreciation of the staging system of musculoskeletal neoplasms (Enneking 1985), the rationale for staging before biopsy (Mankin et al. 1982), and therapeutic options based on location of tumor and histologic diagnosis.

The Relationship Between the Radiograph, Magnetic Resonance Imaging, and Computed Tomography

The radiograph remains not only the least expensive imaging modality but also the most reliable predictor of the histologic nature of a tumor or tumorlike lesion of bone (Sundaram and McLeod 1990). The importance of careful analysis of the radiograph and gleaning from it as much information as possible in conjunction with the patient's age, gender, and clinical presentation cannot be overemphasized. In our practice, further imaging and the choice of imaging procedure stem from the interpretation of the radiograph. If the interpreter is unable to offer a pertinent differential diagnosis from the radiograph, it is unlikely that further imaging will help. Discussion of individual radiographic features of tumor and tumor-like lesions of bone is beyond the scope of this chapter, but broadly speaking the outcome of radiographic interpretation may take one of the following four paths:

1. No further follow-up (examples: nonossifying fibroma, asymptomatic fibrous dysplasia)
2. Repeat radiography following a short interval (examples: simple bone cyst not requiring treatment, eosinophilic granuloma, enchondroma)
3. Immediate biopsy and treatment (examples: chondroblastoma, large symptomatic bone cyst, intracompartmental aneurysmal bone cyst)
4. Further imaging and staging either when the lesion is indeterminate and likely to be biopsied (examples: eosinophilic granuloma vs Ewing sarcoma; acute osteomyelitis vs Ewing sarcoma; enchondroma vs low-grade chondrosarcoma; tibial fibrous dysplasia vs adamantinoma) or when the nature of the lesion demands further staging (all primary malignant tumors of bone, nonmalignant lesions that require local staging such as giant-cell tumors, large aneurysmal bone cysts, and aggressive benign vertebral tumors)

Thus, not every lesion of bone requires further imaging but evaluations of some lesions of bone would be incomplete without further imaging.

If the radiograph suggests a primary malignant tumor of bone, an indeterminate lesion that merits biopsy, or a metastatic lesion, chest radiography, chest CT, and skeletal scintigraphy should be performed principally to establish whether the radiographic lesion is solitary or multiple and, if solitary, whether it is a primary or metastatic lesion of bone. If the scintiscan suggests multiple sites of disease, then appropriate radiographs would need to be obtained and a decision made as to the appropriate site of biopsy to establish a histologic diagnosis. When the solitary nature of a malignant-appearing tumor is confirmed, local staging of the tumor is carried out to determine intracompartmental extent, extracompartmental disease (if any), and the relationship of the tumor to critical neurovascular structures. CT and MRI, with their differing strengths and weaknesses, compete for this role (Sundaram and McLeod 1990).

Until the advent of MRI, CT was unchallenged in its role of staging tumors of bone. CT is superior in demonstrating calcification, periosteal reaction, and endosteal thinning, while MRI's superior contrast resolution has made it the ideal examination for evaluating the soft tissue extent of intramedullary bony disease and depicting the linear extent of intramedullary disease. MRI also has the advantage of providing pluridirectional imaging in axial, coronal, and sagittal planes, rendering a more precise and clinically acceptable set of images than the multiplicity of transaxial images offered by CT.

Uncertainty and unfamiliarity between the strengths and weaknesses of these modalities has resulted in both modalities often being used in

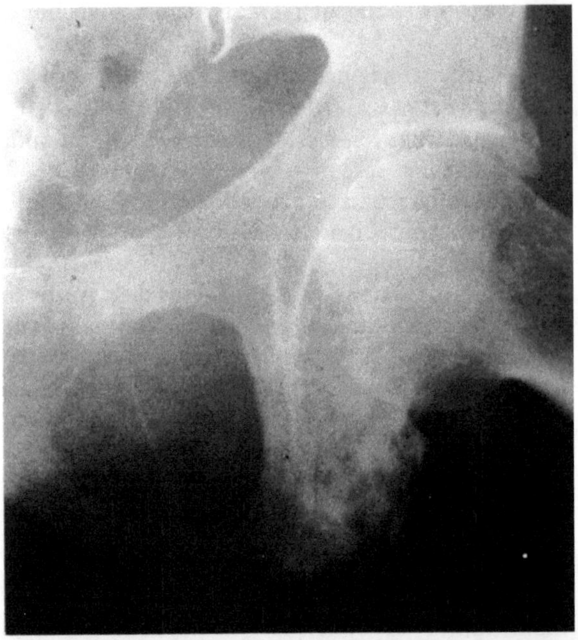

a

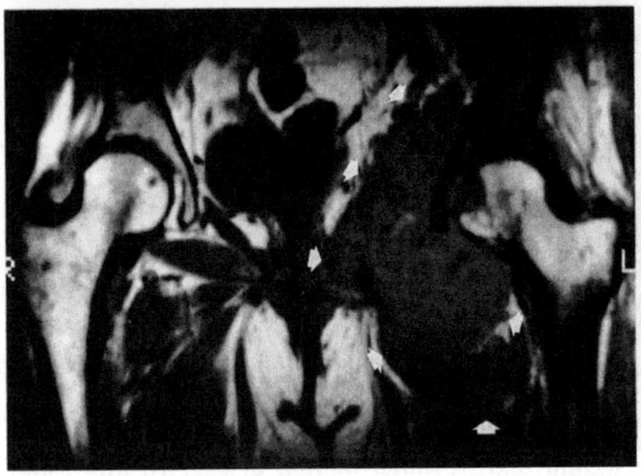

b

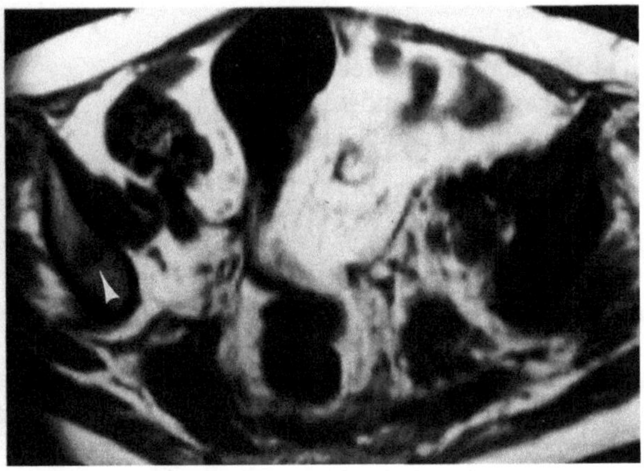

c

Fig. 1a–c. Lymphoma of the ischium. A 55-year-old woman presented with pain in the left hip. **a** Although the radiograph does not permit more than a differential diagnosis, the appearance of a sclerotic lesion in a symptomatic 60-year-old female led to the inclusion of metastases and lymphoma in the differential diagnosis. The lesion required biopsy. MR imaging was chosen to define the extraosseous extent of the lesion, if any. **b,c** Coronal and axial images demonstrate enormous soft tissue mass (*arrows*, *arrowhead*) entirely unsuspected from the clinical examination and radiograph (*arrows* in **b**). In addition, a lesion is seen on the contralateral side (*arrow* in **c**). The entire left iliac wing shows low signal (**b** and **c**) (compare with normal contralateral side), consistent with diffuse infiltration by lymphoma

redundant fashion. It has been our practice to let the radiograph determine which ought to be the next procedure (Sundaram and McGuire 1988; Sundaram and McLeod 1990). If the radiograph permits characterization of the lesion and a reasonably confident differential diagnosis is arrived at and further staging required, MRI is the examination of choice. If the radiograph does not permit adequate characterization of the lesion and probable diagnosis, CT is preferred to MRI because of its superior ability in permitting characterization of the lesion. Radiographic characterization of tumors in long bones is usually reliably made by radiography, whereas those very features appreciated in long bones, such as configuration, matrix, and outline, may only be partially evident when the tumor site is a flat bone, such as the pelvis, sternum, scapula, or rib. In the latter instances, CT is preferred to MRI. If a lesion in a flat bone is well characterized by radiography and requires further staging, MRI is preferred to CT because of its superior contrast resolution of the soft tissue extent of disease and the ease with which pluridirectional images are obtained (Fig. 1).

Computed tomography and MRI are usually competitive rather than complementary examinations despite their quite different imaging qualities and strengths. Although on occasion one examination may complement the other, such a circumstance should be the exception rather than the rule.

Most solitary tumors of bone that require biopsy and treatment occur in the peripheral

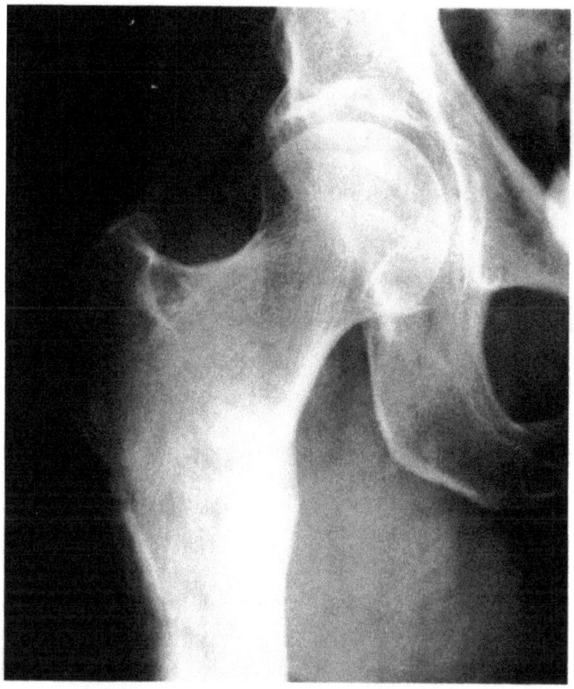

a

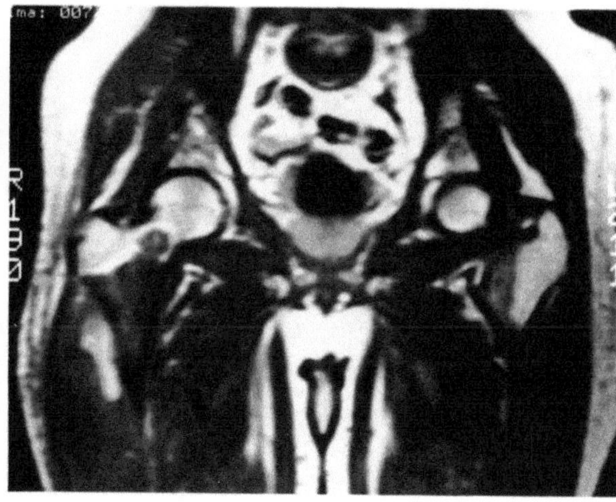

b

Fig. 2a,b. Malignant fibrous histiocytoma of the proximal femur. **a** Radiograph shows an ill-defined aggressive lesion in the proximal femoral shaft. **b** Coronal T1-weighted MR image shows that the proximal portion of the tumor extends into the femoral neck, a finding unsuspected on the radiograph. This feature resulted in the entire proximal femur, including the head, being resected as a part of the limb salvage procedure

skeleton. The optimal staging examination for tumors of the peripheral skeleton is MRI (Sundaram et al. 1986; Bohndorf et al. 1986; Pettersson et al. 1987; Bloem et al. 1988; Sundaram and McGuire 1988). The accuracy of MRI in depicting intramedullary and extraosseous disease and the relationship of tumor to critical neurovascular structures is superior to that of CT, despite CT's superiority in evaluating matrix, fine periosteal reactions, and cortical integrity. For most lesions in the peripheral skeleton, these latter three features are adequately demonstrated by radiography and since the step that follows radiographic diagnosis is staging, the single best examination for a tumor of the peripheral skeleton is MRI (Fig. 2).

In those instances when lesions of long bones are radiographically of indeterminate histology, such as enchondroma vs low grade chondrosarcoma, acute osteomyelitis vs Ewing sarcoma, or the rare instances of aneurysmal bone cyst mimicking telangiectatic osteosarcoma, MRI is undertaken not to aid in the diagnosis but rather to define the extent of intra- and extraosseous disease. In the above-mentioned scenarios, almost always the patient will come to biopsy and the rationale for MRI (staging) to precede biopsy lies in the fact that postbiopsy imaging can result in overestimation of tumor extent. When imaging (MRI or CT) follows biopsy it may be impossible to separate tumor from hemorrhagic tumor and postbiopsy hemorrhage or edema.

All giant-cell tumors of the peripheral skeleton (unless obviously intracompartmental) are staged by MRI (Fig. 3). Treatment of this relatively common tumor is either by aggressive curettage, which has a recurrence rate of approximately 30% (McDonald et al. 1986), or resection of the tumor with insertion of an allograft or prosthesis.

Surface Tumors

Surface tumors are well demonstrated by radiography and the type may be predicted from the radiograph. Surface tumors of the peripheral skeleton that are considered malignant or potentially malignant are staged by MRI (Fig. 4). The commonly encountered tumors are parosteal and periosteal osteosarcomas and juxtacortical chondrosarcomas. The exophytic extent of tumor is usually well demonstrated on the radiograph, but MRI is used to determine whether there is any intramedullary disease and to further define the soft tissue extent of the tumor and establish its relationship to surrounding neurovascular structures. On the basis of this information, limb salvage techniques are planned.

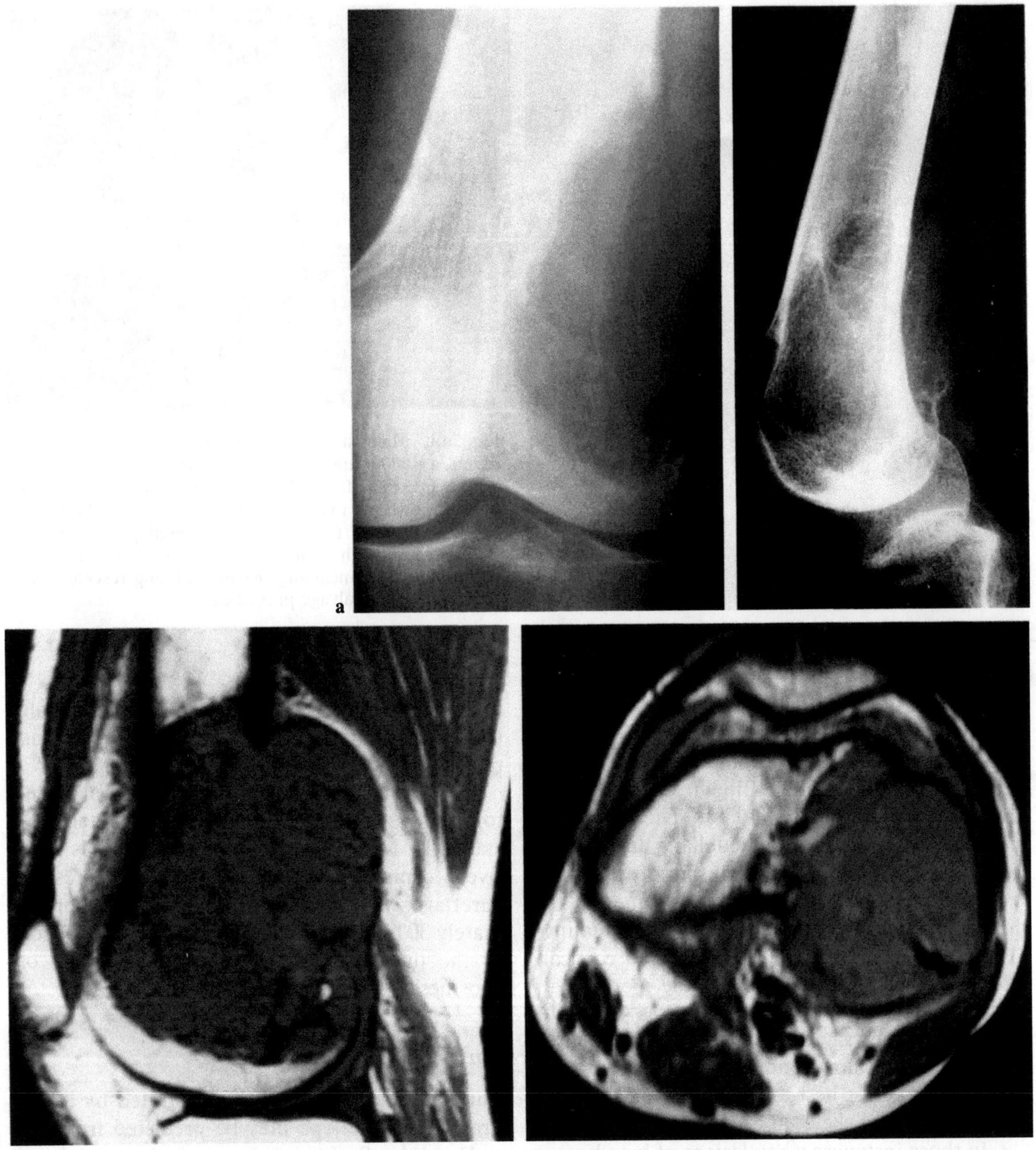

Fig. 3a–d. Giant-cell tumor of the distal femur. **a,b** Anteroposterior and lateral radiographs show an eccentric, aggressive, osteolytic lesion that has breached the cortex. **c,d** Coronal and axial T1-weighted images demonstrate the proximal and distal extent of the tumor and its subarticular location to the patellofemoral joint. The extraosseous component of the tumor appears well contained and has not infiltrated the subcutaneous fat and is separate from the popliteal vessels

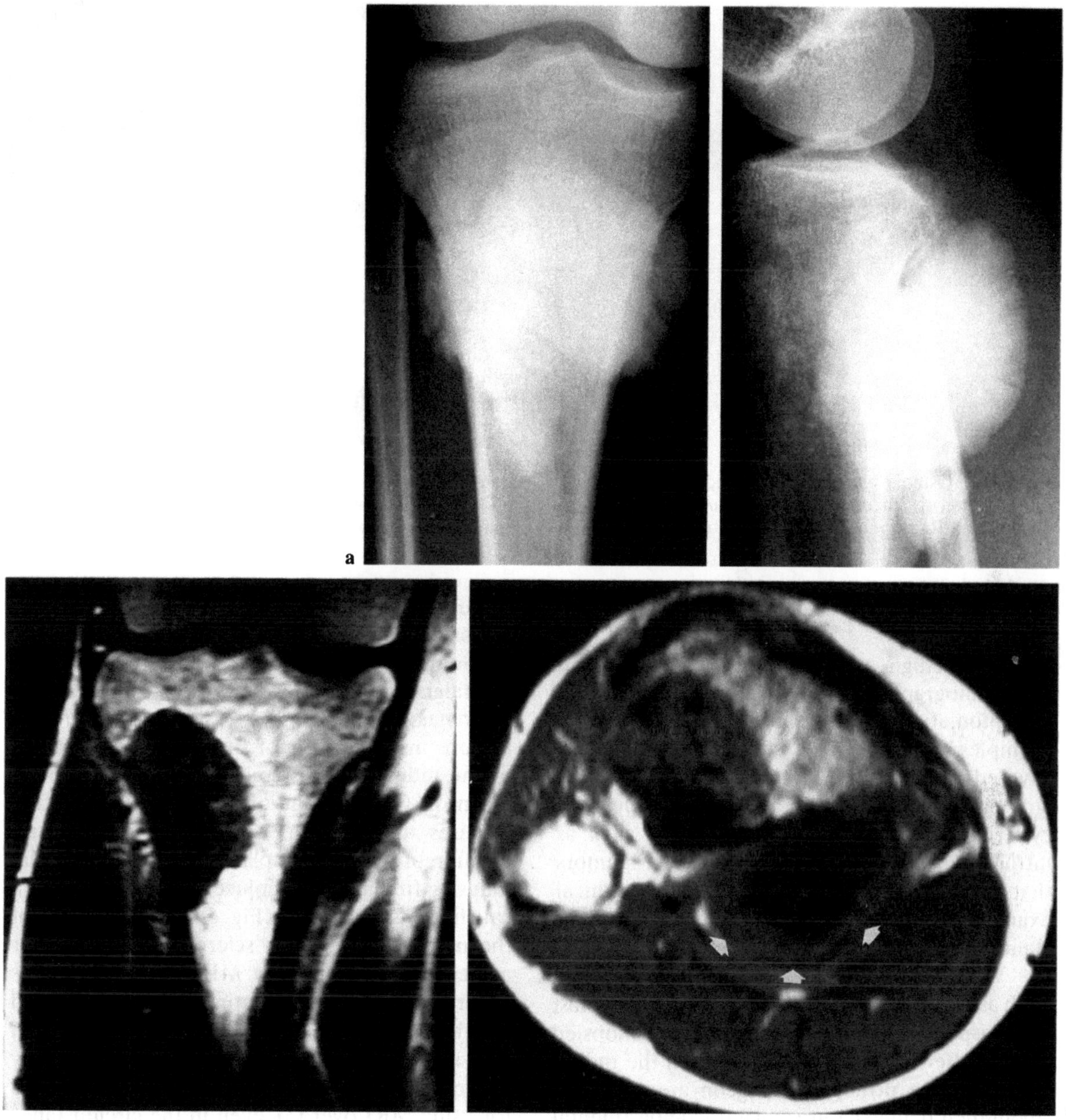

Fig. 4a–d. Surface osteosarcoma with unusual demonstration of intramedullary invasion. **a**,**b** Anteroposterior and lateral radiographs show a large, exophytic tumor with endosteal sclerosis seen on the lateral radiograph and small punctate areas of sclerosis more anteriorly in the medullary cavity of the tibia. The intraosseous extent of this tumor is inadequately defined on the radiographs. **c**,**d** Coronal and axial T1-weighted images demonstrate the intracompartmental extent of the tumor as a sharply defined low signal area against the high signal intensity marrow fat; **d** shows the low signal exophytic component (*arrows*) which is well demonstrated on the radiograph. The anterior extent of tumor involvement in the tibia is well shown on the axial image

a 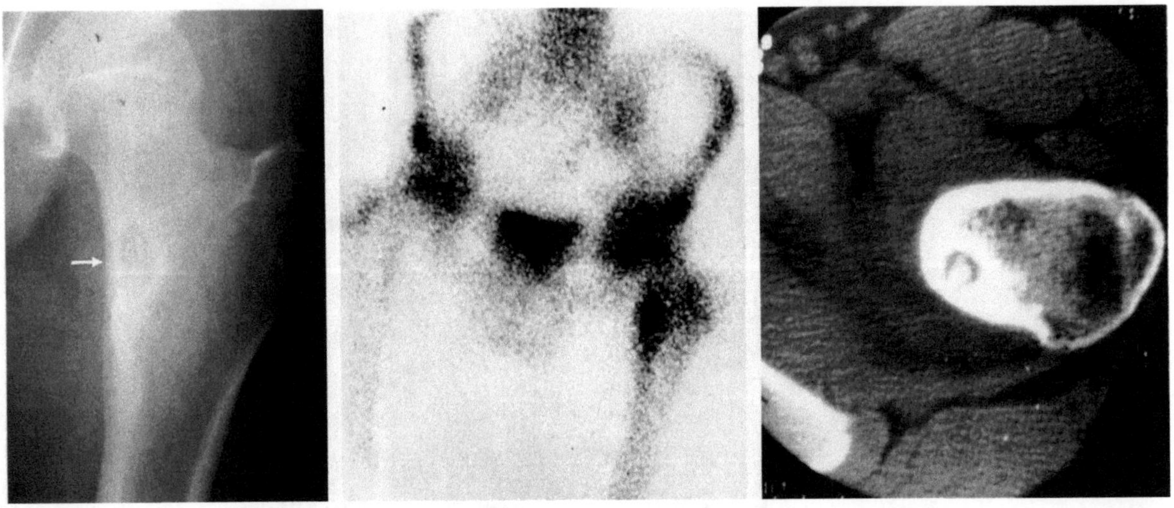 b, c

Fig. 5a–c. Osteoid osteoma of the medial femoral neck. **a** Focal sclerosis surrounding a nidus (*arrow*) suggests the diagnosis. **b** Radiotracer accumulation on the scintiscan is demonstrated at the site of radiographic abnormality. **c** The CT scan shows a calcific center within the radiolucent lesion representing the precise anatomic site of the nidus

Benign Tumors

Not all benign tumors need staging beyond the radiograph. Nonossifying fibromas and asymptomatic fibrous dysplasia are two common examples of bone tumors that often are discovered incidentally. The lesions are frequently ignored and merit no further staging. Simple bone cysts and other benign cystlike lesions such as intraosseous ganglia are examples of tumors that might be periodically observed by clinical examination and radiography and in those instances no further staging is required.

When clearly intracompartmental, lesions such as aneurysmal bone cysts, chondroblastomas, and suspected Brodie's abscess may be biopsied and curetted without further staging if the radiologist and the orthopedic surgeon are confident about their benign nature and intracompartmental confines. If the tumors are to be further staged, whether by CT or by MRI, the purpose is not to further characterize them but rather to determine whether there is extracompartmental disease. In such instances, MRI is the examination of choice. It is as important not to undertake unnecessary imaging as it is to carry out appropriate staging. If further imaging is clearly not going to change management, there is little purpose in an additional test.

In our practice, the sole circumstance where CT is consistently preferred to MRI in the peripheral skeleton is when the radiographic diagnosis of osteoid osteoma is favored. Osteoid osteomas may occur in the cortex, beneath the periosteum, or in the cancellous bone. When they are intracapsular, patients may present with arthralgia and when located in cortical bone, the osteomas may mimic a stress fracture or rarely a more malignant tumor of bone. Identification of the nidus of an osteoid osteoma clinches the diagnosis (Fig. 5). The orthopedic surgeon often requires assistance in ascertaining the precise location of the nidus in planning its removal. The nidus is frequently radiolucent and may have a calcific density within it (Fig. 5c). Identification of the nidus buried within sclerotic bone is better achieved by CT than by MRI because of CT's superiority in demonstrating calcification and also because of the better resolution it affords in demonstrating a radiolucent nidus surrounded by sclerotic bone. If, however, there is a preference for using MRI over CT even in the circumstance of evaluating an osteoid osteoma that certainly is acceptable so long as both imaging modalities are not used routinely.

Tumors in Flat Bones

Unlike the appendicular skeleton, lesions occurring in flat bones such as the pelvis, scapulae, ribs, and vertebrae are not as comprehensively or wholly characterized by radiography as tumors in long bones. This is because the lesion may be difficult to see in its entirety, its matrix may be difficult to examine, and uncertainty may exist

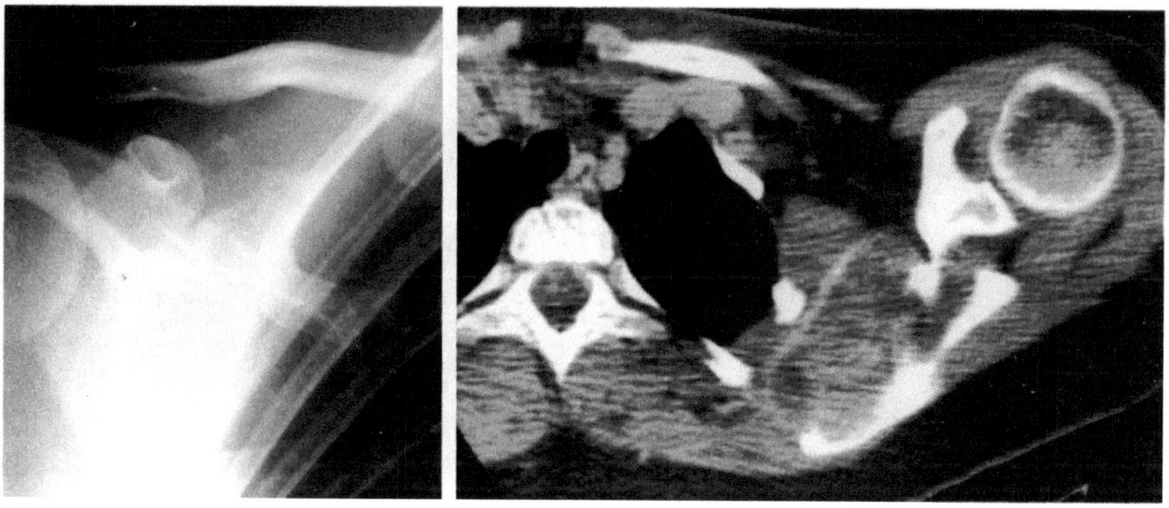

a b

Fig. 6a,b. Aneurysmal bone cyst of scapula. **a** Radiograph shows effacement of the spine of the scapula. The matrix, extent, and morphologic features of the lesion could not be better determined by x-rays. **b** CT scan shows the lesion to have a "blown out" appearance with a bony rim and several bony septa in the tumor. The appearances in an adolescent are consistent with an aneurysmal bone cyst

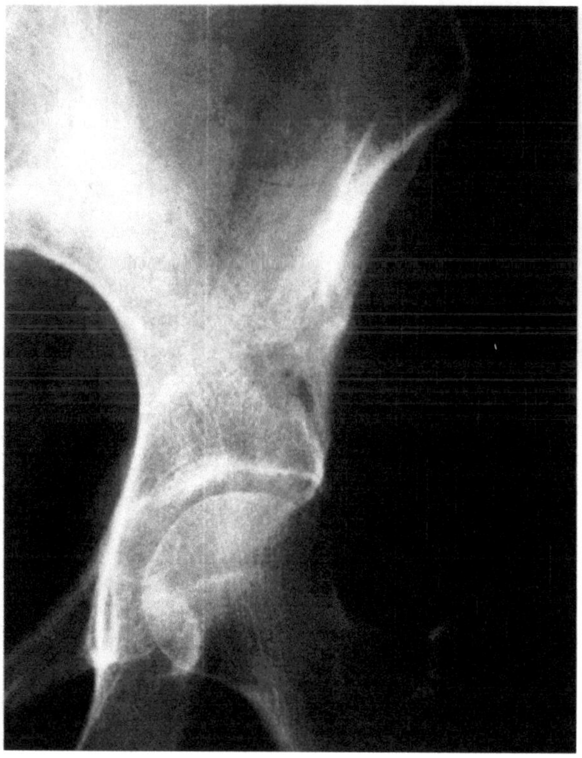

a

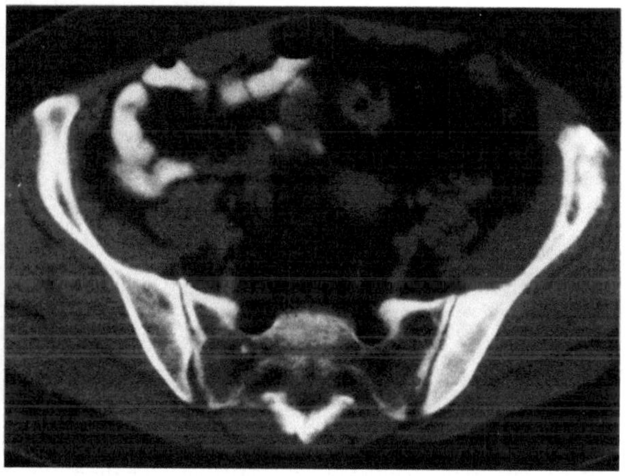

b

Fig. 7a,b. Lymphoma of the iliac wing. **a** Ill-defined lytic lesion is seen in the supra-acetabular region. **b** CT scan shows the lesion to be permeative without calcification and to have breached the cortex laterally

about its extent. When a radiologist is unable to characterize a lesion from the radiographs, it seems virtually impossible to offer a coherent, logical differential diagnosis. In those instances, CT is invaluable not only because of its ability to demonstrate the lesion in the axial plane but also because it permits the radiologist to analyze the matrix of the lesion and to determine whether it is expansile or permeative and whether it has calcification (Figs. 6–8). Once these features are defined and a differential diagnosis arrived at, a biopsy may be undertaken. For tumors in the pelvis, only rarely is MRI required to augment the CT appearances. However, for those rare

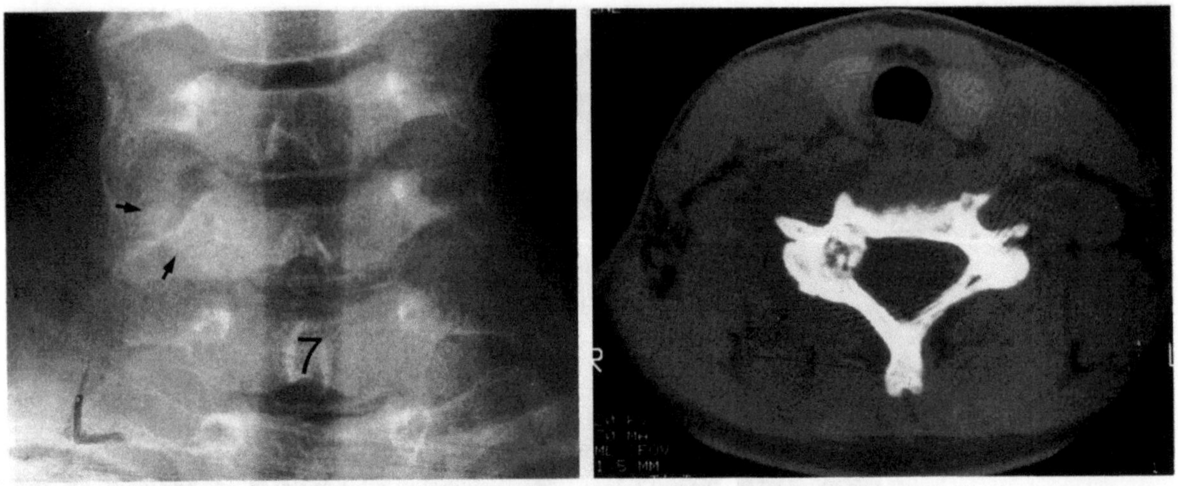

a b

Fig. 8a,b. Osteoblastoma of the cervical vertebra. **a** The pedicle of the right sixth cervical vertebra appears sclerotic. **b** CT scan shows the pedicle to be expanded with calcification within the lesion. This combination of findings favored an osteoblastoma over an osteoid osteoma or aneurysmal bone cyst

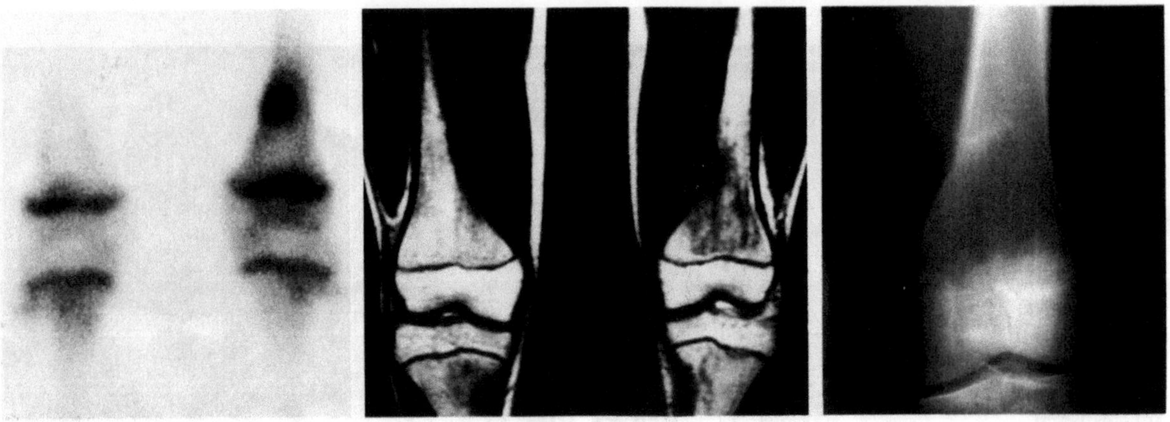

a b, c

Fig. 9a–c. A child was referred with a normal radiograph and an abnormal scintiscan and MRI examination for consideration of biopsy. **a** Focal area of increased radiotracer activity is seen on the scintiscan. **b** MRI demonstrates ill-defined, linear, low-signal areas in distal left femur. The appearances of the MRI and the constellation of findings did not suggest a primary malignant tumor of bone such as Ewing sarcoma. Biopsy was deferred and a repeat radiograph (**c**) shows periosteal reaction and a sclerotic band extending across the femoral shaft, consistent with a healing stress fracture

lesions that occur in vertebrae, ribs, and sternum, CT is augmented by MRI to demonstrate the relationship of extraosseous disease to the major vessels and spinal canal.

Normal or Marginally Abnormal Radiograph with MRI Abnormality

The combination of a normal radiograph, an abnormal scintiscan, and an abnormal MR image in a symptomatic patient can be confusing (Sundaram and McDonald 1989; Sundaram and McLeod 1990). Difficulty arises in knowing which of the examinations to rely on for the exclusion of a tumor. In these instances, the age of the patient, the morphologic appearance of the signal abnormality in the medullary cavity of the bone, and the appearance of soft tissue mass, if present, may all help in arriving at an accurate diagnosis. When the aforementioned constellation of findings (normal radiograph, presence of symptoms, and abnormal scintiscan and MRI examination) occur in an adolescent, the most likely diagnosis is a stress fracture (Fig. 9). Tumors that can present with this constellation of findings in the

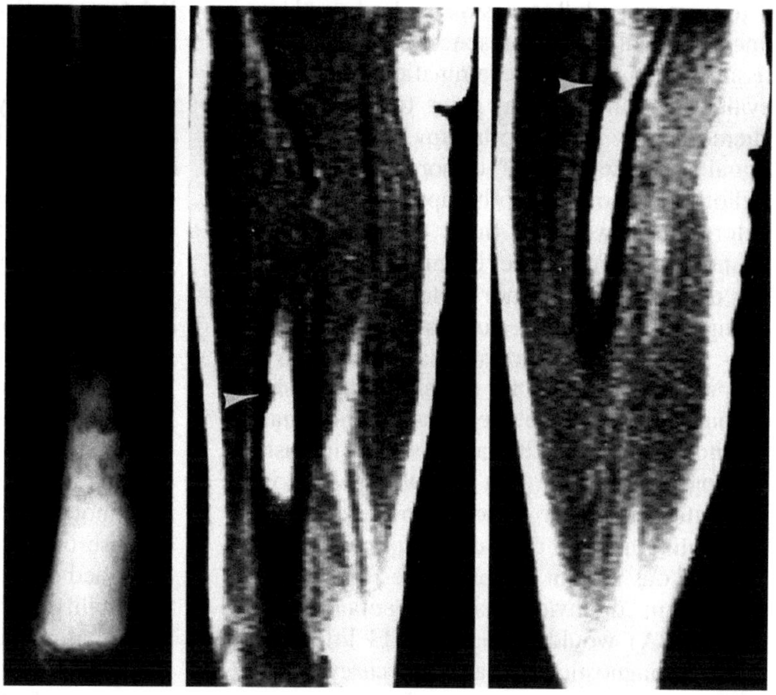

a b, c

Fig. 10a–c. Skip lesions in osteosarcoma. **a** Lateral radiograph demonstrates very sclerotic distal femoral osteosarcoma. **b,c** Sagittal T1-weighted images demonstrate two skip lesions (*arrows*), one in the mid femur (**b**) and the other in the proximal femur (**c**). Low-signal diametaphyseal tumor is seen in **b**. In the evaluation of distally located osteosarcomas or, for that matter, any malignant tumor of bone, the entire compartment (i.e., the entire bone) should be imaged and this can be efficiently done by T_1-weighted images

adolescent are Ewing sarcoma or other round-cell tumors. In this instance, the marrow signal abnormality on T1-weighted images is homogeneously low, with a sharp demarcation between normal marrow fat and abnormal low signal. In stress fractures, the low signal seen in the marrow fat may be inhomogeneous owing to blood and/or edema and may have a linear appearance (Fig. 9b). When there is uncertainty as to the diagnosis, biopsy can be delayed, and a repeat radiograph in a week to 10 days' time may show the characteristic features of a healing fracture (Fig. 9c). The same constellation of findings in an older patient should raise the possibility of a round-cell tumor such as lymphoma, myeloma, or metastases. In such instances, the patient deserves a scintiscan and skeletal survey to determine whether there are any other sites of abnormality.

The MRI Examination

The ideal MR examination is one that is carried out expeditiously and cost-effectively while providing adequate information for planning biopsy and definitive surgery. Imaging time has not been a serious limitation with MRI since most tumors of long bone are adequately staged with either coronal or sagittal T1-weighted and axial T2-weighted images. The value of T1-weighted sequences is for assessing the intraosseous extent of neoplasm, and the T2-weighted imaging sequences highlight the difference in signal intensity between extraosseous tumor and surrounding uninvaded soft tissues. In difficult cases, an axial T1-weighted image could further help in making this differentiation. When evaluating distal long bone osteosarcoma, the entire bone should be imaged in either the coronal or the sagittal plane for "skip lesions," which are clearly demonstrated on T1-weighted pulsing sequences (Fig. 10). A high level of accuracy in depicting tumor extent has been afforded by unenhanced T1- and T2-weighted spin-echo sequences.

Tissue characterization by MRI based on signal intensities is at present unreliable. There is a wide spectrum in the composition of bone tumors of differing histology as well as in tumors of similar histologic diagnosis. The result is either an overlap of signal intensities of histologically different tumors or variability of signal intensities in tumors of the same histology. The MRI examination is sensitive for depicting the extent of disease but is relatively nonspecific.

The single most reliable and reproducible feature of an MR examination for a tumor of bone is the accuracy with which it defines the extent of the tumor. It does this more reliably and accurately than any other modality. It is especially valuable when radiographic appearances suggest a long intramedullary lesion and when there is uncertainty about the presence or absence of soft tissue tumor. It is the examination of choice for evaluating tumor extent prior to and following chemotherapy and radiotherapy. Even if the MR signal characteristics of tumor following either radiotherapy or chemotherapy are tenuous in determining whether there is viable tumor or not, it remains the examination of choice for demonstrating tumor volume, morphologic changes of tumor in the soft tissues, and relationship of tumor to neurovascular structures. The purpose of using MRI for a tumor of bone should primarily be to stage the tumor rather than to diagnose by MR criteria of signal intensities. Radiographs are the best available predictors of the histologic nature of bone tumors.

Unlike in the case of tumors of the central nervous system or spine, the routine use of gadolinium diethylenetriamine-pentaacetic acid (Gd-DTPA) would appear to add little to the routine diagnostic or staging accurcy of MRI examinations of bone tumors. The exception is when MRI is used for estimating tumor necrosis of osteosarcomas and Ewing sarcoma following chemotherapy or radiation therapy (Erlemann et al. 1990). Encouraging results have been reported using Gd-DTPA-enhanced MRI scans in predicting tumor necrosis (Erlemann et al. 1990). If these results are successfully reproduced, Gd-DTPA-enhanced MRI scans may prove to be the single most accurate means of predicting tumor necrosis prior to surgery and would be preferable to random biopsies.

In less than a decade, MRI has achieved a high degree of accuracy in staging tumors of bone and in this role has become virtually indispensable to the orthopedic oncologist. The technology of this modality continues to evolve. With improving resolution, increasing experience, and further modifications of pulsing sequences, it can be relied on to demonstrate with even greater reliability transphyseal spread and cartilage involvement by tumor. Contrast-enhanced MR imaging offers promise in accurately measuring tumor necrosis following neoadjuvant therapy and is expected to be of value in distinguishing recurrent tumor from reactive fibrosis. MR angiography could well replace arteriography in those selected cases where vascular anatomy needs to be displayed prior to a limb salvage procedure.

Polytomography or Linear Tomography and Skeletal Scintigraphy

Polytomography or linear tomography is now rarely used in the evaluation of bone tumors. It may, however, be used to demonstrate the nidus of an osteoid osteoma if there is uncertainty on the radiograph and CT scan.

Scintigraphy and MRI or CT are truly complementary examinations providing quite different staging information in the patient presenting with the tumor of bone that requires biopsy. The main role of scintigraphy is not so much for local staging but for evaluating the remainder of the skeleton. Although scintigraphy provides information on the intraosseous extent of disease, it cannot entirely be relied on for local staging because of the augmented uptake that has been described in osteosarcomas (Hudson et al. 1983), its inability to match MRI in defining normal from abnormal marrow, and its inability to adequately demonstrate extracompartmental disease. Despite these factors, scintigraphy is an extremely important component in the evaluation of the solitary bone tumor.

Before 1970, bone scans were done with strontium 85; because of the high radiation dosage, only patients with known cancer and local areas could be studied. Greater strides were made after 1970, when the short-lived strontium 87m and fluorine 18, and a little later technetium 99m-labeled polyphosphate and technetium 89m-labeled diphosphonate were introduced as bone-scanning agents by Subramanian and others (Subramanian et al. 1972; Subramanian and McAfee 1977).

Increased uptake of radionuclides is highly nonspecific. Any pathologic process in bone resulting in new bone formation (reactive or tumor bone), increased blood flow, or bone turnover, as also normal growth, will show increased radionuclide uptake (Galasko 1969, 1975). Therefore, a bone scan is usually not reliable for identifying the specific type of tumor or for differentiating malignant from benign processes.

Gallium 67 citrate, a "tumor-seeking agent," is deposited in actively functioning and dividing cells as well as in white blood cells. It is therefore picked up by inflammatory lesions, but it is useful and is applied extensively for staging lymphomas. For details on the indications and limitations of radionuclide imaging, the reader is referred to Fordham and Ramachandran's (1977) review article.

Because scintigraphy is the most sensitive examination to evaluate the entire skeleton, it should always be done to determine whether skeletal involvement is solitary or multiple. Metastases are the most common of malignant tumors of bone and can frequently present as a solitary abnormality. In the pediatric age group, as in adults, metastases may mimic solitary tumors of bone. Metastatic neuroblastoma and leukemia may resemble true solitary lesions such as Ewing sarcoma, eosinophilic granuloma, and acute osteomyelitis. Because of synchronous and delayed skeletal metastases, scintigraphy is recommended at the time of presentation and in following patients whose primary Ewing's tumor has been extirpated (Goldstein et al. 1989). In addition to suggesting the presence of disseminated skeletal disease or its absence, scintigraphy in the proper clinical setting can have an appearance that is quite specific for the diagnosis of osteoid osteoma.

Angiography

In previous years angiography was used for planning resection of soft tissue tumors and outlining the extraosseous extent of bone tumors (Chuang et al. 1982; Kumpan et al. 1986).

Angiography now is rarely used as a diagnostic or staging tool. A prospective study (Bloem et al. 1988) has confirmed MRI's superiority to CT and angiography in visualizing the relationship between tumor and large vessels. In centers routinely using intra-arterial chemotherapy for certain malignant tumors there is likely to be a larger role for the pretreatment arteriogram. Arteriography is essential if preoperative embolization of a tumor is being considered. Pre- and post- arteriographic patterns have been found useful in some centers in predicting tumor response to neoadjuvant chemotherapy (Chuang et al. 1982; Kumpan et al. 1986; Bilbao et al. 1990).

The Role of Pathology

The *biopsy* and the *prebiopsy staging studies* are crucial to the treatment outcome of bone tumors. Biopsy should be systematically carried out in all cases, since with few exceptions it is impossible to assure the precise nature of the lesion by other methods. It should not be omitted in any case in which radical surgery, radiotherapy, or chemotherapy is contemplated and should be done *after* performing the necessary staging studies.

Biopsy can be carried out in two ways: (1) by surgical biopsy (incisional or excisional) or (2) by needle or percutaneous biopsy (aspiration or trochar biopsy). Regardless of the procedure used, it should be interpreted by a pathologist who has a good basic knowledge of bone pathology. He must know the exact site of the material submitted and be in possession of the clinical and radiologic information.

Open Surgical Biopsy

Most investigators maintain that surgical biopsy carried out by a competent surgeon under the necessary conditions of asepsis and with the correct techniques (with or without a tourniquet) does not involve any great danger. However, in cartilaginous lesions, an incisional biopsy may result in tumor implantation, often making adequate further surgery difficult.

Open surgical biopsy is the technique usually adopted in most oncology centers; even if competently performed, however, it is still accompanied by a relatively considerable complication rate. Mankin et al. (1982) found 18.2% major errors in diagnosis, and problems in wound healing in 17.3%. The performance of open biopsy may affect adversely the prognosis and successful limb salvage in a further group of patients. The skin incision should be placed in such a manner (longitudinally) as not to compromise subsequent surgery. A generous sample of tissue, preferably from the growing margin of the tumor, should be obtained, care being taken to obtain a representative sample of the lesion, so that the pathologist may be able to perform not only routine techniques but also more sophisticated investigation (electron microscopy, flow cytometry and immunohistochemistry, etc.). For that purpose frozen tissue and special methods of fixation are necessary, besides the routine fixation in neutral formalin. Immediate frozen sections may be prepared, so that the surgeon can judge whether the specimen is adequate and a decision regarding treatment can be made immediately. However, few pathologists have sufficient experience with frozen sections of bone tumors to give an immediate opinion, and most prefer to wait for sections of paraffin-embedded material. In any case biopsy-related problems are from three to five times more frequent when the biopsy is performed in a referring institution rather than in a specialized oncology center.

Percutaneous Needle (Aspiration or Trochar) Biopsy

The value of needle biopsy in diagnosing bone lesions has been discussed widely. One of the main objections to the technique has been the degree of confidence that can be inspired by a diagnosis based on relatively small particles of tissue.

In skilled hands needle biopsy has a definite use, particularly in cases where the site of the lesion (such as vertebrae) or the treatment to be adopted makes open biopsy difficult or undesirable.

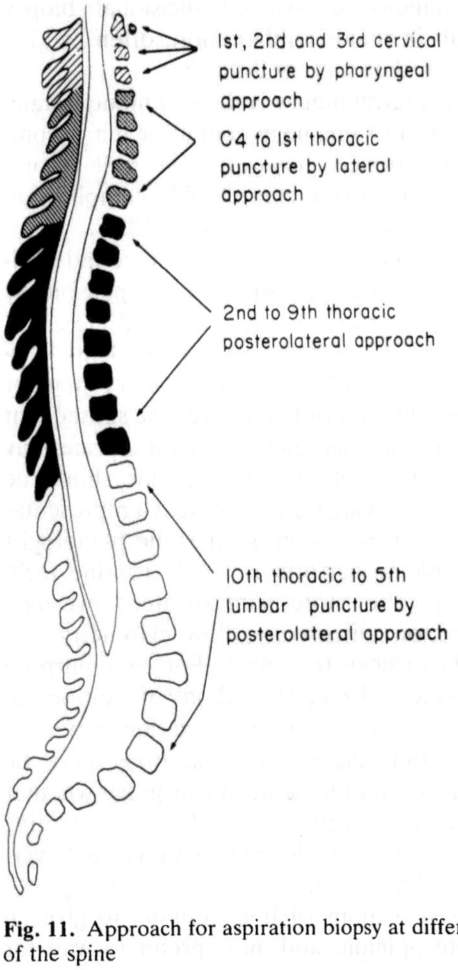

Fig. 11. Approach for aspiration biopsy at different levels of the spine

Aspiration biopsy became the preferred method in the Latin American Registry and Center of Osteoarticular Pathology, Buenos Aires. The technical details, advantages, and disadvantages of this procedure, as well as the approach to lesions involving vertebral bodies at different levels, have been reported in several previous publications by Ray, Valls, Ottolenghi, and myself (Ray 1953; Schajowicz 1955; Valls et al. 1948, 1954; Ottolenghi 1955, 1969; Ottolenghi et al. 1964; Schajowicz and Derqui 1968; Schajowicz and Hokama 1976). More than 9000 needle biopsies had been performed through 1983, including 2500 vertebral punctures with positive results in approximately 75% of the cases (Figs. 11, 12).

Although needle biopsy of the vertebrae is now accepted in many centers, its use in other institutions is restricted or even opposed by the pathologist owing to the aforementioned relatively low degree of confidence in its diagnostic capabilities. Recently, several medical centers in the United States, such as the M.D. Anderson Tumor Institute in Houston (DeSantos et al. 1979; Ayala and Zornosa 1983) and Barnes Hospital in St. Louis (Hardy et al. 1980; Murphy et al. 1981), as well as the Royal National Orthopaedic Hospital in London (Stoker and Kissin 1985), have adopted percutaneous needle biopsy as a valid alternative to open biopsy under certain circumstances. In these institutions the procedure is performed preferably by the radiologist under image amplification (fluoroscopy). In the last few years, the 2-mm needle has frequently been replaced in our institution and others by a Jamshidi needle (3 mm wide) (Jamshidi and Swaim 1971; Shaltot et al. 1982; Berenstein 1984). Recently, CT has been increasingly used with success as a means of guiding skeletal biopsy, especially in deeply located small lesions (Adapon et al. 1981; Gatenby et al. 1984; Frager et al. 1987).

In any case, using either a fine needle, a 2-mm needle, or a Jamshidi needle, we perform the combined cytologic study of the smears and histologic study of the paraffin-embedded material. We consider the smear to be a supplementary method of great value for studying the fine details of cell structure, especially in conditions that involve the hematopoietic system. Moreover, it often permits differentiation of Ewing sarcoma from osteomyelitis and eosinophilic granuloma (Fig. 13). In many cases, however, a smear is not sufficient for accurate

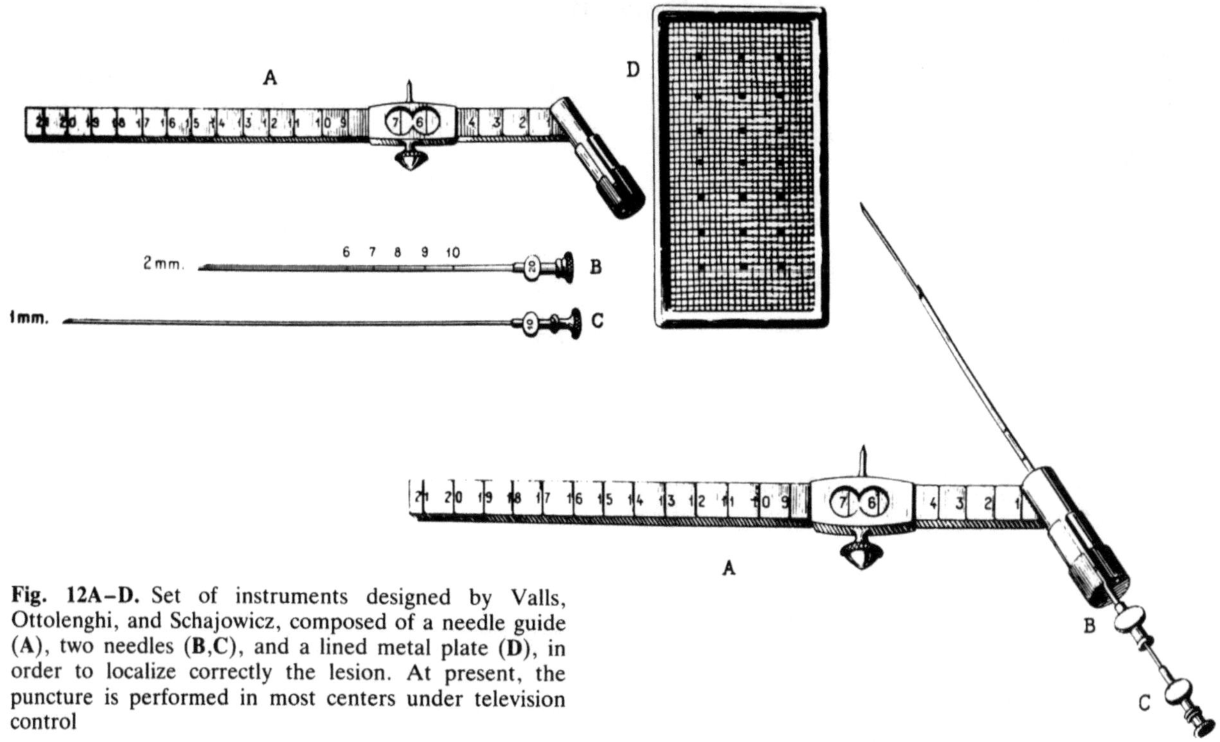

Fig. 12A–D. Set of instruments designed by Valls, Ottolenghi, and Schajowicz, composed of a needle guide (**A**), two needles (**B**,**C**), and a lined metal plate (**D**), in order to localize correctly the lesion. At present, the puncture is performed in most centers under television control

classification of either benign or malignant tumors or for differentiation between primary and metastatic malignant tumors. On the other hand, in some neoplastic growths, in Paget disease, or in other lesions in which the fibrous connective tissue or bone-forming stroma predominates, smears have little or no useful cell content; we do not make smears in these cases.

Moreover, with sufficient material obtained by percutaneous biopsy in adequate condition, bacteriologic and other complementary studies at present utilized and necessary for a more accurate diagnosis (electron microscopy, immunohistochemistry, and others) can be performed. On the other hand, needle biopsy has been used to determine the effect of treatment (chemotherapy or radiation) through repeated punctures, a procedure that has been performed in several oncologic centers (M.D. Anderson Institute in Houston, Texas; Rizzoli Institute in Bologna, Italy; our former center in Buenos Aires; and in St. Louis, Missouri).

Our experience justifies the recommendation of this method: It is technically simple, involves no risk to the patient, and makes it possible to extract material from a tumor at *different depths* and to reach sites that are otherwise only accessible by major surgery. It saves time and money and can usually be carried out in the outpatient department, except in young children, when general anesthesia is often necessary.

When there is little material or it is insufficient for a conclusive diagnosis, the biopsy can be repeated once or twice without any ill-effects. It is always possible to resort to surgical biopsy if the diagnosis remains in doubt. It is rarely difficult or impossible to extract sufficient material; even with dense, sclerosing lesions that the needle cannot penetrate, it is often possible to extract the material after perforation with an electric or manual trephine.

Although technically a simple method, aspiration or needle biopsy nevertheless does require some experience on the part of the surgeon or radiologist. We have observed that results from medical centers where this procedure is used regularly are superior in quantity and value of the material submitted to the results from clinics where lack of opportunity deprives the surgeon of the necessary experience. In our opinion, this is as great a disadvantage as lack of competence in the pathologist, who should of course be experienced in bone pathology. The pathologist must be familiar with the clinical and radiographic evidence if he is to interpret the histopathologic specimen correctly.

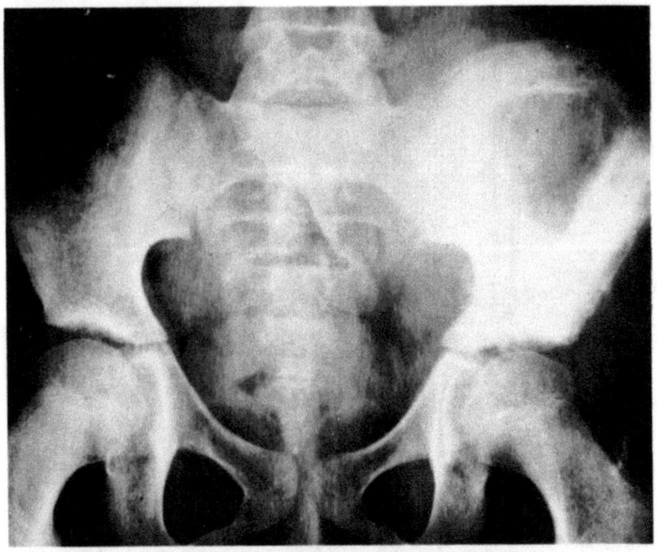

a

Fig. 13a–d. Female, 13 years old, with Ewing sarcoma of the ilium. **a** Radiograph shows a predominantly sclerosing lesion with partial destruction of the cortex. **b** Photomicrograph of a smear showing glycogen granules in the cytoplasm of the tumor cells (PAS strain, ×600). Photomicrographs of a histologic section stained **c** with HE (×400) and **d** with PAS without nuclear counterstain (×400), demonstrating the histologic and histochemical features of Ewing sarcoma, as observed in material obtained with aspiration biopsy

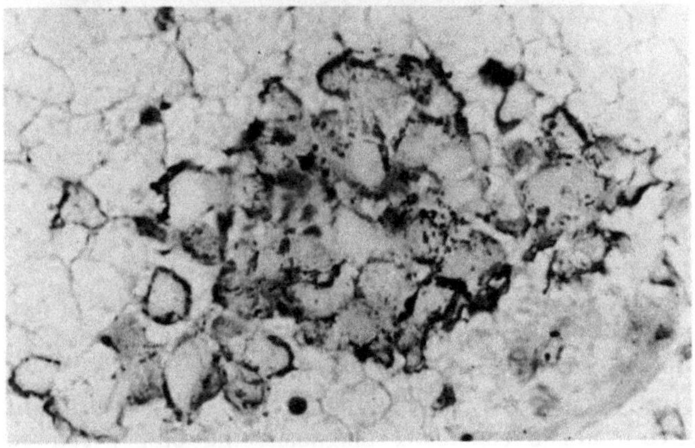

b

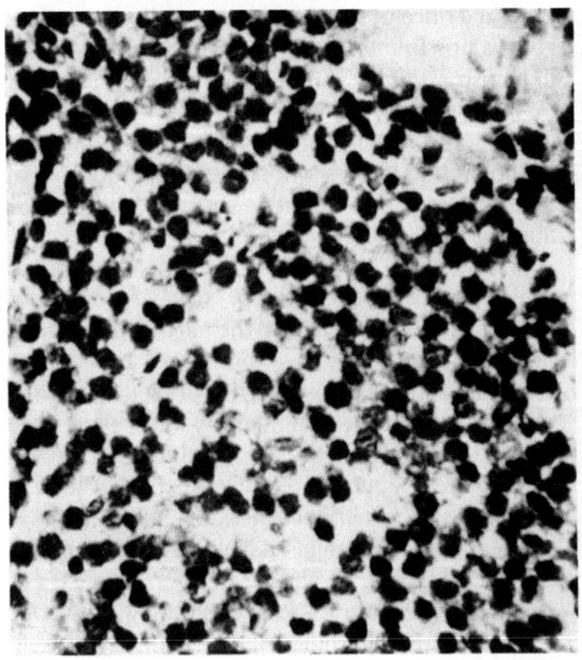

c

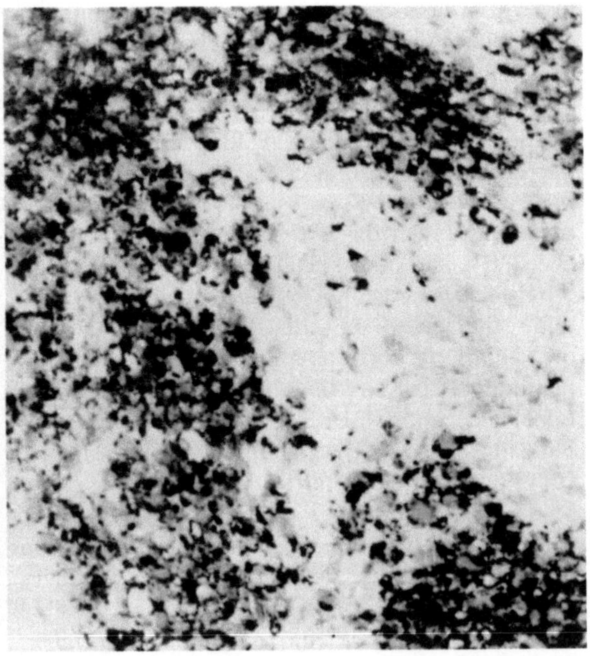

d

Methods of Handling Specimens of Bone Lesions

1. If the diagnosis is to be based on *paraffin sections*, the time can be reduced by selecting material, as for frozen sections, from the *softer parts* of the specimen; these can be studied without decalcification.

2. For the *hard parts of bone specimens*, decalcification is necessary. There are many reports describing different methods that presumably improve the technique of demineralization of bone tissue, by decreasing the time required without altering the morphology and staining reactions of the tissue by varying conditions of temperature, agitation, type of acid, and molarity of the acid bath.

Although Morris and Benton (1956) consider hydrochloric acid in a concentration between 1 and 2 M the best and least harmful demineralizing agent, in our experience decalcification in 5% nitric acid is rapid (generally not more than 24–48 h) and gives excellent results. A temperature of approximately 36°C–40°C and agitation of the specimen decrease the time required for demineralization. Using thin slices (5 mm) and abundant acid solution avoids prolonged treatment. After the acid solution, the slices are placed for several hours (depending on their size) in a solution of 4% sodium sulfate and are then washed in running water for a few hours. The succeeding steps are the same as in the embedding of soft tissue material; a good nuclear staining can be obtained with Hansen's or Harris' hematoxylin.

When there is only a little bony resistance, Bouin's or Rossman's liquid can be used; slightly harder tissues need a stronger acid such as formic acid mixtures (Greep et al. 1948): equal parts of 2% formic acid and a 20% sodium citrate solution. These acids act fairly rapidly, and overtreatment does not seriously interfere with subsequent staining.

Electrolytic decalcification introduced by Richman et al. (1947) can yield good results but must be used carefully and may sometimes destroy the material. Sreebny and Nikiforuk (1951) and Birge and Imhoff (1952) introduced the organic chelating compound ethylenediaminetetraacetic acid (EDTA) at neutral pH, an excellent but slow-acting decalcifying agent. EDTA has little deleterious effect on nuclear staining, even after prolonged periods of treatment, and is especially useful for histochemical studies.

3. *Resection and amputation specimens*, after the soft tissues have been carefully dissected from the affected bone, should be photographed showing the external surface and the cut surface. Radiographs of the entire specimen, the bisected specimen, and a thin slice (5 mm) should be taken, preferably using a source of soft x-rays and a fine-grain film. The resulting radiographs and the selection of blocks for subsequent histologic study provide an important link between the appearance of a lesion in the clinical radiographs and its histologic structure.

4. *Freezing* of the specimen – particularly slow freezing of a bulky specimen – should always be avoided when material is to be taken for histologic study because of the distortion of tissues caused by ice crystal production.

5. In addition to routine HE preparations, sections should be prepared using connective tissue stains, stains for reticulin fibers (preferably on frozen sections), stains for metachromasia, and the periodic acid-Schiff (PAS) procedure.

6. Part of the material may, with advantage, be fixed in 80% alcohol, which permits some histochemical procedures, particularly those for glycogen and alkaline phosphatase.

Histochemistry

The presence of calcified areas has been a serious obstacle to the use of histochemical techniques, and the results obtained should be carefully analyzed in accordance with the method being used. Calcium ions are apt to interfere with the histochemical reactions, and care should be taken when interpreting the results (e.g., metachromasia and acid phosphatase). Various types of buffer solutions that keep the pH within certain limits must be used with the acid decalcifiers. The introduction of chelating agents (EDTA) capable of eliminating calcium salts in a nonacid pH constitutes an advance in the histochemistry of calcified tissues. As a general rule, it is preferable to use uncalcified material when possible.

Histochemical studies supplemented with biochemical and ultramicroscopic methods have been of great value in amplifying concepts of normal osteogenesis (membranous and endochondral) and bone destruction. They have also been helpful in resolving histogenetic problems, specifically, in demonstrating the intense enzymatic activity of osteoclasts and the identical histochemical behavior of giant cells in osteoclastoma, in other giant-cell lesions of bone (so-called variants of giant-cell tumors), and in normal osteoclasts, thus establishing a histogenetic relationship between these elements. The study of the polysaccharide glycogen and of acid mucopolysaccharides permitted the demonstration of similar behavior for the tumor cells and ground substance in chondroblastoma and chondromyxoid fibroma; the cells from both are rich in glycogen, and the ground substance, in metachromatic substances, is the same as in chondromas and chondrosarcomas, thus confirming their cartilaginous derivation.

Histochemistry has not only contributed to our understanding of normal and pathologic ossification, but has also proved to be of *diagnostic value* in some cases. The demonstration of abundant cytoplasmic glycogen granules in Ewing sarcoma and of their absence in lymphoma of bone and most cases of metastatic neuroblastoma provides an important and simple method of differential diagnosis (Schajowicz 1959). The presence of obvious alkaline phosphatase activity makes it possible to detect foci of osteogenesis (osteoblastic activity) that otherwise are difficult to demonstrate with ordinary techniques. In this way, hyalinized connective tissue and cartilage can be differentiated from osteoid (Schajowicz and Cabrini 1954, 1958a,b; Jeffree and Price 1965). Chordoma and mucus-secreting carcinomas are often difficult to differentiate with HE stains; the use of a simple PAS stain permits an easy differential diagnosis, showing the presence of abundant cytoplasmic glycogen granules in chordoma and the existence of mucoproteins resistant to ptyalin digestion in metastatic mucus-secreting carcinomas.

These are a few examples that show the limited but occasionally important diagnostic value of histochemical methods in the study of bone tumors.

Electron Microscopy

Electron microscopy has been of utmost importance in the study of the ultrastructure and function of the different cell components in normal and pathologic conditions. It has also helped greatly in understanding the etiology and pathogenesis of many pathologic processes.

In the field of bone pathology, electron microscopy contributed to establishing the nature and probable histogenesis of certain tumors; it showed that at least some "adamantinomas" of long bones are of epithelial origin, that chordomas are of notochordal origin, and that "osteoid osteomas" and osteoblastoma are closely related processes of osteoblastic derivation. It also demonstrated that the multinucleated giant cells of giant-cell tumors and of the so-called giant-cell variants have cytologic features identical to those of normal osteoclasts; however, it failed to establish the exact mechanism of their formation from the mononuclear stromal cells from which they evidently derive. Despite the great number of studies performed, electron microscopy has not yet resolved the disputed histogenesis of Ewing sarcoma and of other controversial tumor entities of bone and soft tissues, such as malignant fibrous histiocytomas, "clear-cell" sarcomas of tendon, and aponeurosis.

However, under some circumstances electron microscopy may confirm a probable diagnosis based on histologic or histochemical examination, demonstrating the smooth muscle cell character of the tumor cells in leiomyosarcoma and the Birbeck's granules characteristic of histiocytes, the basic element of eosinophilic granuloma (histiocytosis X). Electron microscopy is of value in poorly differentiated myelomas or in some cases of Ewing sarcoma. It may occasionally constitute the only method for establishing the precise diagnosis when the histologic features are not conclusive and/or the biochemical investigation of catecholamines is negative, for example, in some cases of primary neuroectodermal tumor of bone or of metastatic neuroblastoma of bone.

Although these examples show that the application of electron microscopy has contributed to the progress of our knowledge, its use as a routine and essential procedure in the diagnosis of bone tumors and tumorlike lesions is at present still limited, since it is both expensive and time consuming.

The ultrastructural features of various types of tumors as revealed by electron microscopy are discussed in more detail in subsequent chapters, insofar as they have shown aspects of histogenetic or diagnostic importance.

Immunohistochemistry

The application of improved, more sensitive immunohistochemical techniques, and in particular the development of monoclonal antibodies, has simplified the task of solving problems in the diagnosis of tumors in surgical pathology and promises increased diagnostic accuracy.

Undoubtedly many more antibodies with practical applications will soon be discovered. It is evident that monoclonal antibodies will be utilized for identification of increasing numbers of marker substances that have not only diagnostic significance but also possible implications in the treatment of neoplasms, such as coupling different cytotoxic substances with the specific monoclonal antibody.

A variety of methods are available for the detection of antigens in tissue sections. Immunofluorescence techniques on frozen sections have the advantage of superior antigen preservation but are less sensitive than immunoenzyme methods. Moreover, these methods are impractical for the general surgical pathologist because frozen tissue is often not available. For this reason, immunoenzyme methods utilizing either peroxidase-antiperoxidase (PAP) or avidin-biotin complex (ABC), which can be applied to formalin-fixed, paraffin-embedded material, have largely supplanted immunofluorescence methods for routine investigation.

One of the applications with practical importance for the orthopedic surgeon is the development of monoclonal antibodies to human osteosarcoma, produced with success by investigators from various institutions (Farrands et al. 1983; Baldwin and Pimm 1983; Embleton et al. 1983; Wada et al. 1988; Tsai et al. 1990). The initial characterization of six monoclonal antibodies against osteosarcoma used at St. Louis University Medical Center indicated that one of them, TMMR-2, was more specific for osteosarcoma than the others. The results of immunohistochemical and flow cytometric investigation suggest that TMMR-2 is also highly specific for mesenchymal cells of osseous differentiation (osteocytes and osteoblasts), whether normal or neoplastic, and has an inhibitory effect on DNA synthesis in cultured osteosarcoma cells. It is possible that this antibody, when coupled with cytotoxic agents or radioisotopes, could provide a much needed addition to osteosarcoma diagnosis and therapy (Farrands et al. 1983).

Immunohistochemistry has become of fundamental importance in the differential diagnosis of small round-cell tumors of bone (Ewing sarcoma, metastatic neuroblastoma, non-Hodgkin lymphoma, small-cell carcinoma, and the recently identified primary neuroectodermal tumor of bone), especially through the investigation of neuron-specific enolase (NSE) (Tsokos et al. 1984; Thomas et al. 1987) and other neural markers (HNK-1 and HBA7 among others). Other markers such as S-100 (Nakamura et al. 1983; Weiss and Dorfman 1986) are positive in some cartilage tumors, and desmin and actin are important in distinguishing fibrosarcoma from leiomyosarcoma.

In the past decade immunohistologic procedures have been developed for staining tissue sections with antibodies against different collagen types. Accurate definition of material as osteoid is one of the greatest problems in bone pathology. There is no histologic method that clearly differentiates cartilage from osteoid and hyalinized collagen. It was found that cartilage contains mostly type II collagen, whereas bone (osteoid) contains type I collagen. Remberger and Gay (1977) and Gay and Miller (1978) later confirmed these findings, in that they found type I collagen in human osteosarcoma cells and type III collagen in different connective tissues; in contrast, type II collagen was exclusively observed in chondrosarcoma. However, it seems that type II collagen also can be observed in chondroblastic areas of typical osteosarcoma, as well as in typical chondrosarcoma. So this technique seems to be of rather limited value and further investigations are necessary to establish whether these or other immunologic methods such as the use of S-100 protein (positive in cartilage lesions) can be applied in a practical way for the routine diagnosis of bone tumors.

Flow Cytometry

Another new diagnostic method, particularly important for differentiating benign and malignant neoplasms, is the study of cellular DNA content. Initially this was achieved by Feulgen DNA absorption microfluorometry (Schajowicz et al. 1976); however, more recently laser-based flow cytofluorometric analysis by propidium iodide stain has been employed, which has made it possible to perform rapid determinations of DNA content in thousands of cell nuclei. First experiences with this new method as applied to human osteosarcomas and chondrosarcomas were reported by Kreicbergs et al. (1982a,b, 1984) and later by Mankin et al. (1985, 1988) in a series of chondrosarcomas. Classical osteosarcomas and high-grade chondrosarcomas were found to be hyperploid (abnormally increased DNA content) while parosteal osteosarcoma proved to be diploid (normal DNA cotent), the same as chondromas and low-grade chondrosarcomas, as had already been shown by us in 1976 with the older microspectrophotometric method. However, ploidy determinations are not supposed to replace but only to complement conventional histopathologic malignancy grading in osteosarcomas and chondrosarcomas. Their main advantage seems to be the recognition of highly malignant areas among grade I chondrosarcoma by the presence of cells with hyperploid DNA content.

The Pathologist's Role in the Diagnosis of Osteosarcoma

During the last decade new methods of treatment, involving particularly the use of preoperative chemotherapy, have been introduced with the intent of improving the opportunity for surgical extirpation and to perform limb-sparing procedures. These forms of treatment alter profoundly the morphologic features of the tumor, producing varying degrees of tumor destruction, i.e., necrosis, and oblige the pathologist to take a more dynamic part in the planning of treatment.

Determination of necrosis of the primary osteosarcoma was considered useful by Rosen and his colleagues (1982) to evaluate the effect of preoperative chemotherapy. They suggested that patients with complete necrosis have a better prognosis than the nonresponding cases. Several criteria for determining the grade of necrosis have been reported in the last few years. We agree with Raymond and Ayala (1988) and the Rizzoli investigators (Picci et al. 1985) that standardization in percentages of grading is unrealistic and highly subjective, being based principally on the personal experience of the pathologist. It is practically impossible to assess the number of necrotic cells and calculate the exact percentage based generally on the macroscopic and histologic study of 30–40 tissue blocs taken from a longitudinal 5- to 6-mm-thick slab of the tumor, together with some fragments from the surface parts. On the other hand, determining what constitutes *viable* tumor cells or borders is more a "philosophic" than a scientific question. A simple cytomorphologic study of tumor cells does not permit the assessment of the death of a cell or its capacity for continued growth and reproduction. Therefore we agree with Campanacci et al., who suggested dividing tumor destruction into three grades, "good," "fair," and "poor," or with Mazabraud, who suggested "total necrosis" and "subtotal necrosis" with persistence of a few foci of viable tissue – thereby assessing the estimated extent of tumor destruction and thus the efficacy of treatment. On the other hand it is necessary to take into account the fact that on average untreated osteosarcomas present 50% "spontaneous" necrosis (Misdorp et al. 1988), with a range from 10% to 80%.

In an effort to identify the predominant sites of viable and nonviable tumor after treatment with chemotherapy, regional mapping of tumor destruction was performed by the Rizzoli group, using repeated needle biopsies and following the routine used by Ayala and Raymond (M.D. Anderson Institute, Houston, 1988). Thus it was found that the most common sites of persistence of viable tumor were in the extraosseous soft tissue within the cortex and areas adjacent to cartilage or ligaments. This is important in that it indicates the need to obtain wide surgical margins when performing limb-sparing surgery in patients treated with preoperative chemotherapy.

Recently in the Memorial Hospital (Huvos 1991), four different grades of response to preoperative chemotherapy were assigned to osteosarcoma specimens following careful histologic analysis of 20–60 tissue sections. A grade I or II effect is considered no effect or a partial effect, while a grade III or IV effect is considered a near-complete or complete effect, indicating that preoperative chemotherapy is probably going to be curative and that there is no need to add cisplatin and adriamycin chemotherapy to the regimen (high-dose methotrexate). As Huvos stated, only 20% had a grade IV and 21% a grade III response as determined by pathologic examination at the Memorial Hospital. Salzer-Kuntschick et al. (1983), of the Vienna Bone Tumor Registry, divided the tumor response after preoperative chemotherapy into six histologic grades, grades I and II (47%) corresponding to grades III and IV of Huvos' classification (less than 10% or nonviable tumor tissue).

A similar procedure of histologic evaluation and prognostic correlation of the effect of preoperative chemotherapy in the treatment of Ewing sarcoma was also applied by Picci et al. at the Rizzoli Institute (1988).

It is generally agreed that Ewing sarcoma responds very well to chemotherapy and that in most cases the percentage of spontaneous necrosis is high (average 50%–60%). It therefore seems very problematic to accurately evaluate the percentage of necrosis induced by preoperative chemotherapy in this entity. However, Picci et al. found complete tumor necrosis in 40% of their patients and suggested that these cases had a better prognosis that the nonresponding patients. It also shows, as in osteosarcoma, the existence of areas where viable tumor most likely persists: invaded soft tissues, hemorrhagic areas, and the periosteal reaction. However, the small number of cases and the short follow-up of most of Picci et al.'s patients warrants caution in the evaluation of the results.

Classification of Bone Tumors

One of the main reasons for the prevailing difficulties in understanding skeletal tumors is the lack of a common terminology and especially of a classification that is sufficiently complete to cover the different histologic types according to their clinical behavior, and at the same time simple enought to be applied and understood by clinicians and pathologists. This is largely due to the inadequacy of our knowledge of the embryology and histogenesis of normal bone tissue and its possible blastomatous anomalies.

A list of all the attempts at classification would be quite lengthy, so we shall confine ourselves to those which have had a major influence on the knowledge of bone tumors, either because they were based on the study of a large number of cases or because they introduced new ideas.

One of the main contributions to the advancement of our knowledge was the establishment by Codman in 1920 of the Bone Sarcoma Registry under the auspices of the American College of Surgeons. Together with Ewing and Bloodgood, Codman drew up in 1922 the first classification of the Registry, which comprised only three groups of tumors: the osteogenic sarcoma with various subdivisions, the endothelioma, and the myeloma with four variants.

Since then, this classification has been reviewed by several distinguished specialists in pathology and surgery, and has undergone various changes due to the constant increase in material and the resultant advances in our knowledge. Thus, principally as a result of the work of Phemister (1930), chondrosarcoma was separated from osteogenic sarcoma on the strength of its special histologic characteristics

Table 1. Classification of bone tumors (Ewing 1939)

	Malignant	Benign
Osteogenic series	OSTEOGENIC SARCOMA	Exostosis
	Medullary and subperiosteal	Osteoma
	Telangiectatic	
	Sclerosing	
	Periosteal	
	Fibrosarcoma	
	a) Medullary	
	b) Periosteal	
	Parosteal and capsular	
Chondroma series	Chondrosarcoma	Chondrosarcoma
	Myxosarcoma	
Giant-cell tumor series	Malignant	Epiphyseal giant-cell tumor
Angioma series	Angioendothelioma	Cavernous angioma
	Diffuse endothelioma	Plexiform angioma
Myeloma series	Plasma cell	
	Myelocytoma	
	Erythroblastoma	
	Lymphocytoma	
Reticulum-cell lymphosarcoma		
Liposarcoma		

Table 2. Revised W.H.O. classification and incidence of bone tumors

	No. of cases
I. BONE-FORMING TUMORS	
A. Benign	442
1. Osteoma	111
2. Osteoid osteoma and osteoblastoma	262
	69
B. Intermediate	16
1. Aggressive (malignant) osteoblastoma	
C. Malignant	717
1. Osteosarcoma	
a. Central (medullary)	637
b. Surface (peripheral)	80
1. Parosteal	64
2. Periosteal	9
3. High-grade surface	7
II. CARTILAGE-FORMING TUMORS	
A. Benign	1872
1. Chondroma	616
a. Enchondroma	598
b. Periosteal (juxtacortical)	18
2. Osteochondroma (osteocartilaginous exostosis)	1064
a. Solitary	1001
b. Multiple hereditary	63
3. Chondroblastoma (epiphyseal chondroblastoma)	144
4. Chondromyxoid fibroma	48
B. Malignant	381
1. Chondrosarcoma (conventional) (primary-306) (secondary-33)	339
2. Dedifferentiated chondrosarcoma	–
3. Juxtacortical (periosteal) chondrosarcoma	13
4. Mesenchymal chondrosarcoma	22
5. Clear-cell chondrosarcoma	6
6. Malignant chondroblastoma?	1
III. GIANT-CELL TUMOR (OSTEOCLASTOMA)	460
IV. MARROW TUMORS (ROUND-CELL TUMORS)	954
1. Ewing sarcoma of bone	272
2. Neuroectodermal tumor of bone	2
3. Malignant lymphoma of bone (primary-86) (secondary-99)	185
4. Myeloma	495

	No. of cases
V. VASCULAR TUMORS	
A. Benign	65
1. Hemangioma	63
2. Lymphangioma	–
3. Glomus tumor (glomangioma)	2
B. Intermediate or Indeterminate	23
1. Hemangioendothelioma (epithelioid hemangioendothelioma, histiocytoid hemangioma)	15
2. Hemangiopericytoma	8
C. Malignant	12
1. Angiosarcoma (malignant hemangioendothelioma, hemangiosarcoma, hemangioendotheliosarcoma)	12
2. Malignant hemangiopericytoma	–
VI. OTHER CONNECTIVE TISSUE TUMORS	264
A. Benign	24
1. Benign fibrous histiocytoma	14
2. Lipoma	10
B. Intermediate	16
1. Desmoplastic fibroma	
C. Malignant	224
1. Fibrosarcoma	166
2. Malignant fibrous histiocytoma	37
3. Liposarcoma	2
4. Malignant mesenchymoma	4
5. Leiomyosarcoma	3
6. Undifferentiated sarcoma	12
VII. OTHER TUMORS	68
A. Benign	18
1. Neurilemoma	10
2. Neurofibroma	8
B. Malignant	50
1. Chordoma	31
2. Adamantinoma	19
Total benign tumors	2421
Total intermediate tumors	515
Total malignant tumors	2338
TOTAL	5274

Note: Paget sarcoma is not included. Aggressive (malignant) osteoblastoma, giant-cell tumor, desmoplastic fibroma, hemangioendothelioma, and hemangiopericytoma are grouped as intermediate or indeterminate tumors.

and more favorable clinical course. The group of giant-cell tumors, formerly considered as uniformly benign, was divided mainly on the basis of the work of Coley and Higinbotham (1938) and Meyerding (1941) into a benign and a malignant form. In 1939 Parker and Jackson separated primary reticulum-cell sarcoma of bone (classified at present as non-Hodgkin lymphoma) from Ewing sarcoma.

This brings us to the final classification of 1939, as revised by Ewing, which was based on more than 2000 observed cases (Table 1). This classification, which during the years of its development was extremely useful, has since been modified or replaced by others based on embryogenetic or histogenetic concepts (Geschickter and Copeland 1949; Lichtenstein 1952; Johnson 1953; Schajowicz and Mondolfo 1955), despite the fact that histogenetic knowledge is incomplete and possibly misleading.

One histogenetically based classification system that has been widely adopted is that of Lichtenstein (1952). This was the first classification to place Ewing sarcoma in a separate position, based on its direct derivation from the mesenchymal cells [an idea previously suggested by Phemister, whose 1949 classification was adopted by H.L. Jaffe in his book (1958)]. Several authors (Dahlin 1978; Dahlin and Unni 1986; Goidanich 1956; Campanacci 1981; and others) follow Lichtenstein's classification with slight modifications.

The World Health Organization (WHO), which is interested in establishing internationally accepted classification systems that would enable cancer researchers in all parts of the world to compare and collaborate their findings, has since 1958 organized more than 20 International Reference Centers covering almost all tumor types.

The WHO International Reference (IRC) for the Histological Definition and Classification of Bone Tumors was established in 1963 at the Osteo-articular Pathology Center, Italian Hospital, Buenos Aires, Argentina. Under this writer's direction, the IRC prepared and distributed material (clinical information, radiographs, and microscopic slides) from selected cases to seven collaborating centers for histologic typing according to a tentative classification previously established by a group of experts at a meeting in Geneva in 1963.

This classification, together with the definitions, explanatory notes, and color photographs, was published in 1972 by the WHO (Schajowicz et al. 1972). It is based simply on histologic criteria, that is, on the recognizable product of differentiation exhibited by the proliferating tumor cells, because it allows a useful degree of prediction of the properties and behavior of the tumor concerned.

In most instances, tumors apparently arise from the type of tissue they produce, but such an assumption cannot always be proved. There are some neoplasms that are highly undifferentiated without showing any kind of tissue production, e.g., Ewing sarcoma, which can only be classified by the site of most probable origin, i.e., bone marrow.

The classification includes benign and malignant neoplasms primary in bone, together with certain "tumorlike" lesions that are included because of their frequent clinical and histologic similarity to bone tumors, and because of uncertainty with regard to the neoplastic or nonneoplastic nature of some of them.

Since the publication of the first edition of the WHO classification, almost 20 years have elapsed. The introduction of newer cytomorphologic methods, including immunohistochemistry and the study of cellular DNA content by flow cytometry, has greatly improved our diagnostic tools. However, only a few modifications of the classification have been necessary for the introduction of a limited number of new tumor entities, such as the benign and malignant fibrous histiocytoma, the malignant or aggressive osteoblastoma, the primary neuroectodermal tumor of bone, and leiomyosarcoma. The term "primary reticulum-cell sarcoma of bone" coined by Parker and Jackson has been replaced by the term "primary malignant lymphoma" according to the newer classifications of lymphomas.

On the other hand, some entities such as the osteosarcomas have been subdivided into separate variants because of their distinct histopathologic features associated with a different biologic behavior.

In general, the framework and the concept of the original classification, based on widely accepted histologic criteria, remained essentially the same and is now in preparation for publication by this publisher under the auspices of the WHO. This revised WHO classification is reproduced in Tables 2 and 3, and includes the number of cases of each category recorded in our laboratory through the end of 1985. The

Table 3. Tumorlike lesions

Type	No. of cases
1. Solitary bone cyst (simple or unicameral bone cyst)	289
2. Aneurysmal bone cyst	217
3. Juxta-articular bone cyst (intraosseous ganglion)	136
4. Metaphyseal fibrous defect (nonossifying fibroma)	367
5. Eosinophilic granuloma (solitary)	196
6. Fibrous dysplasia and osteofibrous dysplasia	296
7. "Myositis ossificans"	85
8. "Brown tumor" of hyperparathyroidism	32
9. Intraosseous epidermoid cyst	39
10. Giant-cell (reparative) granuloma of hands and feet	8
	1665

tumorlike lesions listed in Table 3 are described in separate chapters, adding to the WHO classification "intraosseous epidermoid cyst" and "giant-cell (reparative) granuloma of hands and feet."

References

General

Adler CP (1983) Knochenkrankheiten. Thieme, Stuttgart
Aegerter E, Kirkpatrick JAJ (1975) Orthopedic diseases: physiology, pathology, radiology, 4th edn. W.B. Saunders, Philadelphia
Bougmill GP, Schwamsu HA (1984) Orthopaedic pathology: a synopsis with clinical and radiographic correlations. W.B. Saunders, Philadelphia
Bullogh P, Vigorita VJ (1984) Atlas of orthopaedic pathology with clinical and radiologic correlations. University Park Press, Gower Medical Publishing, New York, London
Campanacci M (1981) Tumori delle Ossa e delle Parti Molli. 2 volumes. Aulo Gaggi Editore, Bologna, Italy
Campanacci M (1990) Bone and soft tissue tumors. Springer, Vienna New York
Cohen J, Bonfiglio M, Campbell CJ (1990) Orthopedic pathophysiology in diagnosis and treatment. Churchill Livingstone, New York
Dahlin DC (1978) Bone tumors, 3rd edn. Charles C. Thomas, Springfield, IL
Dahlin DC, Unni KK (1986) Bone tumors: general aspects and data on 8542 cases. Charles C. Thomas, Springfield, IL
Dominok GW, Knoch G (1982) Knochengeschwülste und geschwulstähnliche Knochenerkrankungen. Fischer, Jena
Edeiken J, Hodes P (1973) Roentgen diagnosis of bone, 2nd edn, vols I and II. Williams and Wilkins, Baltimore
Edeiken J, Dalinka M, Karasick D (1990) Edeiken's roentgendiagnosis of diseases of bone, 4th edn. Williams and Wilkins, Baltimore
Enneking WF (1983) Musculoskeletal tumor surgery. Churchill Livingtone, New York
Ewing J (1939) A review of the classification of bone tumors. Bull Am Coll Surg 24:290
Ewing J (1940) Neoplastic diseases: a treatise on tumors (3rd edn 1928), 4th edn. W.B. Saunders, Philadelphia
Freyschmidt J, Ostertag H (1988) Knochentumoren: Klinik, Radiologie, Pathologie. Springer, Berlin Heidelberg New York
Greenfield GB (1980) Radiology of bone disease, 3rd edn. J.B. Lippincott, Philadelphia
Hajdu SL (1985) Differential diagnosis of soft tissue and bone tumors. Lea & Febiger, Philadelphia
Hudson TM (1987) Radiologic-pathologic correlation of musculoskeletal lesion. Williams and Wilkins, Baltimore
Huvos AG (1991) Bone tumors: diagnosis, treatment, prognosis. W.B. Saunders, Philadelphia
Jaffe HL (1958) Tumors and tumorous conditions of the bones and joints. Lea & Febiger, Philadelphia
Johnson LC (1953) A general theory of bone tumors. Bull NY Acad Med 29:164
Lichtenstein L (1977) Bone tumors, 5th edn. C.V. Mosby, St. Louis
Mirra JM, Picci P, Gold RH (1989) Bone tumors: clinical, radiologic and pathologic correlations. Lea & Febiger, Philadelphia
Moser RP (1990) Cartilaginous tumors of the skeleton. AFIP atlas of radiologic-pathologic correlations. Fasc II. Hanley & Belfus, Philadelphia
Murray RO, Jacobson HG (1977) The radiology of skeletal disorders, 2nd edn. Churchill Livingstone, Edinburgh
Netherlands Committee on Bone Tumors (1973) Radiological atlas on bone tumors, vols I and II. Williams and Wilkins, Baltimore
Povysil C (1986) Histopathology and ultrastructure of tumours and tumor-like lesions of bones. Acta Univ Carol [Med] (Praha) vol 116
Ranniger K (1977) Bone tumours. In: Diethelm L (ed) Handbuch der medizinischen. Radiologie vol V/6. Springer, Berlin Heidelberg New York
Resnick D, Niwayama G (1988) Diagnosis of bone and joint disorders, 2nd edn, vol 6. W.B. Saunders, Philadelphia
Roessner A (1984) Zur Zyto-und Histogenese der malignen und semimalignen Knochentumoren. Gustav Fischer, Stuttgart
Schajowicz F (1981) Tumors and tumorlike lesions of bone and joints. Springer, New York Berlin Heidelberg
Schajowicz F (1983) Current trends in the diagnosis and treatment of malignant bone tumors. Clin Orthop 180:22
Schajowicz F, Ackerman LV, Sissons HA (1972) Histological typing of bone tumours. World Health Organization, Geneva
Schajowicz F, McGuire MH (1989) Diagnostic difficulties in bone pathology. Clin Orthop 240:281
Sissons HA, Murray RO, Kemp HBS (1984) Orthopaedic diagnosis: clinical, radiological, and pathological coordinates. Springer, Berlin Heidelberg New York
Spjut HJ, Dorfman HD, Fechner RE, Ackerman LV (1971) Tumors of bone and cartilage. Atlas of tumor pathology, 2nd series, Fasc 5. Armed Forces Institute of Pathology, Washington DC
Spjut HJ, Fechner RE, Ackerman LV (1981) Tumors of bone and cartilage. Atlas of tumor pathology. Fascicle 5, Supplement. Armed Forces Institute of Pathology, Washington DC
Uhthoff K (ed) (1984) Current concepts of diagnosis and treatment of bone and soft tissue tumors. Springer, Heidelberg New York Berlin
Unni KK (ed) (1988) Bone tumors. In: Contemporary issues in surgical pathology. Churchill Livingstone, New York
Wilner D (1982) Radiology of bone tumors and allied disorders. W.B. Saunders, Philadelphia
Wold LE, McLeod RA, Sim FH, Unni KK (1990) Atlas of orthopedic pathology. W.B. Saunders, Philadelphia

Diagnosis and Classification of Bone Tumors

Ackermann W (1956) Vertebral trephine biopsy. Ann Surg 143:373–385
Adapon BD, Legada BD, Lim EVA, Silao JV, Dalmacio-Cruz A (1981) CT guided closed biopsy of the spine. J Comput Assist Tomogr 5:73

Awtar K (1975) Rapid flow cytofluorometric analysis of mammalian cell cycle by propidium iodide staining. J Cell Biol 66:188

Ayala AG, Zornosa J (1983) Primary bone tumors: percutaneous needle biopsy. Radiology 149:675–679

Baldwin RW, Pimm MV (1983) Antitumor monoclonal antibodies for radioimmunodetection of tumors and drug targeting. Cancer Metastasis Rev 2:89–106

Battifora H (1984) Recent progress in the immunohistochemistry of solid tumors. Semin Diagn Pathol 1:251–272

Bender CE, Berquist TH, Wold LE (1986) Imaging assisted percutaneous biopsy of the thoracic spine. Mayo Clin Proc 61:942

Berenstein M (1984) Punción biopsia de las lesiones óseas con aguja de Jamshidi. Rev Asoc Arg Ortop y Traumatol 50:393–402

Bilbao JL, Algawa SM, de Negri M et al. (1990) Osteosarcoma: correlation between radiological and histological changes after intra-arterial chemotherapy. Eur J Radiol 11:98

Birge EA, Imhoff CD (1952) Versenate as a decalcifying agent for bone. Am J Clin Pathol 22:192–193

Bloem JL, Taminian AH, Eulderink F et al. (1988) Radiologic staging of primary bone sarcoma: MR imaging, scintigraphy, angiography and CT correlated with pathologic examination. Radiology 169: 805

Bohndorf K, Reiser M, Lochner B et al. (1986) Magnetic resonance imaging of primary tumours and tumour-like lesions of bone. Skeletal Radiol 15:511

Chuang VP, Benjamin R, Jaffe M et al. (1982) Radiographic and angiographic changes in osteosarcoma after intra-arterial chemotherapy. AJR 139:1065

Codman EA (1922) The registry of cases of bone sarcoma. Surg Gynecol Obstet 34:335

Coley BL, Higinbotham NL (1938) Giant cell tumor of bone. J Bone Joint Surg 20:870

Coley BL, Sharp GS, Ellis EB (1931) Diagnosis of bone tumors by aspiration. Am J Surg 13:215–224

Dahlin DC (1978) Bone tumors, 3rd edn. Charles C. Thomas, Springfield, IL

DeSantos LA, Murray JA, Ayala AG (1979) The value of percutaneous needle biopsy in the management of primary bone tumors. Cancer 43:735–744

Dollahite HA, Tatum L, Moinuddin SM, Carnesale PG (1989) Aspiration biopsy of primary neoplasms of bone. J Bone Joint Surg [Am] 71:1166–1169

Eilber FR, Eckhardt J, Morton DL (1984) Advances in the treatment of sarcomas of the extremity: current status of limb salvage. Cancer 54:2695–2701

Ellis F (1947) Needle biopsy in the clinical diagnosis of tumors. Br J Surg 34:240–261

Embleton MJ, Glenn B, Byers VS, Baldwin RW (1981) Antitumour reactions of monoclonal antibody against a human osteogenic sarcoma cell line. Br J Cancer 43:582–587

Embleton MJ, Rowland GF, Simmonds RG et al. (1983) Selective cytotoxicity against human tumour cells by a vindesine-monoclonal antibody conjugate. Br J Cancer 47:43–49

Enneking WF (1985) Staging of musculoskeletal neoplasms. Skeletal Radiol 13:183

Enneking WF, Jewett EL (1982) The issue of biopsy. J Bone Joint Surg [Am] 64:1119–1120

Erlemann R, Sciuk J, Bosse A et al. (1990) Response of osteosarcoma and Ewing's sarcoma to pre-operative chemotherapy: assessment with dynamic and static MR imaging and skeletal scintigraphy. Radiology 175:791

Evarts CMcC (1975) Diagnostic techniques: Closed biopsy of bone. Clin Orthop 107:100–111

Ewing J (1939) A review of the classification of bone tumors. Bull Am Coll Surg 24:290–295

Farrands PA, Perkins A, Sully L, Hopkins JS, Pimm MV, Baldwin RW, Hardcastle JD (1983) Localisation of human osteosarcoma by antitumour monoclonal antibody. J Bone Joint Surg [Br] 65:638–640

Fordham EW, Ramachandran PC (1977) Study of bone tumors with radionuclides. Encyclopedia of medical radiology, vol V, part 6. Springer Berlin Heidelberg New York, pp 603–633

Frager DH, Goldman MJ, Seimon LP et al. (1987) Computed tomography guidance for skeletal biopsy. Skeletal Radiol 16:644–646

Frankel CJ (1954) Aspiration biopsy of the spine. J Bone Joint Surg [Am] 36:69–74

Galasko CSB (1969) The detection of skeletal metastasis from mammary cancer by gamma camera scintigraphy. Br J Surg 56:575

Galasko CSB (1975) The pathological basis for skeletal scintigraphy. J Bone Joint Surg [Br] 57:353–359

Gatenby RA, Mulhern CB, Modofsky PJ (1984) Computed tomography guided thin needle biopsy of small lytic bone lesions. Skeletal Radiol 11:289

Gay S, Miller EJ (1978) Collagen in the physiology and pathology of connective tissue. Fischer, Stuttgart

Geschickter CF, Copeland MM (1949) Tumors of bone, 3rd edn. J.B. Lippincott, Philadelphia

Glass AG, Fraumeni JF (1970) Epidemiology of bone cancer in children. JNCI 44:187–199

Goidanich IF (1956) I tumori primitivi dell'osso. Atti 41st Congr Soc Ital Ortop Traumatol, Bologna

Goldstein H, McNeil BJ, Zufall E et al. (1989) Is there still a place for bone scanning in Ewing's sarcoma? J Nucl Med 21:10

Greep RO, Fischer CJ, Morse A (1948) Alkaline phosphatase in odontogenesis and osteogenesis and its histochemical demonstration after demineralization. J Am Dent Assoc 36:427

Haaga JR, Alfidi RJ (1976) Precise biopsy localization by computed tomography. Radiology 118:603

Hardy DC, Murphy WA, Gilula LA (1980) Computed tomography in planning percutaneous bone biopsy. Radiology 134:447–450

Hudson TM, Enneking WF, Hawkins IF Jr (1981) The value of angiography in planning surgical treatment of bone tumors. Radiology 138:283–289

Hudson TM, Schiebler M, Springfield DS et al. (1983) Radiologic imaging of osteosarcoma: role in planning surgical treatment. Skeletal Radiol 10:137

Jamshidi K, Swaim WR (1971) Bone marrow biopsy with unaltered architecture: a new biopsy device. J Lab Clin Med 77:335–342

Jeffree GM, Price CHG (1965) Bone tumors and their enzymes: a study of the phosphatases, non-specific esterases and betaglucuronidase of osteogenic and cartilaginous tumors, and fibroblastic and giant cell lesions. J Bone Joint Surg [Br] 47:120–136

Jensen RD, Drake RM (1970) Rarity of Ewing's tumors in Negroes. Lancet I:777

Johnson LC (1953) A general theory of bone tumors. Bull NY Acad Med 29:164–171

Katz RL, Silva EG, DeSantos LA, Lukeman JM (1980) Diagnosis of eosinophilic granuloma of bone by cytology, histology, and electron microscopy of transcutaneous bone-aspiration biopsy. J Bone Joint Surg [Am] 62:1284–1290

Kreicbergs A, Boquist L, Borssen B, Larsson SE (1982a) Prognostic factors in chondrosarcoma: a comparative study of cellular DNA content and clinicopathologic features. Cancer 50:577

Kreicbergs A, Brostrom LA, Cewrien G, Einhorn S (1982b) Cellular DNA content in human osteosarcoma: aspects of diagnosis and prognosis. Cancer 50:2476

Kreicbergs A, Silversward C, Tribukait B (1984) Flow DNA analysis of primary bone tumors: relationship between cellular DNA content and histopathologic classification. Cancer 53:129

Kumpan W, Lechner G, Wittich GR et al. (1986) The angiographic response following pre-operative chemotherapy. Skeletal Radiol 15:96

Layfield LJ, Glasgow BJ, Anders KH, Mirra JM (1987) Fine needle aspiration cytology of primary bone lesions. Acta Cytol 31:177–184

Lichtenstein L (1952) Bone tumors. C.V. Mosby, St. Louis

Linden G, Dunn JE (1970) Ewing's sarcoma in Negroes. Lancet I:1171

MacKenzie A, Court Brown W, Doll R, Sissons HA (1961) Mortality from primary tumors of bone in England and Wales. Br Med J I:1782–1790

Mankin HJ, Connor JF, Schiller AL et al. (1985) Grading of bone tumors by analysis of nuclear DNA content using flow cytometry. J Bone Joint Surg [Am] 67:404

Mankin HJ, Lange TA, Spanier SS (1982) The hazards of biopsy in patients with malignant primary bone and soft tissue tumors. J Bone Joint Surg [Am] 64: 1121–1127

Mankin HJ, Matsuno T, Gebhardt MC, Schiller AL, Rosenberg A (1988) Flow cytometry in the management of bone tumors. In: Unni KK (ed) Bone tumors. Churchill Livingstone, New York, pp 85–106

Martin HE, Ellis EB (1934) Aspiration biopsy. Surg Gynecol Obstet 59:578–589

Martin HE, Steward RW (1936) The advantages and limitations of aspiration biopsy. Am J Roentgenol Radium Ther 35:345–347

McDonald DJ, Sim FH, McLeod RA et al. (1986) Giant-cell tumor of bone. J Bone Joint Surg [Am] 68:235

Meyerding HW (1941) Benign and malignant cell tumors of bone. Diagnosis and treatment. J Am Med Assoc 117:1849–1855

Mick CA, Zinrecih J (1985) Percutaneous trephine biopsy of the thoracic spine. Spine 10:737

Miller RW (1976) Etiology of childhood bone cancer: epidemiologic observations. Recent Results Cancer Res 54:50–62

Miller RW, Dalager NA (1974) U.S. childhood cancer deaths by cell types, 1960–68. J Pediatr 85:664–668

Mink J (1986) Percutaneous bone biopsy in the patient with known or suspected osseous metastases. Radiology 161:191

Misdorp W, Hart G, Delemarre JFM et al. (1988) An analysis of spontaneous and chemotherapy-associated changes in osteosarcoma. J Pathol 156:119

Morris RE Jr, Benton RS (1956) Studies on demineralization of bone. Am J Clin Pathol 26:579–595, 596–603, 771–777

Murphy WA (1983) Radiologically guided percutaneous musculoskeletal biopsy. Orthop Clin North Am 14: 233–241

Murphy WA, Destouet JM, Gilula LA (1981) Percutaneous skeletal biopsy 1981: a procedure for radiologists – results, review, and recommendations. Radiology 139:545–549

Nakamura Y, Becker LE, Marks A (1983) S-100 protein in tumors of cartilage and bone: an immunohistochemical study. Cancer 52:1820

Neville AM, Foster CSF, Moshakis V et al. (1982) Monoclonal antibodies in human tumor pathology. Hum Pathol 13:1067–1081

Ottolenghi CE (1955) Diagnosis of orthopaedic lesions by aspiration biopsy. Results of 1061 punctures. J Bone Joint Surg [Am] 37:443–464

Ottolenghi CE (1969) Aspiration biopsy of the spine. Technique for the thoracic spine and results of twenty-eight biopsies of this region. J Bone Joint Surg [Am] 51:1531–1544

Ottolenghi CE, Schajowicz F, DeSchant FA (1964) Aspiration biopsy of the cervical spine. J Bone Joint Surg [Am] 46:715–733

Parker F, Jackson H (1939) Primary reticulum cell sarcoma of bone. Surg Gynecol Obstet 68:45

Pettersson H, Gillespy T III, Hamlin DJ et al. (1987) Primary musculoskeletal tumors: examinations with MR imaging compared with conventional modalities. Radiology 164:237

Phemister DB (1930) Chondrosarcoma of bone. Surg Gynecol Obstet 50:216

Phemister DB (1949) Panel on bone tumors. Proc 1st Natl Cancer Conf, p 217

Picci P, Bacci G, Campanacci M et al. (1985) Histologic evaluation of necrosis in osteosarcoma induced by chemotherapy. Regional mapping of viable and non-viable tumor. Cancer 56:1515

Picci P, Bacci G, Ricci M et al. (1988) Histological evaluation and prognostic correlation in Ewing's sarcoma. In: Kotz R (ed) Proceedings of First Meeting of the European Musculoskeletal Oncology Society (EMSOS). Howmedica International, Vienna, pp 69–70

Ray RD (1953) Needle biopsy of the lumbar vertebral bodies. A modification of the Valls technique. J Bone Joint Surg [Am] 35:760–762

Raymond AK, Ayala AG (1988) Specimen management after osteosarcoma chemotherapy. In: Unni KK (ed) Bone tumors. Churchill Livingstone, New York, pp 157–181

Remberger K, Gay S (1977) Immunohistochemical demonstration of different collagen types in the normal epiphyseal plate and in benign and malignant tumors of bone and cartilage. Z Krebsforschung 90: 95–106

Richman IM, Gelfand M, Hill JM (1947) A method of decalcifying bone for histologic section. Arch Pathol 44:92–95

Robertson WW, Janssen HF, Pugh JL (1984) The spread of tumor-cell sized particles after bone biopsy. J Bone Joint Surg [Br] 66:1243–1247

Roessner A, Mellin W, Hiddemann B, Voss B, Vollmer L, Grundmann E (1984) New cytomorphologic methods in the diagnosis of bone tumors: possibilities and limitations. Semin Diagn Pathol 1:199–214

Rosen G, Caparros B, Huvos AG et al. (1982) Preoperative chemotherapy for osteogenic sarcoma:

selection of postoperative adjuvant chemotherapy based on the response of the primary tumor to preoperative chemotherapy. Cancer 49:1221–1230
Salzer-Kuntschik M, Delling G, Beron G et al. (1983) Morphological grades of regression in osteosarcoma after polychemotherapy – study COSS 80. J Cancer Res Clin Oncol 106:21–24
Schajowicz F (1955) Aspiration biopsy in bone lesions – cytological and histological techniques. J Bone Joint Surg [Am] 37:465–471
Schajowicz F (1959) Ewing's sarcoma and reticulum cell sarcoma of bone. With special reference to the histochemical demonstration of glycogen as an aid to differential diagnosis. J Bone Joint Surg [Am] 41: 185–192
Schajowicz F, Cabrini RL (1954) Histochemical studies of bone in normal and pathological conditions. J Bone Joint Surg [Br] 36:474–489
Schajowicz F, Cabrini RL (1958a) Histochemical studies on glycogen in normal ossification and calcification. J Bone Joint Surg [Am] 40:1081
Schajowicz F, Cabrini RL (1958b) Histochemical localization of acid phosphatase in bone tissue. Science 127:1447–1448
Schajowicz F, Derqui JC (1968) Puncture biopsy in lesions of the locomotor system. Review of results in 4050 cases, including 941 vertebral punctures. Cancer 21:531–548
Schajowicz F, Gimenez IB, Conti CJ, Cabrini RL (1976) Estudio microespectrofotométrico del ADN en condromas y condrosarcomas. Boletín de la Sociedad Argentina de Ortopedia Y Traumatología 24:147
Schajowicz F, Hokama J (1976) Aspiration (puncture or needle) biopsy in bone lesions. Recent Results Cancer Res 54:139–144
Schajowicz F, Mondolfo S (1955) Clasificación de los tumores óseos. Rev Ortop Traumatol Lat-Am 37:266
Shaltot A, Michell PA, Betts JA, Darby AJ, Gishen P (1982) Jamshidi needle biopsy of bone lesions. Clin Radiol 33:193–196
Sicard A, Boureau M, Marsan C (1958) La biopsie transcutanée des corps vertebraux. J Chir (Paris) 76:57–75
Siffert RS, Arkin AM (1949) Trephine biopsy of bone with special reference to the lumbar vertebral bodies. J Bone Joint Surg [Am] 31:146–149
Simon MA (1982) Current concepts review: biopsy of musculoskeletal tumors. J Bone Joint Surg [Am] 64: 1253–1257
Sreebny LM, Nikiforuk G (1951) Demineralization of hard tissues by organic chelating agents. Science 113:560
Stewart FW (1933) The diagnosis of tumors by aspiration. Am J Pathol 9:801–811
Stoker DJ, Kissin CM (1985) Percutaneous vertebral biopsy: a review of 135 cases. Clin Radiol 36:569–577
Subramanian G, McAfee JG (1977) A new complex of ^{99m}TC for skeletal imaging. Radiology 99:192
Subramanian G, McAfee JG, Bell EG et al. (1972) ^{99m}TC labeled polyphosphate as a skeletal agent. Radiology 102:701
Sundaram M, McDonald DJ (1989) The solitary tumor or tumorlike lesion. Top Magn Reson Imag 1(4):17
Sundaram M, McGuire MH (1988) Computed tomography or magnetic resonance for evaluating the solitary tumor or tumor-like lesion of bone? Skeletal Radiol 17:393
Sundaram M, McGuire MH, Herbold DR et al (1986) Magnetic resonance imaging in planning limb-salvage surgery for primary malignant tumors of bone. J Bone Joint Surg [Am] 68:809
Sundaram M, McLeod RA (1990) MR imaging of tumor and tumorlike lesions of bone and soft tissue. AJR 155:817
Taylor SR, Nunez C (1984) Fine-needle aspiration biopsy in a pediatric population. Report of 64 consecutive cases. Cancer 54:1449–1453
Thomas P, Battifora H, Maderino GL, Patrick J (1987) A monoclonal antibody against neuron-specific enolase: immunohistochemical comparison with a polyclonal antiserum. Am J Clin Pathol 88:146
Tsai CC, McGuire MH, Mellitt RJ, Ritter RA III, Xu J, Litwicki DJ, Roodman ST (1990) Monoclonal antibody to human osteosarcoma: a novel M_r 26000 protein recognized by murine hybridoma TMMR-2[1]. Cancer Res 50:152–158
Tsang KY, Warren RQ, Bishop L, Pathak S, Koger B, Lavia MF (1986) Monoclonal antibodies to human osteosarcoma-associated antigen(s). JNCI 77: 1175–1180
Tsokos M, Linnoil RI, Chandra RS, Triche TJ (1984) Neuron-specific enolase in the diagnosis of neuroblastoma and other small round-cell tumors in children. Hum Pathol 15:575
Urban C, Rosen G, Huvos AG et al. (1983) Chemotherapy of malignant fibrous histiocytoma of bone: a report of five cases. Cancer 51:795–802
Valls J, Ottolenghi CE, Schajowicz F (1948) Aspiration biopsy in diagnosis of lesions of vertebral bodies. JAMA 136:376–382
Valls J, Ottolenghi CE, Schajowicz F (1954) La biopsia per aspirazione nella diagnosi delle lesioni dei corpi vertebrali. Chir Organi Mov 4:49–68
Virchow R (1864–1865) Die krankhaften Geschwülste, 2nd vol. Hirschwald, Berlin
Wada T, Uede T, Ishii S, Matsuyama K, Yamawaki S, Kikuchi K (1988) Monoclonal antibodies that detect different antigenic determinants of the same human osteosarcoma-associated antigen. Cancer Res 48: 2273–2279
Weiss AP, Dorfman HD (1986) S-100 protein in human cartilage lesions. J Bone Joint Surg [Am] 68:521
Williams AD (1975) Tumors in childhood in Ibadan, Nigeria. Cancer 36:370–378
Young JL, Miller RW (1975) Incidence of malignant tumors in United States children. J Pediatr 86: 254–258

CHAPTER I

Bone-Forming Tumors

A. Benign

1. Osteoma

Definition, WHO: *"A benign lesion consisting of well differentiated mature bone tissue with a predominantly laminar structure, and showing very slow growth."*

Many investigators regard osteomas as hamartomas rather than as true tumors, but in the classification system adopted in the fascicle of the Armed Forces Institute of Pathology (Spjut et al. 1971) and in most textbooks, osteoma is included in the group of benign bone-forming tumors.

Three different types of osteomas may be distinguished:

1. Conventional classic osteoma ("ivory exostosis")
2. Parosteal (juxtacortical) osteoma
3. Medullary osteoma (enostosis)

Conventional osteoma involves almost exclusively bones of intramembranous (direct) bone formation, preferentially the external table of the skull and the paranasal sinuses, most commonly the frontal and the ethmoid sinuses (Smith and Zavaleta 1952; Andrew 1956). They are often asymptomatic findings and are reported more frequently in the dental (Noren and Roche 1978) and otolaryngologic literature (Teed 1941; Bullough 1965; Graham 1979). The location at the inner table and maxillary bones (Phemister and Grimson 1937) is less frequent, the clavicle being rarely involved.

Many so-called osteomas in long or flat bones represent post-traumatic hyperostosis or long-standing sessile osteochondromas, but we found a number of cases (31) which we classified as parosteal (juxtacortical) osteomas, with microscopic features clearly distinctive from those of periosteal osteosarcoma, despite their radiologic similarities (Tamarit and Pardo 1977).

Both types of osteomas, the cranial osteoma ("ivory exostosis") and the osteomas of long bones, are located almost exclusively at the external surface of a bone. It is difficult to determine whether the origin is periosteal or parosteal, and in the writer's opinion the term "parosteal osteoma" could be applied to both types. These should be distinguished from the intramedullary, radiologically dense, well-delineated nodules known as "enostosis" (Jaffe 1958), as "medullary osteoma," or, in the radiologic literature, as "bone fleck" or "bone islands" (Resnick et al. 1983; Ornitsuka 1977; Simon and Mulligan 1985; Gold et al. 1989; Greenspan et al. 1991). Most enostoses are between 5 mm and 2 cm in size; some exceptional cases of giant bone islands have been reported (Mirra et al. 1989; Stern et al. 1985). Although most authors, including this one, consider "medullary osteomas" (enostosis) as hamartomatous lesions with no clinical significance, it has been reported that exceptionally a "bone island" may increase slowly in size over a period of years (Blank and Lieber 1965; Ngan 1972) (Fig. I.1a–c). In these rare cases, it is mandatory to exclude an osteoblastic metastasis or other sclerosing osteoblastic lesion (osteoblastoma) by means of excisional biopsy. This is especially important in the few histologically proven bone islands exhibiting positive bone scans on scintigraphy (Davies et al. 1979; Greenspan et al. 1991).

Clinical Findings. We have recorded 111 osteomas: 52 conventional osteomas, 31 parosteal osteomas, and 28 medullary osteomas. Osteomas of cranial bones were found in all age groups, but parosteal osteomas of long bone were not observed in the first decade; both were more frequent between the second and fourth decades. They were often asymptomatic or the first complaint was the appearance of a swelling, slowly increasing in size and of hard consistency. An infrequent complication was obstruction of the ostium of a paranasal sinus or proptosis. Conventional osteomas were usually located in the cranium (35 cases); of the remainder, nine were located in the paranasal sinuses and eight in the jaw bones (Figs. I.2–I.4). They were more

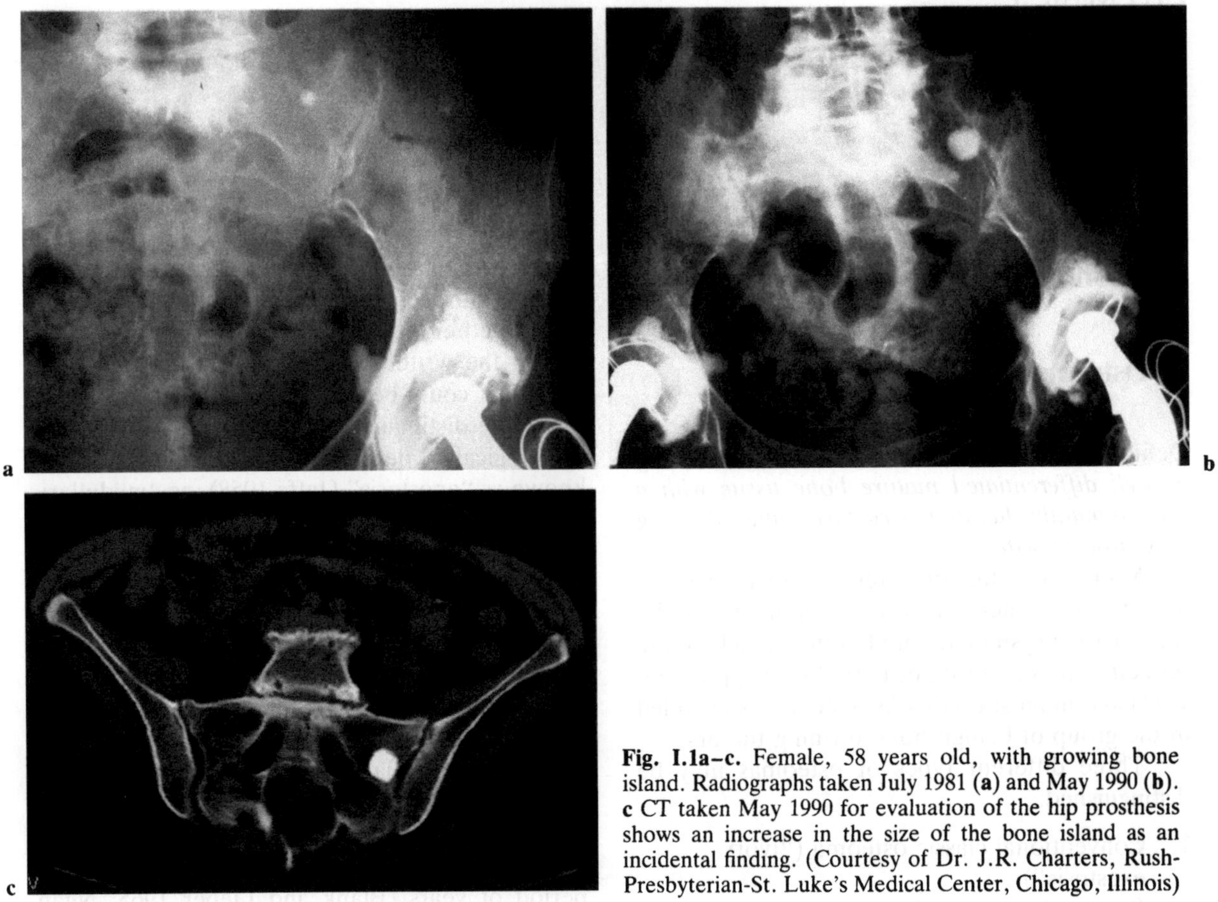

Fig. I.1a–c. Female, 58 years old, with growing bone island. Radiographs taken July 1981 (**a**) and May 1990 (**b**). **c** CT taken May 1990 for evaluation of the hip prosthesis shows an increase in the size of the bone island as an incidental finding. (Courtesy of Dr. J.R. Charters, Rush-Presbyterian-St. Luke's Medical Center, Chicago, Illinois)

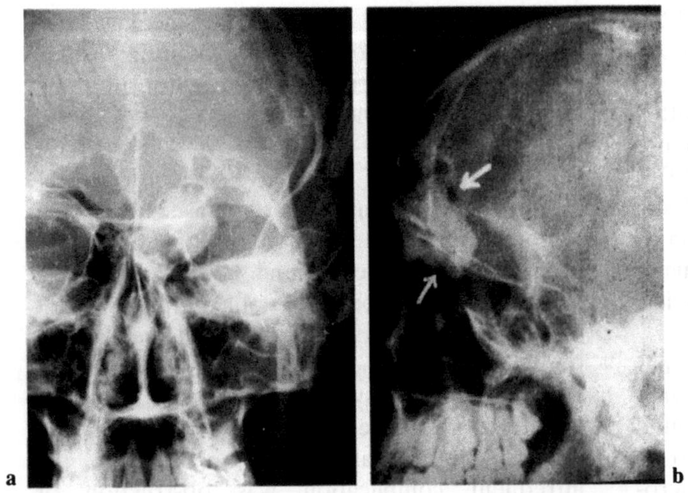

Fig. I.2. a Male, 36 years old, with osteoma of the ethmoid sinus. **b** Female, 40 years old with osteoma of the frontal sinus. Radiographs showing dense, well-circumscribed structureless bony condensation

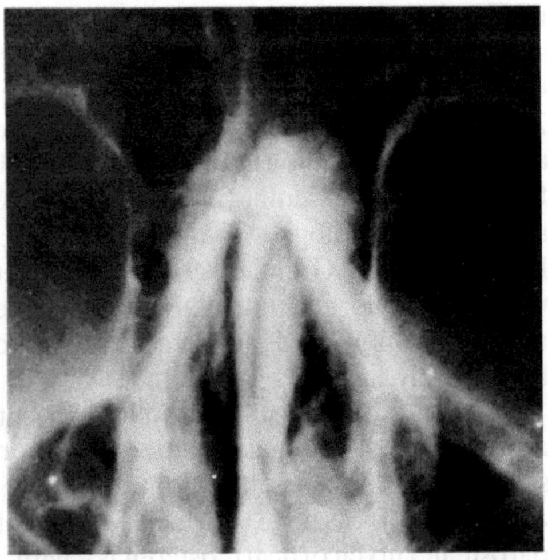

Fig. I.3. Male, 74 years old. Osteoma of the sphenoidal sinus. Radiograph shows compact tumor mass

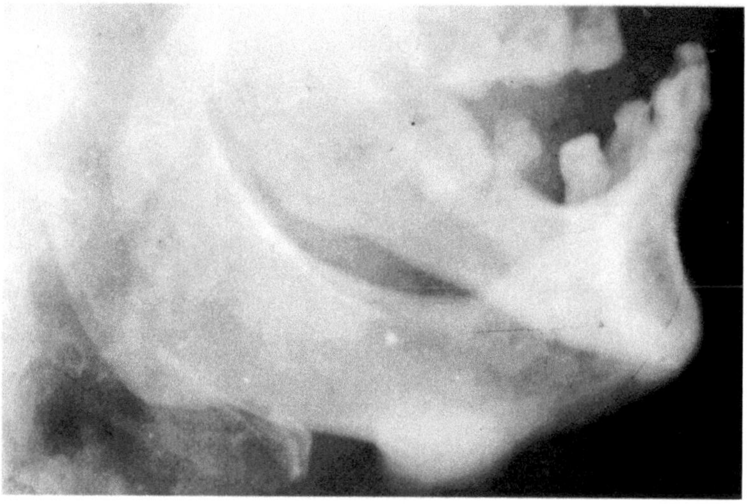

Fig. I.4. Male, 61 years old, with osteoma of the mandible. Radiograph shows a juxtacortical, well-limited sclerotic lesion

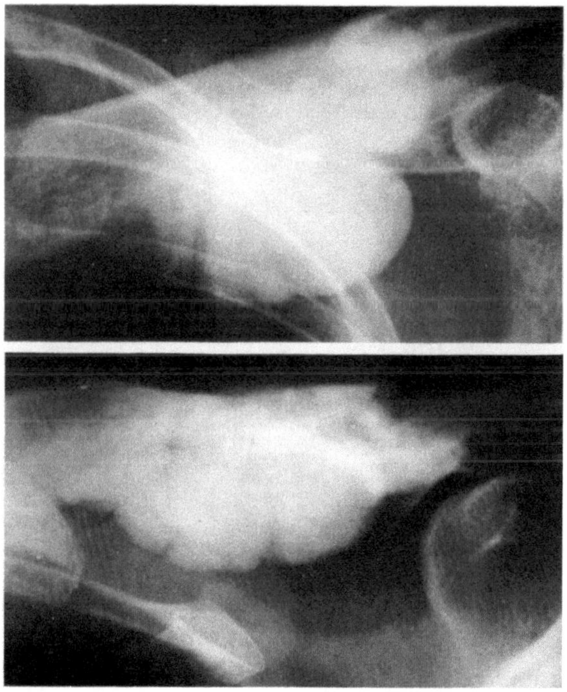

Fig. I.5. Male, 40 years old, with parosteal (juxtacortical) osteoma of the clavicle. Radiographs show a well-limited, dense bony mass, with lobulated surface. A parosteal (juxtacortical) osteosarcoma was suggested, but the histology of the resected specimen did not show any indication of malignancy

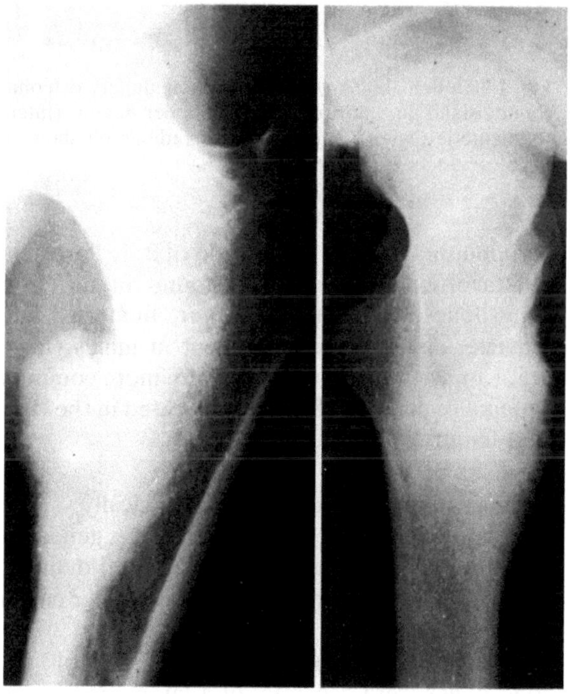

Fig. I.6. Female, 35 years old, with parosteal (juxtacortical) osteoma of the upper femur. Anteroposterior and lateral radiographs show a dense sclerotic juxtacortical lesion

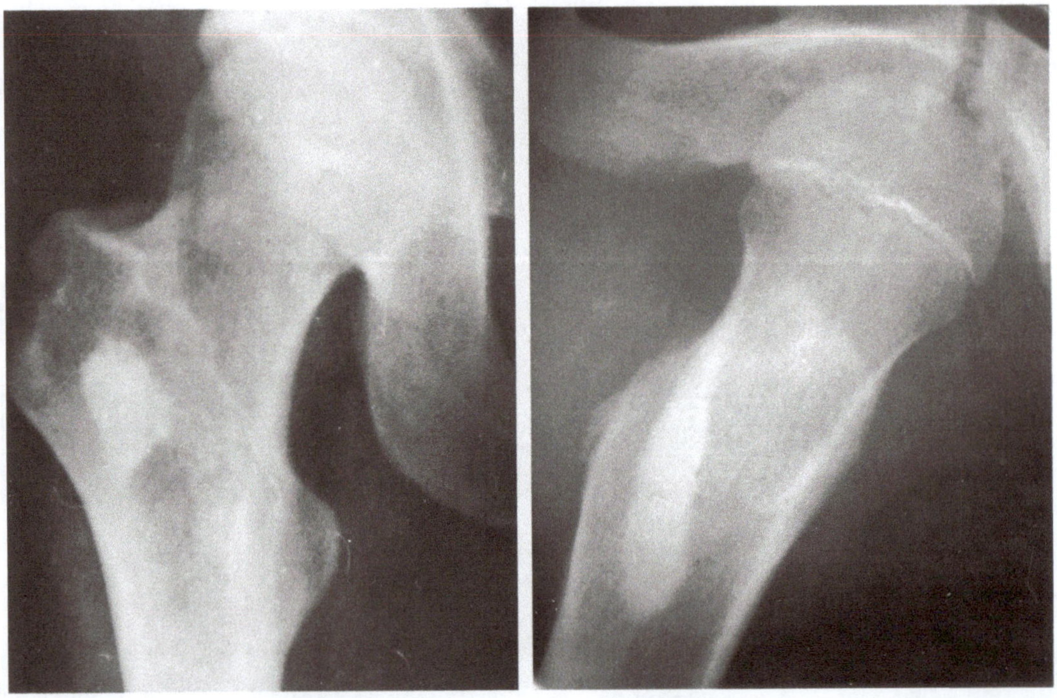

a b

Fig. I.7. **a** Female, 45 years old, with medullary osteoma (bone island or enostosis) of the upper femur (intertrochanteric region); anteroposterior radiograph showing a round dense structureless lesion. **b** A similar ovoid lesion in a 20-year-old male

frequent in females, with a ratio of 2:1. Parosteal (juxtacortical) osteoma was found in different long bones, including the femur, humerus, and clavicle, and was more frequent in males (Figs. I.5, I.6). Medullary osteomas were more common in females and most frequently located in the tibia and femur (Fig. I.7).

Radiographic Features. Radiologically the appearance is a dense, radiopaque, generally structureless bone mass, showing well-defined, often lobular borders, usually less than 3 cm in diameter.

Parosteal (juxtacortical) osteomas of the long bones were generally of a larger size, more elongated, and sometimes more lobulated, as was found in one of our cases located in the clavicle (Fig. I.5).

Osteomas arising from the inner table of the skull (Echlin 1934) should be differentiated from hyperostosis resulting from meningioma, or from hyperostosis frontalis interna.

Occasionally an intensively sclerotized osteoid osteoma or genuine or multifocal osteoblastoma may mimic radiologically a conventional or medullary osteoma (see Fig. I.41). In these cases,

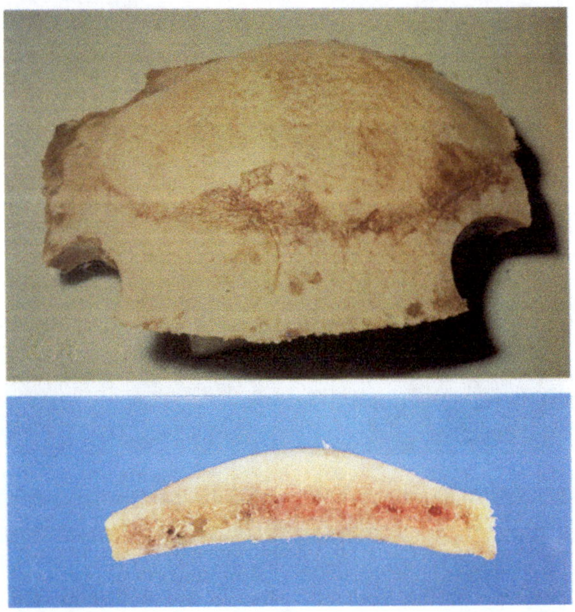

Fig. I.8. Female, 29 years old, with osteoma of the parietal bone. Photographs of the surface and the cut section demonstrate the well-limited, compact juxtacortical bony mass

Fig. I.9. Topographic photomicrograph of an osteoma of the frontal sinus. ×10

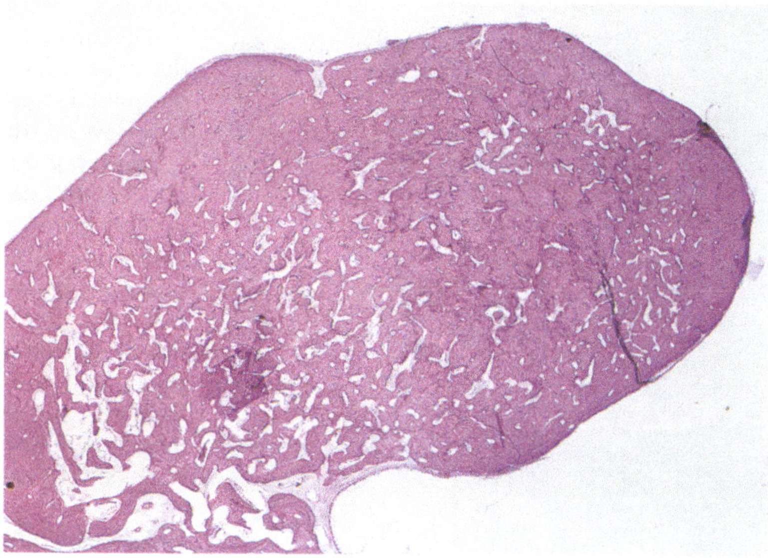

however, CT permits the accurate diagnosis and detection of the nidus.

Pathologic Findings. Most osteomas are dense and compact (ivorylike) bone masses adjacent to the underlying cortex with a well-defined, often lobulated surface, covered by a thin, fibrous membrane that sometimes appears to be in continuity with the periosteum (compact type) (Fig. I.8); rarely, the lesion is more spongious in nature (spongious type).

Histologically, it consists of thick trabeculae of predominantly mature lamellar bone, forming a dense, bony mass, similar to compact cortical bone (Figs. I.9–I.12). The intratrabecular medullary spaces are generally narrow (except in the spongious type) and are occupied by fatty or active marrow, usually without showing osteoblastic or osteoclastic activity (Fig. I.10).

In none of our cases was the surface covered by cartilaginous tissue, which is a characteristic of osteochondromas or of some cases of parosteal osteosarcoma.

Medullary osteoma consists histologically of a dense net of thick compact mature bone trabeculae surrounded by normal spongiosa (Fig. I.13).

Multiple osteomata generally form part of *Gardner's syndrome*, which is a familiar disease with a triad consisting of colonic polyposis, osteomata, and soft tissue tumors (Gardner and

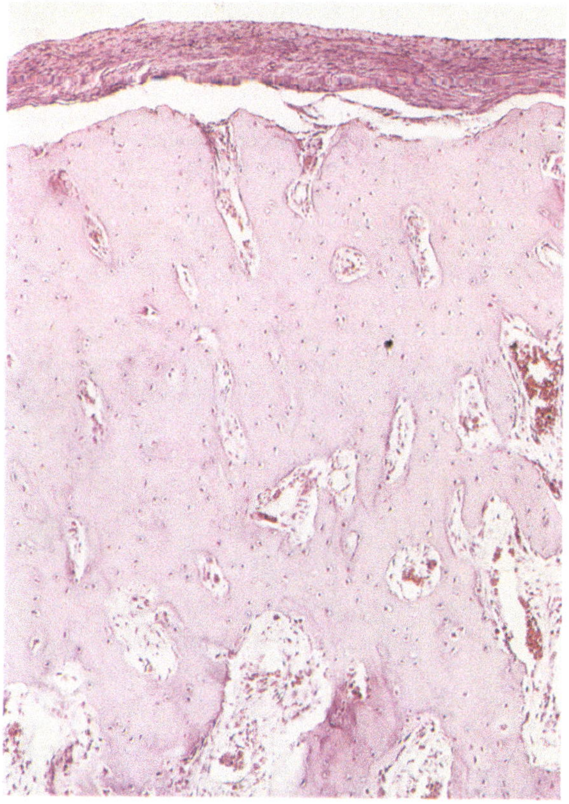

Fig. I.10. Photomicrograph of osteoma reveals newly formed, almost mature bone covered by a layer of fibrous tissue. ×100

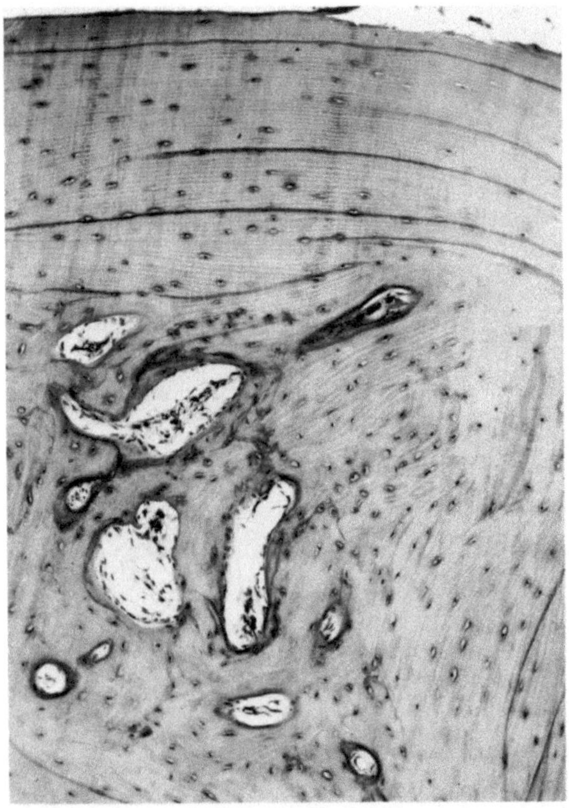

Fig. I.11. Photomicrograph of the periphery of an osteoma, showing dense sclerotic lamellar bone with several cementing lines (bone apposition). ×100; osteoid

Richards 1953). The colonic polyposis is premalignant and colonic cancer may be present at the time of diagnosis. In 1951, Gardner first postulated an autosomal dominant inheritance. In a review of the literature, Jones and Cornell (1966) reported 70 cases of this syndrome. Chang et al. (1968) described a variety of bone lesions, ranging from localized cortical thickening to large osteomas, in 33 members of two families, 4–48 years of age, with this syndrome.

All parts of the skeleton may be involved. In the skull, dense osteomas of the calvaria or the paranasal sinuses, lobulated osteomas arising from the surface of the mandibular angle, and dense pedunculated exostosis of the tubular bones have been observed (Fig. I.14).

Treatment. Treatment is indicated only in patients with clinical symptoms or for aesthetic reasons. It consists of simple excision such as is used for the conventional type of cranial osteoma.

Parosteal osteomas of long bones should be excised in most cases, including the underlying cortex, especially in lesions of larger size, because it is impossible to clinically and radiologically exclude parosteal osteosarcoma. A definite diagnosis can generally be made only after a careful pathologic study of the entire lesion.

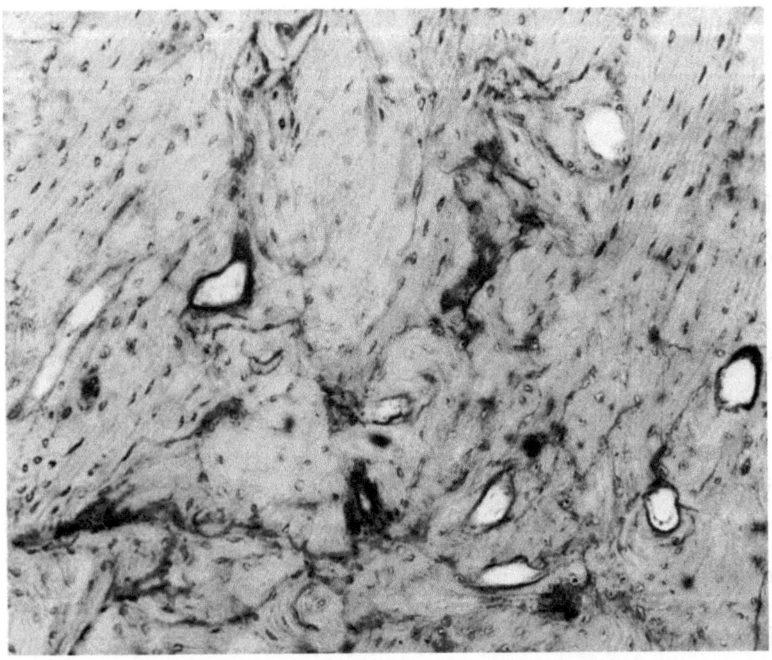

Fig. I.12. Photomicrograph of the central compact part of an osteoma showing irregular distribution and size of bony structures, similar to haversian systems. ×200

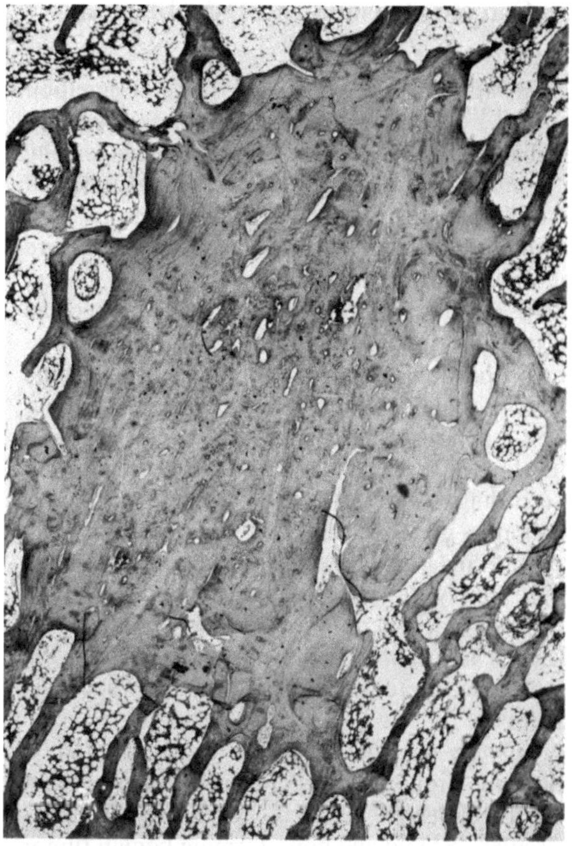

Fig. I.13. Topographic photomicrograph of medullary osteoma ("bone island") of Fig. I.7

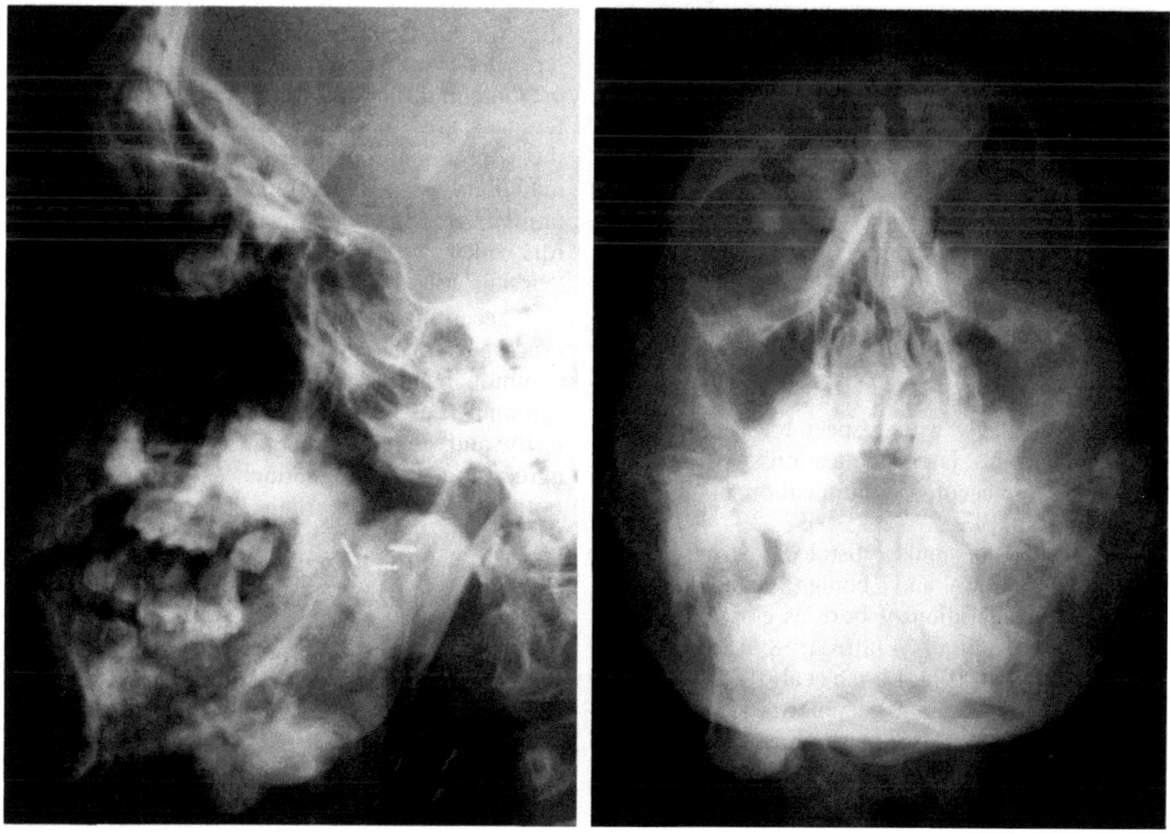

Fig. I.14a,b. Male, 36 years old, with multiple osteomas of the craniofacial bone and intestinal polyposis (Gardner's syndrome). (Courtesy of Dr. J.R. Charters, Rush-Presbyterian-St. Luke's Medical Center, Chicago, Illinois)

2. Osteoid Osteoma and Osteoblastoma

Since Jaffe's classic report (1935), the designation *osteoid osteoma* for a particular bone lesion of probable neoplastic nature has become universally accepted and familiar to orthopedic surgeons and pathologists. The typical osteoid osteoma is a common benign lesion, consisting of a small core or nidus of cellular, highly vascularized tissue, made up of an interlacing network of trabeculae of newly formed bone and osteoid tissue in varying proportions, and, usually, a conspicuous zone of sclerotic bone, the perifocal reactive zone; such a zone is especially typical when the lesion develops in or near a cortical portion of bone. According to Jaffe, the nidus tends not to exceed 1 cm at its greatest diameter but may occasionally reach 2 cm. The reactive perifocal zone is much more likely to be striking when the osteoid osteoma is oriented toward the cortex rather than when it is localized within the spongiosa. In the latter case, there is generally little or no perifocal sclerosis.

Benign osteoblastoma, on the other hand, is the name proposed independently by Jaffe (1956) and Lichtenstein (1956) to designate "a rather vascular, osteoid and bone-forming benign tumor characterized, cytologically, by the abundant presence of osteoblasts"; it also has a larger size (more than 1.5 or 2 cm) and seems to have a predilection for the vertebral column. In a review by Resnick and Niwayama (1988), analysis of 298 benign osteoblastomas reported in the literature revealed the vertebrae to be involved in 30% of the cases.

After Jaffe's first description, this lesion was designated "giant osteoid osteoma" by Dahlin and Johnson (1954) in an attempt to convey the close histologic resemblance to osteoid osteoma and at the same time to indicate a difference especially with respect to size. Dahlin, however, in his later publications favored the more widely accepted denomination of "benign osteoblastoma."

Despite the similar histologic structure of osteoid osteoma and benign osteoblastoma and the consideration of both as closely related lesions, most authors (Jaffe 1958; Lichtenstein 1977; Spjut et al. 1971; Marsh et al. 1975; McLeod et al. 1976) insist upon keeping these tumors as separate entities. This separation is based almost exclusively on clinicoradiologic differences, such as the frequent absence of the characteristic pain pattern and the reactive bone, and the consistently larger size of "benign osteoblastoma" as compared with the limited growth potential of the conventional "osteoid osteoma."

Unfortunately, however, the distinction between these two processes is not always clear, and the problem of differential diagnosis is far from being solved. We have observed an increasing number of borderline lesions with features of both that may be classed in either category according to personal criteria of definition. On the other hand, few cases of spontaneous transition or of local recurrence after incomplete removal of an osteoid osteoma have been published (Campanacci 1990; Bettelli et al. 1991).

In previous publications this writer (Schajowicz and Lemos 1970; 1st edition of this book, 1981) emphasized that osteoid osteoma and osteoblastoma represented closely related processes of osteoblastic derivation without distinguishing histologic and ultrastructural features (Steiner 1976, 1977). Some authors have employed an arbitrary criterion of size, classifying as osteoid osteomas the cases with a maximum nidus size of 1 cm (Byers 1968) or 2 cm (Schajowicz and Lemos 1970). Others (McLeod et al. 1976) have used a dividing line of 1.5 cm for lesions indistinguishable by all other criteria.

Although some clinical and radiologic differences exist between the smaller osteoid osteoma and the larger osteoblastoma, these differences are, in the writer's opinion, probably the consequence of their location (cortical and medullary, respectively). This would explain the limited growth potential of osteoid osteoma, for which we have proposed the designation "circumscribed osteoblastoma."

Accepting in part our criteria, both lesions are reported in the WHO classification under a common heading. However, the term "osteoid osteoma" has been retained because of its familiarity and general acceptance, although it was agreed that the designation "osteoblastoma" for both entities would perhaps be more appropriate.

The writer's concepts have been accepted by Morton et al. (1975) and by De Souza Dias and Frost (1974), who introduced the terms "cortical osteoblastoma" for osteoid osteoma and "spongious osteoblastoma" for genuine osteoblastoma.

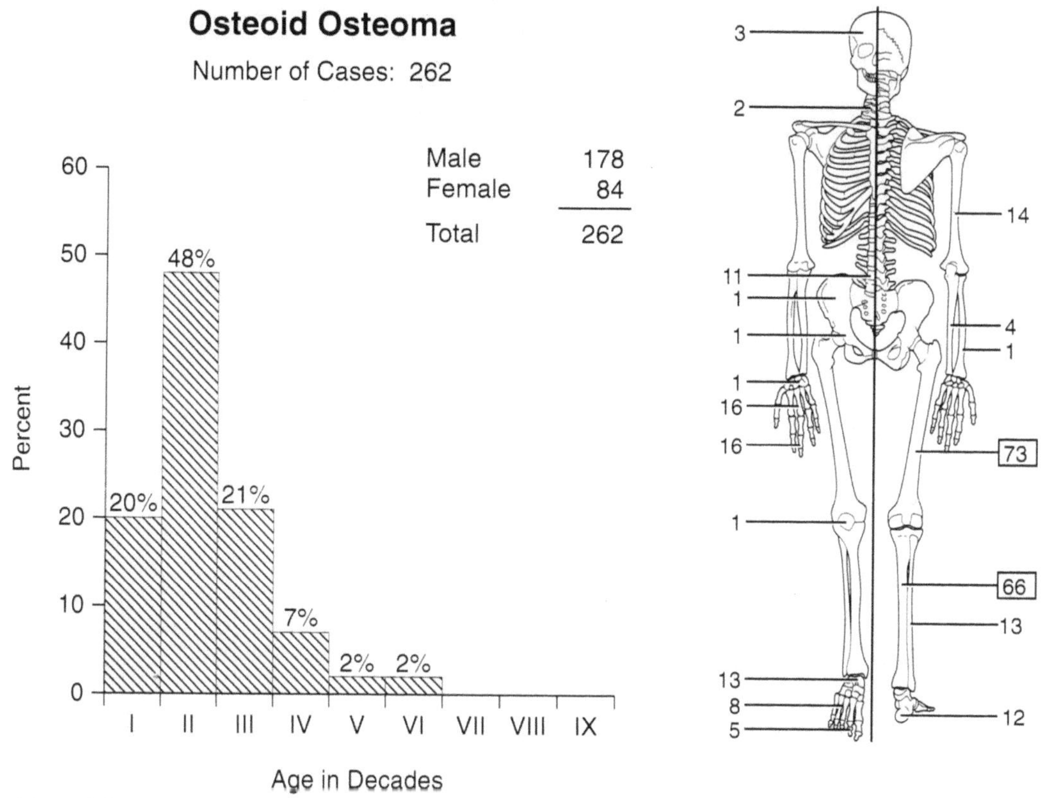

Scheme I.1

Osteoid Osteoma (Circumscribed Osteoblastoma)

Definition, WHO: *"A benign osteoblastic lesion, characterized by its small size (usually less than 1 cm), its clearly demarcated outline and by the usual presence of a surrounding zone of reactive bone formation. Histologically, it consists of cellular, highly vascularized tissue made up of immature bone and osteoid tissue."*

Incidence. The incidence of osteoid osteoma (circumscribed osteoblastoma) is rather high. The 262 cases of our series represented 10.8% of all benign tumors in our material, which is in accordance with other large series (Dahlin and Unni 1986; Campanacci 1990).

Clinical Findings. The data concerning *sex*, *age*, and *localization* coincide, in general, with the data of other authors (Scheme I.1). The tumor occurs more frequently in males (2:1). Almost 50% of the patients were between 11 and 20 years old, and only eight were less than 5 years of age. This tumor occurs rarely in very young children. Our youngest patient was a child of 12 months; other cases reported have been of a 14-month-old (Ponseti and Barta 1947) and of an 8-month-old (Habermann and Stern 1974).

The data concerning anatomic distribution also agree with those of other authors. The femur (73 cases) and the tibia (66 cases) were the most common locations, followed by other long-limb bones. In a review of 661 cases by Resnick and Niwayama, (1988) 57% presented in the femur and tibia, with 71% occurring in long bones. It is interesting to note that 38 of the 73 cases involving the femur were located at the upper end of the femur, principally at the neck and trochanter, and that lesions of the metacarpal, metatarsal, and phalangeal bones were relatively frequent (33 of the hand and 26 of the foot). The carpal bones were rarely involved, but not so the terminal phalanx, contrary to the statements of Caroll (1953), Dunitz et al. (1957), and Rosborough (1966): 21 of our phalangeal tumors were located in a terminal phalanx (16 in the hand and 5 in the foot). Osteoid osteomas of the skull seem to be rare: we have observed only three cases at this location.

Osteoid osteoma of the spine, although less frequent than osteoblastoma, was not uncommon in our experience (13 cases) and in that of others

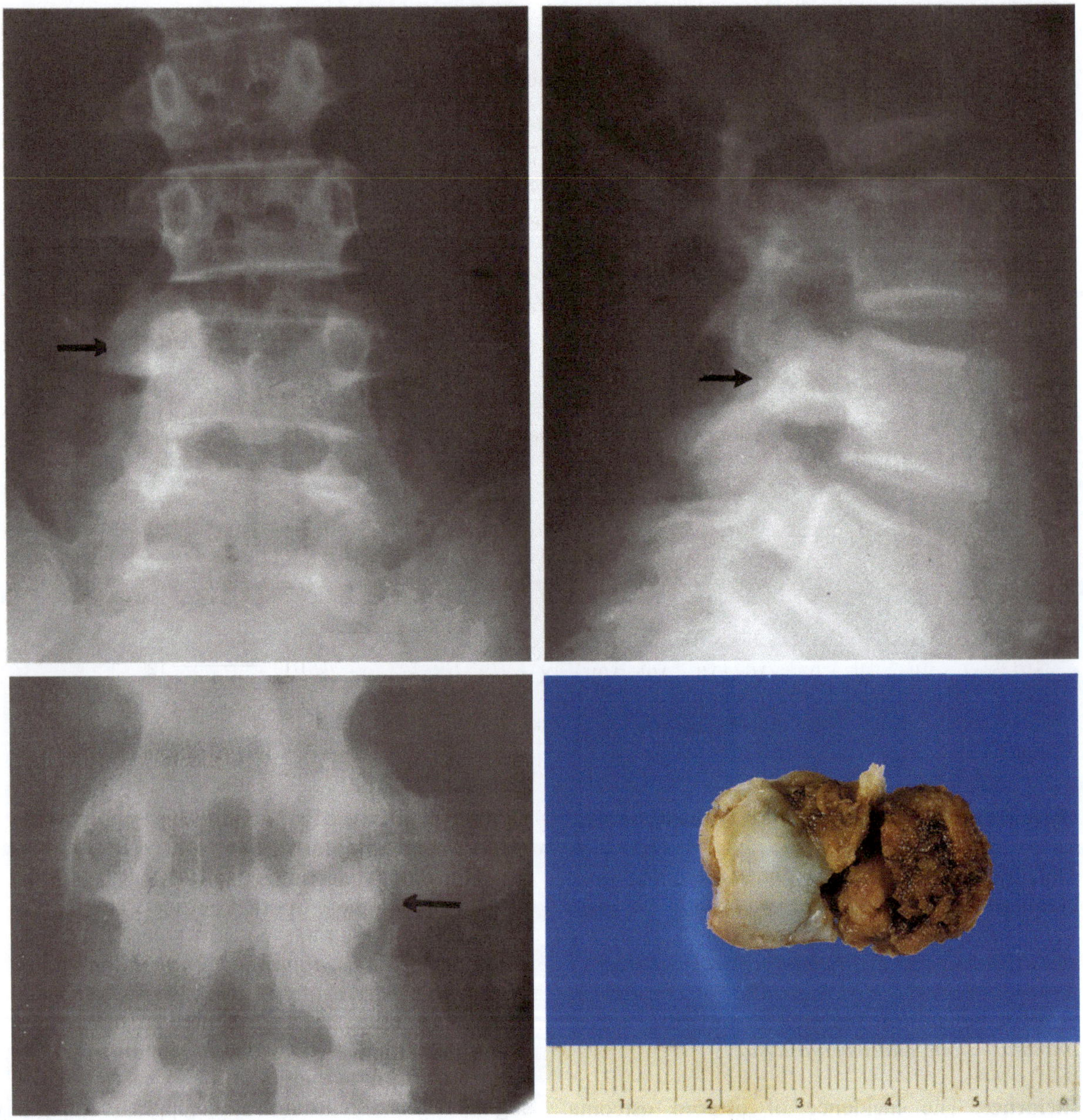

a b c

Fig. I.15. **a** Male, 14 years old. Osteoid osteoma of the pedicle of L4. Anteroposterior and lateral radiographs show sclerotic area and apparent enlargement of the pedicle. **b,c** Female, 18 years old, with a lesion of the pars interarticularis of L3. Radiographs (**b**) demonstrated a sclerotic, poorly delimited lesion. **c** Photograph shows the hyperemic aspect and the size of the lesion (2 cm), which according to the criterion of the pathologist could be classified as osteoid osteoma or osteoblastoma

(Freiberger 1960; MacLellan and Wilson 1967; Keim and Reina 1975; Mehta 1978; Janin et al. 1981; Zwimpfer et al. 1982; Kirwan et al. 1984). It typically occurred in the posterior elements (lamina, the articular facets, and the pedicles). It was usually associated with painful scoliosis with the concavity at the site of the nidus, due to paravertebral muscle spasms, and less frequently with sciatic pain (Keim and Reina 1975; Ransford et al. 1984; Akbarnia and Rooholamini 1981) (Fig. I.15).

Symptoms. The classic, most frequent symptom is pain of increasing severity that is not relieved by rest and is often more intense at night. The pain is sometimes referred to a nearby joint and is

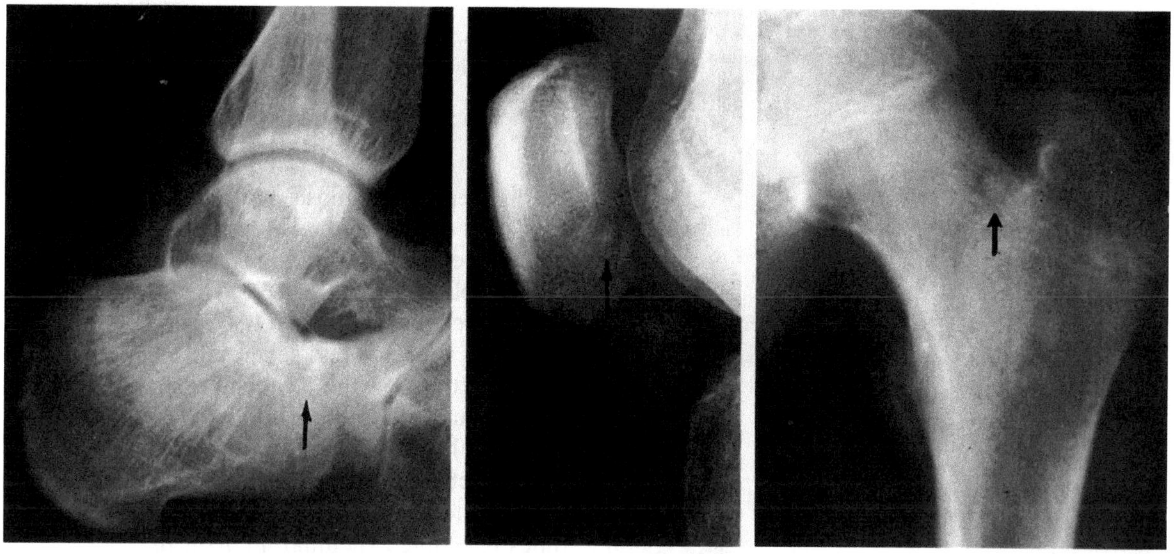
a b, c

Fig. I.16a–c. Three different cases of osteoid osteoma of juxta-articular location, presenting clinically as a synovitis of the involved joint. **a** female, 14 years old; **b** male, 32 years old; **c** male, 20 years old

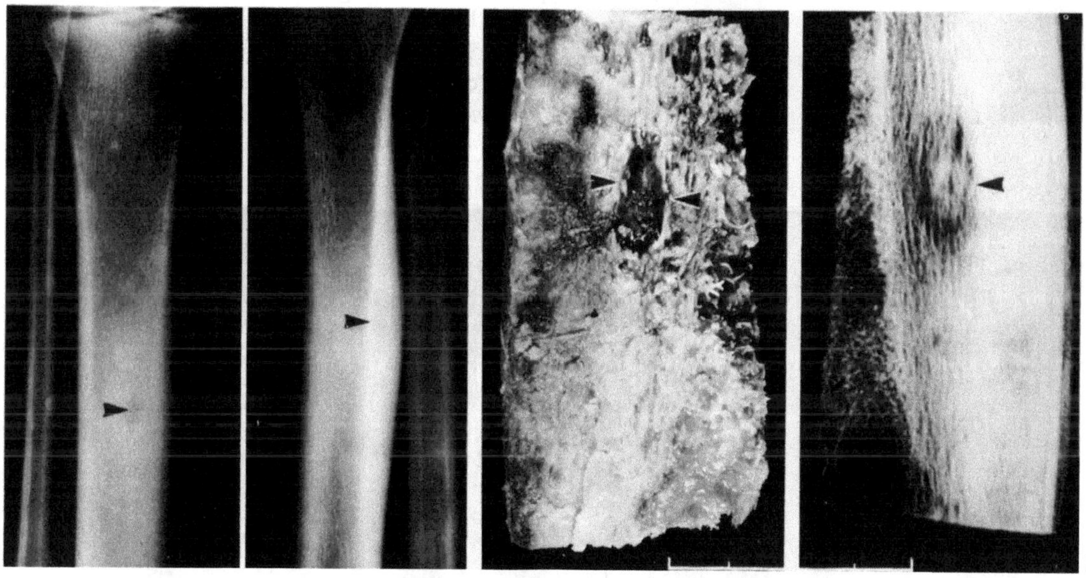
a b, c

Fig. I.17a–c. Male, 9 years old, with osteoid osteoma (circumscribed osteoblastoma) of the shaft of the tibia. **a** Anteroposterior and lateral radiographs showing typical small "nidus" surrounded by reactive bone sclerosis. **b** Photograph of specimen revealing hyperemic aspect of nidus. **c** Radiograph of slab, 5 mm thick, specimen shows a dense calcified zone in the center of the radiolucent nidus

frequently relieved dramatically with aspirin, a fact that was noted early by Jaffe and Lichtenstein (1940). However, this response was not obtained in several of our cases, and Byers (1968) reported negative responses in many cases. A painless osteoid osteoma was also reported by Lawrie and Sinclair (1970). On the other hand, in several of our cases of osteoblastoma and other bone tumors, evident pain relief was obtained with aspirin. The pain may be present for several months before radiographic evidence of the lesion becomes apparent.

Atrophy of muscle, localized swelling, and tenderness were frequent findings in superficial lesions. In several of our cases, osteoid osteoma located adjacent to a joint presented problems

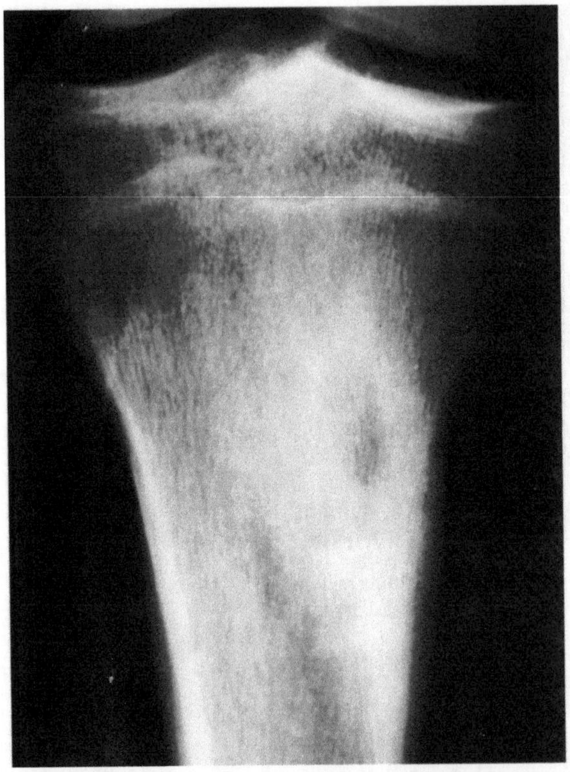

Fig. I.18. Osteoid osteoma. Male, 18 years old. Radiograph showing a radiolucent ovoid "nidus" surrounded by dense sclerotic bone in the upper tibia

of differential diagnosis with an articular process, and the patients were treated for arthritis months before the osteoid osteoma was localized radiographically (Fig. I.16). This fact was first emphasized by Sherman (1947a), who found in two cases more or less severe chronic inflammatory reaction of the synovial membrane with joint effusion. Other authors (Scaglietti and Calandriello 1953; Marcove and Freiberger 1966; Corbett et al. 1974; Snarr et al. 1973) reported similar findings in the adjacent joints that sometimes resembled rheumatoid arthritis.

Radiographic Features. Radiologically, three types may be distinguished according to the location of the nidus (Freiberger et al. 1959; Edeiken et al. 1966): (1) *cortical* (Figs. I.17–I.19), the most frequent, classic type; (2) *medullary or cancellous* (endosteal) (Figs. I.20–I.22); and (3)

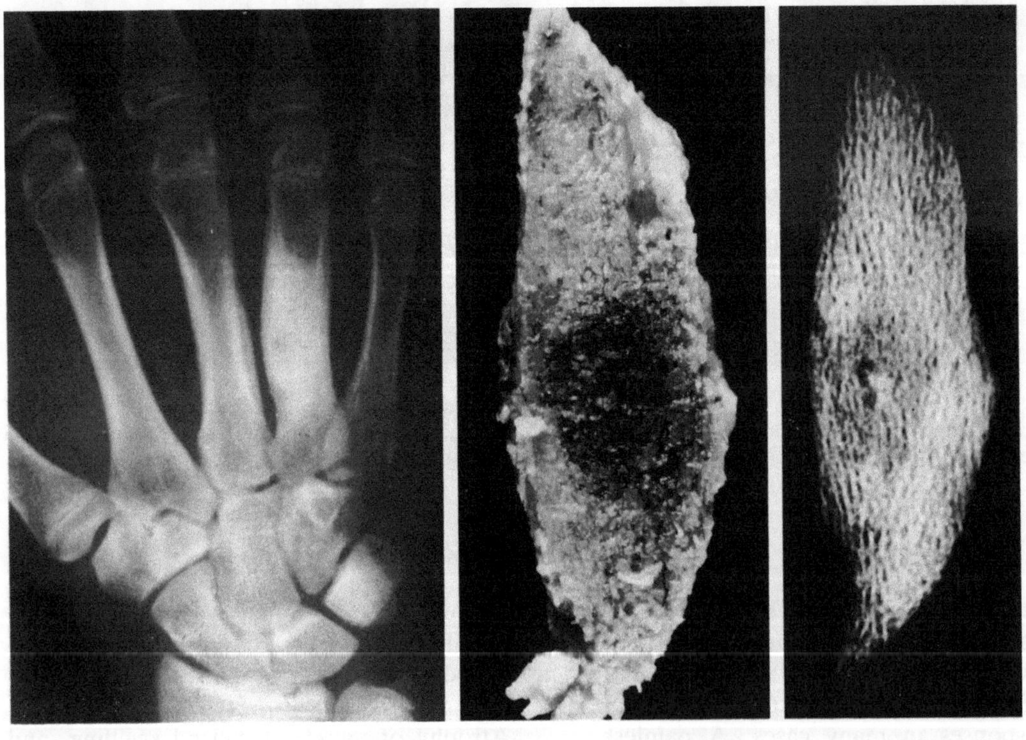

a b, c

Fig. I.19a–c. Male, 15 years old. Osteoid osteoma in the fourth metacarpal bone. **a** Radiograph shows a small nidus surrounded by an extensive area of bone sclerosis. **b** Photograph demonstrates the hyperemic aspect of nidus. **c** Radiograph of a thin slab shows central sclerosis in the nidus surrounded by radiolucent area and reactive sclerosis *subperiosteal or periosteal* (see Fig. I.36), the least frequent type, in which the nidus extends into the soft tissue, raising the periosteum. Rarely, there is reactive bone sclerosis of the underlying cortex; a thin layer of periosteal bone may cover it. These cases are difficult if not impossible to differentiate from the periosteal or peripheral type of "osteoblastoma," their distinction being arbitrary according to size difference. The perifocal reactive sclerosis, which is so characteristic and striking in the cortical type, was mild or completely lacking in 20 of our cases of the intramedullary type (Figs. I.21, I.22). Some of these cases were of juxta-articular location and associated with changes in the adjacent joint (Sherman 1947a). The nidi were osteolytic in the majority of our cases, but in approximately 25% a densely mineralized central part or a ringlike calcified central area (Figs. I.16, I.23) could be observed (Jaffe's "annular sequestrum"). In accordance with other authors (Jaffe 1958; Freiberger et al. 1959), we did not observe any evident correlation between the duration of symptoms and mineralization of the nidus.

It is important to obtain high-quality roentgenograms. The extensive sclerosis may mask the nidus, in which case plain tomography and generally scintigraphy or computed tomography are the most satisfactory methods of depicting the central radiolucent focus (Figs. I.24, I.25) (Gamba et al. 1984). Radioisotope imaging of osteoid osteomas can be very useful both in diagnosis and in anatomic localization (Helms et al. 1984; Smith and Gilday 1980; Sty and Simon 1982; Winter et al. 1977). These lesions avidly take up technetium 99 diphosphonate owing to the intense bone formation within the nidus. Radioisotope imaging can also be useful in the operating room as a technique that can anatomically localize the nidus (Ghelman et al. 1981; Israeli et al. 1983; O'Brien et al. 1984; Papanicolaou 1985) during and after the operation to be certain that the nidus has been fully excised (Ghelman and Vigorita 1983).

Angiography may be useful in demonstrating the hypervascularized nidus in difficult cases (Lindbom et al. 1960; Halpern and Freiberger 1970; O'Hara et al. 1975) and in distinguishing it from the usually less vascularized intracortical bone abscess (Lindbom et al. 1960).

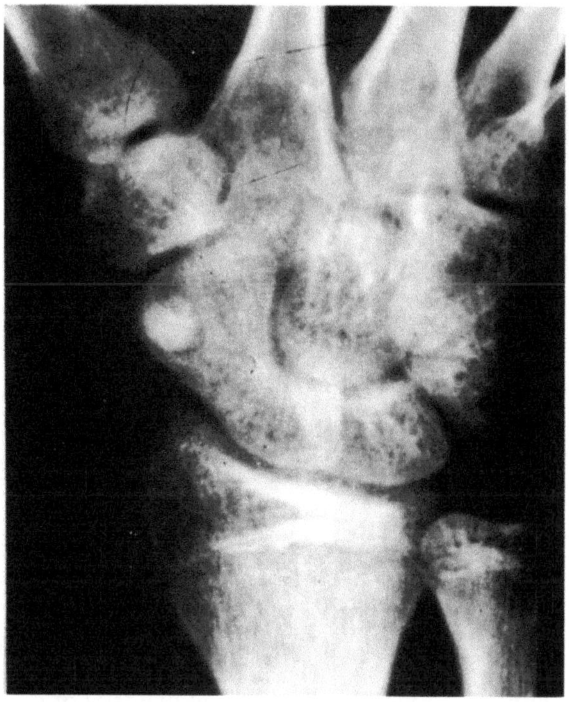

Fig. I.20. Male, 18 years old, with osteoid osteoma in an unusual location in the scaphoid bone, showing a round, almost completely sclerotic "nidus," without surrounding reactive bone sclerosis, which is a common finding in lesions located in cancellous bone

a 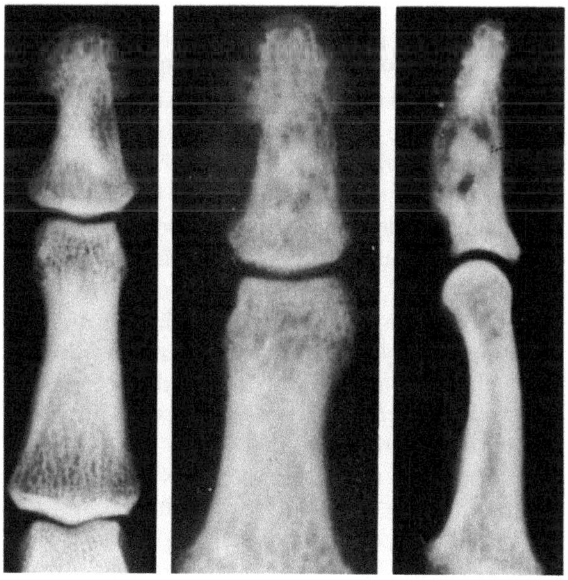 b

Fig. I.21a,b. Two cases of osteoid osteoma of the terminal phalanx. **a** Male, 20 years old. **b** Female, 32 years old. Anteroposterior and lateral radiographs show central sclerosis in the nidus without peripheral reactive sclerosis

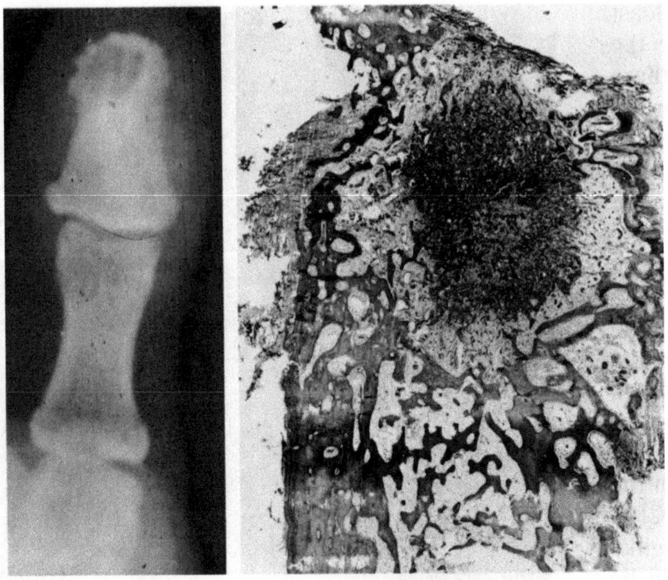

a b

Fig. I.22a,b. Male, 18 years old. **a** Osteoid osteoma of the terminal phalanx of the thumb without striking perifocal sclerosis. **b** Photomicrograph showing the lack of reactive bone sclerosis in the surrounding spongiosa. ×16

Pathologic Findings. In the great majority of our cases, the material received for examination consisted of resection specimens of the nidus included in a more or less extensive block of sclerotic bone; in other cases, fragmented specimens were submitted. To localize the nidus, it is advisable for the pathologist to cut the block longitudinally in sections no more than 5 mm thick (Fig. I.19), taking radiographs in case the nidus is not visible at the cut surface. Using this procedure, the nidus can hardly be missed. As mentioned earlier, the use of a radioisotope probe during the operation can be helpful in localizing the lesion. Other techniques that may be useful include multiplanar fluoroscopy and intraoperative tetracycline fluorescence. The latter technique involves the oral intake of 750–4000 mg tetracycline prior to surgery. Ultraviolet light fluorescence on the resected specimen is used in the operating room to be certain the nidus is excised (Ayala et al. 1986).

In most of our cases, the nidus was less than 1 cm at its largest diameter, reddish in color, and of evident hyperemic aspect (Fig. I.19b). The center of the nidus was often chalky white or grayish, of gritty consistency, surrounded by only a small hemorrhagic ringlike area (Fig. I.23). One patient had osteoid osteomas in two different bones (both upper femurs). Other rare cases with multiple lesions occurring either synchronously or metachronously (Rand et al. 1982) and situated close to each other in the same bone, in adjacent bones, or in two distant locations in widely separated bones have been reported by Glynn and Lichtenstein (1973), Greenspan et al. (1974), McLeod et al. (1976), Uehlinger (1977), and Alcalay et al. (1982), and are referred to as "multicentric osteoid osteoma."

We observed two small nidi adjacent to one another in only two cases. Our other cases with multiple nidi are described in the group of *multifocal osteoblastomas*.

The *histologic picture* (Figs. I.26, I.27) represents a process of dynamic bone remodeling, with alternating areas of active osteoblastic proliferation and formation of osteoid and coarse-fibered (immature or woven), irregularly mineralized bone trabeculae with osteoclastic bone resorption, separated by loose connective tissue rich in hyperemic capillary blood vessels (Fig. I.27). In the central part of the nidus, the immature bone tissue may predominate and accounts for a roentgenographic image generally denser than that of normal bone (Figs. I.23, I.28); on the other hand, the osteoid tissue can be more abundant in this area, causing a translucent image. A central osteoid area sometimes alternates with a woven bone area, followed toward the periphery by another osteoid area. This formation is responsible for the roentgenographic aspect known as "annular sequestrum" (Fig. I.23). Whether the lesion is wholly or partly mineralized at the time of removal depends on the phase at which this cycle is interrupted

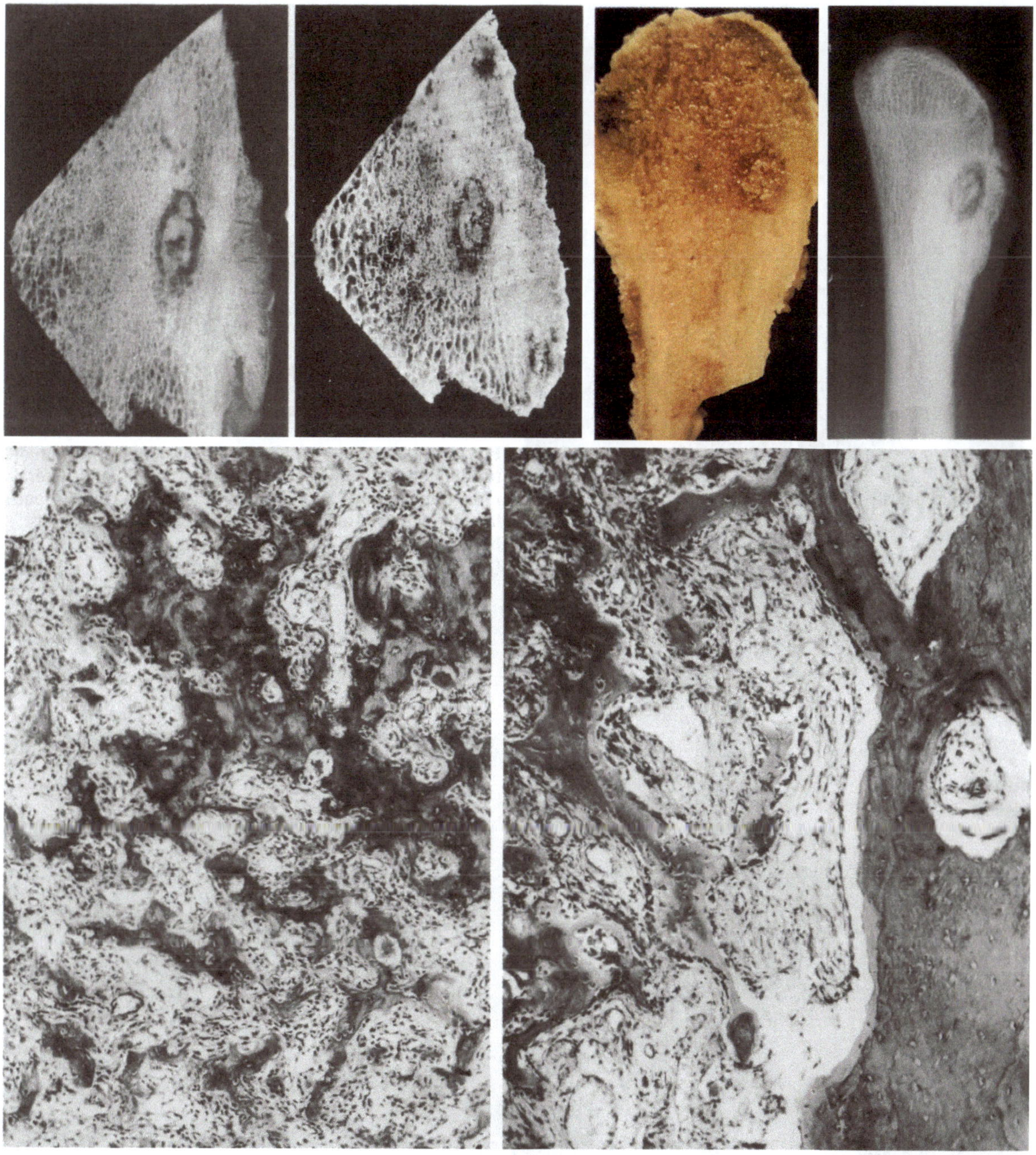

a b c d

Fig. I.23a–d. a,b Photographs and radiographs of two specimens of typical osteoid osteoma (**a** tibia; **b** fibula), the different zones of the central nidus forming a so-called annular sequestrum. **c,d** Photomicrographs showing the central and peripheral zones of the nidus composed predominantly of calcified immature bone, separated by vascular connective tissue. ×120

and not on the total duration of time the nidus was present (Johnston 1962). The surrounding sclerosis may vary from cancellous bone tissue made up of thickened trabeculae separated by richly vascularized connective tissue to a densely sclerotic bone tissue of compact structure, sometimes with genuine haversian systems. It is interesting to note the relationship between capillaries and bone formation in the nidus. It is a common finding for the osteoid trabeculae to form around the hyperemic capillaries, surrounding them like a ring (Fig. I.23). These trabeculae

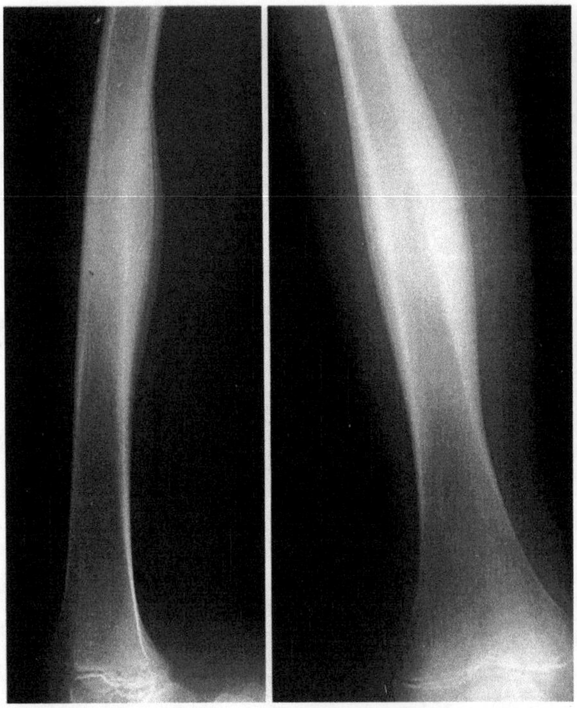

a

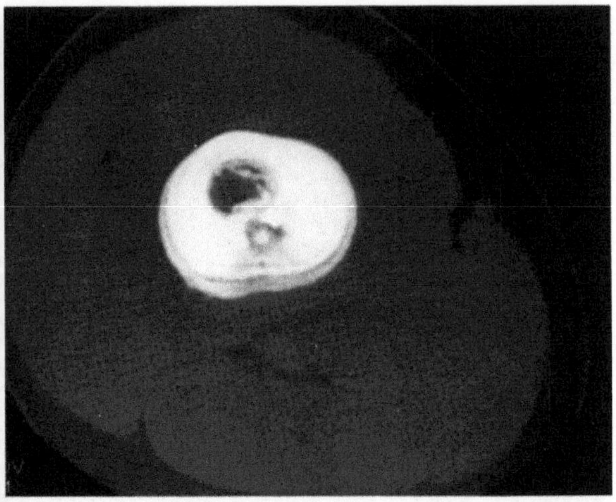

b

Fig. I.24a,b. Male, 16 years old. Osteoid osteoma of the femoral diaphysis. **a** Anteroposterior and lateral radiographs show a conspicuous cortical sclerosis and laminated periosteal reaction without visible "nidus." **b** CT reveals clearly the nidus, showing central sclerosis. (St. Louis University Medical Center)

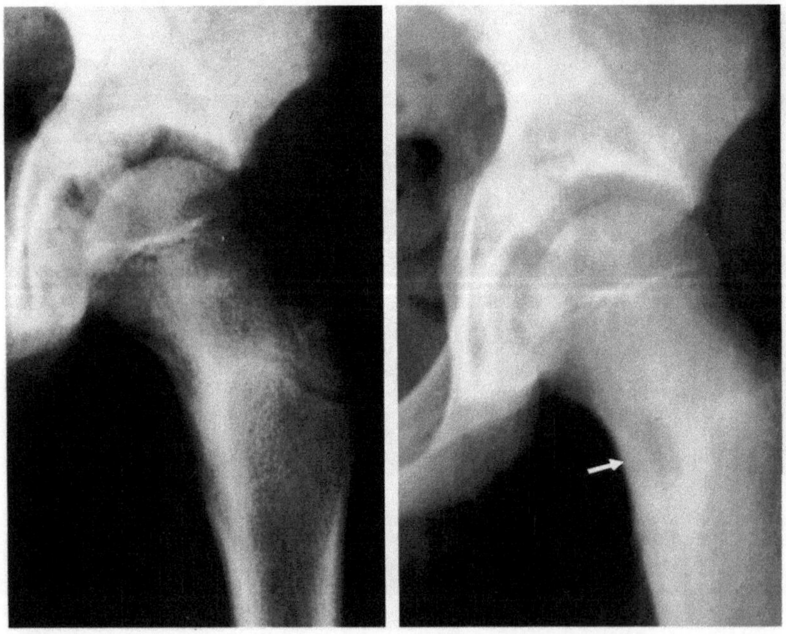

a, b

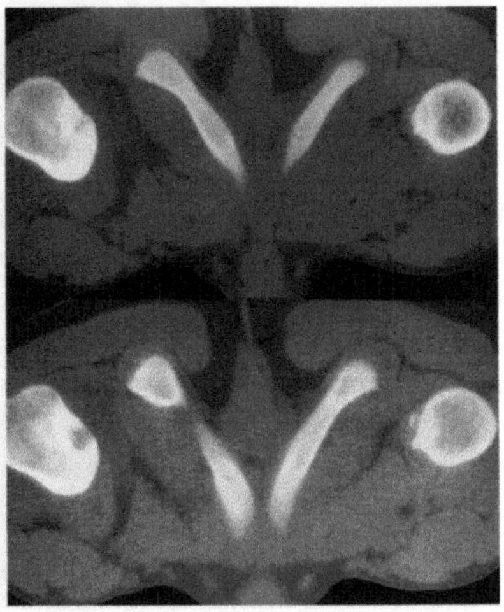

c

Fig. I.25a–c. Male, 11 years old, with growing osteoid osteoma of left femoral neck. **a** Radiograph from 7/22/88. **b** Same patient at 2/14/90. **c** CT showing clearly the nidus surrounded by sclerotic bone. (St. Louis University Medical Center)

Fig. I.26a–d. Photomicrographs showing the characteristic features of typical osteoid osteoma at lower and higher magnification. **a** ×10, **b** ×40, **c** ×100, **d** ×200

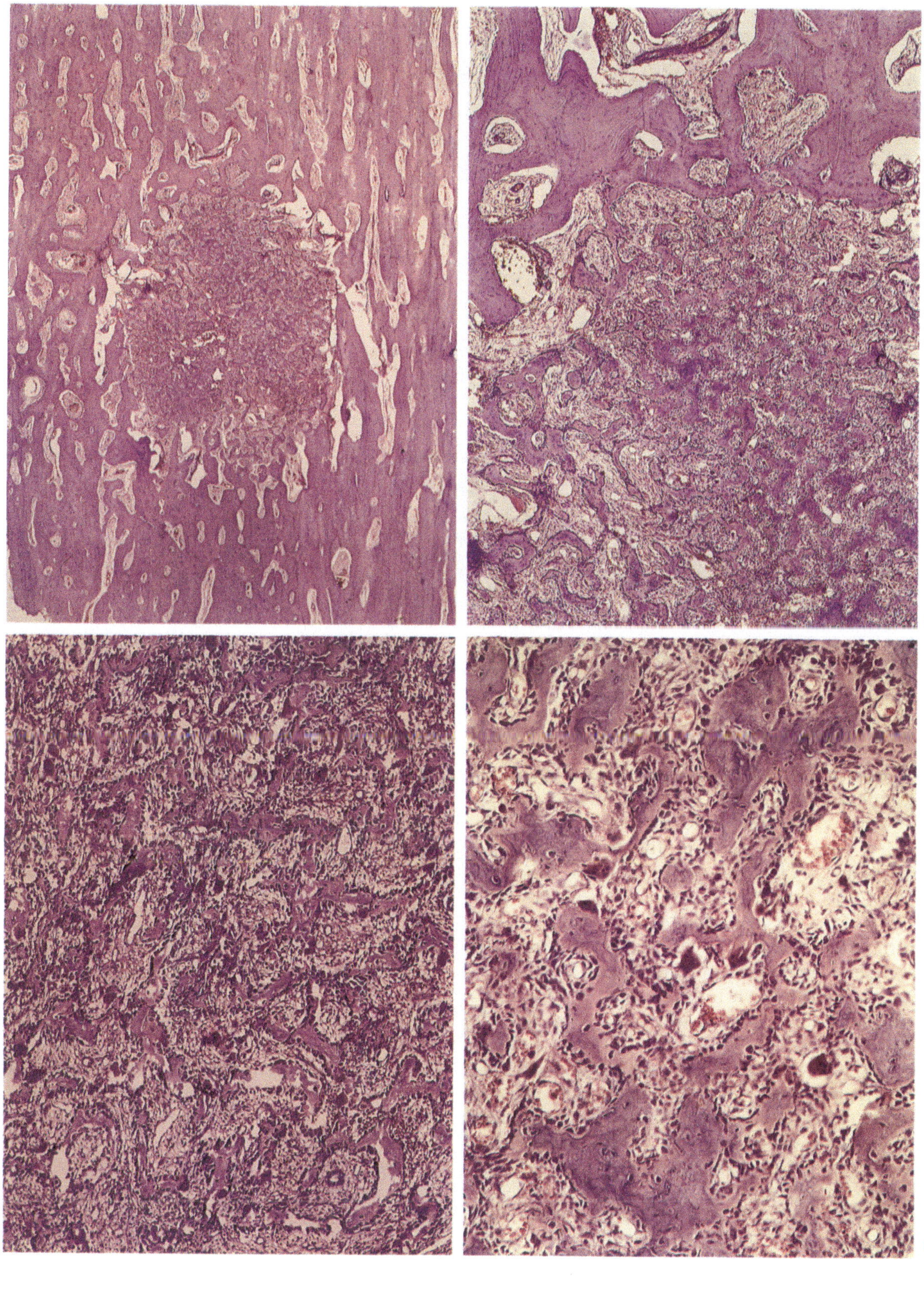

a b c d

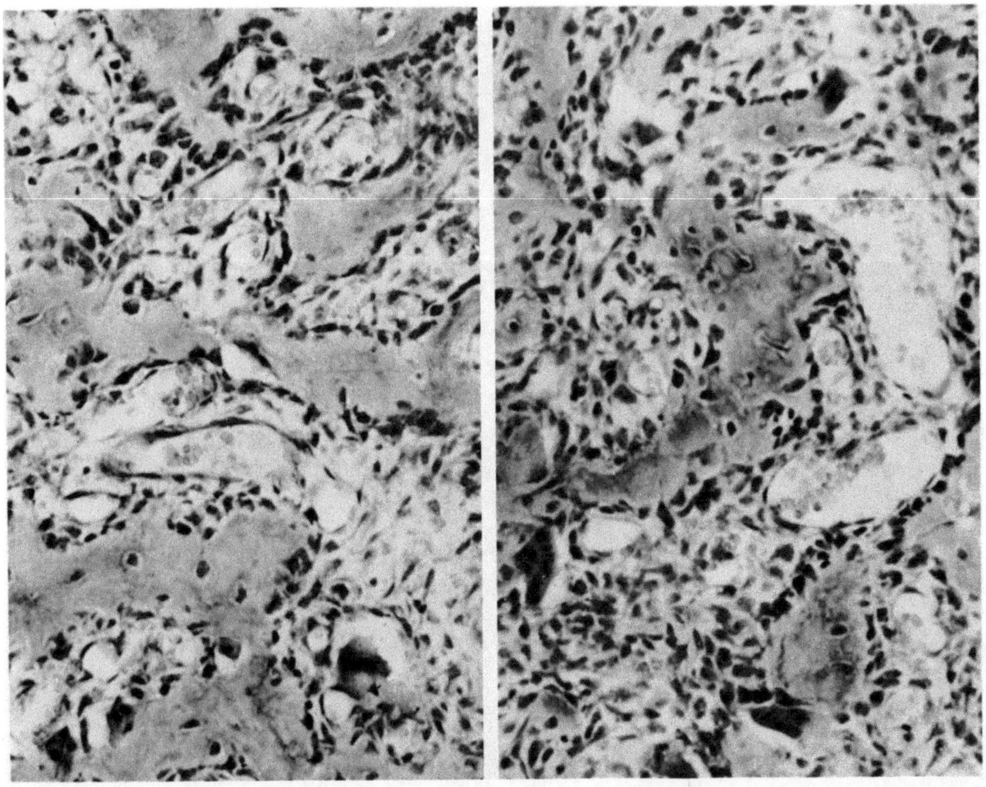

a b

Fig. I.27a,b. Photomicrographs of typical osteoid osteoma of tibia at high magnification. Active new formation of osteoid and incompletely calcified immature bone trabeculae, surrounded by rows of osteoblasts alternating with osteoclast giant cells, separated by connective tissue rich in dilated and hyperemic capillary vessels. ×430

often mature completely from the center to the periphery, becoming larger but maintaining their vascular relationship and becoming more and more similar in shape to the haversian type. Generally, regardless of its stage of development, the nidus of the osteoid osteoma closely resembles a focus of membranous osteogenesis, the difference being that in the former, an anarchic alternation of osteoblastic apposition and osteoclastic bone resorption can be observed, similar to that observed in the active phases of Paget disease. In fact, areas of more mature bone tissue with a typical "mosaic" pattern are occasionally observed. With a few exceptions, we did not observe a predominance of osteoid tissue in the nidus. On the contrary, in most cases, there was a definite predominance of immature, well-mineralized bone tissue.

The mechanism of pain, which is often out of proportion to the small size of the lesion, is presumed to be related to its extremely vascular nature and to the increased tension. Pain is produced by the pressure of local nerves, which, according to Sherman and McFarland (1965), were found singly or in clusters in the fibrous zones *surrounding* the nidus in 15 of 21 cases, usually accompanying one or more blood vessels. Occasionally, a large unmyelinated nerve was observed alone in the spaces of the reactive bone. However, Sherman and McFarland failed to reveal any nerve tissue in the nidus itself. Using the conventional HE stain, the writer obtained similar findings in his material. Byers (1968), Schulman and Dorfman (1970), and Esquerdo et al. (1976), using special silver impregnation techniques, demonstrated axons of nerve fibers associated with blood vessels *within* the matrix of the nidus in most of the cases investigated. Similar findings were evident in two of three genuine osteoblastomas studied by Schulman and Dorfman.

Treatment. The treatment of osteoid osteoma has been well described in the literature and amounts to complete surgical excision of the nidus. This will typically alleviate the pain pro-

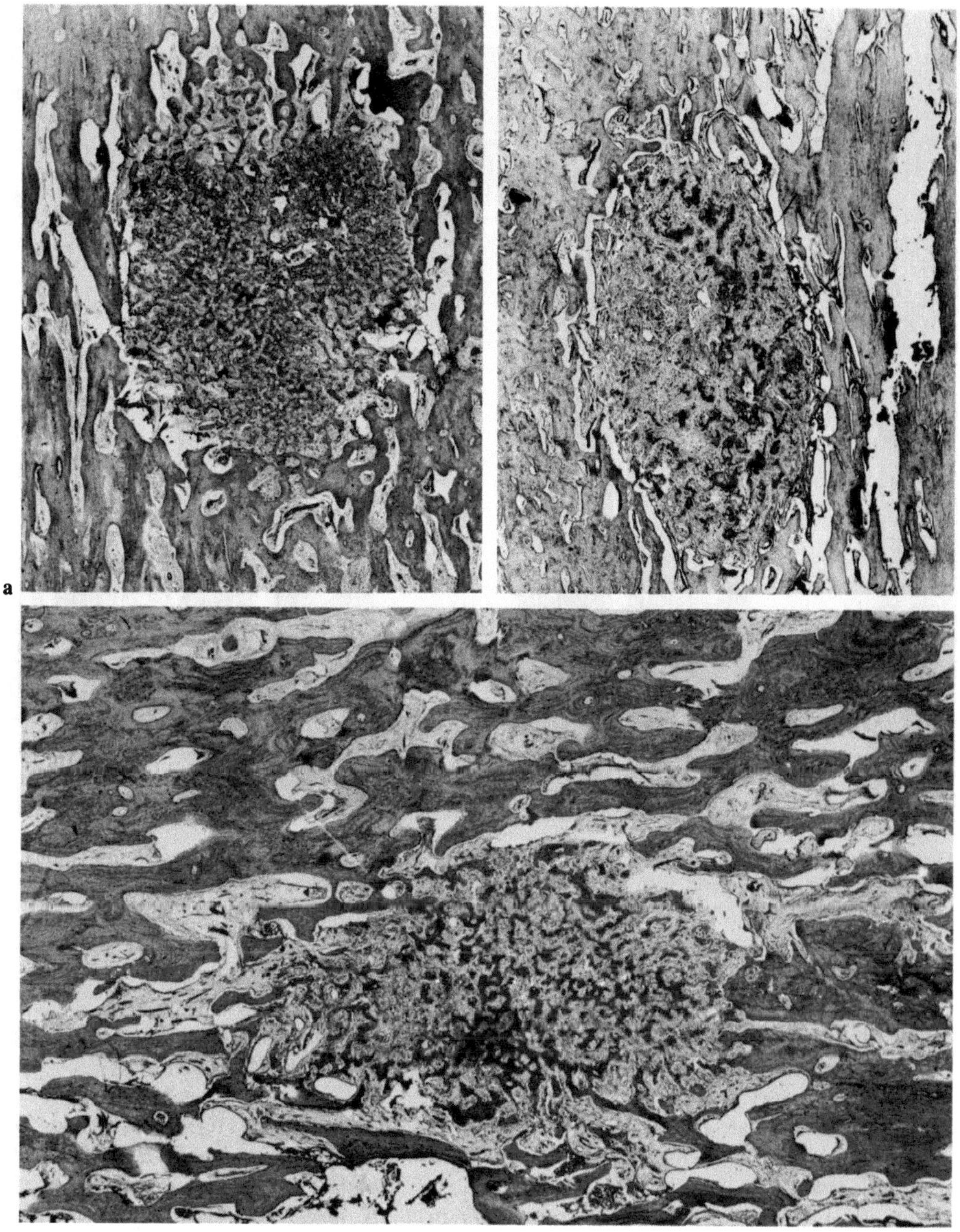

Fig. I.28a–c. Topographic photomicrographs of three different cases of osteoid osteoma (circumscribed osteoblastoma) showing the size and aspect of the central nidus surrounded by a wide area of reactive bone sclerosis. Note the predominance of calcified bone trabeculae and the scarce amount of osteoid tissue in the nidus. ×10

duced by the osteoid osteoma and also eliminate the possibility of local recurrence. The procedure would then be classified as a "wide" en bloc excision. Intralesional procedures, entering the nidus during the excision, are less predictable at curing the pain and eliminating recurrence (Fig. I.29) (Norman 1978). Biopsy prior to surgical excision is rarely needed. Because of the typical clinical, roentgenographic, and radioisotopic imaging of these lesions, a high index of suspicion can be achieved prior to surgical excision. The next question becomes whether the patient can be controlled with long-term salicylates or other nonsteroidal anti-inflammatory medications or needs to be surgically treated. Some patients elect to take drugs for a prolonged period of time,

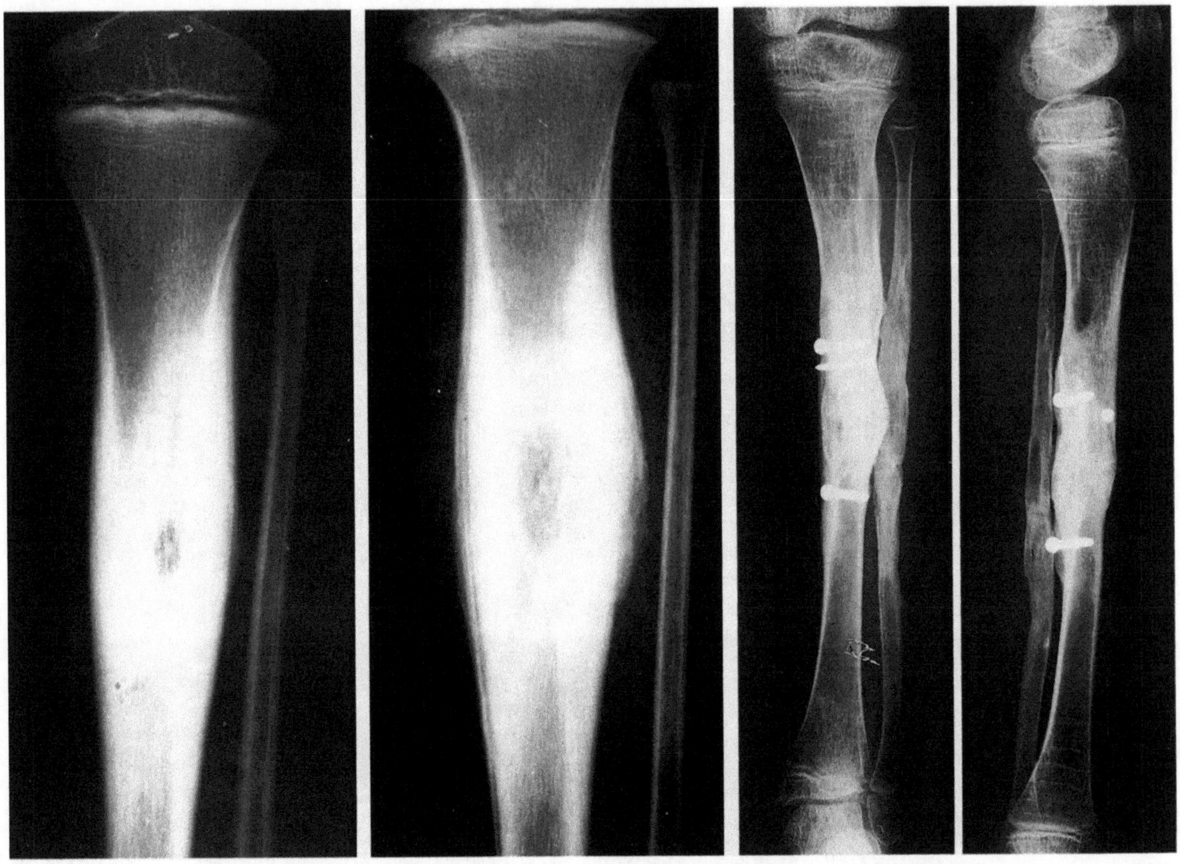

a, b c

Fig. I.29a–c. Male, 8 years old. **a** Radiograph of osteoid osteoma of the tibial shaft with conspicuous reactive sclerosis. **b** Recurrence and increase in size with evident periosteal reactive bone formation 10 months after incomplete excision (curettage). **c** Appearance a year after segmental en bloc resection followed by autograft

especially if they do not encounter the complications of chronic salicylate use. Other patients, however, are very willing to accept a surgical procedure to alleviate the pain that is frequently associated with osteoid osteoma. If the goal of surgery is to remove the nidus en bloc, then one is frequently presented with a large stress riser in a long tubular bone that is at significant risk of fracture. If the lesion is in an area such as the proximal femur, femoral diaphysis, or tibial diaphysis, prophylactic internal fixation along with autogenous bone grafting to prevent the complication of fracture after tumor excision may be indicated (Gitelis and Schajowicz 1989). Metaphyseal osteoid osteomas generally do not present with this problem because of the anatomic location. The lesion can be removed en bloc but because of the rapidity of healing of metaphyseal bone, prophylactic stabilization is usually not necessary.

Genuine Osteoblastoma (Osteoblastoma or Benign Osteoblastoma)

Definition, WHO: "*A benign or locally aggressive lesion presenting a histologic structure similar to that of osteoid osteoma, but characterized by its larger size (usually more than 1 or 2 cm) and the usual absence of a surrounding cone of conspicuous reactive bone formation*".

Osteoblastoma is less common than conventional osteoid osteoma. The majority of cases in this group correspond to the classic forms of osteoblastoma, showing a nidus of more than 2 cm. The incidence of sex, age, and localization of our cases is shown in Scheme I.2.

Comparing our 69 observations of "benign osteoblastoma" with those of other authors, an evident male preference was observed by us (47:20) and by McLeod et al. (1976) and Campanacci (1990). A slight male predominance

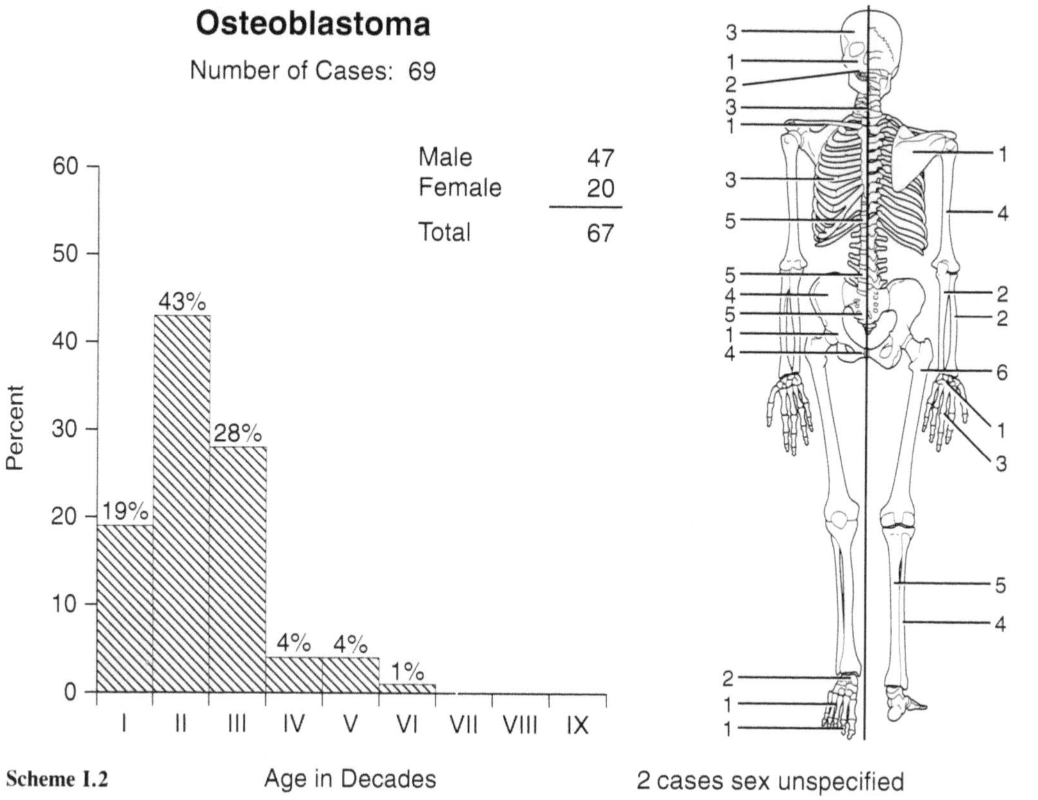

Scheme I.2

was found by some (Giannestras and Diamond 1958; Dahlin and Johnson 1954) and a female predominance by others (Jaffe 1958). The ages varied from 3 to 54 years, more than 60% being under 20 years of age and 14% under 10 years of age.

The localization varied greatly. The most frequent sites were in the spine (coinciding with the findings of other authors), including the sacrum (18 cases), and in the femur (6 cases), tibia (5 cases), ribs (3 cases), ilium (5 cases), and pubis (4 cases).

The duration of symptoms prior to the first consultation varied from 1 week to 2 years, being approximately 6 months in the majority of cases. Osteoblastoma evolves more rapidly than classic osteoid osteoma, which is in accordance with its predominantly lytic nature and less limited growth. It causes pain, swelling, discomfort, and premature functional disability, especially in spine lesions (scoliosis, muscle spasm, and neurologic symptoms), thus requiring earlier medical treatment. Pain was the principal symptom and was generally reported as being intense. Nocturnal intensification of pain or relief by aspirin was mentioned in some cases.

According to the clinicoradiologic manifestation, the following types can be observed.

Medullary (Cancellous) and Cortical Osteoblastoma

This group includes most cases of genuine osteoblastoma, which is characterized by an osteolytic lesion of more than 2 cm, usually localized centrally in the cancellous part of the bone and showing little or no histologic or radiologic evidence of perifocal sclerosis (Figs. I.30, I.38). Ten cases showed a striking reactive sclerosis, developing in or near the cortical portion of bone. We had previously classified several of these lesions as "osteoid osteoma." Lichtenstein denominated such lesions "osteoid osteomas of unusual size" (Fig. I.31). *Microscopically* (Figs. I.32–I.34), they showed new formation of immature (reticular or woven) bone and/or osteoid trabeculae within a richly vascularized connective stroma. The amount of cells (osteoblasts, osteoclasts, and fibroblasts), connective stroma, osteoid, and bone tissue varied widely in these tumors. A comparison of the microscopic features of these lesions with those of conventional "osteoid osteoma" indicated a greater produc-

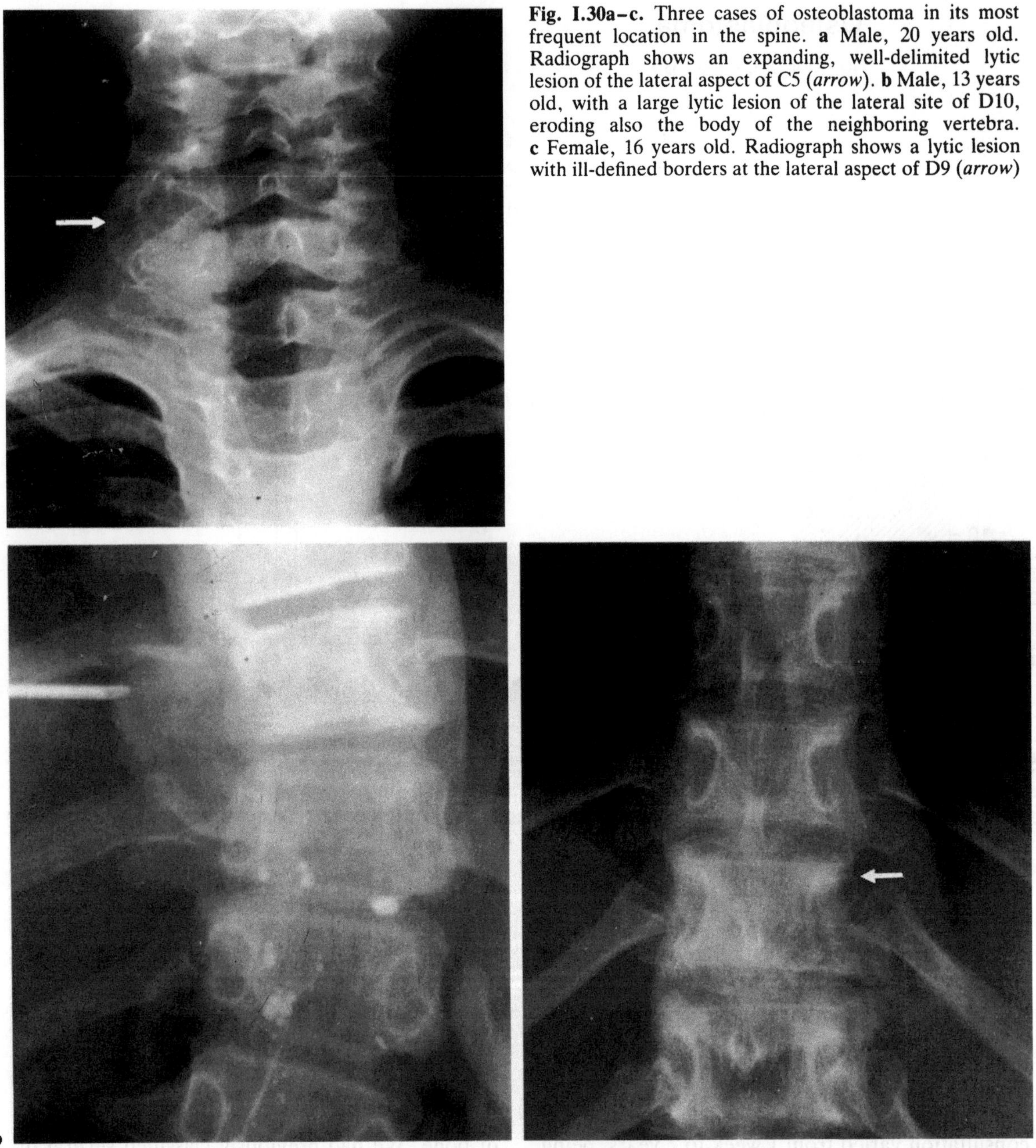

Fig. I.30a–c. Three cases of osteoblastoma in its most frequent location in the spine. **a** Male, 20 years old. Radiograph shows an expanding, well-delimited lytic lesion of the lateral aspect of C5 (*arrow*). **b** Male, 13 years old, with a large lytic lesion of the lateral site of D10, eroding also the body of the neighboring vertebra. **c** Female, 16 years old. Radiograph shows a lytic lesion with ill-defined borders at the lateral aspect of D9 (*arrow*)

tion of osteoid, with only a discrete number of immature (reticular) calcified trabeculae. However, in many cases maturation of the osteoid tissue, tending toward reticular or laminar bone, and heavily mineralized central areas with pagetoid patterns were also observed (Fig. I.34c). Only rarely do conspicuous microscopic differences exist between both tumor types, and these lie principally in their structural organization. Whereas in osteoid osteoma there seems to be a more organized structure with maturation of the nidus toward its periphery, in the genuine osteoblastoma the distribution of osteoid and reticular bone has a less organized pattern. The whole lesion may be found to be in the same stage of development, occasinally showing more conspicuous vascularization accompanied by more evident areas of hypertrophic osteoblasts

Fig. I.31. Male, 11 years old. Osteoblastoma of the ulna with central radiolucent area of almost 3 cm, surrounded by an extensive area of reactive bone sclerosis. Such conditions are classified by Lichtenstein as "osteoid osteoma of unusual size" and are classified by the writer in the group of osteoblastomas

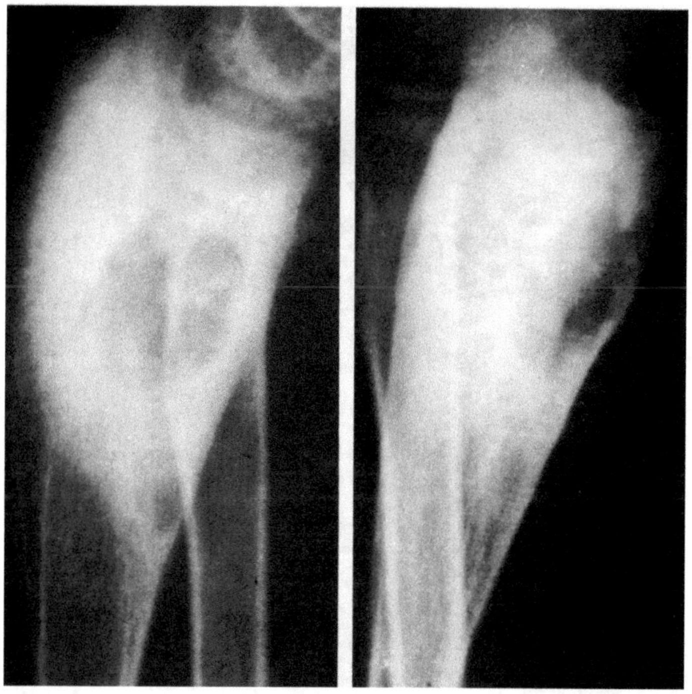

a

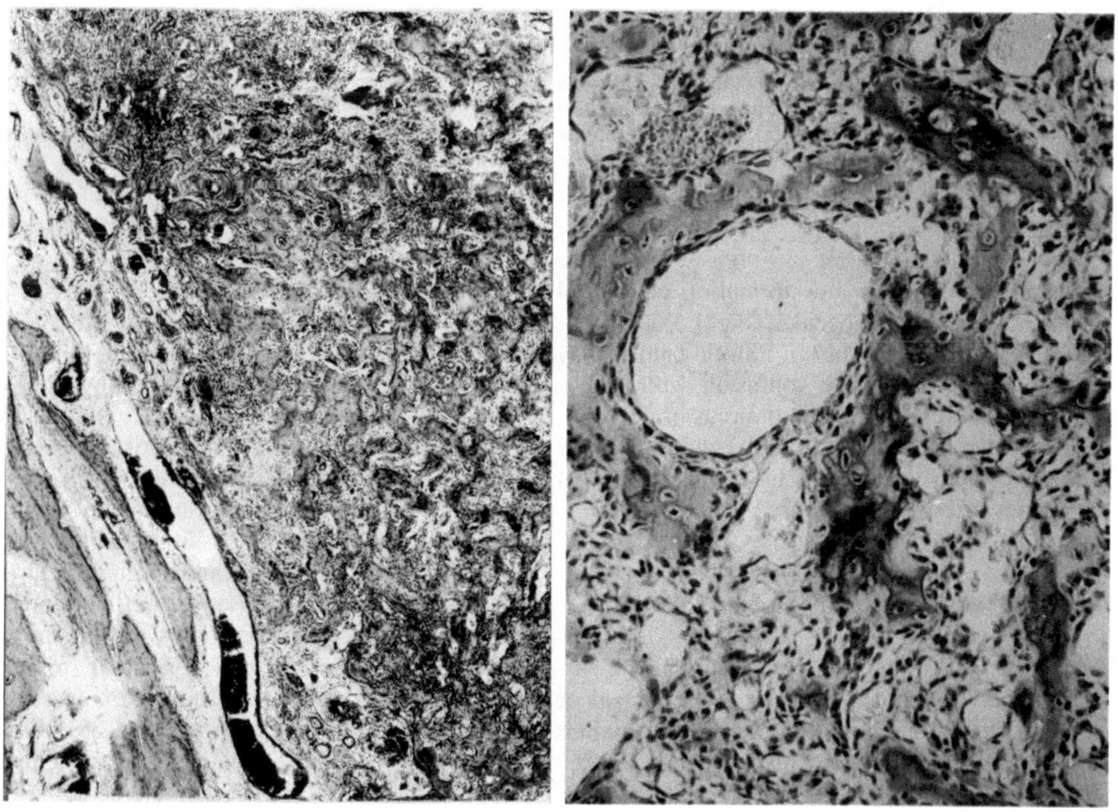

b

Fig. I.32a,b. Photomicrographs showing the microscopic aspect of a genuine osteoblastoma at **a** lower and **b** higher magnification. The histologic pattern is similar to that observed in conventional osteoid osteoma, showing in this case a somewhat more intense vascularization with numerous dilated and hyperemic vessels; perifocal reactive sclerosis is lacking. (Schajowicz and Lemos 1970) **a** ×85; **b** ×170

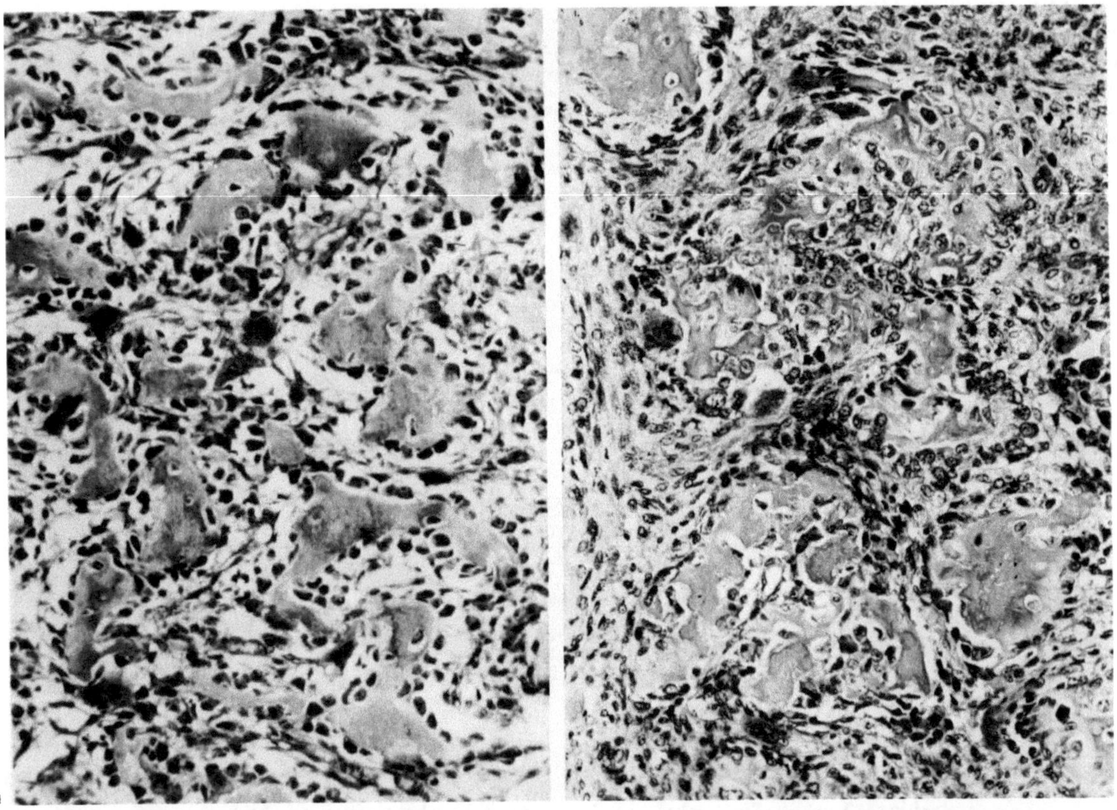

a b

Fig. I.33a,b. Photomicrographs of genuine osteoblastoma showing osteoid and slightly calcified bone trabeculae surrounded by numerous active osteoblasts, alternating with osteoclasts. The connective stroma in **b** is more cellular than commonly seen. ×280

Fig. I.34a–d. Photomicrographs at lower and higher magnification showing the characteristic features of genuine osteoblastoma. **a–c** ×100, **d** ×300

associated with active new formation of osteoid and immature bone trabeculae (Fig. I.35). Exceptionally, a certain number of mitotic figures may appear, causing possible confusion with osteosarcoma. However, the lack of areas of necrosis, of evident cellular pleomorphism, and of atypical mitosis permits one to exclude a diagnosis of malignant osteoblastic tumor.

Periosteal (Peripheral) Osteoblastoma

Nine cases in our series were located at the surface of bone and seemed to be of periosteal or subperiosteal origin (Goldman 1971). Two similar cases were reported by Lichtenstein and Sawyer (1964). This tumor must be differentiated radiologically from osteoma in its cranial localization, myositis ossificans, *parosteal* (juxtacortical) osteoma of long bones, aneurysmal bone cyst, osteochondroma (sessile type), and rarely from a malignant periosteal tumor. Two cases were located in cranial bones, frontal and occipital, respectively, and one in the jaw. The tumor of the jaw, which exhibited a large exophytic growth, recurred after surgical excision. The histologic and roentgenologic characteristics, as well as the evolution, were different from those of osteofibroma (ossifying fibroma). The six remaining cases were localized in the fibula (two), humerus, radius, femur, and the ninth rib (Figs. I.36–I.40). This last tumor showed erosion of the outer part of the cortex, thus raising the question of whether it had a periosteal origin with secondary penetration of the cortex or a cortical origin with exophytic growth (Fig. I.38). All these cases had a similar histologic aspect, identical to that of the other cases of genuine osteoblastoma, but perifocal bone sclerosis was generally lacking, and a thin shell of newly formed periosteal bone covered the lesion.

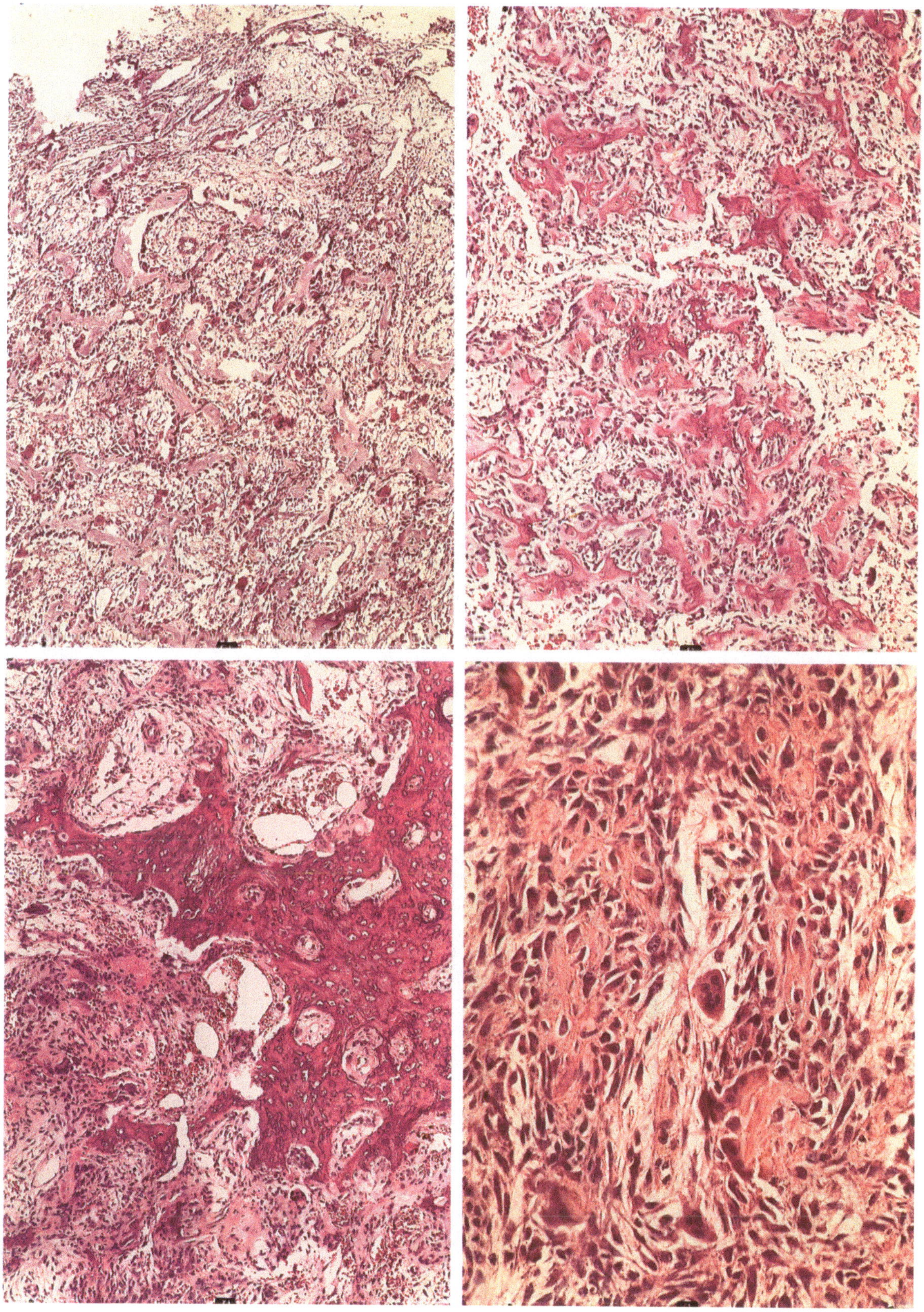

a b c d

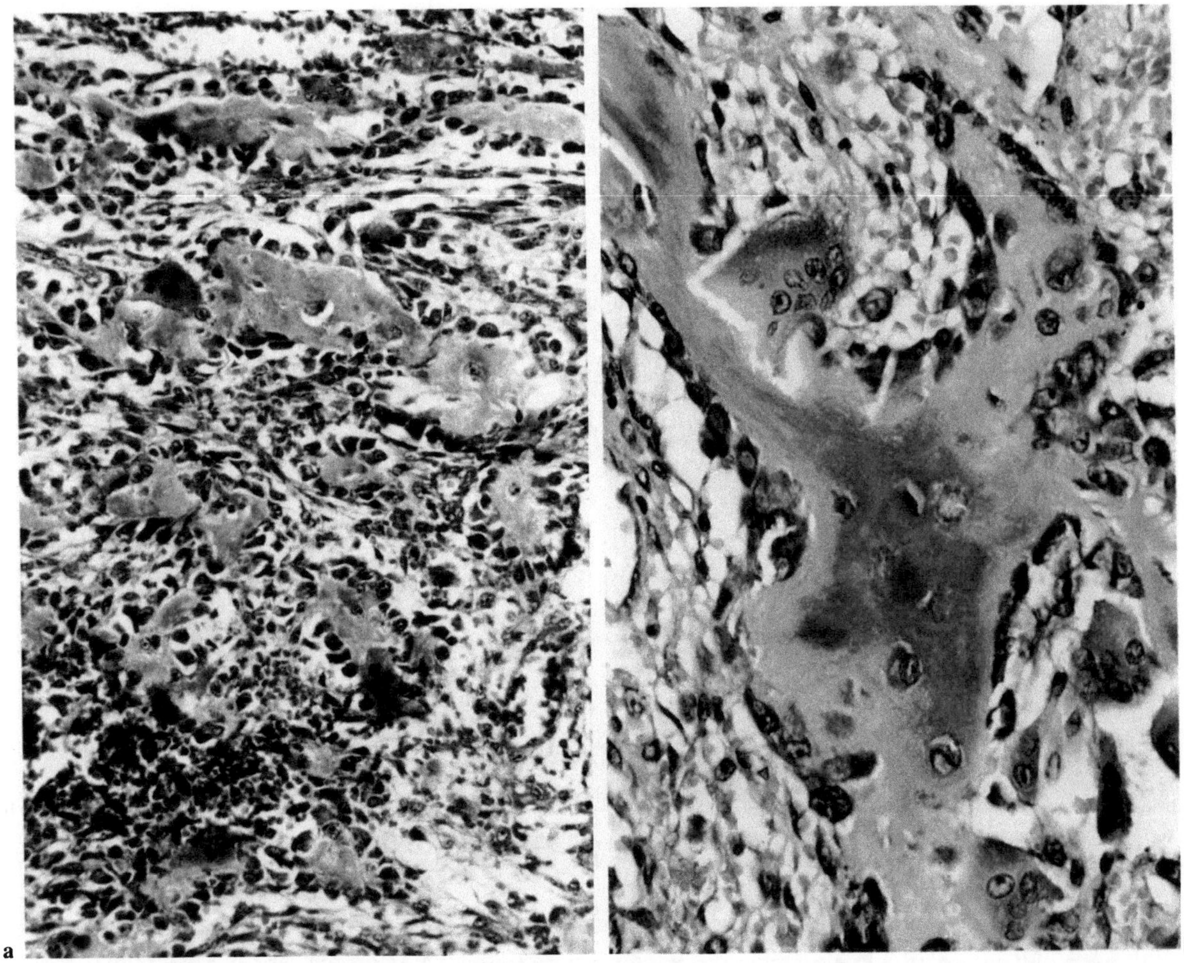

a b

Fig. I.35a,b. Photomicrographs of osteoblastoma showing osteoid and slightly calcified bone trabeculae surrounded by rows of hypertrophic osteoblasts alternating with osteoclasts. a ×200, b ×400

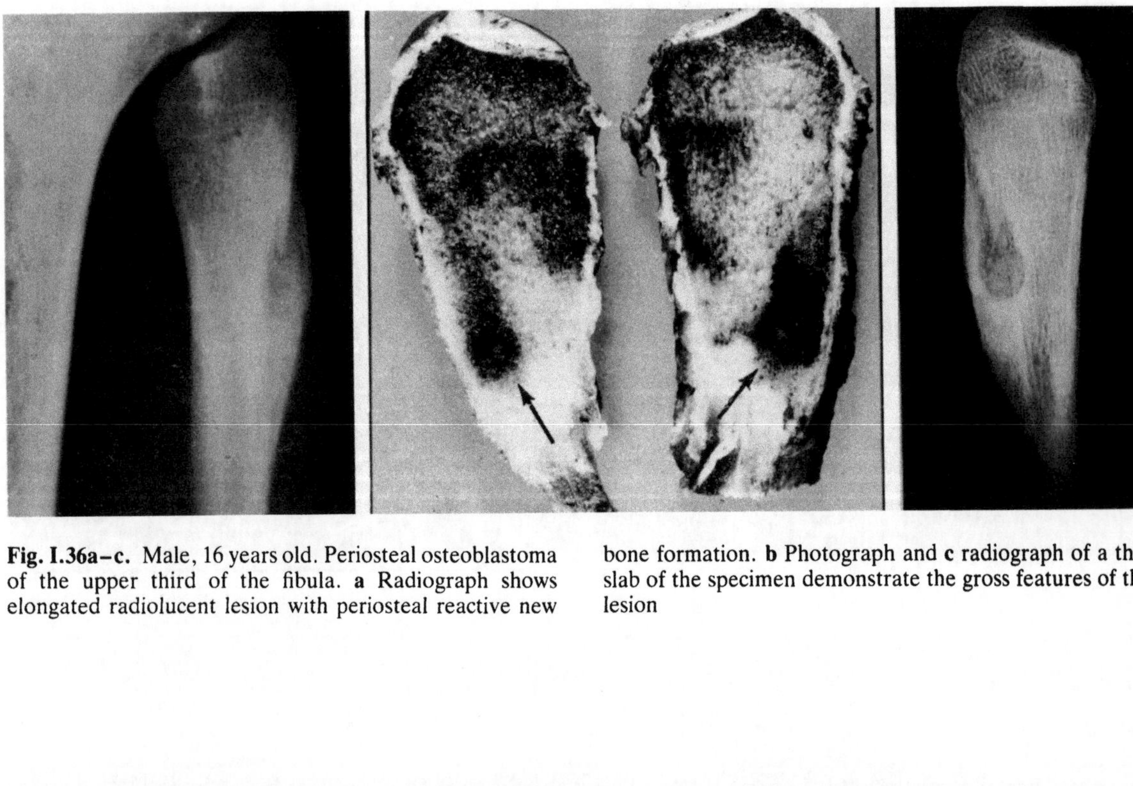

a b, c

Fig. I.36a–c. Male, 16 years old. Periosteal osteoblastoma of the upper third of the fibula. a Radiograph shows elongated radiolucent lesion with periosteal reactive new bone formation. b Photograph and c radiograph of a thin slab of the specimen demonstrate the gross features of the lesion

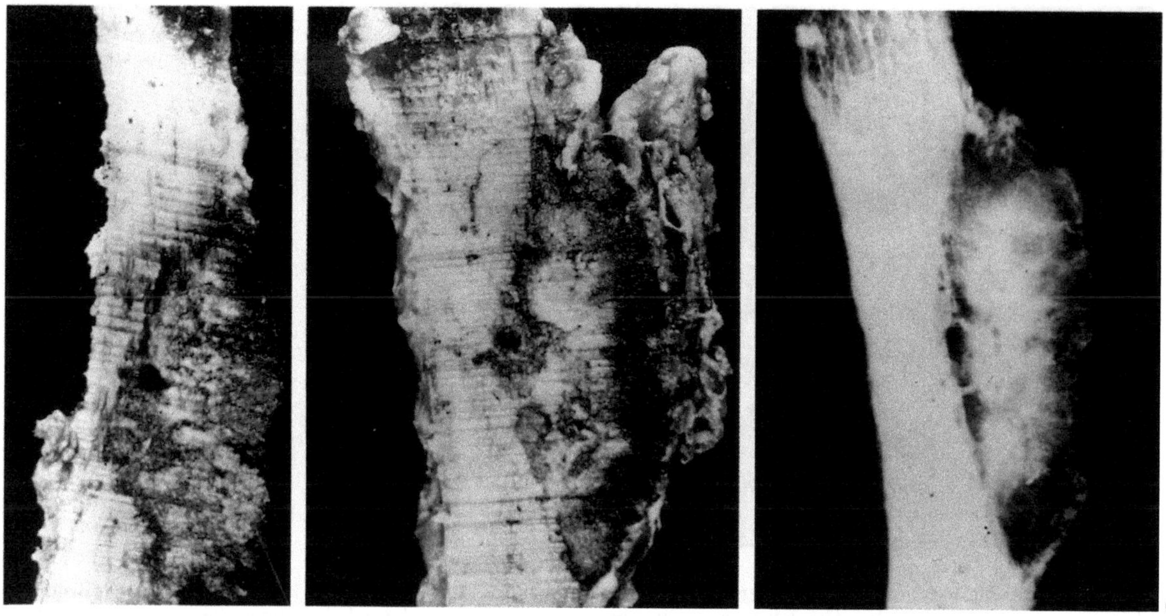

a, b c

▲ **Fig. I.37a–c.** Female 23 years old. **a,b** Photographs and **c** radiograph of a large peripheral lesion of the ninth rib. In this case the periosteal or cortical origin can be questioned

Fig. I.38a–c. Male, 39 years old. Osteoblastoma of the scapula. **a** Radiograph shows a poorly delimited, apparently periosteal lesion, which reveals intense uptake with technetium 99 disphosphonate bone scan (**b**) and is clearly visible with CT (**c**). (Case submitted by Dr. Trias, Barcelona, Spain) ▼

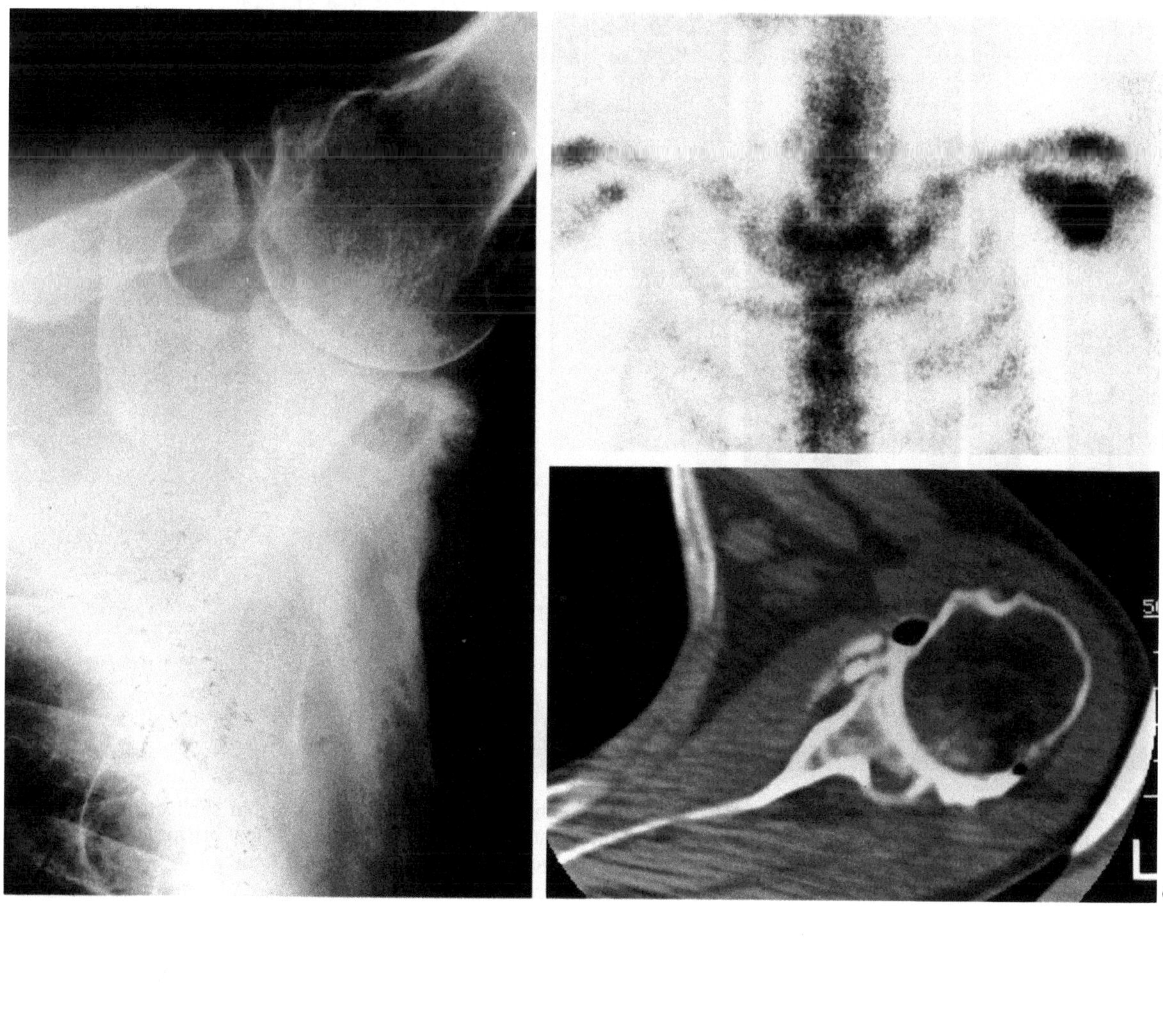

a b c

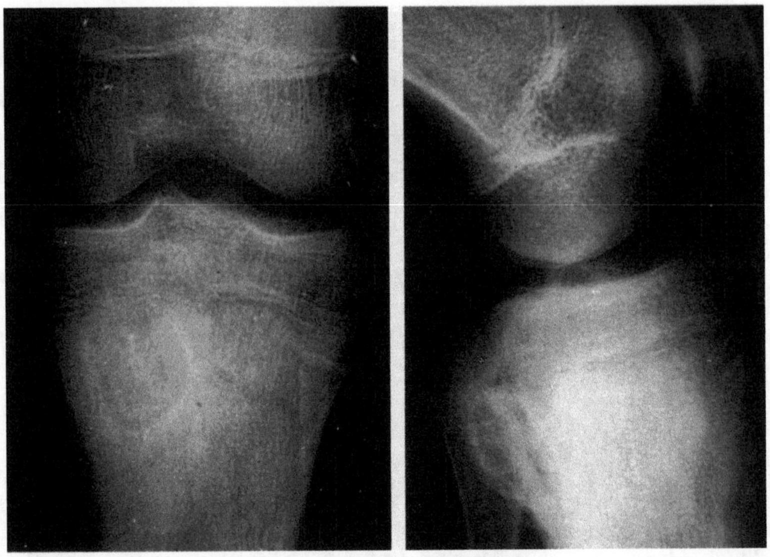

Fig. I.39. Osteoblastoma of the upper metaphysis of the tibia in an 18-year-old male. The appearance on the anteroposterior radiograph, showing a lytic lesion with slightly sclerotic borders, looked similar to a Brodie's abscess, but the lateral view shows the eccentric superficial location.

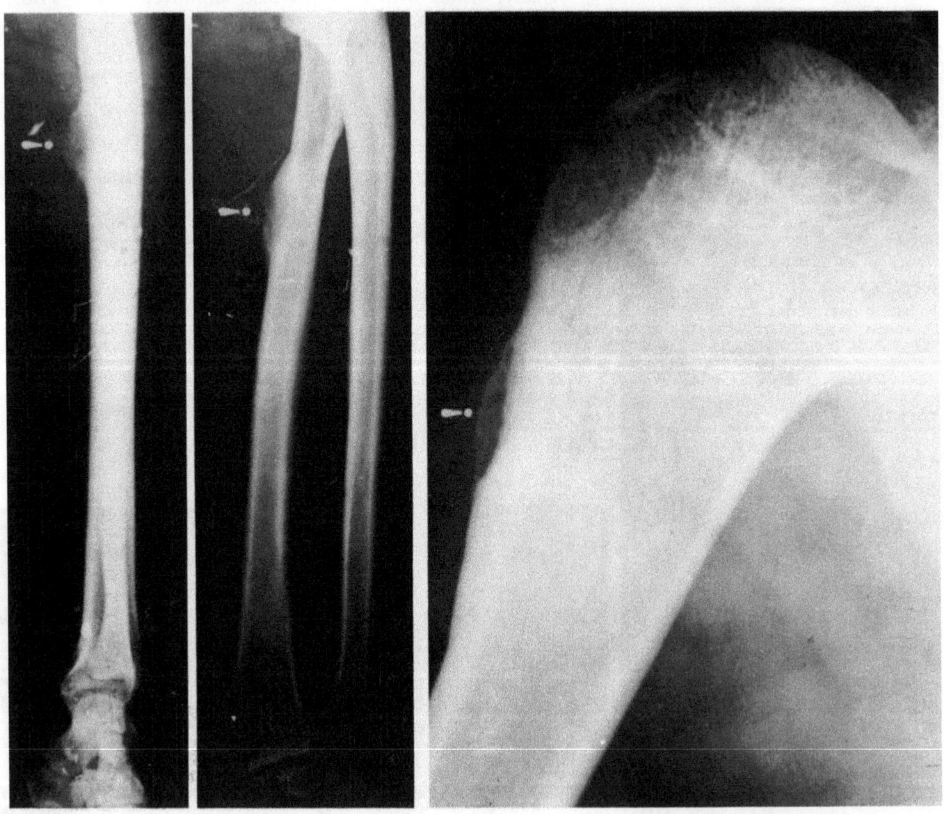

a b

Fig. I.40. a Male, 30 years old. Periosteal osteoblastoma. Lateral and anteroposterior radiographs showing nonsclerosing peripheral lesion of the upper third of the radius. **b** Male, 19 years old. Similar lesion of the upper third of the humerus with a thin shell of newly formed subperiosteal bone. The periosteal origin seems evident in both cases. (Schajowicz and Lemos 1970)

Multifocal Sclerosing Osteoblastoma ("Multifocal Osteoid Osteoma")

This peculiar, relatively rare type of osteoblastoma was described by the writer and Lemos in 1970. The cases reported by Tavernier et al. (1949) under the name "exostosing form of osteoid osteoma" are possibly post-traumatic hyperostosis or "myositis ossificans." We have observed two different types, one *medullary* (central or endosteal), the other *peripheral* (juxtacortical) and of probable periosteal origin, with two cases in each group.

The roentgenologic and especially the macroscopic features showed more than one circumscribed lesion, similar in size to that of a central nidus of osteoid osteoma, all enclosed in a single block of sclerotic bone. One case of the medullary type had three separated, large foci in the sacrum, and the other represented the final stage of a lesion of the humerus after incorrect treatment (curettage).

More interesting are the two cases of juxtacortical (peripheral) location in the ethmoid and in the publis. Roentgenologic and pathologic examination of the resection specimens showed multiple circumscribed images of nidal type, of different sizes, each with a picture both macro- and microscopically identical to that of "osteoid osteoma," surrounded by an extensive block of sclerotic bone (Fig. I.41).

A small number of similar cases with medullary or peripheral multifocal lesions were reported by Sherman (1947b), Goidanich and Battaglia (1959), Meary et al. (1965), Glynn and Lichtenstein (1973), Greenspan et al. (1974), McLeod et al. (1976), and Uehlinger (1977) under the denomination "multifocal or multicentric osteoid osteoma."

According to our observations and those of most authors, it is clear that the so-called osteoid osteoma and benign osteoblastoma constitute closely related processes that may be regarded as members of the same family of benign tumors of osteoblastic derivation. To unify the terminology, we proposed the term "osteoblastoma" for both lesions, which may be classified according to the anatomoclinical types shown in Table I.1.

In our opinion, the adjective 'benign' should be avoided because it is unnecessary and redundant, analogous with the practice in respect of other bone tumors well known to be benign. Even more importantly, our studies demonstrate that with the exception of circumscribed osteoblastoma (osteoid osteoma), osteoblastoma is not as benign as it was once thought to be. We do not have a sufficiently long follow-up of all our cases (a problem common to other reports in the literature), but we have had recurrences in five of them.

Canepa and DeFabiani (1965) reported recurrences in 11 of 54 cases reviewed, with complete data. Other recurrent cases have been published by Dunlop et al. (1970), Gertzbein et al. (1973), and Jackson (1978). Furthermore, the possibility of malignant transformation after conservative (curettage) or incomplete treatment should be considered. Mayer (1967) reported the case of a 43-year-old male who, 13 years after curettage of a lesion at the roof of the acetabulum diagnosed by Jaffe as benign osteoblastoma, developed an osteosarcoma at the same site. We agree with Mayer when he states that "we must accept the fact that the concept of the 'benign osteoblastoma' is still immature. The number of reported cases are too few for us to be dogmatic." The fact that we have observed in two of our cases a possible transformation of a preexisting "benign osteoblastoma" into a low-grade osteosarcoma after incomplete conservative treatment (curettage followed by radiotherapy) seems to confirm Mayer's prediction that "during the next twenty or thirty years, as our experience ripens, additional cases may be discovered and it may be necessary to abandon the term 'benign' as applied

Table I.1. Classification of osteoblastoma

Circumscribed osteoblastoma (osteoid osteoma) – nidus less than 2 cm	Cortical	Sclerosing
	Medullary	With little or no sclerosis
	Periosteal	
Genuine osteoblastoma (benign osteoblastoma) – nidus larger than 2 cm	Medullary (cancellous)	With little or no sclerosis
	Periosteal (peripheral)	
	Cortical	Sclerosing
Multifocal osteoblastoma	Medullary	Sclerosing
	Peripheral (juxtacortical)	

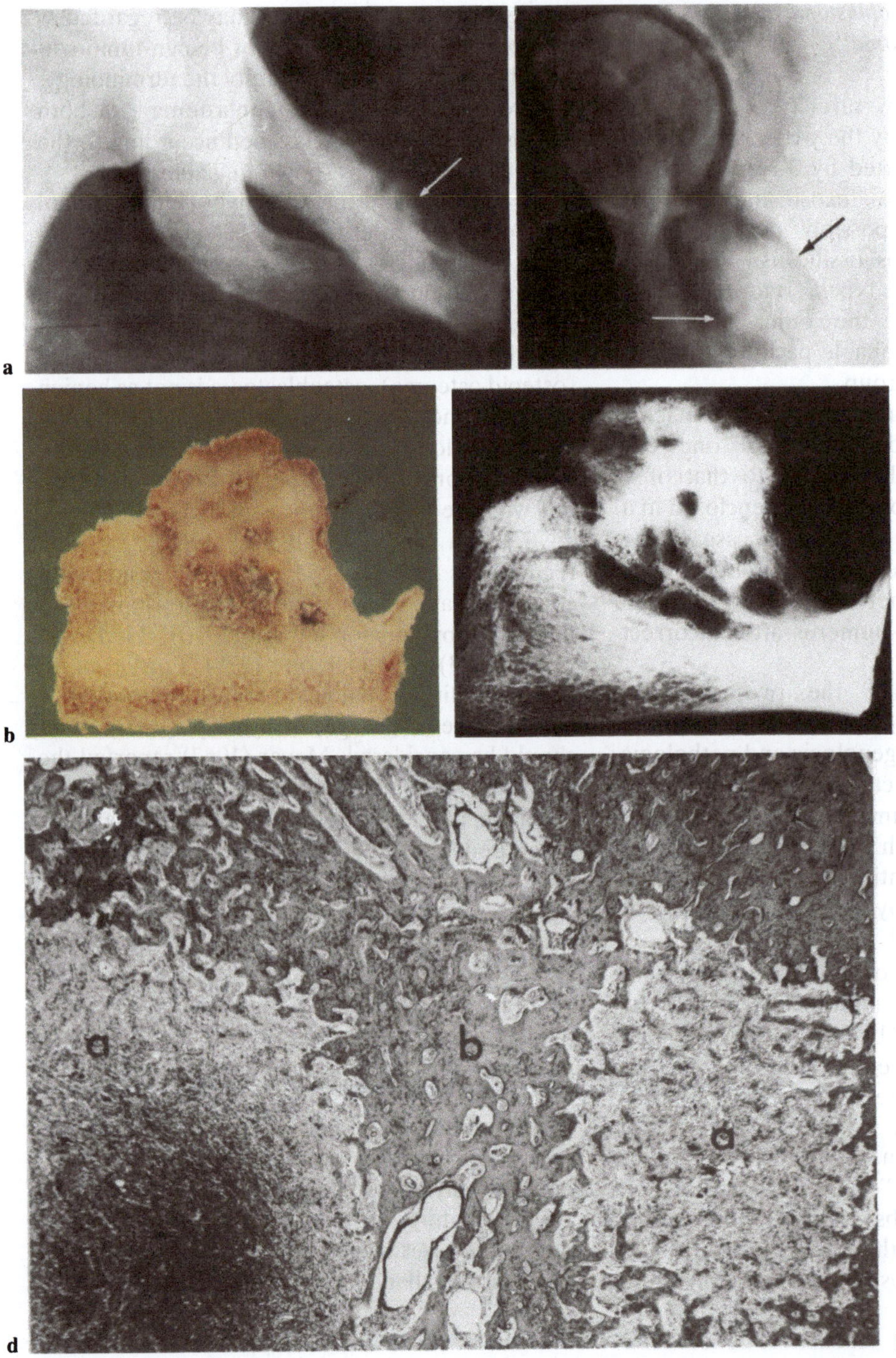

Fig. I.41a–d

to this group of lesions." In fact, we have seen one pertinent case in consultation from England (Merryweather et al. 1980), and another case was reported by McLeod et al. (1976) and is reproduced in the 3rd edition of Dahlin's book (1978, p. 97). We had the opportunity to see the slides of this case, which show clearly the malignant transformation of an osteoblastoma of the tibia after approximately 4 years, following several recurrences after curettage of the lesion. Other similar cases have been published by Seki et al. (1975), Jackson and Bell (1977), Scranton et al. (1975), and Mitchell and Ackermann (1986). On the other hand, an osteoblastoma

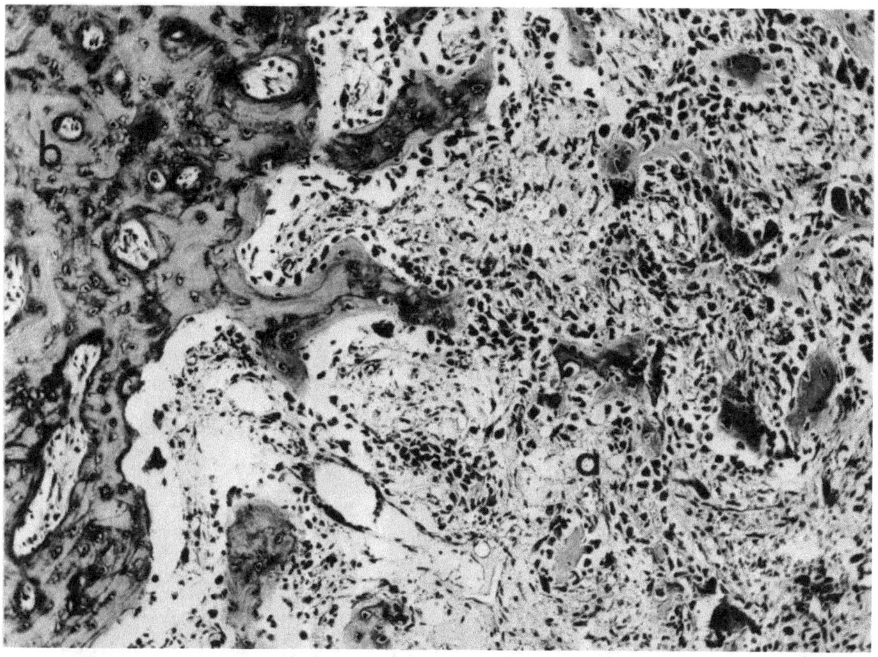

e

▲ **Fig. I.41a–e.** Female, 20 years old. **a** Radiographic appearance of juxtacortical (peripheral) multifocal sclerosing osteoblastoma (*arrows*). **b** Photograph and **c** radiograph of the gross specimen clearly showing the juxtacortical location and the various hemorrhagic foci of different sizes, immersed in a mass of sclerotic bone. The gross aspect of each of the focal lesions is identical to a nidus of conventional osteoid osteoma (Schajowicz and Lemos 1970). **d** Photomicrograph shows two nidi separated by sclerotic reactive bone. **e** Characteristic histologic aspect of one focus. **d** ×40; **e** ×100

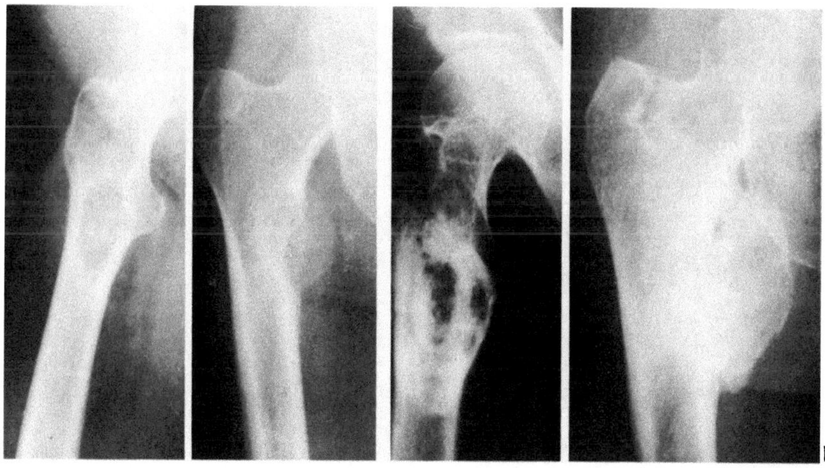

a b

Fig. I.42a,b. Male, 22 years old, with recurrent periosteal osteoblastoma. **a** Radiographs showing the size and location in the upper third of the femur. **b** Radiographs of the recurrent lesion 1 year after incomplete excision

may occasionally show histologically aggressive pseudomalignant features that make it difficult to differentiate it from osteosarcoma (Mirra et al. 1976; Marsh and Choi 1970).

These findings demonstrate that a genuine osteoblastoma may sometimes behave aggressively, especially after incorrect treatment, similar in many respects to a giant-cell tumor (osteoclastoma).

Due to the unpredictable behavior of osteoblastoma, a wide en bloc excision of the lesion is the recommended treatment. Intralesional excisional procedures are less predictable and are associated with a significant recurrence rate for

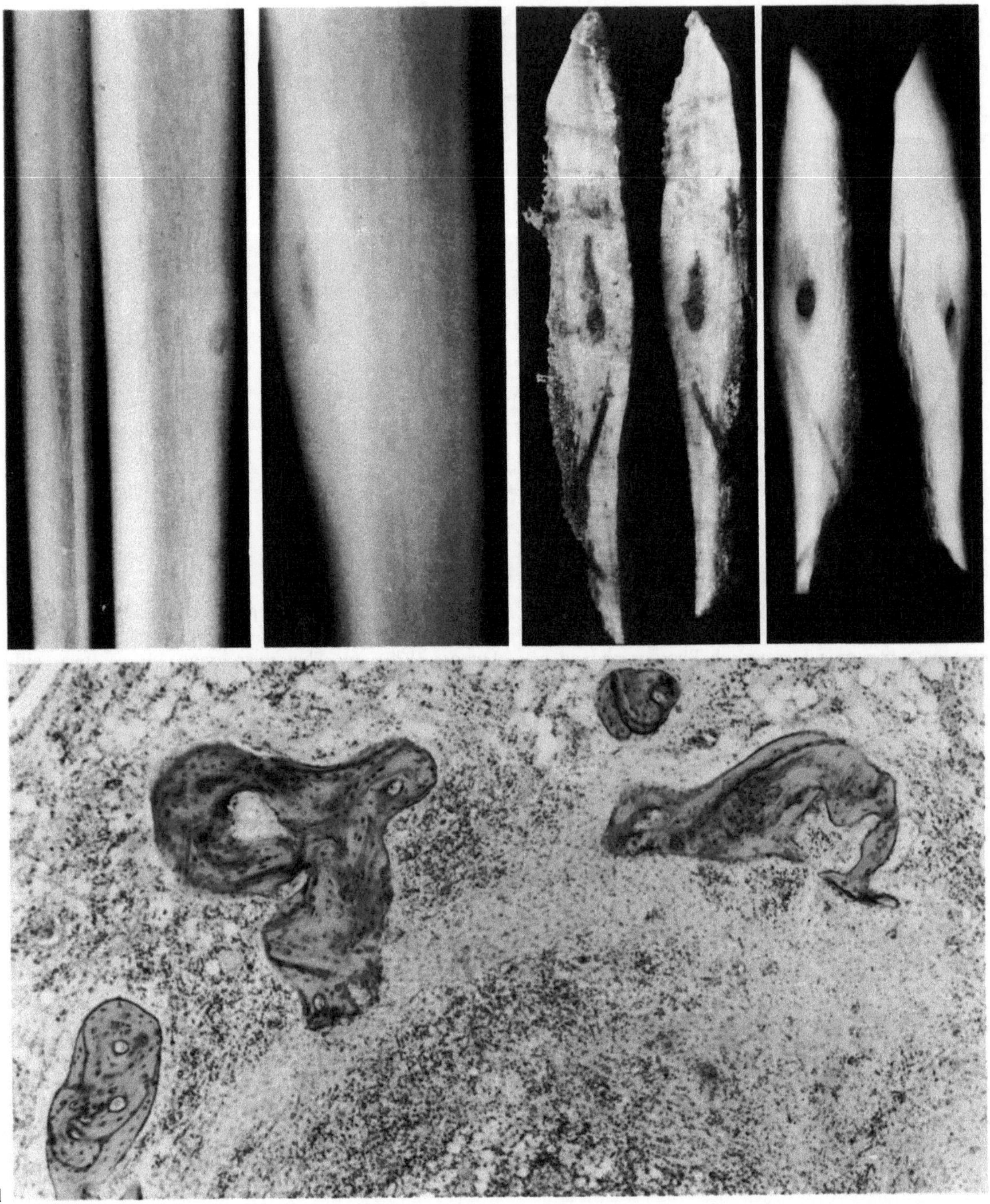

Fig. I.43. **a** Male, 43 years old, with cortical abscess of the tibial shaft. **b** Female, 22 years old, with a similar case of cortical abscess of the femoral shaft. **c** Photograph and radiograph of the resected specimen (case shown in **b**) showing an elongated hyperemic lesion surrounded by reactive bone sclerosis, similar to that observed in osteoid osteoma. **d** Photomicrograph revealing the histologic features of a chronic inflammatory process with central abscess formation. ×120

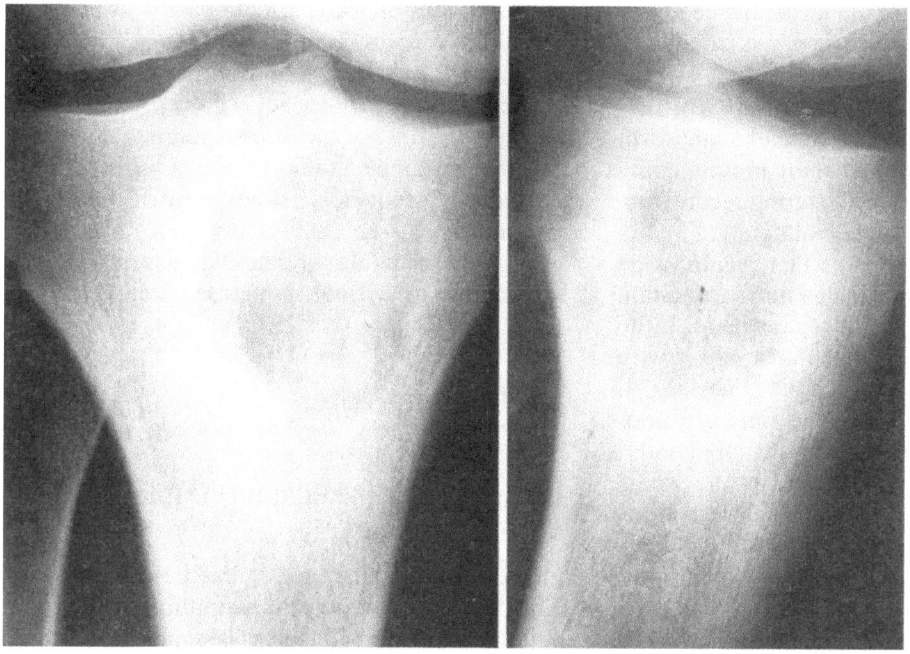

Fig. I.44. Female, 22 years old, with Brodie's abscess. Anteroposterior and lateral radiographs show a large radiolucent lesion at the upper end of the tibia, surrounded by a halo of bone sclerosis

a 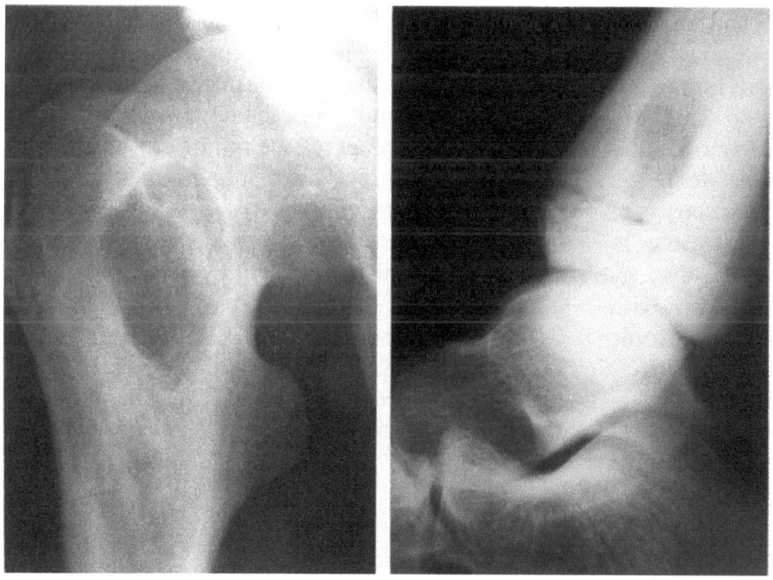 b

Fig. I.45. a Male, 25 years old, with Brodie's abscess in the intratrochanteric region of the femur. **b** Female, 14 years old, with a similar lesion in the lower tibial metaphysis osteoblastoma (Fig. I.42). Due to the need for wide en bloc excision, reconstruction is frequently necessary. Diaphyseal osteoblastoma of long tubular bones may require intercalary reconstruction with allografts or autografts and some form of internal fixation. Tumors that are in the vicinity of joints may require a joint-restoring reconstructive procedure with implant or allograft. Finally, for osteoblastomas in the spine that require wide excision of the posterior elements, a decision regarding spinal stability needs to be made. If the spine is rendered unstable, then arthrodesis with or without internal fixation may be necessary. If wide margins are obtained at the time of tumor excision, then local control is predictably good.

Differential Diagnosis. A few lesions may occasionally simulate osteoid osteoma or osteoblastoma and raise problems of differential diagnosis on a clinicoradiologic basis: chronic bone abscess (intracortical abscess and Brodie's abscess), medullary osteoma (solitary enostosis or "bone island"), or rarely some other lesions of intracortical location, such as hemangioma (Dorfman et al. 1971; Schajowicz et al. 1979).

While an intracortical abscess and osteoid osteoma may appear similar both on plain radiographs and in the gross specimen (Fig. I.43), the angiographic pattern according to Lindbom et al. (1960), Halpern and Freiberger (1970), and O'Hara et al. (1975) distinguishes between the two entities due to the increased vascularity of the osteoid osteoma nidus and its absence in the necrotic inflammatory tissue of the abscess. On the other hand, radioisotope imaging with technetium 99 is generally negative in chronic bone abscess.

Histologically there is no resemblance between the two entities, the intracortical abscess being characterized by a small cavity occupied by partly necrotic inflammatory tissue, rich in neutrophil leukocytes and lymphoplasmacytes (Fig. I.43). Brodie's abscess, on the other hand, is characterized by a larger intramedullary radiolucent lesion surrounded by a rim of bone sclerosis, commonly located in the metaphyseal region (Figs. I.44, I.45). It may raise diagnostic problems in distinguishing it from genuine osteoblastoma or so-called osteoid osteoma of unusual size, but the negative scintigraphy and the histologic appearance, revealing an inflammatory tissue with a predominance of plasmacytes surrounded by thickened cancellous bone trabeculae, support the diagnosis.

The roundish focus of radiopacity observed in medullary osteoma (bone island) may sometimes simulate a radiopaque osteoid osteoma nidus. However, the absence of clinical complaints, especially of tenderness or spontaneous pain, and the negative radioisotope imaging favor medullary osteoma. Histologically it bears no resemblance to an osteoid osteoma nidus, consisting of a nodule of compact lamellar bone surrounded by normal spongiosa (see Fig. I.13).

B. Intermediate

1. Aggressive (Malignant) Osteoblastoma

In the last several years, it has become evident that there is a diversity in the natural history and biologic behavior of osteoblastoma. As stated previously, conventional osteoblastomas have a significant recurrence rate of approximately 15%, especially after intralesional excision (curettage), and on rare occasions present malignant transformation to typical osteosarcoma. In 1976 Schajowicz and Lemos reported under the rubric "malignant osteoblastoma" the clinical, radiographic, and pathologic features of eight cases of a locally aggressive tumor that frequently recurs but does not metastasize. Since the first publication of the eight cases, several others have been referred to this writer. These lesions show some distinct histologic features, such as more abundant and larger hypertrophic osteoblasts with plump or bizarre hyperchromatic nuclei alternating with fields rich in giant cells of osteoclastic type (Figs. I.46–I.49). In addition, there are occasional areas of "blue spiculated"

Fig. I.46a,b. Photomicrographs of aggressive (malignant) ▲ osteoblastoma. Rows of hypertrophic, plump, so-called epithelioid osteoblasts alternating with several osteoclasts, surrounding osteoid or slightly calcified bone trabeculae and separated by a vascular connective stroma. **a,b** ×400

Fig. I.47a,b. Photomicrographs of aggressive (malignant) ▶ osteoblastoma. **a** Irregular woven bone trabeculae ("blue bone spicules") separated by vascular connective stroma. **b** Higher magnification, showing woven bone trabeculae surrounded by hypertrophic, bizarre osteoblasts. **a** ×100, **b** ×400

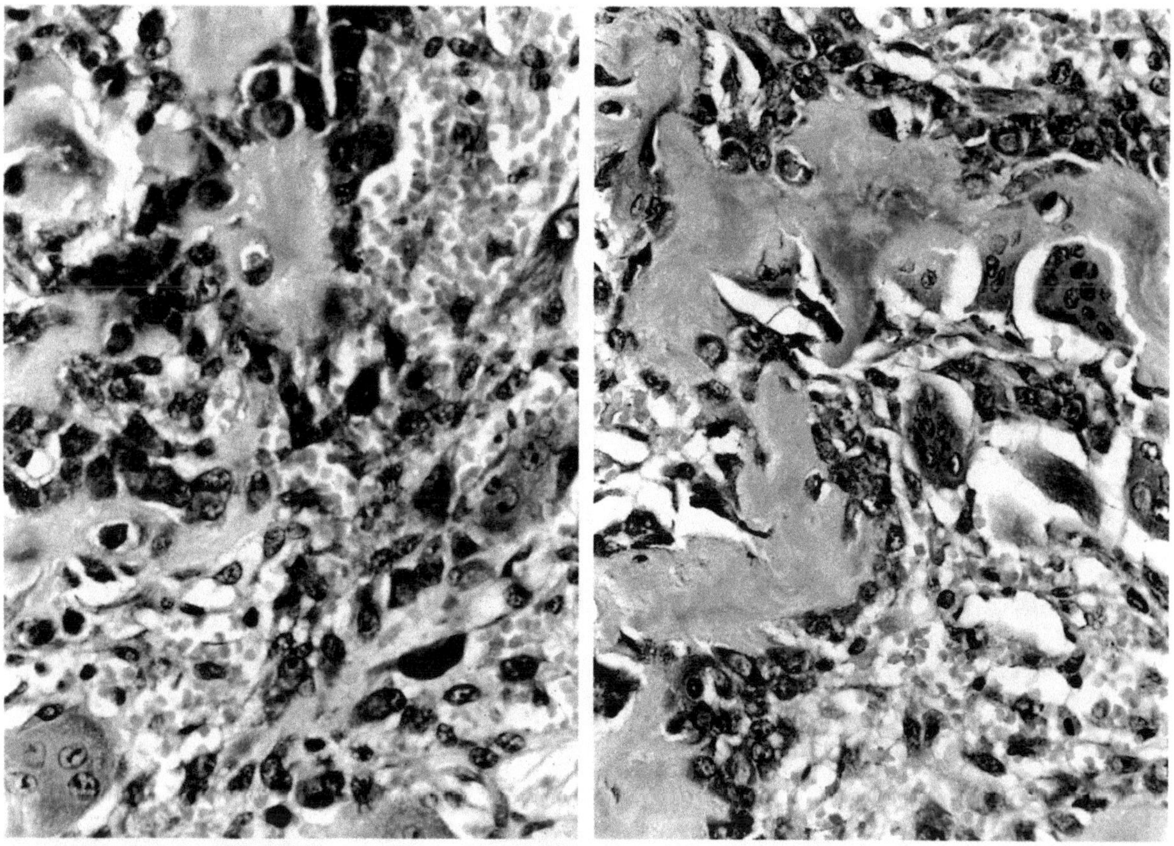

a b

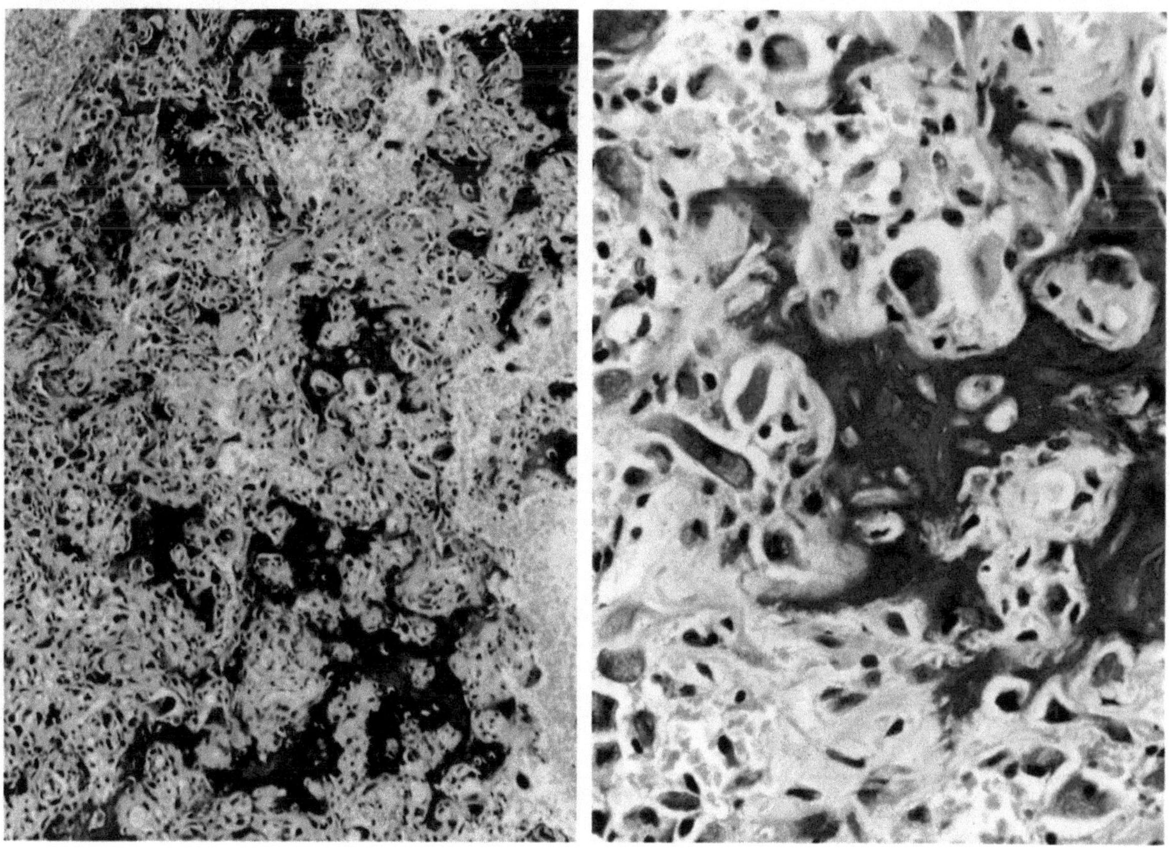

a b

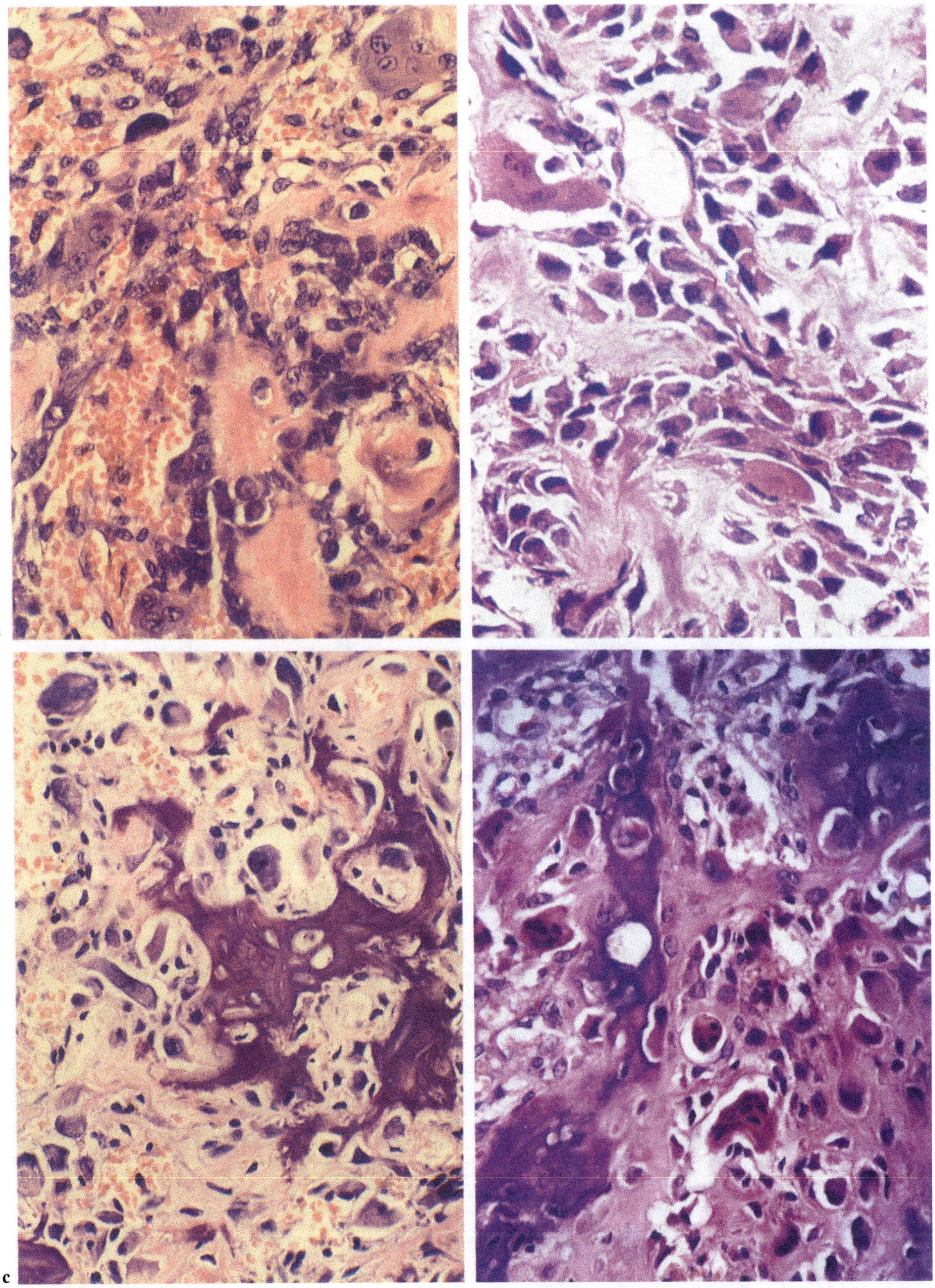

a b c d

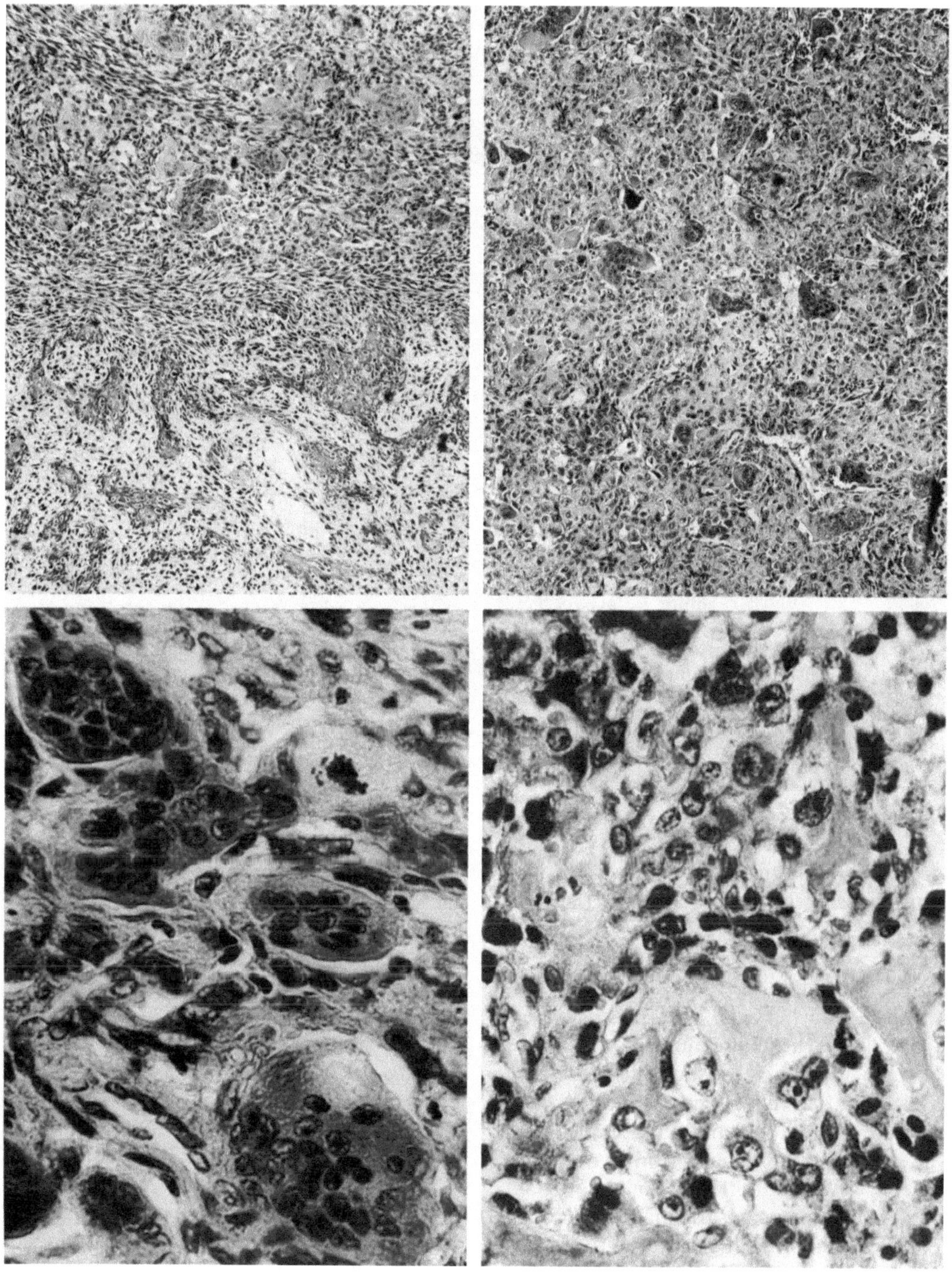

a b c d

◄

Fig. I.48a–d. Photomicrographs showing the characteristic histologic features of different cases of aggressive (malignant) osteoblastoma. **a** ×200, **b–d** ×400

Fig. I.49a–d. Photomicrographs showing other histologic features of malignant osteoblastoma, revealing areas rich in giant cells of osteoclastic type in a cellular stroma, rich in spindle cells (**a**) and hypertrophic osteoblasts which in (**d**) show evident pleomorphism. **c** An exceptional atypical mitosis is seen. Besides osteoid trabeculae, calcified immature and dark-blue-staining immature bone trabeculae are observed in **a**. **a**,**b** ×100; **c**,**d** ×360

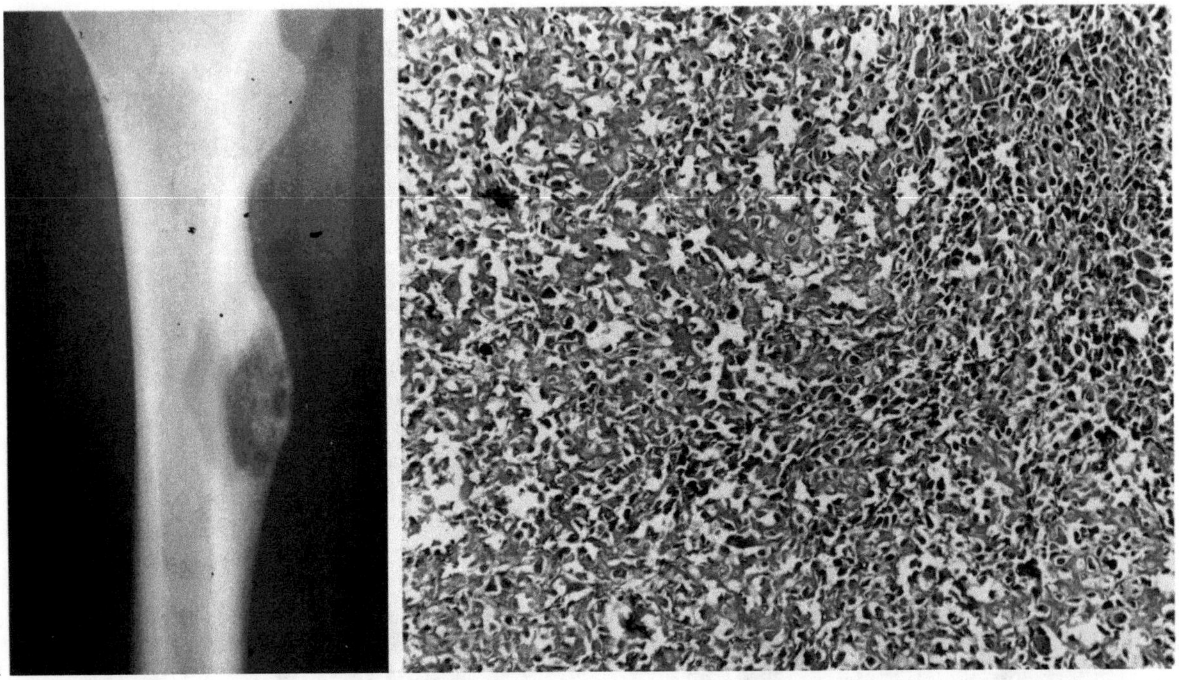

a b

Fig. I.50a,b. Male, 41 years old, with a lesion in the femoral diaphysis, which was diagnosed as malignant osteoblastoma. **a** Radiograph shows a lytic lesion, apparently originating intracortically or subperiosteally, expanding the cortex. There is slight irregular calcification centrally. **b** Photomicrograph reveals a highly cellular lesion with numerous filigree, lacelike osteoid trabeculae, and the histologic features of conventional osteosarcoma. The exact origin (cortical or periosteal) without a CT could not be determined (**b** ×100). (Courtesy of Dr. José Donato de Próspero, São Paulo, Brazil)

bone trabeculae of irregular shape, closely resembling those seen in osteosarcoma, but produced by typical osteoblasts (Fig. I.47). However, special care is necessary in evaluating nuclear atypism because while in some osteoblastomas the osteoblasts can be large with plump hypertrophic and hyperchromatic nuclei, in genuine osteoblastoma the characteristic blue spiculated bone is lacking. The histologic distinction from osteosarcoma may be difficult (Figs. I.50–I.52). However, in malignant osteoblastomas the areas of necrosis, atypical mitosis, and malignant cartilage so evident in osteosarcoma are generally lacking. This tumor was differentiated from conventional osteosarcoma not only because of its peculiar histologic pattern but also because of its different clinical and radiologic features and better prognosis.

The patients' ages varied from 6 to 67 years, with an average of 34 years. In the cases located in long bones, the diaphysis or epiphysis was most frequently affected. Radiologically the appearance was extremely variable and not diagnostic. Most cases were osteolytic with expansion and thinning of the cortex, simulating giant-cell tumor in three cases (Figs. I.53–I.55). Some cases were indistinguishable from conventional osteoblastoma (Fig. I.56). In the more advanced or recurrent lesions destruction of the cortex and inconspicuous invasion of soft tissues were observed (Fig. I.57).

Dorfman (1980) and Dorfman and Weiss (1984) have divided the osteoblastic tumors of

Fig. I.51a,b. Photomicrographs of conventional central osteosarcoma showing numerous irregular or lacelike osteoid trabeculae surrounded by a great number of hyperchromatic and atypical osteoblasts and a stroma rich in anaplastic spindle cells. **a** ×100, **b** ×400 ▲

Fig. I.52a,b. Photomicrographs at **a** lower and **b** higher magnification of a conventional central osteosarcoma, with areas of a predominant hemangiopericytomatous pattern. Capillary vessels surrounded by numerous anaplastic tumor cells, showing formation of osteoid trabeculae. This case has been misdiagnosed as malignant osteoblastoma. **a** ×100, **b** ×400 ▶

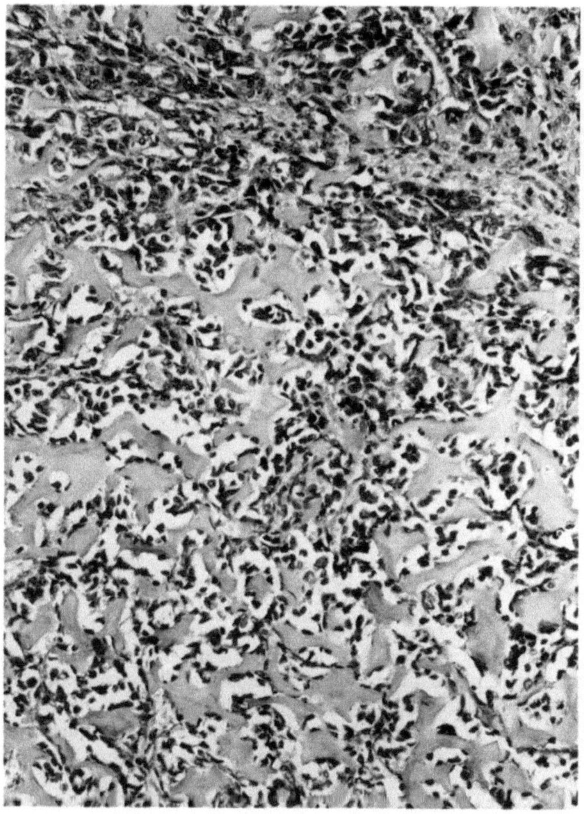

a

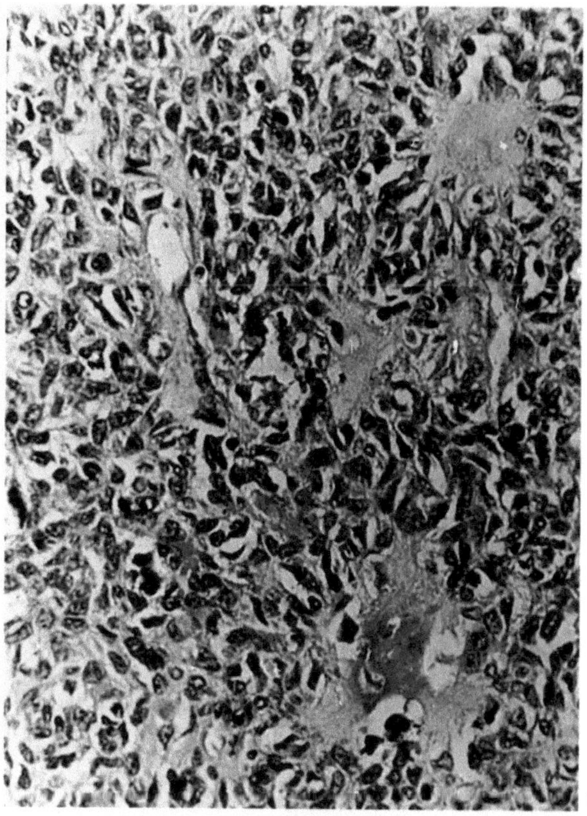

b

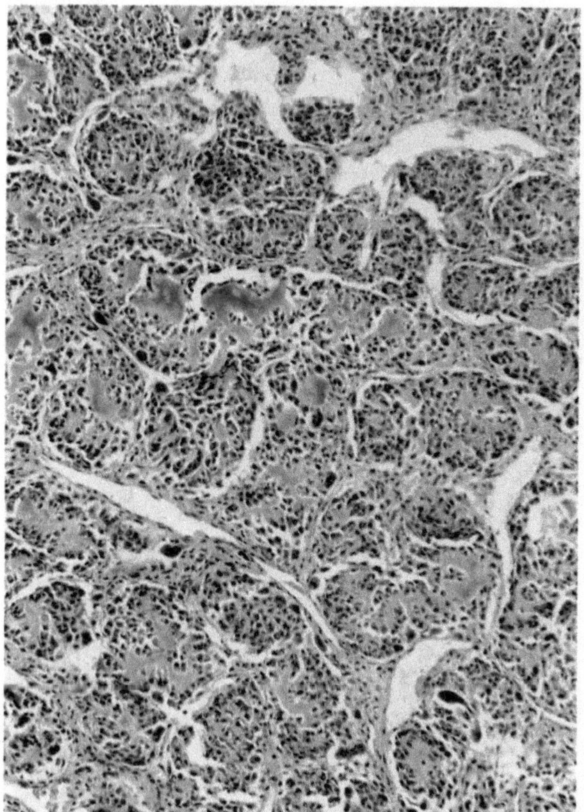

a

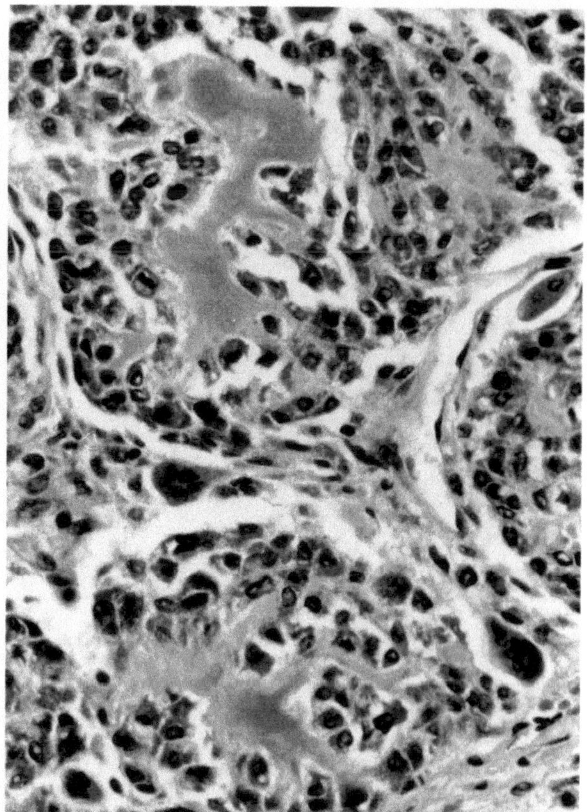

b

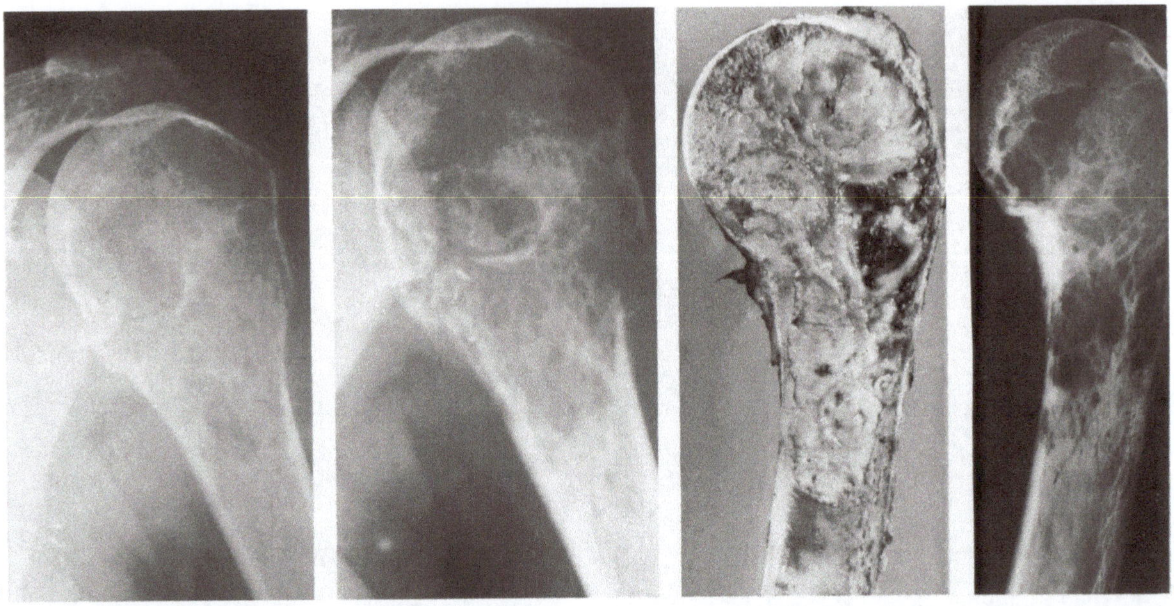

a, b c, d

Fig. I.53a–d. Female, 19 years old. Aggressive (malignant) osteoblastoma of the upper end of the humerus. **a** Radiograph showing an osteolytic lesion of the upper epiphysis extending to the metadiaphyseal region with slight expansion and thinning of the cortex and crossed by several septa. **b** Two months later, the lesion had extended and a pathologic fracture occurred. A wide resection of the upper third of the humerus followed by a fibular graft was performed. **c,d** Photograph and radiograph of the resected specimen showing the tumor, grayish white in color, with some hemorrhagic zones. The patient is in good general health 11 years after the resection of the tumor. (**c,d** Schajowicz and Lemos 1976)

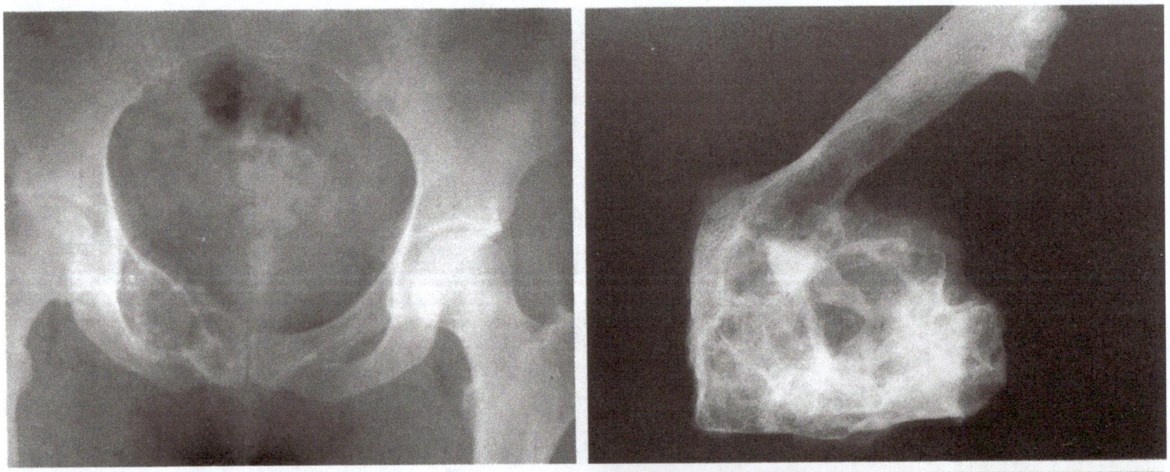

a b

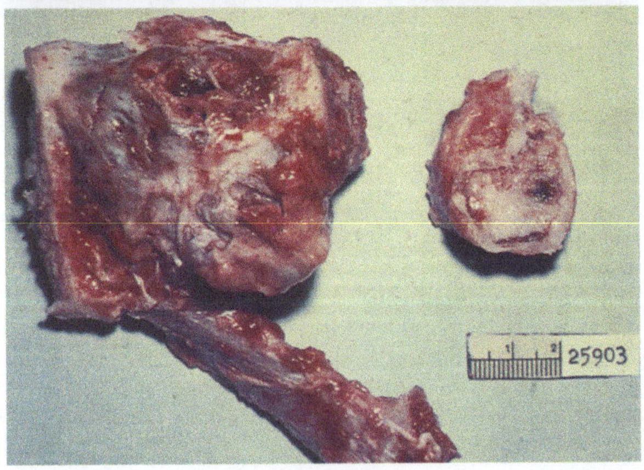

c

Fig. I.54a–c. Female, 28 years old, with aggressive (malignant) osteoblastoma of the iliopubic ramus. **a** Radiograph showing a lytic expanding trabeculated lesion. **b** Radiograph and **c** photograph of the resected specimen. The patient was well and free of disease after 6 years

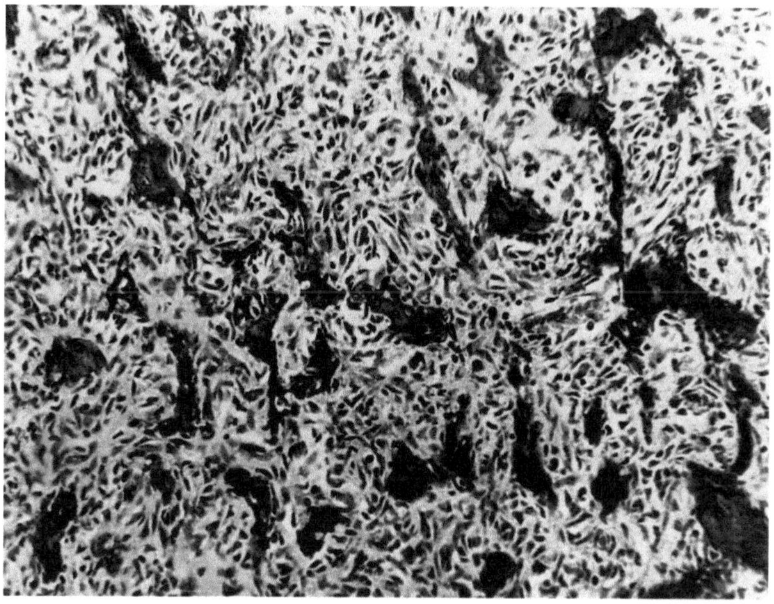

Fig. I.55. Photomicrograph of the case illustrated in Fig. I.54, showing irregular, heavily calcified woven bone trabeculae ("blue bone spicules") described as characteristic of malignant osteoblastoma by Schajowicz and Lemos (1976)

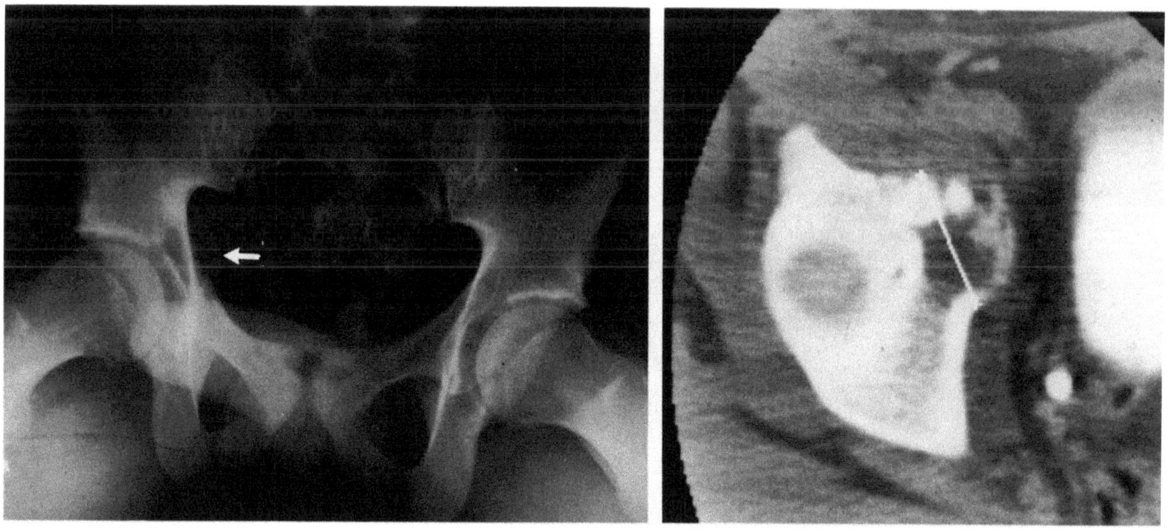

a b

Fig. I.56a,b. Male, 14 years old with an aggressive osteoblastoma of the acetabular region. **a** Radiograph and **b** CT show a radiolucent lesion (*arrow* on **a**) that expanded the thinned cortex, which was partly destroyed

uncertain malignant potential into four groups: (1) low-grade osteosarcoma resembling osteoblastoma (Bertoni et al. 1985) (cf. Fig. I.58); (2) osteoblastoma in which degenerative changes in the osteoblast create a pseudomalignant picture resembling the anaplasia of osteosarcoma, as described by Mirra et al. in 1976; (3) those very uncommon examples of malignant transformation of benign osteoblastic tumors to histologically typical osteosarcomas; and (4) those tumors with features intermediate between osteoblastoma and osteosarcoma. Dorfman and Weiss designated this last group "aggressive osteoblastoma" because of their distinct histologic features and

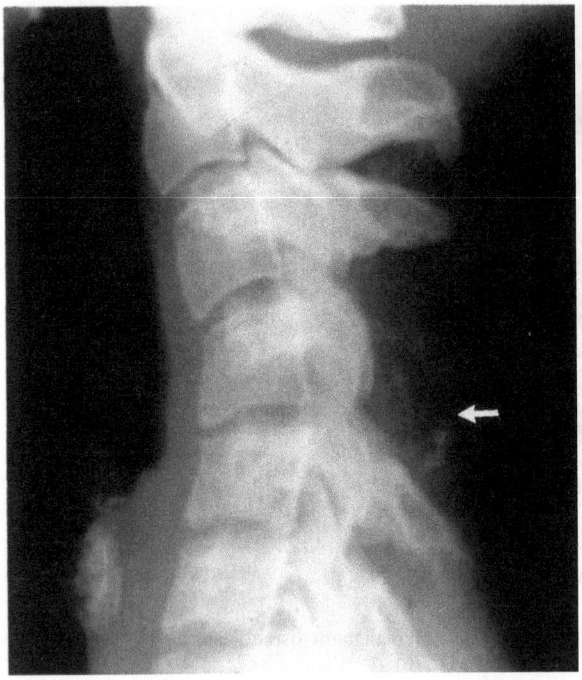

a

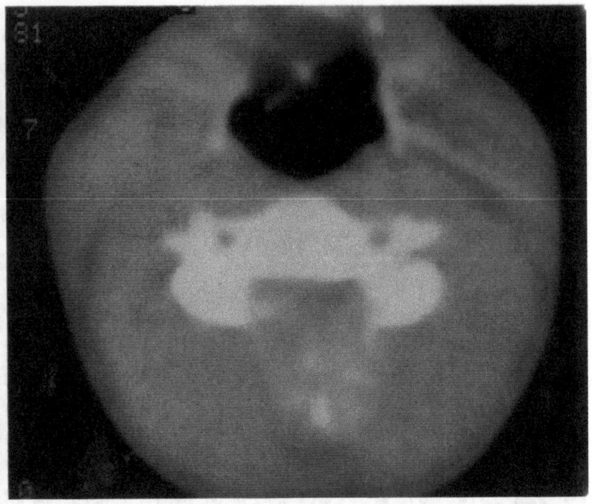

b

Fig. I.57. a Male, 16 years old, with an aggressive (malignant) osteoblastoma of the fourth spinal process showing a radiolucent expanding lesion (*arrow*) that almost completely destroyed the thinned cortex, as is clearly seen with CT (**b**). The patient had fully recovered 4 years after a wide resection, followed by stabilization with a bone graft. (Schajowicz and McGuire 1989)

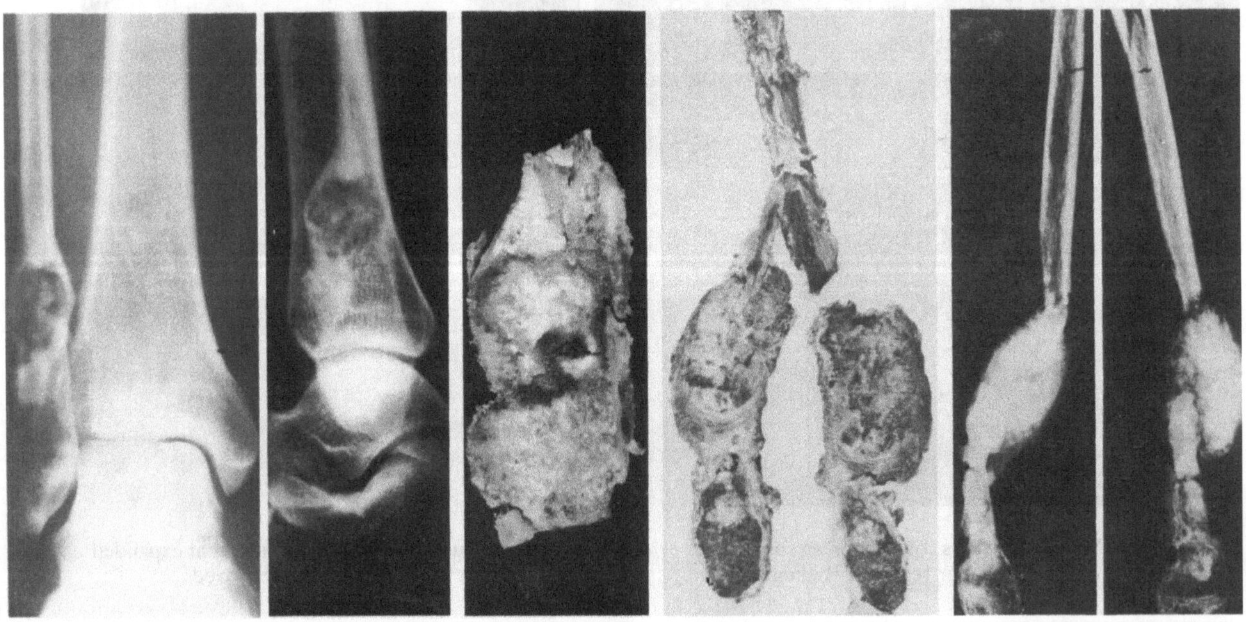

a, b c, d

Fig. I.58a–d. Female, 46 years old. Original diagnosis: malignant (aggressive) osteoblastoma of the fibula. **a** Anteroposterior and lateral radiographs showing an osteolytic lesion in the lower third of the fibula with some spotted areas of calcification in the center and areas of sclerosis in the lower part. **b** Photograph of the cut surface of the resected specimen. The tumor was grayish white in color with an area of hemorrhage in the center. **c** Photograph and **d** radiograph of a local recurrence after 2 years. A resection of the lower fibula was performed. Radiograph shows dense calcification of recurrence. The patient was in good health 10 years after the first resection. After reviewing the histologic slides the lesion was reclassified as well-differentiated (low-grade) osteosarcoma. (Schajowic and Lemos 1976)

Fig. I.59a–c. Male, 25 years old. Osteosarcoma in an exceptional location in the terminal phalanx of the thumb. **a** Lateral radiograph shows the sclerotic lesion with soft tissue extension. **b** Lateral and anteroposterior radiographs demonstrate the sclerotic nodular pattern of the lesion after 8 months. **c** A small dense metastatic nodule in the soft tissues of the same arm

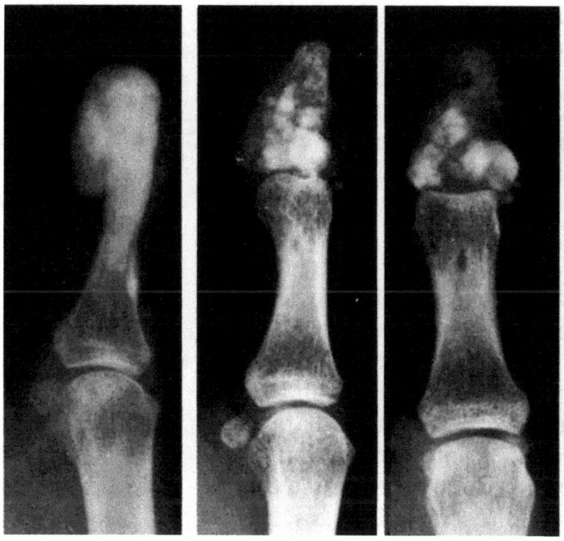

a, b

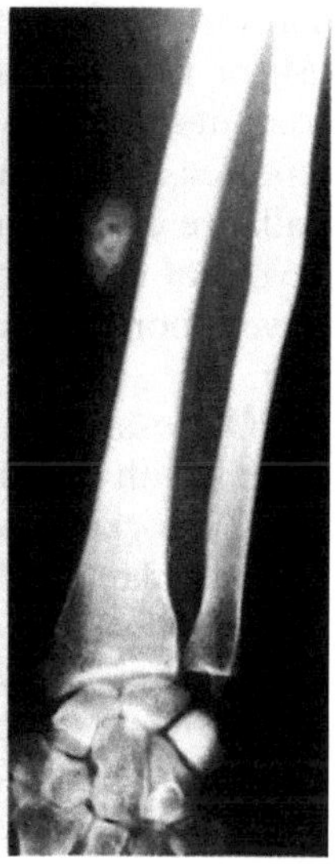

c

more aggressive clinical course. Of 15 cases, seven showed evidence of recurrence, although none metastasized.

The histologic and clinical features of Dorfman's "aggressive osteoblastoma" are similar to those of this author's "malignant osteoblastoma." In spite of their aggressive clinical course and frequent recurrence, none of the 16 cases classified by us as "malignant osteoblastomas," nor the reported cases of "aggressive osteoblastomas," had metastasized (Dorfman and Weiss 1984; Adbelwahab et al. 1986; Kenan et al. 1985; Pieterse et al. 1983; Revell and Scholtz 1979). Since these tumors lack a metastatic potential, we agree with other authors that the term "aggressive osteoblastoma" seems to be more appropriate. It is also less committing to the pathologist, who may feel more comfortable with that diagnosis. Both terms are considered synonymous by Spjut et al. (1981). Mirra (1989) has recently suggested the designation of "osteosarcoma in situ" for these lesions.

The difficulties in the differential diagnosis of benign and malignant or aggressive forms of osteoblastoma may perhaps be overcome by flow cytometry studies, accompanied whenever possible by tissue cultures. These methods appear to be useful in the determination of the tumor's biologic behavior, and in at least one of the author's cases showed a DNA index of 7% aneuploid cells. Tissue cultures of these elements started to grow after 14 weeks and the aneuploidy was at this time much greater. Further studies with these methods associated with more prolonged clinical follow-up studies are necessary to determine whether these procedures could be helpful in predicting the biologic behavior of this tumor.

C. Malignant

1. Osteosarcoma

The term "osteosarcoma" is now used by most authors, replacing the older term "osteogenic sarcoma." It is defined by WHO as "*a malignant tumor characterized by the direct formation of bone or osteoid by the proliferating tumor cells.*"

Tumor bone formation may be present only in small foci, but even when the predominant tissue is cartilaginous or fibroblastic, the lesion should be classified as osteosarcoma. Dahlin (1978) and other authors subdivided osteosarcoma into three categories, depending on the predominant differentiation of the tumor cells. According to Dahlin, about 50% produce tumor bone or osteoid in sufficiently large amounts to be called "osteoblastic osteosarcoma," in about 25% the predominant differentiation is toward cartilage ("chondroblastic osteosarcoma"), and the remaining 25% show a predominant spindle-cell pattern, similar to that seen in fibrosarcoma, and are classified as "fibroblastic osteosarcoma." Recently another variant with predominant fibrohistiocytic differentiation has been added (Mirra 1980; Ballance et al. 1988). This subtype accounts for 5%–10% of all osteosarcomas reported by Mirra. In the six cases reported by Ballance et al., the extraosseous component was devoid of bone elements. Neoplastic osteoid and woven bone were present in the intraosseous part.

Osteosarcoma covers a wide spectrum of lesions with distinct clinical and pathologic features, associated with different biologic behavior. Two fundamental groups can be clearly distinguished, the *central* (*medullary*) and the *surface* (*peripheral*) *osteosarcoma* (Schajowicz 1983). Osteosarcomas of intracortical location seem to be extremely rare, and only isolated cases have been reported (Jaffe 1960; Kyriakos 1980; Picci et al. 1983; Vigorita et al. 1984).

a. Central (Medullary) Osteosarcoma

Osteosarcoma is, with the exception of myeloma, the most common primary malignant bone tumor in all large series. Besides the most frequent conventional or classic osteosarcoma, several variants of central osteosarcoma have been described: the *telangiectatic osteosarcoma*, the *well-differentiated* (*low-grade*) *osteosarcoma*, and the *small-cell* (*round-cell*) *osteosarcoma simulating Ewing sarcoma*. With the exception of the well-differentiated osteosarcoma, all are highly malignant (Table I.2).

Our laboratory's files include 637 cases of central osteosarcoma, its incidence being less than twice that of chondrosarcoma (430 cases) and more than twice that of Ewing sarcoma (272 cases). In the Mayo Clinic files through December 1983 (Dahlin and Unni 1986), covering a period of almost 70 years, 1274 osteosarcomas of bone were identified, together with 635 primary and secondary chondrosarcomas, 207 fibrosarcomas, and 402 Ewing sarcomas during the same period of time. In the Anderson Hospital and Tumor Institute over a 24-year period (1950–1974), 243 cases of primary osteosarcoma of bone were treated (Uribe-Botero et al. 1977). At the Memorial Sloan-Kettering Cancer Center, 1095 patients with osteosarcoma were diagnosed and treated from 1921 through 1979, and 952 cases were identified at the Instituto Ortopedico Rizzoli de Bologna (Campanacci 1990).

An interesting finding is the apparently higher incidence of osteosarcoma in individuals of higher stature (Fraumeni 1967). Veterinarians have long known that giant breeds of dogs (Saint Bernards and Great Danes) have much higher risks for bone cancer (Owen 1969; Miller 1976).

Table I.2. Classification of osteosarcoma

Central (intramedullary)	Surface (peripheral)
1. Conventional (classic)	1. Parosteal (juxtacortical)
2. Telangiectatic	2. Periosteal
3. Well-differentiated (low-grade)	3. High-grade (conventional)
4. With small cells simulating Ewing sarcoma (mesenchymal)	

Clinical Findings. The *age and sex distribution* is shown in Scheme I.3. In our series, the tumor occurred more often in males, with 374 male patients (60%) and 247 females (40%), which agrees with the general male predominance in most other series (Dahlin and Unni 1986; Campanacci 1990; Huvos 1991).

The highest incidence (58%) occurred in the second decade of life, followed by the first and third decades. The tumor was relatively uncommon below the age of 10 (13%) and rare in patients under 5 or over 40 years of age. However, the absolute number of osteosarcoma patients older than 60 years admitted to Memorial Sloan-Kettering Cancer Center abruptly increased in the last 10–15 years (Huvos 1986) and accounted for approximately 10% of all osteosarcoma. Our youngest patient was 2 years old, and the literature contains isolated observations of congenital osteosarcoma.

Most tumors developing after middle age were associated with Paget disease of bone (Wick et al. 1981; Schajowicz et al. 1983; Huvos et al. 1983a) or, more rarely, were secondary to irradiation (Sim et al. 1972) or to fibrous dysplasia (Huvos et al. 1972). These lesions are discussed in separate chapters.

Localization. Although any bone may be affected, osteosarcoma shows a preference for the long bones, with a predilection for the metaphyseal areas of the lower end of the femur (229 cases), the upper end of the tibia (118 cases), and, less frequently, the upper end of the humerus (58 cases), that is, close to the most actively growing epiphyses. Tumors of the first

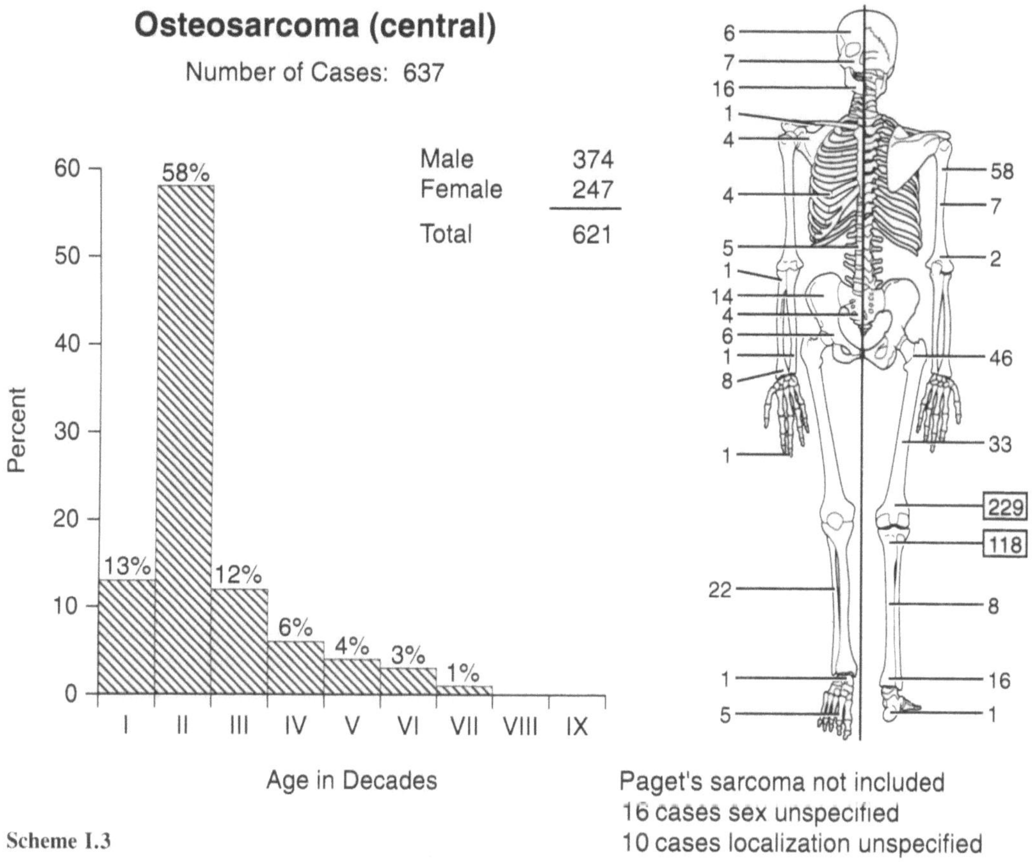

Scheme I.3

two sites, including 16 cases located at the upper fibula, accounted for 363 of our cases, representing 58% of lesions located around the knee.

The upper metaphysis of the femur (46 cases), the inferior metaphysis of the tibia (16 cases), and the upper metaphysis or diaphysis of the fibula (22 cases) were involved less frequently. The diaphyses of other long bones and also of short and flat bones were infrequently affected, among them more commonly the iliac bone (20 cases) and the craniofacial bones, mandible, and maxilla, which accounted for 29 cases. However, the number of craniofacial tumors was higher in the Mayo Clinic series (Dahlin and Unni 1986), which comprises 110 cases (including 26 cases in the skull, 45 in the maxilla, and 39 in the mandible). A similar high percentage (7% of all osteosarcomas) of craniofacial tumors was treated in the Memorial Sloan-Kettering Cancer Center (Huvos 1991). The average age of patients with craniofacial osteosarcoma was generally higher than that of patients with osteosarcoma in other locations. In our series osteosarcoma occurred rarely in the spine (nine cases) and only exceptionally distal to the ankle and wrist joints (seven cases) (Carrol 1957; Fleegler et al. 1980); this is in accordance with most other series (Fig. I.59). A purely epiphyseal location is extremely rare (Tsuneyoshi and Dorfman 1987).

Symptoms. The most common *clinical symptom* was pain at the tumor site, often irradiating to a neighboring joint, which began insidiously, intermittently, and progressed to severe, constant pain which was not relieved by rest, immobilization, or ordinary analgesics. A palpable mass developed later that was associated with limitation of joint motion. However, joint effusion was uncommon, in contrast to tumors involving the epiphysis, such as giant-cell tumors or chondroblastomas.

In advanced lesions, local inflammatory signs and venous stasis occurred frequently. Pathologic fractures were uncommon and were usually found in the predominantly osteolytic lesions. The duration of symptoms prior to diagnosis was extremely variable, averaging not more than a few months.

a, b

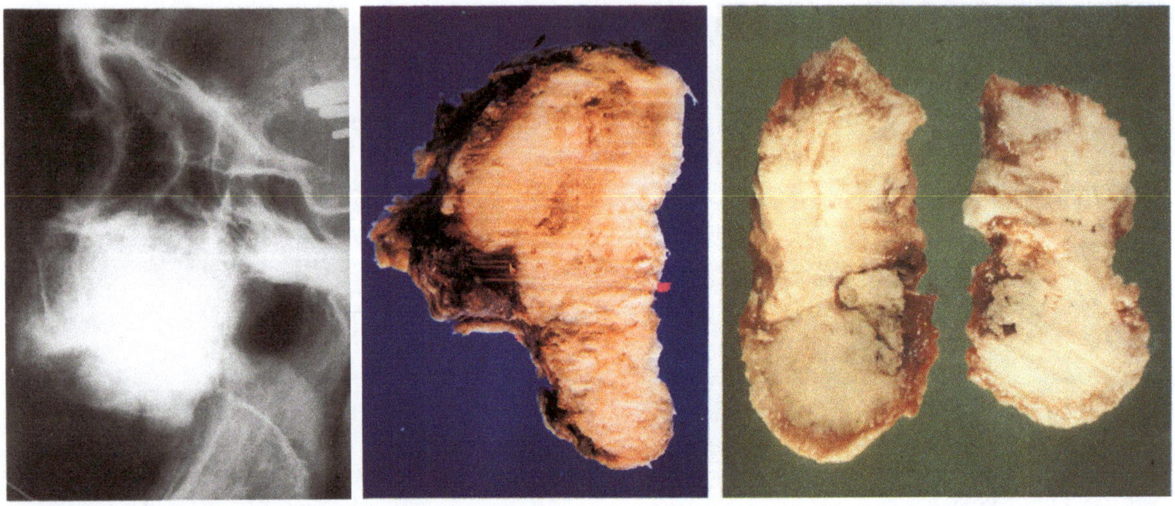

c

Fig. I.60a–c. Two cases of sclerosing osteosarcoma in the maxilla. Both patients were over 30 years of age

An important clinical finding was a moderate to evident increase in alkaline phosphatase activity in the serum, which occurred in the experience of Woodard and Higinbotham (1937), Woodard (1942), and ourselves in a high percentage of cases, and which is related to the osteoblastic activity of the basic tumor cell. However, there was not always an exact quantitative correlation between the phosphatase activity of the tumor tissue and that of the serum. More important than its diagnostic value is the prognostic significance of the fall in the serum alkaline phosphatase to normal levels after the surgical ablation of the tumor. The lack of this response indicates the presence of a metastasis or incomplete removal of the tumor.

Radiographic Features. The conventional (classic) osteosarcoma, in contrast to the surface (peripheral) type, arises *centrally* and, after destroying the cortex, invades the surrounding soft tissues. The extreme variety of tumor-cell differentiation with predominance of bone, cartilage, fibroblastic, or fibrohistiocytic proliferation, associated with more or less conspicuous reactive bone formation, is reflected by the different radiographic patterns of osteosarcoma. In some tumors, bone formation predominates: this variety is generally referred to as *sclerosing type* (Fig. I.60). In more cellular and anaplastic or telangiectatic tumors, bone destruction predominates, and a permeative or motheaten radiolucent pattern with ill-defined margins toward the normal bone is produced (*osteolytic type*). This variety may simulate a non-bone-forming malignant tumor such as a giant-cell tumor or fibrosarcoma, or even a benign lesion such as an aneurysmal bone cyst. However, in most of our cases, the radiographic aspect was of the mixed sclerotic–osteolytic type (Figs. I.61–I.64) (Schajowicz et al. 1972).

The most characteristic features are produced after cortical destruction and extension of the tumor into soft tissues, resulting in the classic reactions exhibited by the periosteum:

1. The *formation of long, thin filiform spicules* of reactive periosteal bone, radiating perpendicularly (hair-on-end pattern) or from a central point, giving the typical "sunburst" pattern (Fig. I.65–I.70). Spiculated periosteal reaction is not specific for osteosarcoma and may be observed in some benign (hemangioma, meningioma) or malignant lesions (Ewing sarcoma). Occasionally, a laminated periosteal reaction may be present (Figs. I.71, I.72).
2. The so-called *Codman's triangle* or *spur*, which is due to formation of reactive bone between the elevated intact periosteum and the underlying cortex at the zone of transition to the extraosseous extension of the tumor (Figs. I.61, I.62, I.73, I.74). Although characteristic, Codman's triangle is not pathognomonic of osteosarcoma and may be found in any aggressive tumoral process, such as in Ewing sarcoma, or even in benign conditions such as osteomyelitis, after infiltration of extraosseous soft tissues.

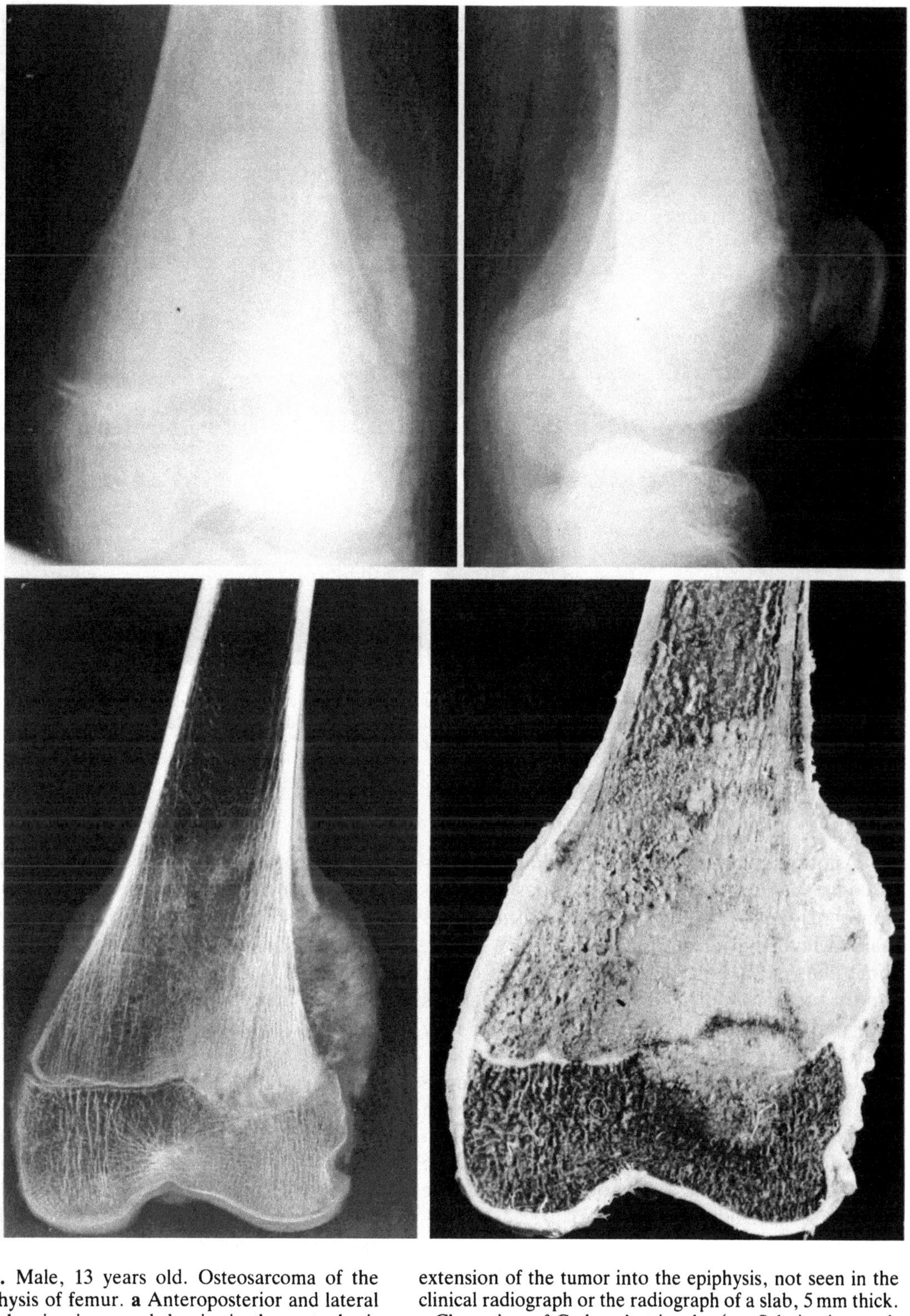

a b c

Fig. I.61a–c. Male, 13 years old. Osteosarcoma of the lower metaphysis of femur. **a** Anteroposterior and lateral radiographs showing increased density in the metaphysis and periosteal new bone formation with a typical Codman's triangle. **b** Photograph of specimen showing the extension of the tumor into the epiphysis, not seen in the clinical radiograph or the radiograph of a slab, 5 mm thick. **c** Clear view of Codman's triangle. (**a**,**c** Schajowicz et al. 1972)

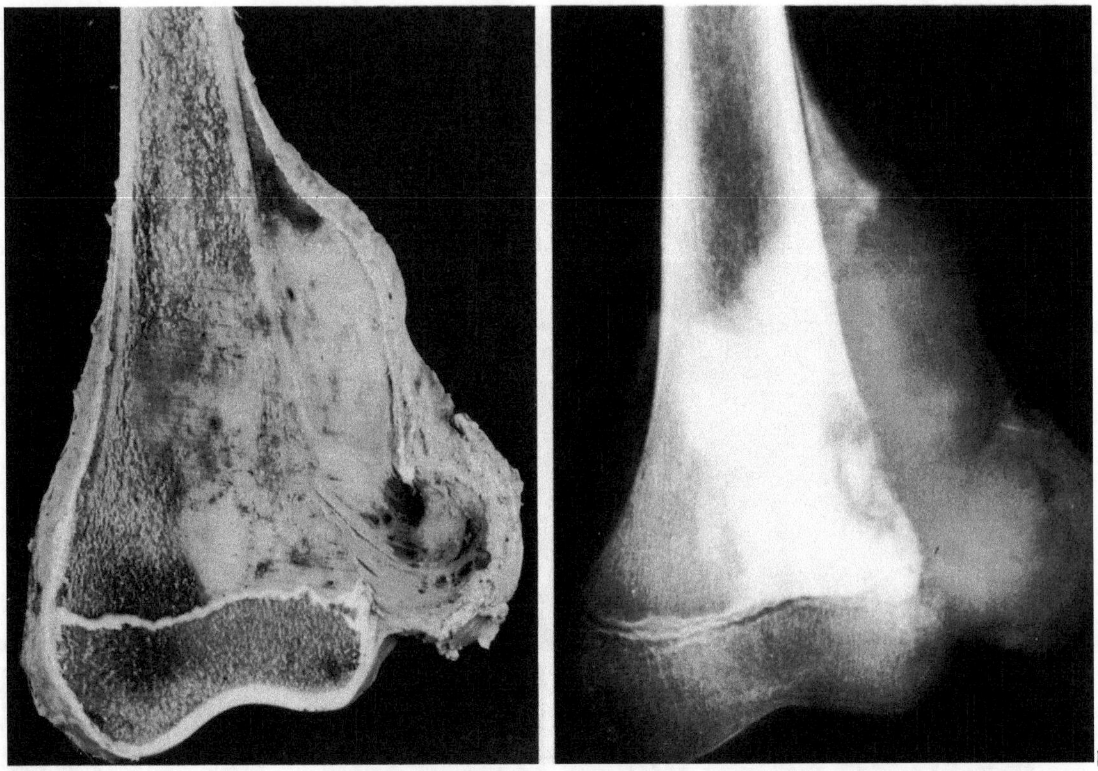

a b

Fig. I.62a,b. Male, 9 years old, with osteosarcoma of the femur. **a** Photograph and **b** radiograph of a longitudinal section of a tumor in the lower metaphysis of the femur with wide extension into the soft tissues and formation of a typical Codman's triangle

Another common radiologic finding in osteosarcoma is the presence of amorphous calcification or irregular ossification of the extraosseous mass, which may be extensive and very dense, sometimes exceeding the density and size of the central tumor; problems of differential diagnosis with parosteal (juxtacortical) osteosarcoma may arise in these cases (Fig. I.75).

Computed tomography, magnetic resonance imaging, and/or angiography are important in determining the intra- and extraosseous extension of the lesion, and isotope scanning may show the presence of metastatic foci or of rare multicentric lesions (see Introduction, p. 3ff.).

Pathologic Findings. *Gross Pathology.* In accordance with its variable radiographic features, osteosarcoma shows considerable diversity in its gross and histologic patterns. The polymorphism of osteosarcoma is due to the fact that the formation of atypical (immature) bone and osteoid by the tumor cells is associated with the destruction and defensive reactive processes of the affected bone, that is, reactive bone formation, centrally and extraosseously.

The author studied more than 200 amputation specimens and performed comparative radiologic and macroscopic examinations. Because many of these are illustrated in the text, a more detailed description is unnecessary.

The various stages of differentiation of the basic pluripotential tumor cell, which in its skeletal evolution may produce different tissue types such as fibroblastic, fibrohistiocytic, myxoid, cartilaginous, and, particularly, immature bone and osteoid, explain, together with the reactive processes described previously, the extremely variable gross patterns and the different subdivisions, that is, fibroblastic, chondroblastic, and osteoblastic (Dahlin 1978), and, more recently, fibrohistiocytic. The neoplasms may vary from soft fleshy grayish-white or reddish, to firm gray or bluish, hard masses of fibrous or cartilaginous material with variable amounts of irregular amorphous calcification or ossification. They often form dense, sclerotic masses that may

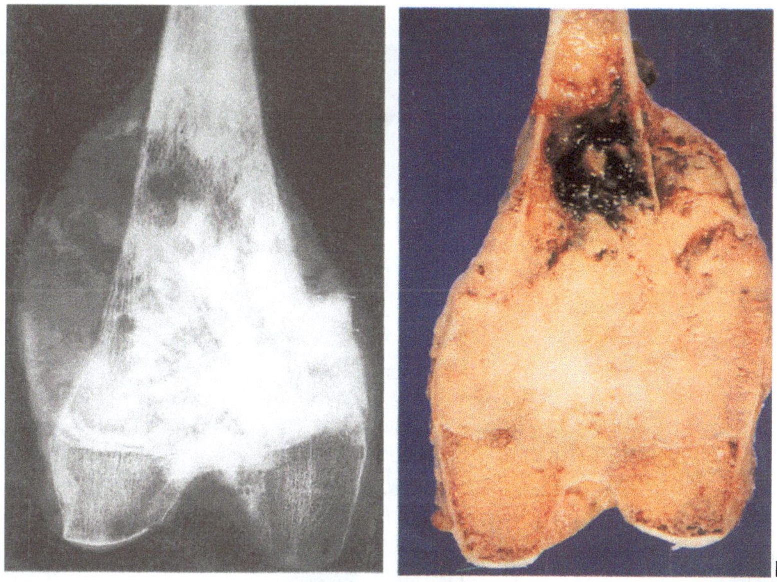

a b

Fig. I.63a,b. Osteosarcoma of the lower femoral metaphysis. **a** Radiograph and **b** photograph demonstrate the mixed osteolytic–osteoblastic pattern and the evident invasion of the epiphysis

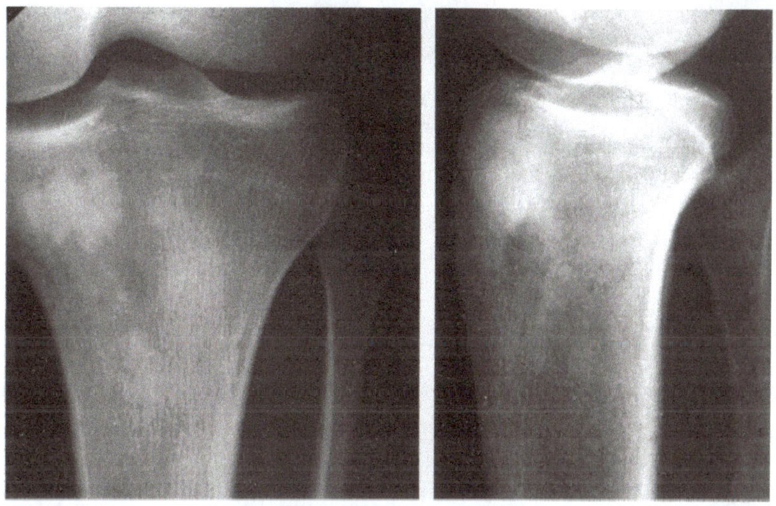

Fig. I.64. Female, 18 years old. Osteosarcoma of the proximal tibial end. Anteroposterior and lateral radiographs show the small size of the osteolytic–osteoblastic lesion, which has not invaded soft tissue (stage IIA)

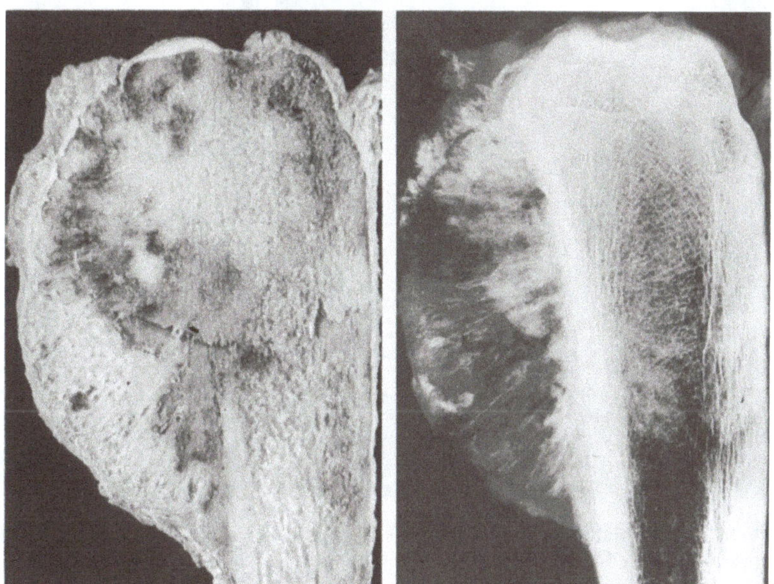

a b

Fig. I.65a,b. Male, 22 years old, with osteosarcoma of the upper tibial end. **a** Photograph and **b** radiograph of the specimen. The epiphyseal plate is already closed and the tumor is invading the epiphysis and soft tissue extensively, showing a sunburst type of periosteal reaction. Small irregular calcifications probably represent tumor new bone formation

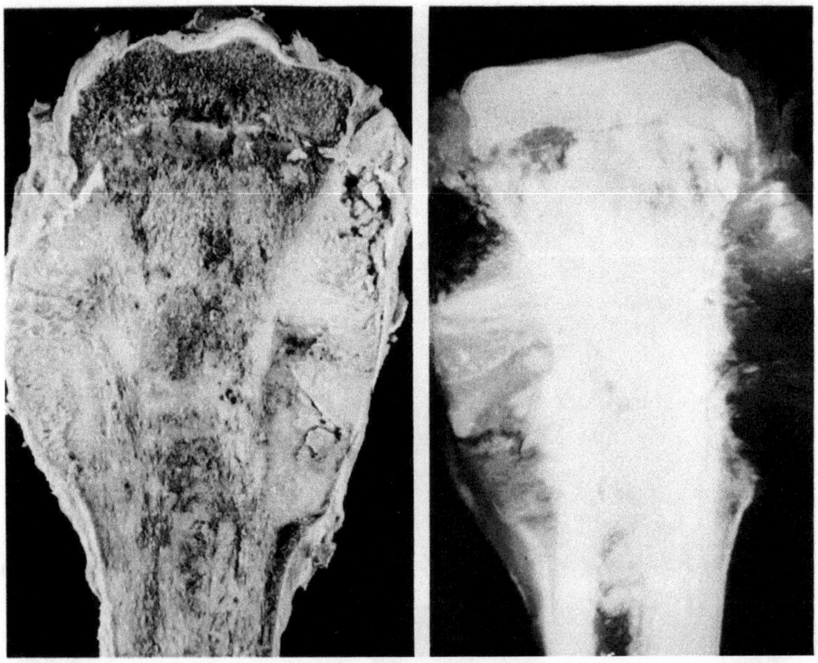

a b

Fig. I.66a,b. Male, 15 years old. Osteosarcoma of the upper metaphysis of tibia. **a** Photograph and **b** radiograph of the specimen. The tumor is predominantly sclerotic with only scarce lytic areas and has partially destroyed the growth plate. There is an extensive soft tissue mass showing spiculated, sunburst-type periosteal reaction and small spotty calcification. Codman's triangles may be seen at the distal aspect of the lesion. (Schajowicz et al. 1972)

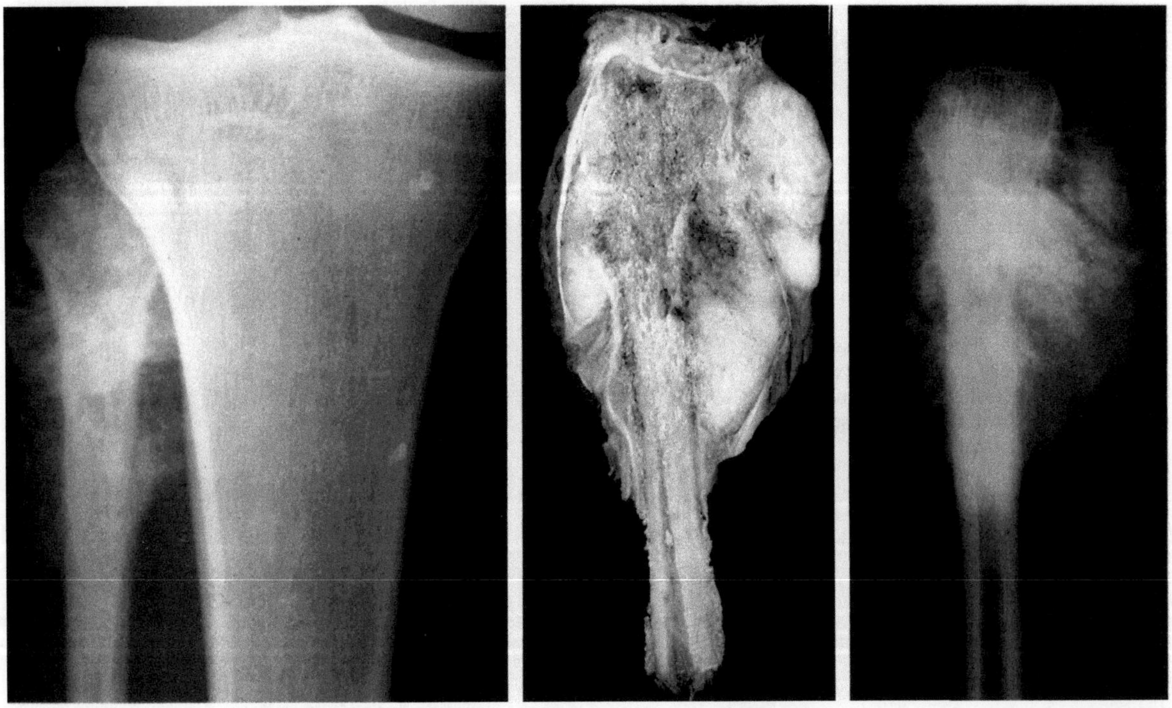

a b, c

Fig. I.67a–c. Male, 19 years old. Osteosarcoma of the upper fibular end. **a** Radiograph, **b** photograph, and **c** radiograph of the specimen show the large soft tissue mass and periosteal "sunburst" new bone formation

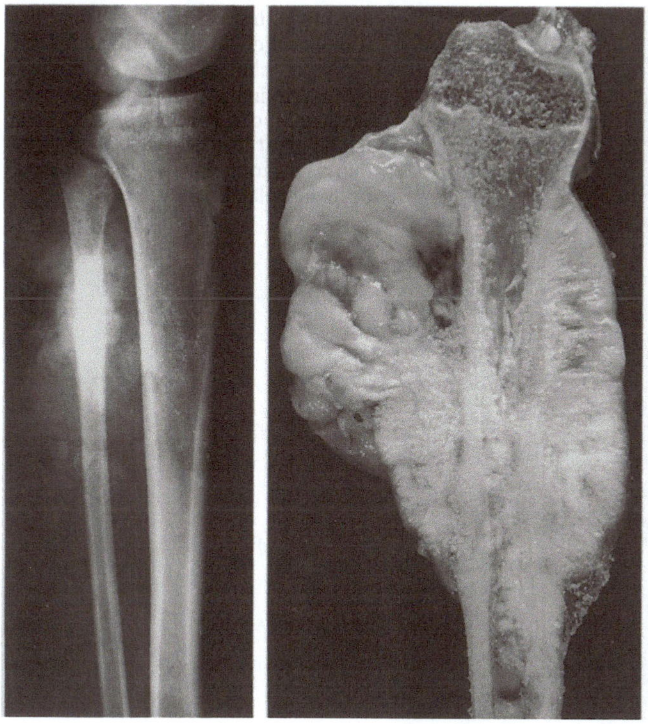

a, b

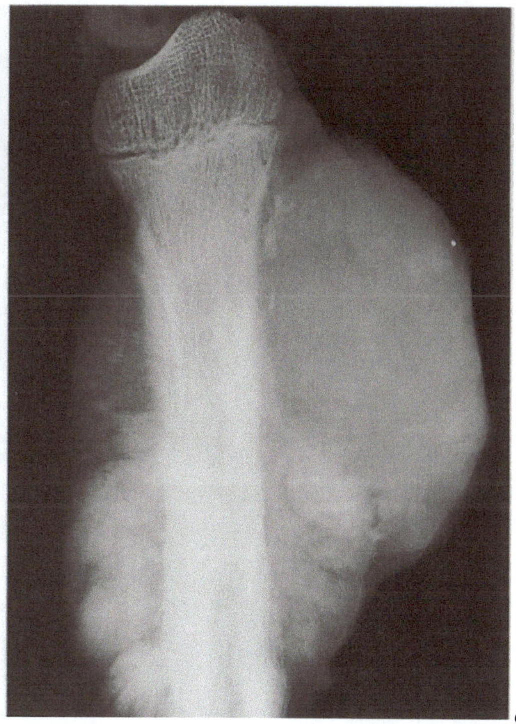

c

Fig. I.68a–c. Female, 17 years old. Osteosarcoma of the upper fibular metaphysis. **a** Radiograph, **b** photograph, and **c** radiograph of the specimen show the extensive soft tissue invasion, but no epiphyseal involvement

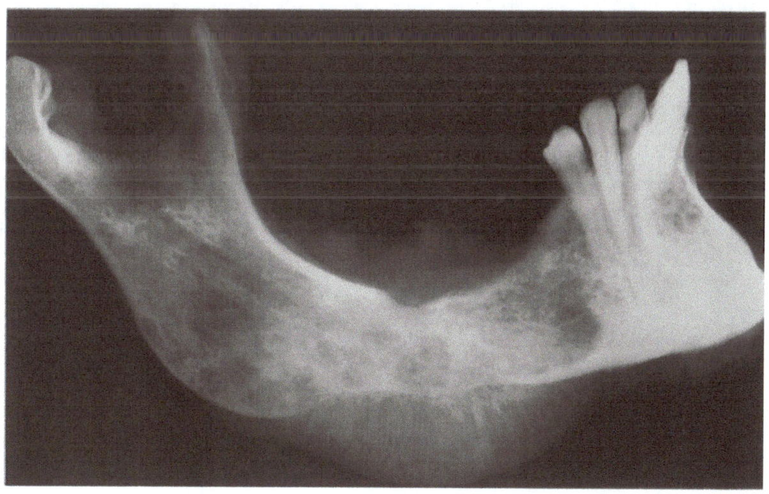

Fig. I.69. Male, 28 years old. Osteosarcoma of the mandible, predominantly radiolucent, showing an evident "sunburst" periosteal reaction

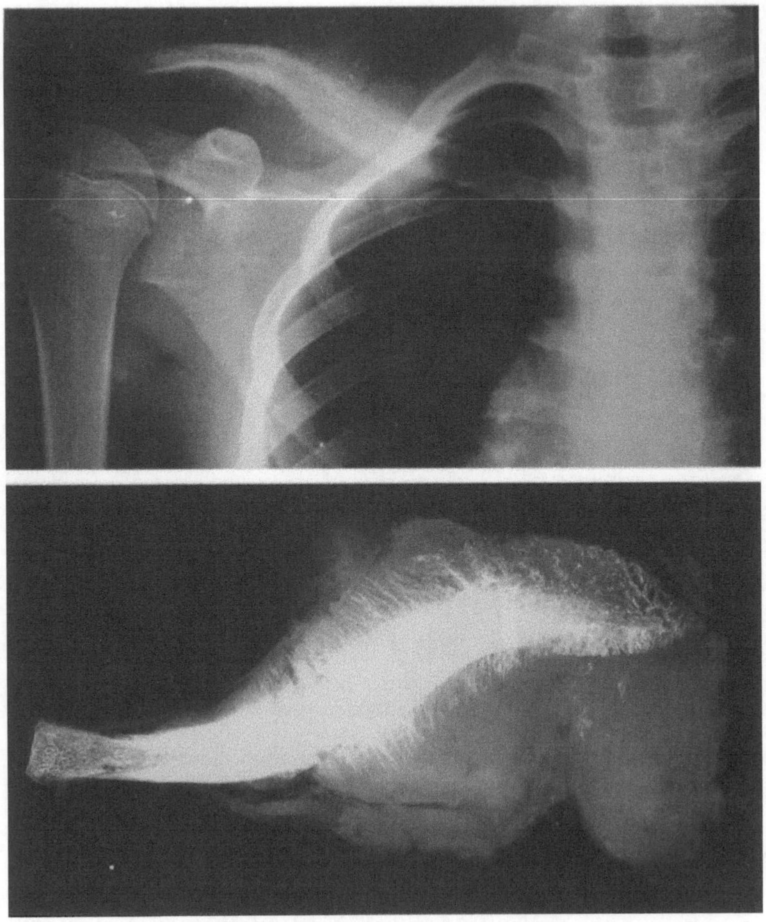

a

b

Fig. I.70a,b. Female, 10 years old. Rare location of osteosarcoma in the right clavicle. **a** Clinical radiograph and **b** specimen radiograph show that the tumor occupies two-thirds of the medial part of the clavicle and produces a conspicuous "hair-on-end" perpendicular periosteal reaction

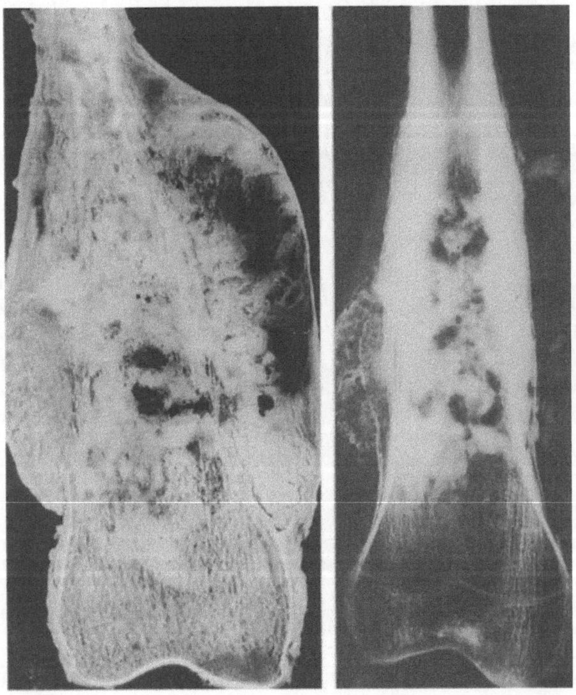

a b

Fig. I.71a,b. Female, 16 years old. Osteosarcoma of the femur. **a** Photograph and **b** radiograph of the specimen show the diaphyseal location of this tumor, patchy destructive changes alternating with spotty or nodular sclerotic areas. Laminated periosteal new bone formation is seen. The radiologic aspect suggested Ewing sarcoma

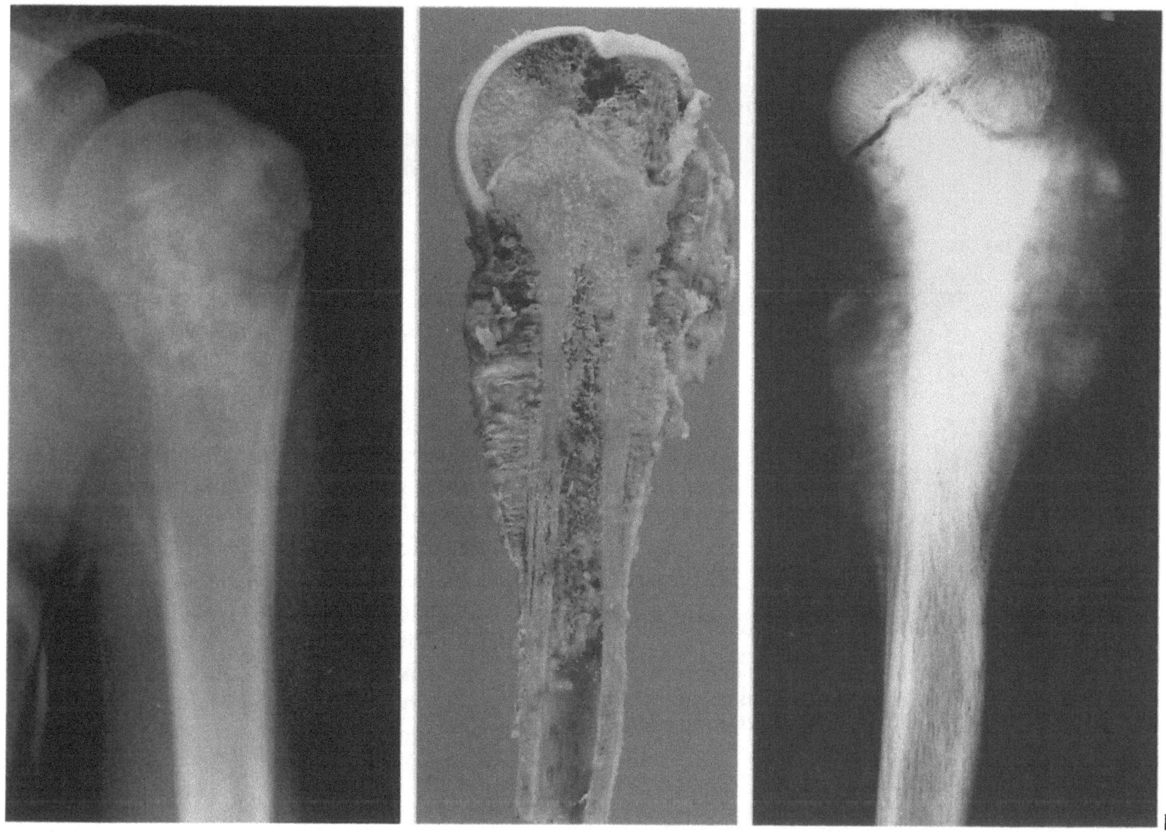

a b, c

▲

Fig. I.72a–c. Male, 16 years old. Osteosarcoma of the upper third of the humerus. **a** Radiograph, **b** photograph, and **c** radiograph of the specimen show the extension of the tumor towards the diaphysis and a partly laminated periosteal reaction, suggesting the possibility of Ewing sarcoma

▶

Fig. I.73a,b. Male, 15 years old. Osteosarcoma of lower third of the femur. **a** Radiograph and **b** photograph of the specimen show the soft tissue extension and typical Codman's triangle

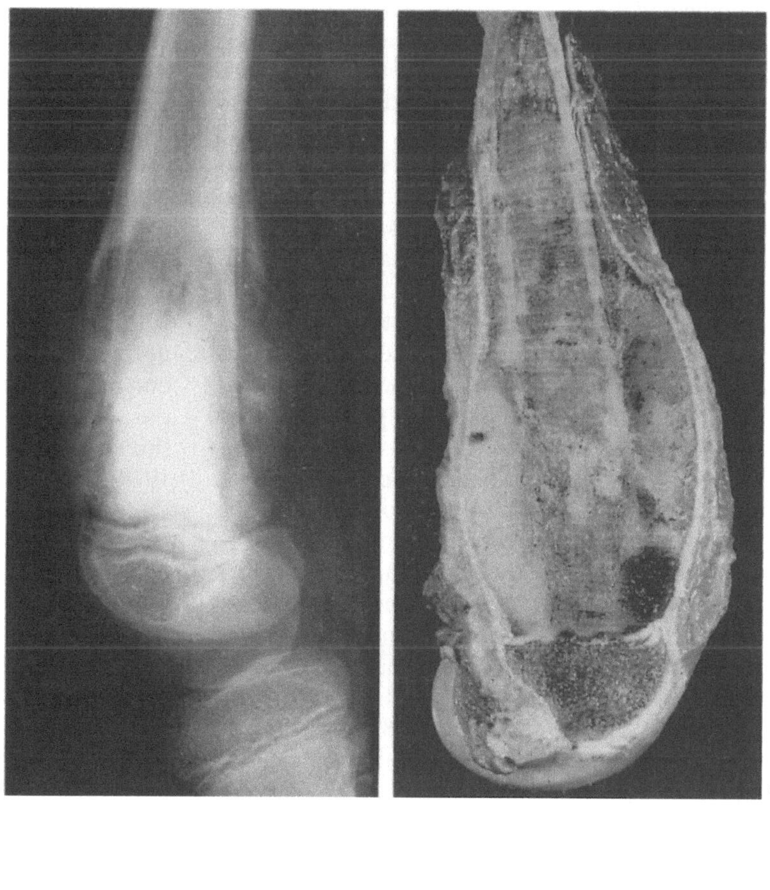

a b

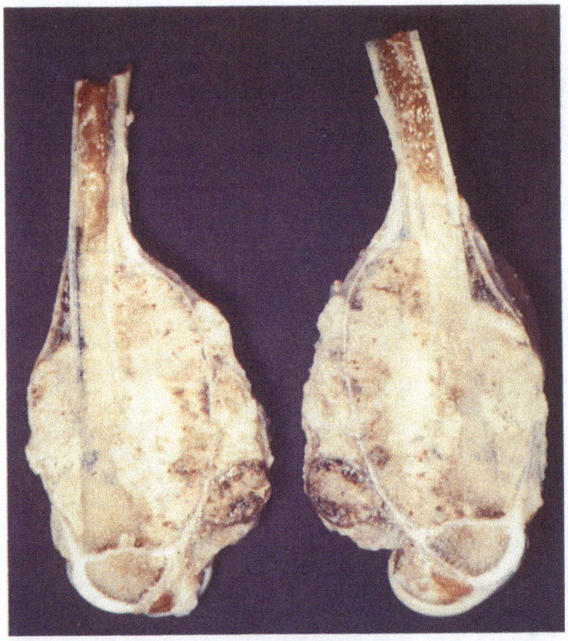

Fig. I.74. Osteosarcoma of the lower metaphysis of the femur, showing typical Codman's triangles at its upper end. In spite of its large size the tumor does not cross the growth cartilage

occupy the major central portion of the tumor (Figs. I.73, I.76, I.77). The picture is further complicated by the presence of intense regressive changes common in any rapidly growing neoplasm, such as abundant hemorrhages and extensive areas of necrosis followed by cystic degeneration (Fig. I.78).

The tumor usually does not spread far into the marrow cavity and generally not beyond the gross or radiologic extraosseous limits of the tumor, in contrast to chondrosarcoma, which extends extensively in the medullary cavity without destroying the overlying cortex. The intramedullary, noncontiguous spread of tumor is referred to as "skip metastases" by Enneking and Kagan, who in 1975 described "skip" lesions in 10 of 40 patients (25%) with osteosarcoma. They defined a "skip" as a solitary separate focus of osteosarcoma, occurring synchronously in the same bone or as a second lesion on the opposite side of a joint, in the absence of anatomic extension, pulmonary metastases, exposure to toxic substances, or Paget disease. From 1972 to 1976, 24 additional primary osteosarcomas were studied by these authors (Enneking and Kagan 1978). They observed two skip lesions (8.3%), bringing the total series to 64 cases with 24 skip metastases. Only 3 of the 12 lesions were evident on initial radiographs. Most lesions (9 of 12) were evident on gross examination of the cut specimen or with tetracycline labeling and examination of the tissue with ultraviolet light. In 3 of 12 cases they were only found following histologic examination of macroslides. The "skips" were intramedullary or involved an adjacent bone (transarticular) and occurred proximal (8 of 12) or distal (4) to the primary osteosarcoma. Six patients had recurrences following ablation proximal to the site of the skip lesions, and all but one patient developed pulmonary metastases within a mean interval of 6 months.

Consequently, it appears that hip disarticulation for the most common location in the lower metaphysis of the femur would be mandatory and more effective in order to avoid stump recurrences after midthigh or upper-thigh amputation. However, the incidence of local recurrences is generally low (Sweetnam 1973) (approximately 2%) with transmedullary amputation.

On the other hand, Upshaw et al. (1949) and Lewis and Lotz (1974) in 50 and 20 cases of long-bone osteosarcomas, respectively, did not observe any intramedullary extension or skip areas. Rohmsdahl and Ayala (1977), who carefully examined 48 surgical specimens at the M.D. Anderson Hospital, found only intraosseous "skip" foci in two disarticulated femora and a third in a transmedullary amputation specimen. They did not observe transarticular metastases in their series. All the patients had large tumors, with pulmonary metastases in two and involved lymph nodes in one, which signifies an evident relationship to exceptionally advanced disease. Following Enneking's and Kagan's (1975a,b) definition of "skip" metastases, the two cases with already present pulmonary metastases are not acceptable as true "skips." Furthermore, in our material, noncontiguous spread of tumor in the affected bone was extremely rare, which was similar to the experience of other authors (Dahlin 1978) (Fig. I.79).

At present, due to the use of newer imaging techniques, particularly MRI and preoperative and/or adjuvant chemotherapy, the risk of leaving microfoci of tumor ("skips") after transmedullary amputation seems to have lost its importance. This is in contrast to a recent report of Wuisman and Enneking (1990), who stated that "it seems quite evident that the use of preoperative or postoperative chemotherapy, or

Fig. I.75a–c. Female, 26 years old. Osteosarcoma of the distal end of the femur. **a** Lateral and anteroposterior radiographs showing a conspicuous sclerotic, well-delimited soft tissue mass in its posterior aspect, suggested a diagnosis of parosteal osteosarcoma. However **b** coronal and sagittal T1-weighted MRI scans and **c** CT scan demonstrated the wide intramedullary involvement of the tumor. A biopsy established the diagnosis of conventional central osteosarcoma, predominantly chondroblastic

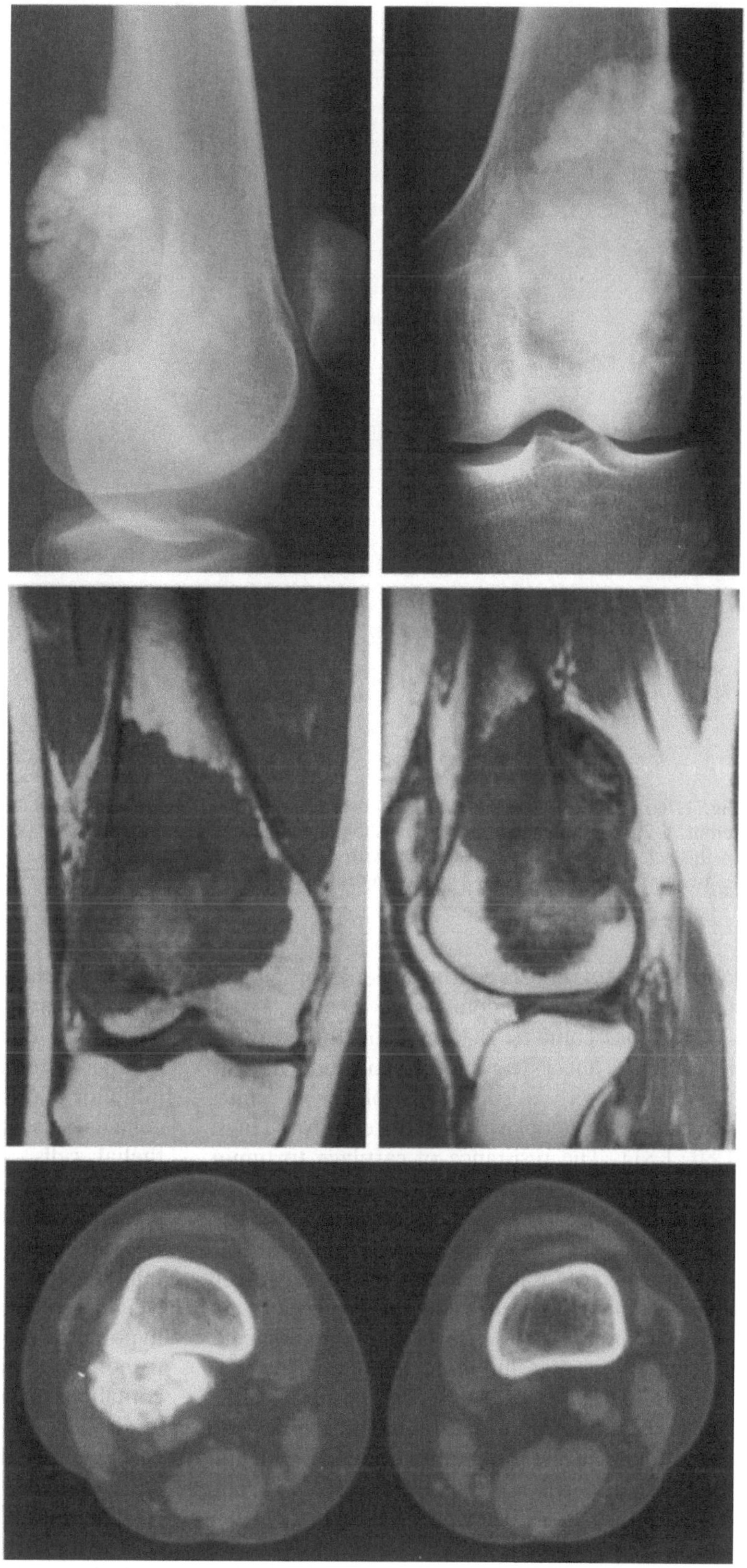

a

b

c

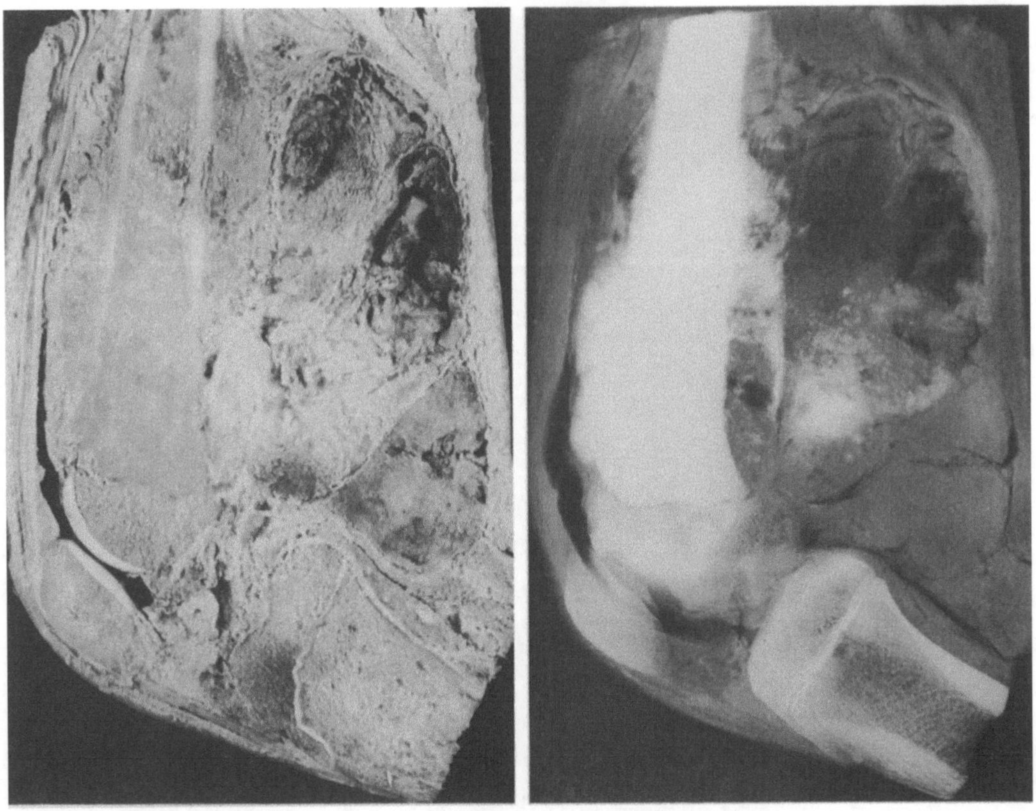

a b

Fig. I.76a,b. Male, 14 years old. Osteosarcoma of the femur. **a** Photograph and **b** radiograph show the large size of this sclerotic type of osteosarcoma with extensive soft tissue mass at its posterior aspect, presenting irregular dense areas of tumor bone formation; however, despite the extension of the tumor, the growth cartilage is not perforated

both, has not improved the adverse prognostic implication of a skip metastasis."

Osteosarcoma is a tumor of the growing individual, most commonly located in the metaphysis with a still-open epiphyseal plate, separating the neoplasm from the epiphysis (Figs. I.80, I.81). The resistance of cartilage to tumor invasion is well known. It was investigated by Kuettner et al. (1978) in osteosarcoma in vitro and in vivo. Cartilage was able to resist the invasion by osteosarcoma cells in the organ-cell culture system as well as in the biopsies of an osteosarcoma. At the growth plate, tumor cells reached only as far into the columnar cartilage as the vascular loops had extended, prior to their removal by trypsin incubation of the explants, to the area of the last hypertrophic chondrocyte and its calcified matrix.

Kuettner et al. showed that cartilage from which low-molecular-weight substances were extracted by selective extraction was invaded not only by endothelial cells but also by osteosarcoma cells. These findings led to the conclusion that cartilage contains an extractable matrix compound that inhibits invasion in an experimental system. It was identified as a protease inhibitor that has the ability to inhibit mammalian collagenases, including those released by endothelial cells. Collagenolytic activity has been demonstrated in both the endothelial and the osteosarcoma lines used in these investigations. Enzyme activity from both these cell lines can be inhibited by a cartilage-derived low-molecular-weight collagenase inhibitor. Therefore, the hypotheses is forwarded that cartilage is resistant to both capillary and tumor-cell invasion since it contains a specific collagenous inhibitor (Kuettner et al. 1976). Inhibition of tumor angiogenesis by cartilage was also shown experimentally by Brem and Folkman (1975).

The intimate causes of the evident resistance of growth cartilage to osteosarcoma penetration and the real incidence of its transepiphyseal extension are still disputed, but it seems much

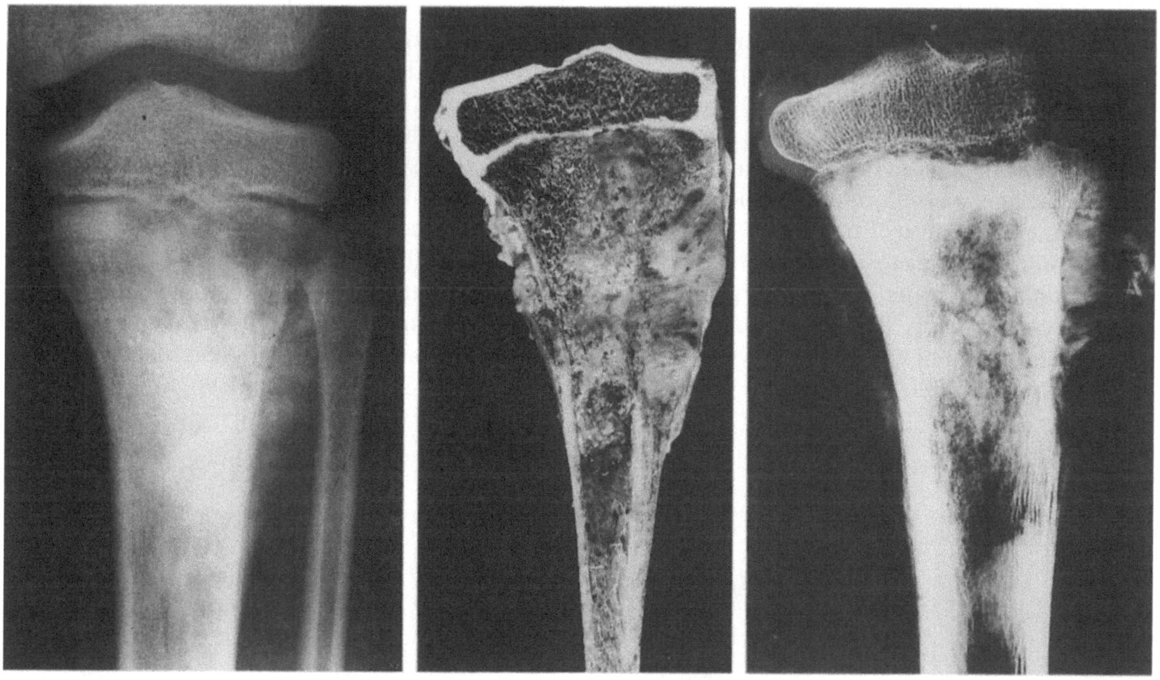

a b, c

Fig. I.77a–c. Male, 14 years old. Osteosarcoma of the upper tibial metaphysis. **a** Radiograph, **b** photograph, and **c** radiograph of a thin slab of the amputation specimen show the characteristic features of this tumor, which has not invaded the epiphysis

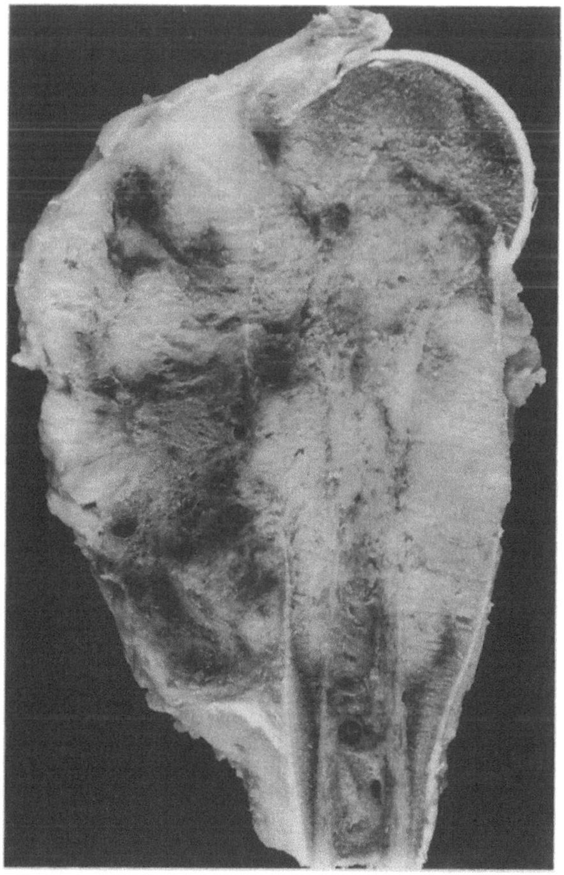

Fig. I.78. Osteosarcoma of the proximal humerus, with extensive soft tissue invasion and destruction of the growth cartilage

more frequent than is evident in preoperative radiographs or bone scans. Enneking and Kagan (1978) studied 45 osteosarcomas for transepiphyseal spread of the lesion because of the present interest in limb-sparing surgery as treatment of this tumor. In 28 cases in which the epiphyseal plate was still open, 21 showed gross or microscopic evidence of transepiphyseal extension of the lesion, the most common being direct penetration through the epiphyseal plate along vascular channels or, less commonly, lateral penetration in continuity with epiphyseal vessels passing through the perichondral ring that anastomose with vessels that supply both the epiphysis and the metaphysis (Spira and Farin 1967). There is still considerable controversy over the existence of vascular channels in the normal epiphyseal plate. Trueta and his school and others deny the presence of vessels crossing the normal growth cartilage in laboratory animals and humans (Trueta and Amato 1960; Trueta and Morgan 1960). However, other authors found such vascular channels in normal laboratory animals and in humans or under pathologic conditions in which the metaphyseal blood supply is interrupted (Spira and Farin 1967).

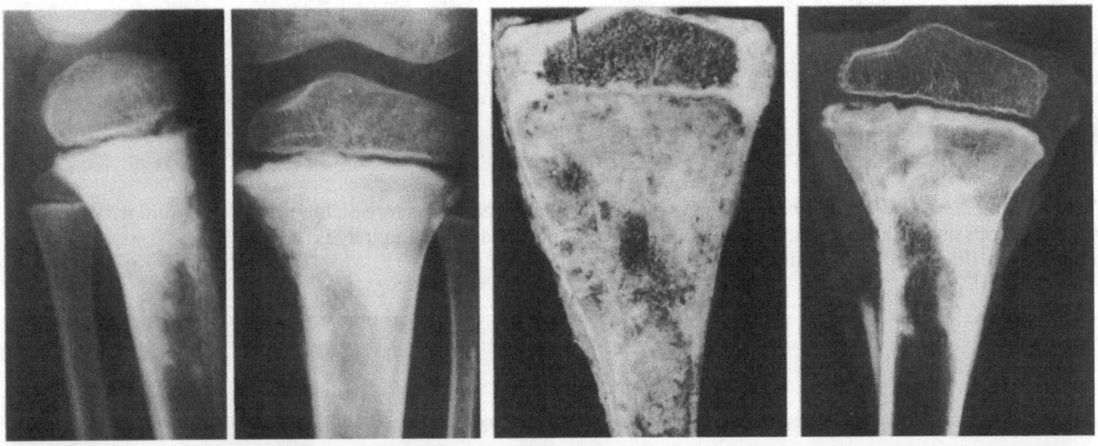

a

b, c

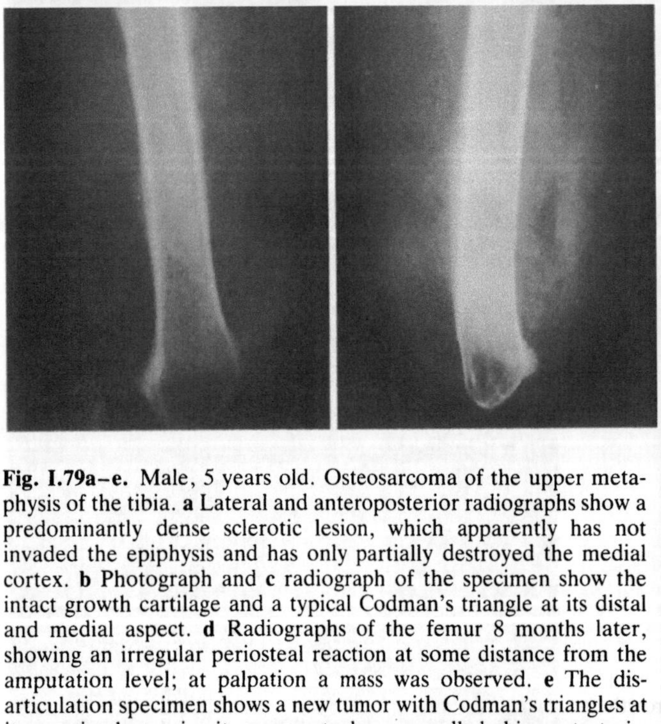

d

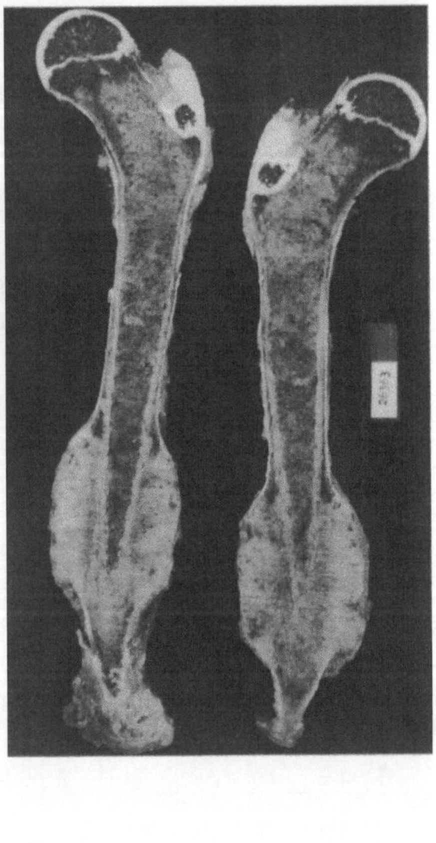

e

Fig. I.79a–e. Male, 5 years old. Osteosarcoma of the upper metaphysis of the tibia. **a** Lateral and anteroposterior radiographs show a predominantly dense sclerotic lesion, which apparently has not invaded the epiphysis and has only partially destroyed the medial cortex. **b** Photograph and **c** radiograph of the specimen show the intact growth cartilage and a typical Codman's triangle at its distal and medial aspect. **d** Radiographs of the femur 8 months later, showing an irregular periosteal reaction at some distance from the amputation level; at palpation a mass was observed. **e** The disarticulation specimen shows a new tumor with Codman's triangles at its proximal margin; it appears to be a so-called skip metastasis; 6 months later the patient died with pulmonary metastases

Fig. I.80a,b. Osteosarcoma of the upper tibial metaphysis. **a** Photograph and **b** radiograph of a thin slab of the specimen show that the tumor does not cross the growth plate. A typical Codman's triangle is seen in **b**

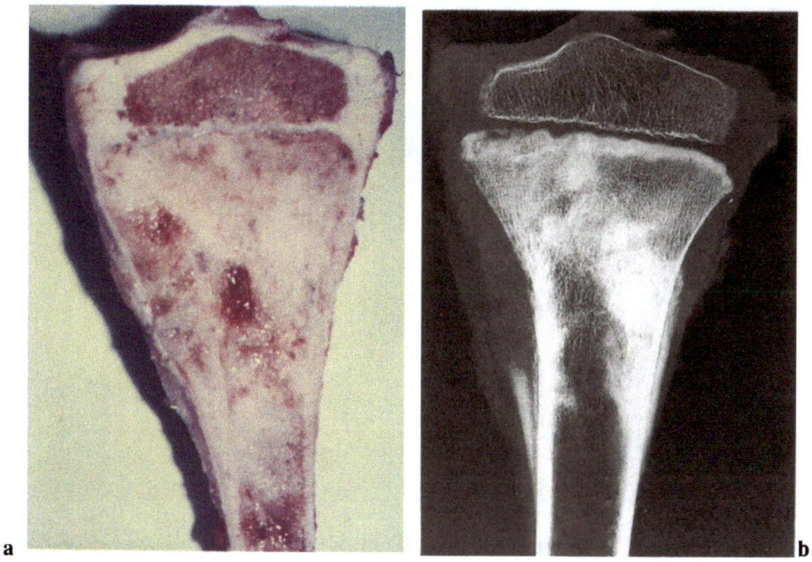

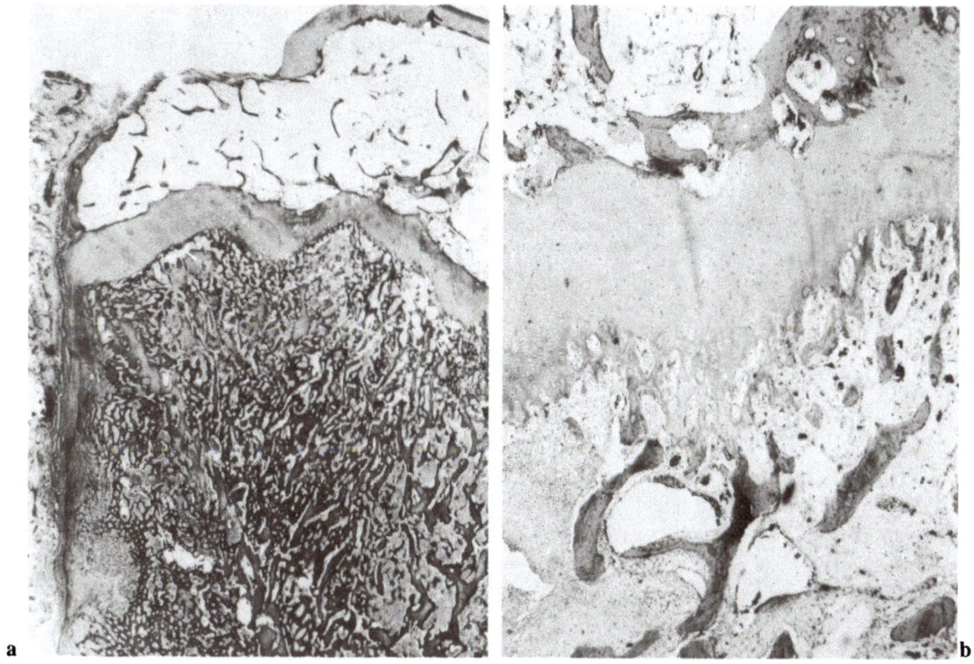

Fig. I.81a,b. Photomicrographs at low and medium magnification show how the growth plate acts in some but not all cases as a barrier to tumor invasion of the epiphysis (*top*); spongiosa invaded by tumor at the *bottom*. **a** ×17, **b** ×85

Enneking and Kagan (1978), using microangiographic techniques, observed open vascular channels between the metaphysis and the epiphysis in normal adolescents with open growth plates, which may provide the route for transepiphyseal extension of the tumor. However, the authors do not mention how often they found crossing vascular channels.

We can confirm that the frequency of this epiphyseal extension with more or less extensive destruction of the growth cartilage is much greater than has been suspected from conventional radiographic studies (Figs. I.61, I.82). With computed tomography and particularly with MRI, more cases of transepiphyseal spread can be documented (Fig. I.75).

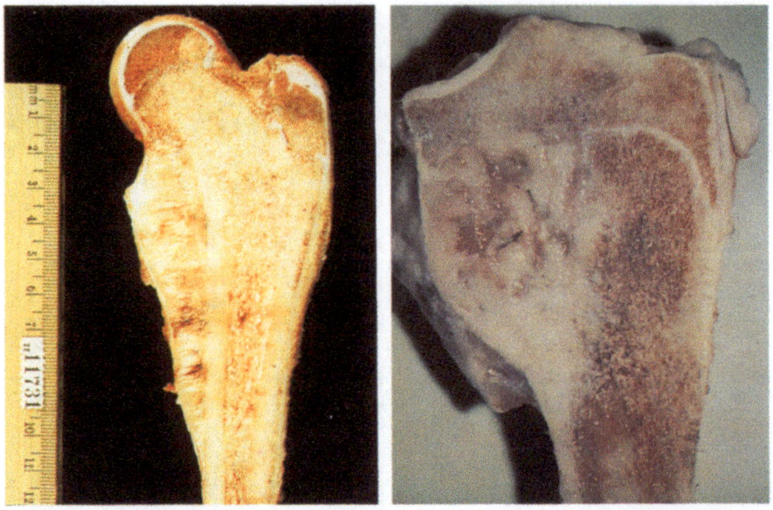

a b

Fig. I.82a,b. Osteosarcoma of **a** the upper end of the femur and **b** the upper metaphysis of the tibia, showing partial destruction of the growth plate and tumor penetration into the epiphysis

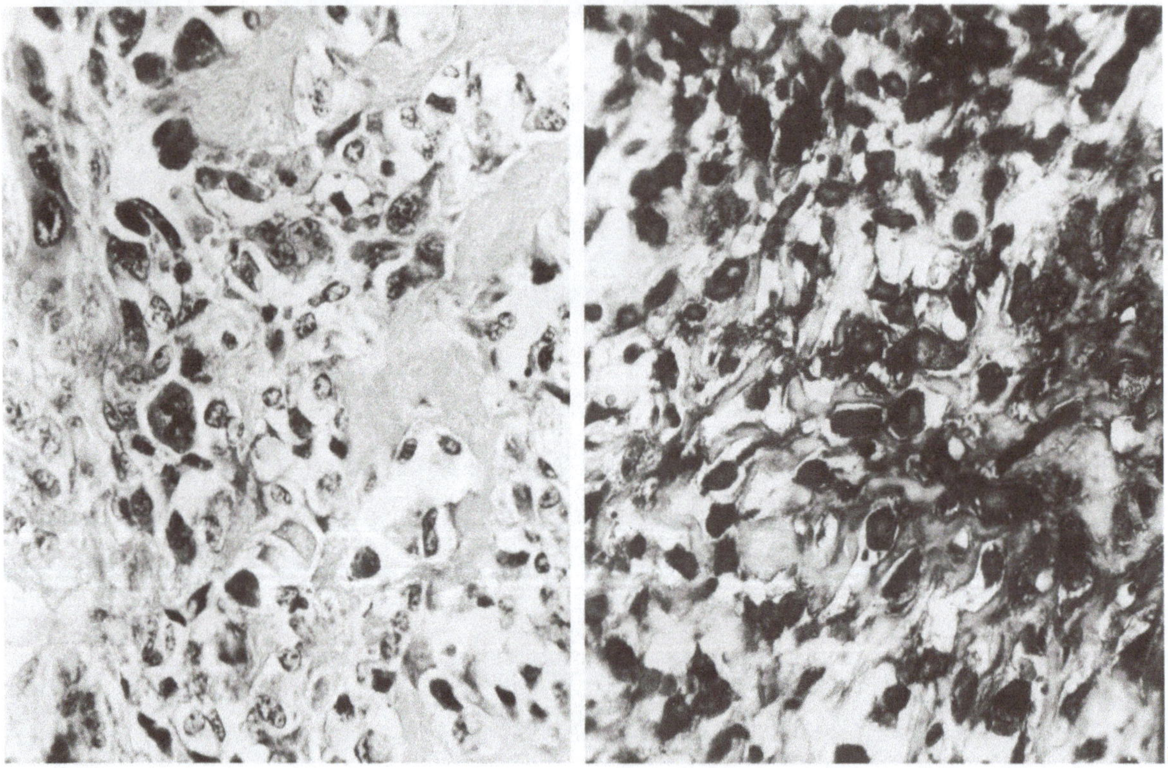

a b

Fig. I.83a,b. Photomicrograph of osteosarcoma illustrating in **a** obviously malignant pleomorphic and bizarre tumor cells, surrounding in part bands of homogeneous tissue, apparently osteoid. **b** Same case showing intense alkaline phosphatase activity of the tumor cells, demonstrating that they are osteoblasts. **a,b** ×400

Histopathology. Osteosarcoma exhibits a wide spectrum in its histologic pattern, reflected by the various stages of differentiation of the multipotential mesenchymal cell during its skeletal evolution, making the *production of osteoid and/or bone by the proliferating tumor cells*, even in only small foci, *essential to the characterization of a neoplasm as osteosarcoma*.

However, Sanerkin (1980) disagreed with the current international histologic definitions of osteosarcoma, chondrosarcoma, and fibrosarcoma, relying instead on the alkaline phosphatase activity for the diagnosis of these sarcomas. He defined osteosarcoma as "a malignant tumor of osteoblasts in which the tumor cells contain abundant alkaline phosphatase, irrespec-

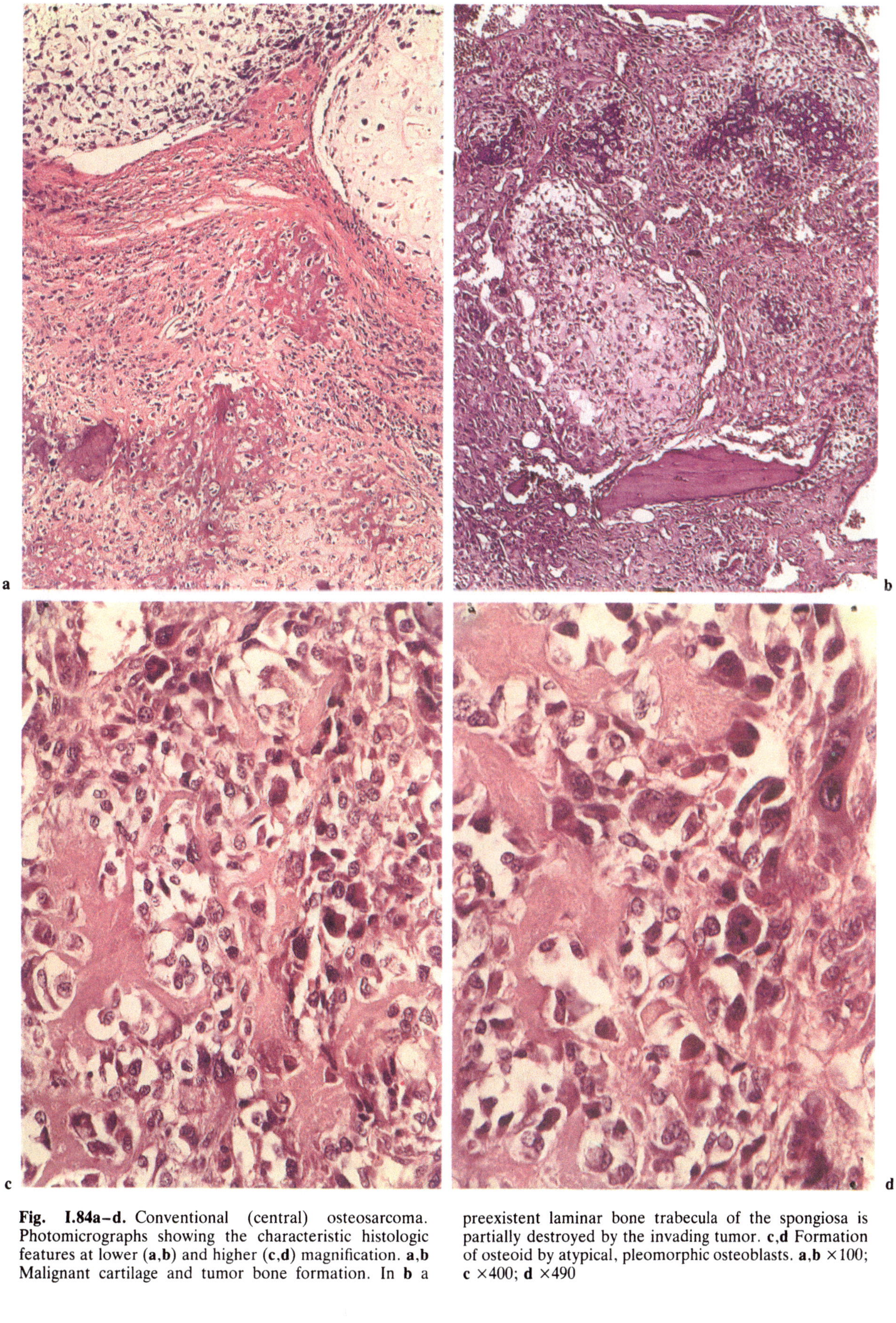

Fig. I.84a–d. Conventional (central) osteosarcoma. Photomicrographs showing the characteristic histologic features at lower (**a**,**b**) and higher (**c**,**d**) magnification. **a**,**b** Malignant cartilage and tumor bone formation. In **b** a preexistent laminar bone trabecula of the spongiosa is partially destroyed by the invading tumor. **c**,**d** Formation of osteoid by atypical, pleomorphic osteoblasts. **a**,**b** ×100; **c** ×400; **d** ×490

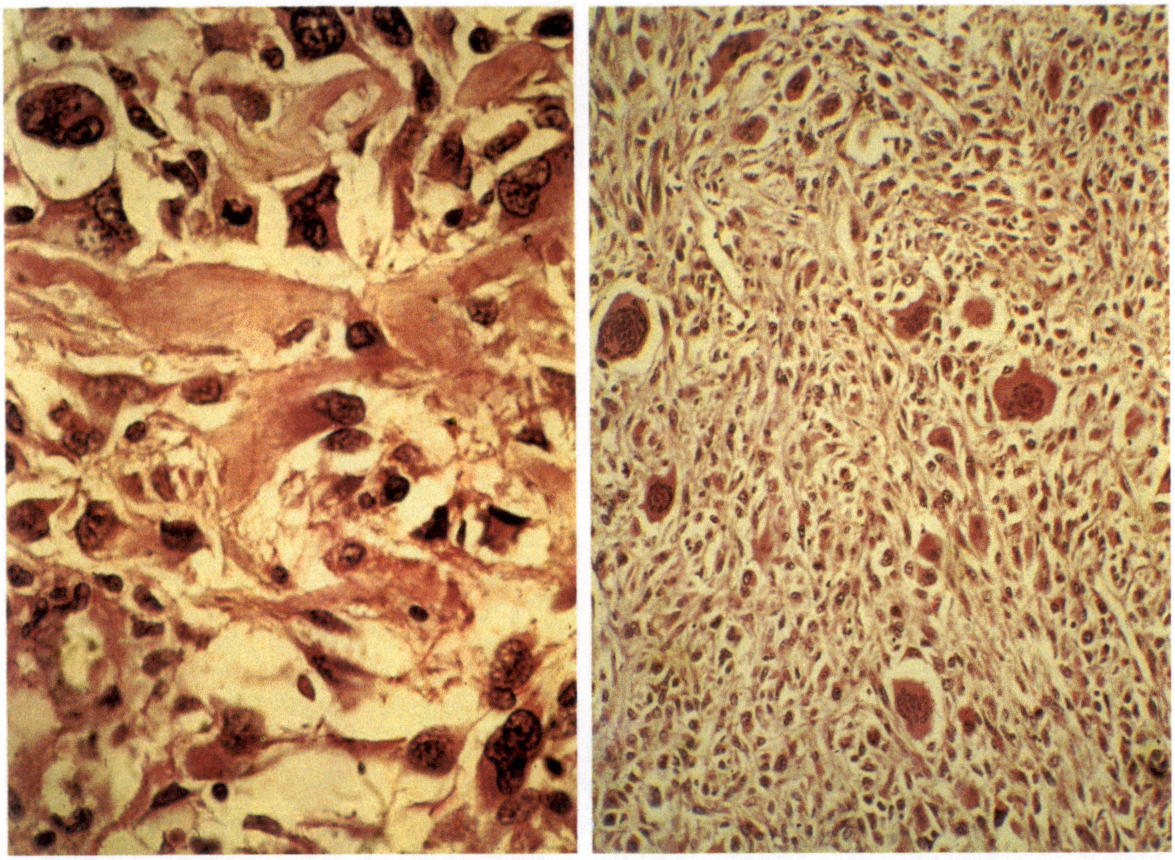
a b

Fig. I.85a,b. Osteosarcoma with a predominant malignant fibrous histiocytoma-like pattern, as shown in microphotograph **a**. However, in some other areas, osteoid formation by the atypical pleomorphic osteoblasts was observed. Such cases, studying only limited biopsy material, especially from the extraosseous soft tissue, can be misdiagnosed as malignant fibrous histiocytoma. **a** ×100, **b** ×400

tive of whether tumor osteoid is present or absent." According to Sanerkin, the tumor cells in osteosarcoma, whether osteoblastic, chondroblastic, fibroblastic, or anaplastic, contain abundant alkaline phosphatase, whereas this enzyme is scanty or absent in chondrosarcoma or fibrosarcoma. This author agrees that tissue alkaline phosphatase is an important marker for the determination of osteoblastic activity and is present even in apparently undifferentiated tumor cells of osteosarcoma. However, while this has allowed differentiation of tumor osteoid from areas of hyaline fibrous tissue and cartilage (Schajowicz and Cabrini 1954), conspicuous alkaline phosphatase activity was not detected within the cartilaginous or fibroblastic areas of osteosarcoma (Fig. I.83).

Cellular pleomorphism is more conspicuous in tumors with scarce tumor bone or osteoid formation, characteristic of the predominantly osteolytic types. In these cases, a compact, richly vascularized mass of cells is observed, showing evident atypism, with hyperchromatic, often bizarre nuclei and prominent nucleoli and many typical and atypical mitoses (Fig. I.84). Cells with several pleomorphic, hyperchromatic, or bizarre nuclei, the so-called malignant giant cells, are a frequent finding. These elements should be differentiated from the multinucleated giant cells of the osteoclast type, which have more numerous and typical nuclei. Both types of giant cells are found in great number in some osteolytic, generally rapidly growing tumors, which are referred to as "giant-cell rich osteosarcoma" (Bathurst et al. 1986) (Figs. I.85, I.86).

These cases may be confounded with "malignant" giant tumors, but the anaplastic, pleomorphic aspect of the stromal cells and the presence of small foci of tumor bone permit the correct diagnosis. We found in several cases of

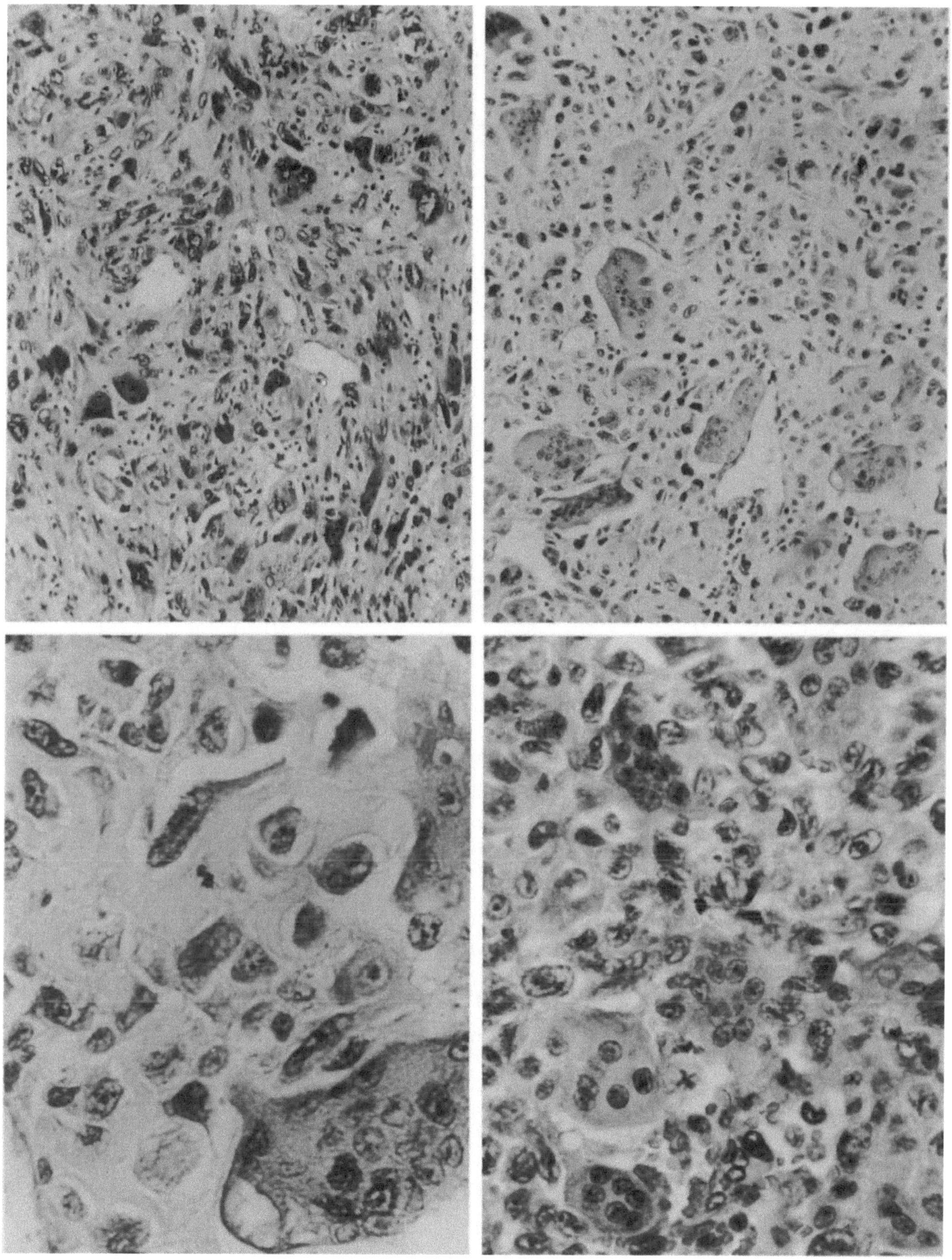

Fig. I.86a–d. Photomicrographs of osteosarcoma, predominantly osteolytic, illustrating the presence of atypical and typical multinucleated giant cells of osteoclast type. Such cases are sometimes classed as malignant giant-cell tumors, but the pleomorphism of the stromal cells and the presence of osteoid tissue, even if scarce, permits the correct diagnosis of osteosarcoma. Cases like those illustrated are referred to as "osteoclast-rich osteosarcoma." **a**,**b** ×120; **c**,**d** ×400

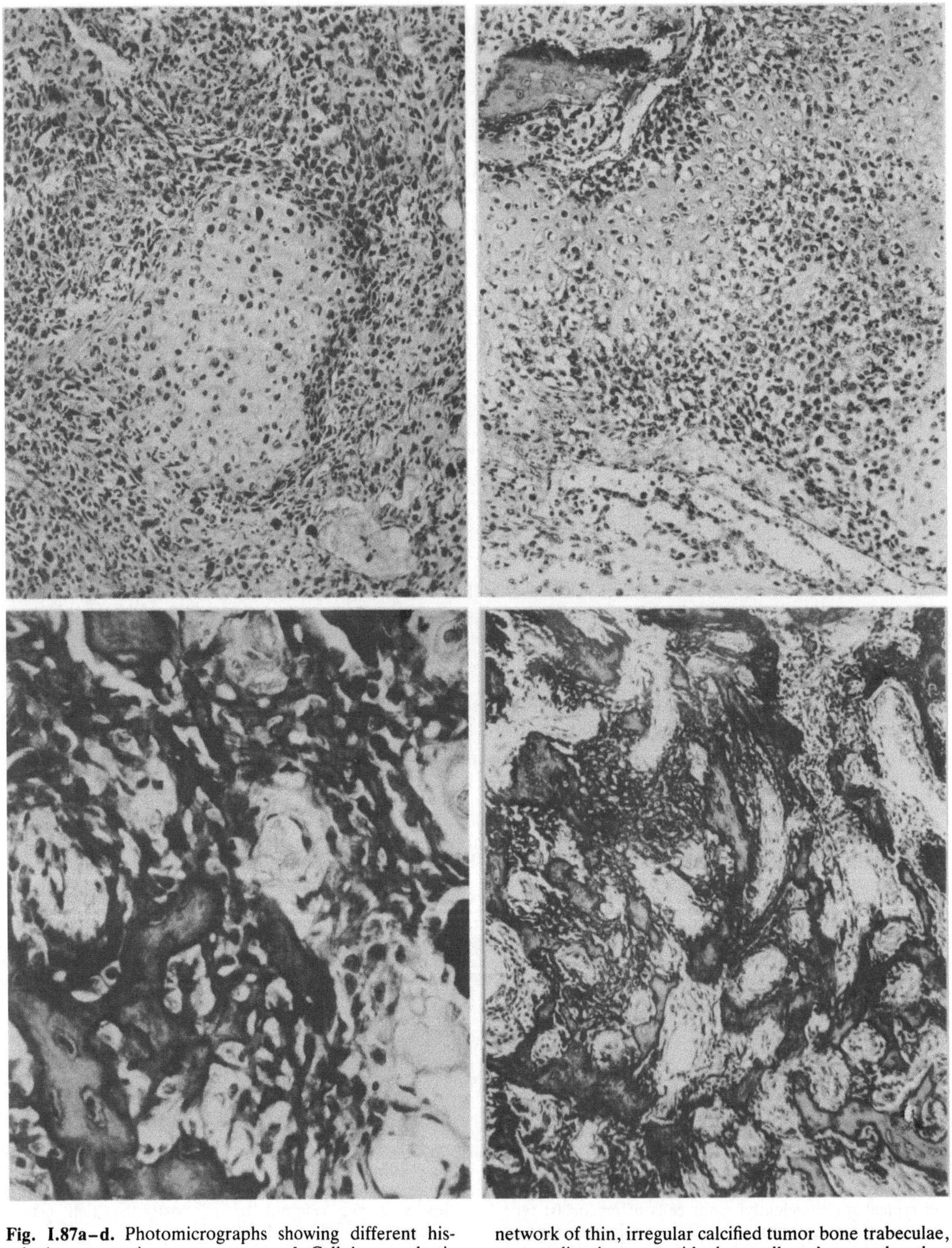

a b c d

Fig. I.87a–d. Photomicrographs showing different histologic patterns in osteosarcoma. **a**,**b** Cellular anaplastic area showing scattered zones of tumor cartilage formation. ×120. **c**,**d** Densely sclerotic zone with formation of a dense network of thin, irregular calcified tumor bone trabeculae, surrounding in part residual cancellous bone trabeculae. **c** ×120, **d** ×250 malignant transformation of Paget disease this particular richness of giant cells of osteoclast and malignant types, which seems to establish a pathogenetic relationship between the neoplasm and the previous Paget disease (see p. 489ff.). Areas of necrosis are frequent and may be extensive (up to 40%) (Misdorp et al. 1988), as are highly vascularized zones rich in newly formed, thin-walled blood capillaries or prominent, blood-filled vascular spaces surrounded by the malignant tumor cells, associated with abundant hemorrhages.

These highly vascularized tumors are often referred to as "telangiectatic osteosarcoma" in spite of lacking the characteristic gross and microscopic features of this tumor type (see p. 96ff.).

In addition to the highly cellular and anaplastic zones, in which tumor bone or osteoid formation is scarce or completely lacking, areas of fibroblastic, fibrohistiocytic, myxoid, or cartilaginous tissue in different grades of evolution and anaplasia may be found, often presenting the most conspicuous features of the neoplasm (Fig. I.87). Although the 5-year survival rate was slightly lower for the osteoblastic than for the chondroblastic and fibroblastic types (Dahlin and Coventry 1967), Dahlin (1978) seems to favor the use of such subdivisions merely to indicate the wide histopathologic variations. It is more important to emphasize the fact that peripheral zones of an osteosarcoma may be composed predominantly or exclusively of cartilaginous, fibroblastic, or fibrohistiocytic tissue, thereby causing one to interpret a biopsy as chondro- or fibrosarcoma or malignant fibrous histiocytoma (Fig. I.85). Such mistakes can be avoided in most cases if the clinicoradiologic information (age, location, etc.) is known.

In the sclerosing type, the new formation of osteoid and bone by the malignant tumor cells is abundant. The atypical osteoblasts produce an irregular, dense or lacelike network of osteoid or immature bone trabeculae of different size and shape, varying from fine to very thick and staining reddish (osteoid) or dark blue with HE, according to the degree of calcification of the immature (reticular or woven) bone (Figs. I.84, I.88).

The newly formed osteoid and bone trabeculae frequently surround remnants of preexistent mature trabeculae (Fig. I.84b). An interesting finding emphasized already by Phemister (1926) and Jaffe (1958) is that the osteoblasts in the densely ossified areas often lose their atypical features, becoming smaller, darker, and regular, particularly those included inside the bone trabeculae as osteocytes (Fig. I.88).

In addition to tumor bone production, the histologic pattern is further complicated by the formation of reactive bone, directly by normal osteoblasts or through endochondral ossification of the cartilaginous areas. This reactive bone formation may be found in the medullary portion of the tumor and also, after the perforation of the cortex, in the subperiosteal or parosteal areas; it forms the substratum of the Codman's triangle (Figs. I.88d, I.89) and the radiating bone spicule.

It is essential to distinguish tumor bone formation from the common reactive bone formation; sometimes, in purely cartilaginous tumors, endochondral ossification or spicules of calcified cartilage can be confused with tumor bone (Figs. I.84, I.122). This distinction is sometimes difficult and requires some experience on the part of the pathologist; it accounts for the fact that, occasionally, a cartilage tumor, which generally has a better prognosis, is classified as an osteosarcoma (see p. 116ff.).

Due to the pleomorphic and variable structure of an osteosarcoma, if we exclude the "well-differentiated variant," histologic grading for determining the degree of malignancy is greatly limited. Price and Dahlin both found it to be of prognostic value (Price and Truscott 1961; Price 1952, 1956; Dahlin and Unni 1986); however, other authors (McKenna et al. 1966, among others) did not confirm the usefulness of grading in this tumor type, which was also attempted by the writer in several cases without satisfactory results.

On the other hand, in most osteosarcomas the gross and histologic patterns, with the exception of the frankly sclerotic tumor, are so variable that it is often impossible to determine the predominant tissue type. For this reason and because of the lack of usefulness as far as prognosis is concerned, we subdivide central osteosarcoma, besides the conventional classic type, only into three varieties, the *telangiectatic* type, the *well-differentiated osteosarcoma*, and the *round-cell osteosarcoma*, which indeed seem to have a different prognostic implication.

The *histochemical* demonstration of alkaline phosphatase, even in apparently undifferentiated tumor cells, may occasionally help in the identification of osteoblasts, which are strongly positive; at the same time it enables one to distinguish tumor osteoid or bone from areas of hyaline

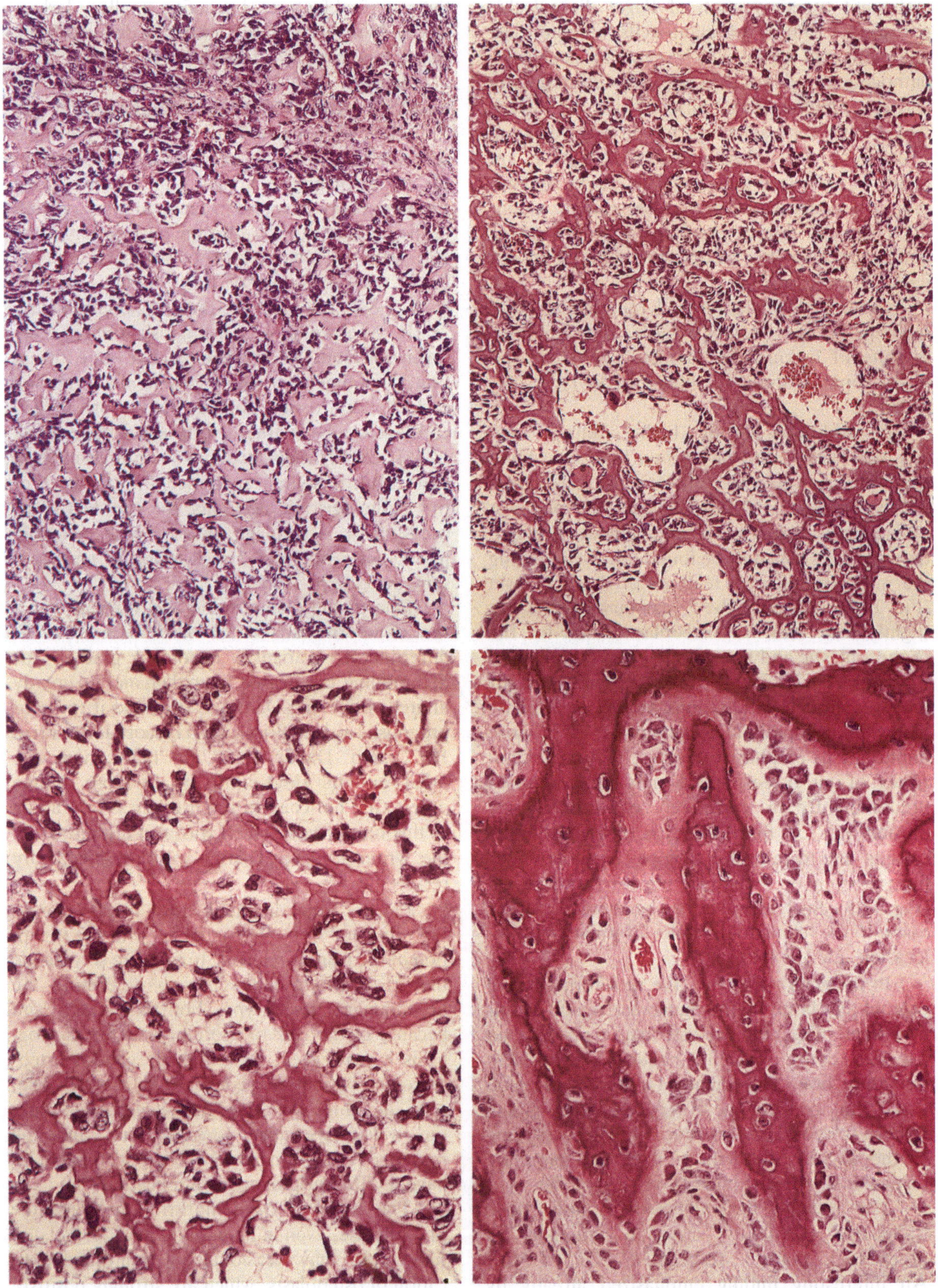

a b c d

Fig. I.88a–d. Conventional (central) osteosarcoma. Photomicrographs showing other histologic aspects of **a** thin lacelike osteoid and **b** calcified bone trabeculae formed by the anaplastic tumor cells. **c** Tumor bone formation by atypical osteoblasts. **d** Reactive periosteal new bone formation. The woven bone trabeculae are surrounded by rows of typical osteoblasts. **a**,**b** ×100; **c**,**d** ×400

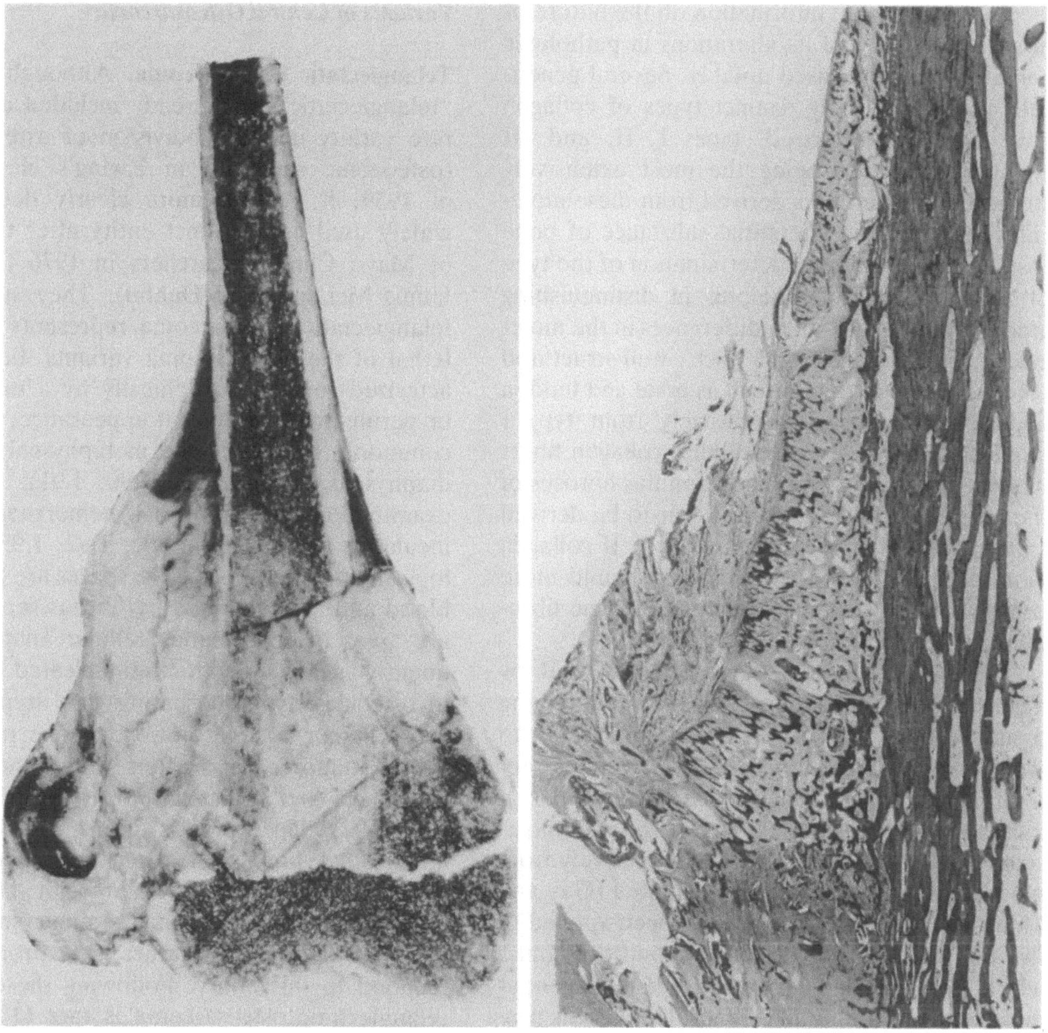

Fig. I.89a,b. Osteosarcoma of the distal metaphysis of femur. **a** Photograph of the specimen shows typical Codman's triangles of the proximal margins of the tumor. **b** Topographic photomicrograph showing periosteal new bone formation, characteristic of Codman's triangle. **b** ×8

fibrous tissue or cartilage (Schajowicz and Cabrini 1954; Jeffree and Price 1965) (Fig. I.83). Several recent *electron-microscopic studies* of single cases (Ghadially and Mehta 1970; Kay 1971) or a major number of cases (Spjut et al. 1971; Paschall and Paschall 1975; Williams et al. 1976; Aparisi et al. 1982; Martínez-Tello and Navas-Palacios 1982; Stark and Ericsson 1983) showed features essentially similar to those seen in normal osteoblasts, with more atypical nuclear structures; in view of the marked ultrastructural similarities of cells from chondrosarcomatous, fibrosarcomatous, and typical osteosarcomatous areas, electron microscopy seems to be of little value in the differential diagnosis of these tumors. No viral particles could be identified in these studies.

Immunohistochemistry. The application of more sensitive immunohistologic techniques, and in particular the development of monoclonal antibodies, has widened the possibilities and accuracy of differential diagnosis of tumors in surgical pathology. One of the applications with practical importance for the orthopedic surgeon is the development of antibodies to human osteosarcoma, produced with success by investigators from England, Japan, and St. Louis University (see Introduction). It is possible that this antibody, when coupled with cytotoxic agents or radioisotopes, could be used in the future as an effective addition to osteosarcoma therapy.

In recent years, information on the nature of normal collagen and its alterations in pathologic conditions has increased notably. Several genetically and structurally distinct types of collagen have been characterized, types I, II, and III collagen molecules being the most extensively studied. Because fibers derived from these molecules make up the interstitial substance of bone (osteoid) and cartilage, determination of the type of collagen could be helpful in distinguishing among these tissues when differences in the molecular structure exist. In fact, well-structured collagen fibers in tissues such as bone and tendon appear to be derived exclusively from type I molecules. However, intercellular collagen fibers of some fibrocartilage, such as annulus fibrosus of the intervertebral disc, also appear to be derived from type I collagen molecules. Type II collagen molecules, forming small fibers, are found more commonly in hyaline cartilage and in some fibrocartilage and notochord.

It is important for the pathologist that by means of immunohistologic procedures (staining tissue sections with anticollagen antibodies to type I or type II collagen, with or without pretreatment with enzymes such as hyaluronidase), cartilage containing mostly type II collagen molecules and bone (osteoid) derived exclusively from type I molecules may be differentiated (Gay and Miller 1978). This procedure has been applied to the study of osteosarcoma and chondrosarcoma, which produce large amounts of collagenous matrix. It was found that osteosarcoma cells produce a matrix containing fibers derived from type I molecules, whereas the fibrous elements of chondrosarcoma are derived from type II molecules (Remberger and Gay 1977). However, further investigations are necessary in order to establish whether this procedure can be used as a secure and practical method, applicable in routine diagnosis of bone tumors. It is highly probable that since most malignant tumors are poorly differentiated, they may synthesize a number of different collagens.

Variants of Central Osteosarcoma

Telangiectatic Osteosarcoma. Although the term "telangiectatic" was already included as a separate variety in the subdivision of osteosarcoma (osteogenic sarcoma) in Ewing's classification of 1939, it became more clearly defined and widely used as a distinct entity after the report of Mayo Clinic researchers in 1976 (Matsuno, Unni, McLeod, and Dahlin). They stated that telangiectatic osteosarcoma represents the most lethal of the osteosarcoma variants, being characterized roentgenographically by a moth-eaten or permeative radiolucent appearance, and most commonly located in the metaphyseal or metadiaphyseal region (Figs. I.90, I.91). On gross examination the tumor is a hemorrhagic multiloculated mass (Figs. I.90c, I.92, I.93). Histologically the numerous large spaces are filled with blood and are separated by fibrous septa. There are areas of conspicuous cellular anaplasia frequently associated with multinucleated giant cells of osteoclast type alternating with atypical giant cells. Tumor osteoid or woven bone production by the tumor cells is often scarce and may be difficult to find in a small biopsy specimen (Figs. I.94–I.97). This lesion is often mistaken for an aneurysmal bone cyst when the characteristic roentgenographic features are not taken into account. Some "malignant aneurysmal bone cysts" of the older literature most probably correspond to this entity. Following these criteria, telangiectatic osteosarcoma is rare (1%–2% of central osteosarcomas). There are, however, differences in the definition of this tumor type. Some authors classify the highly vascularized osteosarcomas or tumors with few dilated blood spaces as telangiectatic osteosarcomas. Huvos et al. (1982) considered telangiectatic osteosarcoma to be more common, representing 11% of all osteosarcomas at his institution. This number is surprisingly high compared with this author's experience and that of Dahlin and Unni (1986). Huvos (1991) found the prognosis similar to, or more favorable than, that of conventional central osteosarcoma. Campanacci and Pizzoferrato (1971), who prefer the term "hemorrhagic osteosarcoma," encountered 21 patients with telangiectatic osteosarcoma out of 170 osteosarcomas (12%). In a later publication (1990), Campanacci reported 48 cases out of 952 osteosarcomas (5%). In contrast, Larsson et al. (1978) found only one example of the telangiectatic type among 242 osteosarcomas.

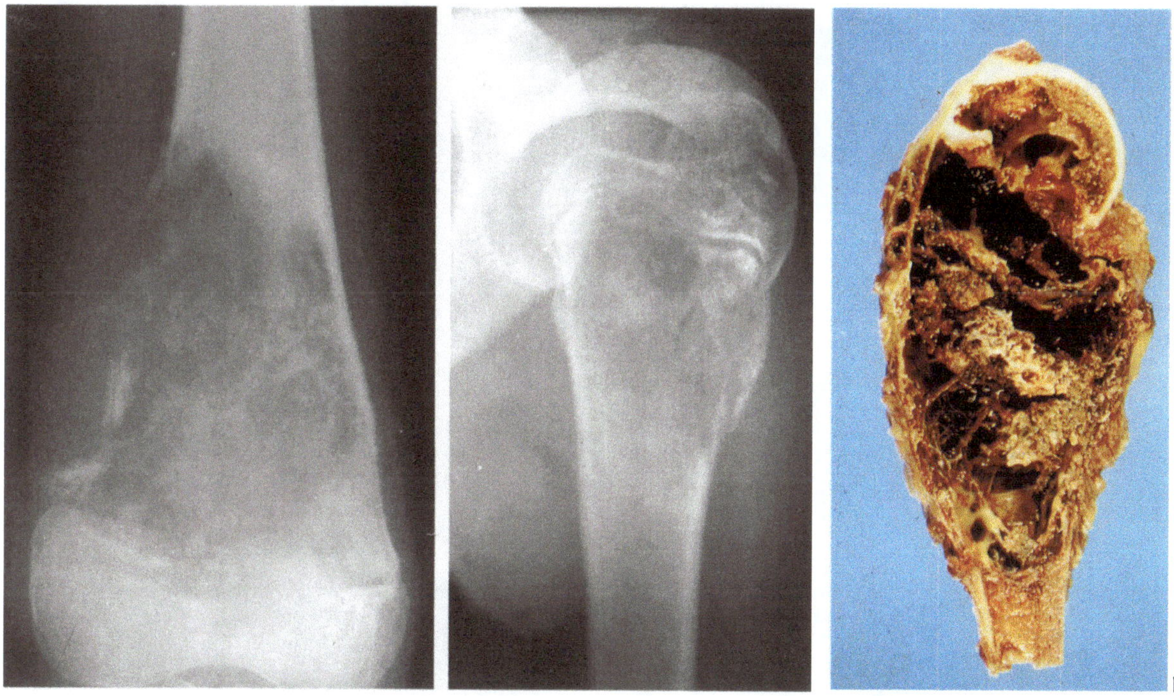

a b, c

Fig. I.90. **a** Male, 16 years old, with telangiectatic osteosarcoma of the lower femoral metaphysis. The osteolytic tumor has destroyed a great part of the inner cortex. **b,c** A 13-year-old girl with telangiectatic osteosarcoma of the upper humerus. **b** Radiograph and **c** photograph show an osteolytic hemorrhagic tumor of the metadiaphyseal region with conspicuous distension and thinning of the cortex. An aneurysmal bone cyst was suspected, but the invasion of the epiphysis and the presence of irregular calcified areas within the tumor inclined the diagnosis toward a malignant osteolytic tumor. (**b,c**, Schajowicz and McGuire 1989)

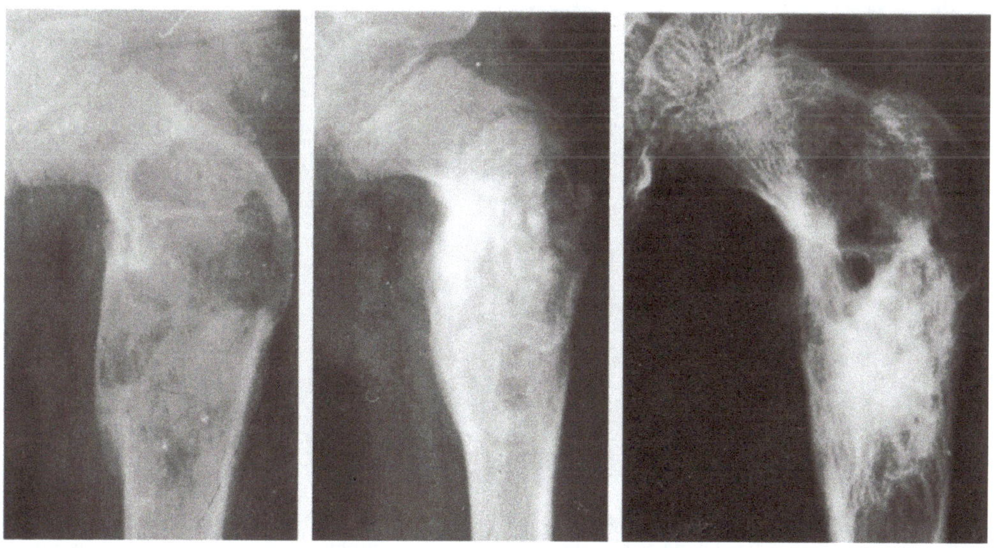

a b, c

Fig. I.91a–c. Male, 8 years old. Telangiectatic osteosarcoma of femur. **a** Radiograph shows radiolucent lesion that expanded and thinned the cortex, producing a pathologic fracture. With the diagnosis of bone cyst, the lesion was curetted, followed by bone graft. At operation a cystic cavity, filled with blood clots, covered by a thin membrane, was found. Histologically, a telangiectatic osteosarcoma was diagnosed (see Fig. I.96). **b** Radiographic aspect 6 months after curettage showing bone partial resorption of the graft and areas of sclerosis; 8 months later, an evident lytic ill-defined lesion appeared, and a new biopsy revealed recurrence of osteosarcoma. A resection of the upper femoral end was performed, followed by prosthesis

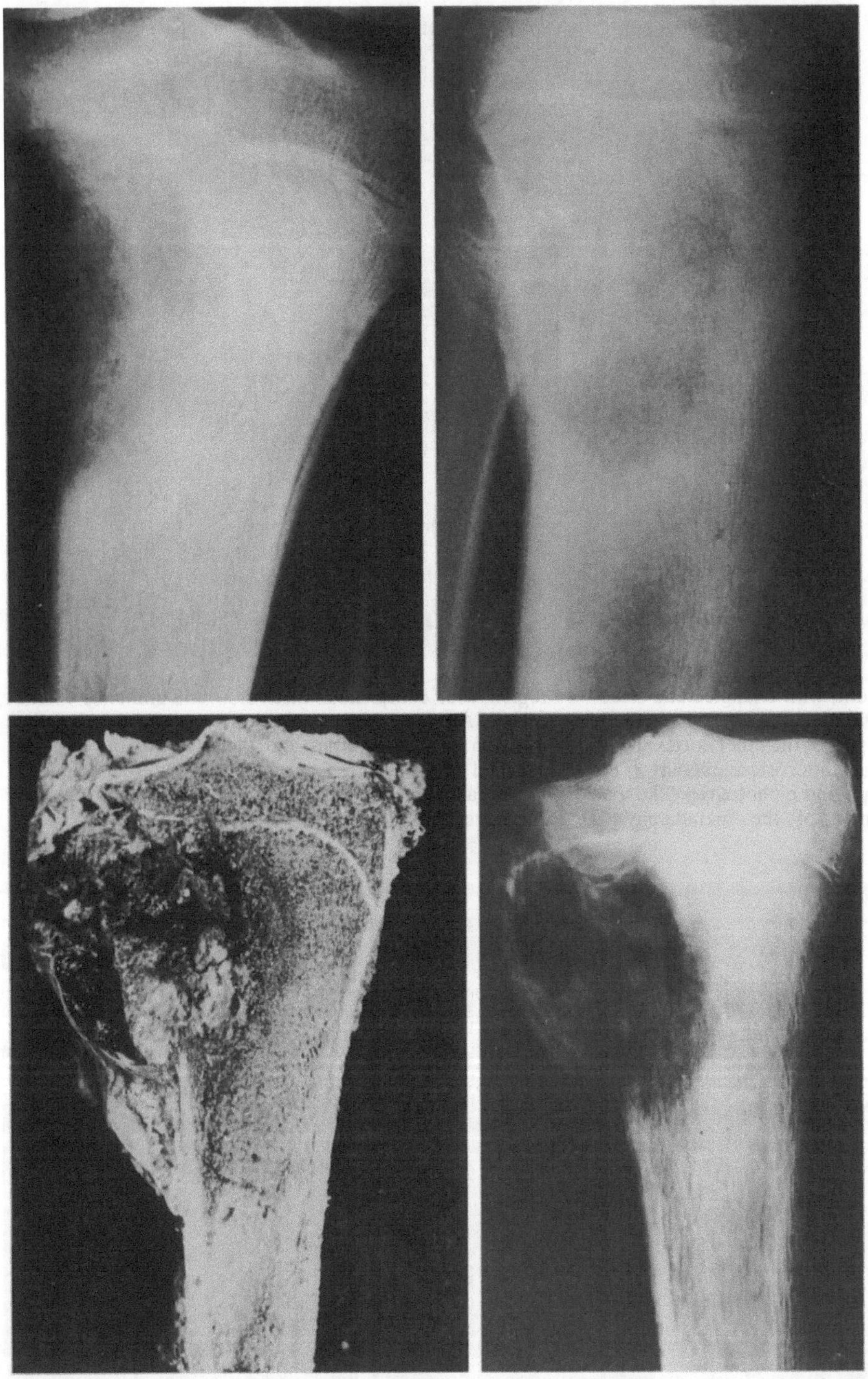

a b c

Fig. I.92a–c. Male, 13 years old. Osteosarcoma of the upper metaphysis of tibia, telangiectatic type. **a** Antero-posterior and lateral radiographs show a purely osteolytic lesion at the posterior aspect of the upper metaphysis with a poorly delimited border and extensive destruction of the cortex. A slight periosteal reaction is seen at the anterior aspect, but a Codman's triangle is not observed. The epiphysis does not appear to be invaded. **b** Photograph and **c** radiograph of the specimen reveal an osteolytic hemorrhagic partially cystic lesion that has destroyed the posterior part of the growth plate

Fig. I.93a,b. Two cases of telangiectatic osteosarcoma. Photographs reveal an osteolytic hemorrhagic multicystic tumor in **a** the lower metaphysis of the femur and **b** the upper end of the tibia

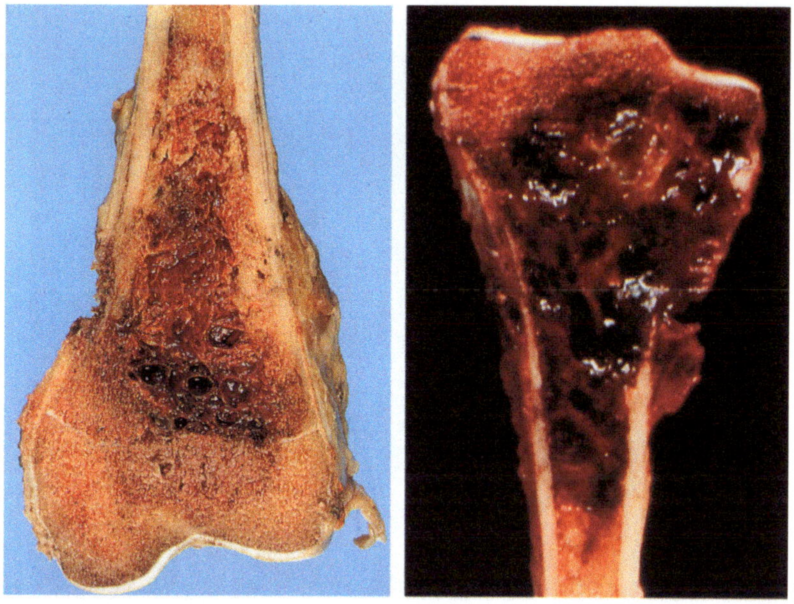

a b

Fig. I.94a–c. Photomicrographs of telangiectatic osteosarcoma, showing large vascular spaces surrounded by septa of different size, often containing anaplastic and pleomorphic tumor cells (**a**, **b**), intermingled with atypical and typical giant cells (**c**). Scarce tumor osteoid trabeculae are seen in **b**. **a** ×100, **b** ×300, **c** ×600

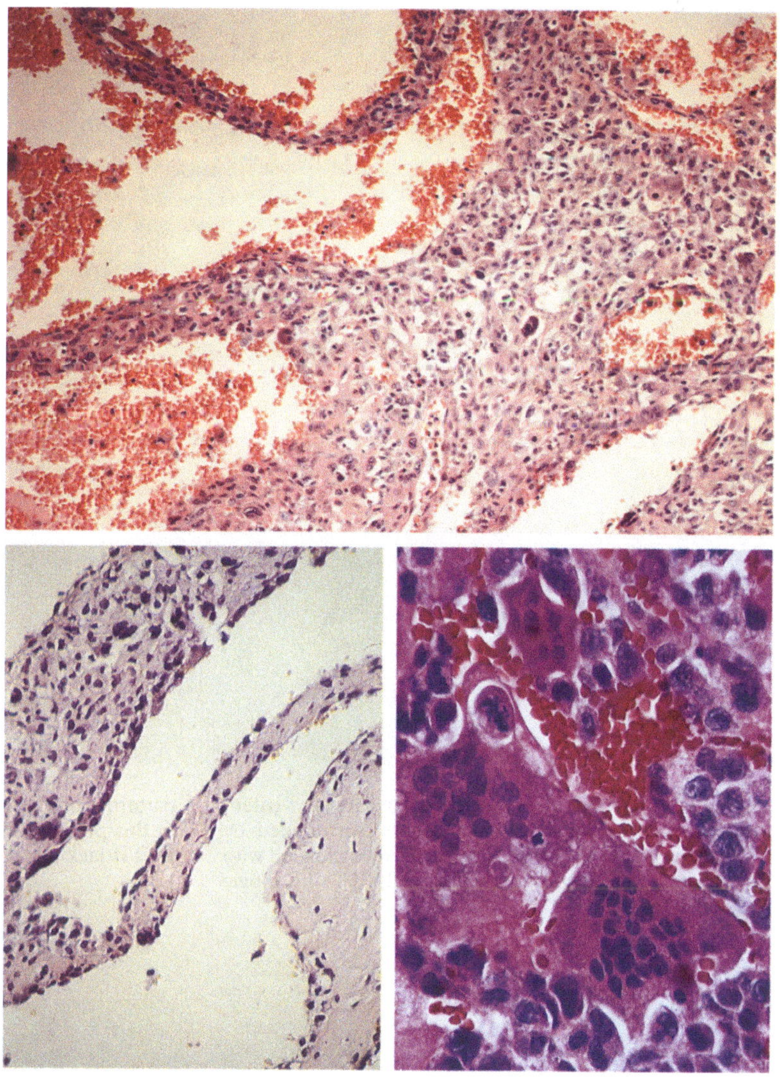

a

b c

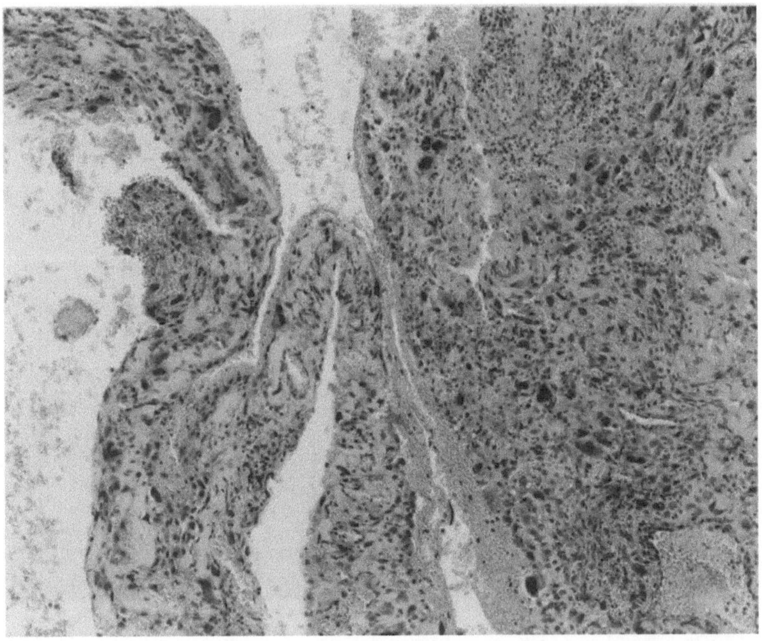

Fig. I.95. Photomicrograph of telangiectatic osteosarcoma showing the fibrous septa containing numerous anaplastic and hyperchromatic tumor cells. ×180

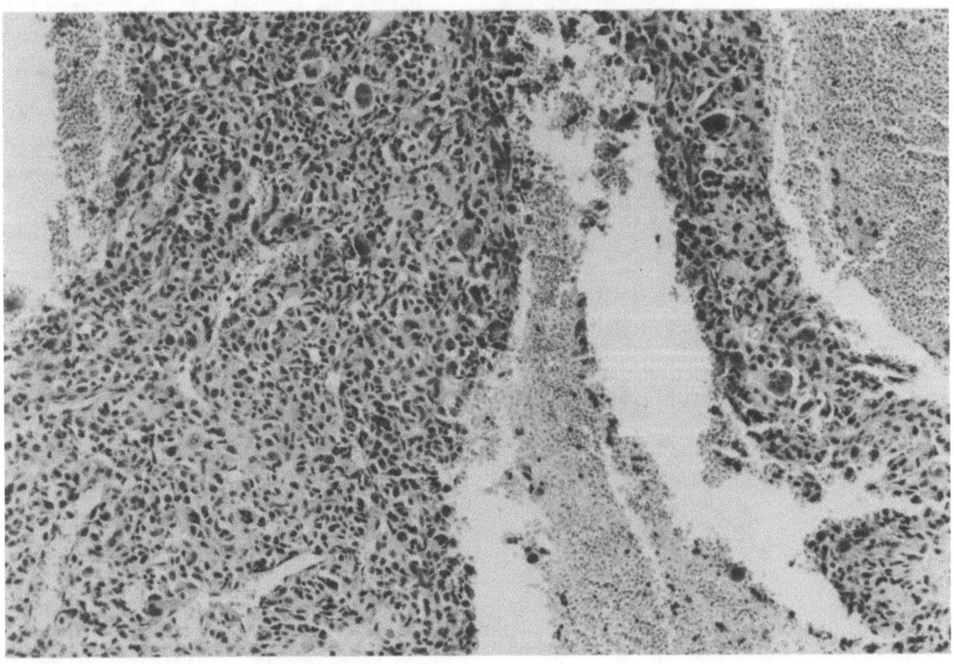

Fig. I.96. Photomicrograph of telangiectatic osteosarcoma, showing large vascular spaces, surrounded by anaplastic and pleomorphic tumor cells, intermingled with atypical and typical osteoclast giant cells. This histologic pattern is often similar to that of aneurysmal bone cyst, but in this process, the evident pleomorphism of the stromal cells is lacking. ×180

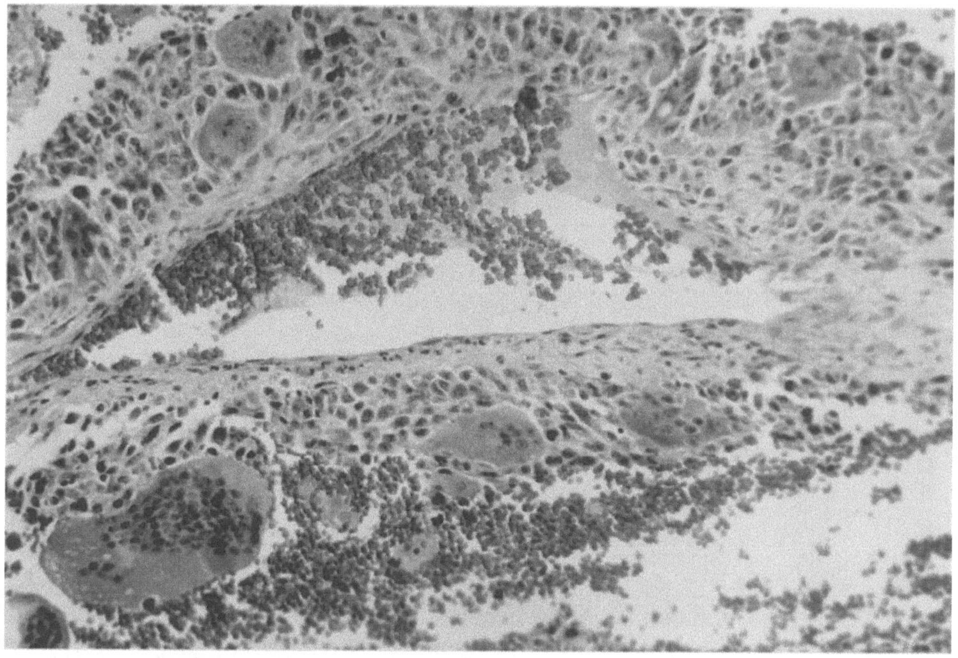

Fig. I.97. Photomicrograph of telangiectatic osteosarcoma showing numerous multinucleated giant cells similar to those seen in genuine giant-cell tumor (osteoclastoma). ×400

In this author's experience, shared by the researchers of the Mayo Clinic, telangiectatic osteosarcoma (as defined by Matsuno et al. 1976) is a rather uncommon lesion which occurs in approximately 2% of the central conventional osteosarcomas. However, the concept that telangiectatic osteosarcoma is a highly malignant tumor with a particularly bad prognosis is no longer maintained by the Mayo Clinic's experience in patients diagnosed since 1976 (Dahlin and Unni 1986), which is also in agreement with the experience at New York's Memorial Hospital and at the M.D. Anderson Cancer Institute in Houston.

This phenomenon may be explained by the exceptional vascularity of the telangiectatic osteosarcoma, resulting in a better perfusion of the lesional tissue by the applied treatment, that is, intravenous or preoperative, preferably intraarterial chemotherapy followed by wide or radical resection and adjuvant chemotherapy. Notwithstanding, the term "telangiectatic" as a distinct variant of central osteosarcoma is still generally maintained because of its particular and characteristic radiologic and, especially, gross and microscopic features.

Intraosseous Well-Differentiated (Low-Grade) Osteosarcoma. Intraosseous well-differentiated (low-grade) osteosarcoma has been identified in recent years (Unni et al. 1977) as a distinct entity with a better prognosis than the conventional high-grade malignant central osteosarcoma. Intraosseous well-differentiated osteosarcoma is composed mainly of fibrous and osseous tissue with little cellular atypia or mitotic activity. This tumor has many histologic similarities with parosteal (juxtacortical) osteosarcoma and shares its biologic behavior. Sometimes the histologic features simulate fibrous dysplasia or aggressive osteoblastoma. For that reason many lesions have been misinterpreted as benign, especially when the clinical and roentgenographic features were not taken into account. This variant of osteosarcoma is rare and represents approximately 1% of all osteosarcomas treated at the Mayo Clinic (Dahlin 1978). It was even less common in the author's files.

Of the 27 patients of Unni et al. (1977), only about 50% were younger than age 30. Many of these patients sought treatment after a long history of pain. Most tumors were located in the femur or tibia. The roentgenographic features are not considered characteristic because some lesions are marginated and sclerotic, whereas

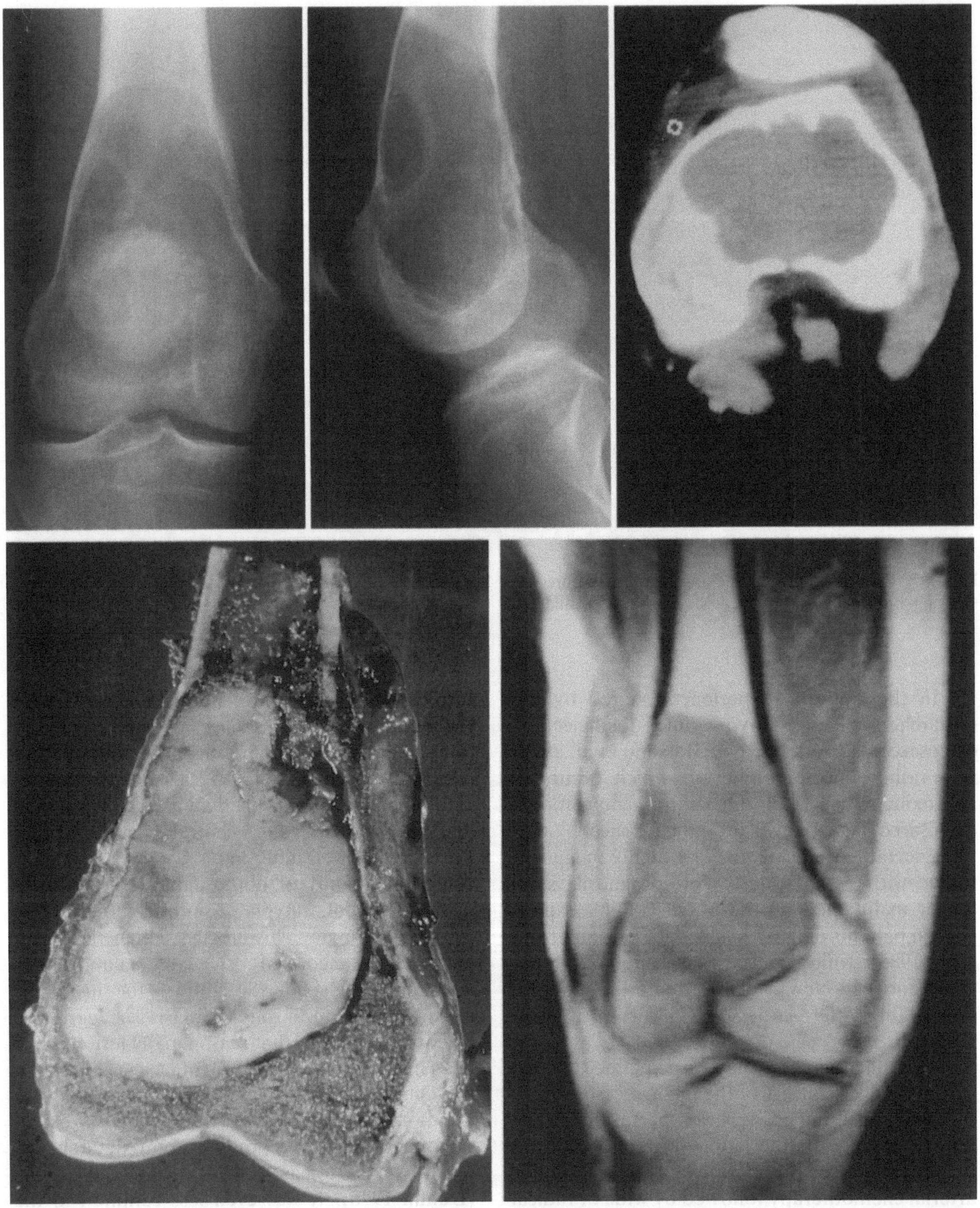

Fig. I.98a–d. Male, 25 years old. Well-differentiated (low-grade) osteosarcoma of the femur. **a** Anteroposterior and lateral radiographs show a radiolucent, well-delimited lesion thinning and slightly distending the cortex, which presents a fissure at its posterior aspect. The lesion does not reach the articular surface. **b** CT scan, **c** photograph of a coronal section of the specimen, and **d** T1-weighted MRI scan show the grayish-white solid aspect and the extension of the tumor, which has only partly destroyed the cortex at the area of the fracture

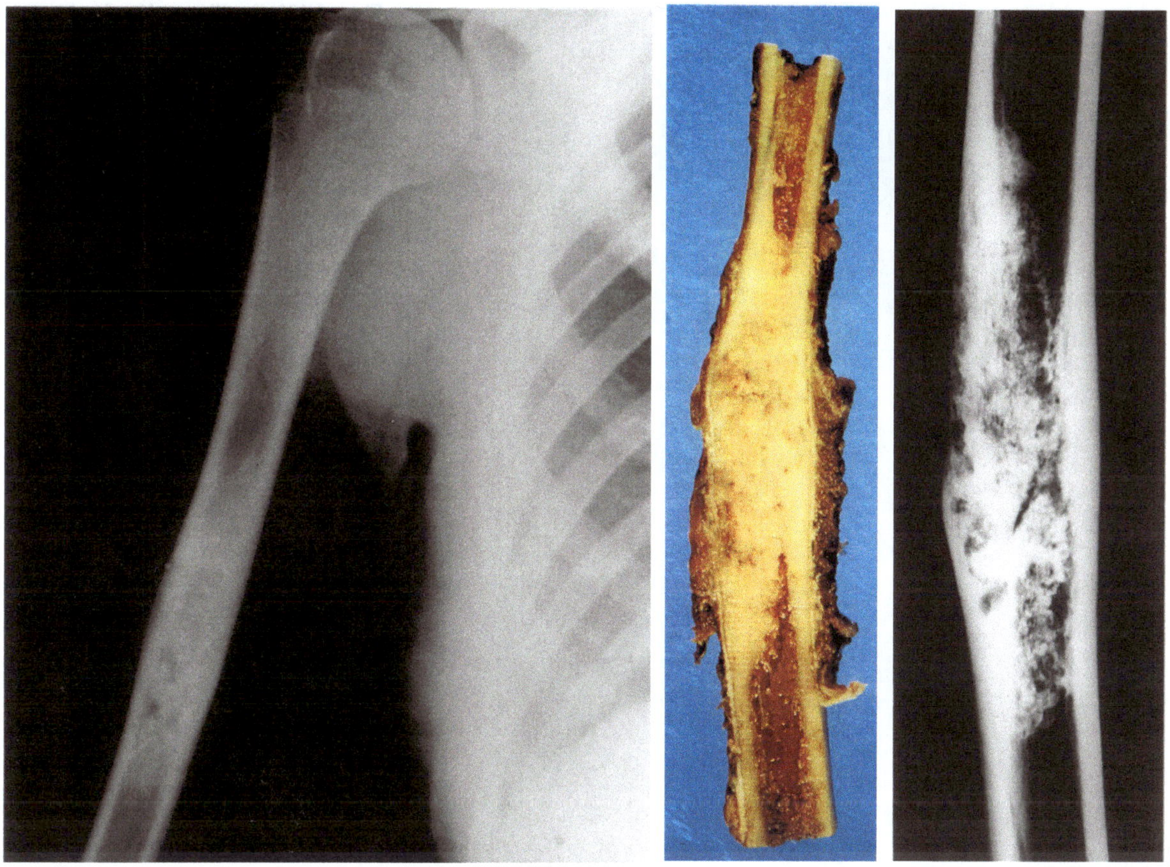

a b, c

Fig. I.99a–c. Female, 15 years old. Well-differentiated osteosarcoma of the humerus. **a** Radiograph shows a sclerotic, irregularly calcified lesion in the midshaft of the humerus. **b** Photograph and **c** radiograph of the resected specimen show the spotty calcification of this sclerotic lesion, which has partly destroyed the cortex at its lateral aspect

others mimic fibrous dysplasia (Figs. I.98–I.100) (Xipell and Rush 1985) or even a giant-cell tumor (Fig. I.98). Some cases of aggressive or malignant osteoblastoma are interpreted as well-differentiated osteosarcoma (Bertoni et al. 1985).

Histologically, the fibrous tissue predominates in some areas (Fig. I.100). It is composed of interlacing bundles of spindle cells separated by dense collagen fibers that are occasionally hyalinized. The nuclei are mostly uniform in size; pleomorphism and/or mitosis are rare. Interspersed with the fibrous tissue are strands of osteoid or mineralized woven bony trabeculae, generally without active osteoblasts on their surfaces. Tumors with more abundant bone production may resemble parosteal osteosarcoma and could be considered its intramedullary counterpart. Small foci of cartilage may be present, though rarely.

Wide en bloc resection as the first procedure seems to be the treatment of choice. Most patients with limited local excision or curettage as the initial therapy had recurrences, and most were treated with amputation between 7 months and 24 years after these procedures. Three of the 27 patients of Unni et al. (1977) died from metastatic tumors.

Small-Cell Osteosarcoma Simulating Ewing Tumor. Twenty-four bone tumors with the histologic features of both Ewing sarcoma and osteosarcoma were labeled "small-cell osteosarcoma simulating Ewing tumor" by Sim et al. (1979). Six additional cases were published by Martin et al. (1982) and 13 by Edeiken et al. (1987). The average patient age was 28 years in the cases of Sim et al.; in those of Martin et al. the patients' ages ranged from 9 to 31 years, and in those of Edeiken et al., from 6 to 28 years. More recently Ayala et al. (1989) and Bertoni et al. (1989) reported similar cases. The roentgenographic features showed a wide variation without

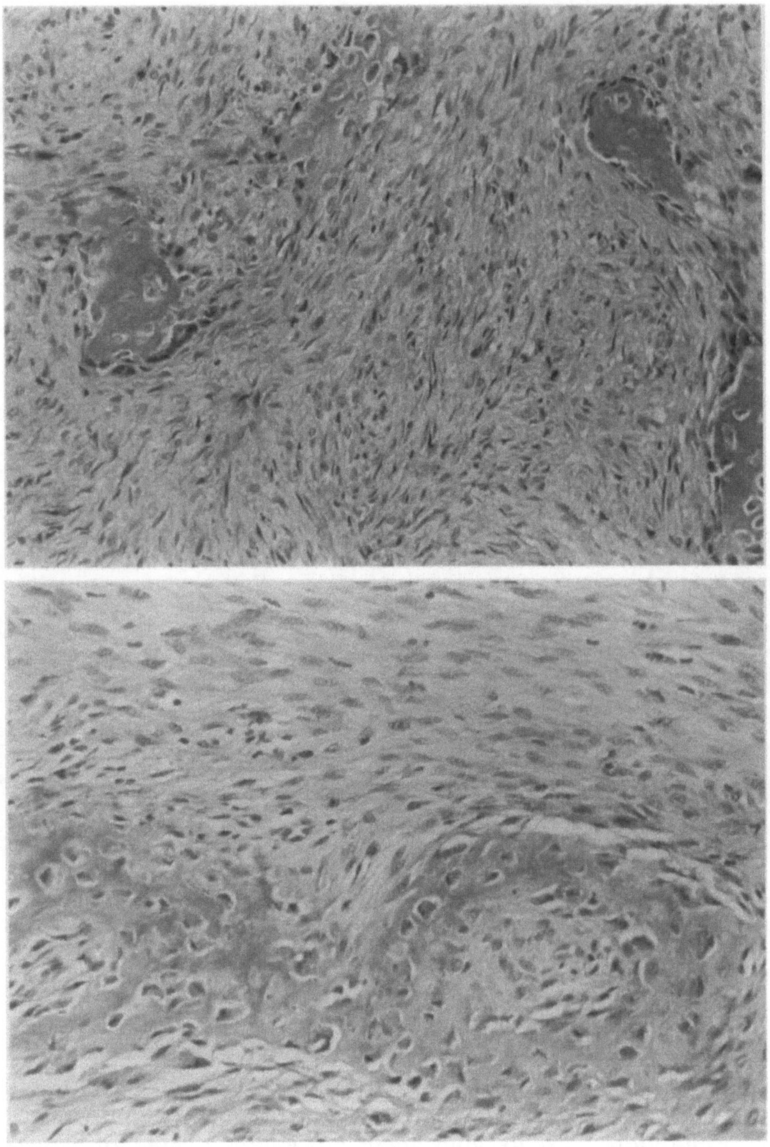

a

b

Fig. I.100a,b. Photomicrographs of well-differentiated osteosarcoma show at **a** lower and **b** higher magnification new formation of osteoid and woven bone trabeculae within a fibrous tissue, similar to the pattern of fibrous dysplasia. However, the lack of a storiform pattern and the herringbonelike distribution of the fibroblasts with only isolated mitotic figures favor a low-grade osteosarcoma. **a** ×200, **b** ×400

a pathognomonic pattern (Fig. I.101). Histologically, the lesions were composed of small cells with round to oval nuclei and indistinct cytoplasmic borders, similar to Ewing sarcoma. A variable amount of osteoid was produced by the tumor cells (Fig. I.102), and in some cases chondroid tissue was also present. Although the periodic acid-Schiff stain (PAS) was negative in the 11 tumors stained with this technique (Sim et al. 1979), cytoplasmic glycogen was present in three of the five cases of Martin et al. for which blocks were available, in 10 of the 27 cases reported by Ayala et al. (1989), and in 6 of the 11 cases from the Rizzoli Institute (Bertoni et al. 1989). Glycogen stains are not mentioned in the article by Edeiken et al. (1987).

This tumor entity is extremely rare. In some Ewing sarcoma cases, reactive osteoid or woven bone formation commonly found in these lesions may have been misinterpreted as tumor bone formation, thus causing an erroneous diagnosis of small-cell osteosarcoma. It is possible that this entity represents a more primitive intermediate stage in the evolution of the undifferentiated cells of Ewing sarcoma toward a skeletongenic tumor (osteosarcoma or chondrosarcoma). A similar hypothesis was postulated by Hutter et al. (1966), who coined the term "primitive multipotential sarcoma of bone," which seems to correspond to Jacobson's (1977) "polyhistioma." Thus, in one of the intermediate stages the undifferentiated mesenchymal tumor cells produce only a

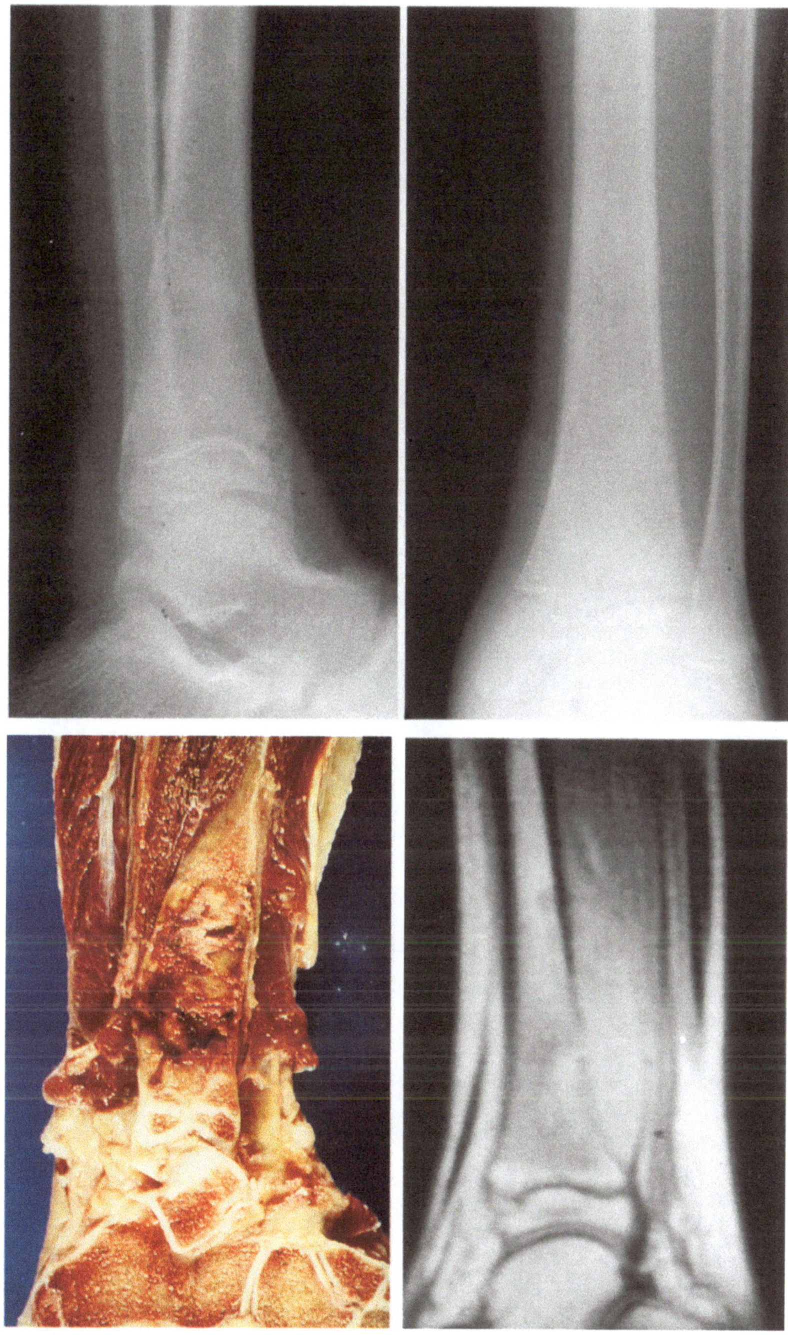

Fig. I.101a–c. Female, 10 years old. Round-cell osteosarcoma of the tibia. **a** Lateral and anteroposterior radiographs show a radiolucent, ill-defined lesion in the lower metaphysis with slight periosteal reaction. **b** Photograph of the amputation specimen and **c** T1-weighted MRI reveal the grayish-white and hemorrhagic aspect of the tumor, which has penetrated widely into the soft tissue (St. Louis University Medical Center)

chondroid matrix; this lesion is classified by most authors as "mesenchymal chondrosarcoma." It would be more logical from a histogenetic viewpoint to classify the small round-cell tumors producing tumor osteoid or bone as *mesenchymal osteosarcoma* (Schajowicz 1983).

Recognizing this rare entity as distinct from Ewing sarcoma could be important because of possible differences of response to treatment. However, the number of cases is too small to determine whether surgery should be combined with chemotherapy only, as Sim et al. suggested, or whether radiotherapy should also be added. Two of the 24 patients of Sim et al. and three of the six patients of Martin et al. who received radiation and adjuvant chemotherapy were alive with no evidence of metastasis after more than 3 years. For this reason a greater number of cases

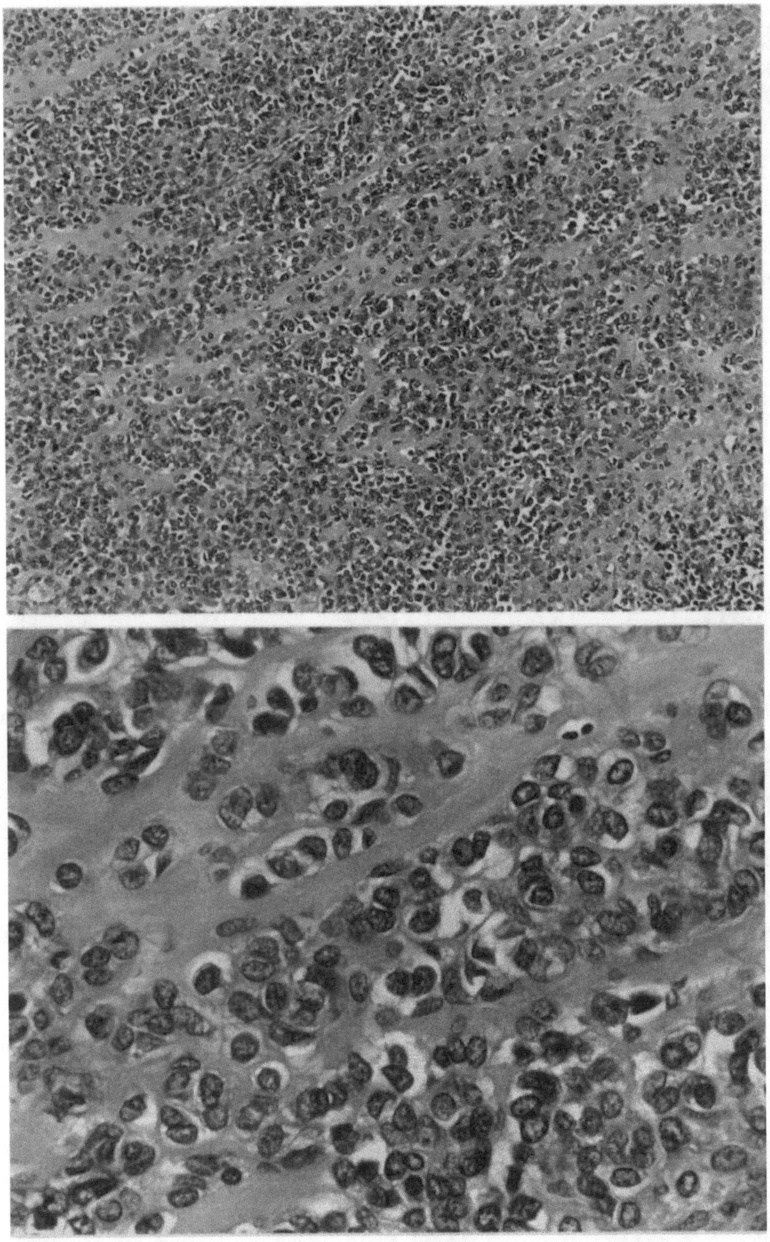

a

b

Fig. I.102a,b. Photomicrographs of same case as in Fig. 101, showing at **a** lower and **b** higher magnification the uniform aspect of the round nuclei without distinct cell borders. The tumor cells were glycogen positive and suggested a primary diagnosis of Ewing sarcoma. However, the finding of osteoid formation by the tumor cells (**b**) inclined the diagnosis towards a round-cell osteosarcoma (osteosarcoma simulating Ewing sarcoma). **a** ×120, **b** ×600

with long follow-up periods are necessary to determine whether the treatment of small-cell osteosarcoma should be different from that of Ewing sarcoma and whether their separation is of practical or only academic importance.

Multifocal (Multicentric) Osteosarcoma. The simultaneous (*synchronous*) occurrence of multiple osteosarcomas, except in Paget disease, is rare; only 3 of our 607 cases of osteosarcoma were of this variety. Our first such case was reported in 1945 by Busso and Schajowicz. Several additional reports, primarily of single cases, appeared later in the literature, which was reviewed extensively by Lowbeer (1968) and Amstutz (1969). A multicentric origin, based on the simultaneous growth and similar gross appearance first postulated by Silverman (1936), as opposed to a metastatic origin, is disputed (Lowbeer 1968).

The typical lesions (type I of Amstutz) occur in childhood and adolescence, with generally symmetric, simultaneously (or nearly so) appearing bone lesions, in most cases without pulmonary involvement. Radiologically, the

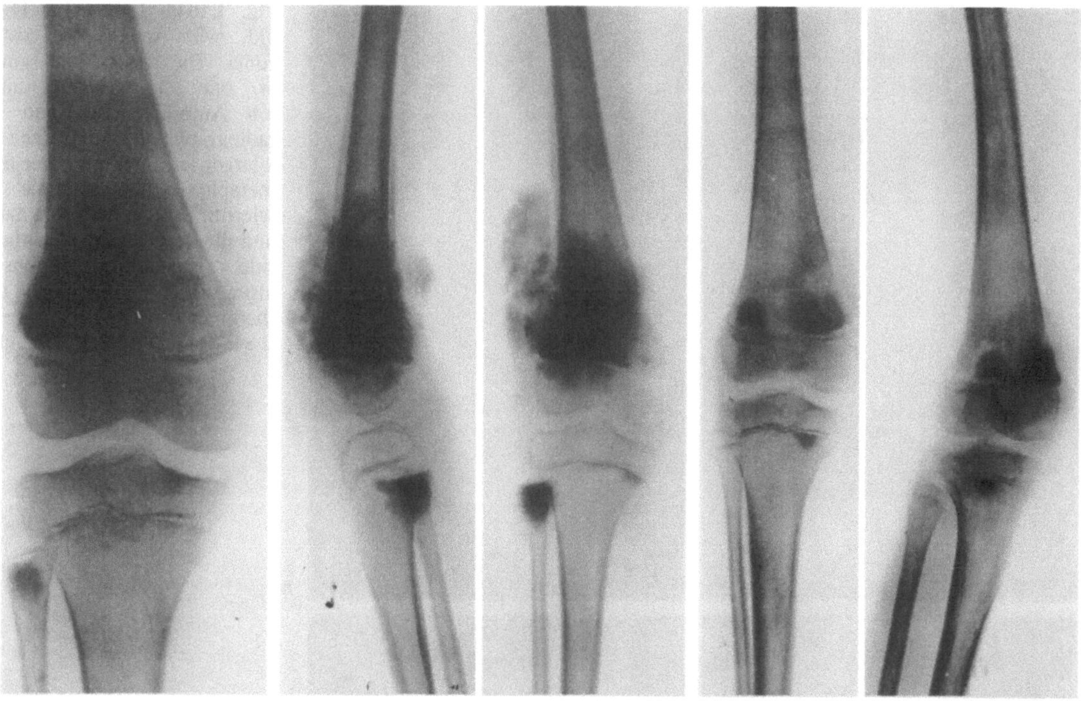
a, b c

Fig. I.103a–c. Female, 5 years old, with multifocal (multicentric) osteosarcoma. Radiographs show multiple osteosclerotic foci in the metaphysis of the distal femur, proximal tibia, and fibula at both extremities

lesions are located preferentially in the metaphysis of long bones and are almost always dense and sclerotic (Figs. I.103, I.104). Grossly and microscopically, the lesions are a densely ossified osteoblastic type of osteosarcoma.

In contrast, multiple *metachronous* osteosarcoma (Fitzgerald et al. 1973) is characterized by skeletal lesions that are asymmetric, variable in size, and not necessarily sclerotic. Patients with this tumor (type II of Amstutz) vary widely in age, but are often adolescents or adults. The prognosis of multifocal (multicentric) synchronous osteosarcoma is poor, most patients surviving only a few months after the diagnosis. Patients with metachronous lesions are potentially curable: surgical treatment produced two long-term survivals in Fitzgerald et al.'s (1973) group of 12 patients.

b. Surface (Peripheral) Osteosarcoma

Malignant bone-forming tumors that arise from the surface of bone, usually long bones, are far less common than those arising from within bone (Schajowicz et al. 1988; Dahlin and Unni 1986). These surface osteosarcomas are clinically and radiologically similar, yet histologically they are quite distinct. In reviewing the literature we classified the tumors into three categories: *parosteal (juxtacortical)*, *periosteal*, and *high-grade surface osteosarcoma*. This division is justified because of evident differences in biologic behavior and widely varying prognoses. Parosteal osteosarcoma is associated with the best prognosis. In contrast, the prognosis for patients with the high-grade surface osteosarcoma is poor, almost identical to that for conventional central osteosarcoma. The prognosis of periosteal osteosarcoma is intermediate.

Parosteal (Juxtacortical) Osteosarcoma

While the name "juxtacortical osteosarcoma" introduced by Jaffe in 1958 was previously the preferred term to designate the largest of the three subgroups of surface osteosarcoma (Schajowicz et al. 1972; Schajowicz 1981), the synonymous designation of "parosteal osteosarcoma" has recently become more popular. To avoid confusion we have adopted the latter term for this lesion, but not for all surface osteosarcomas, which were grouped by Levine et al. (1985) and

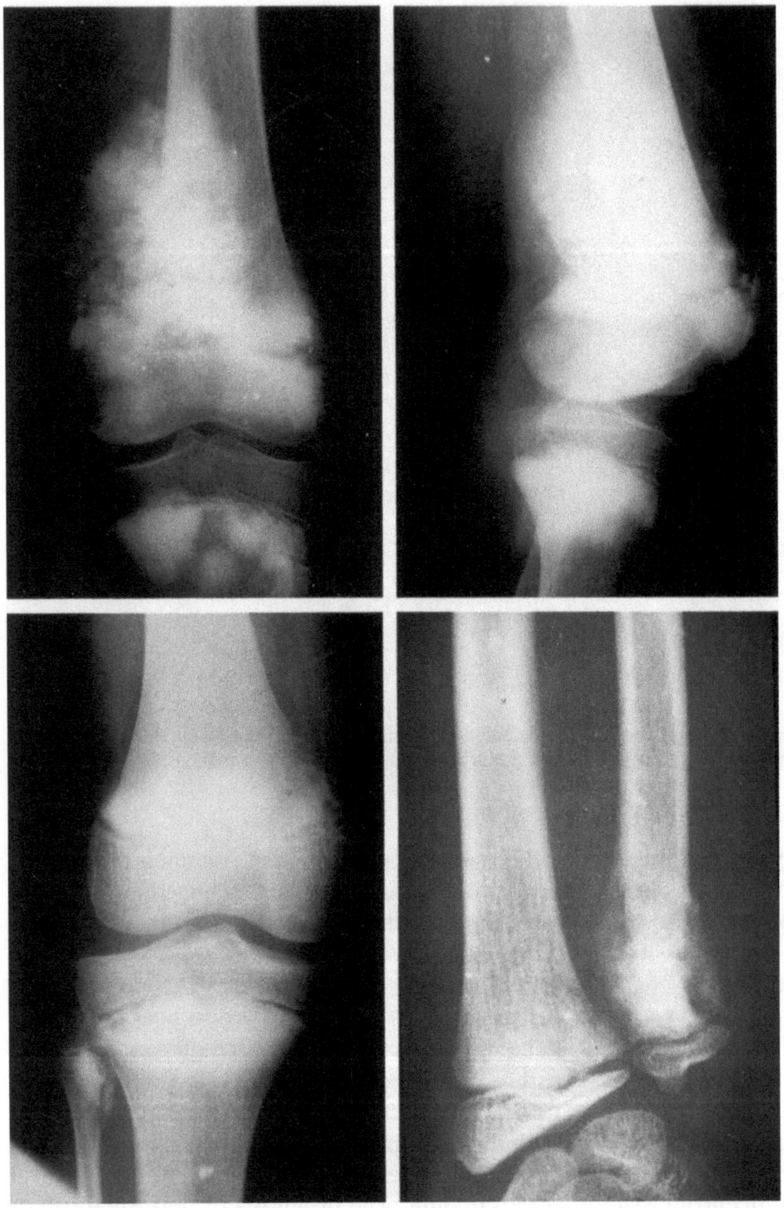

a b c d

Fig. I.104a–d. Female, 11 years old, with multicentric osteosarcoma. The patient had symptoms of only 1 month's duration. **a**,**b** Anteroposterior and lateral radiographs of the left knee reveal a larger lesion in the lower femoral metaphysis and multiple osteosclerotic foci in the proximal tibial and fibular metaphysis of the same side. Osteosclerotic lesions were also present in the proximal tibia of the other extremity (**c**) as well as in the lower metaphysis of the ulna (**d**)

others under the single title of juxtacortical osteosarcoma.

Parosteal (juxtacortical) osteosarcoma is defined by WHO as a distinctive malignant type of osteosarcoma characterized by an origin on the external surface of a bone and a high degree of structural differentiation. These tumors grow relatively slowly and have a better prognosis than the ordinary type of osteosarcoma.

According to the WHO definition, bone-forming tumors of a frankly high degree of histologic malignancy which rarely arise on the surface of a bone are not acceptable as typical parosteal (juxtacortical) osteosarcomas. These lesions are classified by the group at the Memorial Hospital and Hospital for Special Surgery (New York) (Ahuja et al. 1977) and by Campanacci et al. (1984) as grade III juxtacortical osteogenic sarcomas, emphasizing the poor prognosis of this tumor despite early radical surgical treatment. According to Dahlin (1978), osteosarcomas of high-grade malignancy, occasionally seen on the surface of a bone, do not belong to the category under discussion. The writer believes that a better term for this type of tumor would be "high-grade surface osteosarcoma" (Wold et al. 1984a)

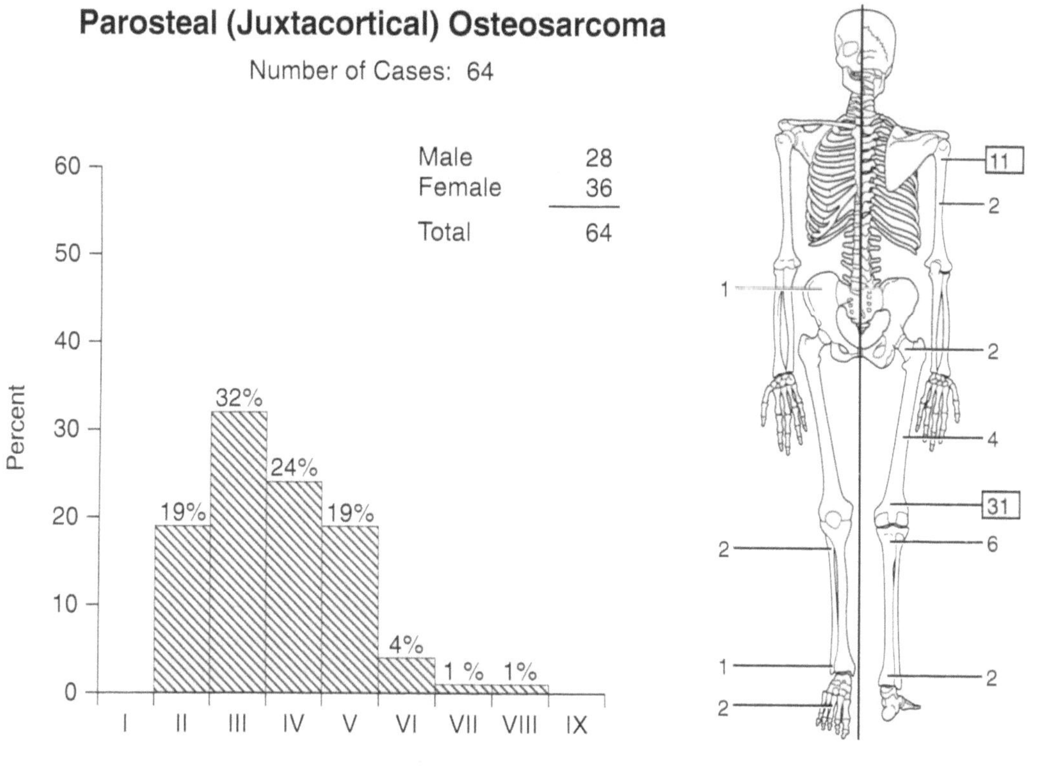

Scheme I.4

or "peripheral conventional osteosarcoma," which comprises the histologically malignant osteosarcomas identical to the central (intramedullary) lesions, but which develop on the external surface of a bone. It also includes some of the more heavily ossified so-called periosteal osteosarcomas described by Unni et al. (1976b), which are discussed later. On the other hand, parosteal (juxtacortical) osteosarcoma was first reported in 1951 by Geschickter and Copeland as "parosteal osteoma," even though these authors realized its malignant potential. Although we accept and have observed cases of completely benign juxtacortical (parosteal) osteomas (see Figs. I.5, I.6), as have Dahlin and Unni (1986: Figs. 6-4, 6-5, p. 86), we have no proof that the malignant counterpart can originate in a previously benign lesion.

Incidence. Parosteal osteosarcoma, although much less frequent than central osteosarcoma (10%), is the most common of the surface osteosarcomas. Our 64 cases represent 2.5% of our series of primary malignant bone tumors, and in Dahlin and Unni's (1986) series of 56 cases, parosteal osteosarcoma represents less than 1% of malignant tumors and approximately 4% of all osteosarcomas. It was somewhat more frequent in the material of the Rizzoli Institute (Campanacci et al. 1984): 41 cases representing 5% of all malignant tumors. Ahuja et al. (1977) collected only 24 cases over a 40-year period in the Memorial Hospital and the Hospital for Special Surgery (New York), including six cases of high-grade malignancy, which in our opinion correspond to high-grade surface osteosarcomas.

Clinical Findings. *Age and Sex.* There was a slight predilection for females in our material (56%), and a greater one in Dahlin and Unni's (1986) series (70%). In other series (Ahuja et al. 1977; Campanacci and Giunti 1976) there was no significant predilection for either sex.

In our and all other statistics, the average age was higher than that for conventional central osteosarcoma. Age ranged in our series from 15 to 78 years, most patients (81%) being more than 20 years old. In many cases, the onset of symptoms started several years before the preoperative diagnosis was made (Scheme I.4).

Localization. Parosteal osteosarcoma was almost exclusively located in long bones and involved preferentially the lower end of the femur (31 cases), especially the popliteal region, in accordance with all other series, followed by the upper end of the humerus (11 cases) and less frequently the tibia, fibula, and upper femur (eight, three, and two cases, respectively). The lesion most commonly arose in the metaphysis and exceptionally in the diaphysis (four cases in the femoral and two cases in the humeral diaphysis).

Symptoms. The common clinical symptom is swelling, sometimes accompanied by pain, which generally is not intense and rarely precedes the swelling. Because of the tumor's slow growth, the symptoms may precede the clinical diagnosis by months or several years. However, in some cases, the duration of symptoms before definite treatment is much shorter, which seems to indicate a faster growth rate and higher malignancy of the tumor.

Radiographic Features. Parosteal osteosarcoma has characteristic radiographic features, showing a densely ossified juxtacortical mass, oval or spherical, attached to the underlying cortex. The lobulated surface is sometimes less dense than the broad base of the tumor. A linear, more translucent zone that separates the bulk of the tumor from the subjacent cortex, except at its site of attachment, is considered a characteristic finding; this was lacking in most of our cases of large tumors, which often encircled the bone (Figs. I.105–I.110).

The surface of the tumor mass is occasionally poorly limited and irregular, being ill-defined with spicules or linear extension; multiple small radiopacities are sometimes seen in the soft tissue separated from the bulk of the tumor, especially in cases of recurrence after local excision. Cortical thickening is occasionally observed under the tumor, but periosteal bone reaction in the form of spicules, a laminated pattern, or a Codman's triangle was not seen in our cases. Cortical destruction and medullary penetration were visible in the clinical radiographs of only a few recurrent and advanced cases (Figs. I.105, I.111).

The radiologic differential diagnosis of so-called myositis ossificans and conventional peripheral or "periosteal" osteosarcoma, as later defined, may present occasional difficulties. In myositis ossificans, however, the most common localization is in the diaphyseal region. The round or oval lesion is limited by a distinct osseous rim at its periphery, whereas the center appears more radiolucent. On the other hand, when a myositis ossificans becomes attached to the underlying bone, it generally does not have the broad base evident in juxtacortical osteosarcoma.

Periosteal and high-grade surface osteosarcomas, when more heavily calcified and ossified, are sometimes difficult to differentiate, but their clinical and radiographic features (age, location, etc.) and especially their histologic features permit one to distinguish them from parosteal osteosarcoma (see Figs. I.123, I.124).

Osteochondroma can easily be differentiated radiographically because the spongiosa of the underlying metaphysis is continuous with the central osseous part of the pedicle of the osteochondroma. However, radiologic distinction from juxtacortical osteoma and subperiosteal ossifying hematoma is generally impossible, a careful histologic study being required for this purpose.

Pathologic Findings. *Gross Pathology.* The tumor is characterized by lobulated masses with generally well-defined limits, varying in size from a few to more than 20 cm. The tumor mass is hard and primarily osseous in nature (Fig. I.107). Irregular, generally small areas of cartilaginous or fibromatous tissue may be visible on a section in most cases, preferentially at the periphery. However, these features do not necessarily indicate a higher grade of malignancy (Enneking et al. 1985). Most of the tumor is ossified and compact, tending to be more sclerotic at its broad base, sometimes encircling the underlying bone in advanced cases. The radiolucent narrow zone, which occasionally separates the tumor from the cortex, corresponds to a fibrous membrane 2–3 mm thick and is thought to represent the periosteum (Fig. I.106b,c).

Histopathology. Most of the tumors are of low-grade malignancy. The histologic diagnosis from a biopsy may be extremely difficult without knowing the clinical and radiologic features, or when the pathologist does not notice the fibrous component that separates the predominant bone tissue (Figs. I.112–I.114). The fibrous stroma is composed of spindle cells, which usually show little pleomorphism and few mitoses and form a moderate amount of collagen fibers similar to a low-grade fibrosarcoma. The extensive bone formation has a well-organized trabecular pattern, composed of immature (woven) bone in different stages of maturation to lamellar bone trabeculae, which predominate in most areas. The osteoblasts surrounding the bone trabeculae are spindle

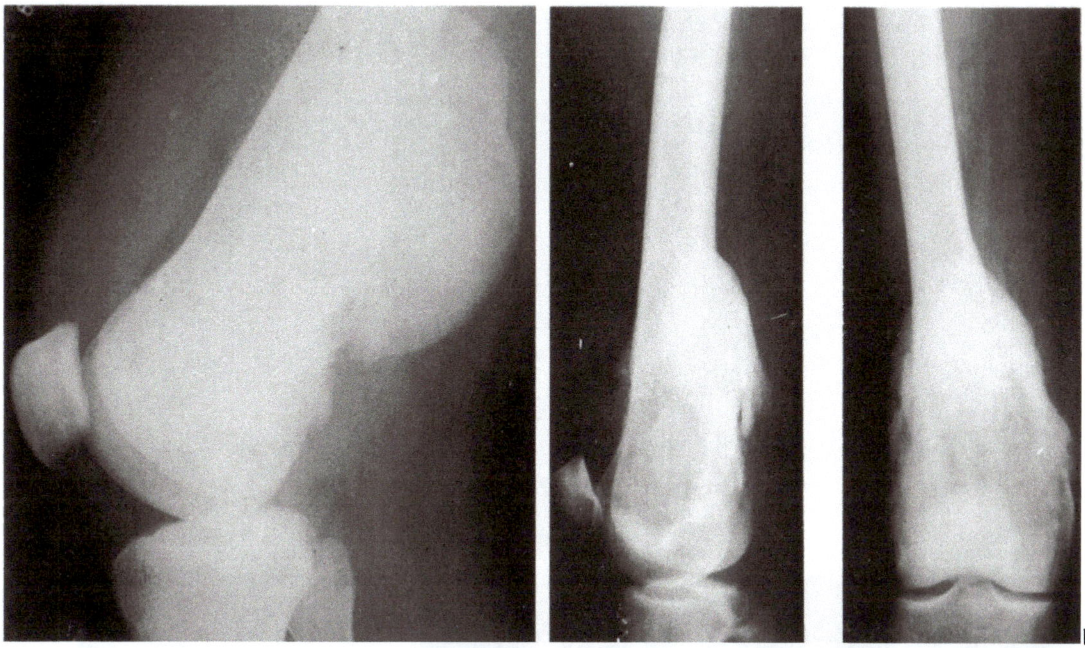

a b

Fig. I.105a–d. Male, 24 years old. Parosteal osteosarcoma of femur. **a** Radiograph shows the juxtacortical location at the posterior aspect of the lower third of the femur and the extreme radiopacity of the well-delineated tumor. The medullary cavity seems not to be involved. An excision was performed, and the tumor recurred twice in the years after local excision. **b** Radiographs 8 years after the first operation, showing recurrence of the tumor, which now evidently involves the medullary cavity. A high-thigh amputation was performed. **c** Photograph and **d** radiograph of the amputation specimen illustrate the densely sclerotic extraosseous components and the extensive invasion of the medullary cavity, where the tumor is predominantly osteolytic

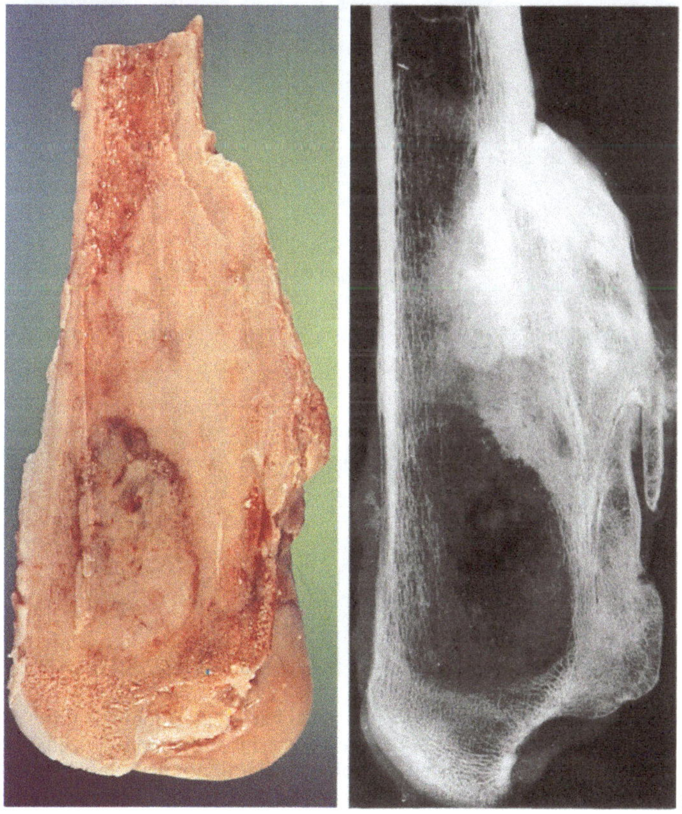

c d

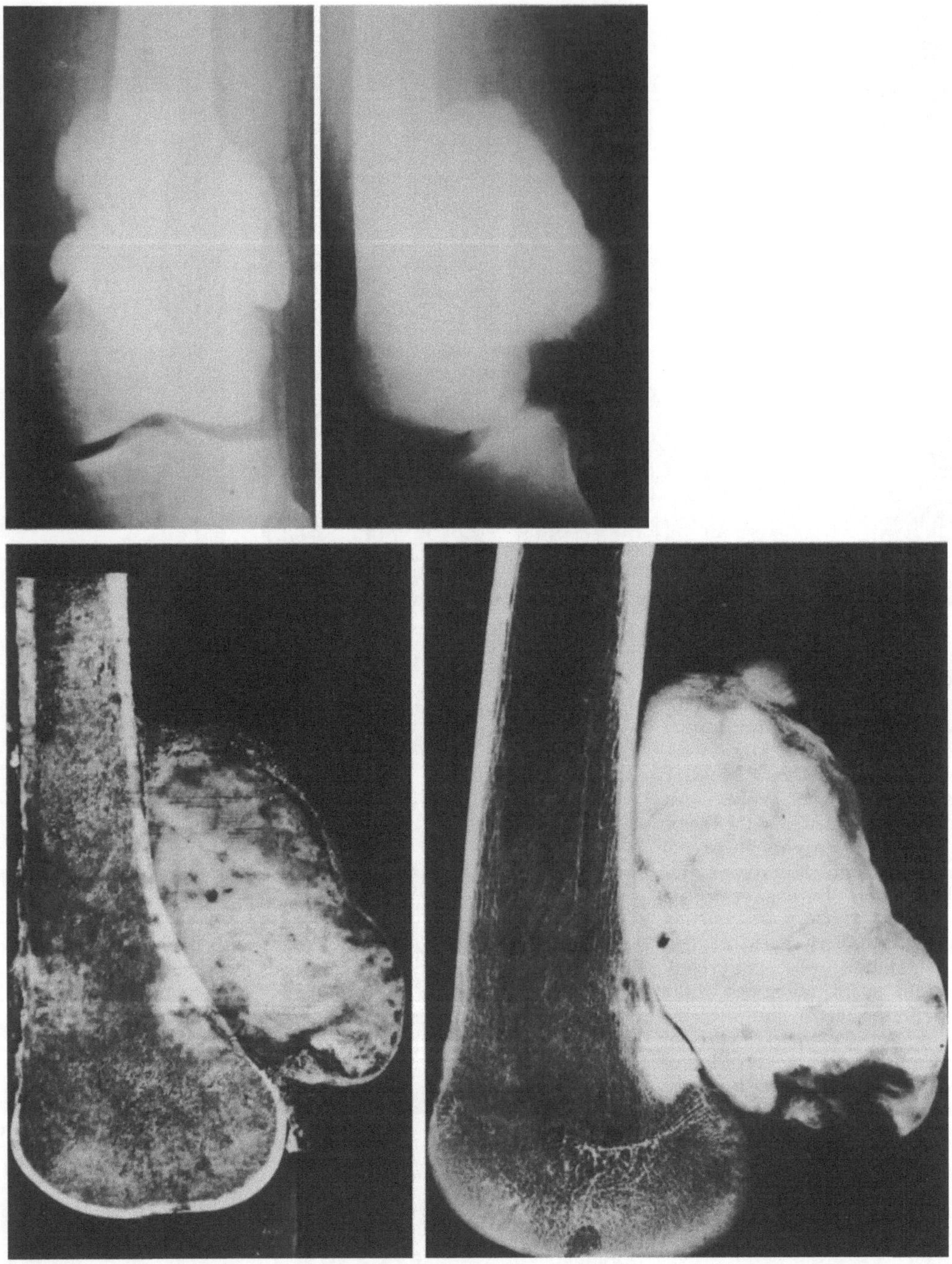

a b c

Fig. I.106a–c. Female, 36 years old. Parosteal osteosarcoma of the distal femur. **a** Anteroposterior and lateral radiographs of the extremely sclerotic, lobular tumor mass located at the posterior part, which appears to envelop the bone. Due to the superimposition of the extracortical tumor mass, it is impossible to determine the involvement of the medullary cavity. A block resection of the lower third of the femur was performed, with replacement by cadaver bone graft. **b** Photograph and **c** radiograph of the resected specimen revealing the juxtacortical location and extreme radiopacity of the tumor with its well-delineated surface. A radiolucent line between the cortex and tumor, a characteristic finding in this tumor type, can be clearly seen, as can the beginning intramedullary penetration

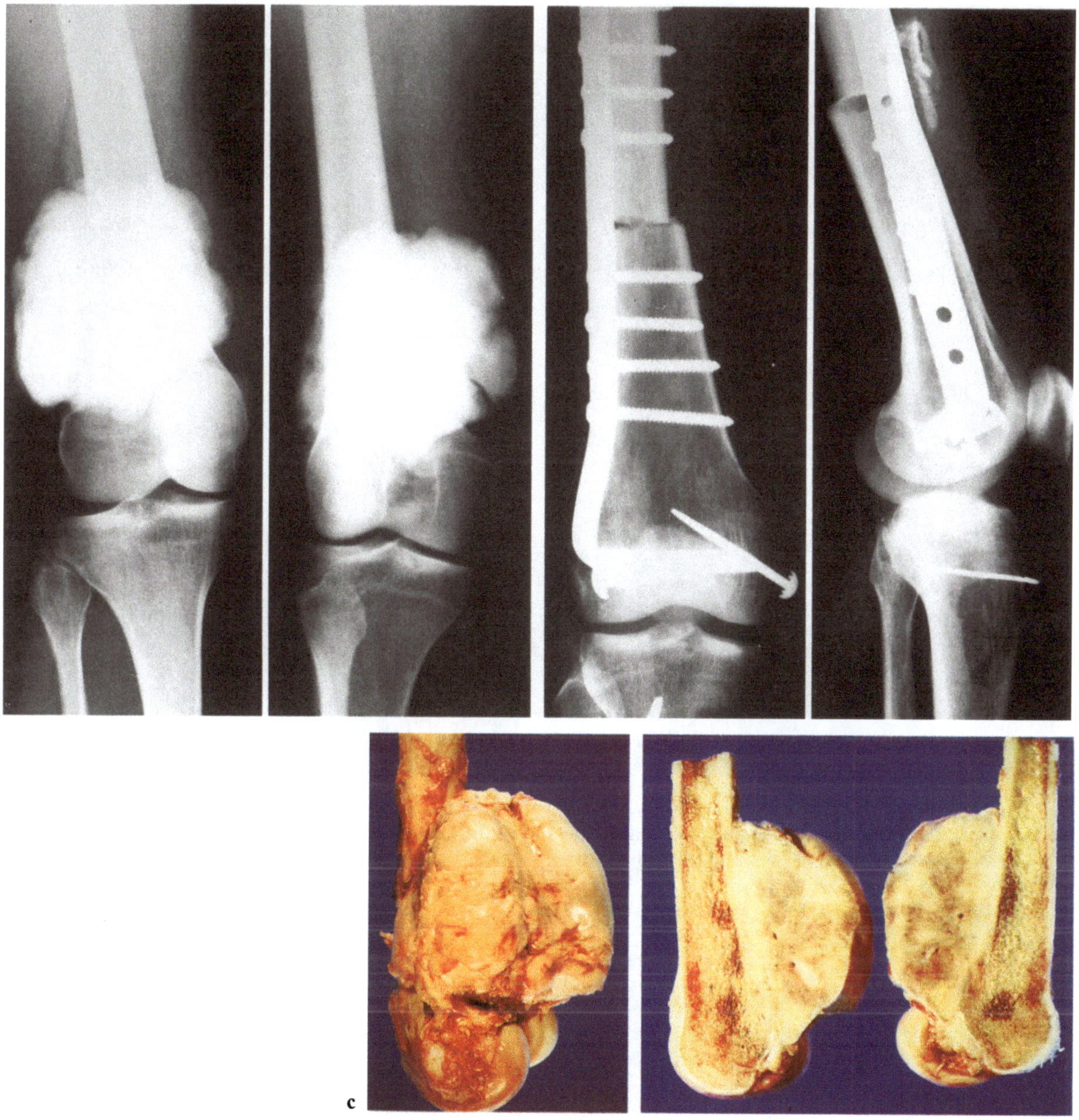

Fig. I.107a–d. Parosteal osteosarcoma of distal femur in a 36-year-old woman. **a** Anteroposterior and oblique radiographs show the juxtacortical location at the posterior aspect and the extreme radiodensity of the well-delineated tumor, which appears to envelop the bone. A segmental en bloc resection followed by an osteoarticular allograft was performed. **b–d** Photographs of the surface and sagittal section demonstrate the juxtacortical location of the sclerotic tumor mass. (Schajowicz and McGuire 1989)

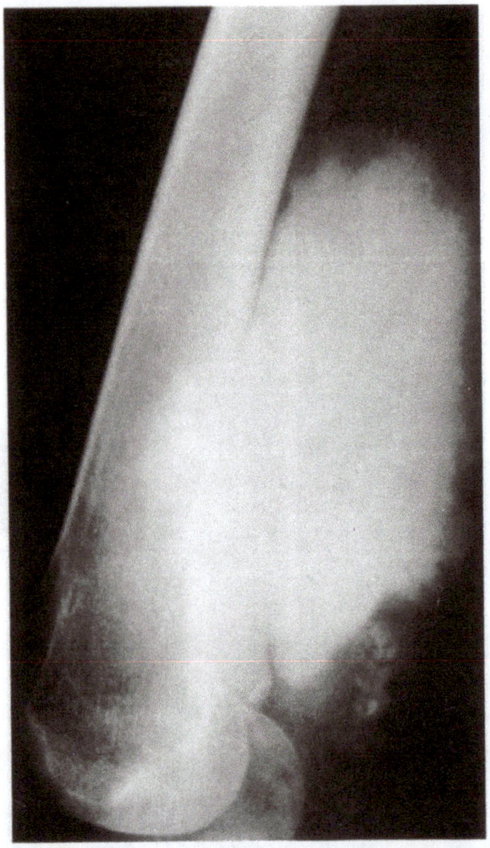

Fig. I.108. Female, 48 years old. Parosteal osteosarcoma of the distal femur. Lateral radiograph illustrates the typical features and location at the posterior and inferior part of the femur

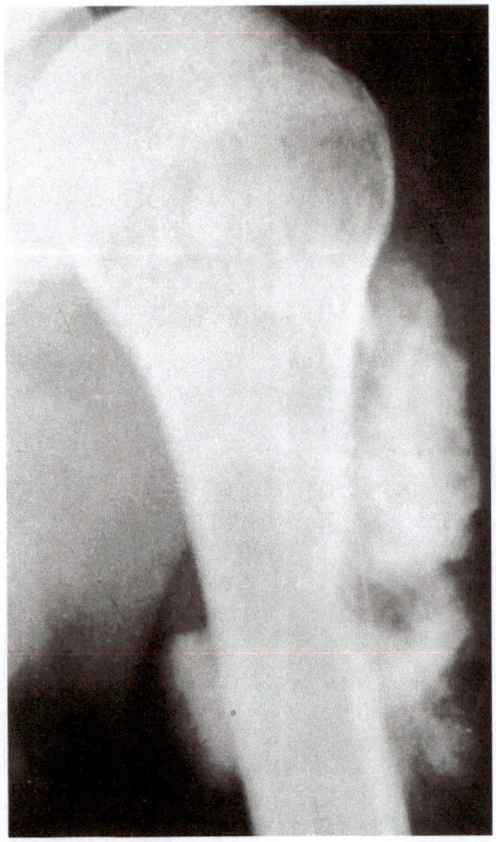

Fig. I.109. Female, 38 years old. Parosteal osteosarcoma of the upper humerus. Radiograph shows the sclerotic aspect and irregular, lobular contour of the tumor

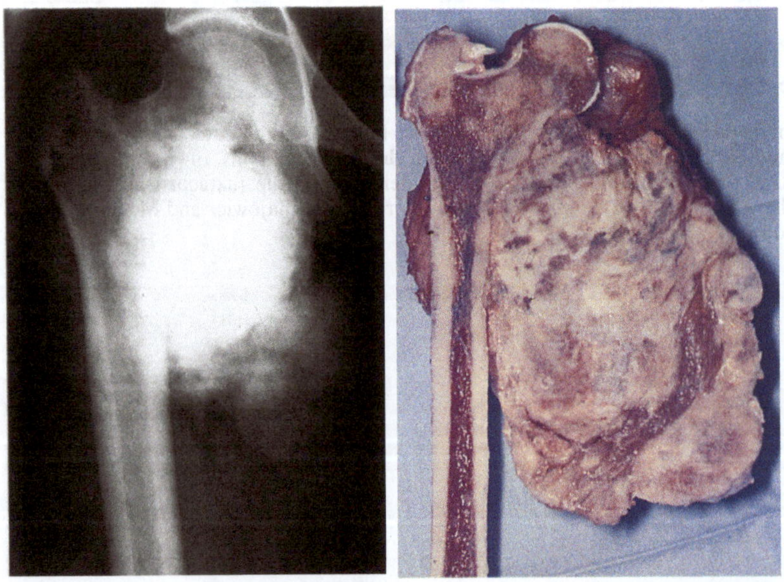

a b

Fig. I.110a,b. Parosteal osteosarcoma of upper femur in a 30-year-old woman. **a** Radiograph shows the large sclerotic lobulated tumor mass. In spite of two recurrences after incomplete excision, the tumor did not penetrate the medullary canal, as shown in **b**

a

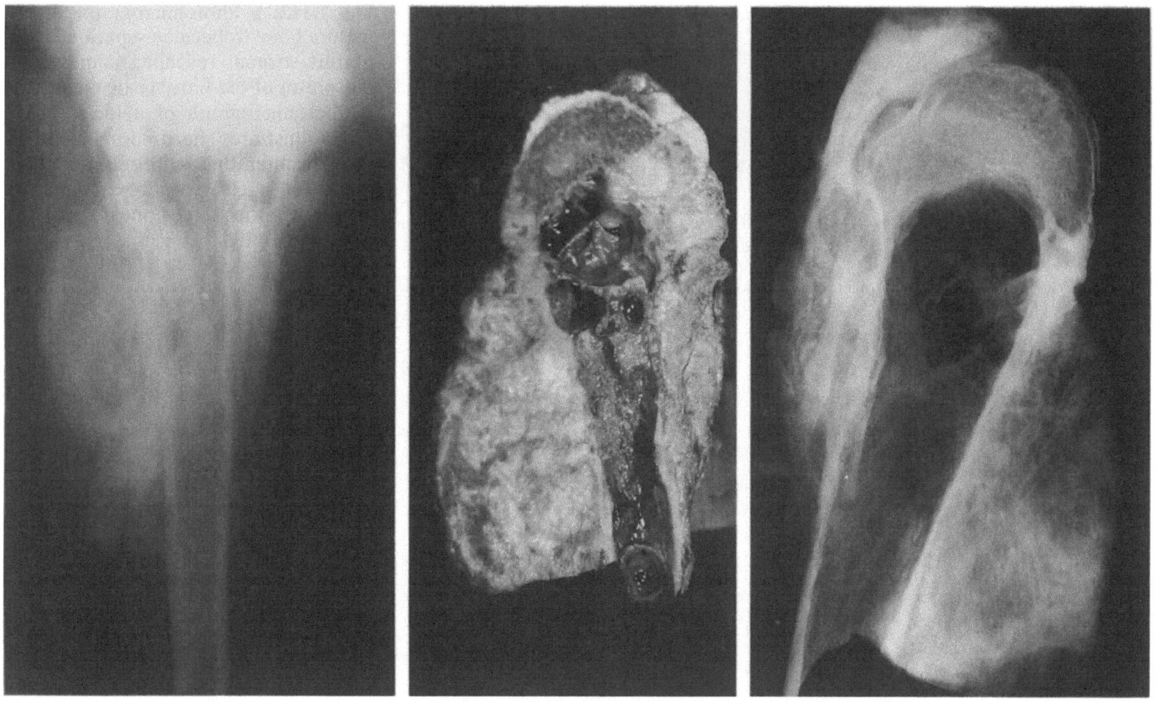

b, c

Fig. I.111a–c. Thirty-year-old female with parosteal osteosarcoma of the upper third of the humerus. **a** Radiograph shows the juxtacortical tumor mass, which appears to envelop the bone. This is more clearly seen in **b** a photograph and **c** a radiograph of a thin slab of the resected specimen

shaped (inactive) and occasionally more hypertrophic and active; however, frankly malignant pleomorphic and hyperchromatic osteoblasts or clearly sarcomatous atypical fibroblasts with abundant mitotic figures are usually absent (Figs. I.113, I.114). The variable number of cartilaginous foci usually show a pattern similar to that of low-grade chondrosarcoma. A superficial, thin cap of cartilage tissue may simulate an osteochondroma, but the discontinuity and irregularity of this cartilage cap and above all the microscopic aspect of the underlying newly formed bone, separated by proliferating fibrous tissues, permit one to discard this diagnosis (Fig. I.115).

We have observed several tumors with radiologic features similar to parosteal osteosarcoma but with no histologic indication of malignancy, which have been classified as parosteal (juxtacortical) osteomas (see p. 29ff.).

Treatment and Prognosis. Radiation therapy and chemotherapy are ineffective; the indicated treatment is surgical ablation of the tumor. In the principal series, the reported survival rate 5 years after the first treatment was 70%–80% (Dwinnel et al. 1954; Scaglietti and Calandriello 1962; Van der Heul and Van Ronnen 1967; Farr and Huvos 1972; Dahlin 1978); in the series of Campanacci et al. (1984), the 10-year survival rate was 55%.

In several of our cases, local excision of small tumors was carried out, and all but one were followed by one or more recurrences within 5–10 years of operation, making amputation necessary because of cortical destruction and/or medullary penetration (Figs. I.105, I.116, I.117). In one of these cases, located at the lower femoral end, a similar tumor developed at the upper end of the humerus a year after amputation; the patient died shortly thereafter of pulmonary and brain metastases.

Wide segmental en bloc resection is the indicated treatment for parosteal osteosarcoma. Amputation should be reserved for patients who have had one or more recurrences or have wide cortical destruction and intramedullary extension, and for cases in which a higher grade of histologic malignancy is suggested (so-called dedifferentiated parosteal osteosarcoma).

It must be emphasized that after repeated recurrences the histologic grade of malignancy often increases, with a greater incidence of pulmonary metastases (Wold et al. 1984b).

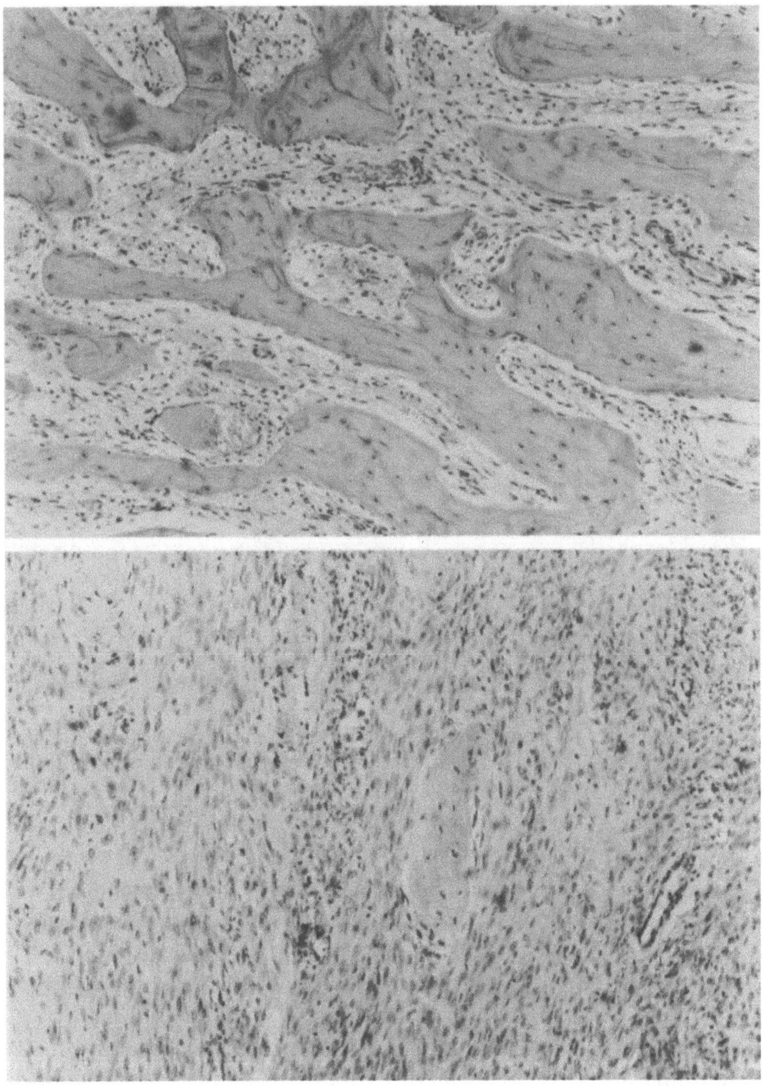

a

b

Fig. I.112. **a** Photomicrograph shows mature bone trabeculae separated by a fibrous stroma, revealing some pleomorphism of the fibroblastic elements. **b** Photomicrograph of a local recurrence illustrates the predominance of the proliferating fibroblastic elements of a clearly fibrosarcomatous aspect over the scarce bone trabeculae. **a** ×120, **b** ×120

Periosteal Osteosarcoma

"Periosteal osteosarcoma" was recognized and included in the classification reviewed by Ewing in 1939 and recorded by Lichtenstein in 1977. He reported three cases, all in children 5–18 years of age, located in the femur and tibia. However, it is only since the appearance of the paper of Unni et al. (1976b) that the lesion has become more widely recognized and clearly defined as a distinct entity.

Unni et al. reported 23 cases under the denomination "periosteal osteosarcoma," 11 of which were from the Mayo Clinic, representing only about 1% of the total of 962 osteosarcomas. This tumor, which they considered a distinct entity, occurred on the surface of bones, with a predilection for the tibia and femur; however, it should be distinguished from parosteal (juxtacortical) osteosarcoma because of its different clinicoradiologic and pathologic features.

In 1977 Spjut et al. reported 13 additional cases from the M.D. Anderson Cancer Institute and consultation cases, confirming the predilection for the tibia and femur. However, several cases were of greater size and in an older age group (14–62 years with an average of 29.3 years) than the cases reported by Unni et al., which were predominantly cartilaginous, small lesions occurring in adolescents. Moreover, 8 of the 13 lesions described by Spjut et al. were highly malignant histologically, and were predominantly osteoblastic or anaplastic rather than chondroblastic. Of these eight patients, four had pulmonary

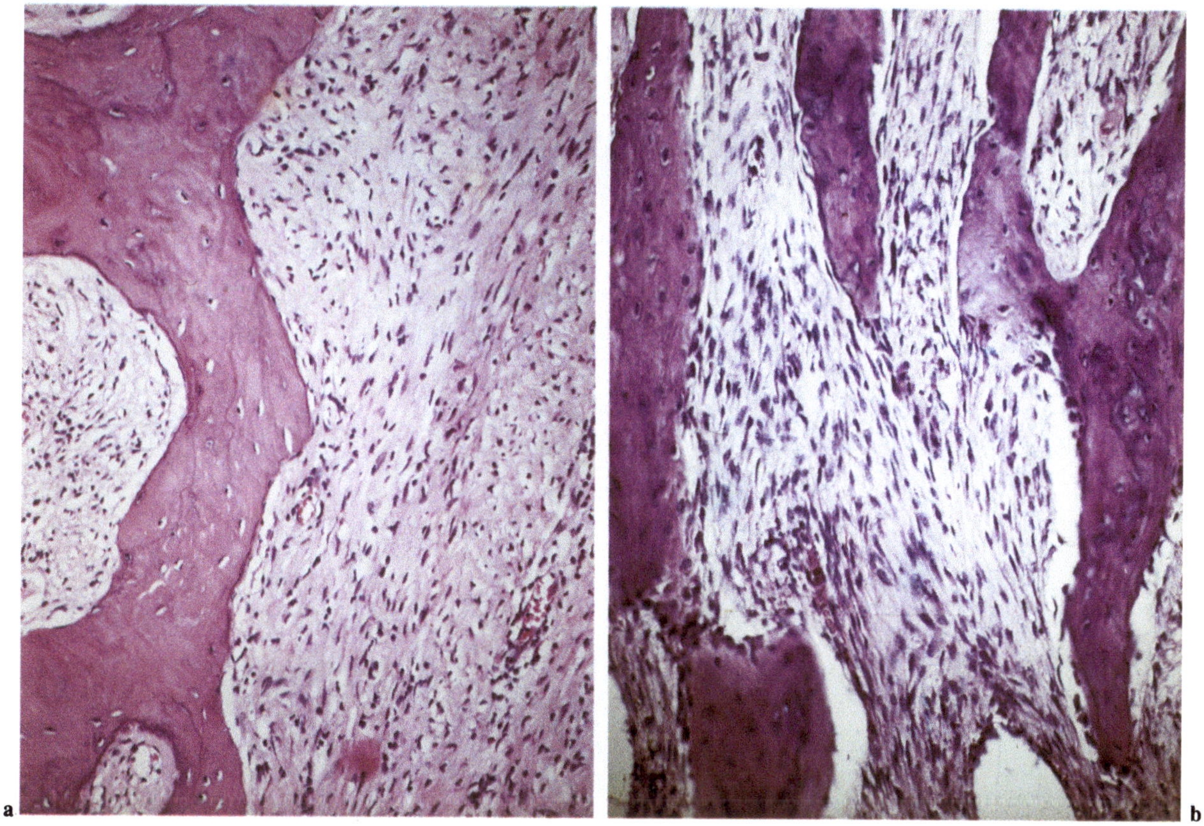

Fig. I.113a,b. Photomicrographs show well-differentiated bony trabeculae separated by a spindle-celled fibrous tissue without evident pleomorphism and scarce mitotic activity, i.e., the features of a well-differentiated fibrosarcoma. a ×100, b ×200

Fig. I.114. Photomicrograph of parosteal osteosarcoma showing at higher magnification the fibrosarcomatous aspect of the stroma. ×200

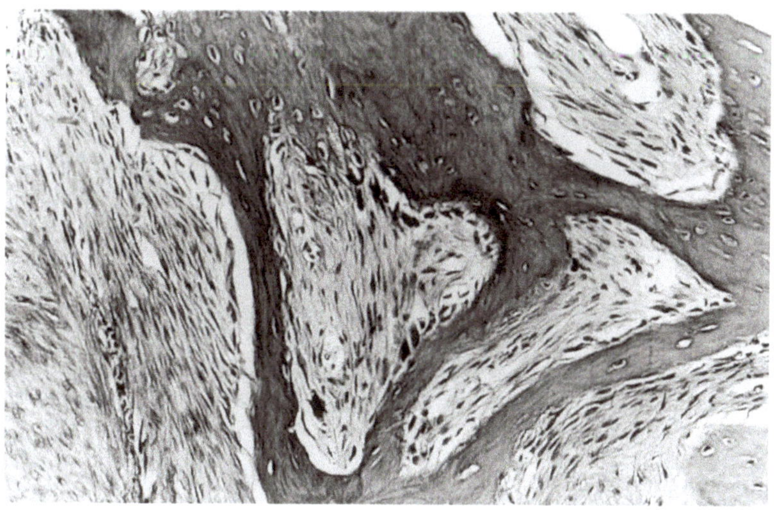

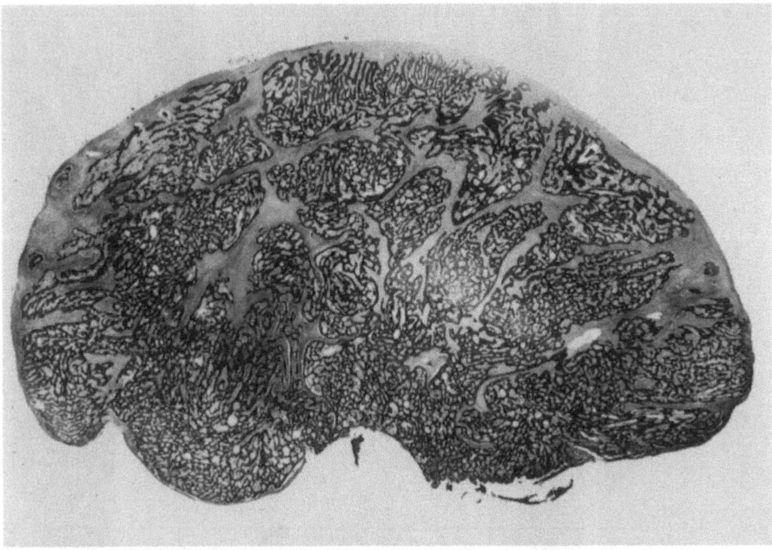

Fig. I.115. Topographic photomicrograph of a parosteal osteosarcoma. An irregular, superficial thin cap of cartilage tissue is present, simulating an osteochondroma. However, the predominance of the underlying newly formed bone and proliferating fibrous tissue supports the diagnosis of parosteal osteosarcoma. ×8

a, b

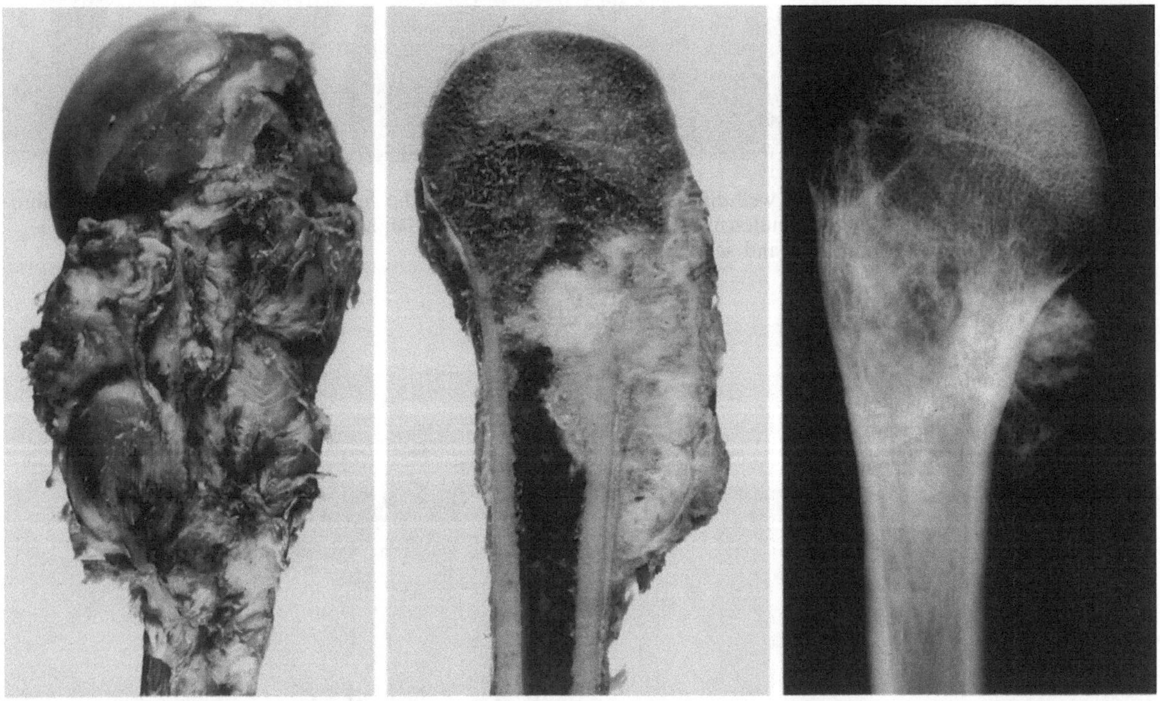

c

Fig. I.116a–c. Parosteal osteosarcoma of the upper humerus. **a,b** Photographs of the surface and a sagittal section of the specimen demonstrate the beginning of medullary penetration by the tumor, not clearly shown in **c** a radiograph of the specimen

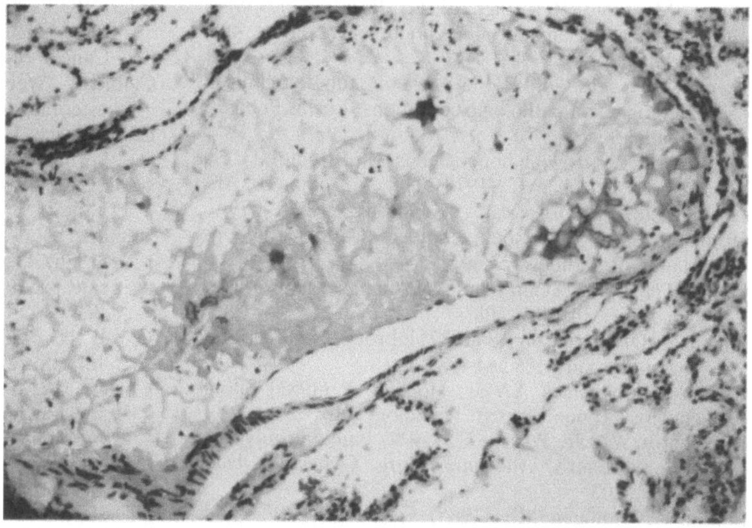
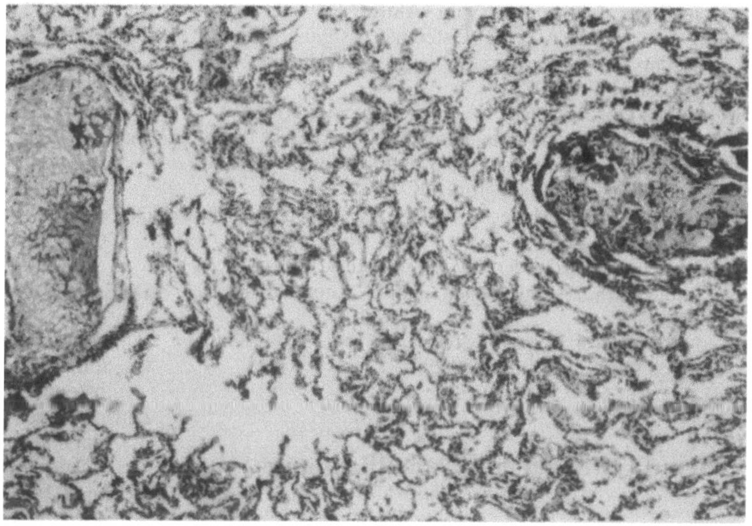
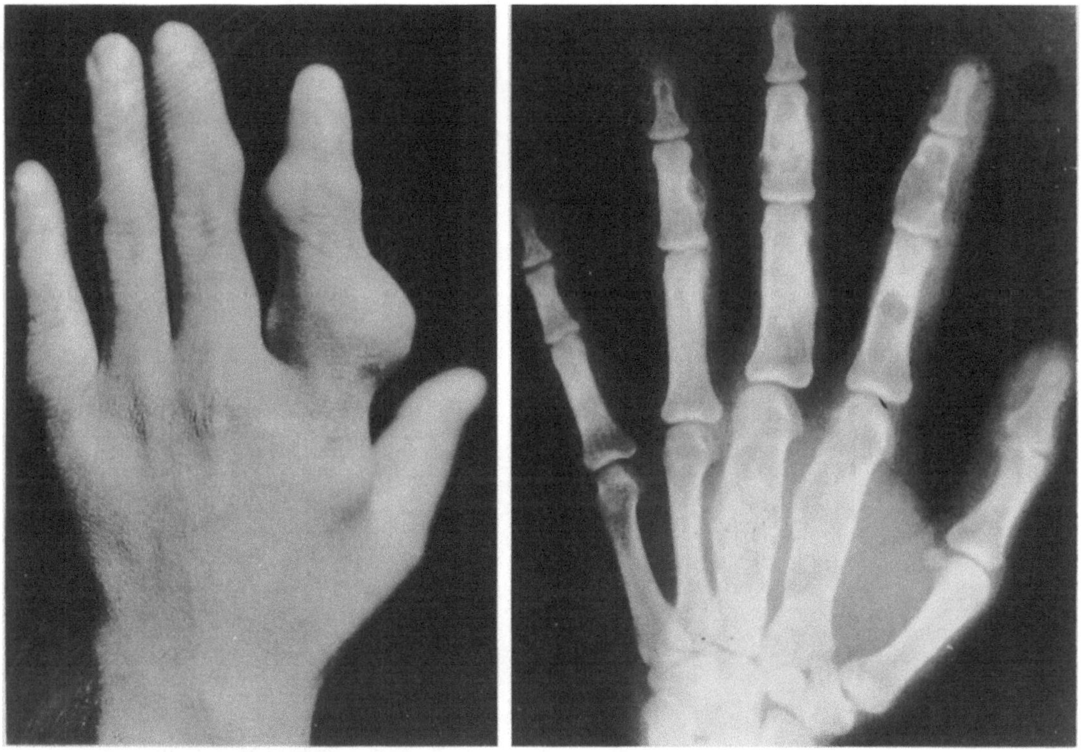

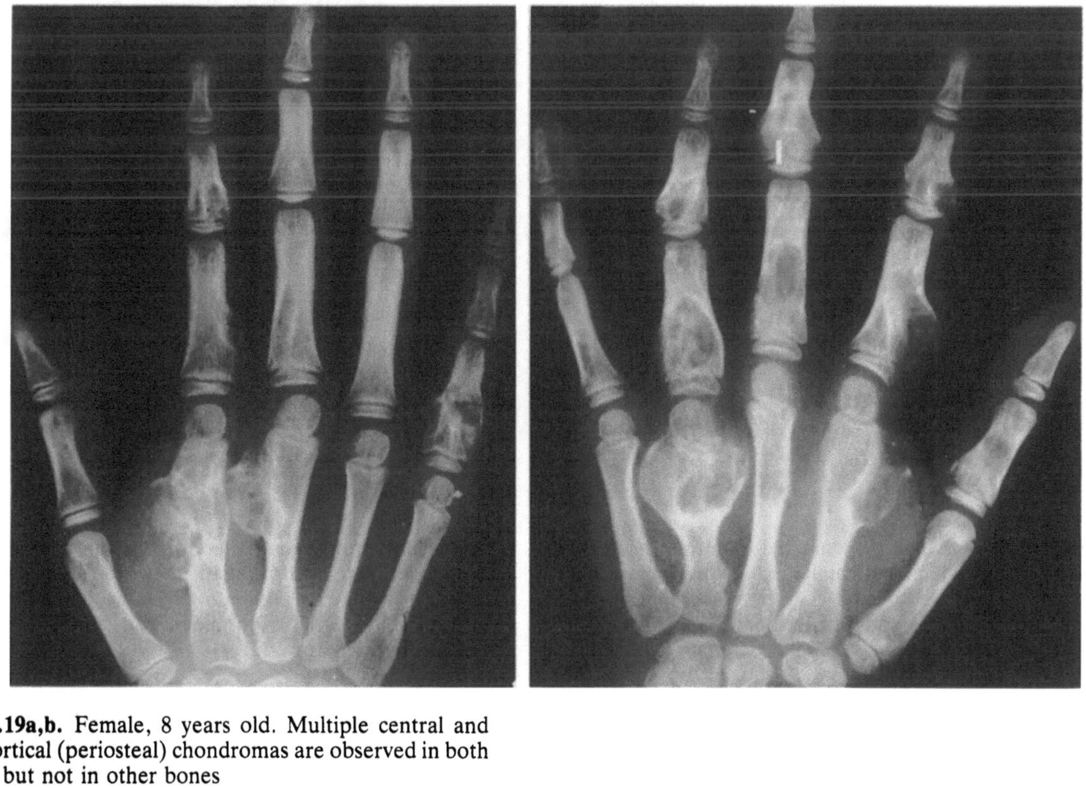

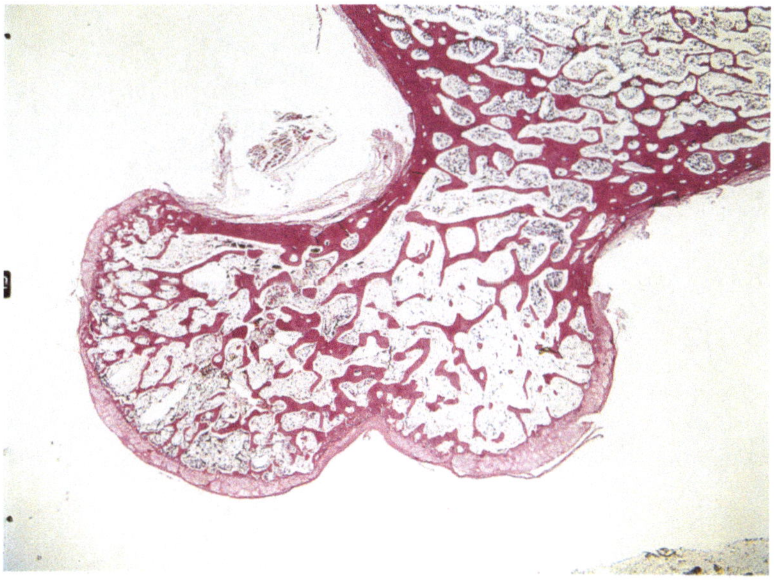

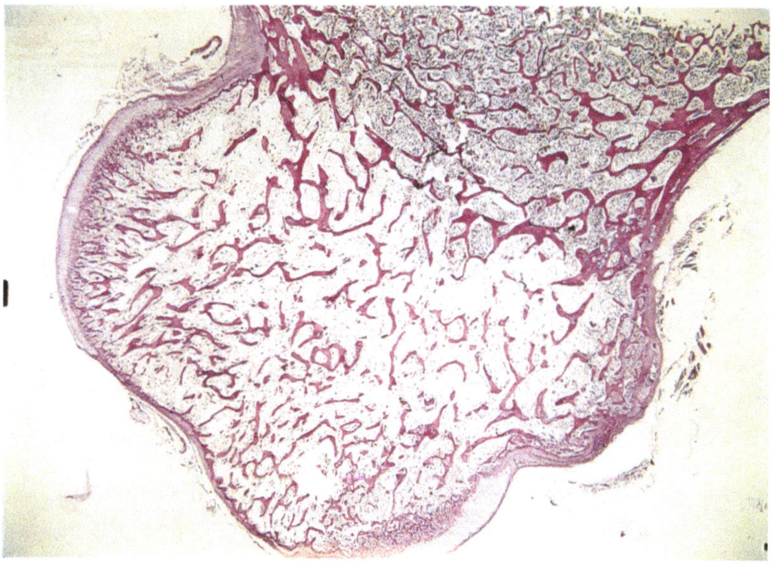

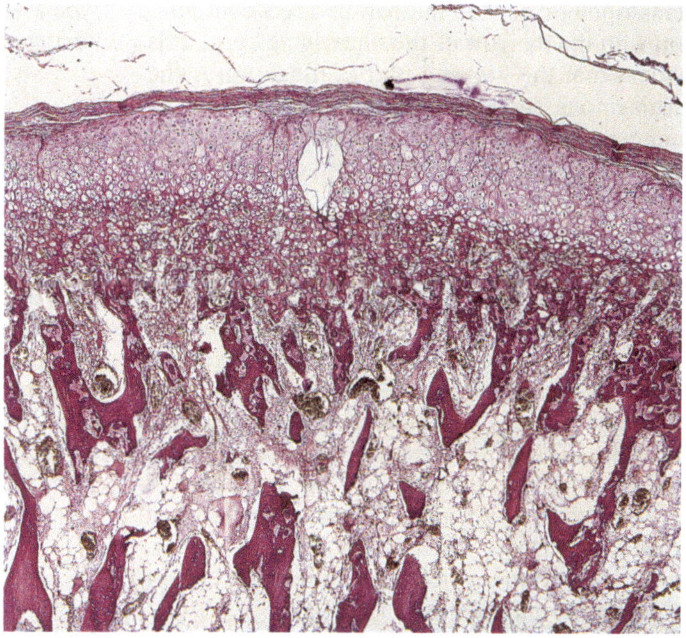

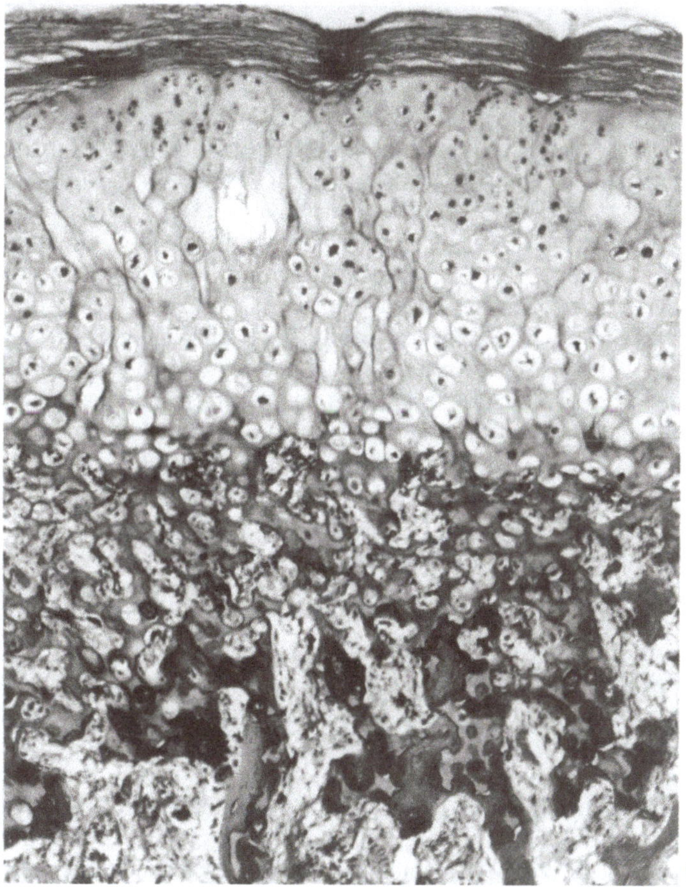

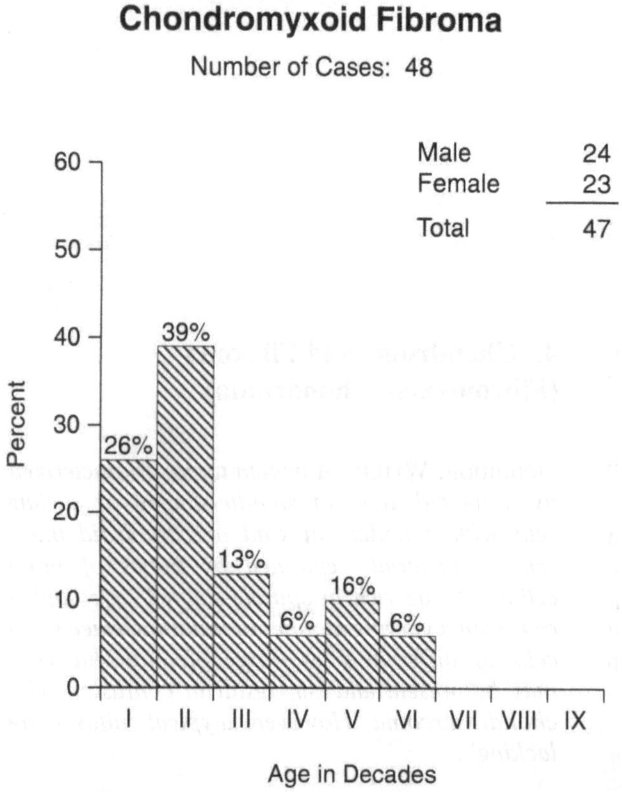

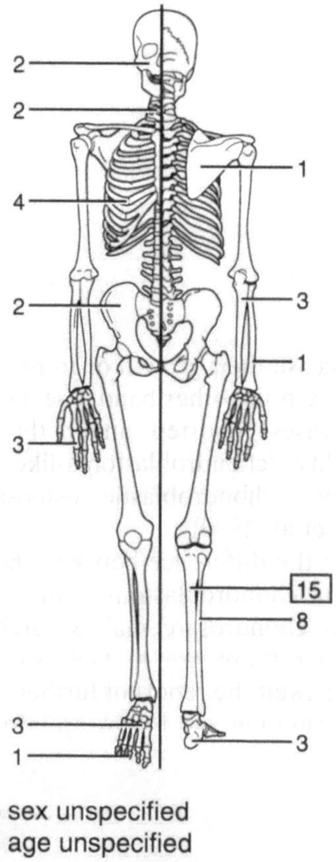

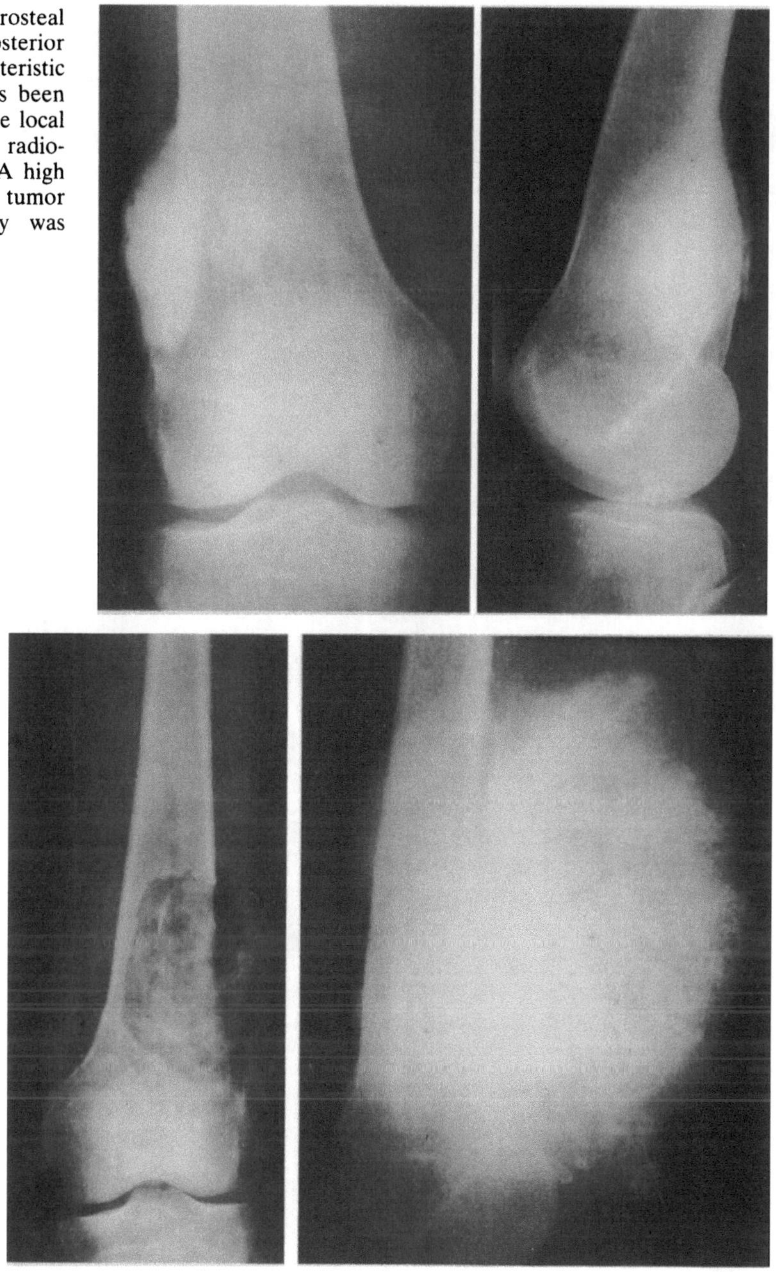

a b c

Fig. I.117a–c. Female, 26 years old. Parosteal osteosarcoma of the femur. **a,b** Anteroposterior and lateral radiographs show the characteristic pattern of this small tumor, which has been excised. **c** Recurrence 14 years after the local excision showing a large, extremely radiopaque tumor with irregular contours. A high thigh amputation was performed; tumor penetration of the medullary cavity was observed

metastases; three of these four died 4–7 months after the diagnosis. These lesions should be classified as high-grade surface osteosarcoma.

In at least some of the cases reported by Unni et al. (1976b) and others (Martínez-Tello and Navas-Palacios 1982; Sundaram et al. 1981), the tumors more closely corresponded to the entity classified by the WHO (1972) and by this author (1977) as juxtacortical (periosteal) chondrosarcoma (see Chap. II). We do not concur with a diagnosis of periosteal osteosarcoma in these patients because despite the clinical and radiographic similarity of these tumors to periosteal osteosarcomas, the histologic features differ (Martínez-Tello and Navas-Palacios 1982; Sundaram et al. 1981; Unni et al. 1976b). Areas that have been interpreted as lacelike osteoid, as shown in some of the published figures, correspond, in our opinion, to strands of cartilage or areas of enchondral ossification rather than to osteoid. Finally, the clinical course of these few patients justifies reclassification of the lesions.

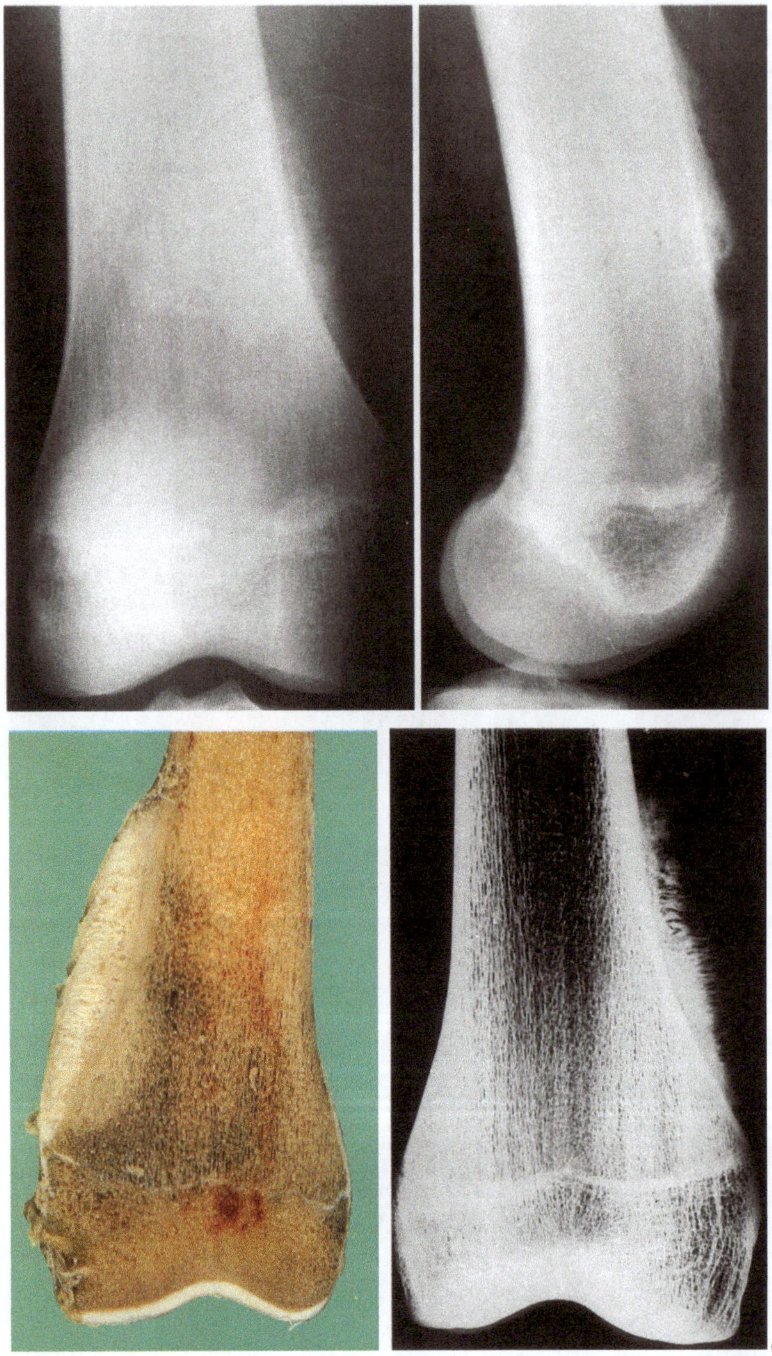

a b c

Fig. I.118a–c. Periosteal (peripheral) osteosarcoma of the femur in a 17-year-old male. **a** Anteroposterior and lateral radiographs show conspicuous periosteal "sunburst" bone formation in the lower diaphysis without involvement of the underlying cortex. **b** Photograph and **c** radiograph of the resected specimen show beginning intraosseous penetration of the predominantly cartilaginous tumor. The lesion recurred locally 14 months after segmental en bloc resection, followed by osteoarticular allograft and adjuvant chemotherapy; a high transfemoral amputation was performed. (Schajowicz 1983)

In periosteal osteosarcoma, the amount of malignant osteoid or bone is often negligible, and a small biopsy specimen may contain no osteoid at all but only cartilaginous tissue. The pathologist may then make a diagnosis of periosteal chondrosarcoma. In other specimens, the presence of strands of clacified cartilaginous foci or enchondral ossification, or of areas in which there is reactive bone formation, may lead to the conclusion that there is osteoid in a juxtacortical chondrosarcoma, resulting in an incorrect diagnosis of periosteal osteosarcoma. It is well known that accurate histologic definition of osteoid is difficult because there is no technique that clearly differentiates cartilaginous matrix tissue from osteoid or hyalinized fibrous tissue (see p. 18ff.).

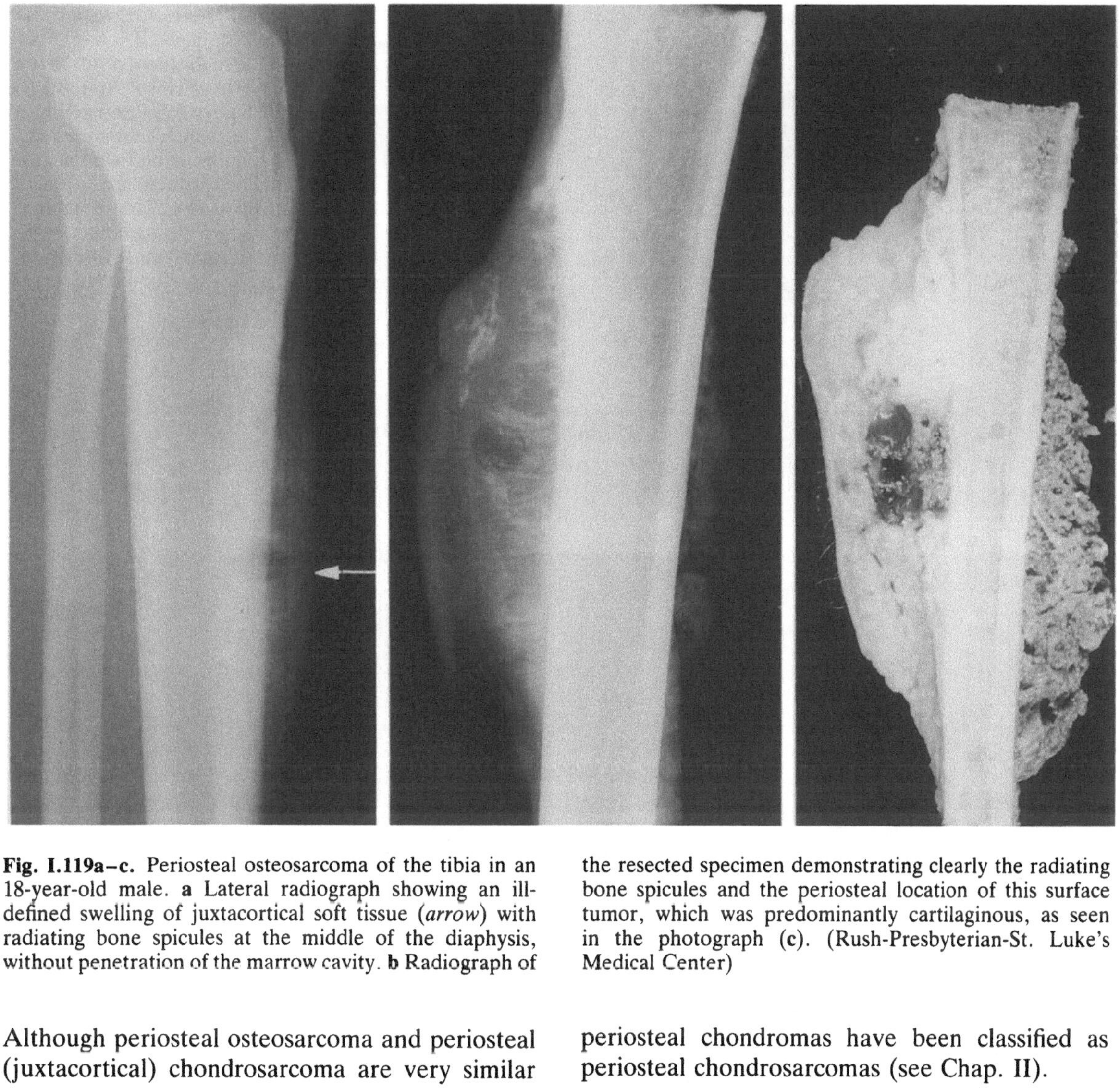

a b, c

Fig. I.119a–c. Periosteal osteosarcoma of the tibia in an 18-year-old male. **a** Lateral radiograph showing an ill-defined swelling of juxtacortical soft tissue (*arrow*) with radiating bone spicules at the middle of the diaphysis, without penetration of the marrow cavity. **b** Radiograph of the resected specimen demonstrating clearly the radiating bone spicules and the periosteal location of this surface tumor, which was predominantly cartilaginous, as seen in the photograph (**c**). (Rush-Presbyterian-St. Luke's Medical Center)

Although periosteal osteosarcoma and periosteal (juxtacortical) chondrosarcoma are very similar both clinically and radiographically and sometimes have been considered identical (Ayala 1978), several investigators (e.g., Bertoni et al. 1982; Nojima et al. 1985) have recently recognized them as distinct entities. This author believes, however, that several of their tumors, especially those located in the metaphysis showing a roentgenographic saucerlike depression with a reactive border towards the cancellous bone and a histologic low-grade malignancy, are actually periosteal chondromas (Fig. II.108b) rather than chondrosarcomas. The periosteal chondromas (Lichtenstein 1955; Schajowicz 1981) are more common than periosteal chondrosarcomas (Ayala 1978) and often show a histologically higher cellularity and more evident pleomorphism than central chondromas. It seems probable that some reported cases of cellular, active, or recurrent periosteal chondromas have been classified as periosteal chondrosarcomas (see Chap. II).

Radiographically, the lesions classified as periosteal osteosarcomas in our series were ill-defined, radiolucent soft tissue swellings with radiating spicules of bone arranged perpendicularly to the underlying bone cortex, usually at the midshaft, with frequent formation of a Codman's triangle (Figs. I.118–I.122). Grossly, the lesions were lobulated, predominantly cartilaginous, with areas of calcification and ossification with no or minimal involvement of the underlying cortex or marrow cavity (Figs. I.118–I.120). Histologically, all cases were *predominantly chondroblastic*, with lobules of malignant cartilage, but showing, in accordance with the classificatory criteria employed by Unni et al. (1976b), production of fine, lacelike osteoid trabeculae toward the center (Figs. I.121, I.122). Only four of Unni et al.'s 23 patients died of metastatic disease, and

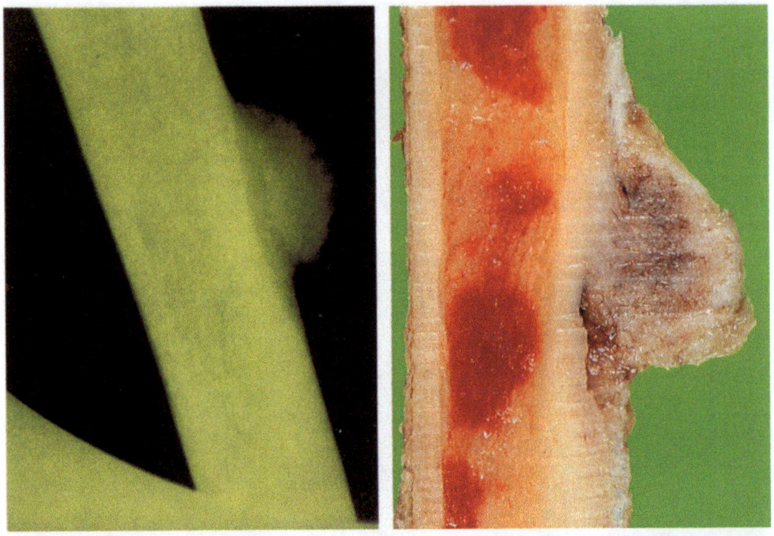

a b

Fig. I.120a,b. Periosteal osteosarcoma of the humerus in a 20-year-old female. **a** Radiograph shows a soft tissue swelling, slightly calcified, on the surface of the diaphysis. **b** Photograph of the resection specimen shows the location of the tumor at the external surface of the bone without involvement of the marrow cavity. The lesion was predominantly cartilaginous with scarce areas of tumor bone formation

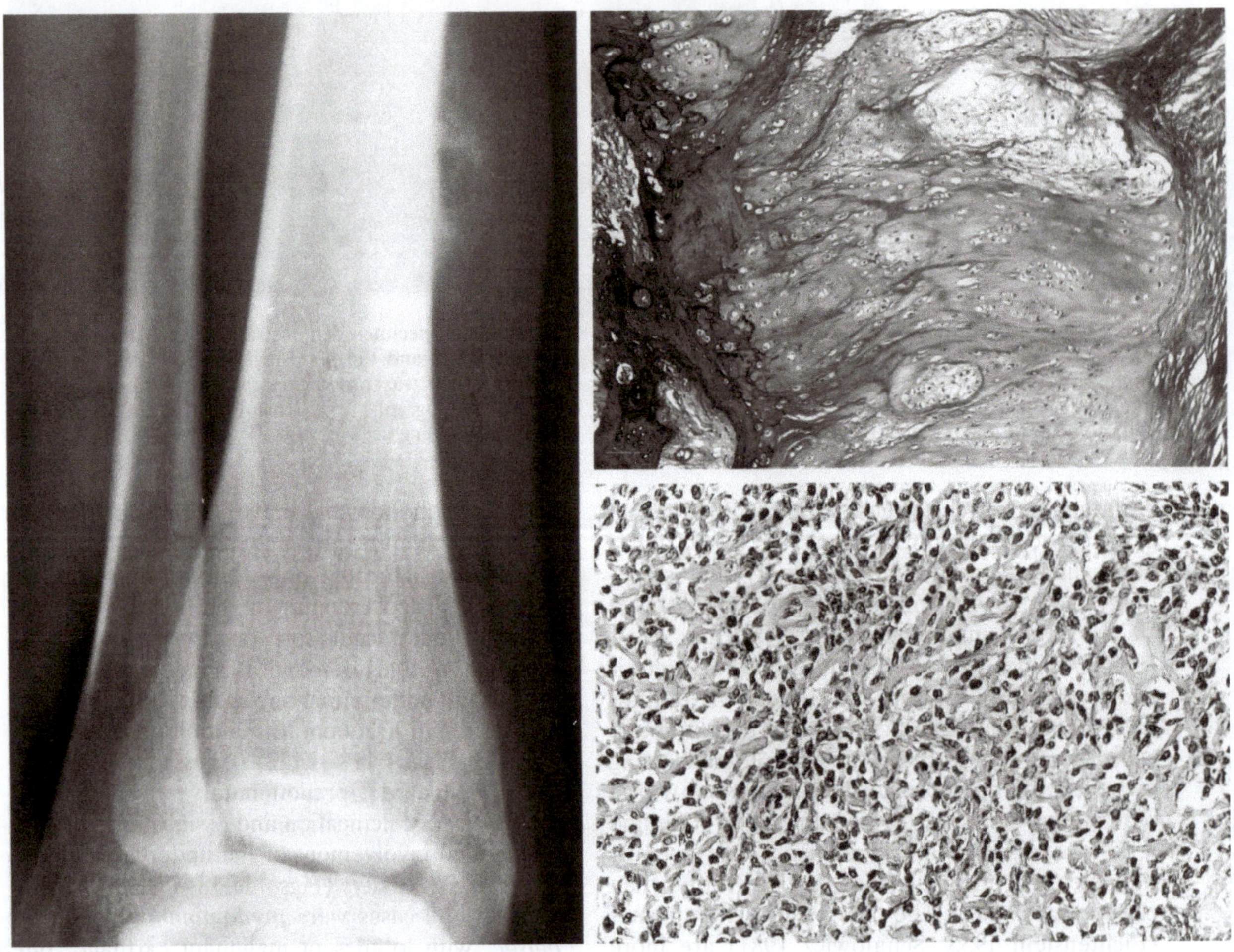

a

Fig. I.121a–c. Periosteal osteosarcoma of the tibia in a 16-year-old girl. **a** Anterolateral radiograph showing an ill-defined radiolucent swelling of soft tissue with radiating bone spicules located at the middle of the shaft, but without involvement of the marrow cavity. The patient was alive and free of disease 12 years after a segmental en bloc resection and subsequent intercalary allograft. **b** Photomicrograph showing the resorbed cortex and the proliferating cartilage (*right*). The cartilage is forming lobules and is covered by periosteum. **c** Photomicrograph of another area showing a network of fine lacelike tumor osteoid trabeculae. (Schajowicz et al. 1988) **b** ×100, **c** ×200

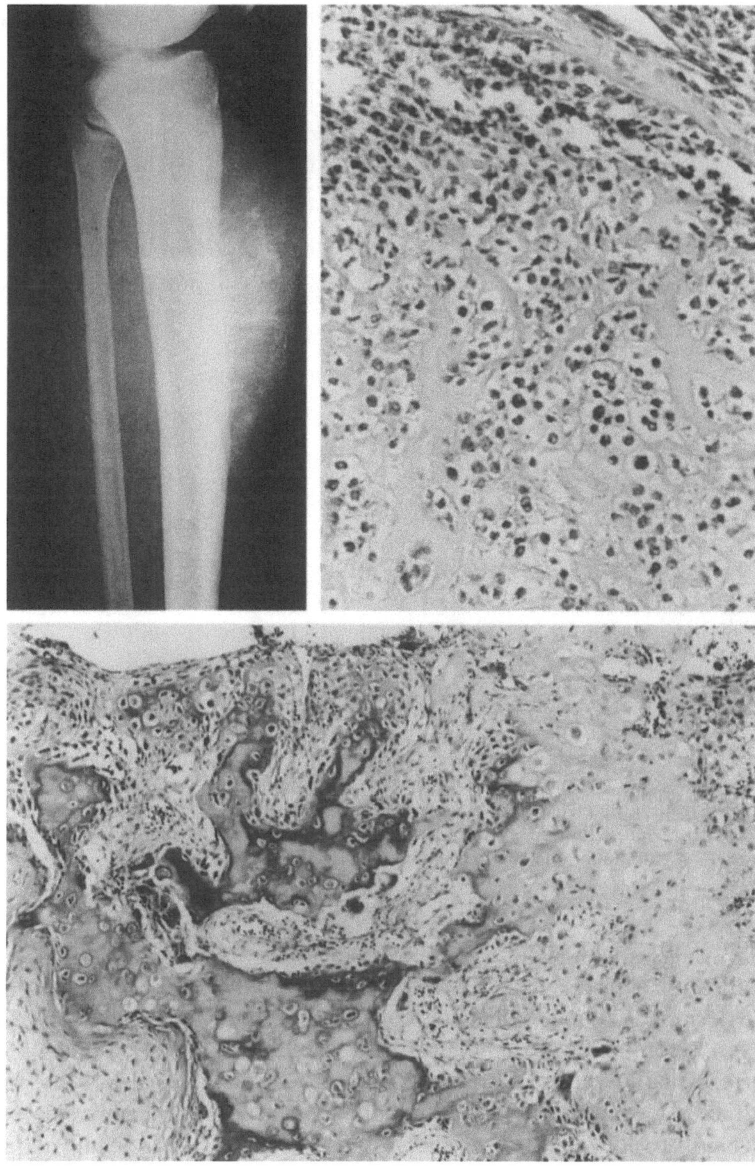

a b c

Fig. I.122a–c. Periosteal osteosarcoma of the tibia in a 17-year-old boy. **a** The lateral radiograph shows a large lesion of the anterior aspect of the diaphysis with radiating bone spicules arranged perpendicularly to the underlying cortex, apparently without penetrating the medullary cavity. An open biopsy followed by a partial resection was performed. **b** Photomicrograph shows that the tumor was predominantly chondroblastic with lobules of actively proliferating cartilage, especially at its periphery. **c** Area of cartilage calcification and enchondral ossification. **b** ×180, **c** ×100

our series had a similar mortality (three of nine patients died). These outcomes suggest that despite the sometimes medium-grade malignant appearance of the chondroblastic tissue, wide en bloc resection can be regarded as appropriate therapy.

As stated above, in periosteal osteosarcoma production of malignant osteoid or bone is often scarce and focal. A small biopsy specimen may miss the malignant tumor bone and show only cartilaginous tissue, misleading the pathologist to make the diagnosis of periosteal chondrosarcoma (Schajowicz 1977; Schajowicz 1981). Conversely, strands of calcified cartilage, enchondral ossification, or reactive bone formation may be misinterpreted by the pathologist as tumor bone or osteoid in a case of periosteal (juxtacortical) chondrosarcoma (Fig. I.122c) and lead to the incorrect diagnosis of periosteal osteosarcoma (see Chap. II).

High-Grade Surface Osteosarcoma

High-grade surface (peripheral conventional) osteosarcoma is indistinguishable histologically from conventional high-grade intramedullary osteosarcoma, but it is much less common (Schajowicz et al. 1988). Radiographically, it appears as a small or moderate-sized lesion (Figs.

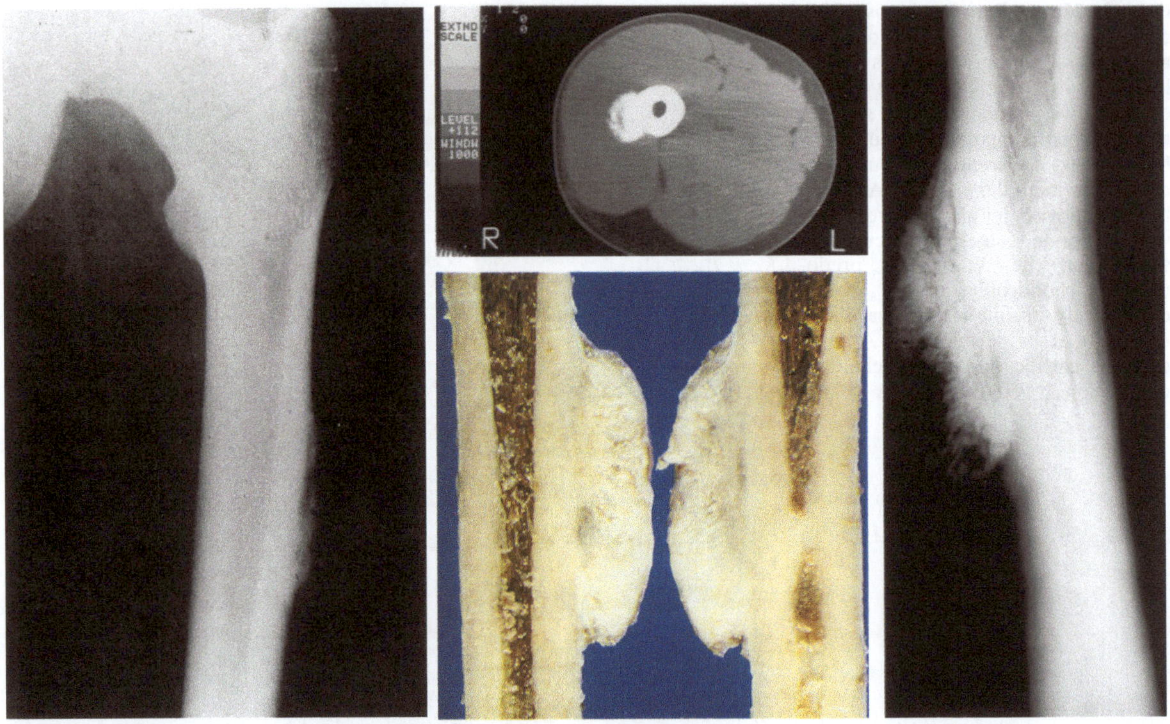

a b–d

Fig. I.123a–d. High-grade surface (peripheral conventional) osteosarcoma of the femoral shaft in a 17-year-old boy. **a** Radiograph showing the small, partly ossified, apparently well-delimited lesion, probably in an early stage. A segmental en bloc resection followed by an intercalary allograft was performed. **b** CT scan, **c** photograph, and **d** radiograph of the specimen reveal clearly the lesion at the surface of the bone without medullary penetration. (Schajowicz et al. 1988)

I.123–I.126), with slight to heavy calcification or ossification (Figs. I.123, I.124). The broad base of the lesion abuts the adjacent cortex, and the lesion is commonly more mineralized close to the cortex. In our series, there were six high-grade surface osteosarcomas, with only slight superficial cortical erosion in three of the lesions. In two lesions, scarce areas of sclerosis adjacent to the inner surface of the cortex were suggestive of medullary penetration. In three cases, there was an evident Codman's triangle at one or both ends of the tumor. The surface border of the tumor was often well defined, but radiating spicules of bone perpendicular to the underlying cortex were rarely seen (cases 1 and 6) (Fig. I.125). The radiographic features were sometimes very similar to those of periosteal osteosarcoma.

The term "peripheral conventional osteosarcoma" (Schajowicz 1983) was proposed for this type of tumor to emphasize that when an osteosarcoma on the surface of a bone is highly malignant histologically, the course will be similar to that of conventional central osteosarcoma. High-grade surface tumors may show extensive intramedullary involvement (two of six patients in our series) and usually carry a poor prognosis. The six surface lesions in the series of Ahuja et al. (1977) and the nine in the series of Campanacci et al. (1984), which were rated as grade III histologically but were included in the category of parosteal (juxtacortical) osteosarcoma, should, in our opinion, be reclassified as high-grade surface osteosarcomas.

In the series reported by Ahuja et al., five of the six patients who had a grade III lesion died of metastatic disease 10 months to 6 years and 10 months after early radical surgical intervention. Four of the eight patients who had a grade III tumor and adequate follow-up in the series of Campanacci et al. died of pulmonary metastases. All four patients had medullary involvement before distant spread. Wold et al. (1984a) reported on nine patients who had a tumor similar to those reported by this author, Ahuja et al., and Campanacci et al. Seven of the nine patients died, despite ablative surgical intervention. The cases of these nine patients were also described by Dahlin and Unni (1986). In our opinion, 8 of the

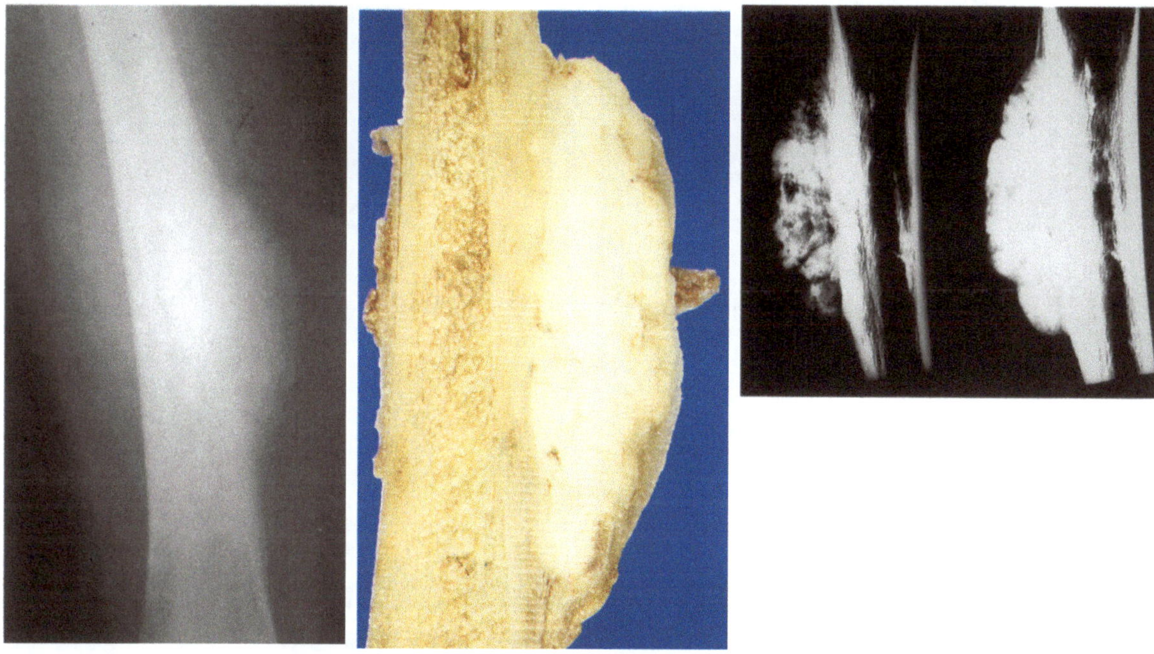

a

b, c

Fig. I.124a–c. High-grade surface (peripheral conventional) osteosarcoma of the femur in a 12-year-old girl. **a** Antero-posterior radiograph shows a dense, sclerotic, apparently well-delineated lesion in the diaphysis. The age of the patient and the site of the lesion were not compatible with a diagnosis of parosteal osteosarcoma. **b** Photograph and **c** radiograph of the resected specimen show the lesion at the external surface of the bone, without involvement of the marrow cavity. The tumor recurred locally, 10 months after a segmental en bloc resection. The patient died of pulmonary metastasis 8 months later. (Schajowicz et al. 1988)

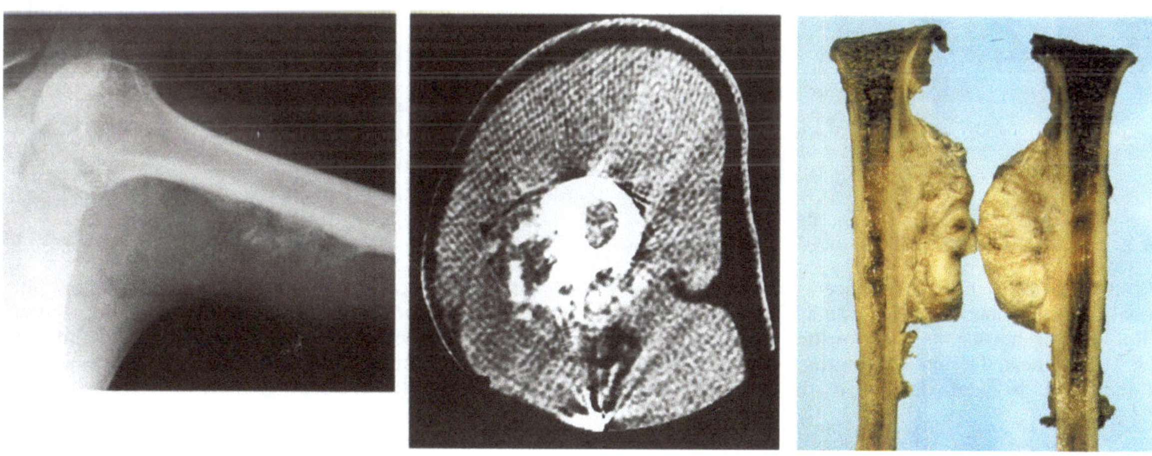

a

b, c

Fig. I.125a–c. High-grade surface (peripheral conventional) osteosarcoma of the humerus in a 14-year-old boy. **a** Radiograph showing the tumor on the surface of the proximal diaphysis with radiating bone spicules. **b** CT scan revealing the juxtacortical location of the poorly delimited tumor, which is also clearly seen in **c** the photograph of the resected specimen. (Schajowicz and McGuire 1989)

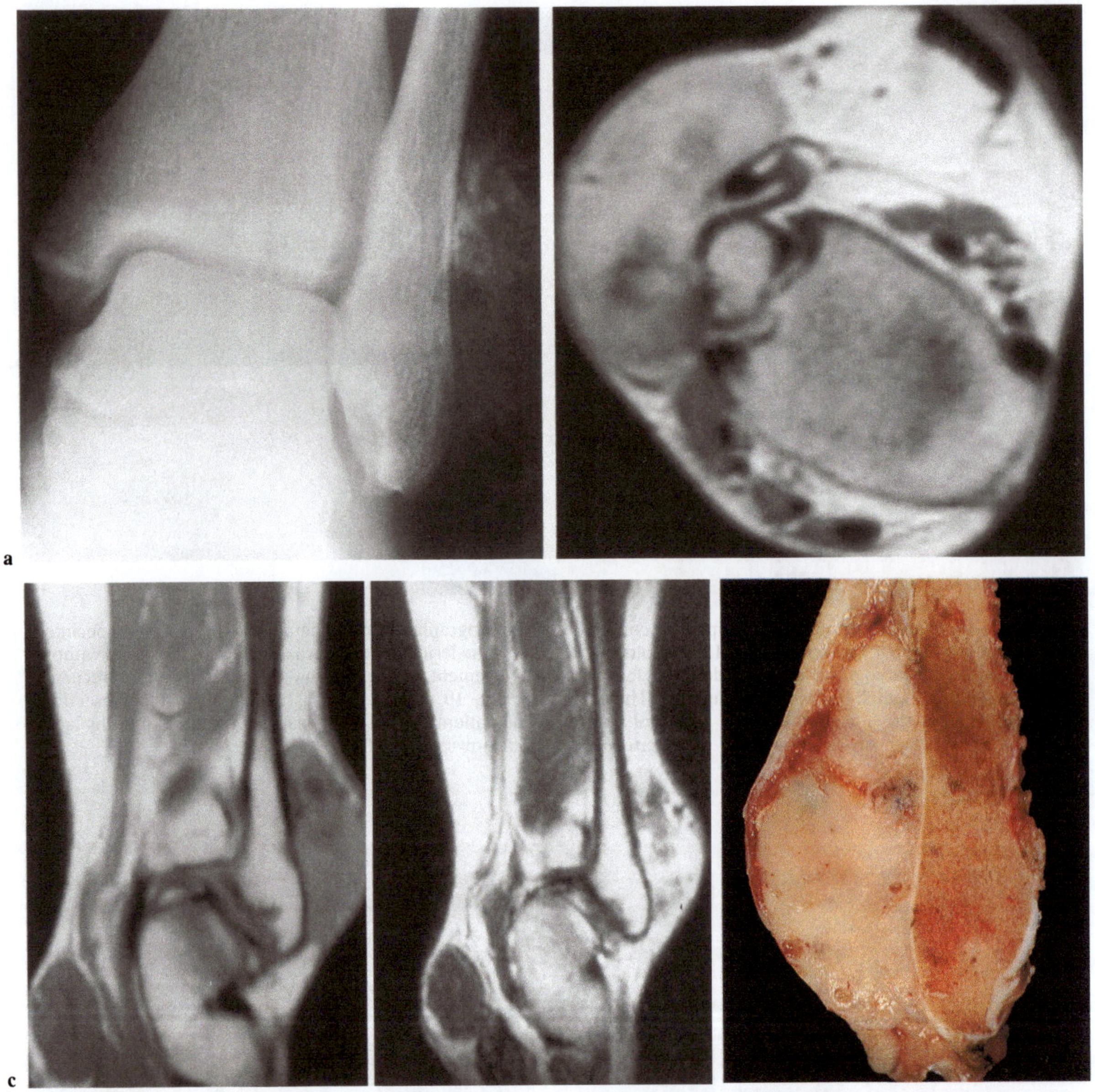

Fig. I.126a–d. High-grade surface (peripheral conventional) osteosarcoma of the fibula in a 35-year-old female. **a** Radiograph showing the partly ossified, apparently small and well-delineated lesion at the surface of the lower third of the bone. **b** Transaxial and **c** coronal T1- and T2-weighted MRI scans show the extent of the tumor, but without penetration of the marrow cavity. **d** Photograph of the resection specimen reveals the large size and the juxtacortical location of the tumor. (St. Louis University Medical Center)

13 periosteal osteosarcomas that were reported by Spjut et al. (1977) should also be reclassified as high-grade surface osteosarcomas because of their prominent osteoblastic and highly malignant histologic features. In that series, four patients died of pulmonary metastases 14 months to 7 years after the diagnosis.

Radiographically, it is often difficult to distinguish the heavily ossified high-grade surface osteosarcoma from parosteal osteosarcoma. However, the young age of the patient, the diaphyseal location, and, above all, the associated histologic features of a high-grade, predominantly osteoblastic lesion permit differentiation from other types of surface osteosarcoma (parosteal and periosteal) (Fig. I.127). In the initial stages of high-grade surface osteosarcoma (Fig. I.123), it may be impossible to differentiate the lesion

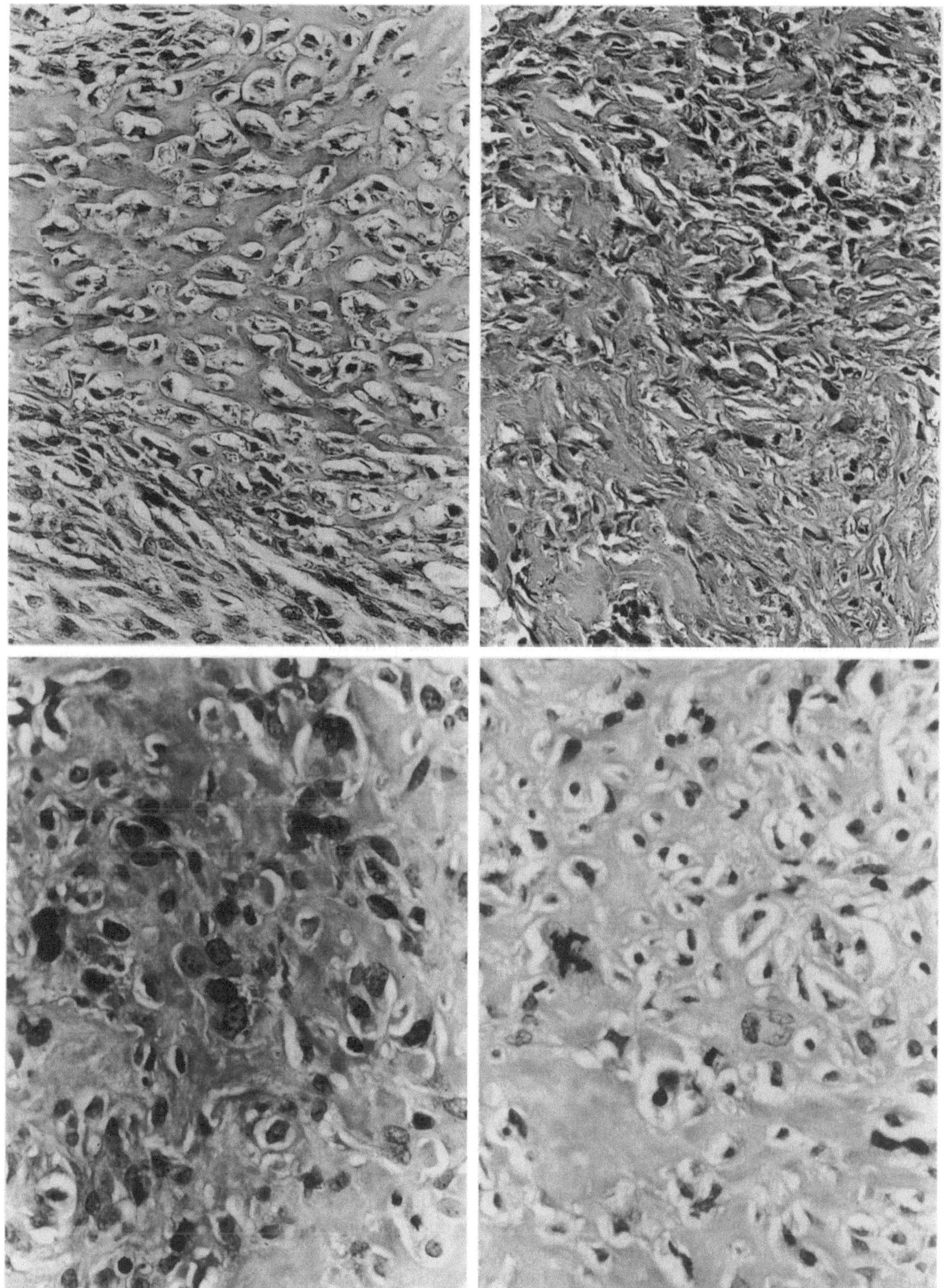

a b c d

Fig. I.127a–d. Photomicrographs of high-grade surface osteosarcoma showing at lower (**a**,**b**) and higher (**c**,**d**) magnification the conspicuous formation of a dense network of thin, lacelike osteoid and bone trabeculae by atypical pleomorphic osteoblasts and atypical mitosis. **a**,**b** ×100; **c**,**d** ×400 clinically or radiographically from periosteal osteosarcoma, and then only histopathologic study allows the correct diagnosis (Fig. I.127). The diagnosis is of fundamental importance, because the two tumors are associated with different prognoses.

Pathogenesis of Osteosarcoma

Despite considerable advances in research on the possible viral etiology and other causes of human osteosarcoma [cytogenetic factors; involvement of the retinoblastoma (RB) gene], the etiology of most osteosarcomas remains obscure.

Several agents are known to induce osteosarcomas in experimental animals, especially chemical products such as methylcholanthrene and particularly beryllium (Janes 1969, and others). Numerous radionuclides that localize in bone (bone seeking) have been reported to induce bone tumors in the laboratory, and all mammals thus far tested with appropriate dosages of either internal or external radiation have developed osteosarcomas.

The older best-known examples of bone tumors induced in humans resulted from exposure to the radiation emitted from the luminous dials in the watch industry (Martland 1931) or from ingestion of radioactive particles of radium 226 by dial painters. Another cause was internal radiation by radium salts or mesothorium administered orally or intravenously for therapeutic purposes in various diseases, especially rheumatoid arthritis.

At present, the best-known examples of osteosarcoma that suggest an apparent pathogenesis include neoplasms arising after exposure to x-ray irradiation and those resulting from a preexisting disease, Paget disease and fibrous dysplasia being the most common examples. Both are precursors of osteosarcoma and fibrosarcoma (and rarely of other tumor types), and are discussed in Chap. VIII.

Numerous attempts have been made to implicate viruses in human bone sarcomas, and some evidence seems to confirm that they do play a role. Finkel and associates (1973) summarized their work and reviewed the evidence obtained in their laboratories for a human osteosarcoma virus. Several viruses that induce bone tumors when injected into newborn mice have been isolated from murine bone tumors, among them FBJ osteosarcoma virus, a C-type RNA virus, originally from a CF_1 osteosarcoma. FBJ tumors contain many virus particles. Evidence for a human bone tumor virus includes the appearance of bone-forming tumors and fibrosarcomas in Syrian hamsters inoculated soon after birth with cell-free extracts of human osteosarcomas, the presence of human sarcoma-specific antigen in some of the experimentally induced hamster tumors, and the presence of C-type particles in both human and hamster tumors.

Although it is now accepted that many tumors are caused by viruses or virus-associated inherited information, there is as yet no unequivocal demonstration of the recovery of a virus from any human osteosarcoma.

The immunofluorescence studies of Morton and Malmgren (1968) and Eilber and Morton (1970) indicated a high incidence of antibodies in the sera of patients with this disease and in those of their family members and close associates, which react with a common antigen (or antigens) in osteosarcomas. The distribution of these antibodies suggests the association of an infectious agent with this neoplasm, capable of producing unrecognized infections in healthy contacts of these patients.

Three additional etiologic agents, although of minor importance, have been mentioned: *genetic factors*, *bone infarcts* (Fig. I.128), and *trauma*. In 1967, the writer, in collaboration with Bessone, reported three siblings affected with chondrosarcomas. Miller and McLaughlin published in 1977 a report of two sisters with osteosarcomas; in a search of the literature since 1935, they found 13 case reports of osteosarcomas in siblings, the most remarkable being that of Harmon and Morton (1966) of osteosarcomas in four siblings. In addition, Epstein et al. (1970) and Swaney (1973) described a family in which both father and daughters died of osteosarcoma, and Schimke et al. (1974) published two cases of osteosarcomas in siblings who had bilateral retinoblastoma in infancy. A genetically transmitted predisposing factor has been suggested in these rare cases.

The role of trauma as an etiologic factor has been extensively discussed in the literature; however, there is no clear evidence that a single trauma, relatively common in children, may produce a bone tumor (Monkman et al. 1974). It appears that trauma calls attention to already existing lesions rather than contributing to their genesis.

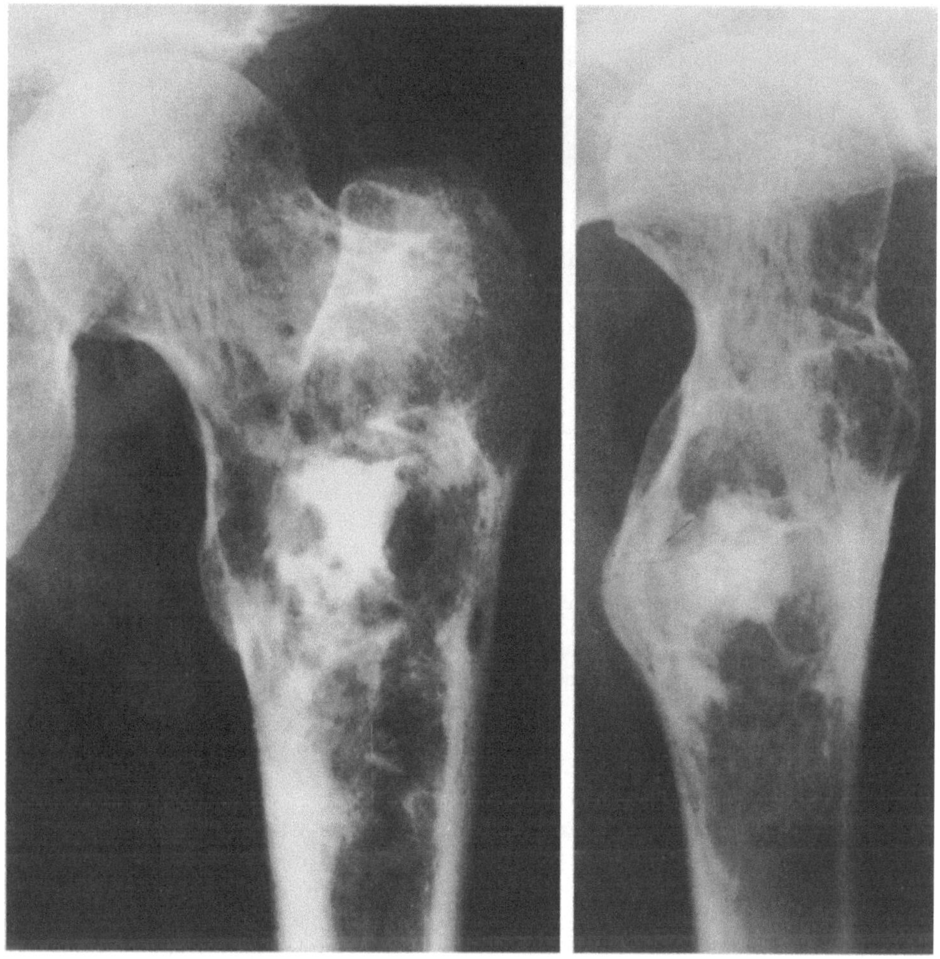

a b

Fig. I.128a,b. Male, 53 years old. Osteosarcoma with bone infarct of femur. Radiographs show a radiolucent permeative lesion of the intertrochanteric region extending into the diaphysis with a central sclerotic calcified mass. A diagnosis could not be made. A curettage was performed, and the histologic study revealed an osteosarcoma associated with bone infarct

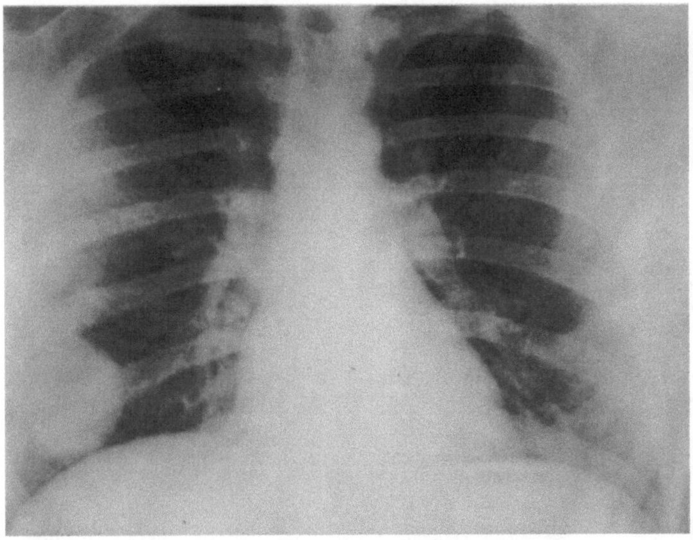
a

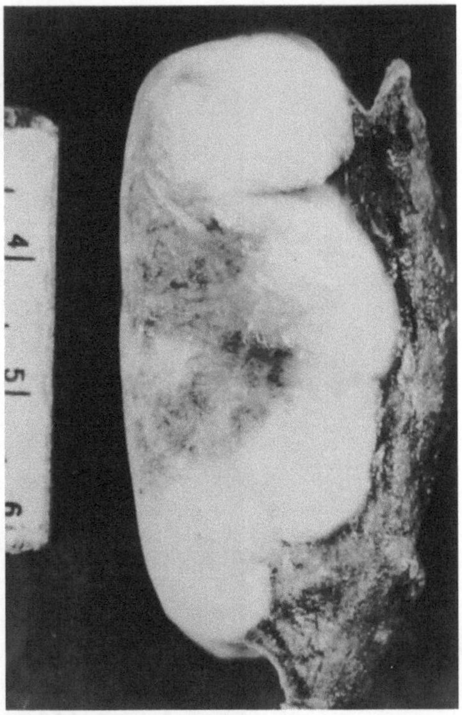

b

Fig. I.129a,b. Male, 20 years old. Osteosarcoma, fibroblastic type with lung metastases. **a** Radiograph showing a single nodule in the left lower lung. **b** Photograph of the subpleural lung metastasis of approximately 5 cm in its largest diameter

Treatment of Conventional Osteosarcoma

See Chap. X.

Metastasis

The common mechanism of metastasis in osteosarcoma is the hematogenous route to the lungs (Figs. I.129, I.130). It is now generally accepted that pulmonary micrometastases already exist when the primary tumor is discovered. Lymphatic metastases are rare and were found in only four of our cases. Similar findings have been reported in the literature (Dahlin and Coventry 1967; Spjut et al. 1971; McKenna et al. 1966). Somewhat more frequent metastases are observed in one or more bones (Dahlin 1978). In 14% of their osteosarcomas, McKenna et al. (1966) observed metastases in other bones in a preterminal stage. At present the more common use of scintigraphy with technetium has demonstrated that bone metastases are more frequent than previously reported.

Uribe-Botero et al. (1977), in a clinicopathologic investigation of 243 cases of primary osteosarcoma of bone, including a detailed analysis of 54 cases with complete postmortem examination from the M.D. Anderson Tumor Institute, found metastases in the following organs in decreasing frequency: lung, 53 cases (98%); bone, 20 cases (37%); pleura, 18 cases (33.3%); heart, 11 cases (20.4%); kidney and liver, 9 cases (11.1%); and other organs (<10%), including lymph nodes, with only 4 cases (7.4%). In the 32 cases in which the primary lesion was located in the femur, metastases were found in the lung in 100% and in bones in 28.1%.

Fig. I.130a,b. Photomicrographs showing micrometastases of osteosarcoma in lung. **a** × 100, **b** ×200

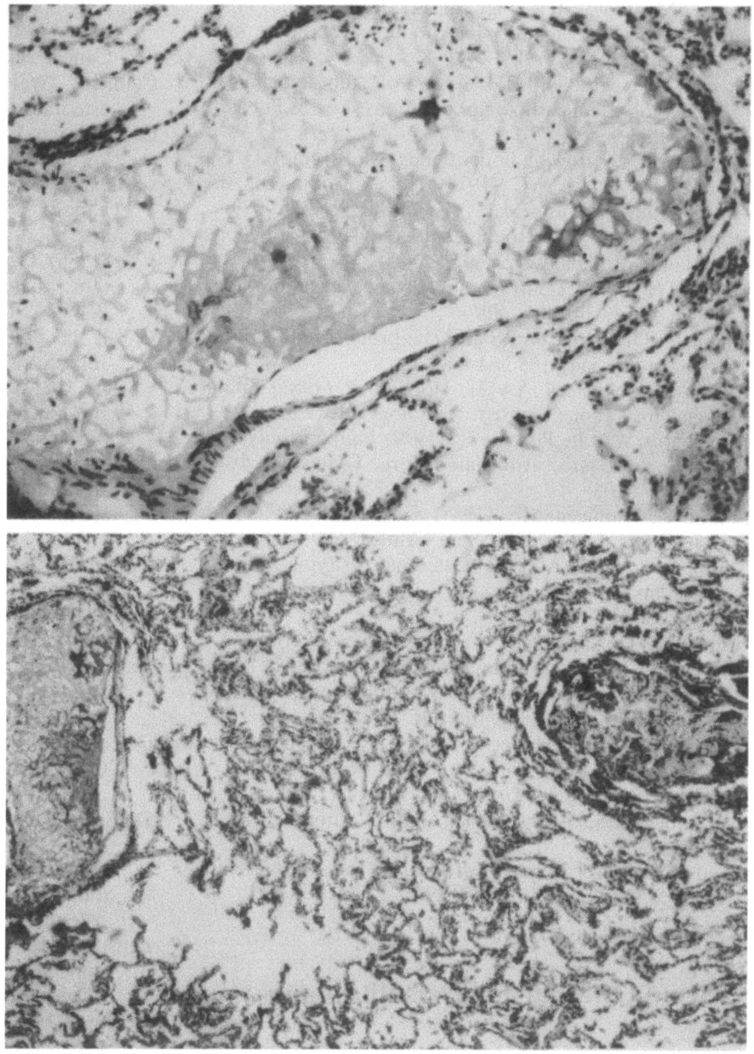

a

b

References

Osteoma

Andrew J (1956) Osteomata of the paranasal sinus. Br J Surg 43:489

Blank N, Lieber A (1965) The significance of growing bone islands. Radiology 85:508–511

Bullough PG (1965) Ivory exostosis of the skull. Postgrad Med J 41:277–281

Chang CH, Piatt ED, Thomas KE, Watne AL (1968) Bone abnormalities in Gardner's syndrome. Am J Roentgenol Radium Ther Nucl Med 103:645

Davies JAK, Mall FM, Goldberg RP et al. (1979) Positive bone scan in bone island. J Bone Joint Surg [Am] 61:943

Echlin F (1934) Cranial osteomas and hyperostoses produced by meningeal fibroblastomas. Arch Surg 28:357

Gardner E (1951) A genetic and clinical study of intestinal polyposis. Am J Hum Genet 3:167

Gardner EJ, Richards RE (1953) Multiple cutaneous and subcutaneous lesions occurring simultaneously with hereditary polyposis and osteomatosis. Am J Hum Genet 5:139–147

Gold RH, Mirra JM, Remotti F et al. (1989) Case report 527. Skeletal Radiol 18:129

Graham MD (1979) Osteomas and exostoses of the external auditory canal. A clinical, histopathological and scanning electron microscopic study. Ann Otol Rhinol Laryngol 88:556–572

Greenspan A, Steiner G, Knotzon R (1991) Bone island enostosis: clinical significance and radiologic and pathologic correlations. Skeletal Radiol 20:85–90

Jaffe HL (1958) Tumors and tumorous conditions of the bones and joints. Lea & Febiger, Philadelphia

Jones EL, Cornell WP (1966) Gardner's syndrome. Review of literature and report on family. Arch Surg 92:287–300

Kim SK, Barry WF (1968) Bone islands. Radiology 90: 77–78

Makrycostas K (1927) Über das Wirbelangiom, Lipom und Osteom. Virchows Arch [A] 265:259–303

Mirra JM, Gold RH, Pignatti G, Remotti F (1988) Compact osteoma of iliac bone: case report 497. Skeletal Radiol 17:437–442
Mirra JM, Picci P, Gold RH (1989) Bone tumors: clinical, radiologic and pathologic conditions. Lea & Febiger, Philadelphia
Ngan H (1972) Growing bone islands. Clin Radiol 23:199
Noren GD, Roche WC (1978) Huge osteoma of the mandible: report of case. J Oral Surg 36:375–379
Ornitsuka H (1977) Roentgenologic aspects of bone islands. Radiology 123:607
Palmer TH Jr (1982) Gardner's syndrome: six generations. Am J Surg 143:405–408
Phemister DB, Grimson KS (1937) Fibrous osteoma of the jaws. Ann Surg 105:564–583
Resnick D, Nemicek AA Jr, Hoglight P (1983) Spinal enostosis (bone islands). Radiology 147:373
Schuchardt WA Jr, Ponsky JL (1979) Familial polyposis and Gardner's syndrome. Surg Gynecol Obstet 148:97–103
Simon K, Mulligan ME (1985) Growing bone islands revisited. J Bone Joint Surg [Am] 67:809–811
Smith A, Zavaleta A (1952) Osteoma, ossifying fibroma, and fibrous dysplasia of facial and cranial bones. Arch Pathol 54:507–527
Spjut HJ, Dorfman HD, Fechner RE, Ackerman LV (1971) Tumors of bone and cartilage. Atlas of tumor pathology, 2nd series, Fasc 5. Armed Forces Institute of Pathology, Washington, DC
Stern PJ, Lim EV, Krieg JK (1985) Giant metacarpal osteoma. J Bone Joint Surg [Am] 67:487–489
Tamarit LV, Pardo J (1977) Parosteal osteoma: a clinicopathologic approach. Pathol Annu 12 (Pt 1): 373–387
Teed RW (1941) Primary osteoma of the frontal sinus. Arch Otolaryngol 33:255–292

Osteoid Osteoma and Osteoblastoma

Adbelwahab I, Frankel VH, Klein MJ (1986) Aggressive osteoblastoma of the third lumbar vertebra. Case report 351. Skeletal Radiol 15:165
Akbarnia BA, Rooholamini SA (1981) Scoliosis caused by benign osteoblastoma of the thoracic or lumbar spine. J Bone Joint Surg [Am] 63:1146
Alcalay M, Clarac JP, Bontaoux D (1982) Double osteoid-osteoma in adjacent carpal bones: a case report. J Bone Joint Surg [Am] 64:779–780
Ayala A, Murray JA, Erling MA et al. (1986) Osteoid-osteoma: intraoperative tetracycline-fluorescence demonstration of the nidus. J Bone Joint Surg [Am] 68:747
Bertoni F, Unni KK, McLeod RA et al. (1985) Osteosarcoma resembling osteoblastoma. Cancer 55:416
Bettelli G, Capanna R, Van Horn JR et al. (1989) Osteoid osteoma and osteoblastoma of the pelvis. Clin Orthop 247:261–271
Bettelli G, Tigani D, Picci P (1991) Recurring osteoblastoma initially presenting as a typical osteoid osteoma. Skeletal Radiol 20:1–4
Bisset GS, Kaufman RA, Towbin R, Bove KE (1987) Recurrent sacral osteoblastoma: case report 452. Skeletal Radiol 16:666–669
Byers PD (1968) Solitary benign osteoblastic lesions of bone. Osteoid osteoma and benign osteoblastoma. Cancer 22:43–57
Caldicott WJH (1969) Diagnosis of spinal osteoid osteoma. Radiology 92:1192
Campanacci M (1990) Bone and soft tissue tumors. Springer, Vienna New York
Canepa G, DeFabiani F (1965) Osteoid osteoma in the hand .J Bone Joint Surg [Am] 35:888–893
Capanna R, Van Horn JR, Ayala A, Picci P, Betteli G (1986) Osteoid osteoma and osteoblastoma of the talus: a report of 40 cases. Skeletal Radiol 15:360–364
Caroll RE (1953) Osteoid osteoma in the hand. J Bone Joint Surg [Am] 35:888–893
Corbett JM, Wilde AH, McCormack J, Evarts CM (1974) Intra-articular osteoid osteoma. A diagnostic problem. Clin Orthop 98:225–230
Cronemeyer RL, Kirchmer NA, DeSmet AA et al. (1981) Intra-articular osteoid-osteoma of the humerus simulating synovitis of the elbow: a case report. J Bone Joint Surg [Am] 63:1172
Dahlin DC (1978) Bone tumors, 3rd edn. Charles C. Thomas, Springfield, IL
Dahlin DC, Johnson EW Jr (1954) Giant osteoid osteoma. J Bone Joint Surg [Am] 36:559–572
Dahlin DC, Unni KK (1986) Bone tumors: general aspects and data on 8542 cases. Charles C. Thomas, Springfield, IL
DeCoster E, Van Tiggelen R, Shahabpour M et al. (1989) Osteoblastoma of the patella: case report and review of the literature. Clin Orthop 234:216–219
De Souza Dias L, Frost HM (1973) Osteoblastoma of the spine: a review and report of eight new cases. Clin Orthop Rel Res 91:141
De Souza Dias L, Frost HM (1974) Osteoid osteoma – osteoblastoma. Cancer 33:1075–1081
Dorfman HD (1973) Malignant transformation of benign bone lesions. Proceedings of the 7th National Cancer Conference. J.B. Lippincott, Philadelphia, p 901
Dorfman HD (1980) Case reports of the Massachusetts General Hospital: case 40. N Engl J Med 303:866
Dorfman HD, Steiner GC, Jaffe HL (1971) Vascular tumors of bone. Hum Pathol 2:349–376
Dorfman HD, Weiss SW (1984) Borderline osteoblastic tumors: problems in the differential diagnosis of aggressive osteoblastoma and low-grade sarcoma. Semin Diagn Pathol 1:215
Dunitz N, Lipscomb P, Ivins J (1957) Osteoid osteoma of the hand and wrist. Am J Surg 94:64
Dunlop JA, Morton KS, Elliott GB (1970) Recurrent osteoid osteoma. Report of a case with a review of the literature. J Bone Joint Surg [Br] 52:128
Edeiken J, DePalma AF, Hodes PJ (1966) Osteoid osteoma (roentgenographic emphasis). Clin Orthop 49:201–206
Eisenbrey AB, Huber PJ, Rachmaninoff N (1969) Benign osteoblastoma of the spine with multiple recurrences. J Neurol 31:468
Esquerdo J, Fernandez CF, Gomar F (1976) Pain in osteoid osteoma. Histological facts. Acta Orthop Scand 47:520–524
Fielding JW, Keim HA, Hawkins RJ et al. (1977) Osteoid osteoma of the cervical spine. Clin Orthop Rel Res 128:163

Freiberger RH (1960) Osteoid osteoma of the spine. A cause of backache and scoliosis in children and young adults. Radiology 75:232–236

Freiberger RH, Lotman BS, Halpern M, Thompson TC (1959) Osteoid osteoma. A report of 80 cases. Am J Roentgenol Radium Ther Nucl Med 82:194–205

Gamba JL, Martinez S, Apple J et al. (1984) Computed tomography of axial skeletal osteoid osteomas. AJR 142:769

Gertzbein SD, Cruickshank B, Hoffman H et al. (1973) Recurrent benign osteoblastoma of the second thoracic vertebra: a case report. J Bone Joint Surg [Br] 55:841

Ghelman B, Thompson FM, Arnold WD (1981) Intraoperative radioactive localization of osteoid osteoma. J Bone Joint Surg [Am] 63:826

Ghelman B, Vigorita VJ (1983) Postoperative radionuclide evaluation of osteoid osteomas. Radiology 146:509

Giannestras NJ, Diamond JR (1958) Benign osteoblastoma of the talus. J Bone Joint Surg [Am] 40:469–478

Gitelis S, Schajowicz F (1989) Osteoid osteoma and osteoblastoma. Orthop Clin North Am 20:313–325

Glynn JJ, Lichtenstein L (1973) Osteoid osteoma with multicentric nidus. A report of two cases. J Bone Joint Surg [Am] 55:855–858

Goidanich IF, Battaglia L (1959) Osteoblastoma (fibroma osteogenico). Neoplasia benigna di tessuto osteoblastico. Chir Organi Mov 46:353–388

Golding JSR (1954) The natural history of osteoid osteoma. With a report of 20 cases. J Bone Joint Surg [Br] 36:218–229

Goldman RL (1971) The periosteal counterpart of benign osteoblastoma. Am J Clin Pathol 56:73

Greenspan A, Elguezabel A, Bruk D (1974) Multifocal osteoid osteoma. A case report and review of the literature. AJR 121:103

Habermann ET, Stern RE (1974) Osteoid osteoma of the tibia in an eight-month-old boy. J Bone Joint Surg [Am] 56:633–636

Halpern M, Freiberger RH (1970) Arteriography as a diagnostic procedure in bone disease. Radiol Clin North Am 8:277–288

Healey JH, Ghelman B (1986) Osteoid osteoma and osteoblastoma: current concepts and recent advances. Clin Orthop Rel Res 204:76–85

Helms CA, Hattner RS, Vogler JB III (1984) Osteoid osteoma: radionuclide diagnosis. Radiology 151:779

Israeli A, Zwas ST, Horozowski H et al. (1983) Use of radionuclide method in preoperative and intraoperative diagnosis of osteoid osteoma of the spine. Case report. Clin Orthop Rel Res 175:194

Jackson JR, Bell MEA (1977) Spurious "benign osteoblastoma": a case report. J Bone Joint Surg [Am] 59:397

Jackson RP (1978) Recurrent osteoblastoma: a review. Clin Orthop 131:229

Jackson RP, Reckling FW, Mantz FA (1977) Osteoid osteoma and osteoblastoma. Similar histologic lesions with different natural histories. Clin Orthop Rel Res 128:303

Jaffe HL (1935) "Osteoid osteoma": a benign osteoblastic tumor composed of osteoid and atypical bone. Arch Surg 31:709

Jaffe HL (1956) Benign osteoblastoma. Bull Hosp Joint Dis 17:141

Jaffe HL (1958) Tumor and tumorous conditions of the bones and joints. Lea & Febiger, Philadelphia

Jaffe HL, Lichtenstein L (1940) Osteoid-osteoma. Further experience with this benign tumor of bone with especial reference to cases showing the lesion in relation to shaft cortices and commonly misclassified as instances of sclerosing non-suppurative osteomyelitis or cortical bone abscess. J Bone Joint Surg 22: 645–682

Jaffe HL, Mayer L (1932) An osteoblastic-osteoid tissue forming tumor of a metacarpal bone. Arch Surg 24:550–564

Janin Y, Epstein JA, Carras R et al. (1981) Osteoid osteoma and osteoblastomas of the spine. Neurosurgery 8:31–38

Johnston AD (1962) Clinical problems in osteoid osteoma. Evidence of osteoclastic aversion to osteoid. Bull Hosp Joint Dis 23:80–94

Kattapuram SV, Kushner DC, Phillips WC et al. (1983) Osteoid osteoma: an unusual case of articular pain. Radiology 147:383

Keim HA, Reina EG (1975) Osteoid-osteoma as a cause of scoliosis. J Bone Joint Surg [Am] 57:159

Kenan S, Floman Y, Robin GC et al. (1985) Aggressive osteoblastoma: a case report and review of the literature. Clin Orthop 195:294

Kirwan EO, Hutton PAN, Pozo JL et al. (1984) Osteoid osteoma and benign osteoblastoma of the spine. J Bone Joint Surg [Br] 66:21

Lawrie TR, Sinclair AM (1970) Painless osteoid osteoma. J Bone Joint Surg [Am] 52:1357–1363

Lichtenstein L (1956) Benign osteoblastoma. Cancer 9:1044

Lichtenstein L (1977) Bone tumors, 5th edn. C.V. Mosby, St. Louis

Lichtenstein L, Sawyer WR (1964) Benign osteoblastoma: further observations and report on twenty additional cases. J Bone Joint Surg [Am] 46:755

Lindbom A, Lindvall N, Soderberg G, Spjut H (1960) Angiography in osteoid osteoma. Acta Radiol 54:327–333

Lindholm TS, Snellman O, Osterman K (1977) Scoliosis caused by benign osteoblastoma of the lumbar spine: a report of three patients. Spine 2:276

Lisbona R, Rosenthall L (1979) Role of radionuclide imaging in osteoid osteoma. AJR 132:77

MacLellan DI, Wilson FC (1967) Osteoid osteoma of the spine: a review of the literature and report of six new cases. J Bone Joint Surg [Am] 49:111

Makeley JT, Dunn MJ (1982) Prostaglandin synthesis by osteoid osteoma (letter). Lancet II:42

Marcove RC, Freiberger RH (1966) Osteoid osteoma of the elbow. A diagnostic problem. Report of four cases. J Bone Joint Surg [Am] 48:1185

Marsh BW, Bonfiglio M, Brady IP et al. (1975) Benign osteoblastoma: range of manifestations. J Bone Joint Surg [Am] 57:1

Marsh HO, Choi C (1970) Primary osteogenic sarcoma of the cervical spine originally mistaken for benign osteoblastoma. J Bone Joint Surg [Am] 52:1467–1471

Mayer L (1967) Malignant degeneration of so called benign osteoblastoma. Bull Hosp Joint Dis 28:4

McLeod R, Dahlin DC, Beabout JW (1976) The spectrum of osteoblastoma. AJR 126:321

Meary R, Merle d'Aubigné R, Mazabraud A (1965) Osteoblastomes benins. Mem Acad pp 911–925

Mehta MH (1978) Pain provoked scoliosis: observations on the evolution of the deformity. Clin Orthop Rel Res 135:58

Merryweather RM, Middlemiss JH, Senerkin NG (1980) Malignant transformation of osteoblastoma. J Bone Joint Surg [Br] 62:381

Mirra JM, Kendrick RA, Kendrick RE (1976) Pseudomalignant osteoblastoma versus arrested osteosarcoma: a case report. Cancer 37:2005

Mirra JM, Picci P, Gold RH (1989) Bone tumors. Clinical, radiologic, and pathologic correlations. Lea and Febiger, Philadelphia

Mitchell ML, Ackerman LV (1986) Metastatic and pseudomalignant osteoblastoma: a report of two unusual cases. Skeletal Radiol 15:213

Moberg E (1951) The natural course of osteoid osteoma. J Bone Joint Surg [Am] 33:166

Morrison GM, Hawes LE, Sacco JJ (1950) Incomplete removal of osteoid-osteoma. Am J Surg 80:476

Morton KS, Vassar PS, Knickerbocker NJ (1975) Osteoid osteoma and osteoblastoma: reclassification of 43 cases using Schajowicz's classification. Can J Surg 18:148–152

Nelson OA, Greer RB III (1983) Localization of osteoid-osteoma of the spine using computerized tomography: a case report. J Bone Joint Surg [Am] 65:263

Norman A (1978) Persistence or recurrence of pain: a sign of surgical failure in osteoid-osteoma. Clin Orthop Rel Res 130:263

Norman A, Abdelwahab IF, Buyon K et al. (1986) Osteoid osteoma of the hip simulating an early onset of osteoarthritis. Radiology 158:417

O'Brien TM, Murray TE, Malone LA et al. (1984) Osteoid osteoma: excision with scintimetric guidance. Radiology 153:543

O'Dell CW Jr, Resnick D, Niwayama G et al. (1976) Osteoid osteomas arising in adjacent bones: report of a case. J Can Assoc Radiol 27:298

O'Hara JP III, Tegtmeyer C, Sweet DE, McCue FC (1975) Angiography in the diagnosis of osteoid osteoma of the hand. J Bone Joint Surg [Am] 57:163–166

Orlowski JP, Mercer RD (1977) Osteoid osteoma in children and young adults. Pediatrics 59:526

Papanicolaou N (1985) Osteoid osteoma: operative confirmation of complete removal by bone scintigraphy. Radiology 154:821–822

Pettine KA, Klassen RA (1986) Osteoid-osteoma and osteoblastoma of the spine. J Bone Joint Surg [Am] 68:354–361

Pieterse AS, Vernon-Roberts B, Paterson DC et al. (1983) Osteoid osteoma transformed to aggressive (low grade malignant) osteoblastoma: a case report and literature review. Histopathology: 7:789

Ponseti I, Barta LK (1947) Osteoid osteoma. J Bone Joint Surg 29:767–776

Rand JA, Sim FH, Unni KK (1982) Two osteoid-osteomas in one patient. A case report. J Bone Joint Surg [Am] 64:1243

Ransford AO, Pozo JL, Hutton PAN et al. (1984) The behavior pattern of the scoliosis associated with osteoid osteoma or osteoblastoma of the spine. J Bone Joint Surg [Br] 66:16

Resnick D, Niwayama G (1988) Diagnosis of bone and joint disorders, 2nd edn, vol 6. W.B. Saunders, Philadelphia

Revell PA, Scholtz CL (1979) Aggressive osteoblastoma. J Pathol 127:195

Rinsky LA, Goris M, Bleck EE et al. (1980) Intraoperative skeletal scintigraphy for localization of osteoid-osteoma in the spine. Case report. J Bone Joint Surg [Am] 62:143

Roessner A, Metze K, Heymer B (1985) Aggressive osteoblastoma. Pathol Res Pract 179:433

Rosborough D (1966) Osteoid osteoma. Report of a lesion in the terminal phalanx of a finger. J Bone Joint Surg [Br] 48:484–487

Scaglietti O, Calandriello B (1953) Sulla vasietá asticolare del granuloma osteoide. Arch Putti 12:9–28

Schajowicz F, Lemos C (1970) Osteoid osteoma and osteoblastoma: closely related entities of osteoblastic derivation. Acta Orthop Scand 41:272

Schajowicz F, Lemos C (1976) Malignant osteoblastoma. J Bone Joint Surg [Br] 58:202

Schajowicz F, Rebecchini AC, Bosch-Mayol G (1979) Intracortical hemangioma simulating osteoid osteoma. J Bone Joint Surg 61:94

Schulman L, Dorfman HD (1970) Nerve fibers in osteoid osteoma. J Bone Joint Surg [Am] 52:1351

Scranton PE Jr, De Cicco FA, Totten RS et al. (1975) Prognostic factors in osteosarcoma. Cancer 36:2179

Seki T, Fukada H, Ishi Y et al. (1975) Malignant transformation of benign osteoblastoma. J Bone Joint Surg [Am] 57:424

Seruzier E, Simonin JL, Ducastelle C et al. (1976) Osteome osteoide avec synovite. A propos de deux observations. Rev Rhum Mal Osteoartic 43:521

Sherman MS (1947a) Osteoid osteoma associated with changes in adjacent joints. Report of two cases. J Bone Joint Surg 29:483

Sherman MS (1947b) Osteoid osteoma: review of the literature and report of thirty cases. J Bone Joint Surg 29:918

Sherman MS, McFarland G (1965) Mechanism of pain in osteoid osteoma. South Med J 58:163

Sim FH, Dahlin DC, Beabout JW (1975) Osteoid-osteoma: diagnostic problems. J Bone Joint Surg [Am] 57:154

Smith FW, Gilday DL (1980) Scintigraphic appearances of osteoid osteoma. Radiology 137:191–195

Snarr JW, Abell MR, Martel W (1973) Lymphofollicular synovitis with osteoid osteoma. Radiology 106:557–560

Spjut HJ, Dorfman HD, Fechner RE, Ackerman LV (1971) Tumors of bone and cartilage. Atlas of tumor pathology, 2nd series, Fasc 5. Armed Forces Institute of Pathology, Washington, DC

Spjut HJ, Fechner RE, Ackerman LV (1981) Tumors of bone and cartilage. Atlas of tumor pathology, Fasc 5, Supplement. Armed Forces Institute of Pathology, Washington, DC

Steiner GC (1976) Ultrastructure of osteoid osteoma. Hum Pathol 7:309

Steiner GC (1977) Ultrastructure of osteoblastoma. Cancer 39:2127

Stutch R (1975) Osteoblastoma – a benign entity? Orthopaed Rev 4:27

Sty J, Simon G (1982) Intraoperative ^{99m}technetium bone imaging in treatment of benign osteoblastic tumors. Clin Orthop Rel Res 165:223

Swee RG, McLeod RA, Beabout JW (1979) Osteoid osteoma. Detection, diagnosis, and localizations. Radiology 130:117

Tavernier L, Guillemenet M, Faysse R (1949) Forme espéciale d'ostéome osteoide à point de départ cortical et à évolution paraosseuse. L'ostéome ostéoide a forme exostosante. Mem Acad Chir 75:267–274
Tonai M, Campbell CJ, Ahn GH et al. (1982) Osteoblastoma: classification and report of 16 patients. Clin Orthop Rel Res 167:222
Uehlinger E (1977) Multizentrisches Osteoid Osteom des Tibioschaftes mit atypischem Roentgenbild. Arch Orthop Unfall-Chir 89:101–107
Winter PF, John PM, Hilal SK et al. (1977) Scintigraphic detection of osteoid osteoma. Radiology 122:177
Worland RL, Ryder CT, Johnston AD (1975) Recurrent osteoid-osteoma. Report of a case. J Bone Joint Surg [Am] 57:277
Zwimpfer TJ, Tucker WS, Faulkner JF (1982) Osteoid osteoma of the cervical spine: case reports and literature review. Can J Surg 25:637–641

Osteosarcoma

Allan CJ, Soule EH (1971) Osteogenic sarcomata of the somatic soft tissues. Clinico-pathologic study of 26 cases and review of literature. Cancer 27:1121–1133
Amstutz H (1969) Multiple osteogenic sarcomata – metastastic or multicentric? Report of two cases and review of literature. Cancer 24:923–931
Aparisi T, Stark A, Ericsson JLE (1982) Human osteogenic sarcoma. Study of the ultrastructure, with special notes on the localization of alkaline and acid phosphatase. Int Orthop 6:171–179
Ayala AG, Raymond AK, Jaffe N (1984) The pathologist's role in the diagnosis and treatment of osteosarcoma in children. Hum Pathol 15:258–266
Ayala AG, Ro JY, Raymond AK et al. (1989) Small cell osteosarcoma: a clinicopathologic study of 27 cases. Cancer 64:2162–2173
Bacci G, Picci P, Orlandi M et al. (1987) Prognostic value of serum alkaline phosphatase in osteosarcoma. Tumori 73:331–336
Ballance WA Jr, Mendelsohn G, Carter JR et al. (1988) Osteogenic sarcoma. Malignant fibrous histiocytoma subtype. Cancer 62:763–771
Barwick KW, Huvos AG, Smith J (1980) Primary osteogenic sarcoma of the vertebral column. A clinicopathologic correlation of ten patients. Cancer 46:595–604
Bathurst N, Sanerkin N, Watt I (1986) Osteoclast-rich osteosarcoma. Br J Radiol 59:667–673
Bertoni F, Boriani S, Laus M, Campanacci M (1982) Periosteal chondrosarcoma and periosteal osteosarcoma: two distinct entities. J Bone Joint Surg [Br] 64:370–376
Bertoni F, Unni KK, McLeod RA et al. (1985) Osteosarcoma resembling osteoblastoma. Cancer 55:416–426
Bertoni F, Present D, Bacchini P et al. (1989) The Istituto Rizzoli experience with small cell osteosarcoma. Cancer 64:2591–2599
Brem H, Folkman I (1975) Inhibition of tumor angiogenesis by cartilage. J Exp Med 141:427–439
Busso MG, Schajowicz F (1945) Sarcoma osteogénico a localización multiple. Rev Ortop Traumatol 15:85–96
Cade S (1955) Osteogenic sarcoma. A study based on 133 patients. J R Coll Surg Edinb 1:79–111
Camblin JG, Enneking WF (1979) Immunotherapy in osteosarcoma. In: Jaffe N (ed) Bone tumors in children. PSG, Littleton, Massachusetts, pp 215–231
Campanacci M (1990) Bone and soft tissue tumors. Springer, Vienna New York
Campanacci M, Cervelleti G (1975) Osteosarcoma. A review of 345 cases. Ital J Orthop Traumatol 1:5–22
Campanacci M, Giunti A (1976) Periosteal osteosarcoma. Review of 41 cases, 22 with long-term follow-up. Ital J Orthop 1:23–25
Campanacci M, Pizzoferrato A (1971) Osteosarcoma emorragico. Chir Organi Mov 60:409–421
Campanacci M, Bertoni F, Capanna R et al. (1981) Central osteosarcoma of low grade malignancy. Ital J Orthop Traumatol 7:71–78
Caron AS, Hajdu SI, Strong EW (1971) Osteogenic sarcoma of the facial and cranial bones. A review of 43 cases. Am J Surg 122:719–725
Carroll RE (1957) Osteogenic sarcoma in the hand. J Bone Joint Surg [Am] 39:325–331
Clark JL, Unni KK, Dahlin DC, Devine KD (1983) Osteosarcoma of the jaw. Cancer 51:2311–2316
Coley BL (1960) Neoplasms of bone and related conditions, 2nd edn. Harper, New York
Cremin BJ, Heselson NG, Webber BL (1976) The multiple sclerotic osteogenic sarcoma of early childhood. Br J Radiol 49:416–419
Dahlin DC (1978) Bone tumors, 3rd edn. Charles C. Thomas, Springfield, IL
Dahlin DC, Coventry MB (1967) Osteogenic sarcoma. A study of six hundred cases. J Bone Joint Surg [Am] 41:101–110
Dahlin DC, Unni KK (1977) Osteosarcoma of bone and its important recognizable varieties. Am J Surg Pathol 1:61–72
Dahlin DC, Unni KK (1986) Bone tumors: general aspects and data on 8542 cases, 4th edn. Charles C. Thomas, Springfield, IL
Dahlin DC, Unni KK, Matsuno T (1977) Malignant (fibrous) histiocytoma of bone – fact or fancy? Cancer 39:1508–1516
Delling G, Krumme H, Salzer-Kuntschik M (1983) Morphological changes in osteosarcoma after chemotherapy-COSS 80. J Cancer Res Clin Oncol 106 [Suppl]:32–37
Dryja TP, Rapaport JM, Epstein J et al. (1986) Chromosome 13 homozygosity in osteosarcoma without retinoblastoma. Am J Hum Genet 38:59–66
Edeiken J, Raymond AK, Ayala AG et al. (1987) Small-cell osteosarcoma. Skeletal Radiol 16:621–628
Eilber FR, Morton DL (1970) Immunologic studies of human sarcomas: additional evidence suggesting an associated sarcoma virus. Cancer 26:588–596
Enneking WF, Kagan F (1975a) The implications of "skip" metastases of osteosarcoma. Clin Orthop 111: 33–41
Enneking WF, Kagan A (1975b) "Skip" metastases in osteosarcoma. Cancer 36:2192–2205
Enneking WF, Kagan A (1978) Transepiphyseal extension of osteosarcoma – incidence, mechanism and implications. Cancer 41:1526–1537
Enneking WF, Springfield DS (1977) Osteosarcoma. Orthop Clin North Am 8:785–803

Enneking WF, Spanier SS, Goodman MA (1980) Current concepts review: the surgical staging of musculoskeletal sarcoma. J Bone Joint Surg [Am] 62:1027–1030

Epstein LI, Bixler D, Bennett JE (1970) An incident of familial cancer. Including 3 cases of osteogenic saroma. Cancer 25:889–891

Ewing J (1939) A review of the classification of bone tumors. Bull Am Coll Surg 24:290–295

Farr GH, Huvos AG, Marcove RC, Higinbotham NL, Foote FW (1974) Telangiectatic osteogenic sarcoma. A review of twenty-eight cases. Cancer 34:1150–1158

Ferguson RJ, Yunis EJ (1978) The ultrastructure of human osteosarcoma. A study of nine cases. Clin Orthop 131:234–246

Fine G, Stout AP (1956) Osteogenic sarcoma of the extraskeletal soft tissues. Cancer 9:1027–1043

Finkel MP, Reilly CA Jr, Biskis BO, Greco IL (1973) Bone tumor viruses. Proc Symp Colston Res Soc 24:353–364

Fitzgerald RH Jr, Dahlin DC, Sim FH (1973) Multiple metachronous osteogenic sarcoma: report of twelve cases with two long-term survivors. J Bone Joint Surg [Am] 55:595–605

Fleegler EJ, Marks KE, Sebek BA et al. (1980) Osteosarcoma of the hand. Hand 12:316–322

Fraumeni JF (1967) Stature and malignant tumors of bone in childhood and adolescence. Cancer 20:967

Friedlaender GE, Mitchell MS (1976) A virally induced osteosarcoma in rats. A model for immunological studies of human osteosarcoma. J Bone Joint Surg [Am] 58:295–302

Fudenberg HH (1976) Dialyzable transfer factor in the treatment of human osteosarcoma: an analytical review. Ann NY Acad Sci 277:545–557

Garrington GE, Scofield HH, Cornyn J et al. (1967) Osteosarcoma of the jaws: analysis of 56 cases. Cancer 20:377–391

Gay S, Miller EJ (1978) Collagen in the physiology and pathology of connective tissue. Fischer, Stuttgart

Ghadially FN, Mehta PN (1970) Ultrastructure of osteogenic sarcoma. Cancer 25:1457–1467

Ghandur-Mnaymneh L, Mnaymneh WA, Puls S (1983) The incidence and mechanism of transphyseal spread of osteosarcoma of long bones. Clin Orthop 177: 210–215

Gherlinzoni F, Antoci B, Canale V (1983) Case report 250. Diagnosis: multicentric osteosarcomata (osteosarcomatosis). Skeletal Radiol 10:281–285

Gilman PA, Wang N, Fan SF et al. (1985) Familial osteosarcoma associated with 13;14 chromosomal rearrangement. Cancer Genet Cytogenet 17:123–132

Haibach H, Farrell C, Dittrich FJ (1985) Neoplasms arising in Paget's disease of bone: a study of 82 cases. Am J Clin Pathol 83:594–600

Harmon TP, Morton KS (1966) Osteogenic sarcoma in four siblings. J Bone Joint Surg [Br] 48:493–498

Heater K, Collins PA (1987) Osteosarcoma in association with infraction of bone: report of two cases. J Bone Joint Surg [Am] 69:300–302

Hudson TM, Schiebler M, Springfield DS et al. (1983) Radiologic imaging of osteosarcoma: role in planning surgical treatment. Skeletal Radiol 10:137–146

Hutter RVP, Foote FW, Francis KC et al. (1966) Primitive multipotential primary sarcoma of bone. Cancer 19: 1–25

Huvos AG (1986) Osteogenic sarcoma of bones and soft tissues in older persons. A clinicopathologic analysis of 117 patients older than 60 years. Cancer 57:1442–1449

Huvos AG (1991) Bone tumors: diagnosis, treatment, prognosis. W.B. Saunders, Philadelphia

Huvos AG, Higinbotham NL, Miller TR (1972) Bone sarcomas arising in fibrous dysplasia. J Bone Joint Surg [Am] 54:1047–1056

Huvos AG, Rosen G, Bretsky SS et al. (1982) Telangiectatic osteogenic sarcoma: a clinicopathologic study of 124 patients. Cancer 49:1679–1689

Huvos AG, Butler A, Bretsky SS (1983a) Osteogenic sarcoma associated with Paget's disease of bone: a clinicopathologic study of 65 patients. Cancer 52: 1489–1495

Huvos AG, Butler A, Bretsky SS (1983b) Osteogenic sarcoma in the American black. Cancer 52:1959–1965

Huvos AG, Woodard HQ, Cahan WG et al. (1985a) Postirradiation osteogenic sarcoma of bone and soft tissue: a clinico-pathologic study of 66 patients. Cancer 55:1244–1255

Huvos AG, Sundaresan N, Brestsky SS et al. (1985b) Osteogenic sarcoma of the skull. A clinicopathologic study of 19 patients. Cancer 56:1214–1221

Huvos AG, Butler A, Bretsky SS (1985c) Osteogenic sarcoma in pregnant women. Prognosis, therapeutic implications and literature review. Cancer 56:2326–2331

Jacobson SA (1977) Polyhistioma. A malignant tumor of bone and extraskeletal tissues. Cancer 40:2116–2130

Jaffe HL (1958) Tumors and tumorous conditions of the bones and joints. Lea & Febiger, Philadelphia

Jaffe HL (1960) Intracortical osteogenic sarcoma. Bull Hosp Joint Dis 21:189–197

Jaffe N (ed) (1979) Bone tumors in children. PSG, Littleton, Massachusetts

Janes JM (1969) The influence of splenectomy on the induction of osteogenic sarcoma in rabbits. J Bone Joint Surg [Am] 51:1432

Jeffree GM, Price CHG (1965) Bone tumors and their enzymes: a study of the phosphatases, non-specific esterases and betaglucuronidase of osteogenic and cartilaginous tumors, and fibroblastic and giant cell lesions. J Bone Joint Surg [Br] 47:120–136

Kaufman RA, Towbin RB (1981) Telangiectatic osteosarcoma simulating the appearance of an aneurysmal bone cyst. Pediatr Radiol 11:102–104

Kay S (1971) Ultrastructure of an osteoid type of osteogenic sarcoma. Cancer 28:437–445

Kolodny A (1927) Bone sarcoma. Surg Gynecol Obstet [Suppl] 44:1

Kragh LV, Dahlin DC, Erich JB (1958) Osteogenic sarcoma of the jaws and facial bones. Am J Surg 96:496–505

Kreicbergs A, Broström LA, Cewrien G et al. (1982) Cellular DNA content in human osteosarcoma. Aspects on diagnosis and prognosis. Cancer 50: 2476–2481

Kuettner KE, Hiti J, Eisenstein R, Harper E (1976) Collagenase inhibition by cationic proteins derived from cartilage and aorta. Biochem Biophys Res Commun 72:40–46

Kuettner KE, Pauli BU, Soble L (1978) Morphological studies on the resistance of cartilage to invasion by

osteosarcoma cells in vitro and in vivo. Cancer Res 38:277–287
Kurt AM, Unni KK, McLeod RA, Pritchard DJ (1990) Low-grade intraosseous osteosarcoma. Cancer 6: 1418–1428
Kyriakos M (1980) Intracortical osteosarcoma. Cancer 46:2525–2533
Larsson SE, Lorentzon R, Boquist L (1978) Telangiectatic osteosarcoma. Acta Orthop Scand 49:589–594
Levine AM, Triche T, Rosenberg SA (1980) Osteosarcoma cells in tissue culture: II. Characterization and localization of alkaline phosphatase activity. Clin Orthop 146:259–268
Lewis RJ, Lotz MJ (1974) Medullary extension of osteosarcoma. Implications for rational therapy. Cancer 33:371–375
Lindbom A, Soderberg G, Spjut HJ (1961) Osteosarcoma. A review of 96 cases. Acta Radiol 56:1–19
Lowbeer L (1968) Multifocal osteosarcomatosis – a rare entity. Bull Pathol 9:52–53
Marcove RC, Mike V, Hajek JV, Levin AG, Hutter RVP (1970) Osteogenic sarcoma under the age of 27. A review of 145 operative cases. J Bone Joint Surg [Am] 52:411–423
Marsh HO, Choi CB (1970) Primary osteogenic sarcoma of the cervical spine originally mistaken for benign osteoblastoma: a case report. J Bone Joint Surg [Am] 42:1467–1471
Martin SE, Dwyer A, Kissane JM et al. (1982) Small-cell osteosarcoma. Cancer 50:990–996
Martínez-Tello FJ, Navas-Palacios JJ (1982) The ultrastructure of conventional, parosteal, and periosteal osteosarcomas. Cancer 50:949–961
Martland HS (1931) The occurrence of malignancy in radioactive persons. Am J Cancer 15:2435–2515
Matsuno T, Unni KK, McLeod RA, Dahlin DC (1976) Telangiectatic osteogenic sarcoma. Cancer 38:2538–2547
Mazabraud A, Gongora R, Gongora G et al. (1982) Value of the study of the kinetics of 85 strontium for the classification of osteogenic sarcomas. Sem Hop Paris 58:1664–1667
McDonald I, Budd JN (1943) Osteogenic sarcoma. I. A modified nomenclature and a review of 118 five-year cures. Surg Gynecol Obstet 76:421–423
McKenna RJ, Schwinn CP, Soong KY, Higinbotham NL (1964) Osteogenic sarcoma arising in Paget's disease. Cancer 17:42–66
McKenna RJ, Schwinn CP, Soong KY, Higinbotham NL (1966) Sarcomata of the osteogenic series (osteosarcoma, fibrosarcoma, chondrosarcoma, periosteal osteogenic sarcoma and sarcomata arising in abnormal bone). An analysis of 552 cases. J Bone Joint Surg [Am] 48:1–26
Miller CW, McLaughlin RE (1977) Osteosarcoma in siblings. Report of two cases. J Bone Joint Surg [Am] 59:261–262
Miller RW (1976) Etiology of childhood bone cancer: epidemiologic observations. Recent Results Cancer Res 54:50–62
Mirra JM (1980) Bone tumors: diagnosis and treatment. J.B. Lippincott, Philadelphia
Misdorp W (1980) Skeletal osteosarcoma. Animal model: canine osteosarcoma. Am J Pathol 98:285–288
Misdorp W, Hart AAM (1979) Some prognostic and epidemiologic factors in canine osteosarcoma. J Natl Cancer Inst 62:537–545
Misdorp W, Hart G, Delemarre JF, Voute PA, Van der Eijken JW (1988) J Pathol 156:119–128
Mnaymneh W, Brown M, Tejada F et al. (1979) Primary osteogenic sarcoma of the second cervical vertebra: case report. J Bone Joint Surg [Am] 61:460–462
Monkman GR, Orwoll G, Ivins JC (1974) Trauma and oncogenesis. Mayo Clin Proc 49:157
Morton DL, Malmgren RA (1968) Human osteosarcoma: immunologic evidence suggesting an associated infection agent. Science 162:1279
Neff JR, Enneking WF (1975) Adoptive immunotherapy in primary osteosarcoma. An interim report. J Bone Joint Surg [Am] 57:145–148
Nosanchuk JS, Weatherbee L, Brody GL (1969) Osteogenic sarcoma. Prognosis related to epiphyseal closure. JAMA 208:2439–2441
Ohno T, Abe M, Tateishi A et al. (1975) Osteogenic sarcoma. A study of 130 cases. J Bone Joint Surg [Am] 57:397–404
Owen LN (1969) Bone tumors in man and animals. Butterworths, London
Paschall HA, Paschall MM (1975) Electron microscopic observations of 20 human osteosarcomas. Clin Orthop 111:42–56
Patel DV, Hammer RA, Levin B et al. (1984) Primary osteogenic sarcoma of the spine. Skeletal Radiol 12:276–279
Phemister DB (1926) A study of the ossification in bone sarcoma. Radiology 7:17–23
Picci P, Gherlinzoni F, Gerra A (1983) Intracortical osteosarcoma: Rare entity or early manifestation of classical osteosarcoma? Skeletal Radiol 9:255–258
Polednak AP (1985) Primary bone cancer incidence in black and white residents of New York State. Cancer 55:2883–2888
Poretta CA, Dahlin DC, Janes JN (1957) Sarcoma in Paget's disease of bone. J Bone Joint Surg [Am] 39:1314–1329
Pratt CB, Rivera G, Shanks E (1977) Osteosarcoma during pregnancy. Obstet Gynecol 50 [Suppl]:24s–26s
Price CHG (1952) The grading of osteogenic sarcoma. Br J Cancer 6:46–68
Price CHG (1956) The grading of osteogenic sarcoma and its bearing upon survival and prognosis. J Fac Radiol 7:237–241
Price CHG, Truscott DE (1957) Multifocal osteogenic sarcoma. Report of a case. J Bone Joint Surg [Br] 39:524–533
Price CHG, Truscott DE (1961) Osteogenic sarcoma. An analysis of survival and its relationship to histological grading and structure. J Bone Joint Surg [Br] 43:300–313
Pritchard DJ, Finkel MP, Reilly CA (1975) The etiology of osteosarcoma. A review of current considerations. Clin Orthop 111:14–22
Remberger K, Gay S (1977) Immunohistochemical demonstration of different collagen types in the normal epiphyseal plate and in benign and malignant tumors of bone and cartilage. Z Krebsforsch 90:95–106
Rohmsdahl MM, Ayala AG (1977) Surgical management of osteosarcoma. In: Dybala LW, Freitag SB,

Culhane DC (eds) Management of primary bone and soft tissue tumors. Year Book Medical, Chicago
Rosen G, Marcove RC, Caparros B, Nirenberg A, Kosloff C, Huvos AG (1979) Primary osteogenic sarcoma: the rationale for preoperative chemotherapy and delayed surgery. Cancer 43:2163–2177
Rosen G, Caparros B, Huvos AG et al. (1982) Preoperative chemotherapy for osteogenic sarcoma: selection of postoperative adjuvant chemotherapy based on the response of the primary tumor to preoperative chemotherapy. Cancer 49:1221–1230
Rosen G, Huvos AG, Marcove R, Nirenberg A (1986) Telangiectatic osteogenic sarcoma: improved survival with combination chemotherapy. Clin Orthop 207:164–173
Salzer-Kuntschik M, Delling G, Beron G et al. (1983a) Morphological grades of regression in osteosarcoma after polychemotherapy – study COSS 80. J Cancer Res Clin Oncol 106 [Suppl]:21–24
Salzer-Kuntschik M, Grand G, Delling G (1983b) Bestimmung des morphologischen Regressionsgrades nach Chemotherapie bei malignen Knochentumoren. Pathologe 4:135–141
Sanerkin NG (1980) Definitions of osteosarcoma, chondrosarcoma, and fibrosarcoma of bone. Cancer 46:178–185
Schajowicz F (1977) Juxtacortical chondrosarcoma. J Bone Joint Surg [Br] 59:473–480
Schajowicz F (1983) Current trends in the diagnosis and treatment of malignant bone tumors. Clin Orthop 180:22
Schajowicz F, Bessone JE (1967) Chondrosarcoma in three brothers. J Bone Joint Surg [Am] 49:129–141
Schajowicz, F, Cabrini RL (1954) Histochemical studies of bone in normal and pathological conditions. J Bone Joint Surg [Br] 36:474
Schajowicz F, Oleaga Alarcon F (1945) La transformación sarcomatosa de la osteitis deformante de Paget. Bol Trab Soc Argent Cirug Ortop 10:116–130
Schajowicz F, Ackerman LV, Sissons HA (1972) Histological typing of bone tumours. International histological classification of tumors, No. 6. World Health Organization, Geneva
Schajowicz F, Santini Araujo E, Berenstein M (1983) Sarcoma complicating Paget's disease of bone. A clinicopathologic study of 62 cases. J Bone Joint Surg [Br] 65:299–307
Schimke R, Lowman J, Cowan GAG (1974) Retinoblastoma and osteogenic sarcoma in siblings. Cancer 34:2077–2079
Scranton PE, DeCicco FA, Totten RS, Yunis EJ (1975) Prognostic factors in osteosarcoma. Cancer 36:2179–2197
Siegel RD, Rayan LM, Antman KM (1989) Osteosarcoma in adults: one institution's experience. Clin Orthop 240:261–269
Silverman G (1936) Multiple osteogenic sarcoma. Arch Pathol 21:88–95
Sim FH, Cupps RE, Dahlin DC, Ivins JC (1972) Postradiation sarcoma of bone. J Bone Joint Surg [Am] 54:1479–1489
Sim FH, Unni KK, Beabout JW, Dahlin DC (1979) Osteosarcoma with small cells simulating Ewing's tumor. J Bone Joint Surg [Am] 61:207–215
Simon MA, Bos GD (1980) Epiphyseal extension of metaphyseal osteosarcoma in skeletally immature individuals. J Bone Joint Surg [Am] 62:195–204
Spanier SS, Shuster JJ, Vander Griend RA (1990) The effect of local extent of the tumor on prognosis in osteosarcoma. J Bone Joint Surg [Am] 72:643–653
Spira E, Farin I (1967) The vascular supply to the epiphyseal plate under normal and pathological conditions. Acta Orthop Scand 38:1–22
Spjut HJ, Dorfman HD (1981) Florid reactive periostitis of the tubular bones of the hands and feet. A benign lesion which may simulate osteosarcoma. Am J Surg Pathol 5:423–433
Spjut HJ, Dorfman HD, Fechner RE, Ackerman LV (1971) Tumors of bone and cartilage. Atlas of tumor pathology, 2nd series, Fasc 5. Armed Forces Institute of Pathology, Washington, DC
Spjut HJ, Ayala AG, DeSantos LA, Murray JA (1977) Periosteal osteosarcoma. In: Dybala LW, Freitag SB, Culhane DC (eds) Management of primary bone and soft tissue tumors. Year Book Medical, Chicago, pp 79–95
Springfield DS, Schakel ME Jr, Spanier SS (1991) Spontaneous necrosis in osteosarcoma. Clin Orthop Rel Res 263:233–237
Stark A, Ericsson JLE (1983) Human osteogenic sarcoma: fine structure of the osteoblastic type. Ultrastruct Pathol 4:311–329
Steiner GC (1965) Postradiation sarcoma of bone. Cancer 18:603–612
Sundaram M, McGuire MH, Herbold DR (1987) Magnetic resonance imaging of osteosarcoma. Skeletal Radiol 16:23–29
Swaney JJ (1973) Familial osteogenic sarcoma. Clin Orthop 97:64–68
Sweetnam R (1973) Amputation in osteosarcoma. Disarticulation of the hip or high thigh amputation for lower femoral growths? J Bone Joint Surg [Br] 5:189–192
Thomson AD, Turner-Warwick RT (1955) Skeletal sarcomata and giant cell tumors. J Bone Joint Surg [Br] 37:266–303
Tjalma RA (1966) Canine bone sarcoma: estimation of relative risk as a function of body size. J Natl Cancer Inst 36:1137–1150
Trifaud A, Meary R (1972) Prognostic et traitment des sarcomes ostéogeniques. Masson, Paris
Trueta J, Amato VP (1960) The vascular contribution to osteogenesis. (3) Changes in the growth plate caused by experimentally induced ischemia. J Bone Joint Surg [Br] 42:571–587
Trueta J, Morgan JD (1960) The vascular contribution of osteogenesis. Studies by the injection method. J Bone Joint Surg [Br] 42:97–109
Tsuneyoshi M, Dorfman HD (1987) Epiphyseal osteosarcoma: distinguishing features from clear cell chondrosarcoma, chondroblastoma and epiphyseal enchondroma. Hum Pathol 18:664–651
Unni KK, Dahlin DC (1984) Grading of bone tumors. Semin Diagn Pathol 1:165–172
Unni KK, Dahlin DC, Beabout JW (1976) Periosteal osteogenic sarcoma. Cancer 37:2476–2485
Unni KK, Dahlin DC, McLeod RA et al. (1977) Intraosseous well-differentiated osteosarcoma. Cancer 40:1337–1347

Upshaw JE, McDonald JR, Ghormley RK (1949) Extension of primary neoplasm of bone to bone marrow. Surg Gynecol Obstet 89:704

Uribe-Botero G, Russel WO, Sutow WW, Martin RG (1977) Primary osteosarcoma of bone. A clinicopathologic investigation of 243 cases, with necropic studies in 54. Am J Clin Pathol 67:427–435

Vanel D, Tcheng S, Contesso G et al. (1987) The radiological appearances of telangiectatic osteosarcoma: a study of 14 cases. Skeletal Radiol 16:196–200

Vigorita VJ, Jones JK, Ghelman B, Marcove RC (1984) Intracortical osteosarcoma. Am J Surg Pathol 8: 65–71

Wick MR, Siegal GP, McLeod RA, Greditzer HC III, Unni KK (1981) Sarcomas of bone complicating osteitis deformans (Paget's disease): fifty years' experience. Am J Surg Pathol 5:47–59

Williams AH, Schwinn CP, Parker JW (1976) The ultrastructure of osteosarcoma. A review of twenty casese. Cancer 37:1293–1301

Wold LE, Unni KK, Beabout JW, Pritchard DJ (1984) High-grade surface osteosarcomas. Am J Surg Pathol 8:181–186

Woodard HG (1942) Acid and alkaline glycerophosphate in tissue and serum. Cancer Res 2:407

Woodard HQ, Higinbotham NL (1937) The correlation between serum phosphatase and roentgenographic type in bone disease. Am J Cancer 31:221–237

Wuisman P, Enneking WF (1990) Prognosis for patients who have osteosarcoma with skip metastasis. J Bone Joint Surg [Am] 72:60–68

Xipell JM, Rush J (1985) Well-differentiated intraosseous osteosarcoma of the left femur. Skeletal Radiol 14: 312–316

Surface (Peripheral) Osteosarcoma

Ahuja SC, Villacin AB, Smith J et al. (1977) Juxtacortical (parosteal) osteogenic sarcoma. Histological grading and prognosis. J Bone Joint Surg [Am] 59:632–647

Ayala AG (1978) Periosteal osteosarcoma [letter]. Radiology 129:836

Bertoni F, Boriani S, Laus M, Campanacci M (1982) Periosteal chondrosarcoma and periosteal osteosarcoma: two distinct entities. J Bone Joint Surg [Br] 64:370–376

Bertoni F, Present D, Hudson T et al. (1985) The meaning of radiolucencies in parosteal osteosarcoma. J Bone Joint Surg [Am] 67:901–910

Campanacci M, Giunti A (1976) Periosteal osteosarcoma; review of 41 cases, 22 with long-term follow-up. Ital Orthop 1:23–25

Campanacci M, Picci P, Gherlinzoni F et al. (1984) Parosteal osteosarcoma. J Bone Joint Surg [Br] 66: 313–321

Dahlin DC (1978) Bone tumors, 3rd edn. Charles C. Thomas, Springfield, IL

Dahlin DC, Unni KK (1986) Bone tumors: general aspects and data on 8542 cases, 4th edn. Charles C. Thomas, Springfield, IL

Dunham WK, Wilborn WH, Zarzour RJ (1979) A large parosteal osteosarcoma with transformation to high-grade osteosarcoma: a case report. Cancer 44:1495–1500

Dwinnel LA, Dahlin DC, Ghormley RK (1954) Parosteal (juxtacortical) osteogenic sarcoma. J Bone Joint Surg [Am] 36:732–744

Edeiken J, Farrell C, Ackerman LB, Spjut HJ (1971) Parosteal sarcoma. Am J Roentgenol Radium Ther Nucl Med 111:579–583

Enneking WF, Springfield D, Gross M (1985) The surgical treatment of parosteal osteosarcoma in long bones. J Bone Joint Surg [Am] 67:125–135

Ewing J (1939) A review of the classification of bone tumors. Bull Am Coll Surg 24:290–295

Farr GH, Huvos AG (1972) Juxtacortical osteogenic sarcoma. An analysis of fourteen cases. J Bone Joint Surg [Am] 54:1205–1216

Gay S, Miller EJ (1978) Collagen in the physiology and pathology of connective tissue. Fischer, New York

Geschickter CF, Copeland MM (1951) Parosteal ostema of bone: a new entity. Ann Surg 133:790–806

Gravanis MB, Whitesides TE (1970) The unreliability of prognostic criteria in osteosarcoma. Am J Clin Pathol 53:15–20

Hall FM (1978) Periosteal osteosarcoma [letter]. Radiology 129:835

Hall R, Robinson L, Malawer M, Dunham W (1985) Periosteal osteosarcoma. Cancer 55:165–171

Huvos AG (1979) Bone tumors: diagnosis, treatment, and prognosis. WB Saunders, Philadephia, p 100

Jacobson SA (1968) Early juxtacortical osteosarcoma (parosteal osteoma). J Bone Joint Surg [Am] 40:1310–1328

Jaffe HL (1958) Tumors and tumorous conditions of the bones and joints. Lea and Febiger, Philadelphia

Junqueira LC, Montes GS (1983) Biology of collagen-proteoglycan interaction. Arch Histol Jpn 46:589–629

Levine E, DeSmet AA, Huntrakkon M (1985) Juxtacortical osteosarcoma: a radiologic and histologic spectrum. Skeletal Radiol 14:38–46

Lichtenstein L (1955) Tumors of periosteal origin. Cancer 8:1060–1069

Lichtenstein L (1977) Bone tumors, 5th edn. C.V. Mosby, St Louis

Lorentzon R, Larsson SE, Boquist L (1980) Parosteal (juxtacortical) osteosarcoma: a clinical and histopathological study of eleven cases and a review of the literature. J Bone Joint Surg [Br] 62:86–92

Martínez-Tello FJ, Navas-Palacios JJ (1982) The ultrastructure of conventional, parosteal, and periosteal osteosarcomas. Cancer 50:949–961

Merle d'Aubigné R, Meary R, Mazabraud A (1959) Sarcome ostéogenique juxtacortical, Rev Chir Orthop 45:873–884

Nojima T, Unni KK, McLeod RA, Pritchard DJ (1985) Periosteal chondroma and periosteal chondrosarcoma. Am J Surg Pathol 9:666–677

Picci P, Campanacci M, Bacci G et al. (1987) Medullary involvment in parosteal osteosarcoma: a case report. J Bone Joint Surg [Am] 69:131–136

Pintado SO, Lane J, Huvos AG (1989) Parosteal osteogenic sarcoma of bone with coexistent low- and high-grade sarcomatous components. Hum Pathol 20:488–491

Ritts GD, Pritchard D, Unni KK et al. (1987) Parosteal osteosarcoma. Clin Orthop 219:299–307

Scaglietti O, Calandriello B (1962) Ossifying parosteal sarcoma. Parosteal osteoma or juxtacortical osteogenic sarcoma. J Bone Joint Surg [Am] 44:635–647

Schajowicz F (1977) Juxtacortical chondrosarcoma. J Bone Joint Surg [Br] 59:473–480

Schajowicz F (1981) Tumors and tumorlike lesions of bone and joints. Springer, New York Berlin Heidelberg

Schajowicz F (1983) Current trends in the diagnosis and treatment of malignant bone tumors. Clin Orthop 180:220–252

Schajowicz F, Ackerman LV, Sissons HA (1972) Histological typing of bone tumours. International histological classification of tumors, No. 6. World Health Organization, Geneva

Schajowicz F, McGuire M, Santini Araujo E et al. (1988) Osteosarcomas arising on the surfaces of long bones. J Bone Joint Surg [Am] 70:555–564

Spjut HJ, Ayala AG, DeSantos LA, Murray JA (1977) Periosteal osteosarcoma. In: Management of primary bone and soft tissue tumors. Yearbook Medical, Chicago, pp 79–95

Sundaram M, Burdge RW, Martin SA, Wolverson MK (1981) Case report 142. Skeletal Radiol 6:131–133

Unni KK, Dahlin DC, Beabout JW, Ivins JC (1976a) Parosteal osteogenic sarcoma. Cancer 37:2466–2475

Unni KK, Dahlin DC, Beabout JW (1976b) Periosteal osteogenic sarcoma. Cancer 37:2476–2485

Unni KK, Dahlin DC, McLeod RA, Pritchard DC (1977) Intraosseous well-differentiated osteosarcoma. Cancer 40:1337–1347

Van der Heul RO, Van Ronnen JR (1967) Juxtacortical osteosarcoma. Diagnosis, differential diagnosis, treatment, and an analysis of eight cases. J Bone Joint Surg [Am] 49:415–439

Weston WY, Redi JD, Saunders JH (1958) Parosteal osteogenic sarcoma of bone. J Bone Joint Surg [Am] 40:722–724

Wold LE, Unni KK, Beabout JW, Pritchard DJ (1984a) High-grade surface osteosarcomas. Am J Surg Pathol 8:181–186

Wold LE, Unni KK, Beabout JW, Sim FH, Dahlin DC (1984b) Dedifferentiated parosteal osteosarcoma. J Bone Joint Surg [Am] 66:53–59

CHAPTER II

Cartilage-Forming Tumors

Cartilaginous lesions are the most common tumors in our and other series. More than with any other lesions, close interdisciplinary cooperation is of utmost importance.

There are often evident discrepancies between the biologic behavior and the histologic appearance, depending on age, clinical symptoms, multiplicity, and overall site of the lesion. Thus, some periosteal (juxtacortical) or solitary tumors in the tubular bones of hands and feet and certain cartilaginous tumors and tumorlike lesions involving the soft tissues, for example, synovial chondromatosis, although often showing cytologic features that would indicate low-grade malignancy in other locations, generally behave in a benign fashion. Although the diagnosis of high-grade cartilaginous tumors generally does not present problems to the diagnostic pathologist, the differentiation between entirely benign and low-grade malignant lesions may be extremely difficult or impossible based on study of cytology or histopathology alone. Associated with that difficulty is the danger of underdiagnosis by the pathologist, with the disastrous result that the lesion is undertreated. Similarly, there is a danger of "overdiagnosing" benign lesions of this family such as "chondromyxoid fibromas" or "chondroblastomas."

A. Benign

Benign cartilage-forming tumors are divided into the groups shown in Table II.1, with the number of cases corresponding to each tumor type.

1. Chondroma

Definition: *Chondroma is a relatively common neoplasm and is accepted as such by most authors and by WHO, who defined it as "a benign tumor characterized by the formation of mature cartilage but lacking the histological characteristics of chondrosarcoma (high cellularity, pleomorphism and presence of large cells with double nuclei or mitosis)."*

Most chondromas are located centrally within the medullary cavity (enchondroma). When they rarely occur outside the bone, in close contact with the underlying cortex, they have been described as "periosteal chondroma" (Lichtenstein and Hall 1952) or as "juxtacortical chondroma" (Jaffe 1956). Although the periosteal or subperiosteal origin cannot always be proven, the term "periosteal chondroma" is now generally preferred.

Table II.1. Benign cartilage-forming tumors

Solitary	No. of cases	Multiple	No. of cases
Chondroma	576	Multiple chondromas (enchondromatosis)	25
Enchondroma	558		
Periosteal (juxtacortical)	18		
Osteochondroma (osteocartilaginous exostosis ecchondroma)	1001	Enchondromatosis, predominantly unilateral (Ollier's disease or dyschondroplasia, Maffucci's syndrome)	15
Chondroblastoma (epiphyseal chondroblastoma, benign chondroblastoma)	144	Multiple osteochondromas, osteochondromatosis, hereditary multiple exostosis, hereditary deforming chondrodysplasia, diaphyseal or metaphyseal aclasis, maladie osteogénique	63
Chondromyxoid fibroma (fibromyxoid chondroma)	48		

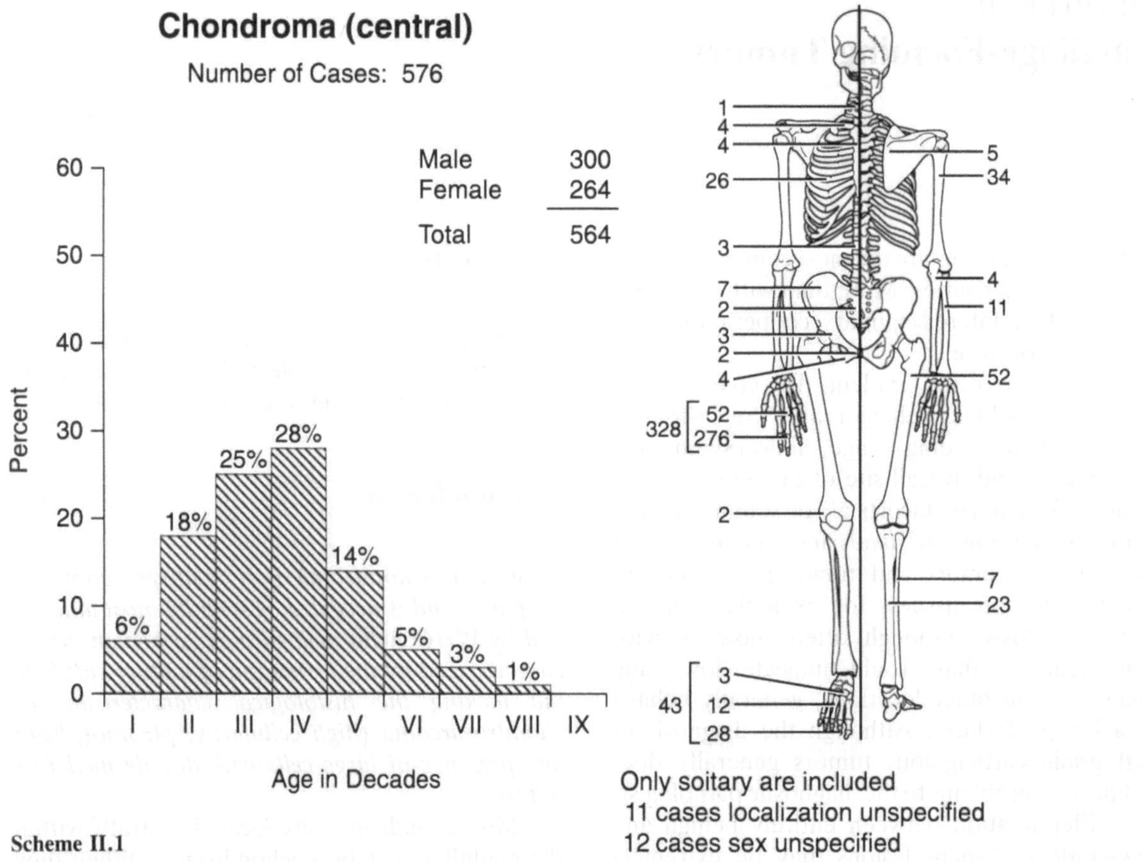

Scheme II.1

Enchondromas are most frequently solitary but may affect few or many bones, preferentially of hands, resulting in the condition called *enchondromatosis*. Cases with a tendency toward predominantly unilateral involvement are generally referred to as "Ollier's disease" or "dyschondroplasia" (Fairbank 1948).

The writer prefers the term "Ollier's syndrome" because the pathologic basis of this disorder is only a special skeletal distribution of multiple enchondromata. The same syndrome associated with soft tissue hemangiomas and phleboliths is called "Maffucci's syndrome" (Maffucci 1881). Both syndromes are apparently congenital disorders due to some failure of endochondral ossification (Fairbank 1948; Aegerter and Kirkpatrick 1975).

Incidence. In our series chondroma was less common than osteochondroma. We recorded 576 cases of solitary lesions (558 of which were enchondromas), that is, 24% of benign tumors and 11% of all tumors. In addition, 25 cases of multiple chondroma and 15 cases of enchondromatosis were recorded. Dahlin and Unni (1986) reported 245 chondromas, including 41 cases of multiple enchondromatosis, that is, 12% of the benign tumors in the Mayo Clinic series. The archives of the Department of Radiologic Pathology of the Armed Forces of Pathology (AFIP) contain records of 880 solitary osteochondromas, as compared with 725 solitary chondromas, 248 chondroblastomas, and 173 chondromyxoid fibromas (Moser 1990).

Clinical Findings. *Age and Sex.* Enchondroma frequently occurred in an older age group than osteochondroma, with an evident predominance after the second decade (76%) and an average age of 32 years. There was no clear sex predominance in our series, as in other large series (Scheme II.1).

Localization. Anatomically, as in all other statistics, the great majority were located in the tubular bones of hands (58%) and much less frequently in feet. Other frequent sites of involvement were in the long bones, such as the femur, humerus, and fibula, and in the ribs. In contrast to chondrosarcoma, enchondromas of flat bones

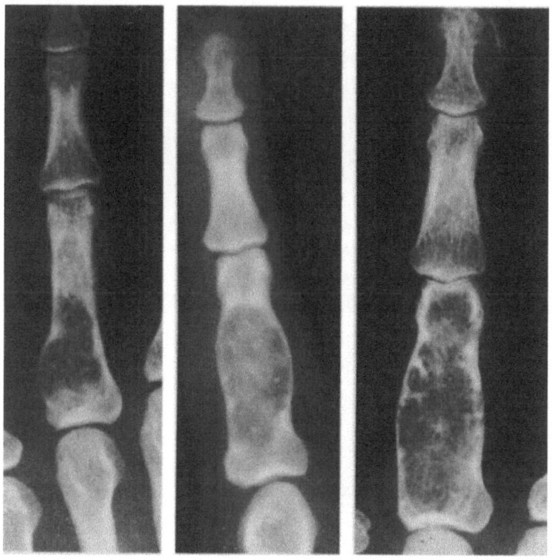

a, b, c

Fig. II.1a–c. Three different chondromas of patients aged 25 (**a**), 30 (**b**), and 65 (**c**) years. Radiographs show radiolucent lesions, located in the proximal phalanges. The cortex is thinned and slightly expanded. Scarce areas of spotty calcification may be seen

(ilium, scapula, and sternum) were relatively rare, as were those located in the spine, especially the vertebral bodies. The distal phalanges were affected more often than reported in the literature, there being 26 such cases in our series. In this location, the differential diagnosis with intraosseous epidermoid cysts was often difficult and possible only with pathologic study.

Radiologic Features. Enchondromas are frequently asymptomatic and are discovered incidentally after a pathologic fracture or on a radiograph taken for other reasons. Sometimes pain with accompanying swelling led to a roentgenographic examination, which revealed a radiolucent, often well-delineated round or ovoid lesion, expanding and slightly thinning the cortex (Figs. II.1, II.2). The lesion was usually located either in the metaphysis extending toward the diaphysis or in the diaphysis, and less frequently in the epiphysis. In the not-infrequent cases of involvement of the terminal phalanx (Fig. II.3) (Schajowicz et al. 1970), the lesion often involved the entire extension of the affected bone and was radiologically generally indistinguishable from the somewhat more frequent intraosseous epidermoid cysts (see Chap. IX).

Conspicuous mottled calcification is characteristic for cartilaginous tumor, benign or malignant, but may be absent in several cases. The mineral deposits may show different patterns, varying from discrete, finely stippled foci scattered through the lesion (Figs. II.4, II.5) to larger, coarse conglomerates with a floccular or "popcorn ball" appearance. This last pattern is frequently observed in the heavily calcified enchondromas, occurring in the metaphyseal region of the long bones, often without symptoms. Such lesions have been referred to as "calcifying and ossifying chondromas." They are probably chondromatous hamartomas and not true neoplasms (see Fig. II.13).

Enchondromas of long bones may occasionally involve an extensive portion of the shaft, without evident expansion of the sometimes slightly thickened cortex, but pressure erosion on its endosteal surface associated with pain is generally lacking.

Fig. II.2a–c. Female, 70 years old. **a** Enchondroma of the proximal phalanx of the middle finger. This is a recurrence 2 years after curettage. The tumor expanded widely the thinned cortex, which is interrupted at one side. The lesion was diagnosed as malignant and the finger was amputated. **b** Photograph and **c** radiograph illustrate the features of the amputation specimen and show the cartilaginous aspect of the tumor mass with extensive hemorrhagic areas. Histologically, the tumor was benign

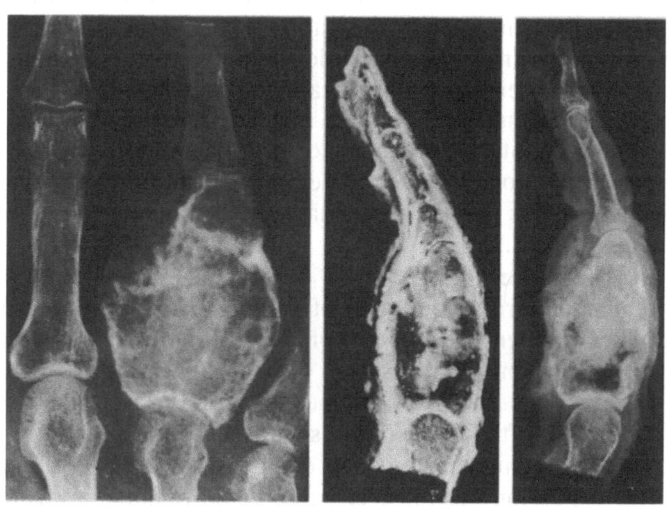

a b, c

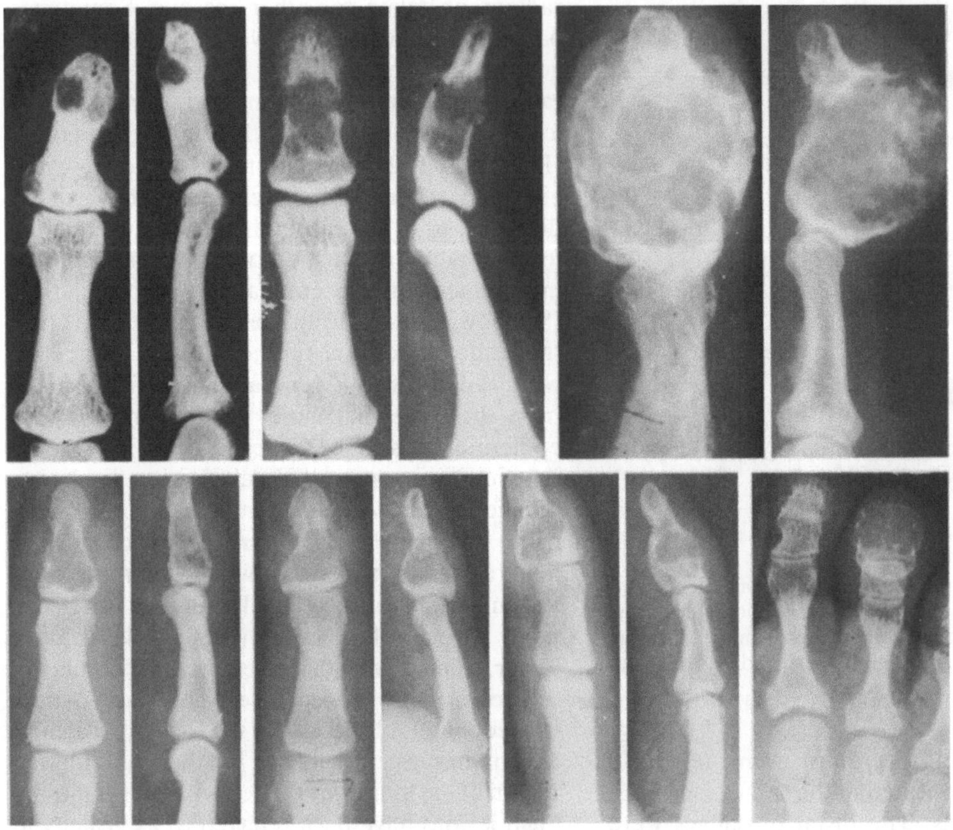

a, b c

d, e f, g

Fig. II.3a–g. Radiographs of seven different cases of enchondromas of terminal phalanges of the hand. These radiographs illustrate the radiolucent aspect of the lesions, generally lacking spotty calcification; this makes them impossible to differentiate radiologically from epidermoid cysts located in the terminal phalanx (see Chap. IX). Location of enchondroma in distal phalanges appears to be not so uncommon as generally supposed. (Schajowicz et al. 1970)

Pathologic Findings. *Gross Pathology.* The material submitted generally consisted of fragments of different sizes, of bluish-white cartilaginous aspect, alternating with areas of necrosis and relatively conspicuous calcification of yellowish color, sometimes showing reddish spots, corresponding to enchondral ossification. Frequently, some fragments were frankly myxoid. On rare occasions, intact specimens of a phalanx or metacarpal bone or resected segments of a long bone, such as the fibula or ulna, were submitted (Figs. II.4, II.5).

These specimens showed the characteristic lobular pattern with lobules of varying size and shape, frequently confluent, or penetrating into the neighboring marrow spaces without showing a definite bone shell toward the spongiosa. The cortex was often thinned and slightly expanded, through pressure erosion on its endosteal surface. This expansion was more conspicuous in tumors of the fingers, especially in cases with multiple lesions. In the long bones, the cortex was sometimes slightly thickened, but it remained generally intact; its partial destruction, especially when accompanied by extraosseous extension of the tumor, was usually an indication of malignancy.

Histopathology. The histologic features and the cytologic details of the cartilage cells are of fundamental importance for the diagnosis. All fragments should be studied carefully, because the structure may vary from fragment to fragment, and some tumors of long bones, which had been interpreted as benign in other institutions, recurred, showing the microscopic features of low-grade chondrosarcoma. Reviewing the original sections, few zones of chondrosarcomatous aspect were observed. These findings explain why it is generally so difficult to determine the true incidence of a possible malignant transformation

II.4a,b

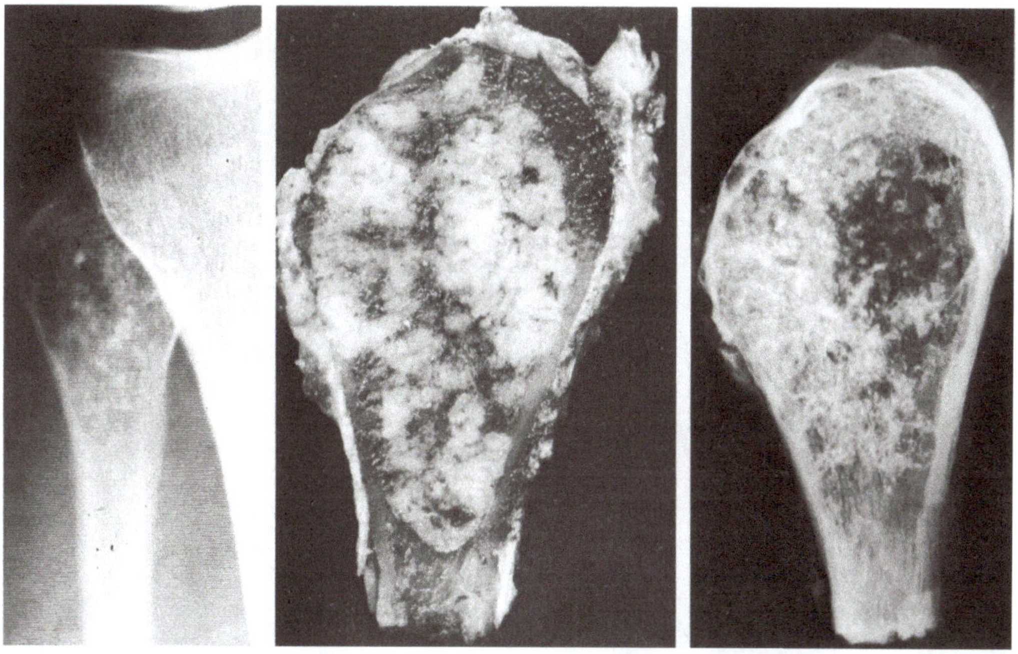

c

II.5a

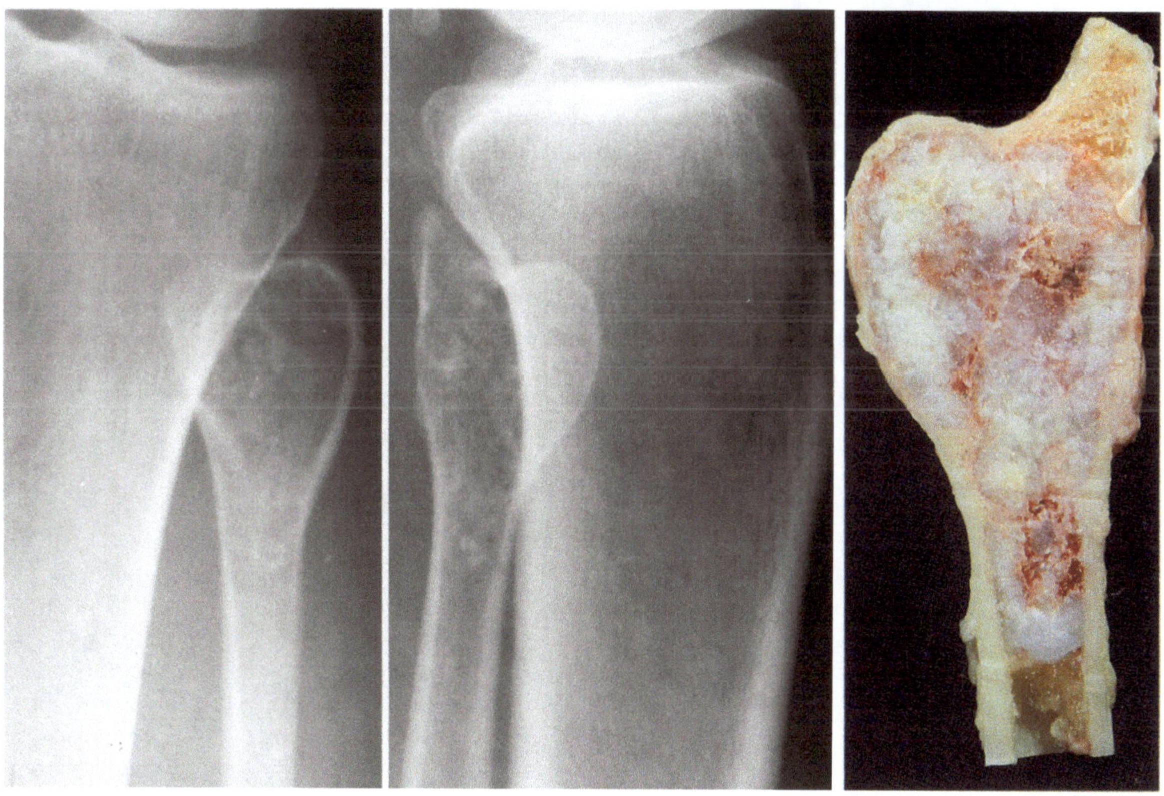

b

Fig. II.4a–c. Female, 58 years old. Enchondroma of the fibula. **a** Radiograph shows an irregular radiolucent central lesion with small calcifications, which expands the cortex only slightly. **b** Photograph of the resection specimen reveals the lobulated cartilaginous aspect of bluish-gray color with small areas of calcification and endochondral ossification (dark reddish) that are seen clearly in the radiograph (**c**)

Fig. II.5a,b. Female, 38 years old. Enchondroma of the fibula. **a** Anteroposterior and lateral radiographs showing a radiolucent lesion, slightly expanding the cortex with spotty granular calcification. **b** Photograph of the resection specimen shows the lobulated cartilaginous pattern of bluish-white color with central yellowish areas of calcification and enchondral ossification (reddish)

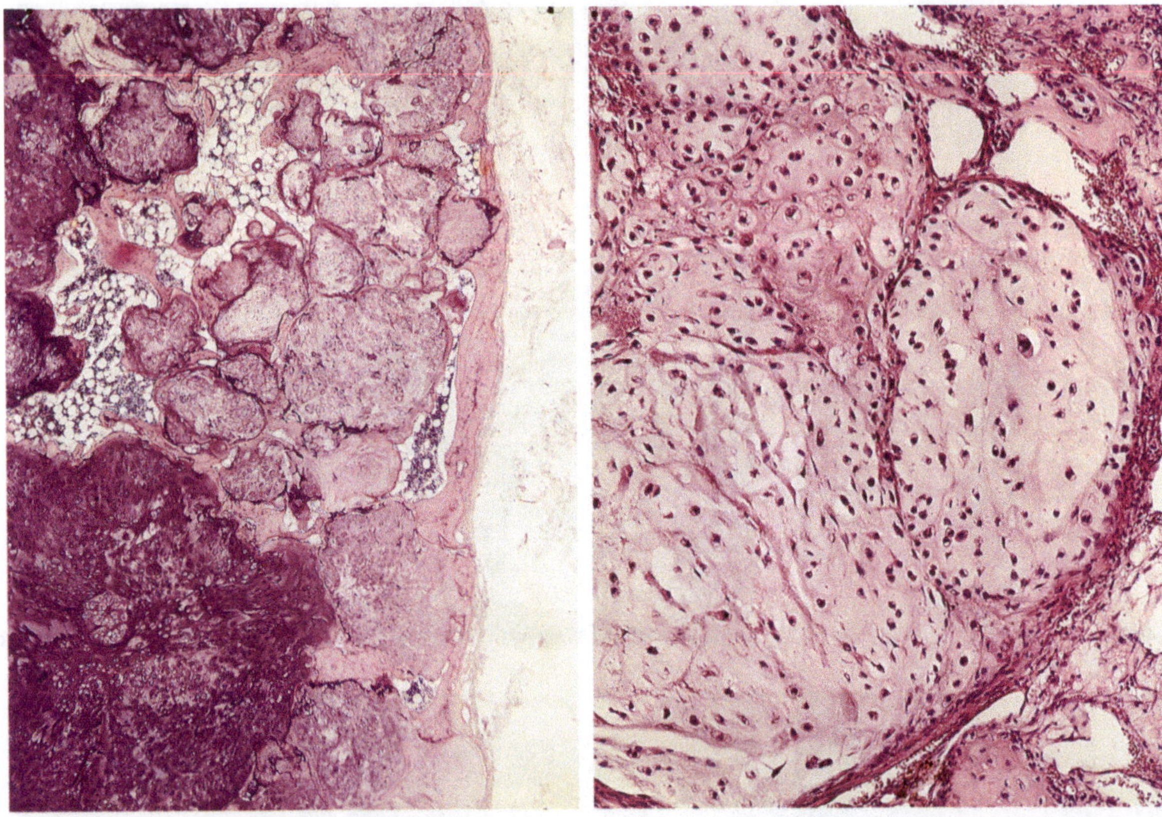

II.6a b

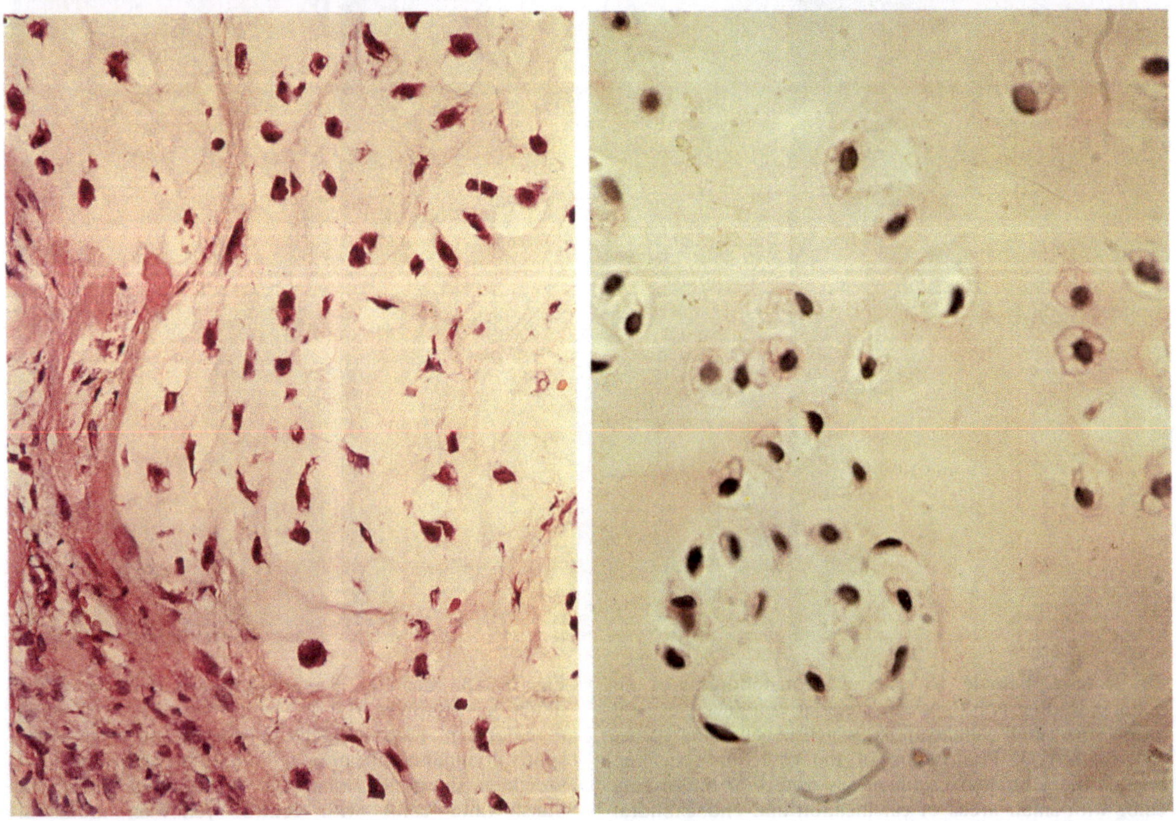

II.7a b

of an enchondroma, which seems to be much lower than suggested by some authors (Wilner 1982; Mirra et al. 1989).

The cartilage cells are generally of small and uniform size with one or occasionally two small dark round nuclei, which lay in typical lacunae, separated by more or less abundant hyaline ground-substance-forming lobules, often separated by septa of connective tissue (Figs. II.6, II.7). Some areas may be much more cellular but the greater cellularity, sometimes more evident in younger patients, or zones of myxoid aspect are not indicative of malignancy.

Regressive changes such as mucinous degeneration and areas of necrosis, associated or not with more or less conspicuous granular amorphous calcification that is followed by enchondral ossification, are a common finding in benign and malignant cartilage tumors.

If one searches for indications of malignancy, that is, the presence of cells with one or more large, plump, hyperchromatic nucleus, then fields without these regressive changes (especially calcified areas) must be studied. Although these cytologic criteria are applied by most pathologists, they are highly subjective; therefore, the structural features of the histopathologic appearance have been suggested as an aid to the differential diagnosis of enchondroma and chondrosarcoma (Sanerkin 1980; Mirra et al. 1989) (see Sect. B.I).

Enchondromas of the long bones of the hands and feet often show a cellular pleomorphism, with frequent double nuclei and more cellular areas, but in this location these features do not imply malignant biologic behavior (Fig. II.7); furthermore, chondrosarcomas are extremely rare at these sites. However, the same histologic pattern observed in a tumor of a long bone or in the pelvic and shoulder girdle should arouse the suspicion of malignancy.

Fig. II.6a,b. Photomicrographs of enchondroma showing **a** at lower magnification cartilage lobuli of different size, surrounded frequently by cancellous bone trabeculae. **b** At higher magnification the cartilage lobules, separated by vascular-connective septa, show the generally uniform size of the small hyperchromatic nuclei, with occasional binucleated or plump nuclei. This is not an uncommon feature in enchondromas of the long bones of the hands and feet; in this location it does not imply malignant biologic behavior. **a** ×20, **b** ×125

Fig. II.7a,b. Photomicrographs showing **a** at higher magnification the cytologic details of the case illustrated in Fig. II.6b. **b** Enchondroma showing the uniform size of the small hyperchromatic nuclei in a background of hyaline cartilage matrix. **a** ×300, **b** ×250

Treatment and Prognosis. Curettage was the treatment of choice for most enchondromas of the tubular bones of hands and feet, in some cases followed by insertion of bone chips; it was generally curative. In a few cases of recurrence, a new curettage cured the lesion. Exceptionally, in large lesions with or without destruction of the cortex and penetration into neighboring soft tissues, a wide block resection or amputation of the corresponding bone was necessary.

In other small long bones, such as the fibula, radius, ulna, and ribs, en bloc resection was the treatment of choice. It was also the preferred treatment in several tumors located in flat or long bones even if this procedure signified loss of function, because it was often extremely difficult to exclude a low-grade chondrosarcoma. The resulting bone defects were repaired by cadaver bone grafts or exceptionally by prosthetic devices. This treatment was also performed in some recurrences after a previous curettage in these locations. Wide excision followed by bone grafts or cementation is at present the treatment of choice in most institutions.

The risk of local recurrence or implantation of tumor tissue in all cartilage tumors, benign or malignant, is so high that wide excision, including the areas of previous biopsy (surgical or even the tract of aspiration biopsy), is always preferable to curettage in bones other than the tubular bones of hands and feet.

Although we have no personal experience with cryosurgery or curettage followed by introduction of liquid nitrogen into the resulting cavity (Marcove et al. 1977), we do not believe that this method is convenient for cartilage tumors of the extremities.

Periosteal (Juxtacortical) Chondroma

Under the denomination "periosteal chondroma," Lichtenstein and Hall (1952) reported six cases as a distinct entity. Jaffe (1956) reported another nine cases and proposed the term "juxtacortical chondroma." Although the latter term is more descriptive and a periosteal or subperiosteal origin cannot always be established, most authors prefer the denomination "periosteal chondroma." This is a slowly growing, distinctly eccentric tumor that develops within or beneath the periosteal or

II.8
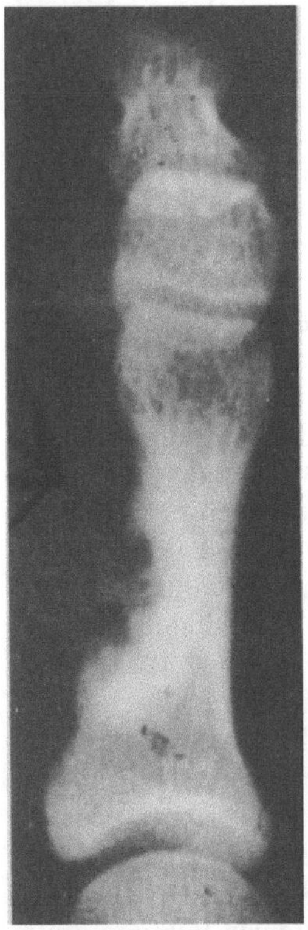

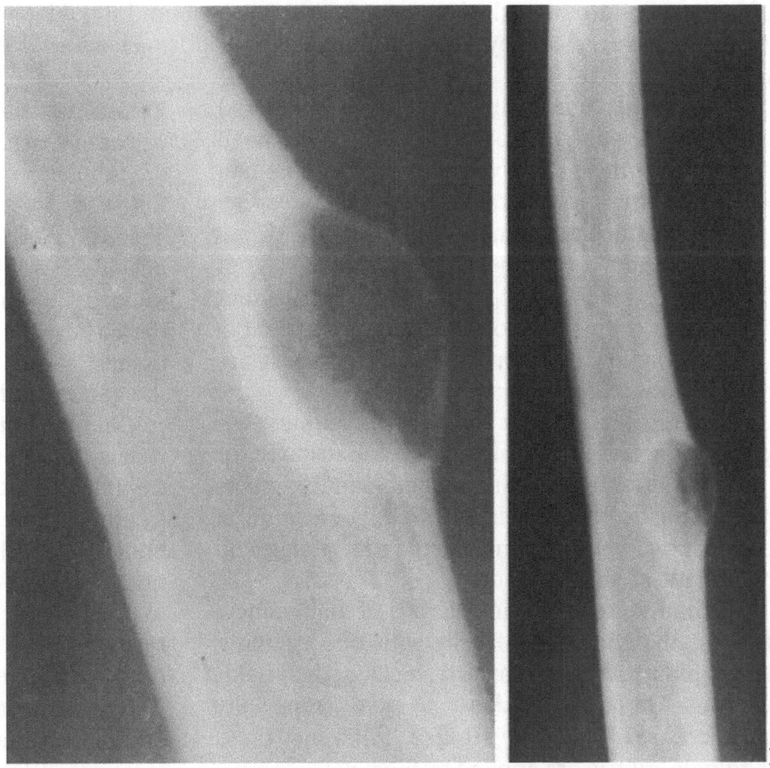
II.9

Fig. II.8. Female, 15 years old. Juxtacortical (periosteal) chondroma of phalanx. Radiograph shows eccentric lesion with cortical indentation and marked sclerosis

Fig. II.9. Juxtacortical (periosteal) chondroma of shaft of the humerus, showing a well-circumscribed eccentric lesion with a sclerotic base separating it from medullary activity. The periphery was well defined by a thin, newly formed bone membrane of apparently periosteal derivation. (Courtesy of Dr. Lemos, Rio de Janeiro, Brasil)

parosteal connective tissue. It typically erodes the underlying cortex and induces a saucer-shaped defect limited by sclerotic bone, accompanied by a localized swelling with or without pain. A moderate number of cases have been reported (Marmor 1964; Merlino and Nixon 1964; Rockwell et al. 1972; Fornasier and McGonigal 1977; Bauer et al. 1982; Boriani et al. 1983; DeSantos and Spjut 1981; Nojima et al. 1985; Lewis et al. 1990); we ourselves have only 18 cases in our files. The preferred locations are tubular bones of hands and feet (Fig. II.8), the metaphysis of long bones, especially the humerus (Figs. II.9–II.11), and the femur. There seems to be no sex predilection, and the lesion occurs more frequently in younger or middle-aged adults, with 52% between 20 and 40 years of age.

Radiographically, a small soft tissue mass (2–3 cm), adjacent to the bone cortex, often showing irregular focal calcification, and a characteristic, semilunar-shaped cortical concavity with a reactive sclerotic base are characteristic and diagnostic findings.

Grossly, the lesion shows a lobular cartilaginous aspect with some small foci of irregular spotty calcification, sometimes followed by enchondral ossification, starting from the underlying cortex (Figs. II.11, II.12).

Histologically, some of these tumors show a higher grade of cellularity and more evident pleomorphism, ordinarily not found in most enchondromas. In the writer's view, some cases of cellular or "active" periosteal chondromas (Dahlin 1978) or cases that have recurred (Nosanchuk and Kaufer 1969), are possibly periosteal (juxtacortical) chondrosarcomas. This problem is discussed in more detail later.

Because of these histologic features, the danger of local recurrence following curettage, and possible confusion with a malignant tumor, the preferred treatment is en bloc excision, including the underlying cortex, or segmental

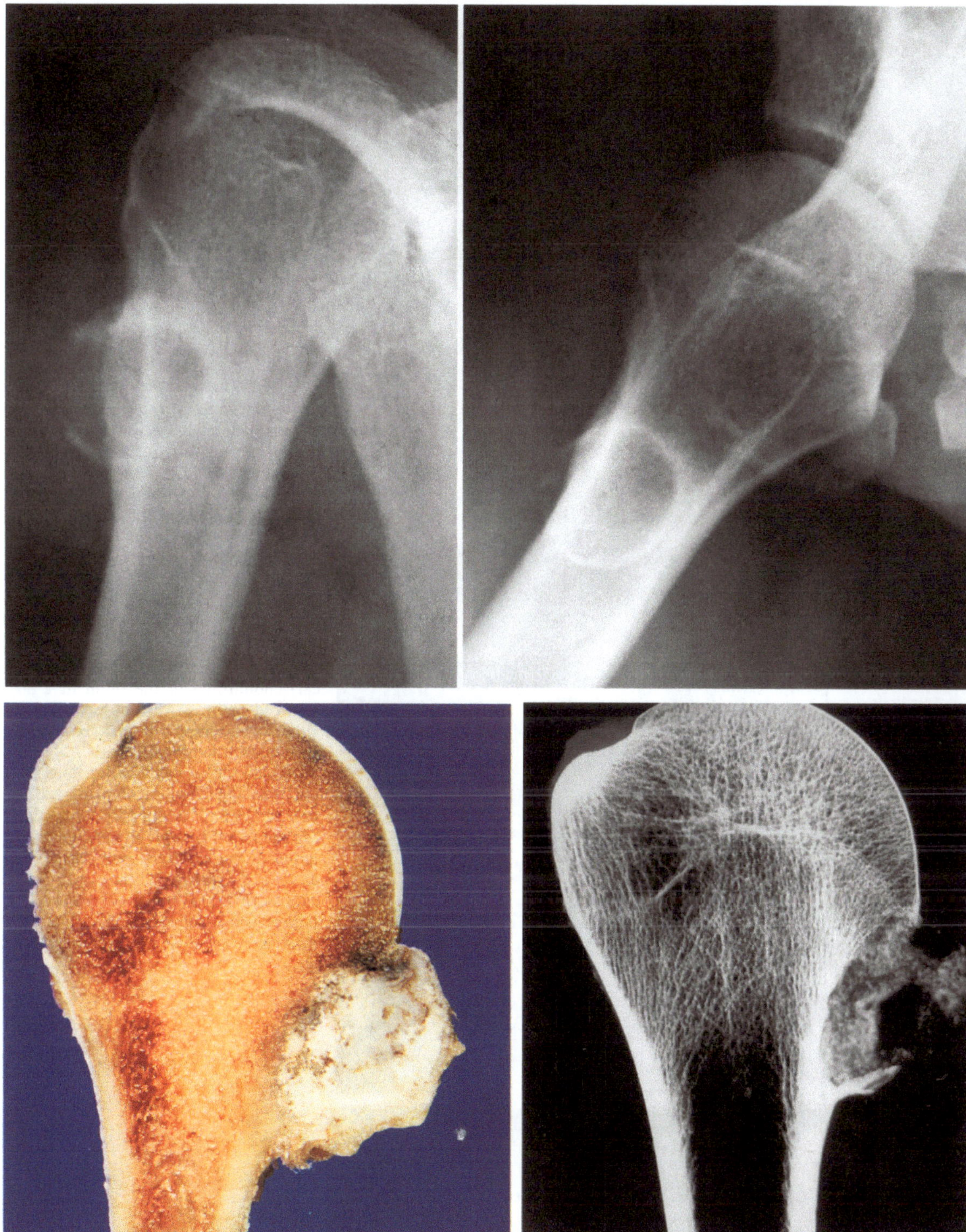

a

b

c

Fig. II.10a–c. Periosteal (juxtacortical) chondroma of the upper humerus. **a** Anteroposterior and lateral radiographs show a well-circumscribed, eccentric lesion surrounded by a thin sclerotic rim. **b** Photograph and **c** radiograph of the resected specimen show a well-circumscribed, eccentric, subperiosteal lesion with scalloping of the underlying cortex. The cartilaginous aspect with spotty calcification can be appreciated

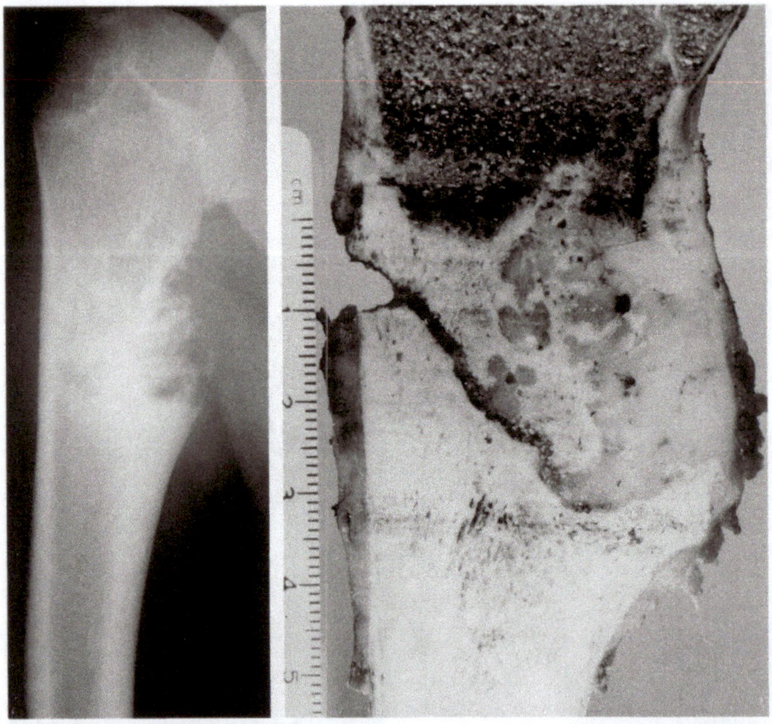

a, b

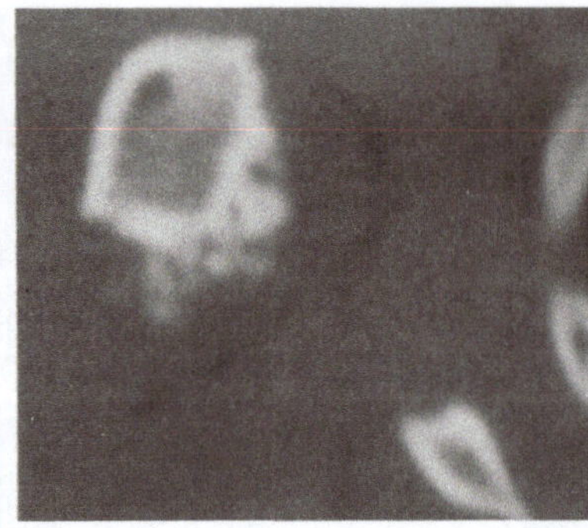

c

Fig. II.11a–c. Periosteal (juxtacortical) chondroma of the humerus in an 18-year-old male. **a** Radiograph shows the eccentric lesion of the upper metaphysis scalloping the underlying cortex, where it is limited by a sclerotic rim. The tumor presents conspicuous areas of calcification of the cartilage, as is shown in **b** the photograph and **c** the CT scan. (Rush-Presbyterian-St. Luke's Medical Center)

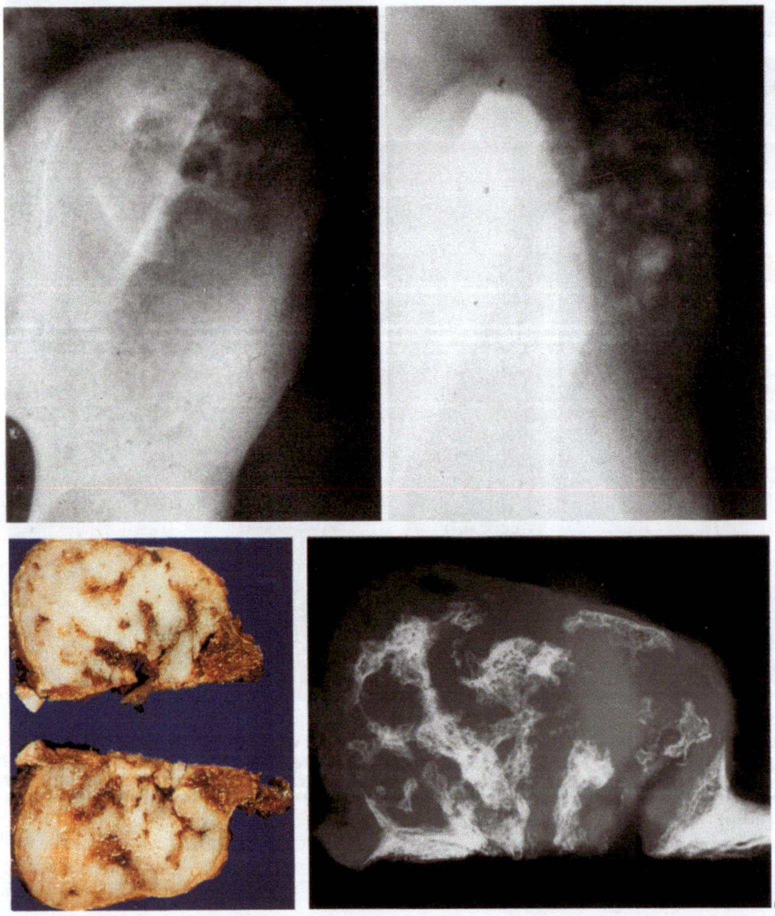

a

b

c

Fig. II.12a–c. Periosteal (juxtacortical) chondroma of the ilium in a 30-year-old male. **a** Anteroposterior and lateral radiographs show a large juxtaosseous tumor mass with areas of coarse flocculent calcification, suggesting the diagnosis of osteochondroma or peripheral secondary chondrosarcoma. **b** Photograph and **c** radiograph of the resected specimen reveal an entirely cartilaginous tumor with extensive areas of calcification and enchondral ossification. Histologically there were no signs of malignancy resection in cases located in small bones, such as the ribs, fibula, or ulna.

Calcifying and Ossifying Enchondroma

An enchondroma located in the metaphyseal region of a long bone sometimes shows radiographically dense, ringlike, or flocculent agglomerated radiopacities that correspond to heavily calcified and ossified cartilaginous tissue (Fig. II.13). The writer reported two cases (Slullitel et al. 1954), describing the clinical and pathologic features of this entity, whose biologic behavior is different from that of ordinary enchondroma at the same location. In our series of 558 (solitary) enchondromas, 30 lesions were of this type. Most were asymptomatic and were discovered incidentally after a radiographic examination of a knee or shoulder, performed because of joint problems. The most common locations were in the upper humerus (8 cases) and distal femoral metaphysis (11 cases). The lesion occurred with greatest frequency in adults 30 years of age or

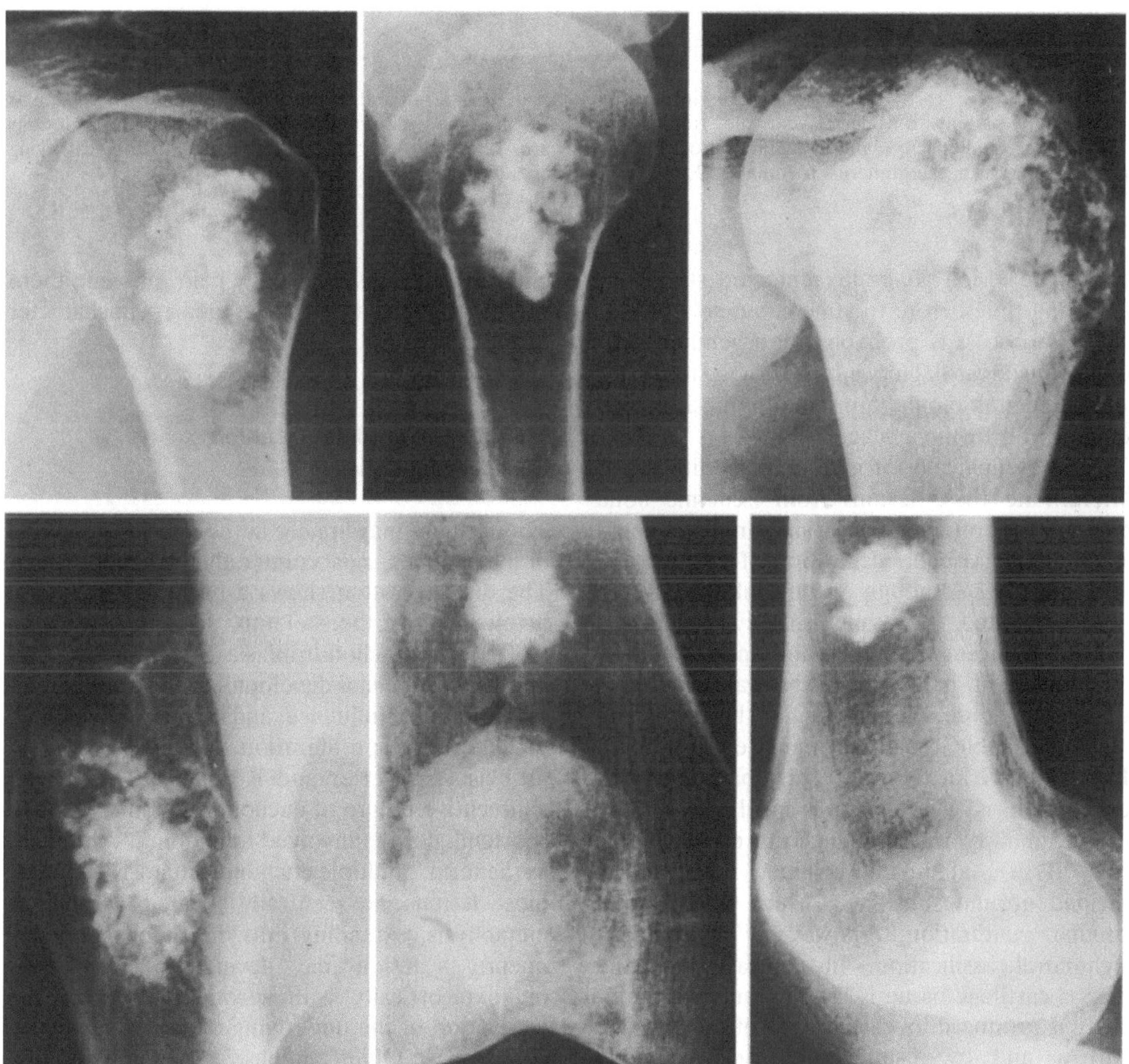

a b c d

Fig. II.13a–d. Radiographs of four different cases of so-called calcifying and ossifying chondroma. **a** Female, 64 years old, anteroposterior and lateral radiographs show asymptomatic patient with heavily calcified, centrally located metaphyseal lesion with coarse flocculent calcifications, with irregular contours. **b** Female, 52 years old, with a larger, heavily calcified lesion. **c** Female, 45 years old. Radiograph illustrates centrally located lesion in the upper femoral metaphysis. **d** Female, 60 years old. Anteroposterior and lateral radiographs reveal a small densely calcified lesion in the lower third of the femur. All lesions were cured by curettage

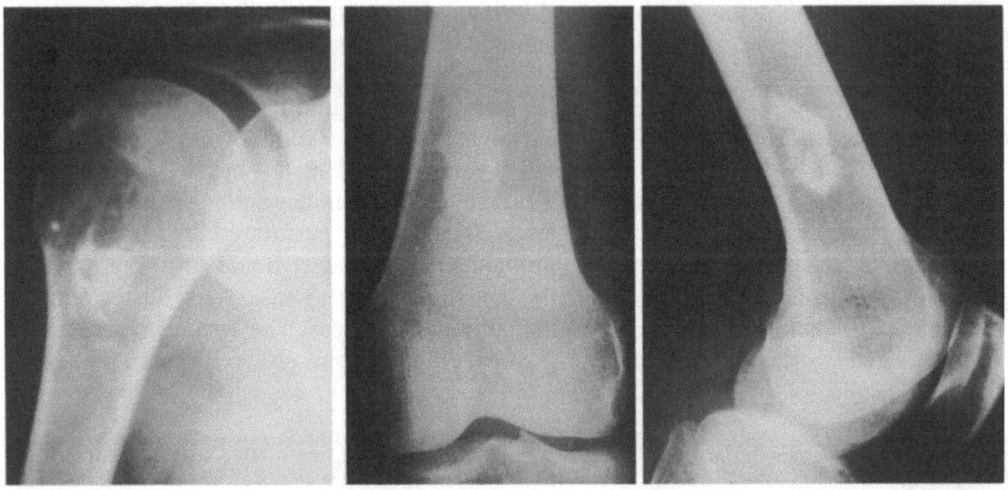

Fig. II.14a,b. Two cases of ischemic bone infarcts in asymptomatic patients. **a** Male, 71 years old. Radiograph shows a dense radiopacity, with irregular contours in the upper metaphysis of the humerus. **b** Female, 52 years old. Anteroposterior and lateral radiographs illustrate a similar lesion in the lower metaphysis of the femur. These lesions are often difficult to differentiate from "calcifying chondroma"

older. The lesion generally remained stationary for a long time before treatment was sought.

This process is probably not a genuine neoplasm, but a cartilaginous hamartoma, that is, a developmental anomaly, originating in displaced remains of growth cartilage.

Radiographically, it is sometimes difficult to differentiate these lesions from ischemic bone infarct, which often exhibits a similar location and heavy circumscribed calcification of the necrotic bone marrow. Although a bone infarct is often more elongated, sometimes sharply marginated with radiolucent centers, and most heavily mineralized at its borders, the calcification is sometimes dense, with irregular borders, and indistinguishable from calcifying enchondroma (Figs. II.14, II.15). However, histopathologic differentiation is easy, mature cartilage showing scarce, small, typical, often necrotic cartilage cells (Fig. II.16), abundant hyaline, and heavily calcified ground substance, which often shows vascular penetration, followed by conspicuous enchondral ossification. In contrast, in bone infarct, cartilage tissue is lacking, and the radiopacity is produced by calcification of the necrotic marrow and by disintegrating necrotic bone trabeculae (Fig. II.15b). Similar cases have been interpreted by Milgram (1983) as intraosseous lipomas.

In some of our patients, curettage was performed, and we had no recurrences. Surgical treatment was indicated only in lesions with clinical symptoms, especially pain, or when there was the slightest doubt about the benign character of the process.

Multiple Chondromas (Multiple Enchondromatosis)

Chondromas may appear in the interior of several or many bones, most commonly the hands or feet. The disorder often shows a preferred unilateral involvement of the skeleton, described by Ollier (1900) as "dyschondroplasia." It represents an anomaly of skeletal development, without hereditary or familial influence, and is apparently related to heterotopic proliferation of epiphyseal chondroblasts (Aegerter and Kirkpatrick 1975) with consecutive failure of enchondral ossification and shortening of the involved long bones. Although, as the term "multiple enchondromatosis" implies, most lesions are centrally located within the metaphysis, extending into the diaphysis, infrequently a lesion may develop subperiosteally or juxtacortically with secondary erosion and excavation of the underlying cortex.

Because Ollier emphasized the unilaterality, most writers use the name Ollier's disease to designate those cases in which the lesions are entirely or predominantly in one side of the skeleton. The association of enchondromatosis with multiple hemangiomas of soft tissue, reported in 1881 by Maffucci (18 years before Ollier), is

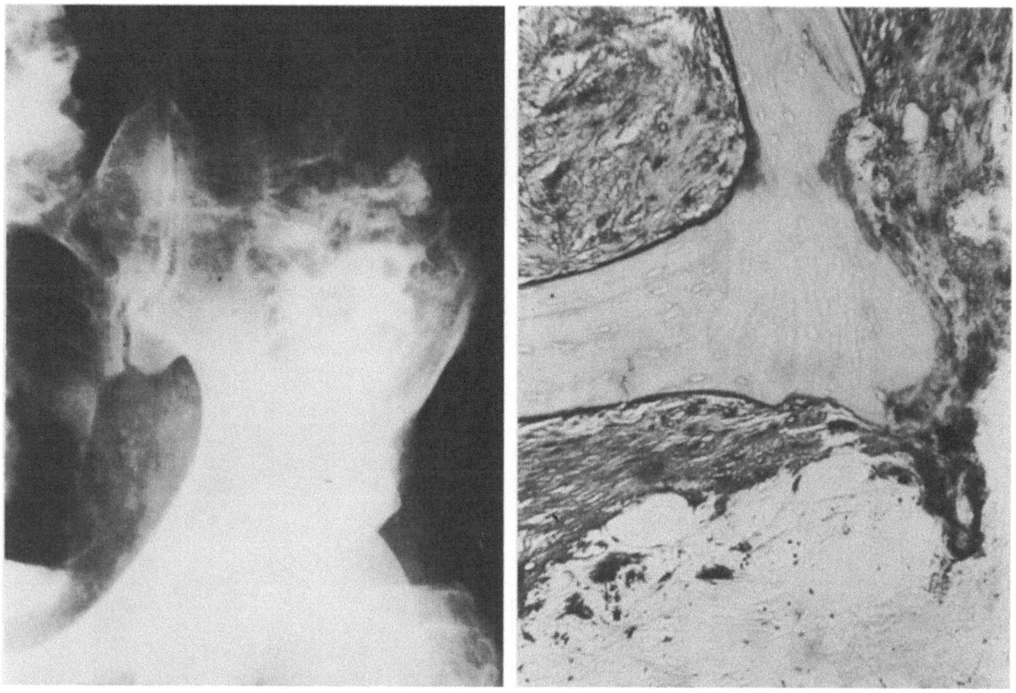

a b

Fig. II.15a,b. Male, 46 years old. **a** Radiograph shows dense, heavily calcified lesion in the ilium, with irregular contours, partly surrounded by a radiolucent area. **b** Photomicrograph shows necrotic bone surrounded by necrotic and calcified fat marrow. The histologic aspect is similar to that observed in radiation osteitis. ×100

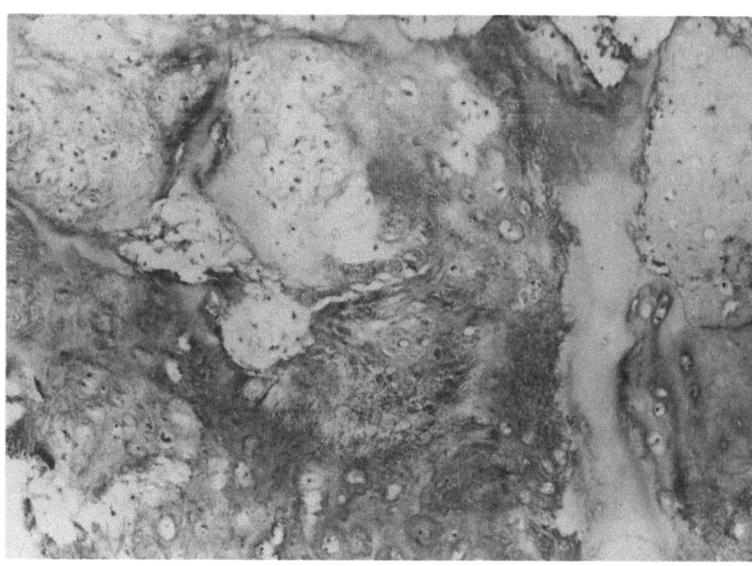

Fig. II.16. Photomicrograph illustrating the histologic features of "calcifying chondroma." The cartilage tissue is poorly cellular and shows extensive areas of calcification. ×80

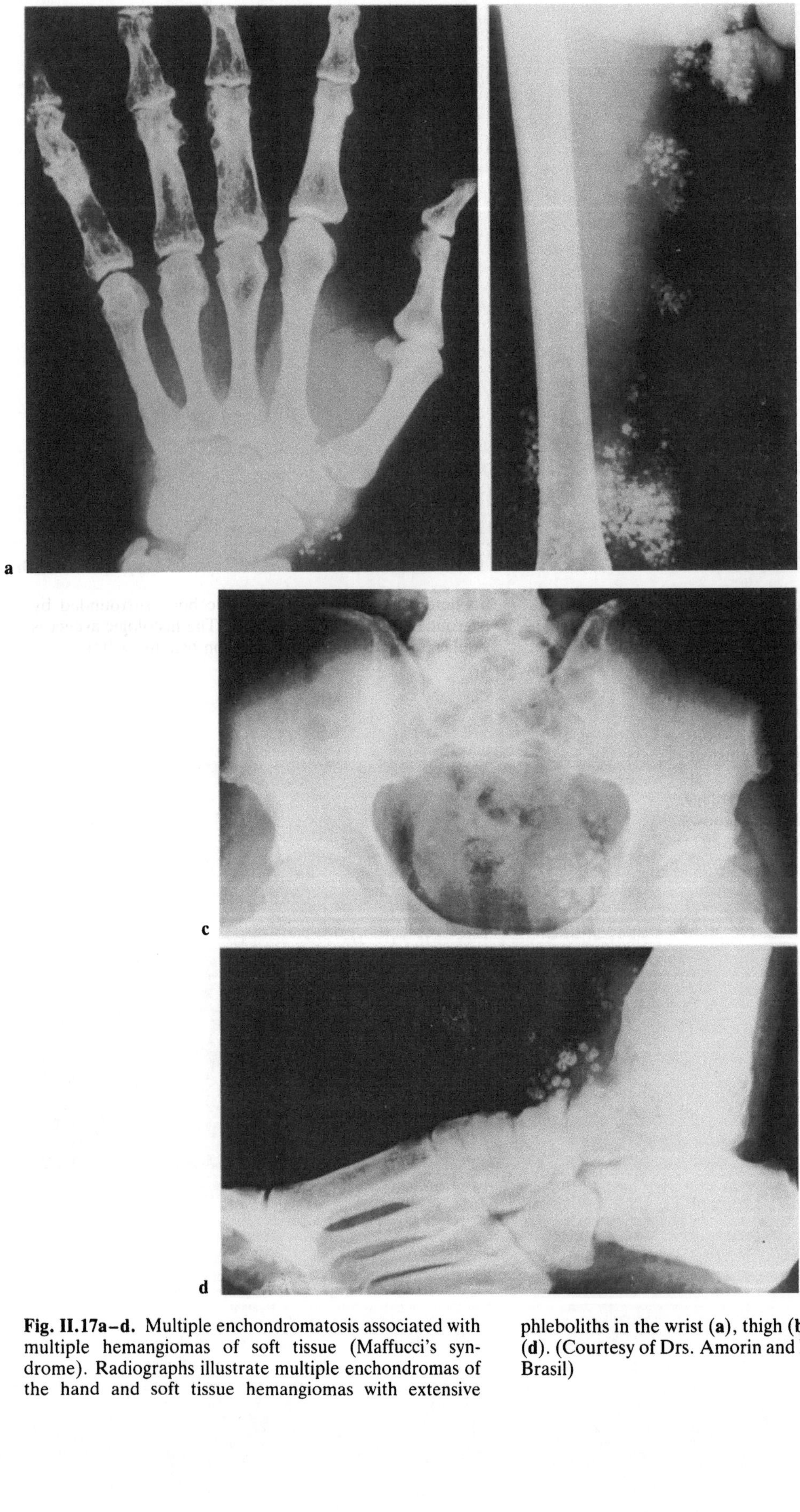

Fig. II.17a–d. Multiple enchondromatosis associated with multiple hemangiomas of soft tissue (Maffucci's syndrome). Radiographs illustrate multiple enchondromas of the hand and soft tissue hemangiomas with extensive phleboliths in the wrist (**a**), thigh (**b**), pelvis (**c**), and ankle (**d**). (Courtesy of Drs. Amorin and Lemos, Rio de Janeiro, Brasil)

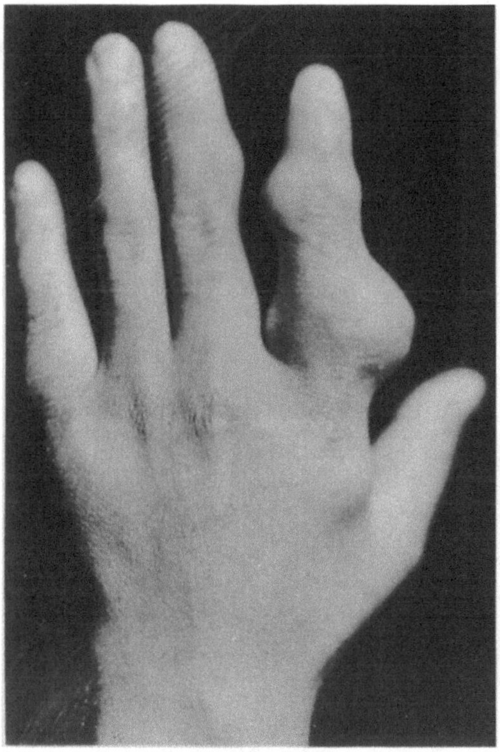
a

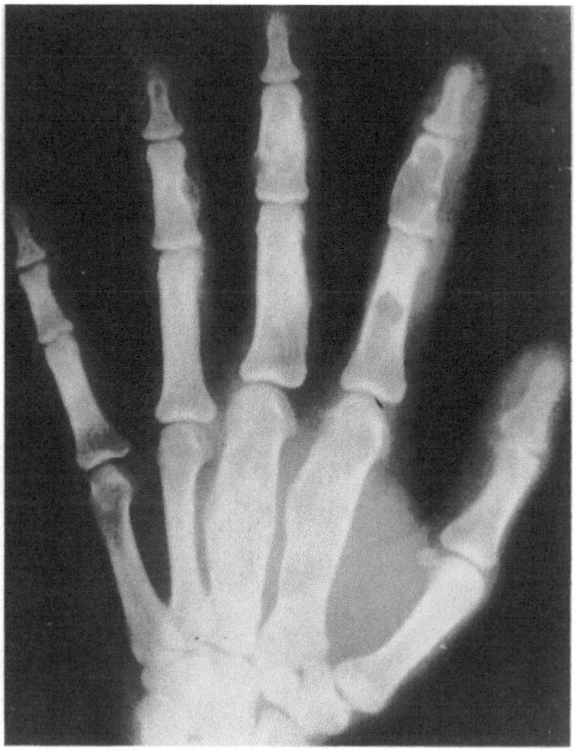
b

Fig. II.18a,b. Multiple chondromatosis of the hand without Ollier's syndrome. **a** Photograph showing deformities of fingers. **b** Radiograph reveals multiple central chondromas of metacarpal and phalangeal bones. A small juxtacortical chondroma is seen in the second phalanx of the ring finger. No chondromas were found in the other bones

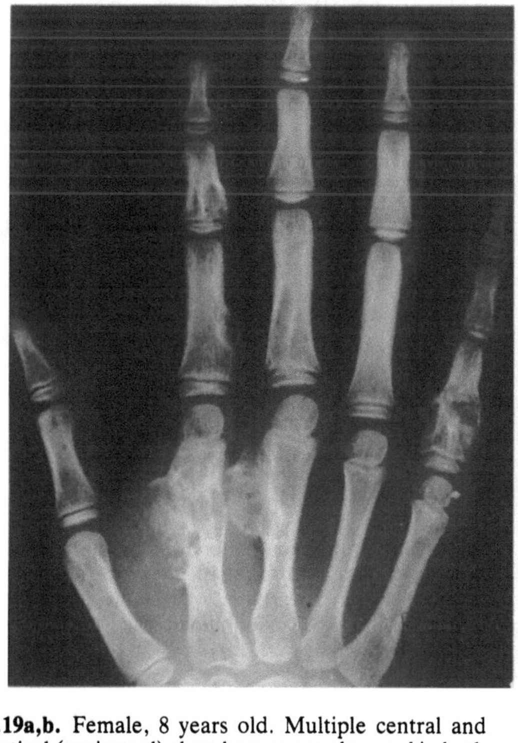
a

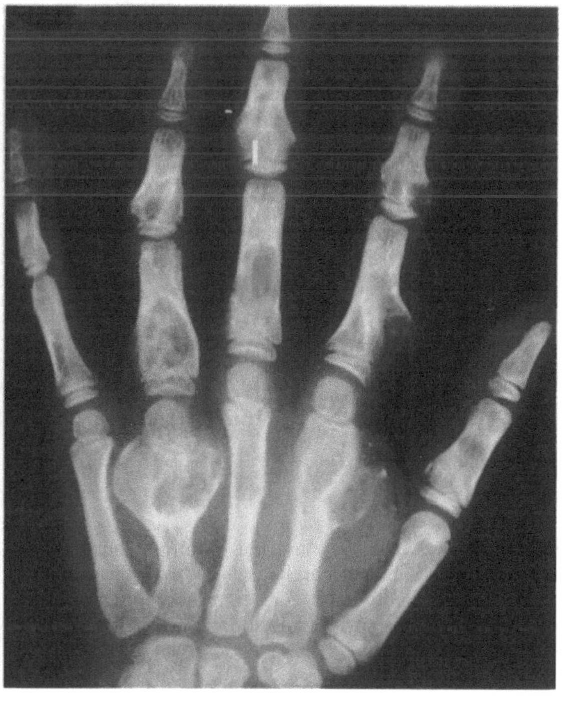
b

Fig. II.19a,b. Female, 8 years old. Multiple central and juxtacortical (periosteal) chondromas are observed in both hands, but not in other bones

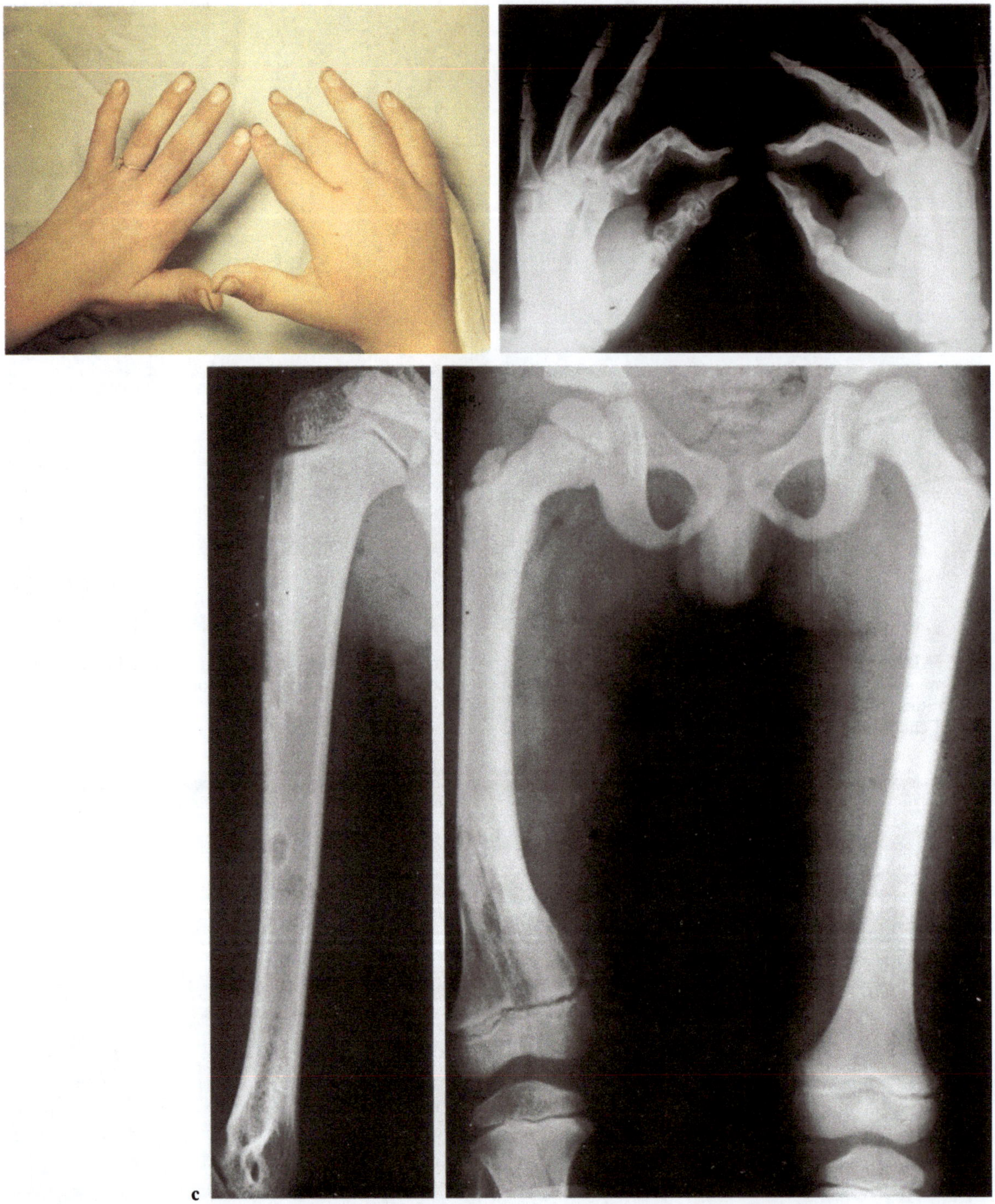

a b c d

Fig. II.20a–e. Male, 9 years old. Multiple enchondromatosis of predominantly unilateral involvement (Ollier's syndrome). **a** Photograph and **b** radiograph show the predominant unilateral involvement of the hand. **c–e** Radiographs illustrate the characteristic longitudinal radiolucent strands that extend a variable distance from the growth plate into the shaft; they are clearly visible in **c** the upper humerus, **d** the lower femur, and **e** the upper part of the ilium. A small radiolucent lesion is seen in the shaft of the humerus

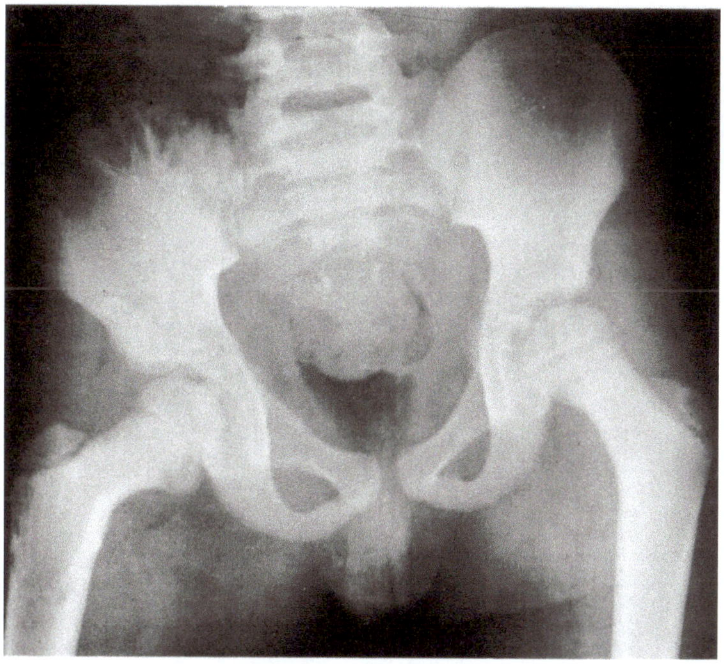

II.20e

Fig. II.21a,b. Ollier's syndrome. Photographs showing the characteristic longitudinal cartilage columns extending from the growth cartilage into a the shaft of the femur and b the tibia. Small isolated, separated cartilage nodules are seen in the spongiosa

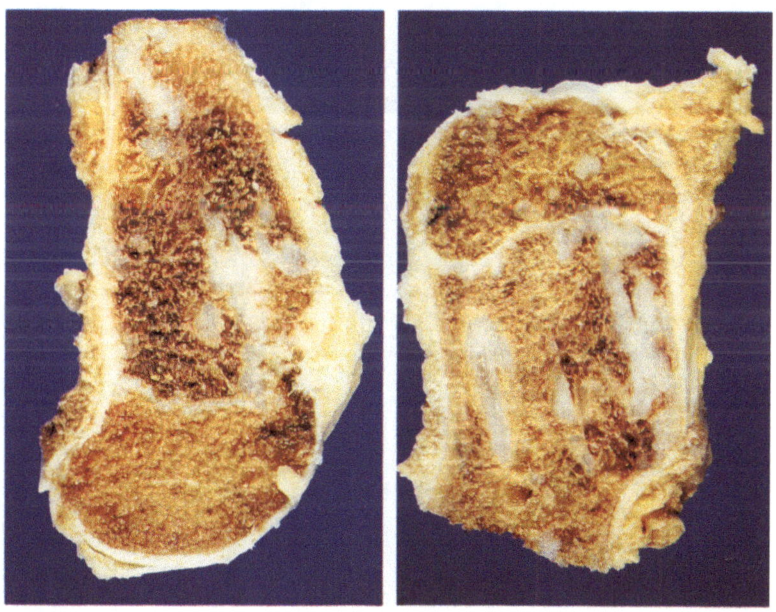

generally referred to as "Maffucci's syndrome" (Fig. II.17). Lewis and Ketcham (1973) found in 96 of 103 cases from the literature cavernous or capillary hemangiomas of phlebectasia, most commonly subcutaneous and rarely visceral with or without phleboliths. In others, they also found venous plus lymphatic lesions or lymphangiomas. The bone lesions are enchondromas and not intraosseous hemangiomas, and we agree with Spjut et al. (1971) that the cases reported by André et al. (1963) should be classified as hemangiomatosis of bone and not as Maffucci's syndrome.

Clinical Findings. Multiple enchondromatosis first becomes manifest in early childhood, with deformities and distortion of the growth length of the involved bones as a result of the failure

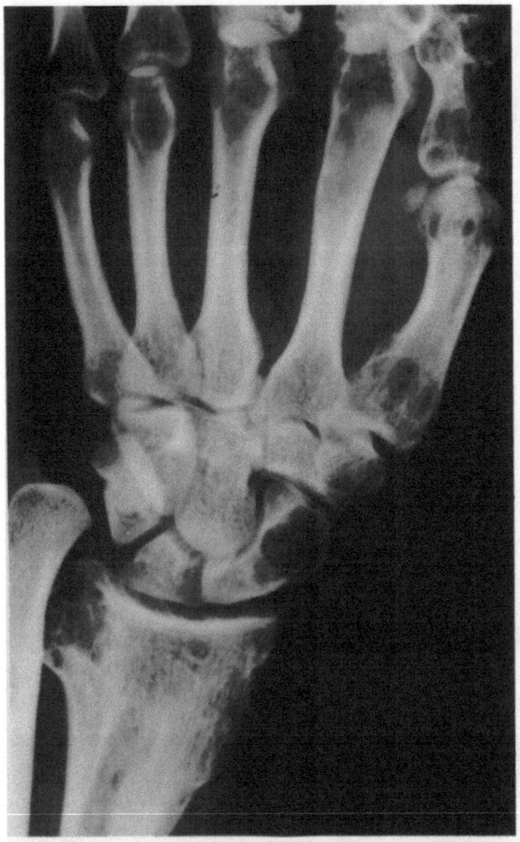

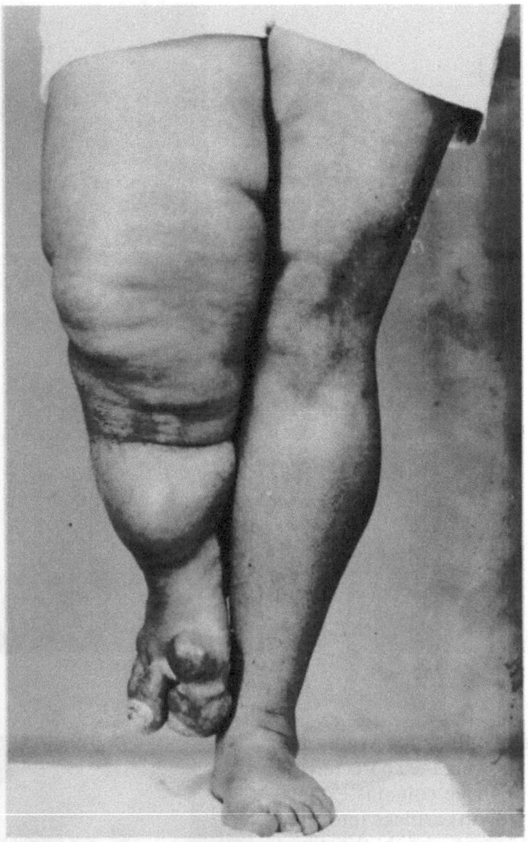

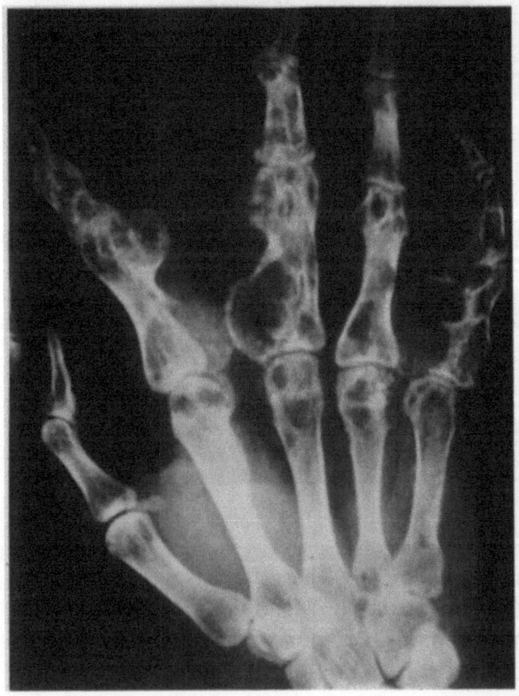

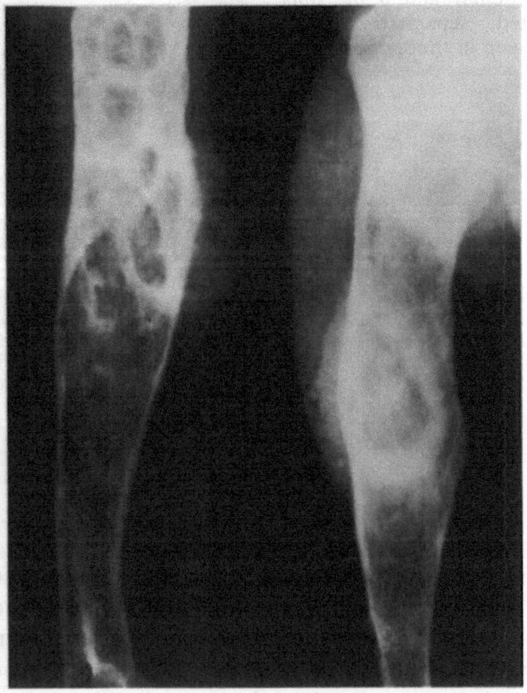

Fig. II.22. a,b. Female, 16 years old. Multiple enchondromatosis with sarcomatous transformation. **a** Radiograph showing multiple enchondromas in the phalanges, scaphoid, and lower end of the radius. **b** Photograph showing marked shortening of one extremity and the malignant tumor of the foot. **c–e** Male, 21 years old. Ollier's syndrome with sarcomatous transformation. **c** Radiograph of hand with multiple enchondromas. **d** Radiograph of humerus with chondrosarcoma.

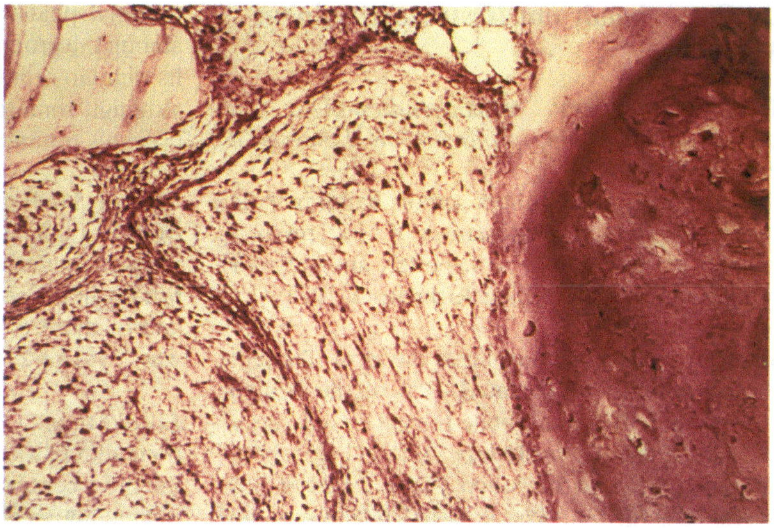

e

Fig. II.22e. Photomicrograph showing areas of enchondroma (*right*) besides others of chondrosarcoma, predominantly myxoid. ×125

of normal enchondral ossification. The lesion is often apparent at an early age, especially because of evident swelling of the fingers (Figs. II.18, II.19), followed by bowing and growth distortion, with resulting deformities such as genu valgum and retarded growth, commonly of the lower extremities. As in multiple osteochondromatosis, the ulna frequently displays a greater degree of shortening than the radius; in these circumstances, the shaft of the radius may be curved and the radial head dislocated. Fractures are rare, except in severely affected phalanges.

Radiographic Features. Areas of radiolucency of varying size and shape but with a marked tendency toward a columnar arrangement are observed in the metaphyses of the most rapidly growing ends of long bones, except in the hands and feet. Longitudinal radiolucent strands are produced which extend varying distances from the growth cartilage into the shaft (Fig. II.20). The density of bone between the cartilage columns is sometimes increased, giving a characteristic striated appearance of the involved, often enlarged and deformed, metaphysis. In the digits, distension and bulging of the thinned and sometimes interrupted cortex over one or more chondromas are common, with less preference for the metaphysis and rarely a tendency toward columnar arrangements (Figs. II.19, II.21). Some of the lesions are evidently eccentric, apparently of periosteal origin. Another common location is the ilium, near the crest, where one observes typical columns radiating in a fanlike manner toward the crest (Fig. II.20).

Grossly and microscopically, the lesions are similar to those of solitary enchondroma, but are often predominantly myxoid and more cellular, with larger and more common double nuclei, that is, more ominous looking. In fact, the risk of malignant transformation is greater than with any other benign cartilage lesion (Fig. II.22). However, the exact incidence of this complication, which may affect one or rarely more bones, is difficult to establish. Dahlin (1978) reported eight cases complicated by chondrosarcoma in 26 patients with skeletal enchondromatosis (32%), which is more in accordance with our experience (20%) than the estimated 50% of Jaffe (1958). A lower incidence (15%) of sarcomatous transformation in the enchondromas associated with Maffucci's syndrome was reported in a review of the literature by Lewis and Ketcham (1973). On the other hand, Sun and Swee (1985) gave a higher number of cases of malignant transformation in Maffucci's syndrome.

Treatment and Prognosis. Sometimes the disorder ceases to progress after puberty; in other cases, the lesions continue growing, with development of monstrous deformities, especially of the fingers and feet (Fig. II.22b).

There is no indication for radiotherapy. Surgery may be required to correct deformities of the extremities or to remove large tumors of the fingers in order to improve hand function.

2. Osteochondroma (Osteocartilaginous Exostosis)

Definition, WHO: *Osteochondroma is "a cartilage-capped bony projection on the external surface of a bone."*

Although most authors and the writer include this lesion in their classification of bone tumors, others consider it a congenital anomaly or hamartoma (Aegerter and Kirkpatrick 1975).

Incidence. Osteochondroma is the most frequent bone tumor; it represented 41% of the benign tumors and 19% of all bone tumors in our series of 1001 cases (considering solitary osteochondromas only). In the Mayo Clinic series of 640 cases (Dahlin and Unni 1986), it represented 35.8% of the benign tumors and 8.5% of all tumors. In the AFIP files, 880 cases of solitary osteochondromas were recorded as compared with 725 enchondromas. In Huvos' series (1991) osteochondromas constituted approximately 50% of benign tumors and 10%–15% of all bone tumors. In contrast to other authors (Dahlin and Unni 1986), we included the so-called subungual exostosis, which arises from the distal portion of a terminal phalanx, particularly of the great toe, among the group of osteochondromas, because of its similar radiographic and pathologic aspects, although some cases may possibly be related to previous traumas.

Clinical Findings. *Age and sex.* Most patients (69%) in our and other series were less than 20 years of age at the time of diagnosis or removal, usually in the second decade (47%). In our series and in those of others, the male-to-female ratio was 1.5:1 or 2:1 (Scheme II.2).

Localization. Osteochondroma may occur in any bone that has been preformed from cartilage, but the most common locations are the long bones at the metaphyseal region of the most active growth cartilage, that is, the upper end of the humerus (146 cases), the lower end of the femur (215 cases), and the upper end of the tibia (140 cases), with an incidence of 36.4% around the knee.

Other bones often involved are the ilium (38 cases), scapula (41 cases), fibula (32 cases), and phalanges of hands and feet. In patients over 20 years old, an osteochondroma may be located in the shaft of a long bone.

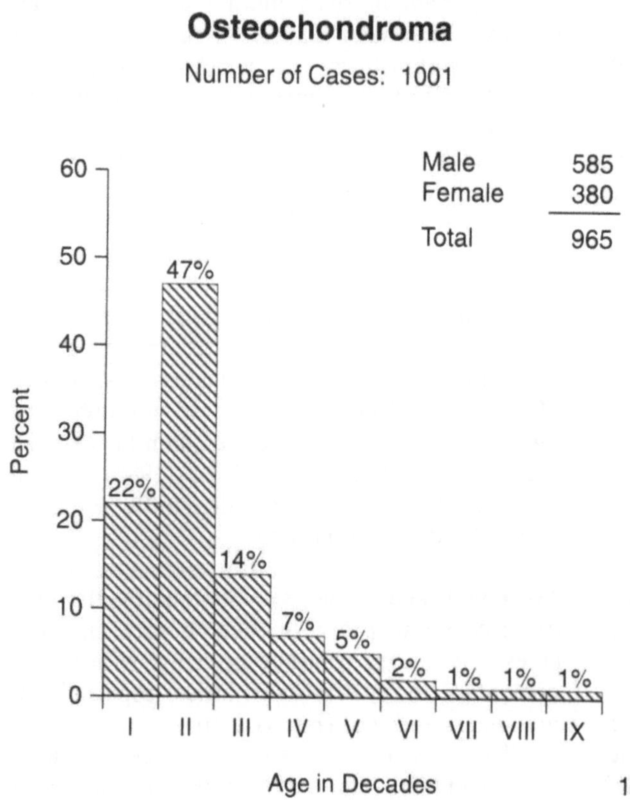

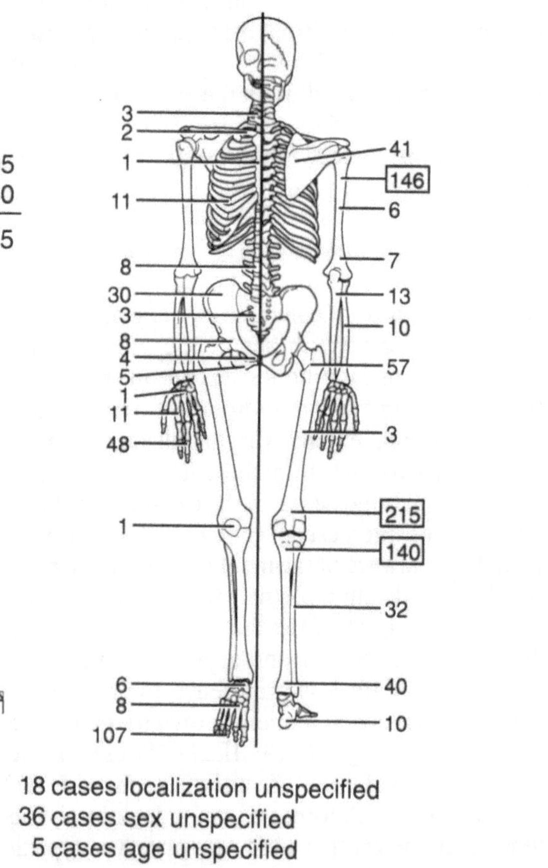

Scheme II.2

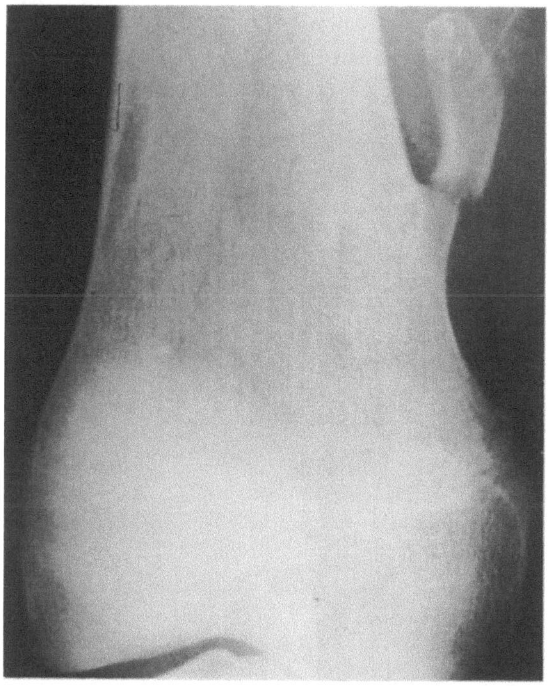

Fig. II.23. Male, 15 years old. Pedunculated osteochondroma of the lower metaphysis of the femur with fracture of the large pedicle. Cortex and spongiosa of the exostosis blend with those of the shaft

Symptoms. Osteochondroma may be asymptomatic and is frequently discovered in an incidental radiographic study or because of a painless bony mass. In several cases, the lesion was accompanied by pain due to pressure on neighboring structures, most commonly bones or vascular-nervous elements. In some cases, the development of a bursa on the top of the cartilage cap, accompanied by an inflammatory reaction, led to the discovery of a previously silent lesion. In several others, sudden pain was due to a fracture of the long stalk of a pedunculated osteochondroma (Fig. II.23). Rarely, the rupture of a major blood vessel may result in formation of a false aneurysm (Anastasi et al. 1963; Clark and Keokarn 1965; Hershey and Lansden 1972; Ferriter et al. 1983).

Radiographic Features. Osteochondromas may have a narrow or a broad base, that is, they may be either *pedunculated* or *sessile* (Figs. II.24–II.31). The radiographic aspect of the pedunculated type is characteristic, showing a bony projection of different thickness or longitude, continuous with the underlying cortex and spongiosa and showing irregular calcification of

a

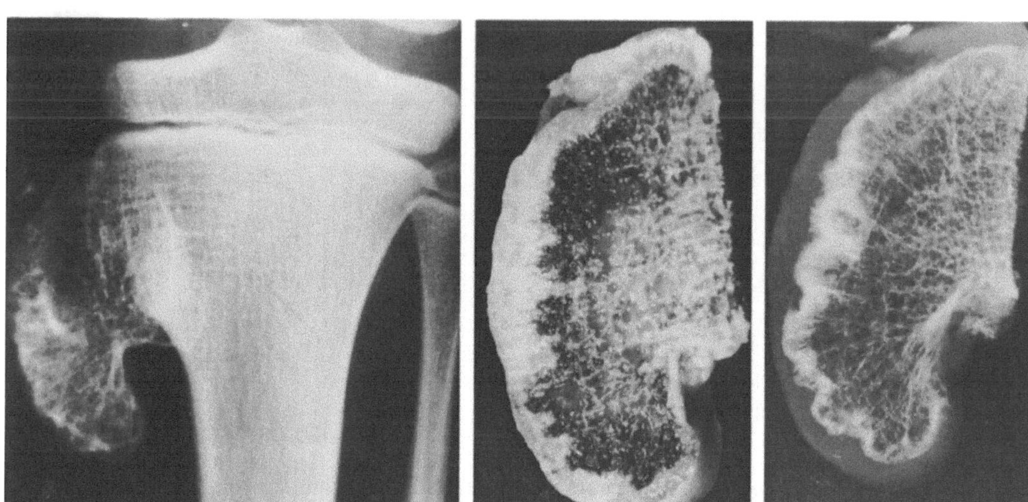

b, c

Fig. II.24a–c. Male, 10 years old. Osteochondroma of the upper metaphysis of the tibia. **a** Radiograph shows the short pedicle with broad base and areas of calcification at its surface. **b** Photograph and **c** radiograph of the specimen illustrate the variable thickness of the cartilage cap and a more radiodense zone at the osteocartilaginous limit, corresponding to areas of calcification

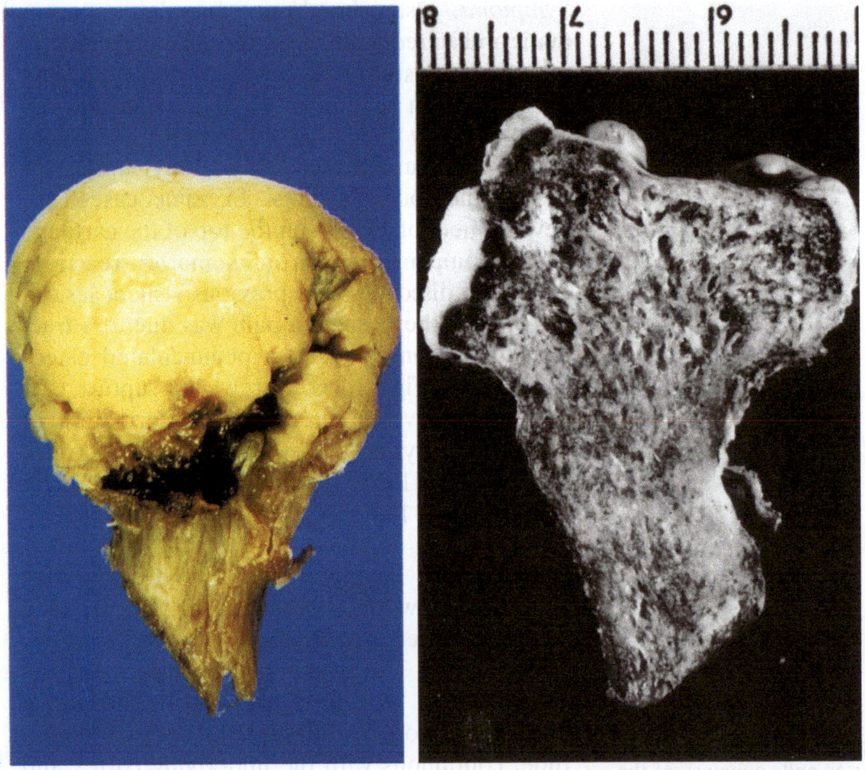

Fig. II.25a,b. Female, 21 years old, with osteochondroma of the femur. Photographs of the surface and cut section showing the smooth lobulated cartilage cap and the stalk of the lesion that contains normal cancellous bone

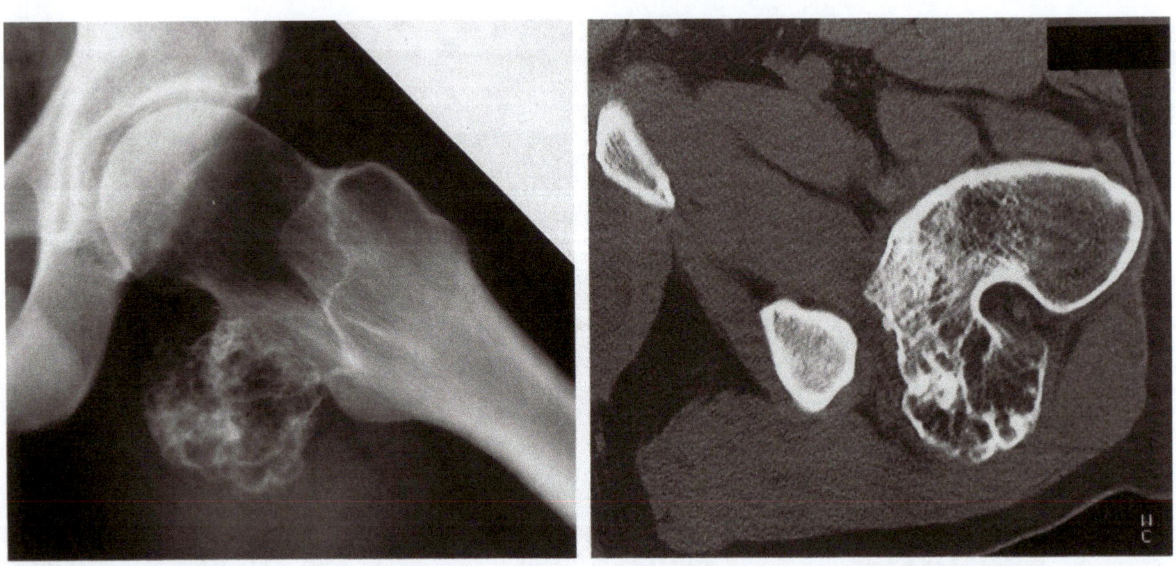

Fig. II.26a,b. Male, 44 years old. Osteochondroma of the femoral neck. **a** Radiograph shows the short pedicle and lobulated, well-defined surface, clearly seen with **b** CT scan, illustrating the continuity of the spongiosa of the exostosis with that of the femoral neck. The patient consulted because of moderate pain, apparently due to an overlying bursitis. (St. Louis University Medical Center)

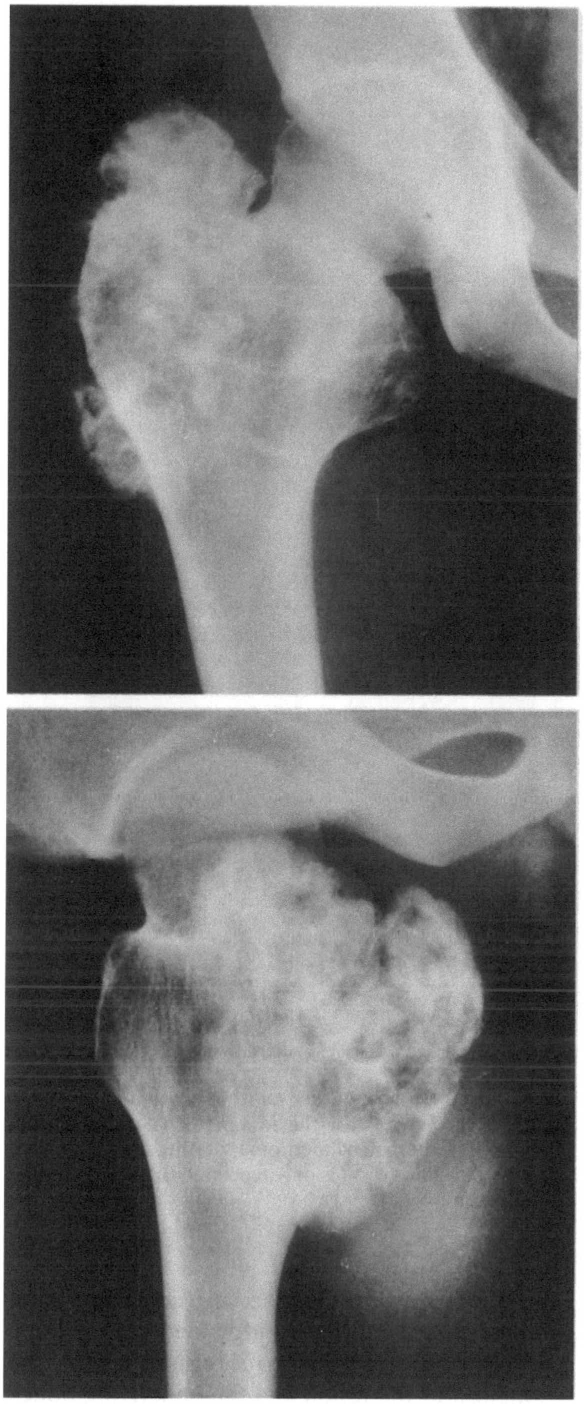

a

b

Fig. II.27a,b. Female, 18 years old. Osteochondroma of femur. **a** Anteroposterior and **b** lateral radiographs show a large lesion of the upper metaphysis with a well-delineated lobular surface. Histologically the lesion was benign

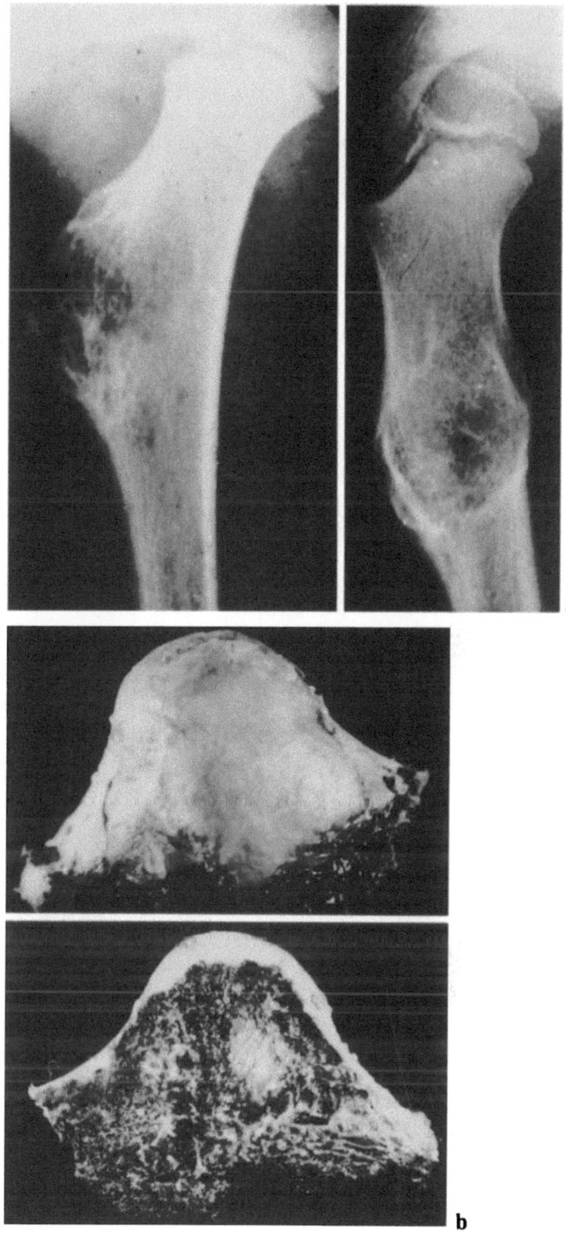

a

b

Fig. II.28a,b. Male, 6 years old. Osteochondroma of the upper metaphysis of the humerus, sessile type. **a** Anteroposterior and lateral radiographs showing the continuity of the spongiosa and the cortex of the humerus with those of this sessile osteochondroma. The lateral radiograph simulates a solitary bone cyst. Abnormal width of the bone at level of osteochondroma due to failure of normal remodeling. **b** Photographs of the surface and cut section showing the smooth cartilage cup that covered only part of the exostosis. The bulk of the lesion is cancellous bone containing red marrow extending into the spongiosa of underlying bone

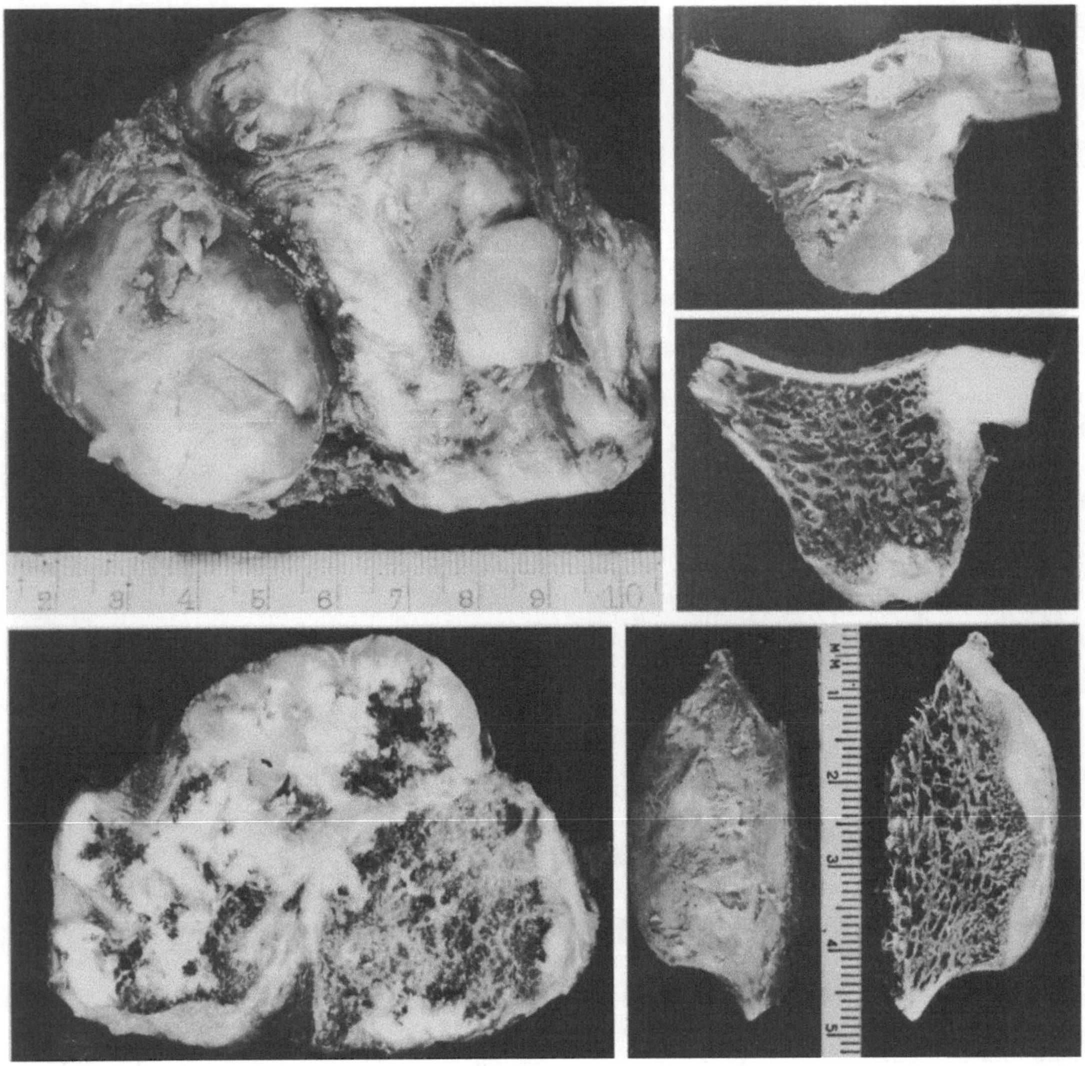

Fig. II.29. a,b. Male, 26 years old. Large osteochondroma of the ilium, sessile variety. Photographs showing the lobulated surface (**a**) and the cut section (**b**), which reveals the variable thickness of the cartilage that is in part more than 2 cm thick; however, histologically, there were no signs of malignancy and the patient was free of disease 6 years after resection of the lesion. **c** Male 15-year-old. Photographs of osteochondroma of the rib. **d** Female 14-year-old. Photographs of osteochondroma of the upper tibial metaphysis

the cartilage-capped surface. This distal part is often enlarged and may show a cauliflowerlike aspect (Figs. II.25, II.26). The widening of the metaphyseal region, commonly observed in multiple osteochondromas, due to a lack of bone remodeling and tubulation, is generally absent in solitary osteochondroma. The diagnosis of an osteochondroma with a broad base (sessile type) is sometimes more difficult; it may be misdiagnosed as parosteal osteoma or hyperostosis, but the presence of a superficial zone of irregular calcification covering the bony part inclines the diagnosis toward osteochondroma (Fig. II.27).

If only one projection is used, the radiographic aspect may be confounded with a bone cyst (Fig. II.28), due to continuity with the spongiosa of the lesion and the underlying bone.

Pathologic Findings. *Gross Pathology.* The presence of a cartilage cap of variable thickness (generally less than 1 cm) in different areas depending on its growth activity is a characteristic finding. Especially in elderly patients, the cartilage cap may be thin or almost lacking. The size of the tumor varies from a few centimeters to more than 10 cm (Fig. II.27), but in our experience the size

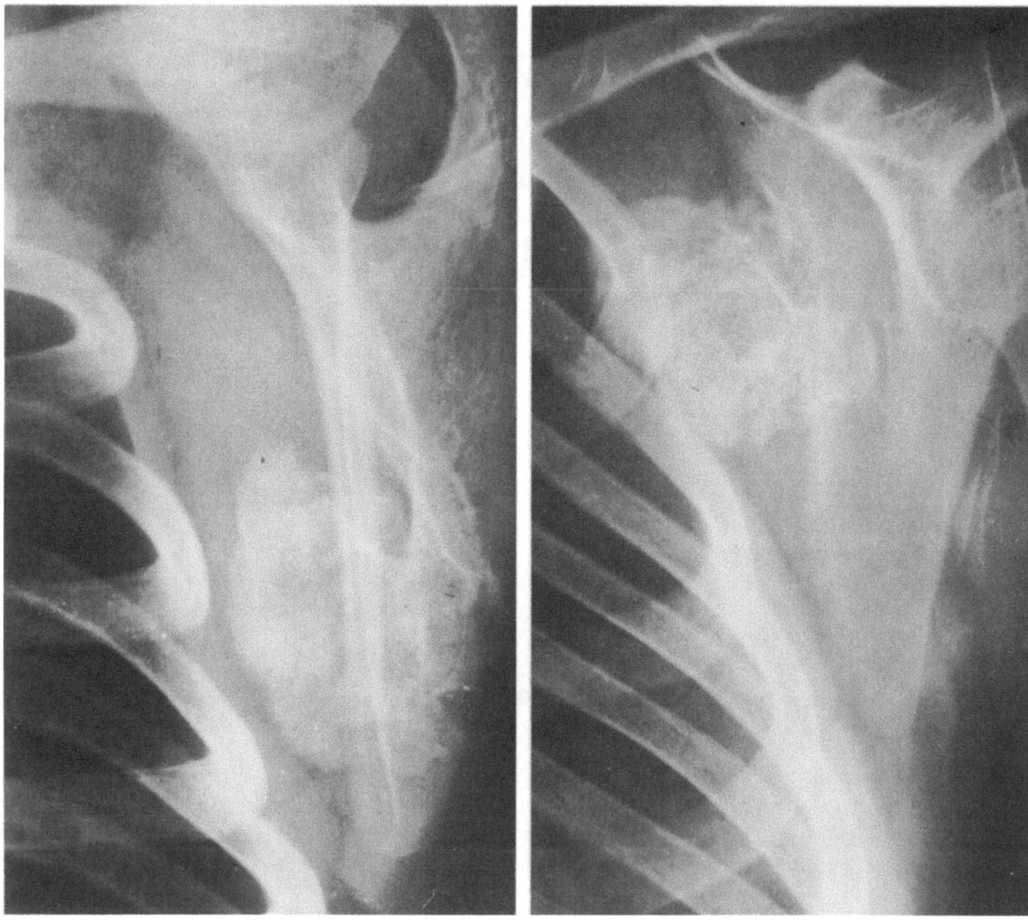

Fig. II.30. Male, 11 years old. Osteochondroma, scapula. Tangential and anteroposterior radiographs show a large, well-defined lesion, abutting the rib cage directly

Fig. II.31a,b. Two cases of osteochondroma of tibia with resorption due to compression of the fibula. **a** Male, 25 years old. Broad-based pedunculated osteochondroma of the upper metaphysis of the tibia. **b** Male, 12 years old. Sessile osteochondroma of the lower metaphysis of the tibia

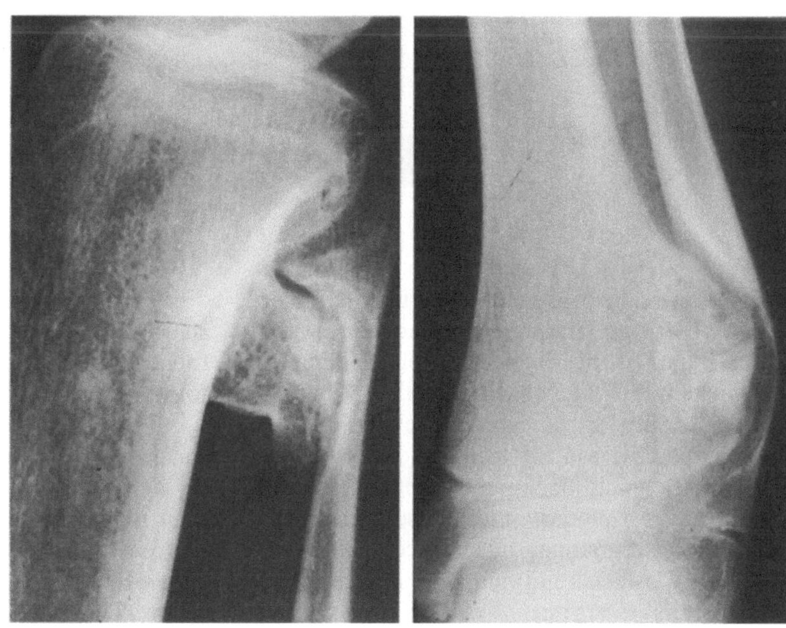

a b

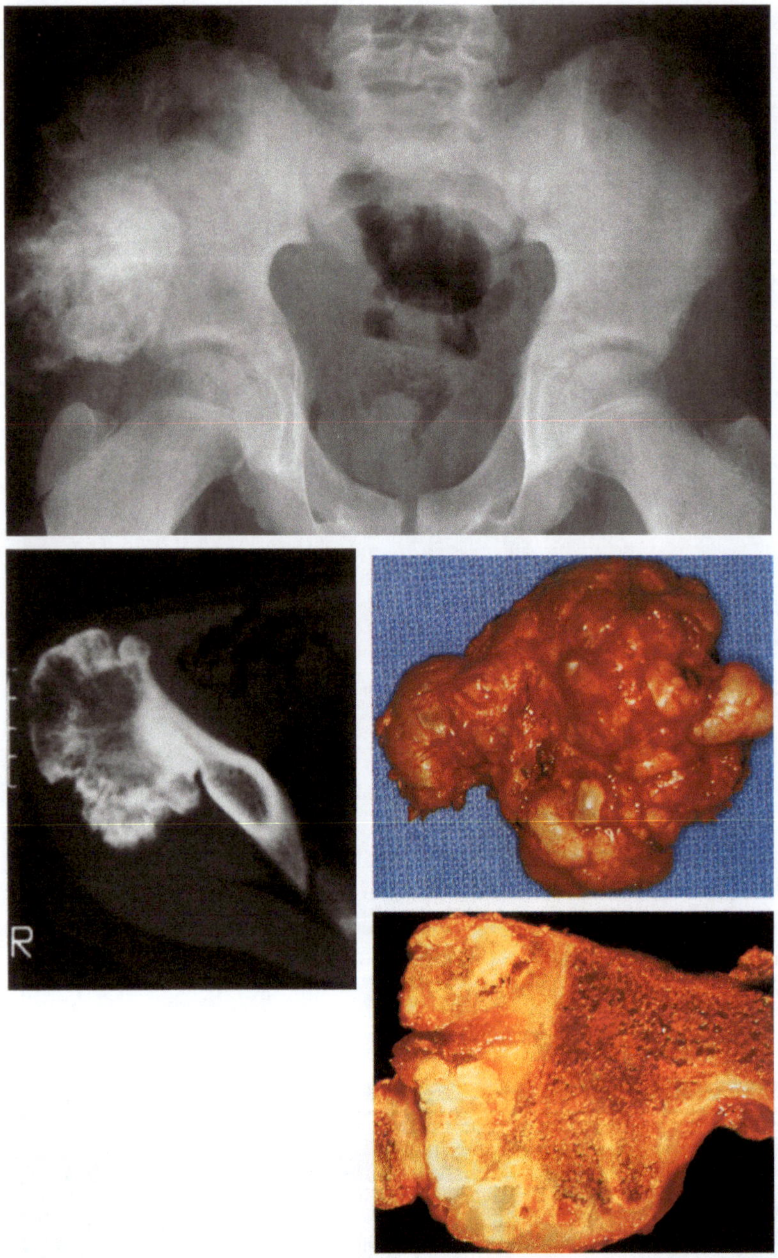

a b c d

Fig. II.32a–d. Female, 11 years old. Osteochondroma of ilium. **a** Radiograph shows a large calcified lesion with apparently ill-defined margins. However, CT scan **b** reveals the sharply defined, lobulated surface of this sessile lesion. **c,d** Photographs of the specimen illustrate the lobulated surface. At the cut section the variable thickness of the cartilage cap, which in part exceeds 2 cm, is seen. However, histologically the lesion was benign. (St. Louis University Medical Center)

of the lesion or the presence of a cartilaginous cap of more than 1 cm (frequent in osteochondromas of the ilium) is not indicative of malignancy (Lichtenstein 1977) (Figs. II.29, II.32). There is no absolute rule for the cap thickness that serves as a reliable criterion for malignancy. However, these lesions should be studied carefully in order to rule out a secondary chondrosarcoma (peripheral chondrosarcoma), which occurred rarely in a solitary osteochondroma (1.4%) in our and other authors' experience.

Furthermore, when an osteochondroma starts to become painful or starts growing after the end of the growth period, malignant transformation should be suspected.

The cartilage cap shows a smooth or lobulated surface of grayish-blue color and is covered by a thin, fibrous membrane (perichondrium) that represents a continuation of the adjacent periosteum. The spongious trabeculae of the exostosis blend with those of the shaft via the base (Figs. II.28, II.29, II.32). In some of our cases, an

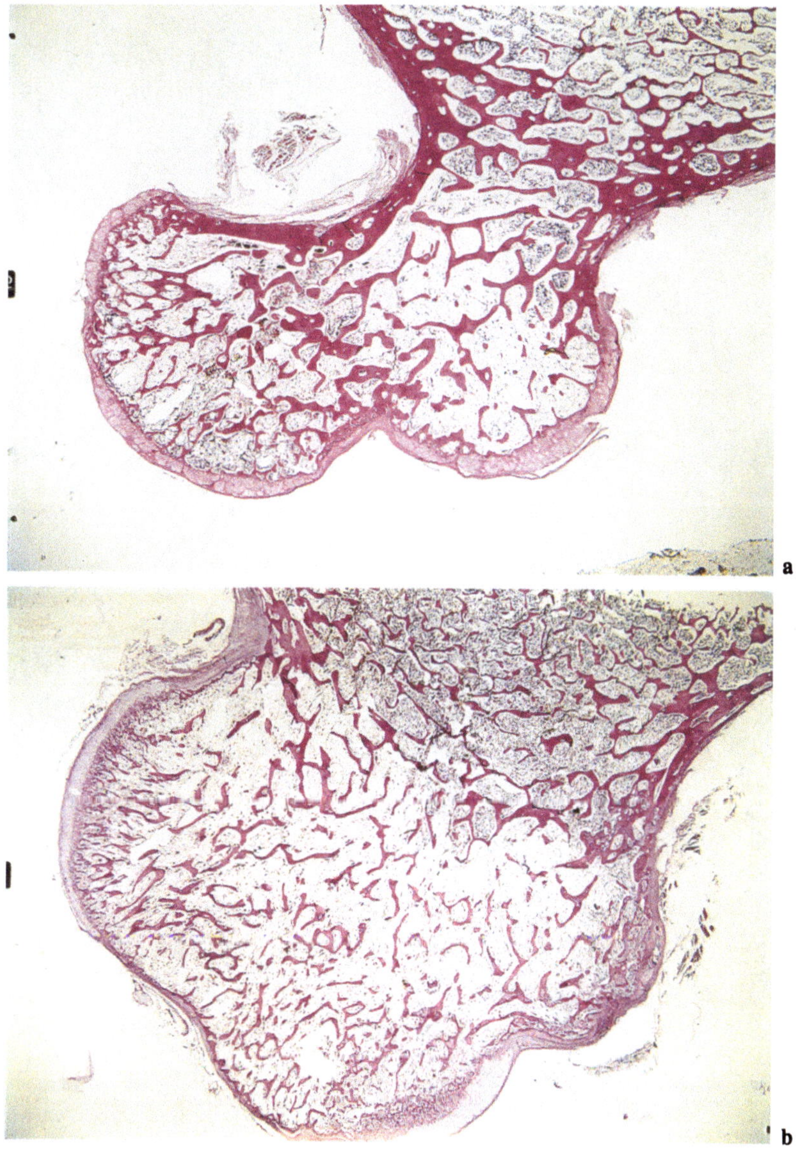

Fig. II.33a,b. Topographic photomicrograph of two different cases of osteochondroma, pedunculated type, showing the continuity of the cancellous bone and cortex of the stalk of the lesion with that of the underlying bone. **a,b** ×10

occasional bursa, developed on the top of the exostosis, showed an inflammatory reaction of the covering synovium, containing loose osteocartilaginous bodies in two patients. Borges et al. (1981) recorded a similar case.

Histopathology. The histologic aspect of the cartilage cap is similar to that seen in normal growth cartilage, although somewhat more irregular, especially in the deeper zone of hypertrophic and calcified cartilage (Figs. II.33, II.34). This zone is often much wider and of variable thickness. Since the process of active enchondral ossification is more irregular, it is common to find calcified cartilage rests, often surrounded by spongious bone trabeculae, at a certain distance from the irregular osteocartilaginous limit. The cartilage cells of the cap show small, single, dark nuclei and occasionally binucleated cells; cells with large, plump nuclei are generally absent (Fig. II.35). The bony component of the tumor consists of normal spongiosa that contains active

a
b
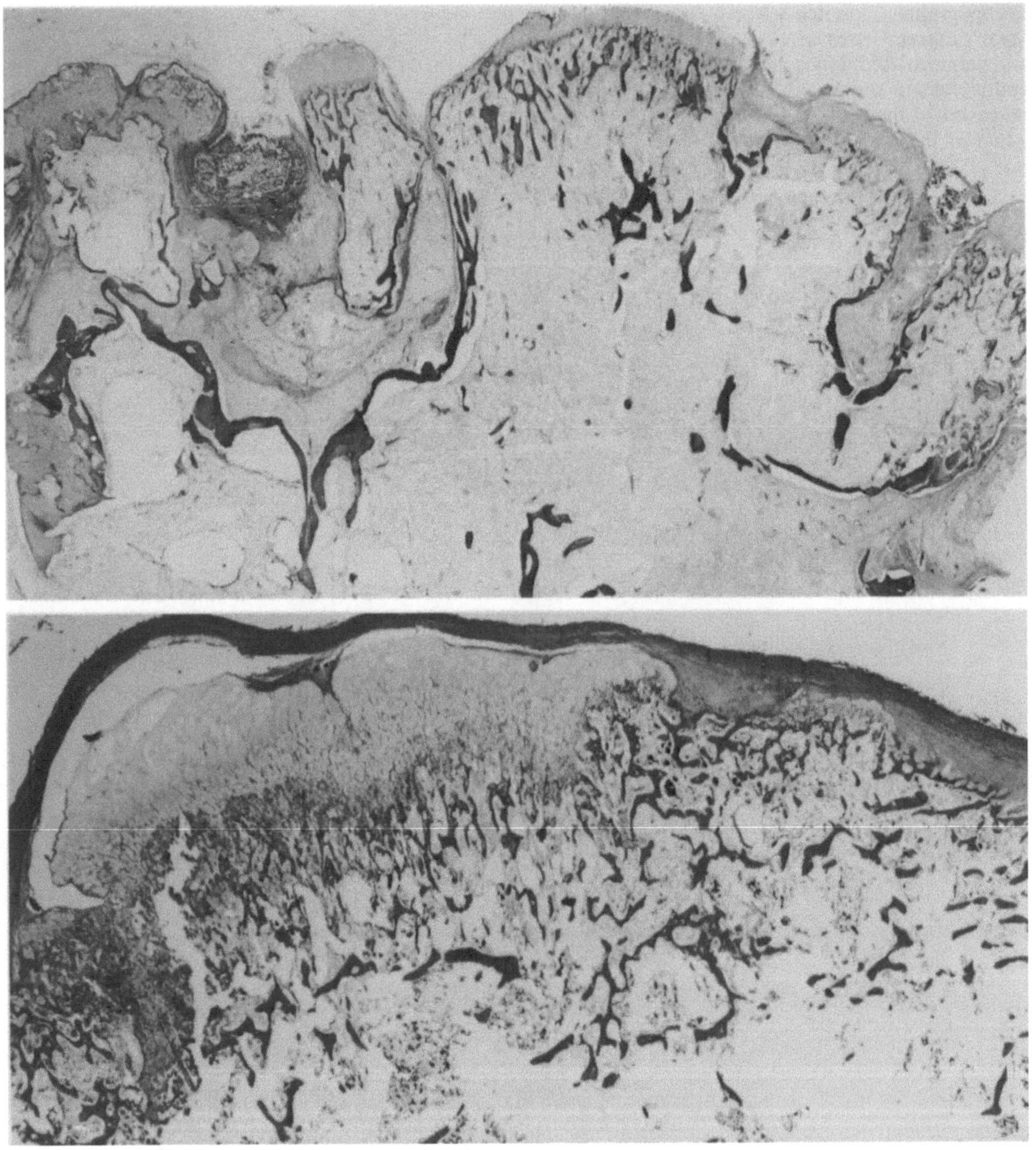

Fig. II.34a,b. Photomicrographs of two different cases of sessile osteochondroma. **a** Cartilage cap of variable thickness, partly lobulated with irregular osteocartilaginous limits. The cancellous bone is osteoporotic and occupied by predominantly fatty marrow. **b** Thick calcified area between the cap and cancellous bone. The superficial fibrous membrane (perichondrium) is partly detached (artifact). **a,b** ×6

Fig. II.35a,b. Photomicrographs of the cartilage cap and the underlying bone at lower (a) and higher (b) magnifications. The lower part is calcified and in the process of endochondral ossification. The underlying cancellous bone contains predominantly fatty marrow. The cartilage cap is covered by a fibrous tissue layer (perichondrium). a ×30, b ×100

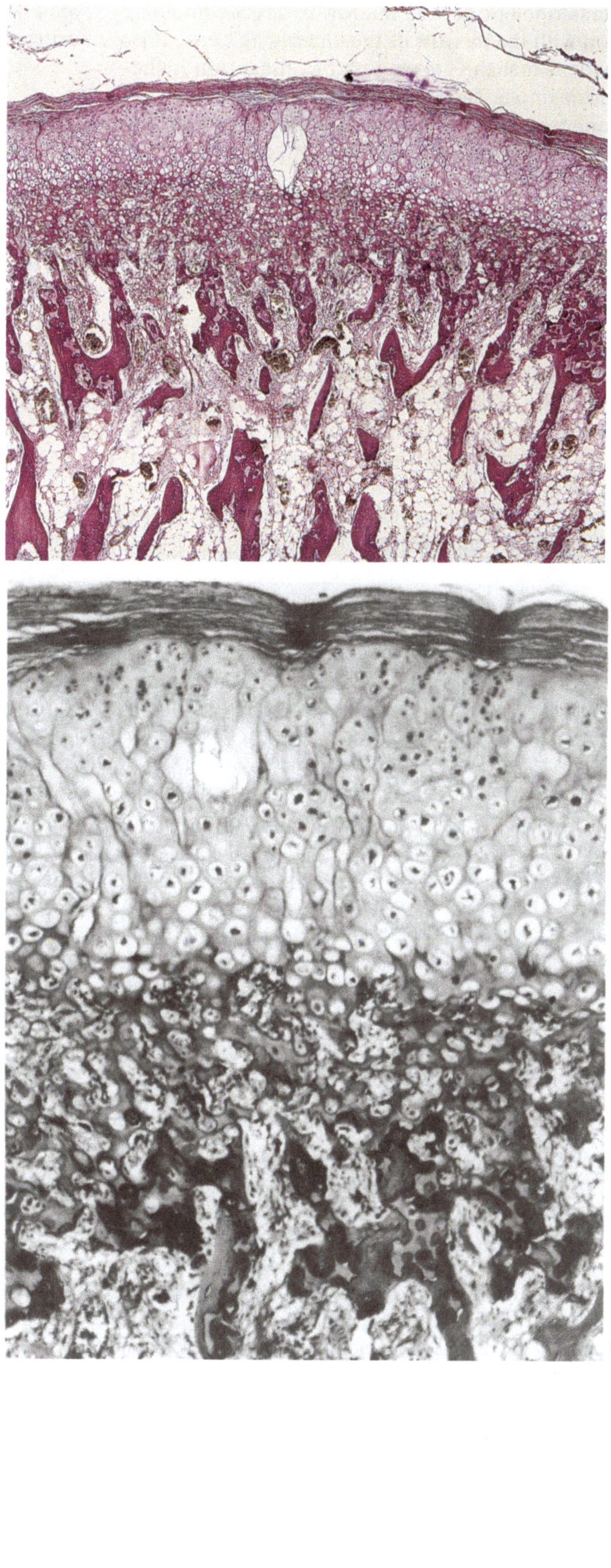

a

b

hematopoietic or fatty marrow in direct continuation with the marrow of the underlying bone. It is evident that the growing part of the lesion is the cartilaginous surface, which is often thicker in younger children, becoming thinner and sometimes disappearing completely in adults.

Pathogenesis. Since Virchow's (1891) hypothesis that a displaced fragment of growth cartilage rotates 90° and grows transversely to the long axis of the shaft under the periosteum of the juxtaepiphyseal-metaphyseal area, the genesis has remained disputed (Bethge 1963). Other authors suggested abnormal activity of periosteum (Scherer 1928), the presence of cartilage rests beneath the periosteum, or the presence of periosteal defects with herniation of segments of growth cartilage. Virchow's hypothesis seems to be supported by the experimental work of D'Ambrosia and Ferguson (1968).

On the other hand, there have been reports of the appearance of osteochondroma after intervals of several years in children exposed to radiation therapy at doses of 10–60 Gy and always involving bones adjacent to the irradiated area (Murphy and Blount 1962; Libshitz and Cohen 1982).

Treatment and Prognosis. Surgical removal is indicated only in those cases that present symptoms, especially pain due to neurovascular compression or the presence of bursitis. Surgical removal is also indicated in osteochondromas that have increased in size or become painful after the end of the epiphyseal growth period or when the radiologic aspect arouses suspicion of malignant transformation (Hudson et al. 1984). This complication is fortunately rare in solitary osteochondroma (Garrison et al. 1982) and had an incidence of only approximately 1% in our and in Dahlin's Mayo Clinic series (1978). The malignant tumor arising in osteochondroma is generally a chondrosarcoma (peripheral or exostotic chondrosarcoma), although cases of secondary osteosarcoma have been observed (Dahlin 1978, two cases; Slullitel et al. 1971, one case).

Recurrence in the pedunculated type is rare, because its complete excision is usually not difficult. The complete removal of a sessile osteochondroma is more difficult. In several cases, rests of the cartilage cap or the perichondrium remained, leading to recurrences of the lesion, but without malignant transformation or change in the histologic pattern. Therefore, in the sessile type a wider excision, including part of the neighboring cortex, is advised.

Subungual Osteochondroma (Subungual Exostosis)

Despite its histologic similarity, several authors (Jaffe 1958; Dahlin 1978) do not consider this painful lesion, located in the subungual zone of the distal phalanx, usually of the great toe, a genuine osteochondroma because of the frequent antecedent trauma and/or an associated infection. The cases with the pathologic features of osteochondroma and a definite cartilage cap (107 cases) were included in our statistics of osteochondromas.

Multiple Osteochondromas (Hereditary Osteochondromatosis)

Osteochondromatosis is an autosomal dominant hereditary disorder, transmitted by both parents (Shapiro et al. 1979; Peterson 1989). This condition was mentioned by Virchow, but it was Ehrenfried who reported 12 cases and reviewed the literature in 1915 and 1917, proposing the term "hereditary deforming chondrodysplasia." In the English literature "diaphyseal aclasis," introduced by Keith in 1919–1920, is the term of preference (Fairbank 1948). It emphasizes a characteristic of this condition, namely the greater widening and deformation of the metaphyseal as compared with the diaphyseal region due to a failure of remodeling or tubulation of this region. Therefore, in our opinion, the term "metaphyseal aclasis" would be preferable. The denomination "multiple hereditary osteochondroma or exostosis" is most commonly used.

The pathogenesis and the radiologic and pathologic features are similar to those of the solitary osteochondroma. However, a greater circumference of the bones and less usual sites are frequently involved. In our series of 63 cases, there was a slight predilection for males, and the disorder was often first discovered at a younger age than the solitary lesion (30% under 10 years of age). Frequently, growth disturbances such as shortness and marked deformities of the involved long bones were observed (Fig. II.36). As in enchondromatosis, shortening of the ulna, associated with marked bowing of the radius, is a

Fig. II.36. Female, 18 years old. Multiple osteochondromas (osteochondromatosis). Photographs show the limitation of joint movement (flexion) of the right leg and the multiple deformities in the metaphyseal region of both extremities

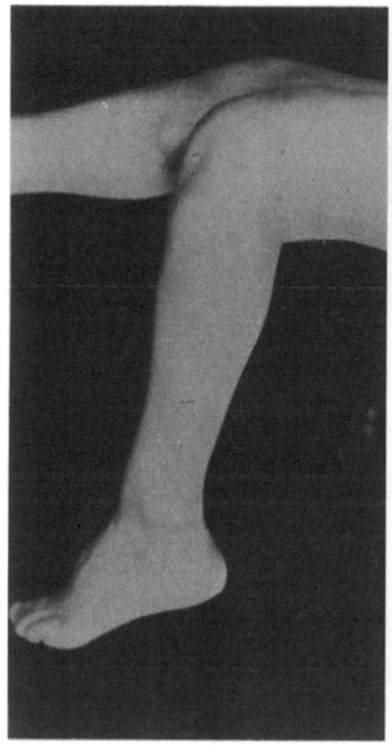

a

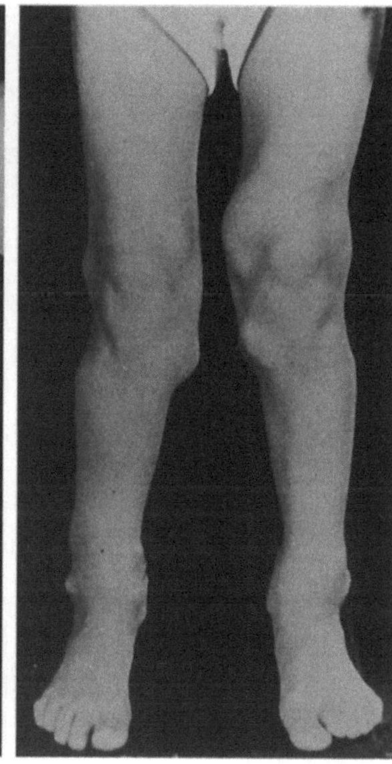

b

frequent finding, producing the so-called pseudo-Madelung deformity.

The most commonly involved sites are the metaphyseal regions around the knee, hip, and shoulder joints; however, flat bones, especially the scapula and the innominate bone, are also frequently involved. All bones of cartilaginous preformation may be the site of an exostosis; no lesions in bones of membranous origin (skull) were observed in our series (Figs. II.37, II.38).

Treatment and Prognosis. The treatment should be selective: That part of the large exostosis that causes unaesthetic deformities or functional disturbances, such as reduction of joint motion and/or pain due to pressure phenomena or bursae formation, should be removed. On the other hand, the risk of chondrosarcomatous transformation is higher than in solitary osteochondroma. Exact figures on the real incidence of malignant change are unknown, because many cases are not followed long enough, and only selected cases come to specialized centers. The percentage varies in different publications from 11% (Jaffe 1958) to approximately 20% (Dahlin 1978). In the writer's material, it was approximately 15%.

Dysplasia Epiphysealis Hemimelica

This developmental nonhereditary disorder, also referred to as "Trevor disease," is characterized by an asymmetric overgrowth at one side of one or more epiphyses, with predilection for one side of the limb. Fairbank (1956) reported 14 cases and introduced the term "dysplasia epiphysealis hemimelica." Kettlekamp et al. (1966) found multiple lesions in more than two-thirds of 56 cases. However, though more than one epiphysis may be involved, the lesions are usually located in one extremity. The talus and distal femoral and tibial epiphyses are the most common sites (Keats 1957; Fairbank 1956). The most frequent complaint is restricted motion, especially in the ankle joint due to the cartilaginous overgrowth. Radiologically, one sees several irregular radiopacities adjacent to one side of the involved epiphysis, often separated at the beginning and later fusing with the neighboring bone (Fig. II.39).

Pathologically, with the exception of its location in relation to an *epiphysis* or to carpal or tarsal bones, the lesion is indistinguishable from an osteochondroma and has also been called "epiphyseal osteochondroma."

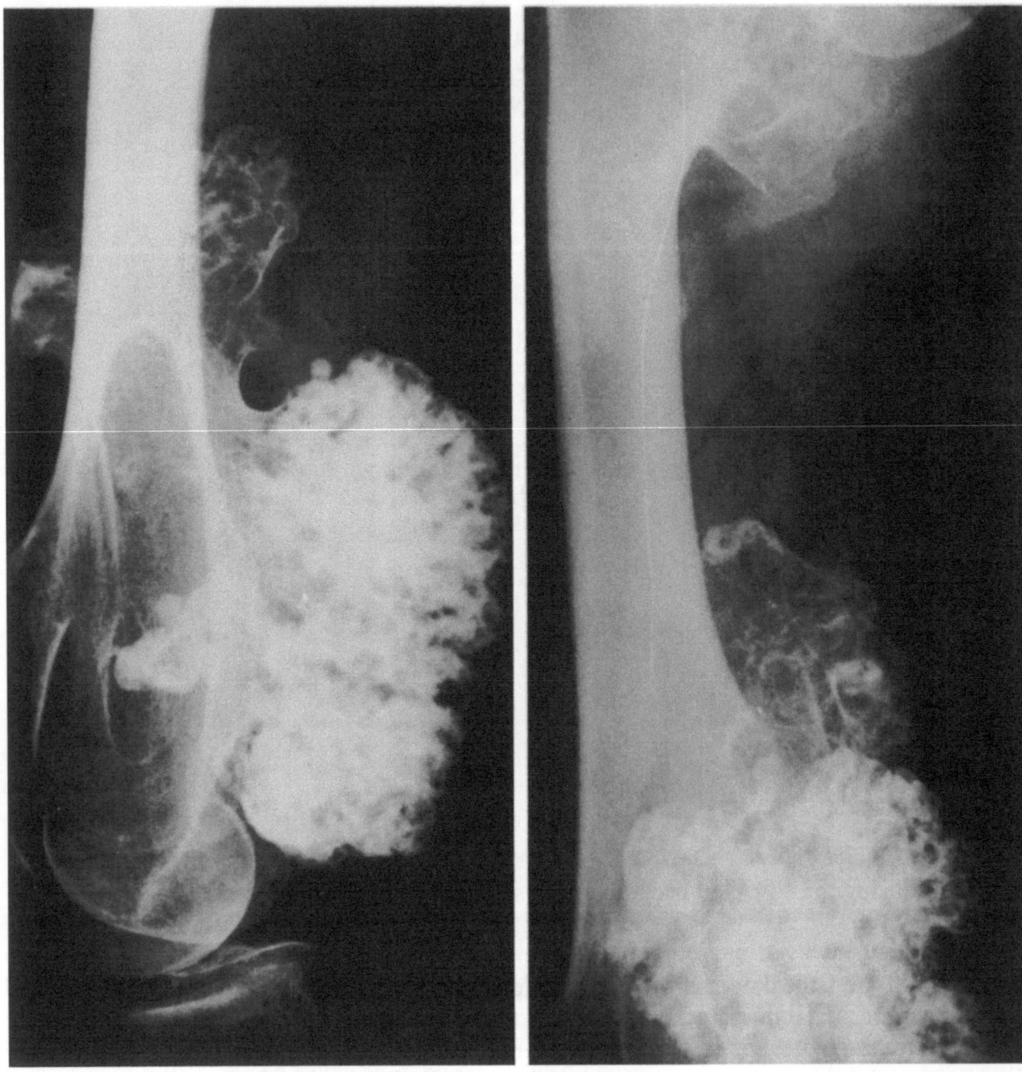

II.37a b

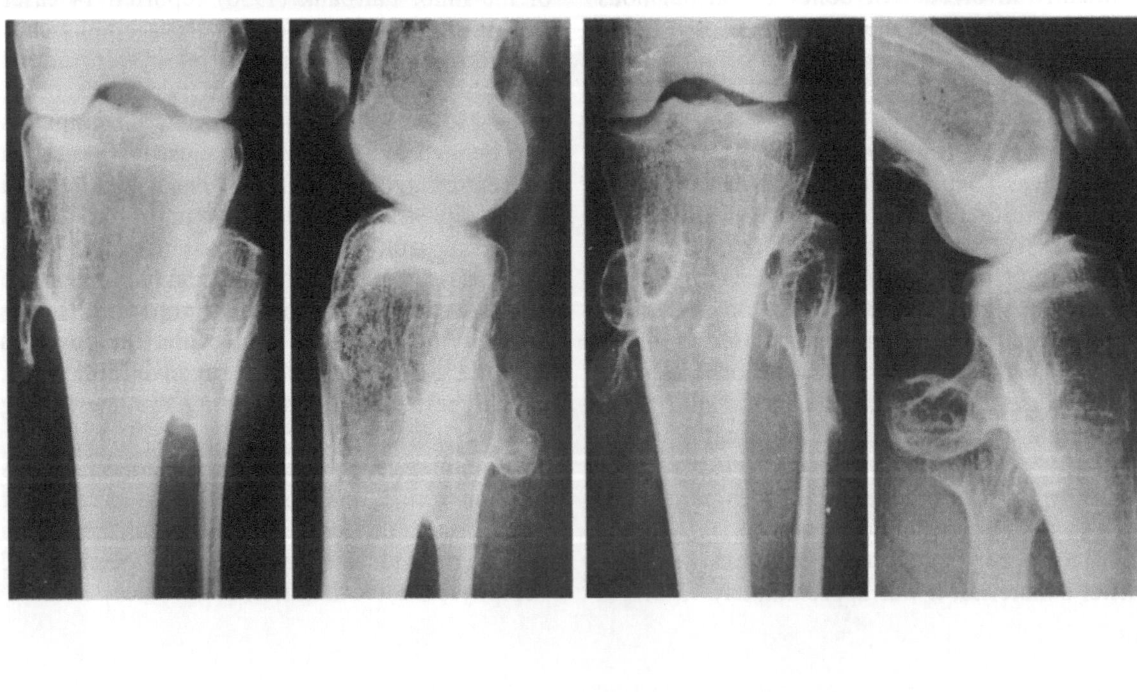

II.38a b

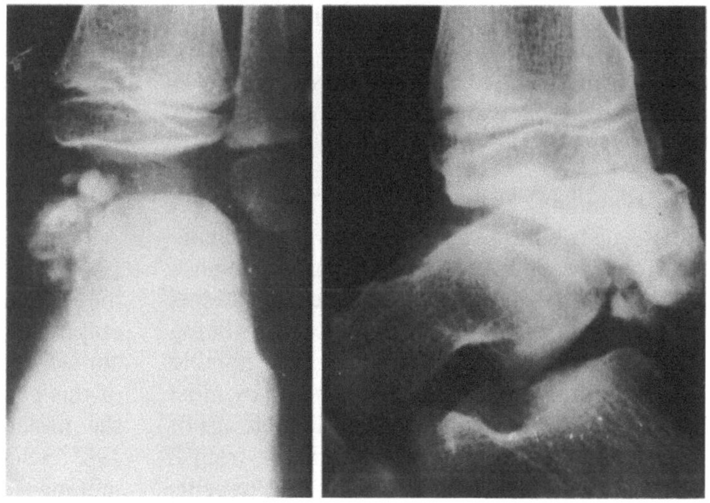

a b

Fig. II.39. Male, 4 years old, with dysplasia epiphysealis hemimelica, tarsus. Anteroposterior and lateral radiographs show heavily calcified lobulated lesions at the medial aspect of the talus. The histologic features are those of osteochondroma

3. Chondroblastoma (Epiphyseal Chondroblastoma, Benign Chondroblastoma)

Definition, WHO: *"An uncommon benign tumor, characterized by highly cellular and relatively undifferentiated tissue composed of rounded or polygonal chondroblast-like cells with distinct outlines, together with multinucleated giant cells of osteoclast type arranged either singly or in groups. The presence of cartilaginous intercellular matrix with areas of focal calcification is typical."*

This tumor, which was formerly regarded as "calcifying giant cell tumor" by Ewing (1928) and as an "epiphyseal chondromatous giant-cell tumor" by Codman (1931), was separated by Jaffe and Lichtenstein in 1942 as a distinct entity from the so-called giant-cell tumor variants under the designation "benign chondroblastoma."

◄

Fig. II.37. Male, 34 years old. Multiple osteochondromatosis of long duration. Lateral and anteroposterior radiographs show the enormous size of the exostosis of the lower femoral end, which is heavily calcified, but the contours are still well defined. The widening of the upper and lower femoral ends is clearly visible. The large tumor mass and two other osteochondromas of the lower femur metaphysis were resected, but no signs of malignancy were observed

Fig. II.38a,b. Male, 20 years old. Multiple osteochondromatosis. **a,b** Anteroposterior and lateral radiographs illustrating the presence of multiple sessile and pedunculated exostoses in the upper metaphysis of the tibia and fibula of both extremities. The bone ends are only slightly widened and flask shaped, owing to failure of normal metaphyseal remodeling ("aclasis")

The writer proposed in 1947 the name "epiphyseal chondroblastoma," a denomination that emphasized not only its most common location but also its possible origin from cellular structures at the epiphyseal site of the growth cartilage.

The fact that its pathogenesis is still disputed notwithstanding, the significant clinical features – the predilection for adolescents in the second decade and the characteristic radiographic picture showing a well-defined osteolytic area with foci or mottled calcification, located in the great majority of cases in the epiphysis of a long bone – usually permit a correct diagnosis after one has had the opportunity to see several cases. However, some cases are still incorrectly diagnosed and classified as genuine giant-cell tumors or as malignant tumors, especially chondrosarcomas, the result being the application of unnecessary treatment. This error was relatively frequent before Jaffe and Lichtenstein's publication, but it is not exceptional even now, especially with lesions that present atypical features of site, age, and sex. Almost all authors accept the benign behavior of epiphyseal chondroblastoma, which in most cases is cured by conservative treatment (curettage or radiotherapy, either alone or combined).

Incidence. Chondroblastoma is relatively uncommon, and there are only a few reports of more than 30 fully documented cases (Huvos et al. 1972; Campanacci et al. 1977; Bloem and Mulder 1985; Springfield et al. 1985; Dahlin and Unni 1986; Moser 1990). In our laboratory we observed 144 well-documented cases over a 45-year period. Feldman (1977) reviewed 691 cases reported in the world literature. Chondroblastoma accounted for 79 (i.e., less than 1%) of all benign tumors in the Mayo Clinic series (Dahlin and Unni 1986), and 6% in our files. The AFIP files contain 248 cases collected over a period of 40 years (Moser 1990).

Clinical Findings. *Age and Sex.* The sex, age, and site distribution data are shown in Scheme II.3. There was an evident male predominance (2:1). The tumor occurred most often in patients in the second decade (76%), most patients being 5–25 years of age, which confirms the notable predilection for this age group reported by most authors. In the AFIP collection the average age of presentation was 18 years, with a range from 8 to 65 years. Approximately 65% of the patients presented during the second decade (Moser 1990).

The number of patients over 25 years is small; only a few cases in elderly patients have been published (Hatcher 1945; Coley 1960; Wright and Sherman 1964; Lichtenstein 1965; Huvos et al. 1972; Dahlin and Unni 1986) or observed by us.

The oldest patient was a 73-year-old woman reported by Wright and Sherman, in whom a slowly growing mass appeared at age 14 and remained unchanged and symptomless until she was 72; during the next year, the mass enlarged slowly and caused slight pain. Dahlin (1978) reported a symptomless lesion in the medial condyle of the femur of a 54-year-old man, found incidentally during angiography. Our oldest patient was 60 years of age.

Localization. The tumor was always related to the growth cartilage of a primary or accessory epiphyseal nucleus (Figs. II.40–II.43), and was almost invariably situated at the epiphyseal side of this cartilage but occasionally penetrating into the underlying metaphysis (Bloem and Mulder 1985; Schajowicz and Gallardo 1970). A primarily metaphyseal location is exceptional and has been observed in three of our cases. About 15 such cases have been reported in the literature (Fechner and Wilde 1974; Aronson et al. 1976; Sotelo-Avila et al. 1986), although Copeland and Geschickter (1965) stated that the tumors were usually situated on the metaphyseal side of the epiphyseal line in long bones.

The most frequent sites affected were the epiphysis of long bones and, in descending order, the femur (27 cases), upper end of the tibia (26

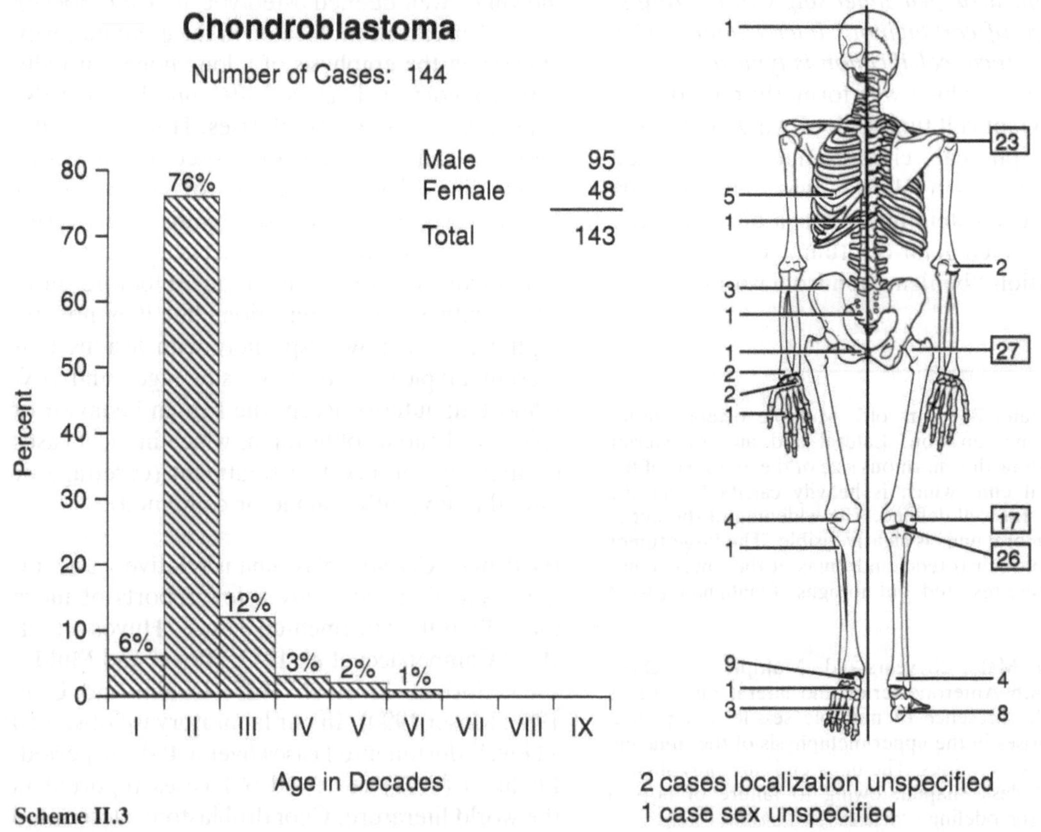

Scheme II.3

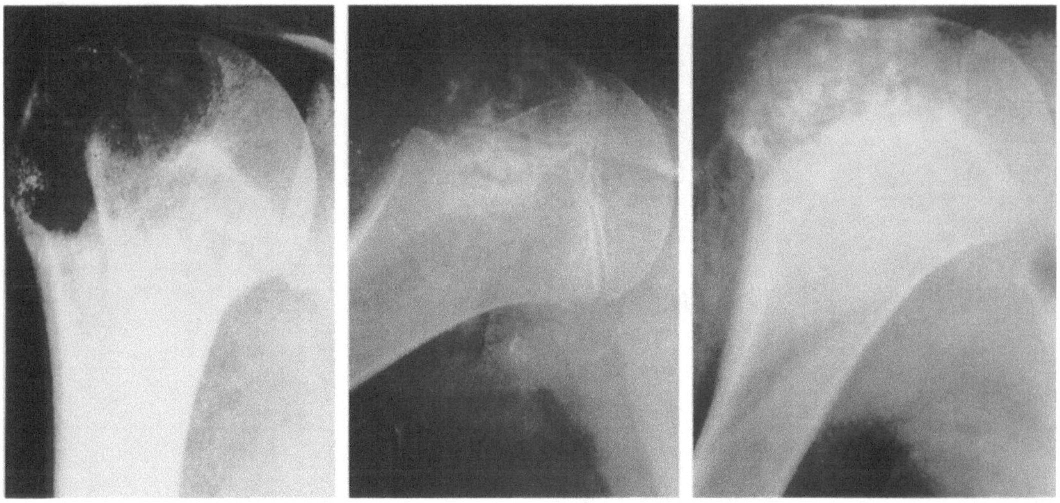

a b, c

Fig. II.40. a. Male, 11 years old. Chondroblastoma of the humerus. Well-defined osteolytic lesion of the upper humeral epiphysis showing spotty calcification and extending a little toward the metaphysis. **b,c** Female, 10 years old. Chondroblastoma of the humerus. **b** Large osteolytic lesion of the great tuberosity of the right humerus. An incomplete curettage was done. **c** Radiograph 8 months later showing recurrence of the tumor, which has enlarged in size and extended into the epiphysis. Heavy spotty calcification is seen. A wide excision was performed. (Schajowicz and Gallardo 1970)

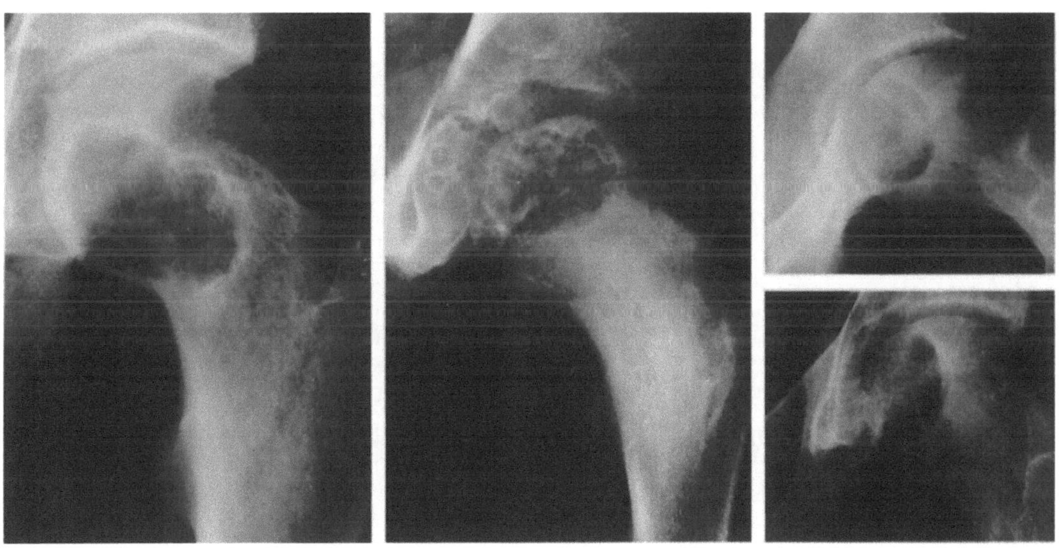

a, b c d

Fig. II.41a–d. a Male, 32 years old. Chondroblastoma. Osteolytic lesion in the femoral head and neck with well-defined sclerotic borders. **b** Male, 11 years old. Lesion in the femoral head showing fuzzy mottled appearance. A secondary villous synovitis developed, producing cystic changes in the acetabulum. **c,d** Female, 22 years old. Radiographs showing well-defined radiolucent lesion in the femoral head. (**a,b**, from Schajowicz and Gallardo 1970)

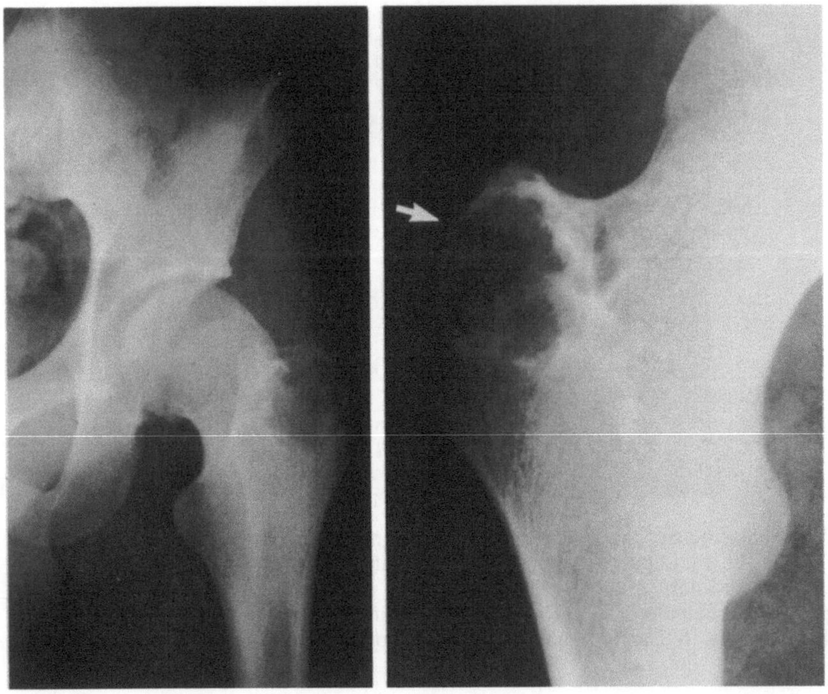

a b

Fig. II.42a,b. Two different cases of chondroblastoma in teenagers, showing radiolucent lesions in the trochanteric region

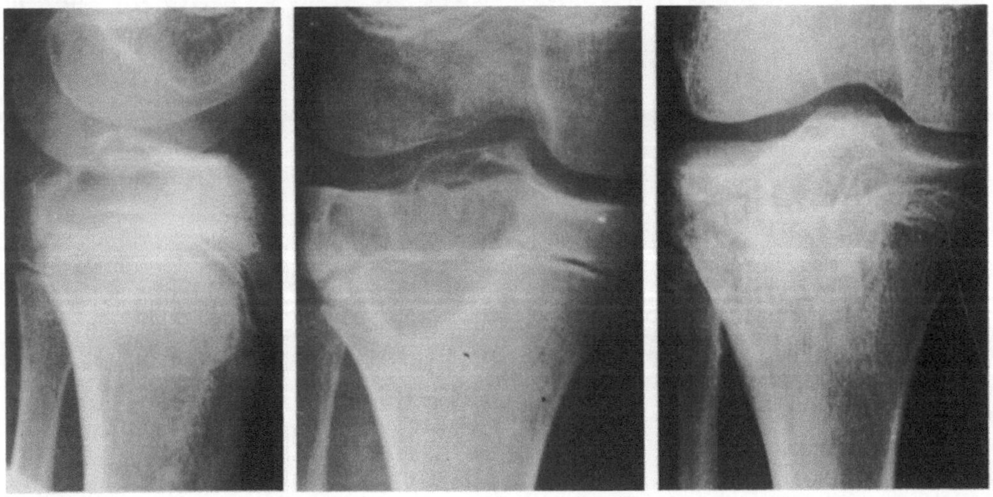

a b, c

Fig. II.43a–c. Female, 11 years old. **a,b** Anteroposterior and lateral radiographs showing osteolytic lesion of the upper tibial epiphysis, extending toward the joint and the adjacent metaphysis. **c** Radiograph 4 years after curettage. (Schajowicz and Gallardo 1970) cases), the humerus (23 cases), and the lower end of the femur (17 cases). Our experience, like that of Jaffe and Lichtenstein, did not confirm the impression given by Codman's paper of a predominant location in the upper end of the humerus. Codman was, after all, confining his attention to the shoulder. Chondroblastoma was rare in the small bones of the hands and feet; however, it was not uncommon in the talus and calcaneus. We found only one case in the spine and only one in the cranial bones. Instances in these bones have only rarely been reported (Denko and Krauel 1955; Sherman and Uzel 1956; Buraczewski et al. 1957; Wright and Sherman 1964; Dahlin and Unni 1986; Bertoni et al. 1987).

Symptoms did not present a constant pattern. Pain with local tenderness was the most frequent complaint, followed by swelling and limitation of movement of the adjacent joint. In 25 cases there was effusion into the joint, caused undoubtedly by the location of the tumor in the epiphyses and sometimes by actual destruction of articular cartilage, with reactive changes in the synovial membrane. Enlargement of lymph nodes was present in five cases. There was no disturbance of general health: the usual laboratory analyses gave negative results in the majority of cases, though in some with secondary articular manifestations there was a slight elevation of the sedimentation rate.

Radiographic Features. In most cases, the radiographic appearance was characteristic: There was an oval or rounded, sharply limited area of osteolysis, generally of moderate size, located eccentrically in the epiphysis; it sometimes expanded the cortex (Fig. II.40), not infrequently causing periosteal bone production, particularly in the more advanced cases. Often, a slight area of bone condensation delimited the tumor toward the medullary cavity (Figs. II.41–II.44), but on other occasions, the border of the lesion was irregular or vague. The fuzzy mottled appearance described since Codman's paper as a characteristic finding (Fig. II.32) was lacking in almost half of our cases. The tumor was located in most cases on the epiphyseal side, but in several cases it penetrated secondarily into the metaphysis (Figs. II.41, II.43) and less often invaded the joint (Figs. II.43, II.45). In three cases, the tumor was confined to the metaphyseal side; in one case with an apparently long evolution in a 60-year-old man, the lesion extended widely into the diaphysis of the humerus (Fig. II.46). A cystic trabecular

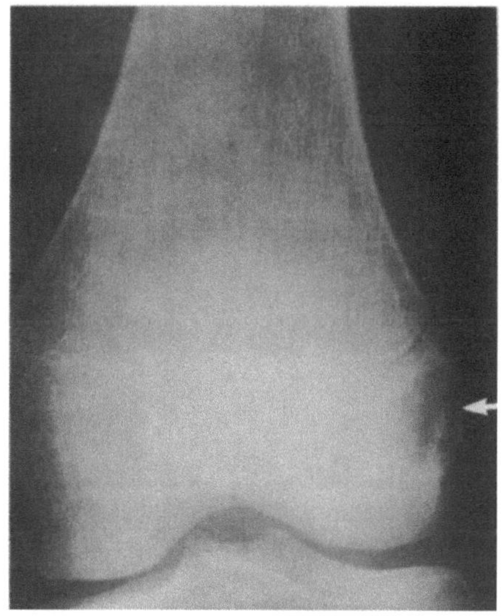

Fig. II.44. Male, 11 years old. Small, radiolucent, well-defined lesion located eccentrically in the lower femoral epiphysis

appearance with cortical expansion like that of giant-cell tumors was observed in only four cases (Figs. II.47, II.48).

Pathologic Findings. *Gross Pathology.* The ordinary surgical material obtained by curettage consisted of numerous small, irregular, grayish-pink or hemorrhagic soft fragments, alternating with gritty calcified yellowish material or bluish-gray nodules corresponding to chondroid tissue.

In addition to this fragmented material, we had ten complete and intact resection specimens, which gave us an excellent opportunity to observe the gross aspects of this tumor. Some of the tumors had been resected because of their location in an expendable bone (patella and rib) (Fig. II.49); others, because of the mistaken diagnosis of malignancy (three cases) or because conservative treatment was no longer possible due to the extent of the lesion (Fig. II.45). The smallest tumor was in the patella (Fig. II.49a,b); it measured 2 cm in its largest diameter and was irregularly rounded and of grayish or bluish color with only a few particles of yellowish calcified material. No cystic or evident hemorrhagic areas were observed in this case. In another, much larger example in a patella (Fig. II.49c,d), more than half of the lesion was cystic and hemorrhagic. In two resection specimens from the tibia (Fig. II.45), the tumor was located posteriorly in the epiphysis and was adjacent to the epiphyseal plate

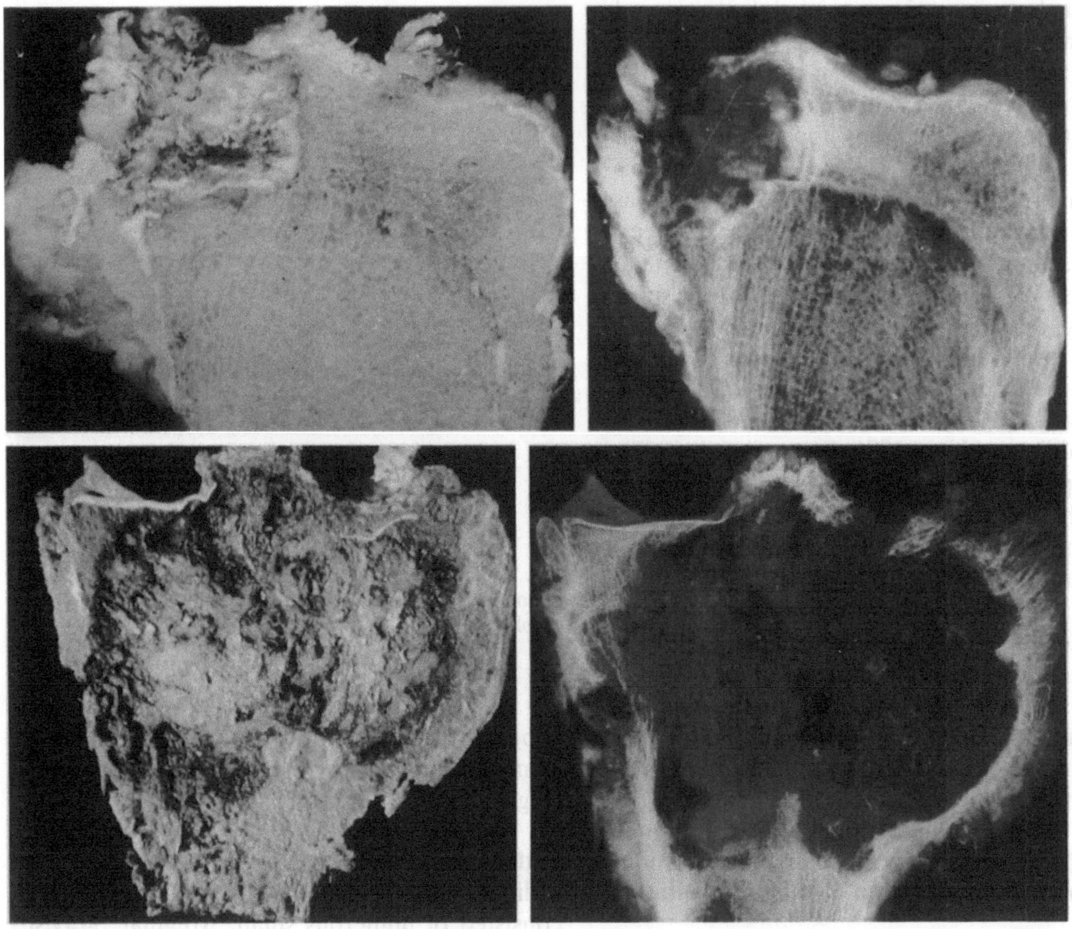

a b c d

Fig. II.45

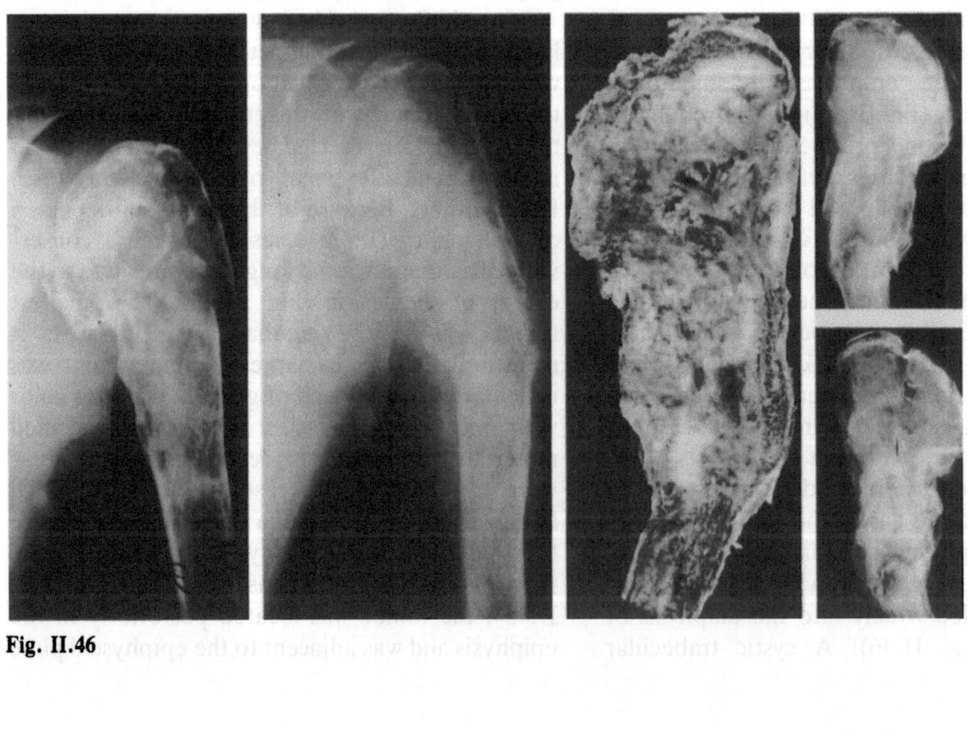

a,b,c d e

Fig. II.46

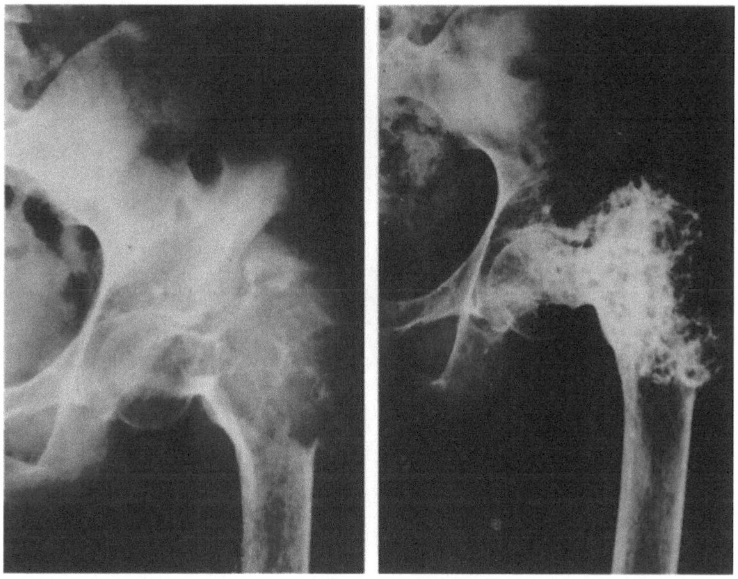

a b

Fig. II.47a,b. Male, 20 years old. **a** Large osteolytic lesion of the trochanteric region with a trabeculated appearance, simulating giant-cell tumor or aneurysmal bone cyst. **b** Radiograph 2 years after radiotherapy shows heavy calcifications of the lesion. The patient was free of symptoms 25 years after treatment. (Schajowicz and Gallardo 1970)

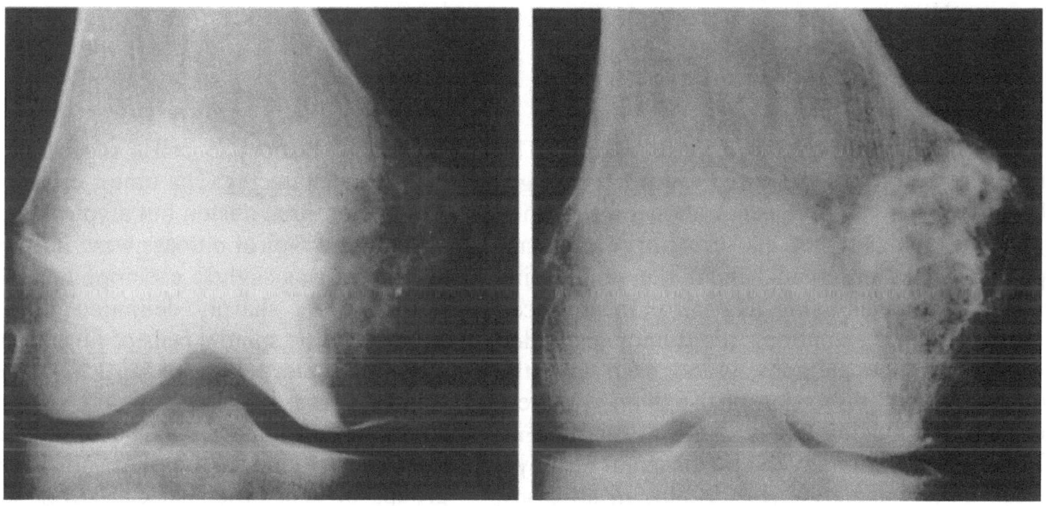

a b

Fig. II.48a,b. Female, 12 years old. **a** Extensive radiolucent lesion of the medial femoral condyle with slight spotty calcification. **b** Ten years after curettage the patient was free of symptoms. (Schajowicz and Gallardo 1970)

◀———

Fig. II.45a–d. Female, 16 years old. Photographs and radiographs of thin slabs of two different chondroblastomas of the upper tibial epiphysis, which were resected because of their size and because of misdiagnosis with malignant cartilage lesion (**a,b**) or giant-cell tumor (**c,d**). The relation of the tumor to the epiphyseal plate is clearly seen. (**a,b** from Schajowicz and Gallardo 1970)

Fig. II.46a–e. Male, 60 years old. **a** Radiograph showing an unusually large chondroblastoma of the upper end of the humerus extending into the diaphysis at a very unusual age, with a pathologic fracture. **b** Two months later, after new fracture. **c–e** Photograph and radiographs of coronal section and thin slab

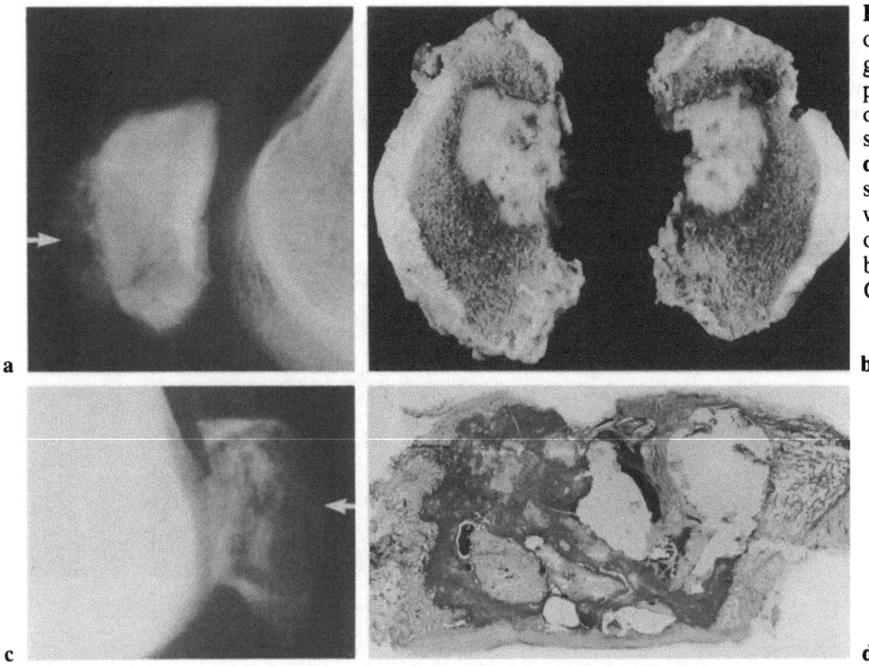

Fig. II.49. a,b. Female, 21 years old. Radiograph and photographs of the lesion in the patella. c,d Female, 20 years old, with lesion of the patella showing spotty calcification. d Topographic photomicrograph showing solid areas alternating with large cystic spaces, typical of "cystic type" of chondroblastoma. (Schajowicz and Gallardo 1970)

from which it appeared to have originated. The tumor was not well delimited toward the neighboring spongiosa, and penetration of the knee joint by lobular tumor masses of hyperemic appearance was observed behind the tibial spine or posteromedially (Fig. II.45a,b). In advanced cases of long evolution, the tumor extended widely into the metaphysis and even into the diaphysis, with distension of the thinned cortex, in one case looking like a giant-cell tumor (Fig. II.45c,d). Occasionally the tumor might occupy a small bone completely (Fig. II.50). In all cases, the solid bluish-gray, grayish-pink, or yellowish areas, of different firmness or friability, alternated with more or less frequent hemorrhagic areas, which sometimes showed cystic softening. Areas of necrosis with or without spotty calcification were common.

Histopathology. The histologic features in our present series did not differ substantially from those described in our previous papers (Valls et al. 1951; Schajowicz and Gallardo 1970) and in the literature. The predominant tissue was generally composed of a compact cellular mass, formed by roundish or polyhedral cells of moderate but variable size (Fig. II.51). The nuclei were relatively large and often of different shape (round, oval, reniform, or cleaved), sometimes similar to histiocytic cells, suggesting a rather malignant character. The tumor cells occasionally had two or three nuclei, but atypical mitoses were absent, and typical mitoses were infrequent. The cytoplasm was slightly eosinophilic, and the cell borders were sharply delimited, thus differing from the basic spindle cells of fibroblastic type of giant-cell tumors (Figs. II.51, II.52). The compact cellular areas did not show any interstitial substance with ordinary stains, but abundant reticulin fibers were found surrounding individual or small groups of cells when special silver stains were used. Using, as in our previous work, the Del Rio Hortega technique for basic tumor cells, the tumor cells stained positively for reticuloendothelial elements, showing the characteristic ramified or ameboid aspect (Fig. II.53). The basic tumor cells showed an evident chondroblastic evolution, being separated by a small but increasing amount of cartilaginous ground substance (Fig. II.51). In the septa that separated the tumor cells of chondroblastic appearance, calcium granules, which were always extracellular, might appear, thus starting irregular foci of calcification (Figs. II.51, II.52), sometimes producing necrosis of the cells. This aspect is generally referred to as "chicken wire" pattern. However, relatively extensive areas of cartilage tissue were often present without showing calcification, or

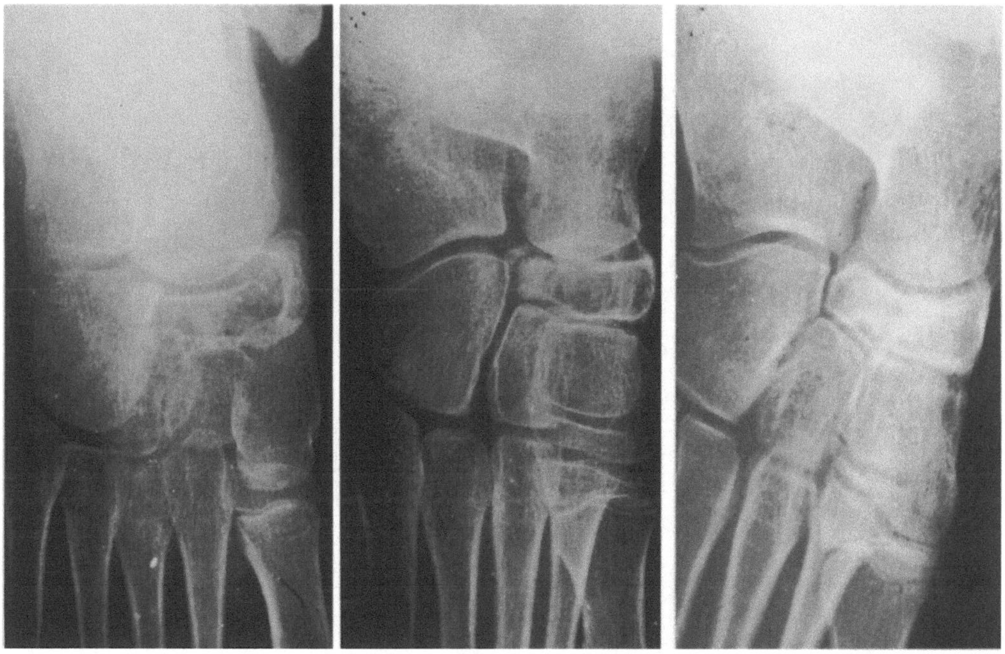

a b

Fig. II.50a,b. Male, 20 years old. **a** Anteroposterior and lateral radiographs showing a radiolucent, slightly expanding lesion in the tarsal scaphoid. **b** Two years after curettage with full recovery

areas of necrosis might occur that only later became calcified.

Another characteristic pattern was the occurrence of multinucleated giant cells, generally small or of medium size, containing less than 20 nuclei (Fig. II.51). However, it was not rare to find groups of large giant cells with a greater number of nuclei, resembling those observed in genuine giant-cell tumors (Figs. II.52, II.54c). However, their distribution was irregular, generally in smaller groups, and they were found not only in relation to and secondary to necrosis or hemorrhages, as Jaffe and Lichtenstein (1942) maintained, but also independently, dispersed between the mononuclear cells. The tumor cells occasionally had two or three nuclei, and intermediary stages with giant cells could be observed. Areas with only moderate vascularization were observed in addition to others rich in blood vessels, generally of the capillary type, with frequent hemorrhages and cystic spaces. These cystic spaces, which usually lacked an endothelium and were lined by tumor cells, occurred in approximately 20% of our cases and gave rise to a multiloculated cavitary appearance, often indistinguishable from aneurysmal bone cyst. We suggested the name "cystic chondroblastoma" for the lesions with this special pattern (Fig. II.54).

In a few cases, areas of myxoid appearance, similar to those observed in chondromyxoid fibroma, were found; most such cases were more advanced lesions, but in one case the areas were so extensive that it was difficult to decide in which category the tumor should be placed. However, the abundant cartilage and calcified areas were suggestive of the classification of chondroblastoma. Similar cases with transitional stages between chondroblastoma and chondromyxoid fibroma have also been observed by others (Dahlin 1956), and they occasionally make the exact classification of these lesions difficult. Hemorrhages and necrosis may cause secondary modifications such as organization and replacement by irregular masses of hyalinized collagenous tissue, resembling chondroid or osteoid substance. Sometimes the newly formed tissue is difficult or impossible to differentiate from cartilage or osteoid, and seems to be a transitional stage between both ("chondro-osteoid").

New formation of scarce bone was found as a secondary change in areas of endochondral ossification of calcified cartilage or as reactive bone in fibrous septa, separating or surrounding tumor lobules.

Histochemistry and Immunohistochemistry. In adequately fixed material, we found abundant

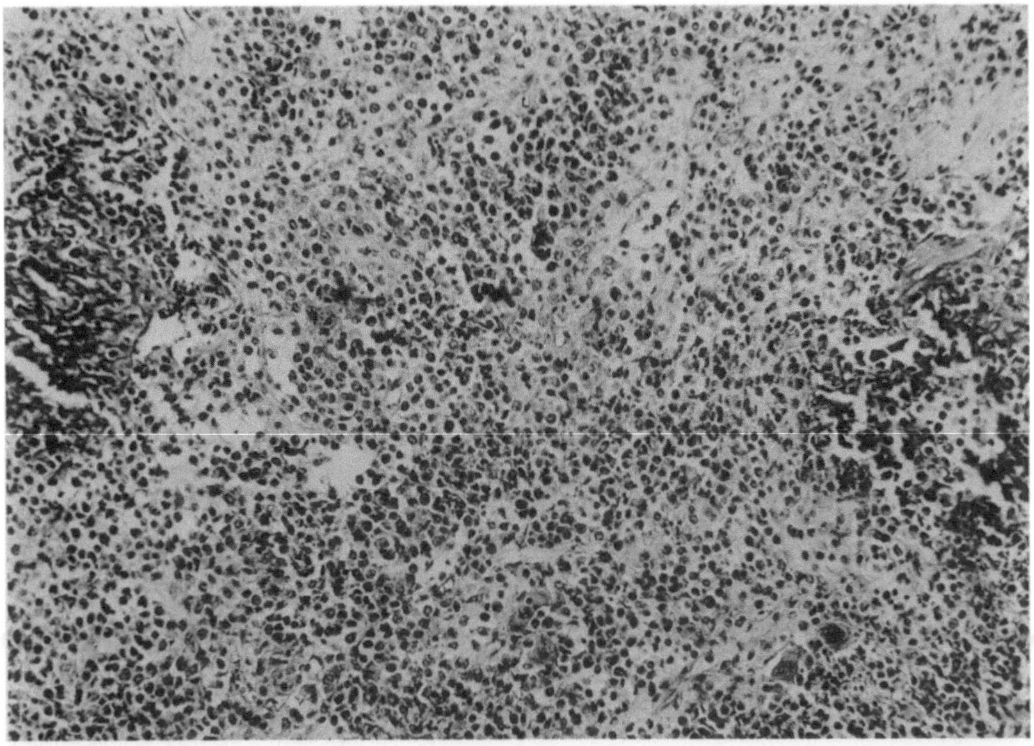

a

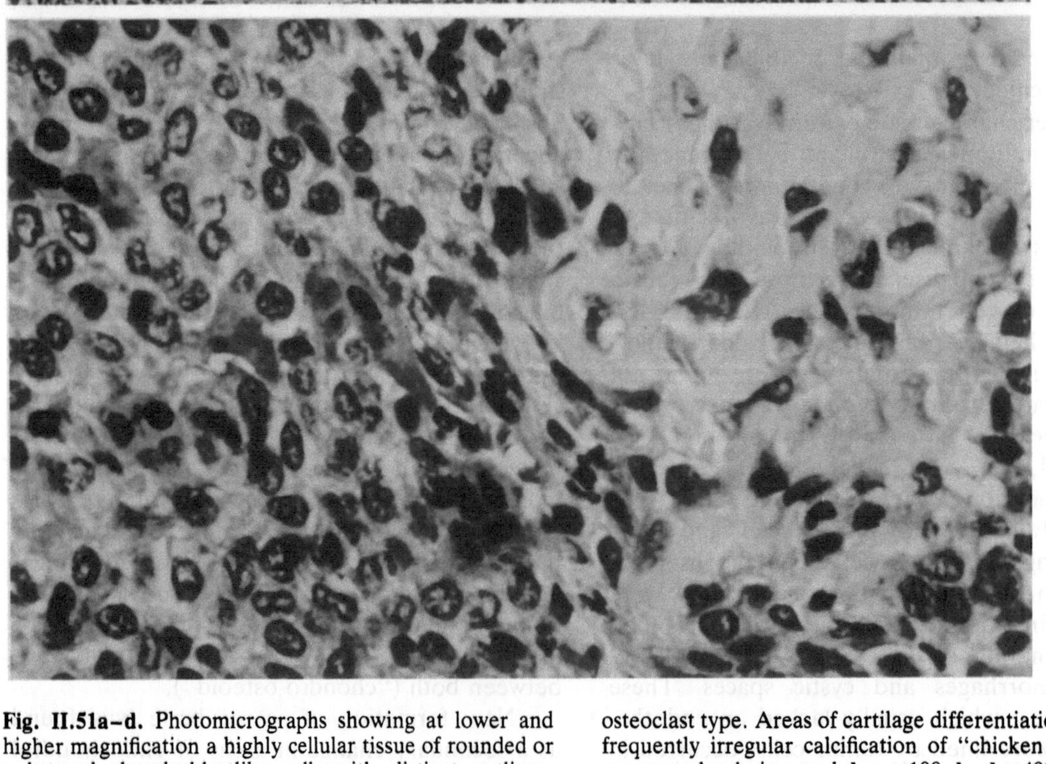

b

Fig. II.51a–d. Photomicrographs showing at lower and higher magnification a highly cellular tissue of rounded or polygonal chondroblastlike cells with distinct outlines, intermingled with a variable number of giant cells of osteoclast type. Areas of cartilage differentiation, showing frequently irregular calcification of "chicken wire" type are seen clearly in **c** and **d**. **a** ×100, **b–d** ×400

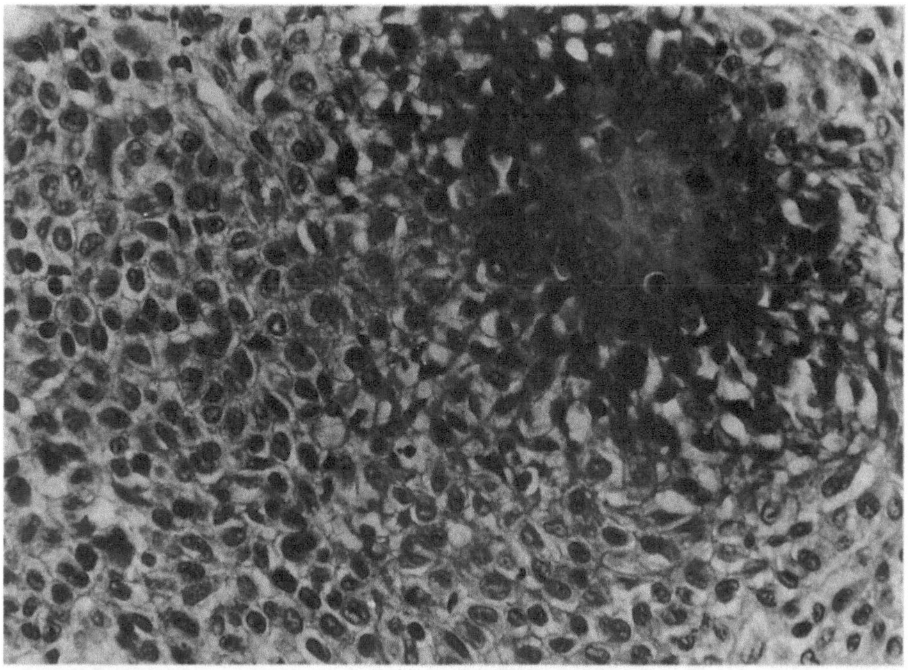

c

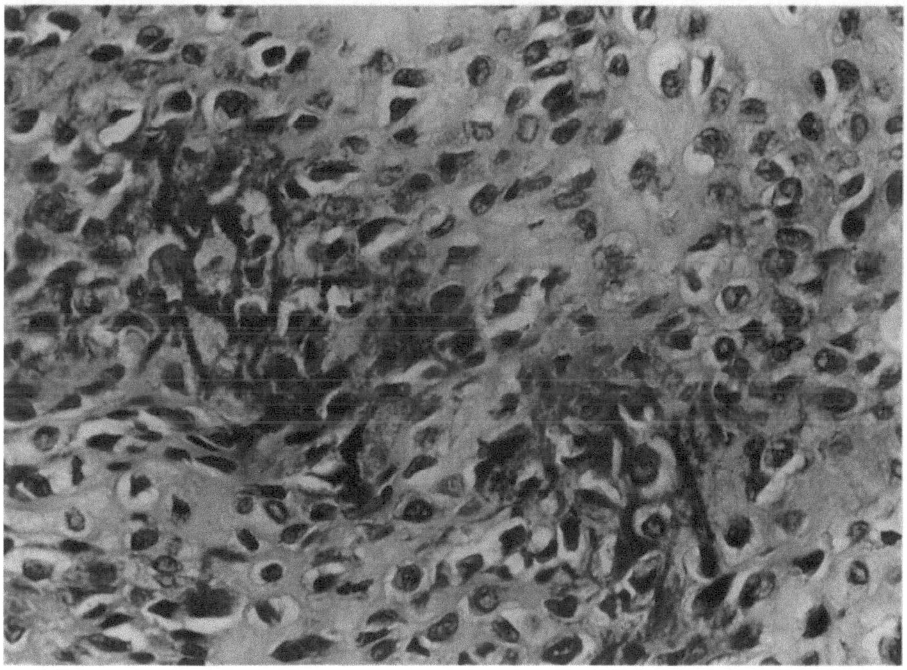

d

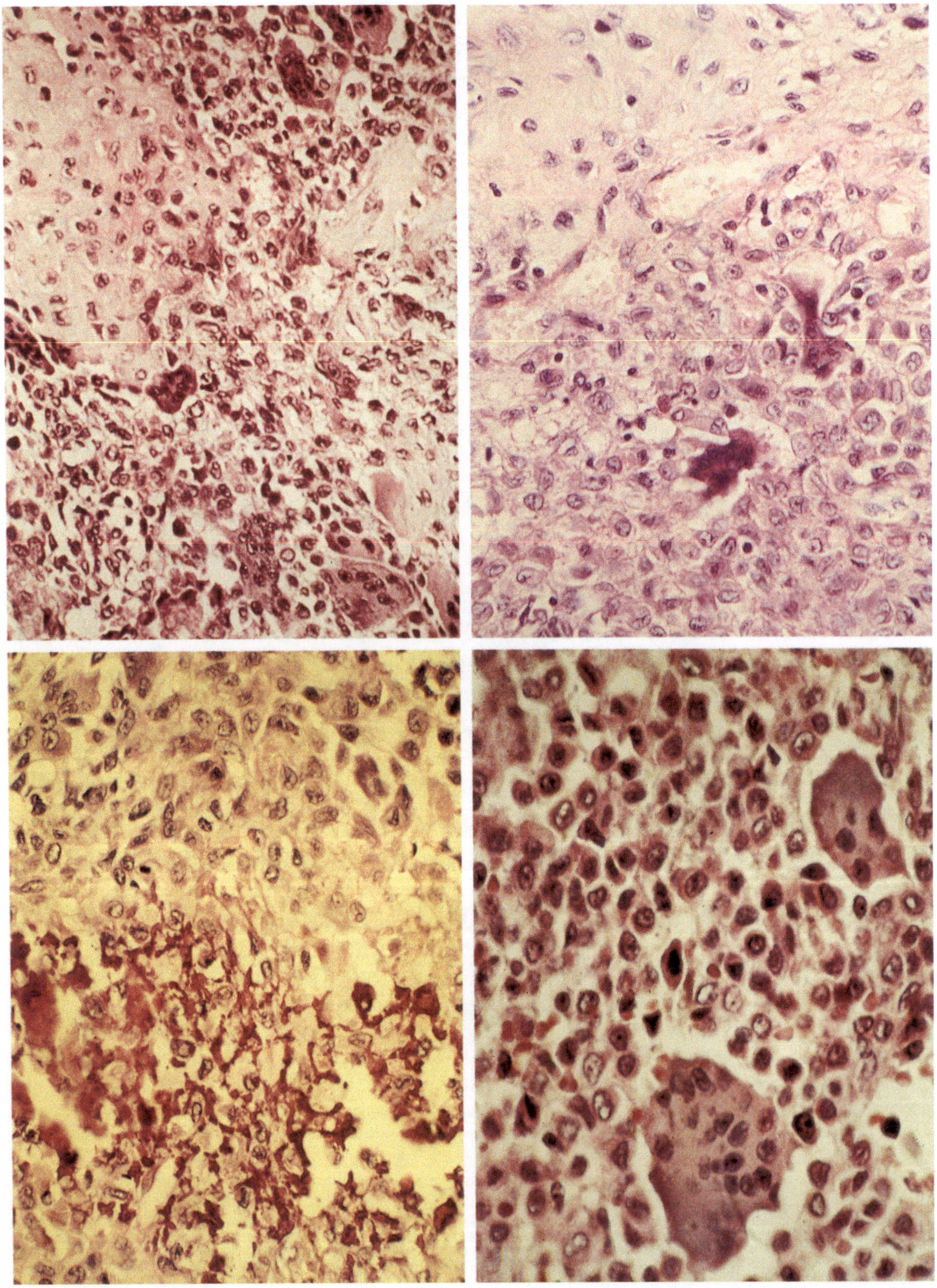

a b c d

Fig. II.52a–d. Photomicrographs showing different histologic features of chondroblastoma. **a,d** "Chicken wire" cartilage calcification. **b,c** Multinucleated giant cells between compact mass of round or ovoid tumor cells with distinct cytoplasmic outlines, a pattern distinct from giant-cell tumor. **b,d** Cartilage differentiation of the tumor cells. **a** ×100, **b–d** ×400

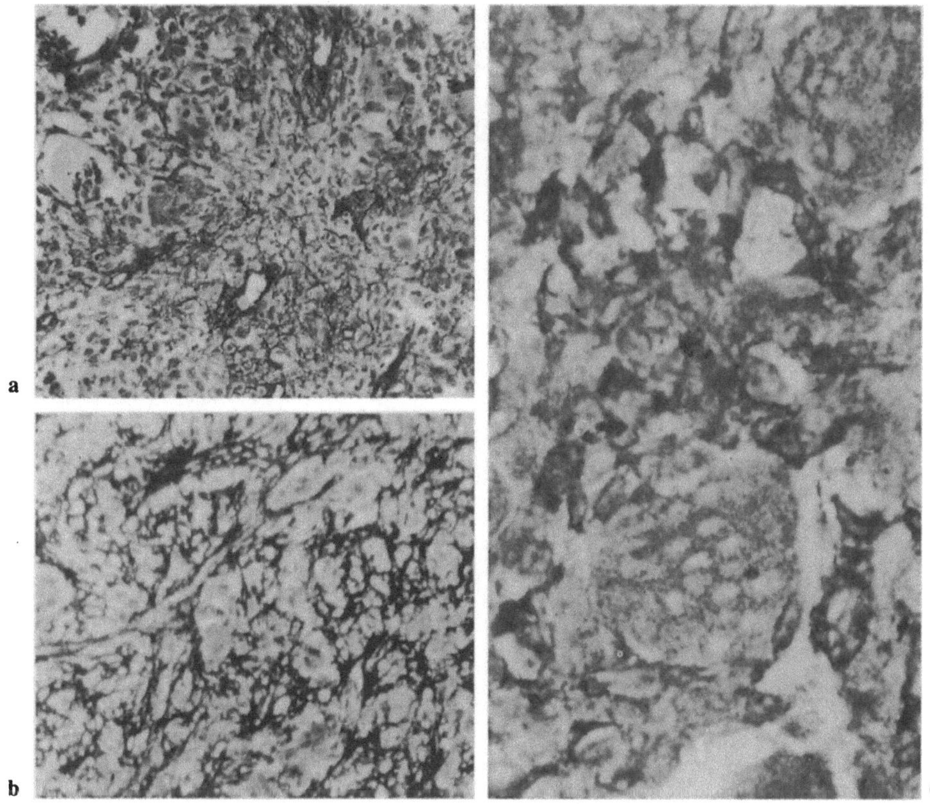

Fig. II.53a–c. Photomicrographs showing **a,b** the richness of reticulin fibers (Del Rio Hortega's silver stain) and **c** the reticulohistiocytic nature of the stromal cells, ramified or ameboid in form (Del Rio Hortega's stain for reticuloendothelial elements). (Schajowicz and Gallardo 1970) **a,b** ×55; **c** ×335

granules of glycogen in the rounded tumor cells of histiocytic appearance and in chondroblastic evolution, which reached a maximum at the young chondroblastic stage and were separated by a small amount of cartilaginous ground substance. The glycogen content diminished as the ground substance increased and disappeared completely in the extensive areas of necrosis and calcification so common in these tumors.

The multinucleated giant cells showed discrete amounts of periodic acid-Schiff-positive granulations that were nearly always smaller than those of glycogen and did not disappear with digestion by ptyalin. Metachromatic stains were positive in the chondroid and myxoid areas, and the chondroid areas were resistant to digestion with hyaluronidase.

Immunohistochemical methods specific for histiocytic elements, such as α_1-antitrypsin and nonspecific esterase, were applied in some of our cases and reacted positively only inconstantly. The proliferating stromal cells in seven of the nine chondroblastomas stained for S-100 protein, as did the lacunar chondrocytes in enchondromas and chondrosarcomas (Monda and Wick 1985). Weiss and Dorfman (1986), who studied the immunoreactivity of several cartilaginous tumors, as well as normal epiphyseal growth cartilage, stated that in chondroblastoma the "chondroblasts" were less reactive than the chondrocytes in the areas of chondroid matrix production.

Electron Microscopy. The reported ultrastructural studies showed similar findings (Welsh and Meyer 1964; Wellman 1969; Huvos et al. 1972) and tended to support Jaffe and Lichtenstein's original view of cartilage germ-cell origin. Chondroblasts show ultrastructural features somewhat distinct from chondrocytes seen in normal human cartilage and the cells seen in chondrosarcoma (Schajowicz et al. 1974). The cells have cytoplasmic blunted microvillous processes, continuous dense bands of nuclear substance along the inner nuclear membrane, and frequent multilobulated or indented nuclei. Glycogen granules and fine cytoplasmic filaments are frequent findings. Welsh and Meyer (1964) supported the view that the tumor cells resemble normal

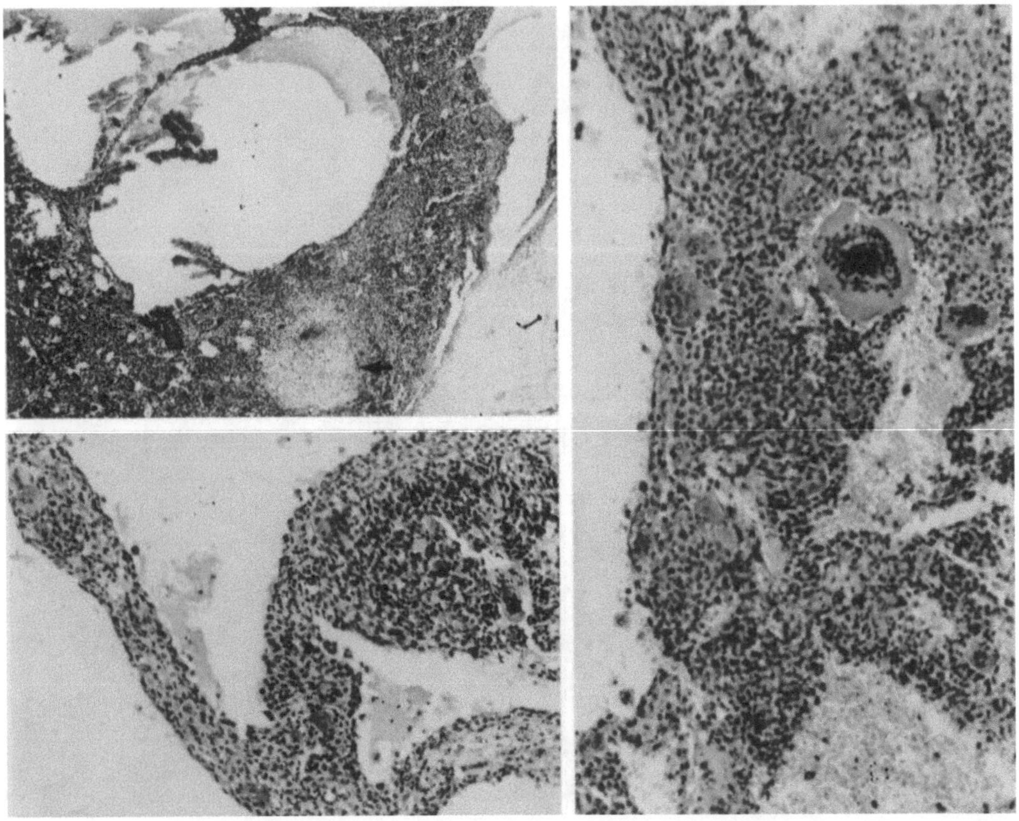

a b c

Fig. II.54a–c. Cystic chondroblastoma. **a** Topographic photomicrograph showing large cystic spaces surrounded by cellular tissue containing small cartilage nodules. **b,c** Other zones, showing large cavities, separated by cellular septa rich in giant cells. These features are similar to those observed in aneurysmal bone cyst. (Schajowicz and Gallardo 1970) **a** ×40, **b** ×100, **c** ×150

epiphyseal growth cartilage cells growing in tissue cultures. Wellman (1969) maintained that they originate from cartilage-forming matrix cells, whereas Huvos et al. (1972) concluded that the basic cells are "most likely immature chondrocytes." Levine and Bensch (1972) felt that the chondroblastoma cells show features of fetal and adult cartilage cells, thereby questioning the contention that chondroblastoma is made up of embryonic cells, and they suggested that the term "chondroblastoma" may be a misnomer.

Pathogenesis. Most authors suggest, without being able to confirm it, that chondroblastoma is related to the absorption of misplaced islands of cartilage by newly formed cartilage cells (Kolodny 1927) derived from cartilage germ cells (Jaffe 1958) or cartilage-forming connective tissue (Lichtenstein 1952), occurring as a perversion or acceleration of a normal endochondral ossification process. Lichtenstein (1965) suggested the hypothetical possibility of an origin from an anomalous or accessory epiphyseal cartilage center that was stimulated to growth at the time of puberty by sex hormones or unknown factors. These views seem to be supported by electron microscopic studies of Welsh and Meyer (1964), Wellman (1969), and others who maintained that the tumor cells strongly resembled normal epiphyseal cartilage cells growing in tissue culture or originating from cartilage-forming matrix cells.

Our findings confirm that chondroblastoma is a cartilage-forming tumor originating in close relationship to the growth cartilage, probably from cellular elements on the epiphyseal side of this cartilage. In the writer's opinion, the basic tumor cells could be reticulohistiocytic elements possessing a definite potentiality and tendency to develop into poorly differentiated chondroblastic tissue and then into more mature cartilage. They may correspond to Jaffe's cartilage germ cells and may be identical to "resting or reserve cells," normally situated at this area of the growth cartilage, facing the epiphysis.

This interpretation, already put forward by the writer in previous papers, was based primarily on the observation of all stages of transition of the basic tumor cells towards the young chondroblast and more mature cartilage, and the evidence of the tumor's probable reticulohistiocytic character, demonstrated by the specific silver stain of Del Rio Hortega and by the abundance of reticular fibers surrounding the tumor cells in the undifferentiated areas. In three cases, in vitro cultures seemed to confirm the histiocytic character of the basic tumor cells, which in addition to chondroblastic differentiation also showed the formation of multinucleated giant cells. This confirms our finding of transitional stages between the mononuclear tumor cell and giant cells commonly observed in ordinary histologic sections. Immunohistochemical techniques using nonspecific esterase and α_1-antitrypsin, applied in a few of our cases, only yielded positive reactions in scarce tumor cells.

Although most authors (Welsh and Meyer 1964; Wellman 1969; Huvos et al. 1972) favor a cartilage cell origin, based especially on ultrastructural studies, the true nature of the basic tumor cell is, in the writer's opinion, still not completely resolved despite extensive histochemical, tissue culture, electron microscopic, and autoradiographic studies (Levine and Bensch 1972; and others). Additional studies using more specific techniques, particularly immunohistologic studies, for demonstrating histiocytic origin, such as determination of nonspecific esterase, α_1-antitrypsin, S-100, and membrane-bound immunofluorescence, should be performed in a greater number of cases in order to confirm or rule out a possible reticulohistiocytic derivation of the basic tumor cell.

The statement of Levine and Bensch that "while an origin from reticulo-histiocytic elements cannot be entirely excluded, the tumor cells are most likely truly cartilaginous in nature" demonstrates that the problem of histogenesis of the basic tumor cell is still unresolved.

Treatment and Prognosis. The follow-up of the writer's cases indicated the benign character of this neoplasm. Conservative treatment and preferably curettage, often followed by packing of the cavity with cancellous bone chips, or local excision or resection in lesions of the patella (three cases) or the rib (four cases), have generally been sufficient for successful treatment.

In exceptional cases, when a surgical approach was impossible or not accepted, radiotherapy cured the lesion. Although we had five cases of local recurrence after curettage, the subsequent evolution of these cases was favorable; the same was true for several other cases reported in the literature (Castleman and McNeill 1966; Coleman 1966; Sundaram 1966). This finding is in agreement with those of most authors, who recorded only rare instances of verified aggressiveness and none of spontaneous malignant transformation. Some cases of local aggressiveness (Huvos et al. 1977; Dahlin 1978) and of autopsy-verified malignant transformation with pulmonary metastases were reported by Kahn et al. (1969) and were observed in the writer's series in two cases. In the first case, reported later in detail by Sirsat and Doctor (1970), the patient died 6 years after four unsuccessful curettages, possibly with pulmonary metastases. In our second case, it was difficult to establish with certainty whether the original lesion, which was located in a metatarsal head and had recurred twice after curettage and resection, and which produced multiple soft tissue metastases during the following 4 years, was an atypical chondroblastic tumor (malignant chondroblastoma) rather than a benign chondroblastoma that became malignant. Reviewing the slides of the original lesion, we came to the conclusion that the histologic features, the same as those of the recurrent lesion, corresponded to a clear-cell chondrosarcoma. This patient died 6 years after the first curettage, possibly with pulmonary metastases (Figs. II.55, II.56).

Finally, it is interesting to point out that, exceptionally, a chondroblastoma may metastasize to the lungs as a benign tumor, as reported by Green and Whittaker (1975), Huvos et al. (1977), Riddell et al. (1973), and Dahlin (1978). These metastases usually develop subsequent to surgery. With the exception of one case of Kyriakos et al. (1985), the reported cases have behaved in a relatively benign fashion.

The existence of a "primary malignant chondroblastoma" remains questionable. The question must be answered affirmatively if the term "malignant chondroblastoma" means, as quoted by Kyriakos et al. (1985), "a tumor with benign-appearing histological features capable of aggressive behavior with metastases and death of the patient" (Kahn et al. 1969). Unfortunately there are as yet no histologic parameters that permit determination of which metastases are

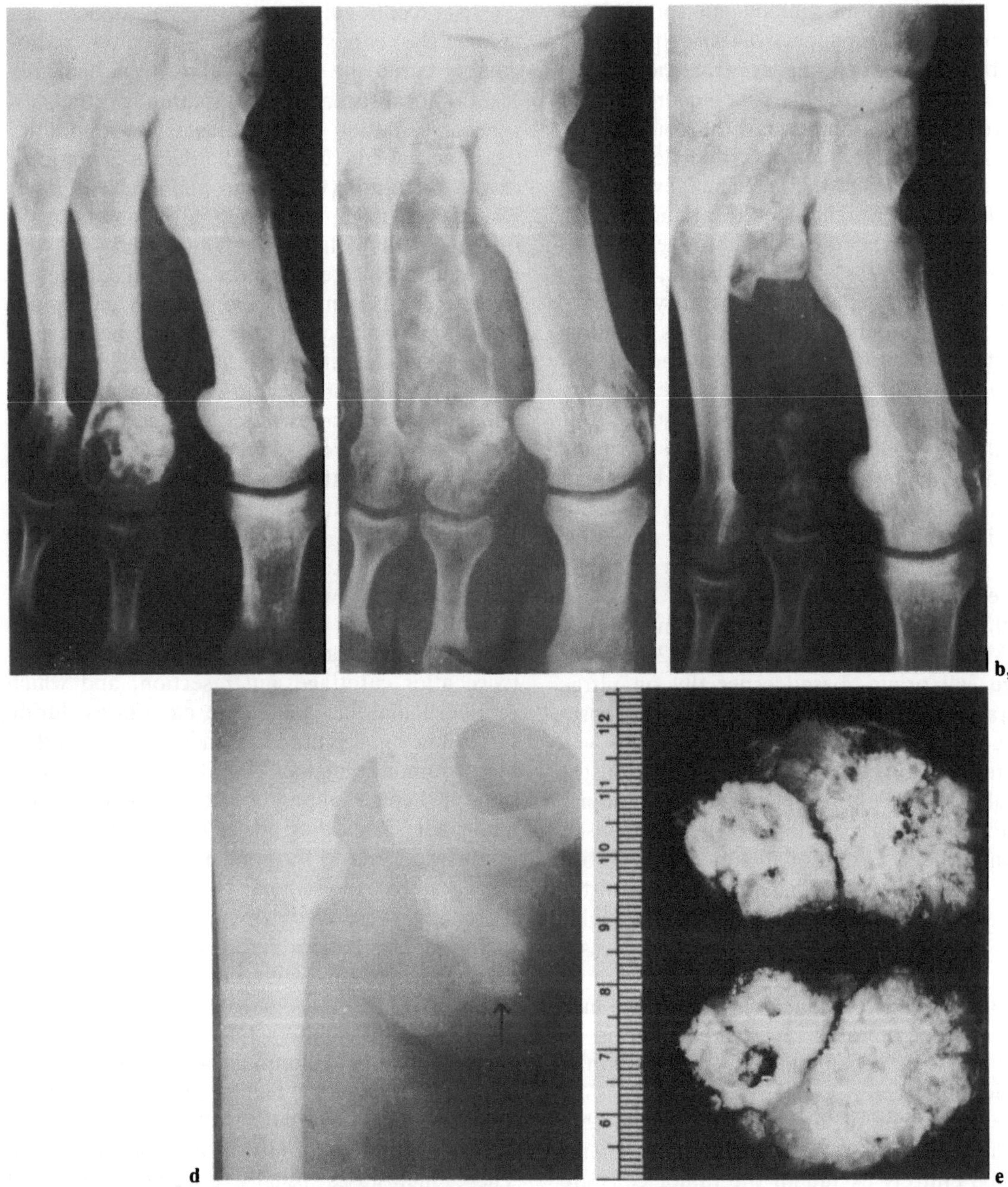

Fig. II.55a–e. Female, 32 years old. **a** Radiograph showing an osteolytic, heavily calcified lesion in the head of the second metatarsal bone. The histologic diagnosis was that of chondroblastoma. **b** Five months after curettage. The lesion involves the whole metatarsal bone. **c** Local recurrence 18 months after resection of metatarsal bone. **d** A metastatic calcified nodule appeared 1 year later in the upper thigh. **e** Photograph of the cut surface of the heavily calcified tumor nodule of the thigh. (**a–c** from Schajowicz and Gallardo 1970)

Fig. II.56a,b. Photomicrographs at lower and higher magnification of a recurrence of the same case as in Fig. II.55, showing the pleomorphic aspect of the cartilage-cell areas with spotty calcification and spindle-cell proliferation in the septa, indicating a malignant cartilage tumor. Some histologic features were identical to those of clear-cell chondrosarcoma. Reviewing the slides of the original lesion, we rectified our diagnosis to that of clear-cell chondrosarcoma. **a** ×100, **b** ×360

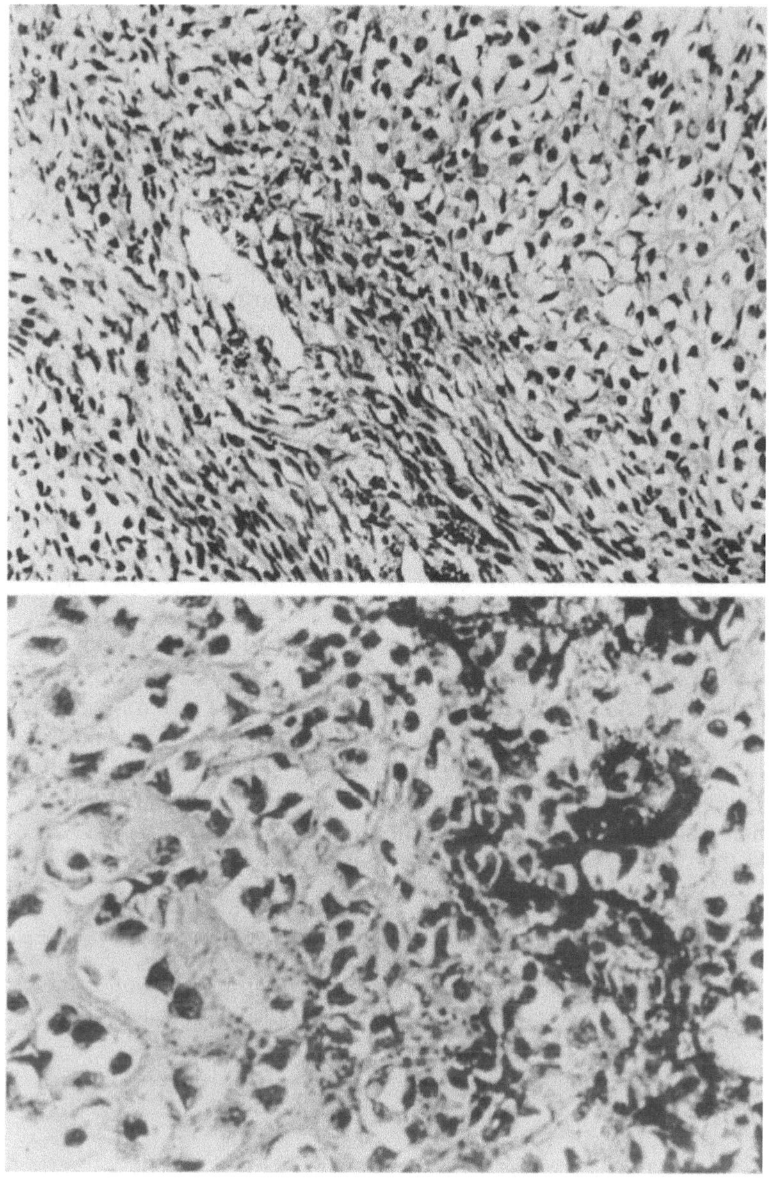

a

b

destined to cease their growth or to progress and kill the host. On the other hand it seems possible that some cases reported under this heading were in reality "chondroblastoma-like chondrosarcoma" or "chondroblastic osteosarcomas" (Schajowicz et al. 1990).

Whether the difference between the concept of "malignant chondroblastoma" and "chondroblastoma-like chondrosarcoma" is purely semantic or whether there are in fact two different entities must await the report of further cases with good documentation and follow-up information.

4. Chondromyxoid Fibroma (Fibromyxoid Chondroma)

Definition, WHO: *"A benign tumor characterized by lobulated areas of spindle-shaped or stellate cells with abundant myxoid or chondroid intercellular material, separated by zones of more cellular tissue rich in spindle-shaped or rounded cells with a varying number of multinucleated giant cells of different sizes; large pleomorphic cells may be present and can result in confusion with chondrosarcoma. However, atypical mitoses are lacking".*

Chondromyxoid fibroma, which is the least common benign tumor of cartilage derivation, was described in 1948 by Jaffe and Lichtenstein as a distinct entity; it was formerly regarded as a myxoma (Bloodgood 1924) or a myxomatous variant of giant-cell tumor, or mistaken for a malignant lesion, especially chondrosarcoma, chondromyxosarcoma, or myxosarcoma (Ottolenghi and Petracchi 1953). In fact myxomas of bone seem to be peculiar to the jaws and of odontogenic origin and apparently have no counterpart or at least are exceptional in other bones of the skeleton; the few such cases reported in the literature as myxomas or myxofibromas (Bauer and Harell 1954; Scaglietti and Stringa 1956; Marcove et al. 1964; Perou et al. 1967; McLure and Dahlin 1977) are probably mostly chondromyxoid fibromas in which the chondroid tissue and septa containing giant cells have been overlooked or are lacking (Gherlinzoni et al. 1983). Because of the relative rarity of chondromyxoid fibroma, only a small number of publications exist dealing with more than 20 cases (Rahimi et al. 1972; Gherlinzoni et al. 1983; Zillmer and Dorfman 1989). The major textbooks of Jaffe (1958) (25 cases), Lichtenstein (1977) (60 cases), and Aegerter and Kirkpatrick (1975) do not include precise statistical details. Feldman (1977) tabulated 367 cases reported in the literature.

Incidence. The incidence in our series of 48 cases was approximately 1% of all tumoral lesions filed in our laboratory and was one-third of the chondroblastomas observed by us over the same period.

Clinical Findings. *Age and Sex.* As reported by other authors, there was no evident sex predominance, unlike in chondroblastoma, in which there was a 66% male predominance. However, Dahlin and Unni (1986) found a definite male predominance in their series of 39 chondromyxoid fibromas.

There was a predilection for the second decade of life (39%), and 68% occurred in patients between 5 and 25 years old (compared with a figure of 88% for chondroblastoma). Our youngest patient was 6 years old, and the oldest patient was 58 years of age. The number of cases after 25 years is frankly higher than in chondroblastoma. However, Scaglietti and Stringa (1961) and Ralph (1962) reported several cases in children under 10 years, the youngest being 5 years old (Scheme II.4).

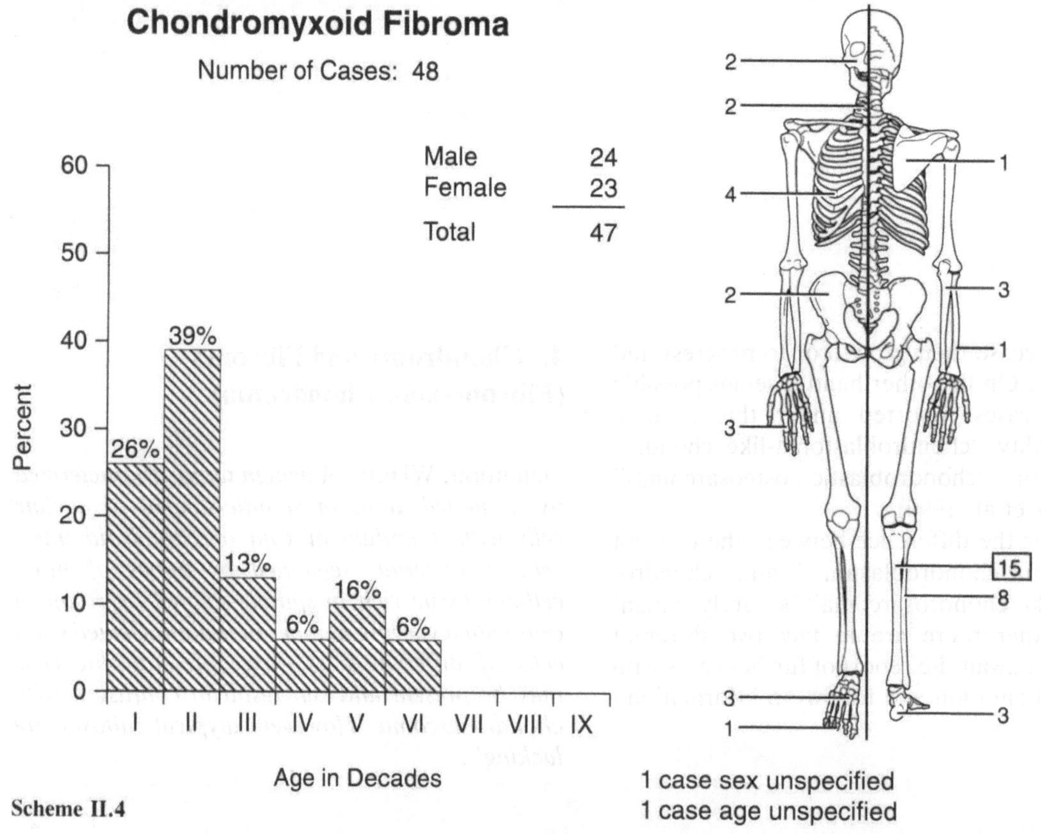

Scheme II.4

Localization. Anatomically, the most common site was the *metaphyseal* region of a large tubular bone of the lower limb at variable distances from the growth cartilage, but often in close contact with it. The preferred site was the upper end of the tibia (15 cases), which was also the most common site in other reports (Jaffe 1958; Lichtenstein 1977; Dahlin and Unni 1986). In our series, the other bones frequently involved were the fibula (eight cases) and bones of the foot (seven cases), yielding an incidence of 62.5% in the lower limb. Surprisingly, we had no case in the femur, which most authors consider to be one of the most common sites. Involvement of bones of membranous origin seems to be rare; in the English literature only one case has been reported in a parietal bone (Aegerter and Kirkpatrick 1975) and one in the mastoid apophysis (Jaffe 1958). A few cases have been reported in the maxilla and mandible, and only one in the sternum (Teitelbaum and Bessone 1969). A rare location in our series was in the spinous process of the third cervical vertebra. Benson and Bass (1955) reported a similar case in which the uppermost part of the thoracic spine was involved.

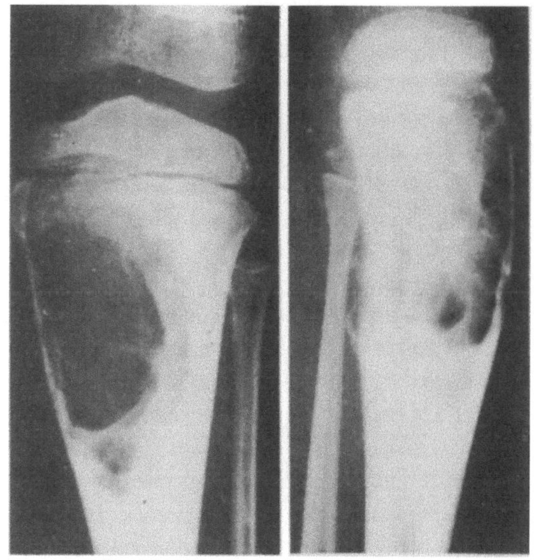

Fig. II.57. Male, 10 years old. Chondromyxoid fibroma. Anteroposterior and lateral radiographs showing an extensive radiolucent lesion located eccentrically in the upper metaphysis of the tibia. A scalloped margin of sclerosed bone is observed at the medullary side. The cortex is expanded, thinned, and interrupted on its posterolateral surface. (Schajowicz and Gallardo 1971)

Symptoms. The patient's symptoms were not specific. Usually there was pain and slowly increasing local swelling, occasionally accompanied by a palpable tumor. Sometimes, there was limping and slight limitation of movement, but because of the position of the tumor in the metaphysis of a long bone, irritation of the joint, so often seen in chondroblastoma, was lacking. A pathologic fracture occurred in only one case. Previous history of injury was rare; as in other bone tumors, trauma does not seem to be related to the pathologic process.

Radiographic Features. The radiographic aspect was characteristic in cases involving long bones, where the lesion appeared as a radiolucent area of variable size, located eccentrically in the metaphysis (Fig. II.57). Only rarely and in advanced lesions did the tumor cross the epiphyseal line. When it involved a small tubular bone such as the fibula (Fig. II.58), the ulna (Fig. II.59), a metatarsal, or a phalanx (Fig. II.60), it generally occupied the entire width of the affected bone and produced a fusiform expansion and thinning of both cortices, often making the differential diagnosis with fibrous dysplasia or chondroma difficult. Three cases of small size and with predominant cortical involvement were reported by this author in 1987 (Fig. II.61).

The internal border of the tumor tended to be scalloped and well defined by a narrow rim of bone sclerosis toward the marrow cavity (Figs. II.57, II.60). On its outer surface, it was delimited by a thinned cortex, replaced in great part by a thin, blown-up shell of newly formed periosteal bone, often partially absent (Figs. II.62, II.63), similar to the radiologic picture of an aneurysmal bone cyst. In only one case were areas of conspicuous spotty calcification visible on the radiograph; more often, bone septa traversing the tumor and producing a trabecular appearance were seen. However, study of the gross and microscopic specimens shows that this is usually only a pseudotrabeculation caused by ridges and corrugations of the sclerotic border at the inner surface, similar to the pseudotrabeculation observed in solitary (unicameral) bone cysts.

Pathologic Findings. *Gross Pathology.* Besides the numerous irregular fragments obtained by curettage, we examined a number of entire resection specimens and large fragments obtained from wide excision of tumors of appreciable size, one of which was located in the innominate bone and

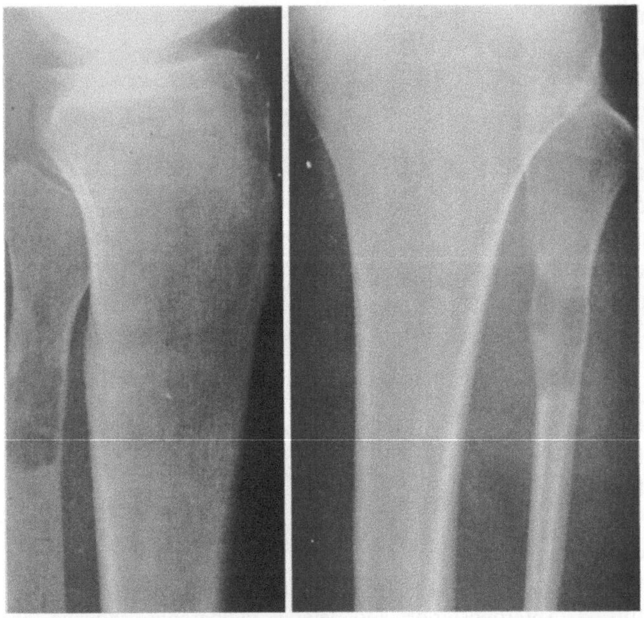
a

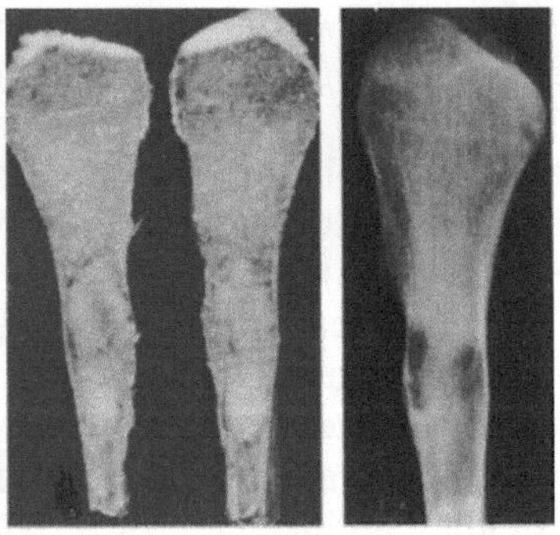
b, c

Fig. II.58a–c. Female, 32 years old, with chondromyxoid fibroma. **a** Lateral and anteroposterior radiographs showing a translucent well-delimited lesion in the upper third of the fibular shaft. **b** Photograph and **c** radiograph of the resection specimen. (Schajowicz and Gallardo 1971)

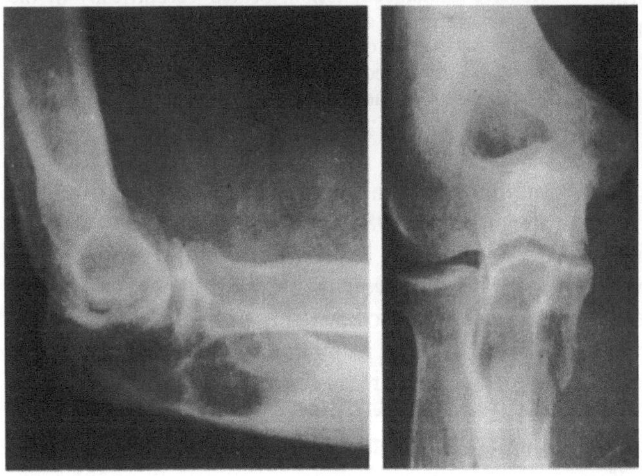

Fig. II.59. Male, 49 years old. Osteolytic, somewhat trabeculated lesion in the upper end of the ulna. (Schajowicz and Gallardo 1971)

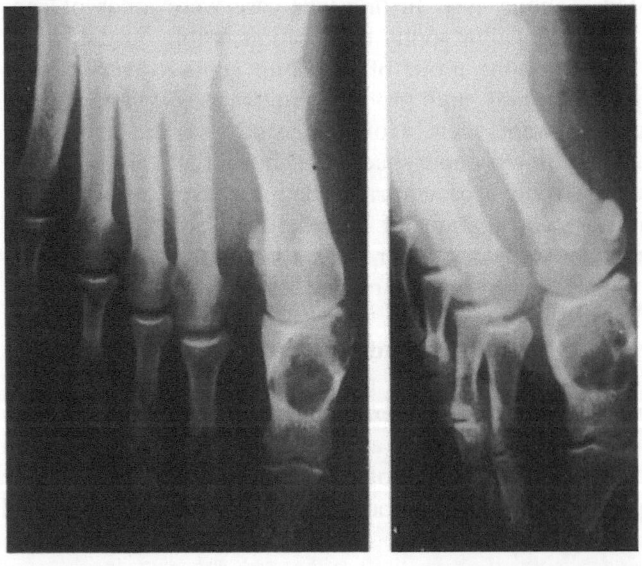

Fig. II.60. Male, 22 years old. Anteroposterior and lateral radiographs showing a centrally, slightly trabeculated osteolytic lesion in the first phalanx of the great toe. (Schajowicz and Gallardo 1971)

Fig. II.61a,b. Male, 30 years old. Chondromyxoid fibroma of tibia. **a** Anteroposterior and lateral radiographs illustrate an unusually small (2 × 1.5 cm), ovoid, apparently intracortical lesion in the upper diaphysis, sharply outlined by a thin sclerotic rim. **b** Photograph and radiograph of the resected specimen reveal the bluish-white color and the intracortical location of the round 2 × 1.5 cm tumor nodule, which expanded the periosteum, producing a thin shell of newly formed bone and a Codman's triangle. (Schajowicz 1987)

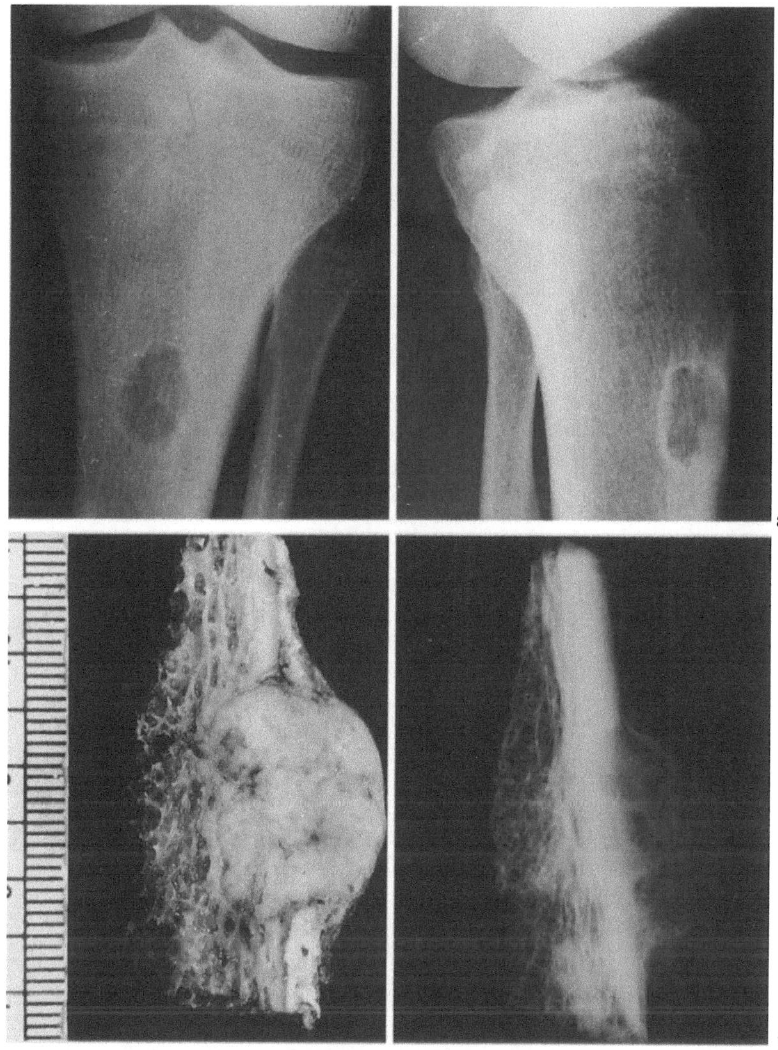

a

b

Fig. II.62a,b. Fourteen-year-old girl with chondromyxoid fibroma of fibula. **a** Lateral radiograph shows a large, eccentric radiolucent lesion in the upper metaphysis. Scalloped sclerotic borders are observed at its medullary side. The thinned cortex is widely expanded and partly interrupted. A Codman's triangle is present at the lower end. A diagnosis of aneurysmal bone cyst was suggested. **b** The photograph of the resected specimen showed the solid nature and grayish-white color of the tumor

a

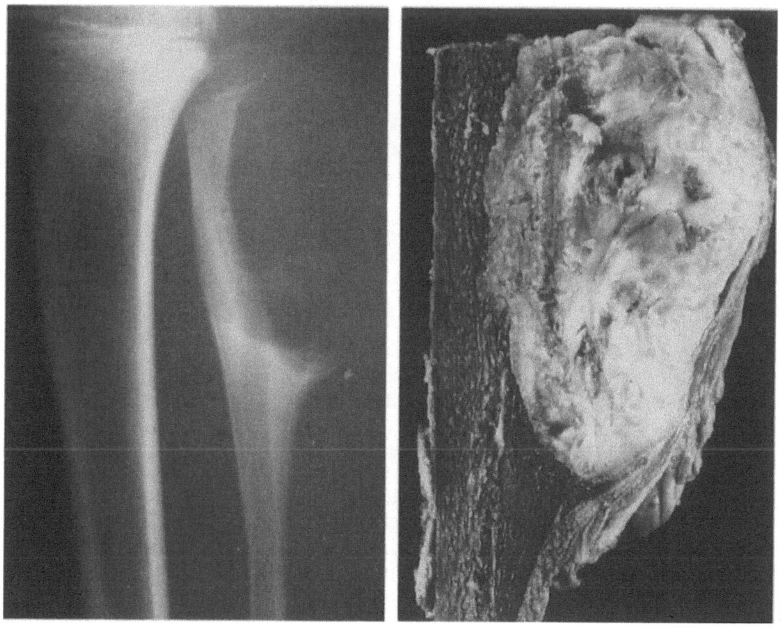

b

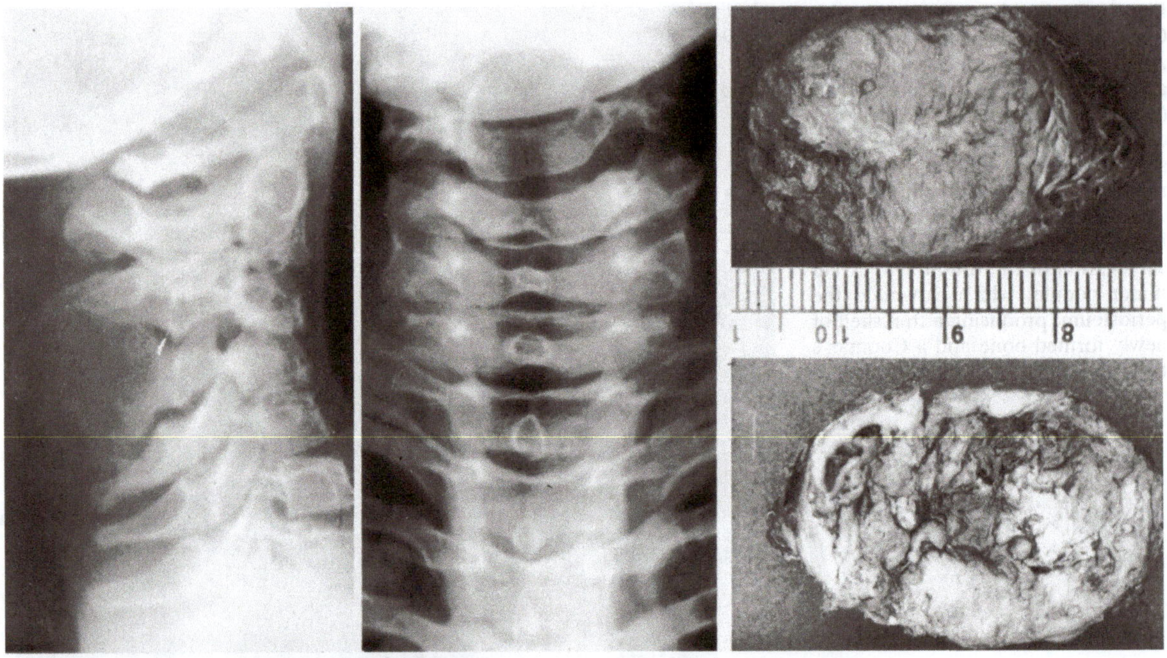

II.63a b c

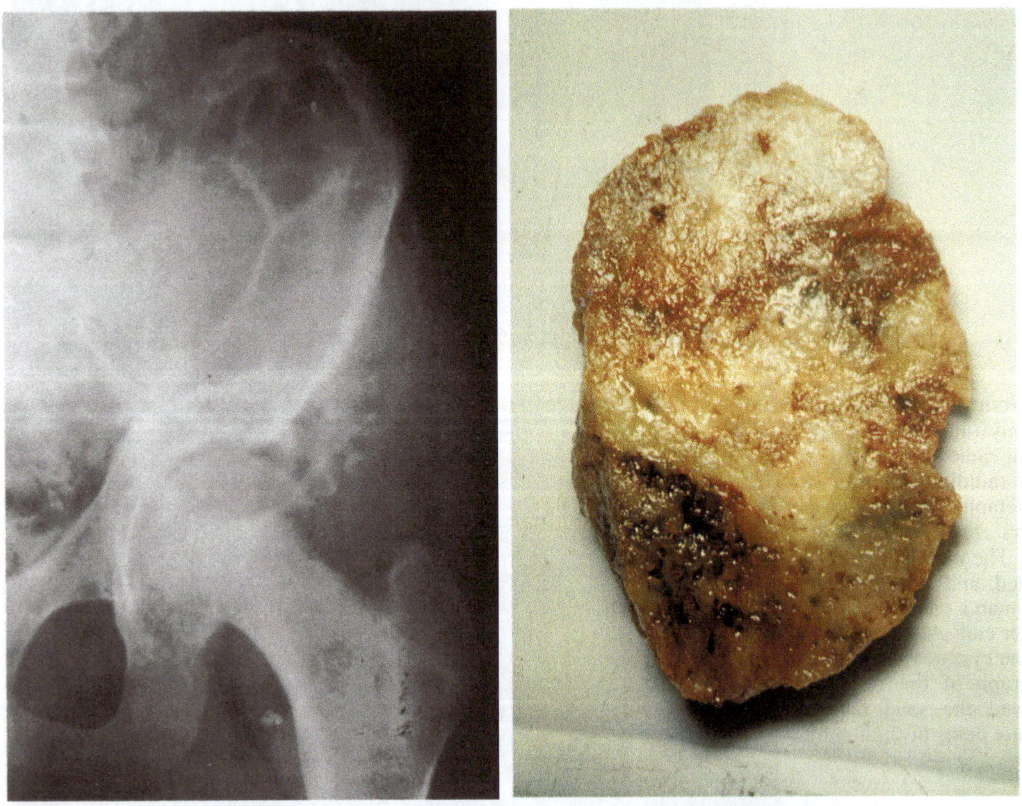

II.64a b

Fig. II.63a–c. Female, 6 years old. **a** Lateral and anteroposterior radiographs showing distension of the spinous process of the third cervical vertebra, suggesting an aneurysmal bone cyst. **b,c** Photographs of the entire and the cut surface of the specimen, which is mainly solid, though there are some irregular cystic hemorrhagic areas. (Schajowicz and Gallardo 1971)

Fig. II.64a,b. Female, 13 years old. **a** Radiograph shows a large trabeculated lesion in the ilium with penetration into the soft parts, surrounded in part by a thin shell of new bone. **b** Photograph of the specimen of bluish-gray color and myxoid aspect. (**a**, Schajowicz and Gallardo 1971)

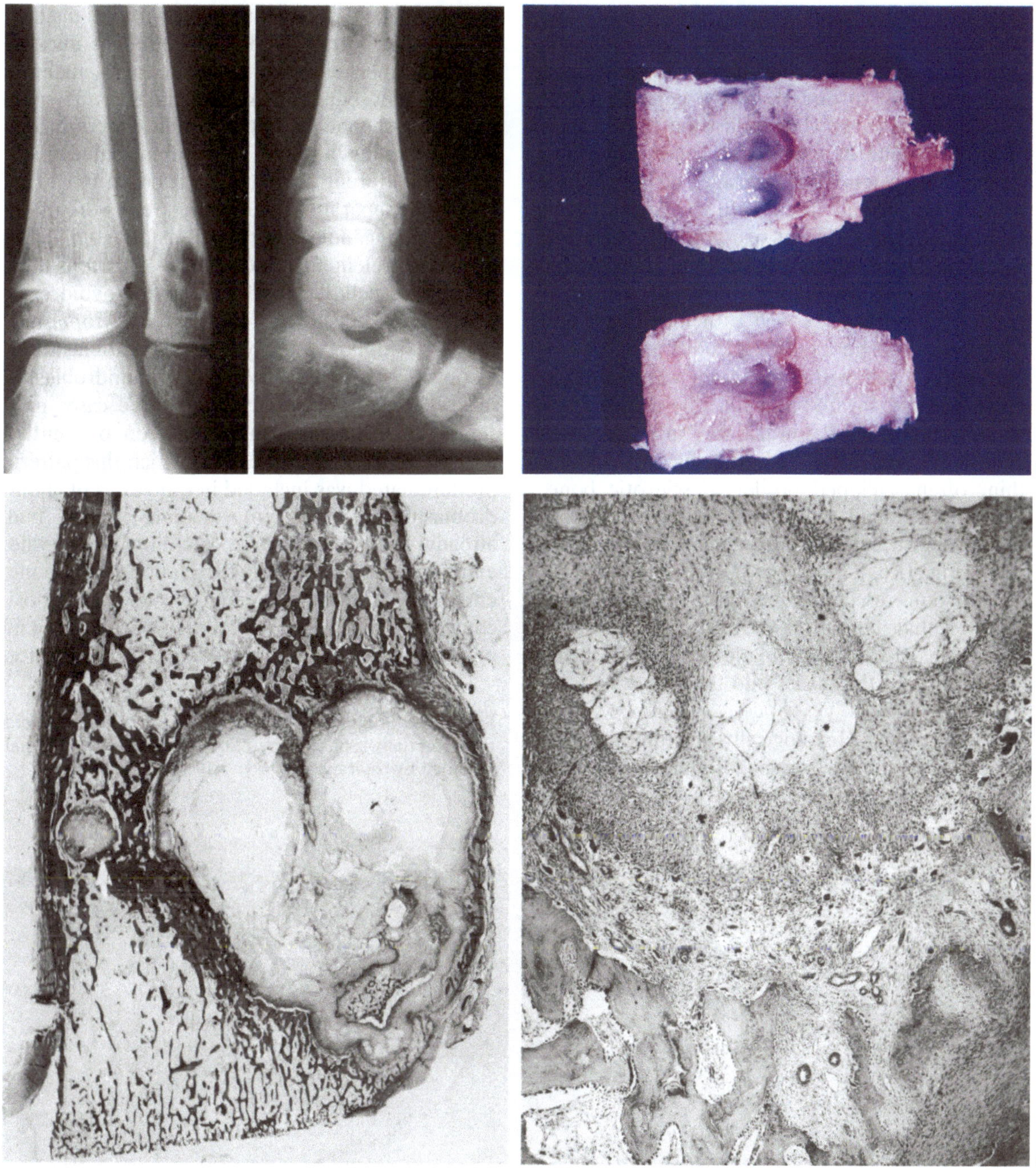

Fig. II.65a–d. Male, 9 years old. **a** Anteroposterior and lateral radiographs showing a radiolucent lesion located eccentrically in the lower metaphysis of the fibula, with a scalloped sclerotic inner border. **b** Macroscopic aspect of the specimen showing several cystic cavities and some small tumor lobules separated by normal marrow from the bulk of the tumor. **c** Topographic photomicrograph showing the thinned distended cortex, formation of cystic cavities, and the slceotic border toward the medullary cavity. A small tumor nodule separated by sclerotic bone from the main neoplasm is seen. **d** Photomicrograph showing formation of small irregular cystic spaces in the tumor, which shows a well-defined limit toward a small ring of vascular loose connective tissue separating the tumor from the sclerotic bone border. (Schajowicz and Gallardo 1971) **c** ×3, **d** ×40 measured more than 10 cm (Fig. II.64). The tumor was generally well limited on its outer surface and covered by a thin shell of newly formed periosteal bone or directly by the periosteum.

The cut surface showed a solid tumor mass of grayish-white or bluish-gray color, somewhat translucent, resembling cartilage; however, in a few frankly mucoid cases there was formation of small cavities of different size produced by cystic softening of the mucoid tissue (Fig. II.65). The consistency was usually firm, although soft areas could be observed, as well as hemorrhages and foci of blood pigment. Conspicuous areas of calcification of yellowish-white color were found in only one case, located in a rib. The demarcation of the tumor mass toward the spongiosa was generally sharp, lobulated, and surrounded by a thin, often scalloped border of sclerotic bone. Sometimes, small tumor lobules were found in the spongiosa, separated from the principal tumor mass (Fig. II.65).

In our resection specimens, we did not observe that bony septa traversing the tumor tissue caused true trabeculation, nor did we find penetration of the tumor into the epiphysis.

Histopathology. Histologically, the tumor is composed of lobulated or pseudolobulated areas of spindle-shaped or stellate cells without distinct cytoplasmic borders and with abundant myxoid or sometimes chondroid intercellular material separated by bands of more cellular tissue, rich in spindle-shaped or rounded cells, intermingled with a varying number of multinucleated giant cells of different sizes (Figs. II.66–II.69). The septa that separated the myxoid areas were often rich in collagenous fibers with a fair number of fibroblastic elements, but on many occasions they were more cellular with roundish or ovoid cells predominating, showing conspicuous cytoplasmic borders, similar to the young chondroblastic or histiocytic elements observed in chondroblastomas. This pattern was clear in three cases presenting intermediate stages between one entity and the other; a fourth case in which this pattern predominated was included in our series of chondroblastomas. Such intermediate stages had already been observed by Dahlin (1956), who emphasized the morphologic relationship of bone entities. Multinucleated giant cells were an almost constant finding (Fig. II.69); they were lacking in only two cases, and appeared later in a recurrence

Fig. II.66. Photomicrograph showing lobules of myxoid tissue partially separated by more cellular septa. Material obtained by aspiration biopsy. ×100
▼

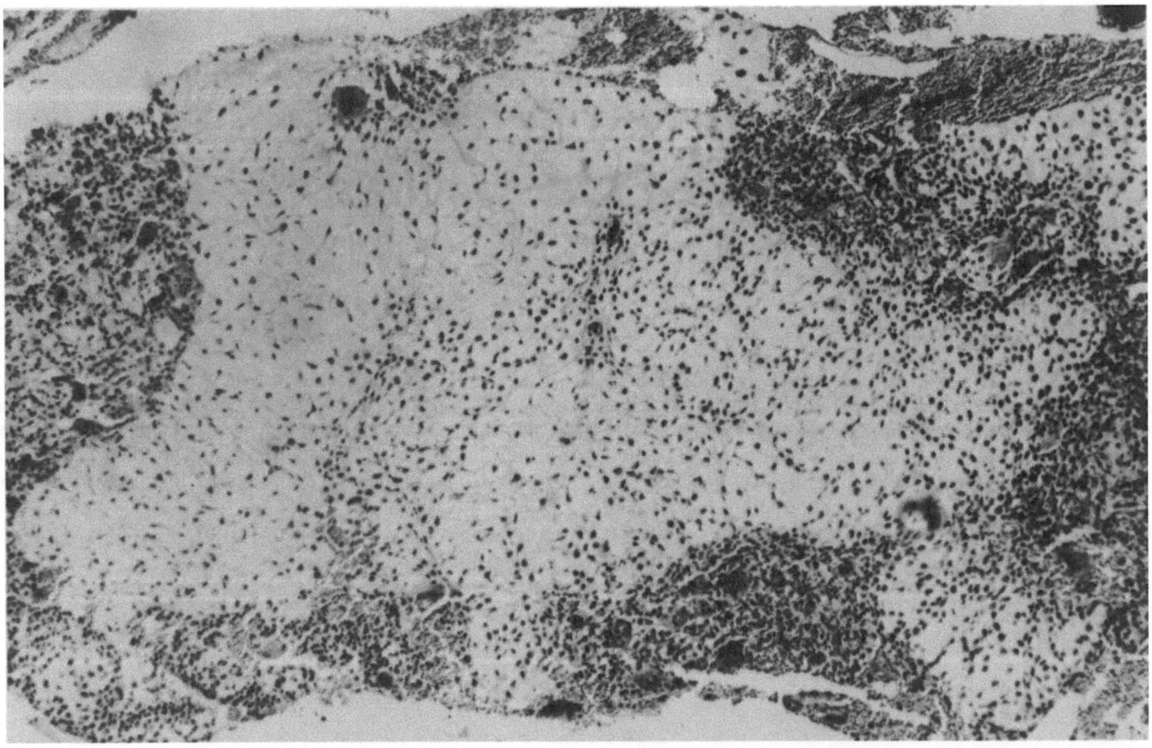

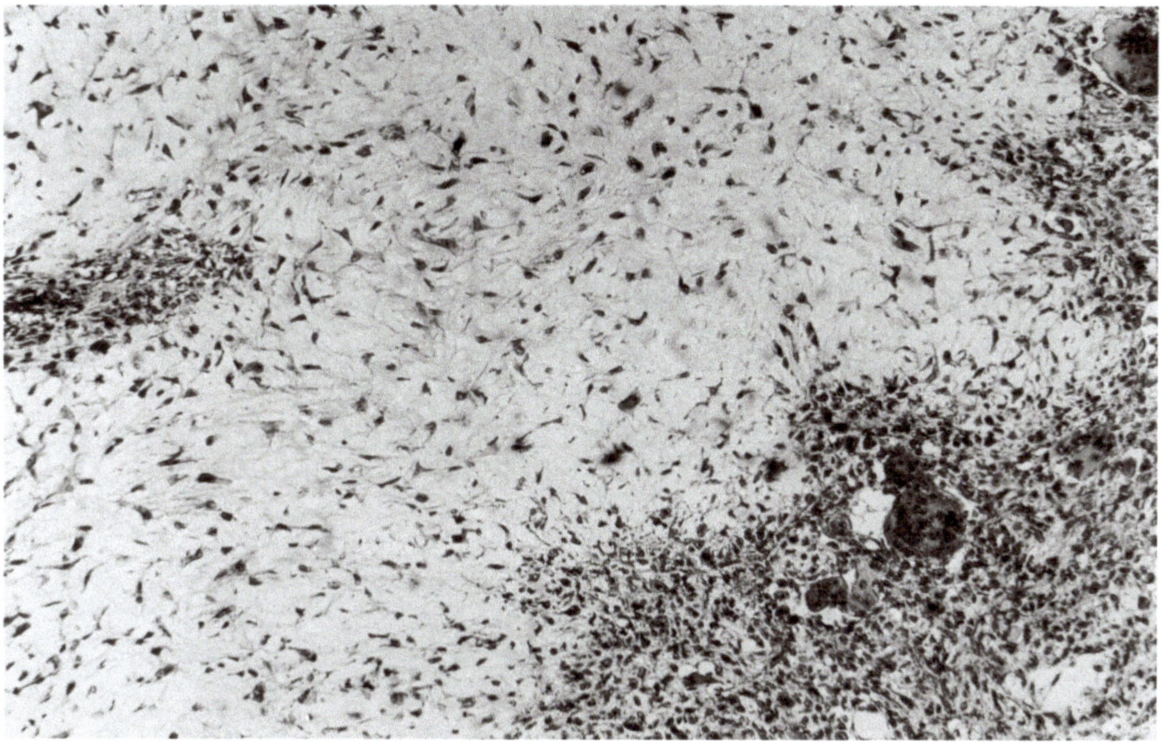

II.67

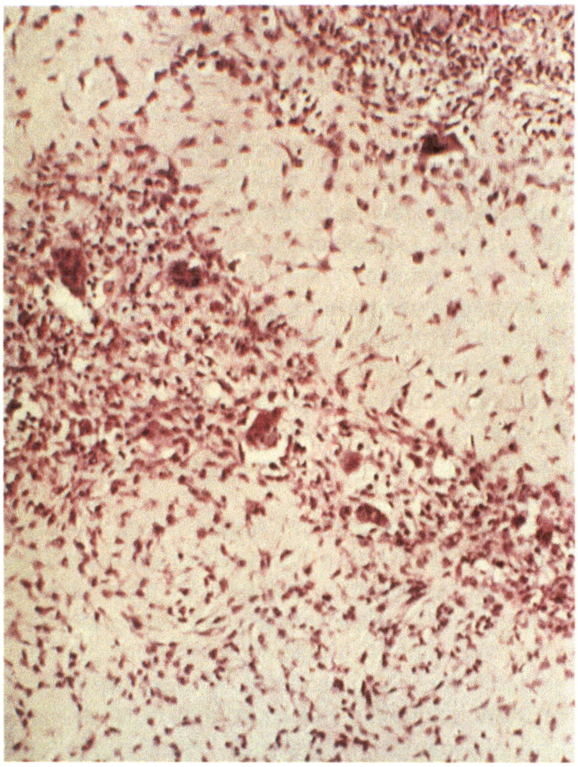

II.68a

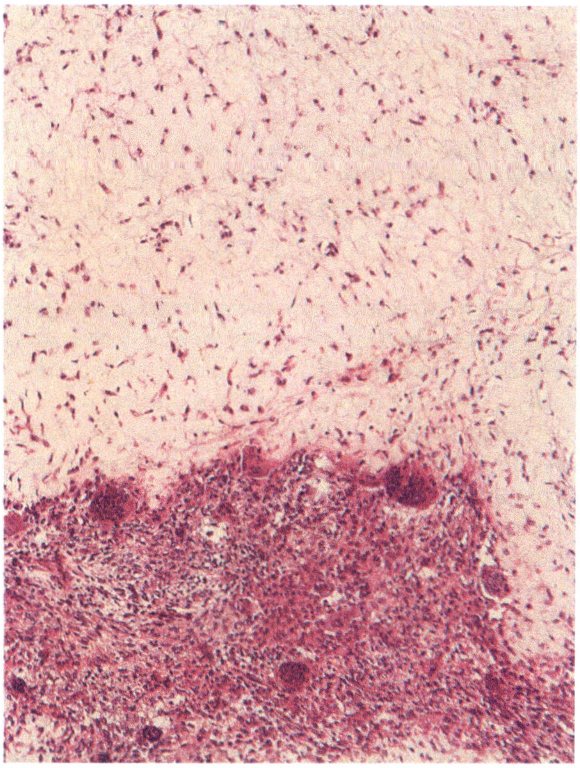

b

Fig. II.67. Photomicrograph shows the myxoid aspect with its stellate cells and the more cellular septa containing some multinucleated giant cells. ×180

Fig. II.68a,b. Photomicrographs show cellular septa containing several multinucleated giant cells, separating the myxoid lobules **a** ×100, **b** ×150

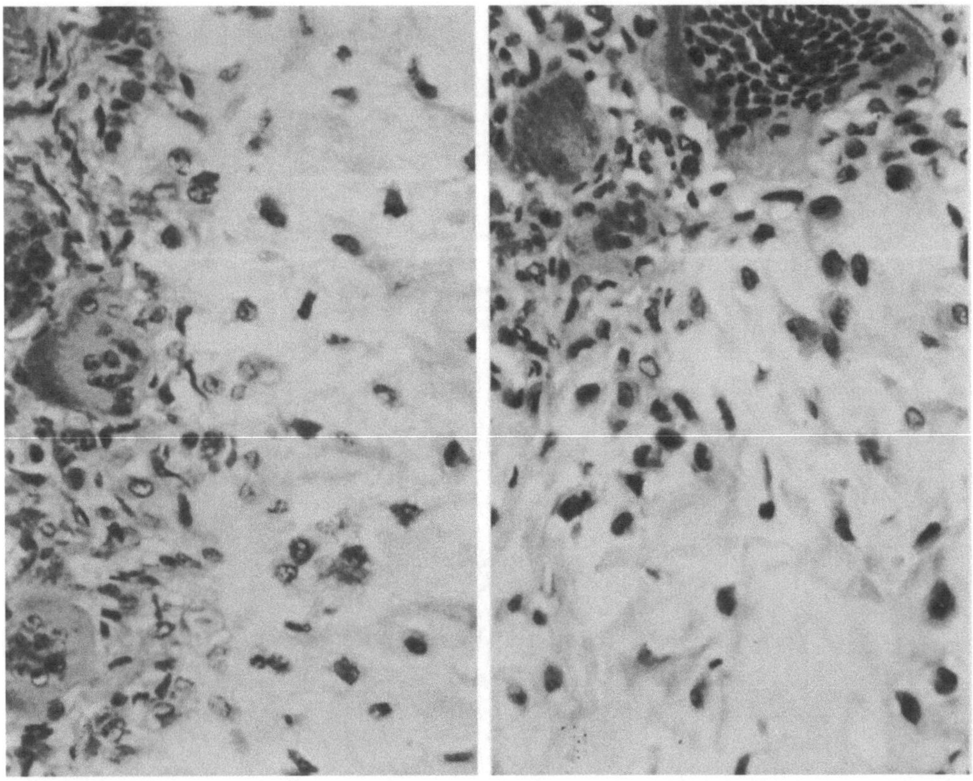

a b

Fig. II.69a,b. Photomicrographs showing at higher magnification the myxoid tissue and the multinucleated giant cells of the septa. **a,b** ×400

of one of these cases. A characteristic feature was the lobular aspect of the tumor borders, with an evident increase in cells, thus distinguishing this process from the myxoma of the mandible.

Between this lobular surface and the surrounding rim of spongiosa, a narrow zone of richly vascularized, loose connective tissue was a regular finding (Fig. II.65e). With silver stains, a loose net of reticular fibers was observed in the myxoid zones; it was much more dense, and it surrounded individual chondroblastic and histiocytic elements of the septa. Some myxoid lobules showed increased collagenization, and in several cases areas of frank chondroid differentiation with formation of lobules of hyaline cartilage were observed. In approximately one-third of the cases, we observed large pleomorphic cells with one or more hyperchromatic nuclei, often plump or monstrous, in the myxoid areas (Fig. II.70), particularly at the periphery of the tumor, which led to confusion with chondrosarcoma in one of our cases before Jaffe and Lichtenstein's (1948) publication. However, mitotic figures were generally lacking. Conspicuous foci of amorphous calcification sufficiently abundant to be visible in the radiographs were found in only one case located in a rib. The interlobular septa were generally richly vascularized, and recent or old hemorrhages with abundant blood pigment, partly phagocytized by histiocytic elements, were common findings. Trabeculae of newly formed bone were rarely found.

The histochemical studies demonstrated glycogen granules in many chondroblastic elements as well as in the stellate cells of the myxoid areas. The multinucleated giant cells of osteoclast type showed a discrete amount of periodic acid-Schiff-positive material in their cytoplasm, resistant to ptyalin digestion, and were strongly acid phosphatase-positive, as in other giant-cell lesions (Schajowicz and Cabrini 1958a,b).

The myxoid and chondroid areas gave, in most parts, a positive metachromatic reaction with toluidine and Alcian blue, which disappeared almost completely in the myxoid areas after

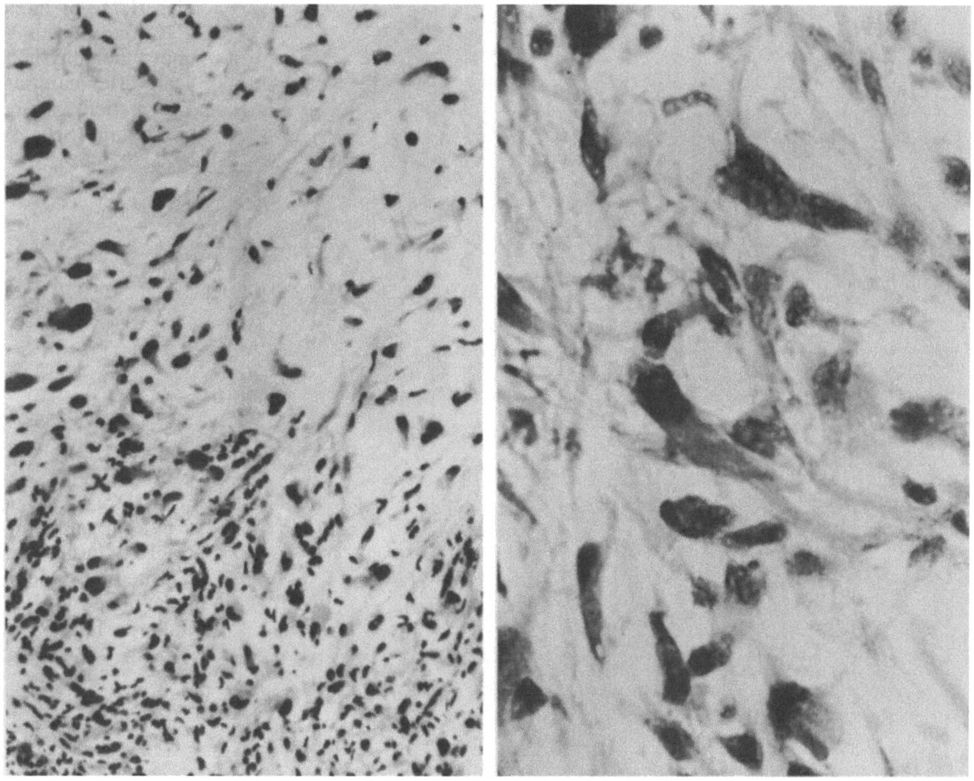

Fig. II.70a,b. Photomicrographs showing marked cellular atypism with one or more hyperchromatic nuclei; no atypical mitoses are observed. These cytologic features are frequently encountered in chondromyxoid fibroma and apparently have no prognostic significance. **a** ×200, **b** ×600

hyaluronidase digestion (Schajowicz and Gallardo 1971). We did not find immunohistologic studies in this tumor type in our search of the literature, except for a brief mention of the presence of S-100 protein positivity in a few cases studied by Monda and Wick (1985) and Weiss and Dorfman (1986).

Pathogenesis. The presence of transitional types between this tumor and chondroblastoma, the evidence of areas of chondroid differentiation, and the similar histochemical behavior [particularly the demonstration of metachromatic substances in the myxoid and chondroid areas, also found by others (Benedetti et al. 1962; Scaglietti and Stringa 1956, 1961)] indicate a cartilaginous derivation of this process. Despite the agreement that it belongs to the general group of cartilage tumors, it is designated as a "fibroma," which in the writer's opinion appears illogical; the term "fibromyxoid chondroma" would be much more appropriate. This was also pointed out by Aegerter and Kirkpatrick (1975).

Treatment and Prognosis. Although a certain percentage of chondromyxoid fibromas can be cured by thorough intralesional excision (Figs. II.71, II.72), the incidence of recurrence after this treatment is relatively high, varying from 12.5% in Ralph's (1962) review of the published cases up to 25% in Dahlin's report (1967) (Fig. II.73). The tendency toward local recurrence after initial curettage seems to be even higher in young children (Scaglietti and Stringa 1961; Ralph 1962). A more radical surgical treatment (marginal excision or en bloc resection) is indicated in these patients. In our opinion, the presence of small tumor lobules in the spongiosa, separated from the bulk of the tumor by a rim of sclerotic bone, probably impedes adequate and complete extirpation of the lesion by curettage. Thus, en bloc resection should be the treatment of choice whenever possible (such as in expendable bones, fibula, ribs). The low incidence of local recurrences in our series (one case) is possibly due to our preference for wide excision or en bloc resection as the *initial* treatment. The presence of a 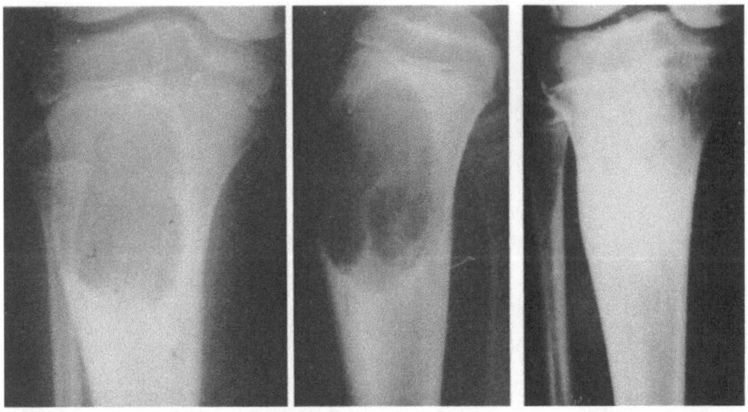 b

Fig. II.71a,b. Female, 12 years old. a Chondromyxoid fibroma of the upper metaphysis of the tibia. b Four years after curettage and bone graft. The patient is well 16 years after operation. (Schajowicz and Gallardo 1971)

a b 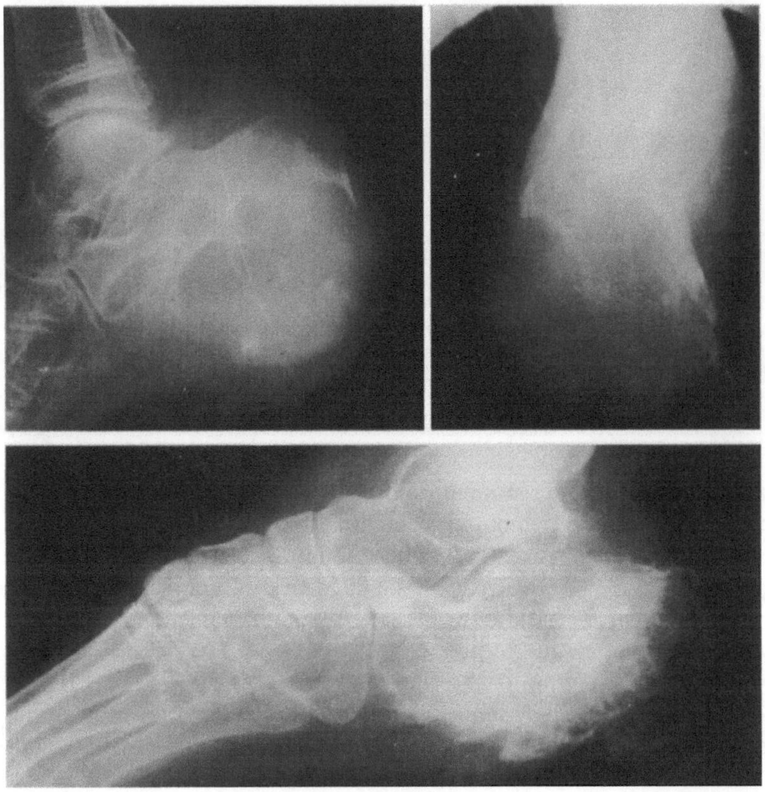

Fig. II.72a,b. Male, 16 years old. a Lateral and anteroposterior radiographs of large expanding lesion of the calcaneus. b One year after curettage and bone graft. (Schajowicz and Gallardo 1971)

evident nuclear atypism with one or more hyperchromatic nuclei, often plump or monstrous, but with only exceptional mitotic figures, was a frequent finding in our and in virtually all other publications. The evolution of our cases, that is, the complete absence of malignant transformation, and the extreme rarity of reported malignant behavior confirm that this finding has no prognostic significance. The isolated cases of malignant change reported in the literature by Iwata and Coley (1958), Gilmer et al. (1963), and Dahlin (1978) have demonstrated that this complication is extremely rare.

a 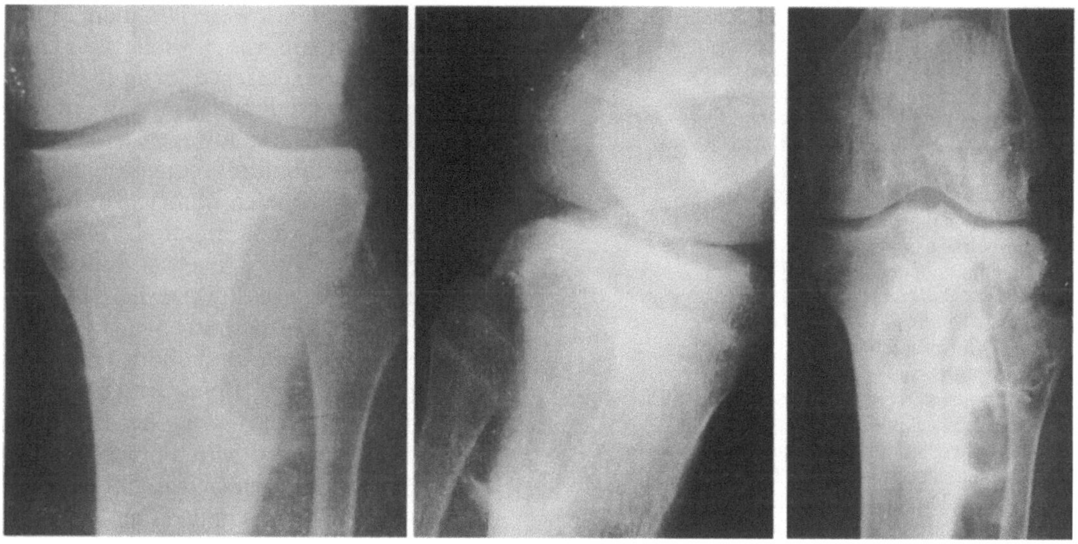 b

Fig. II.73. a Chondromyxoid fibroma of the upper tibial metaphysis showing wide expansion of the cortex. **b** Recurrence 2 years after curettage. (Schajowicz and Gallardo 1971)

B. Malignant

1. Chondrosarcoma

Definition, WHO: *"A malignant tumor characterized by the formation of cartilage, but not of bone, by the tumor cells. It is distinguished from chondroma by its higher cellularity and greater pleomorphism, and by appreciable numbers of plump cells with large or double nuclei. Mitotic cells are infrequent."*

Chondrosarcomas exhibit a wide spectrum of clinicopathologic features and biologic behavior, and several different variants, in addition to the most common conventional central chondrosarcoma, may be observed. They may be either *primary*, apparently originating de novo in a previously normal bone, or *secondary* to some preexistent benign cartilage tumor, most frequently to multiple hereditary osteochondromatosis (peripheral or exostotic chondrosarcoma) and enchondromatosis.

Keiller (1925) and Phemister (1930) were the first to separate chondrosarcoma as a distinct entity from the group of "osteogenic sarcomas" not only because of its distinct morphologic and clinicoradiologic appearance, but also because of its generally slower course and better prognosis (Phemister 1930). This separation was accepted later by the Committee of the Bone Tumor Registry in their revised classification (Ewing 1939). However, the morphologic criteria for the definition of chondrosarcoma as an entity distinct from osteosarcoma remained imprecise, because Phemister and later Thomson and Turner-Warwick (1955) based their differentiation on the *predominance* of cartilage present and accepted cases containing small amounts of tumor bone as chondrosarcomata. Lichtenstein and Jaffe (1943) were the first to make a clear distinction between chondrosarcoma and osteosarcoma. They considered that a chondrosarcoma develops from full-fledged cartilage, and although it might become calcified or ossified, it never, in contrast to osteosarcoma, shows neoplastic osteoid or bone evolving directly from the sarcomatous stroma, that is, formed by the tumor cells.

According to their origin, we divided chondrosarcomas into primary and secondary, and according to their position in the affected bone, into central and peripheral or exostotic (Table II.2).

Secondary chondrosarcomas were also observed as a rare complication of Paget disease and fibrous dysplasia (Price and Goldie 1969; Huvos et al. 1972), in association with bone infarct and unicameral bone cyst (Grabias and Mankin 1974), or after radiotherapy of benign cartilage tumors (Hatcher and Campbell 1951) or intravenous injection of thorium dioxide sol (Thorotrast) (Schajowicz et al. 1967).

Table II.2. Classification of chondrosarcomas

Primary chondrosarcomas (348 cases)
1. Central (conventional) (306 cases)
2. Dedifferentiated chondrosarcoma: these cases are included with poorly differentiated central chondrosarcomas
3. Juxtacortical (periosteal) (13 cases)
4. Mesenchymal (22 cases)
5. Clear-cell (6 cases)
6. Malignant chondroblastoma? (1 case)

Secondary chondrosarcomas (33 cases)
Central chondrosarcoma
1. Enchondroma
2. Multiple enchondromatosis with or without Ollier's disease (8 cases)

Peripheral (exostotic) chondrosarcoma
3. Solitary osteochondroma (14 cases)
4. Multiple hereditary osteochondromas (osteochondromatosis) (10 cases)
5. Periosteal (juxtacortical) chondroma (1 case)

Primary Chondrosarcomas

Central (Conventional) Chondrosarcoma

Incidence. Chondrosarcoma accounted for 14.5% of malignant bone tumors and 6.4% of all bone tumors in our files, which agrees with the statistics of most other series (Jaffe 1958; Lindbom et al. 1961; Barnes and Catto 1966; Lichtenstein 1977). The 635 cases of primary chondrosarcoma in the Mayo Clinic series account for 11% of the malignant tumors (Dahlin and Unni 1986).

Among 493 cases of chondrosarcoma, including all variants, diagnosed and treated at the Memorial Hospital in New York (Huvos 1991) from 1928 through 1982, 305 (64.5%) arose de novo (primary chondrosarcoma) and 168 (35.5%) proved to be secondary to preexistent benign cartilage lesions.

Clinical Findings. *Age and Sex.* The sex, age, and site distribution data are shown in Scheme II.5. According to the sex distribution data, more males than females presented with central chondrosarcoma in our series (65%) and in Dahlin and Unni's 1986 series (60%); this predominance of males was slightly more evident than in other series (Huvos 1991).

Chondrosarcoma is a tumor of adulthood or old age; the peak incidence in Henderson and Dahlin's (1963) series of 288 cases was between 30 and 60 years of age; only ten patients were under 20 years of age. Only four patients in Dahlin and Unni's series (1986) were less than 10 years old, and the youngest was 3 years old. Our results confirmed the experience of most other authors by revealing a predominance between the second and seventh decades; however, a small number of conventional chondrosarcomas in children and adolescents have been reported in the literature (Gitelis et al. 1981; Aprin et al. 1982; Huvos and Marcove 1987). Sixty-seven of our patients were 20 years of age or less, six of them being 10 years of age or less. Furthermore, most authors agree, as we do, that central chondrosarcomas in children generally have a poor prognosis, as bad as that of osteosarcoma. On the other hand, the differential diagnosis with a predominantly chondroblastic osteosarcoma was difficult and could sometimes be made only after a careful study of the amputation specimen. This distinction, which was formerly considered of only academic interest, has assumed a definite importance because of its role in the selection of the appropriate therapy, which is different for osteosarcoma.

Localization. Central chondrosarcoma may arise in any bone of cartilaginous preformation, and was found in our series most frequently in the femur (96 cases). In the trunk the most common sites were the pelvis (63 cases), ribs (14 cases), and the scapula (10 cases). Chondrosarcoma was located infrequently in the vertebral column (8 cases) and sternum (4 cases). As in other major statistics, the involvement of short tubular bones of hands and feet was uncommon.

Symptoms. Pain, which was sometimes severe, was usually the first symptom of central chondrosarcomas, whereas the peripheral (eccentric or exostotic) tumors were sometimes painless. A firm swelling was noticed first in many cases. In accord with the degree of malignancy, the duration of complaints may range from a few weeks to years. In highly malignant central tumors, destruction of the cortex with presence of a palpable soft tumor mass, associated with generally severe pain, was a common feature; occasionally a pathologic fracture was the first symptom. Some cases with these features may correspond to the variant referred to as "dedifferentiated chondrosarcoma" (see later in this chapter).

The role of hereditary or familial factors in the *genesis* of chondrosarcoma is not proved. A few cases of familial occurrences have been reported, one of them by Schajowicz and Bessone

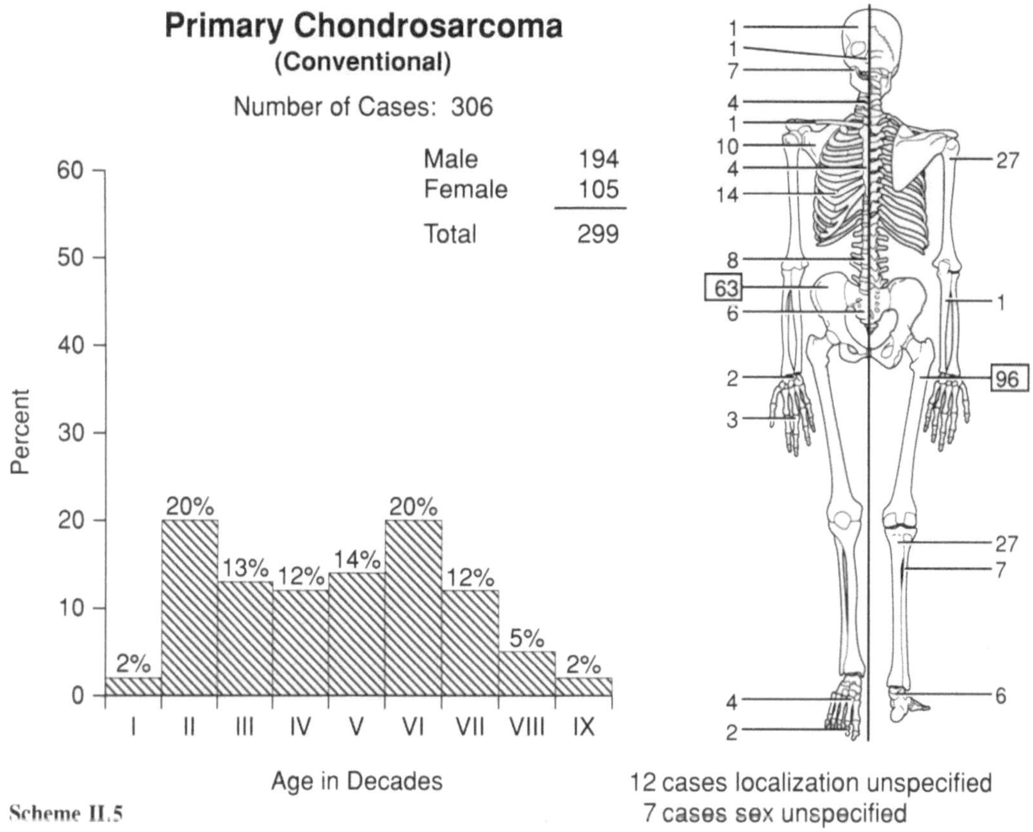

Scheme II.5

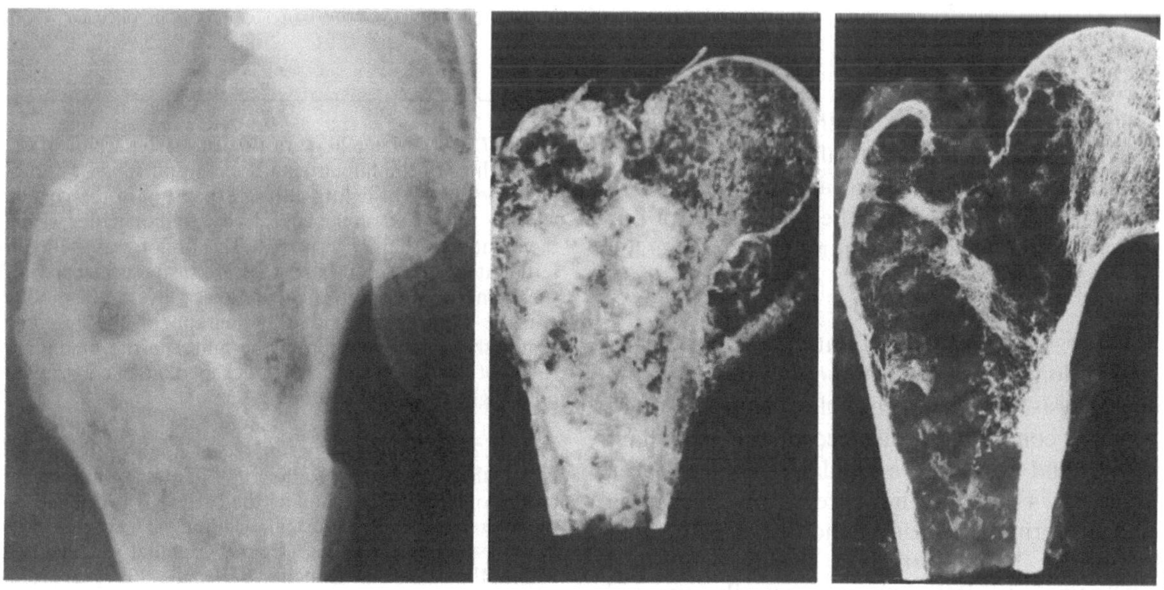

a b, c

Fig. II.74a–c. Female, 36 years old. Chondrosarcoma of the femoral neck. **a** Radiograph shows radiolucent lesion of the femoral neck extending toward the diaphysis, with ill-defined borders. The absence of calcification did not suggest the diagnosis on a radiographic basis. Aspiration biopsy showed a poorly differentiated chondrosarcoma. Disarticulation of the hip was performed. **b** Photograph of the specimen reveals the characteristic aspect of chondrosarcoma, which has partly destroyed the upper cortex of the femoral neck. This is seen in the radiograph of the specimen, which also shows slight spotty calcification and endosteal scalloping of the lateral cortex

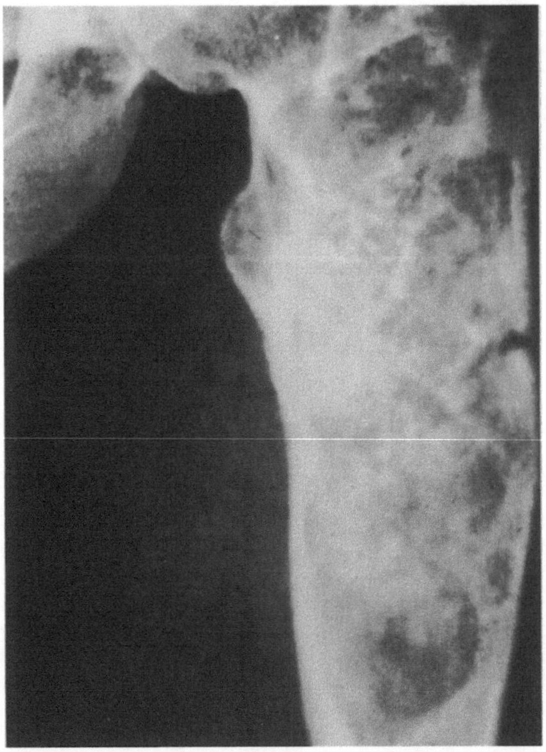

Fig. II.75. Male, 38 years old. Chondrosarcoma of upper third of the femur. Radiograph shows a large lesion involving the metaphysis and diaphysis and expanding into the thinned cortex. Coarse granular "popcorn ball" and ringlike calcification within the tumor is evident

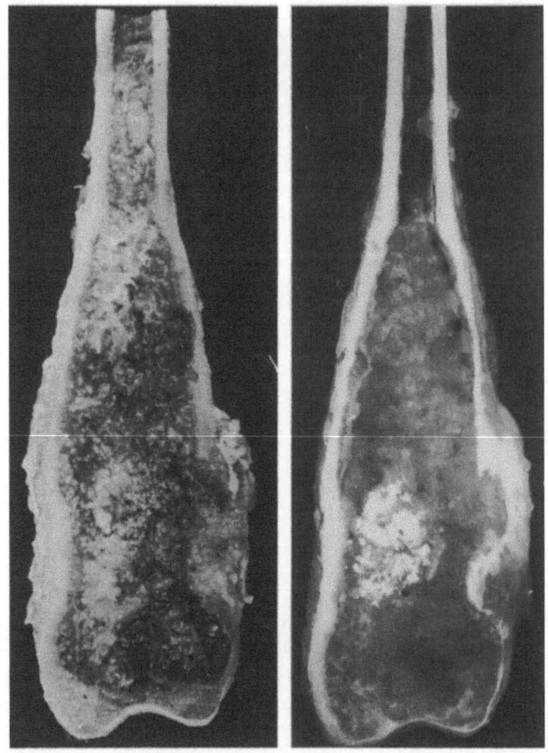

a, b

Fig. II.76a,b. Male, 48 years old. Chondrosarcoma of the lower end of the femur. a Photograph and b radiograph of a longitudinal section of the specimen, demonstrating the expansion of the cortex, which is partly thickened and only partly destroyed, and a central, heavily calcified area within the predominantly radiolucent lesion

(1967) in three teenage brothers, two of whom had periosteal (juxtacortical) chondrosarcoma and one central chondrosarcoma. A fourth brother died 3 years after the publication of our article with a high-grade central chondrosarcoma of the mandible.

Radiographic Features. Central chondrosarcomas of long bones are commonly situated in the metaphysis, extending into the diaphysis, often along a considerable distance of the medullary cavity, and producing a lobular radiolucent area (Figs. II.74–II.77). They often show thickening and fusiform expansion of the cortex with slight periosteal bone formation and/or endosteal scalloping. In later stages, centrally situated stippled or ringlike areas of calcification (Lodwick 1965) appear in the radiolucent areas, which may be extensive and dense, especially in low-grade tumors (Figs. II.75, II.76, II.78a, II.79, II.84) (O'Neal and Ackerman 1952; Barnes and Catto

Fig. II.77a–d. Male, 20 years old. Chondrosarcoma of the upper third of the humerus. **a** Radiograph shows a radiolucent lesion with slightly diffuse expansion of the cortex, which is thickened on the lateral side. Radiopacities within the tumor are hardly visible. **b** The tumor was well differentiated, and an en bloc resection of the upper half of the humerus was performed, followed by cadaver bone graft. **c** Photograph and **d** radiograph of the resected tumor show the extension of the tumor in the medullary cavity of the diaphysis and the thickened intact cortex with only slight endosteal scalloping

Fig. II.78. a Male, 40 years old. Chondrosarcoma of upper shaft of femur. Radiograph shows a radiolucent lesion, only slightly expanding the cortex. It is thinned on the lateral side, with endosteal scalloping. The cortex at its inner aspect is thickened. Coarse granular calcification within the tumor is evident. **b** Female, 31 years old. Chondrosarcoma of radius. Anteroposterior and lateral radiographs illustrate a radiolucent, diaphyseal lesion expanding the thinned cortex, which shows scalloping at its inner aspect. Calcifications are hardly visible. The case was first classified as enchondroma, but after review, modified to well-differentiated (low-grade) chondrosarcoma

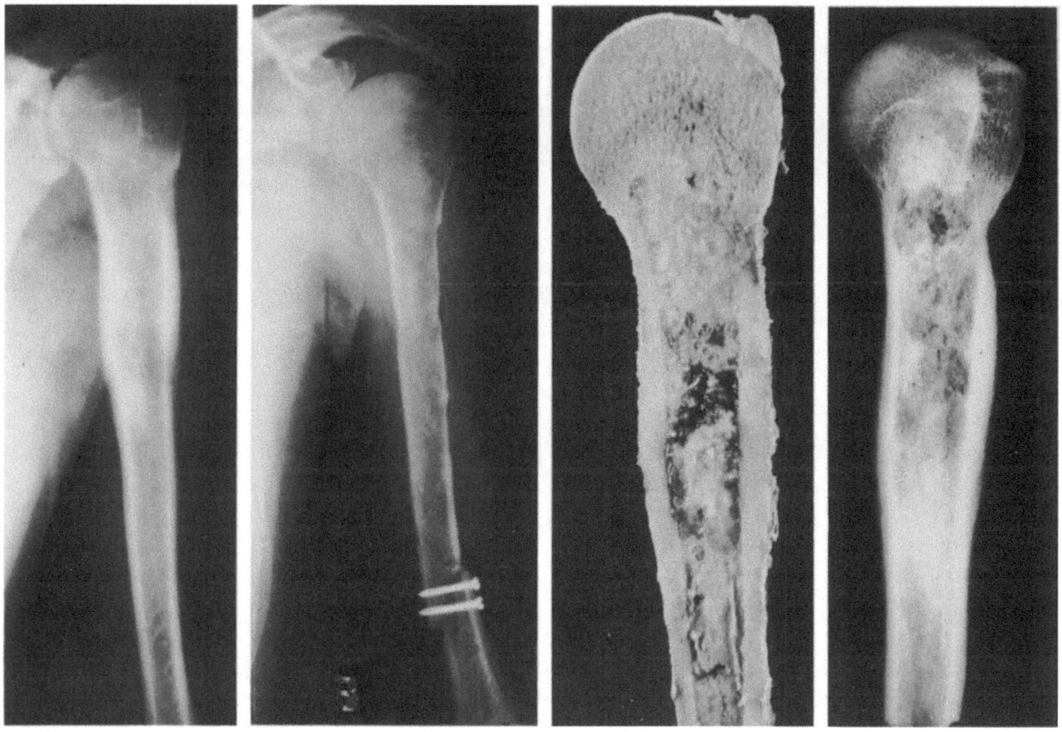

II.77a,b c, d

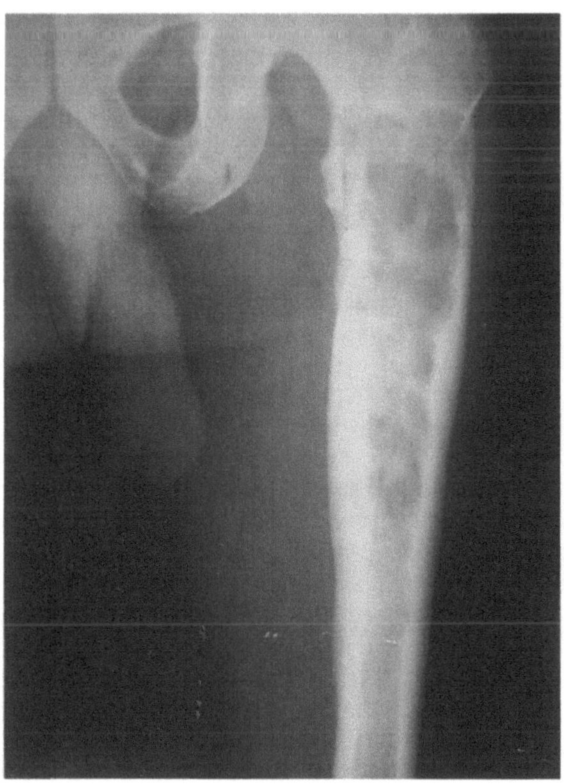

II.78a

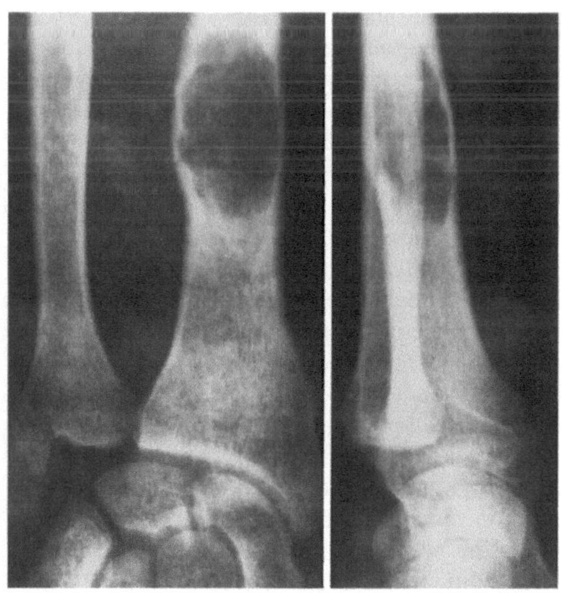

b

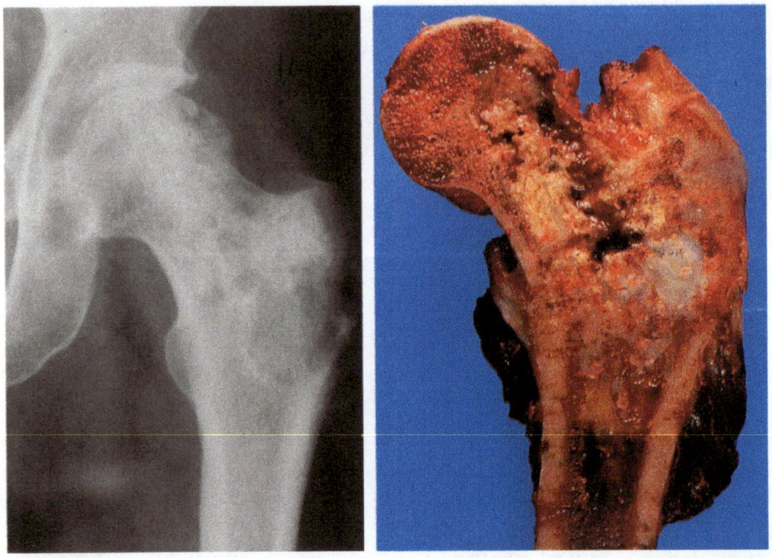

Fig. II.79a,b. Male, 50 years old. Chondrosarcoma of femur. **a** Radiograph shows the heavily calcified radiolucent tumor of the upper femoral end, which has partially destroyed the cortex in the trochanteric region. **b** Photograph reveals the bluish-white cartilage with extensive areas of calcification of yellowish color

1966), or more poorly mineralized in aggressive lesions. Some chondrosarcomas may show ballooned-out expansion of the thinned cortex with minimal or no calcification, or they may rapidly disrupt the cortex, extending, more or less widely, into extraosseous soft tissues, almost certainly indicating high-grade malignancy (see Figs. II.93–II.95) or so-called dedifferentiation (progression of malignancy).

Computed tomography is a superior method for defining extraosseous involvement, particularly in pelvic and scapular tumors, as is MRI in the detection of the intramedullary extension of the tumor (Fig. II.84).

Pathologic Findings. *Gross Pathology.* The gross pattern is similar to that of enchondroma, with a characteristic lobulated aspect separated by thin vasculoconnective septa, frequently producing scalloping of the endosteal surface of the often thickened or extended cortex. The tumor is bluish-white, showing scarce or more abundant yellowish foci of calcification. As in other cartilaginous tumors, regressive phenomena are common, including mucoid degeneration with formation of irregular cavities containing thick viscid fluid, and areas of necrosis (Figs. II.79–II.84), followed in some cases by amorphous calcification and secondary endochondral ossification, which are visible grossly as reddish areas.

The more malignant types, which frequently perforate the cortex and invade the soft tissues (Figs. II.80–II.84), may appear well defined and covered by an apparent capsule; they often present a fleshy aspect of soft consistency and grayish-white color, losing the characteristic chondroid pattern. This pattern is more frequent in the so-called dedifferentiated chondrosarcoma (see Figs. II.93–II.95).

Histopathology. The histologic features of cartilaginous tumors cover a wide range, varying from clearly benign to frankly malignant. There are no problems in the histologic diagnosis of the frankly malignant types, but great difficulties in the cases of low-grade malignancy, which are frequently "underdiagnosed" by the pathologist, especially if the clinicoradiologic features are not considered.

Keiller (1925) first emphasized the importance of nuclear changes in the diagnosis of chondrosarcoma; however, the fundamental importance of cytologic features, which usually correspond to clinical behavior, was generally recognized only after Lichtenstein and Jaffe's paper (1943). According to their criteria, a cartilage tumor should be regarded as malignant when viable noncalcified areas, even scattered fields, show "(1) many cells with plump nuclei, (2) more than an occasional cell with two such nuclei, and especially (3) giant cartilage cells with large simple and multiple nuclei or with clumps of chromatin" (Figs. II.85–II.89). Furthermore, most authors agree that mitotic figures are uncommon in chondrosarcoma, but when they are numerous, they indicate high-grade malig-

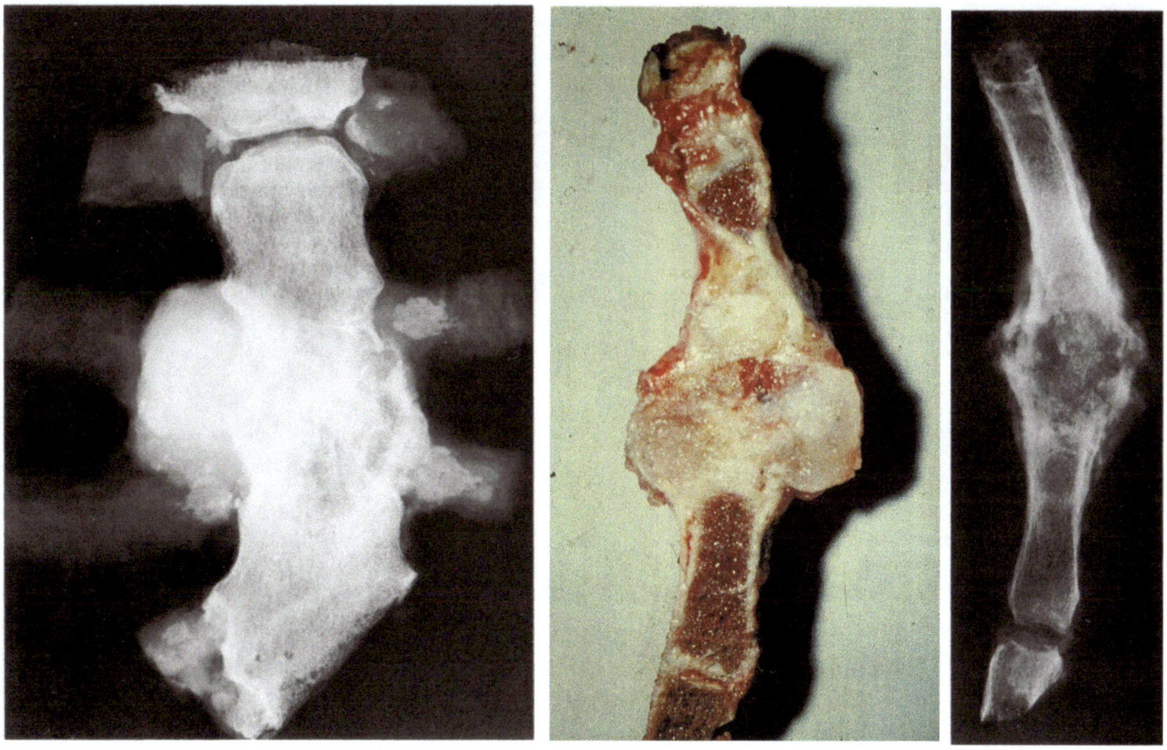

a b, c

Fig. II.80a–c. Female, 36 years old. Chondrosarcoma of the sternum. **a** Radiograph of the entire operation specimen, involving a great part of the sternum and part of three ribs, demonstrates extensive cortical destruction with a large soft tissue mass. **b** Photograph and **c** radiograph of a longitudinal section show the gross pattern and the bone lysis. Despite the wide excision, the tumor recurred three times locally and killed the patient by wide invasion of thorax and lungs after 4 years

Fig. II.81a–c. Male, 67 years old. Chondrosarcoma of the metacarpal bone of the thumb. **a** Radiograph shows a radiolucent, ill-defined lesion that has widely destroyed the cortex and invaded soft tissues. Coarse granular calcifications are seen within the tumor. **b** Photograph and **c** radiograph of the amputation specimen illustrate the large size and destructive tendency of this tumor, which histologically was of high-grade malignancy. The patient died 2 years later with pulmonary metastases

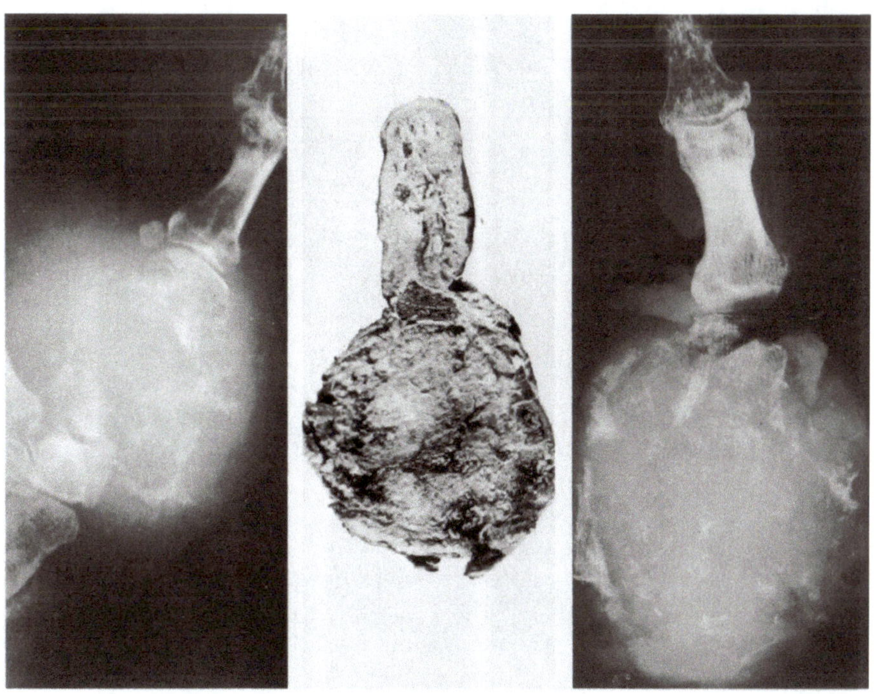

a b, c

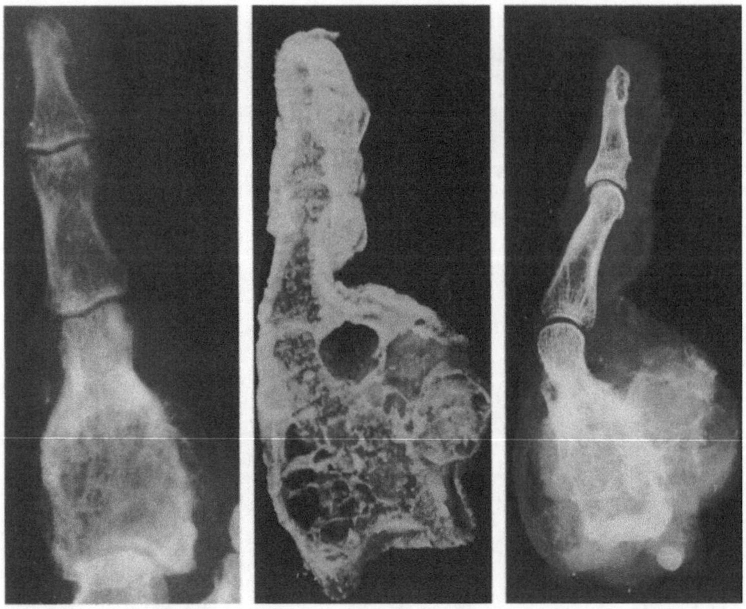

a, b c

Fig. II.82a–c. Male, 48 years old. Chondrosarcoma of the first phalanx. **a** Radiograph shows a radiolucent lesion with expanded and thinned cortex, which is destroyed at one side, better visible on the photograph and radiograph (**b,c**) of the specimen. This tumor previously was curetted after a diagnosis of chondroma. Reviewing the slides, a diagnosis of well-differentiated chondrosarcoma was made. The file was amputated

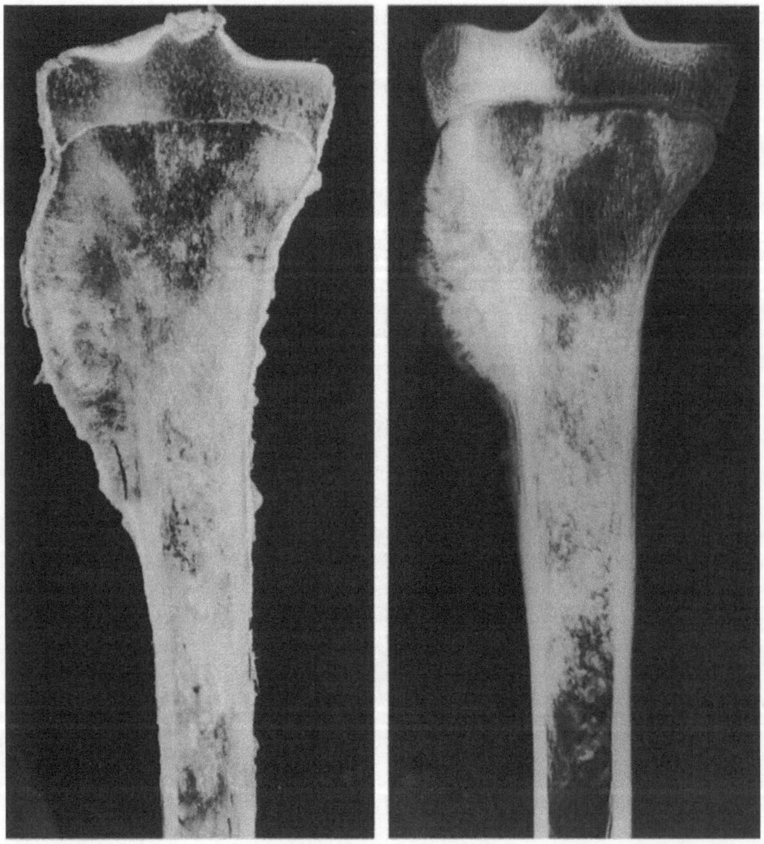

a b

Fig. II.83a,b. Female, 13 years old. Chondrosarcoma of the tibia. Photograph (**a**) and radiograph (**b**), of amputation specimen of an exceptional case of chondrosarcoma in a young child, which on the basis of the clinical radiographs and a biopsy was diagnosed as osteosarcoma, chondroblastic type. The radiograph shows the extension into the medullary cavity of the diaphysis and the coarse granular aspect of the calcifications within the tumor. The histologic study revealed a chondrosarcoma of high-grade malignancy; the patient died 16 months after the amputation with pulmonary metastases

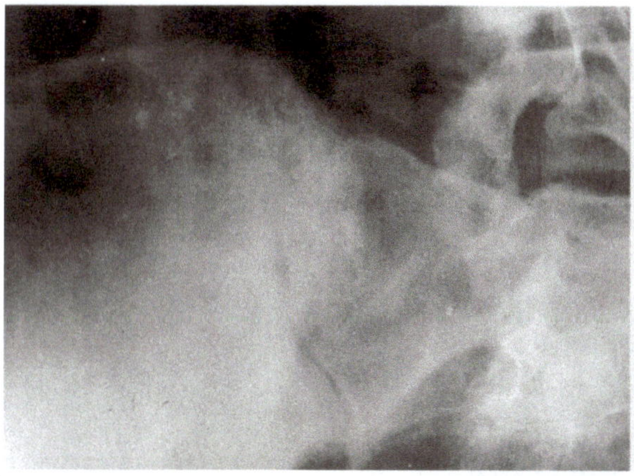

a

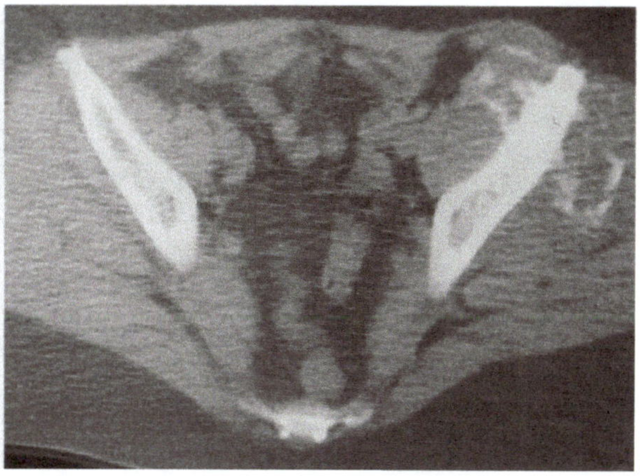

b

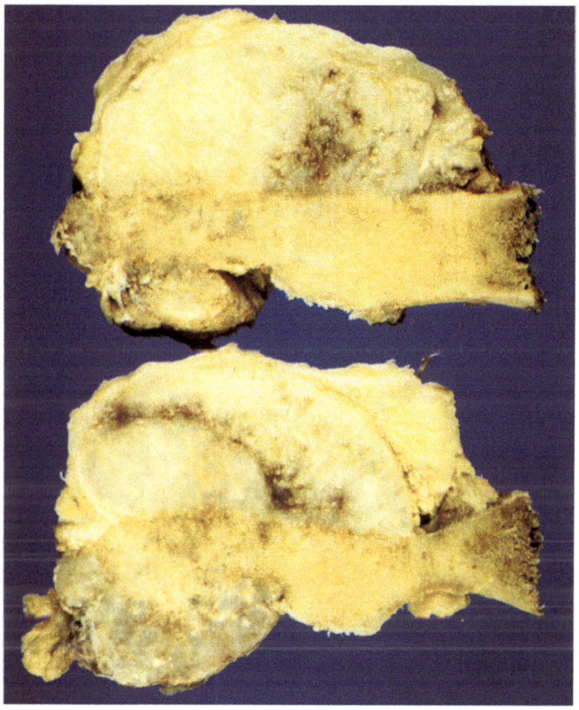

c

Fig. II.84a–c. Female, 42 years old. Chondrosarcoma of the ilium. **a** Radiograph shows a poorly delimited radiodense lesion; its location and extension into the extraosseous soft tissue could only be appreciated in the CT scan (**b**). **c** Photograph of the specimen show the cartilaginous aspect and the spotty calcificaton of this tumor of intraosseous origin

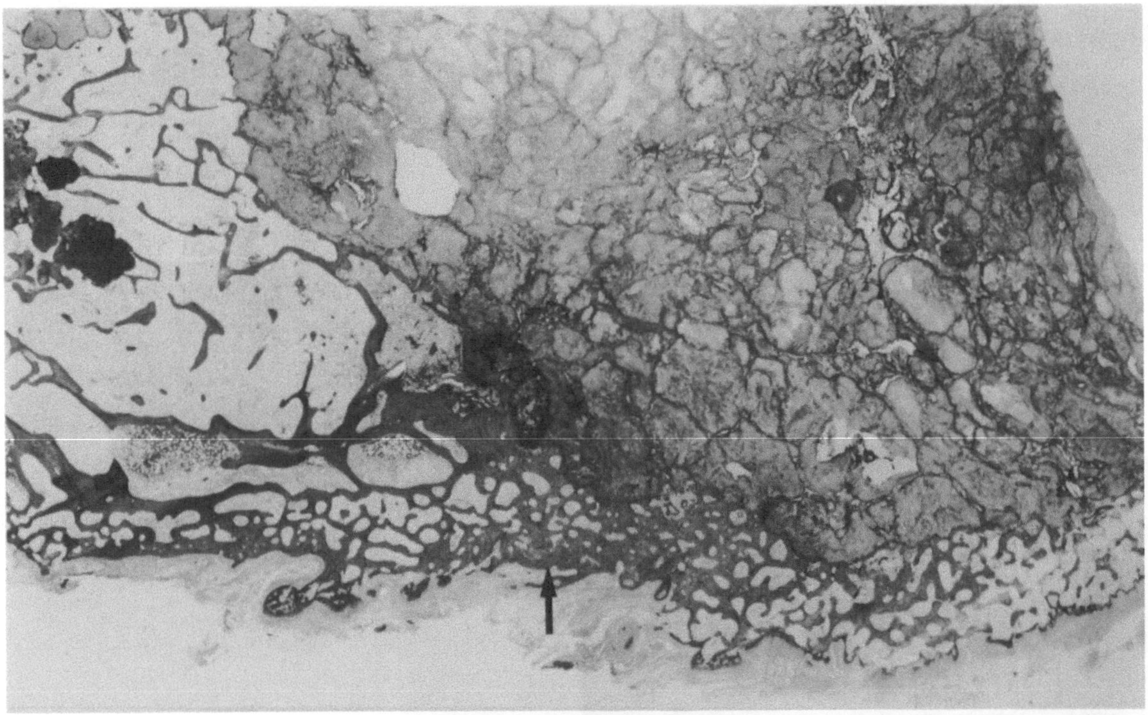

a

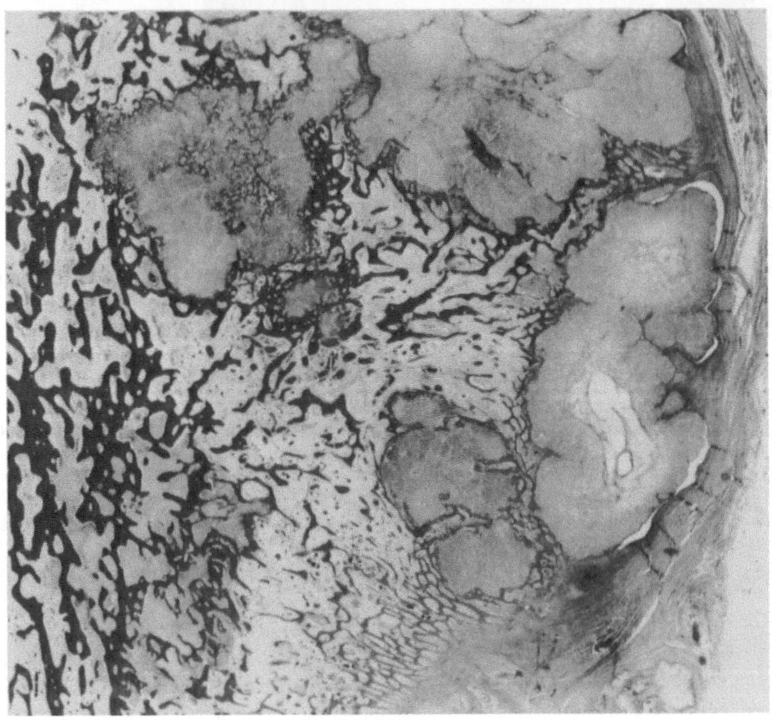

b

Fig. II.85a,b. Photomicrographs of chondrosarcoma showing the lobulated pattern of the chondroid tissue with small, separated nodules within the spongiosa. **a** Tumor is covered by a thick shell of newly formed bone. **b** Tumor lobules are covered by a fibrous membrane (periosteum). **a** ×20, **b** ×30

Fig. II.86a–c. Photomicrographs of well-differentiated chondrosarcoma (grade I) showing a fairly cellular chondroid tumor, with a moderate number of cells with one or two plump nuclei. In **a** and **b** some woven bone and calcified cartilage trabeculae are seen. **a** ×60, **b** ×120, **c** ×400

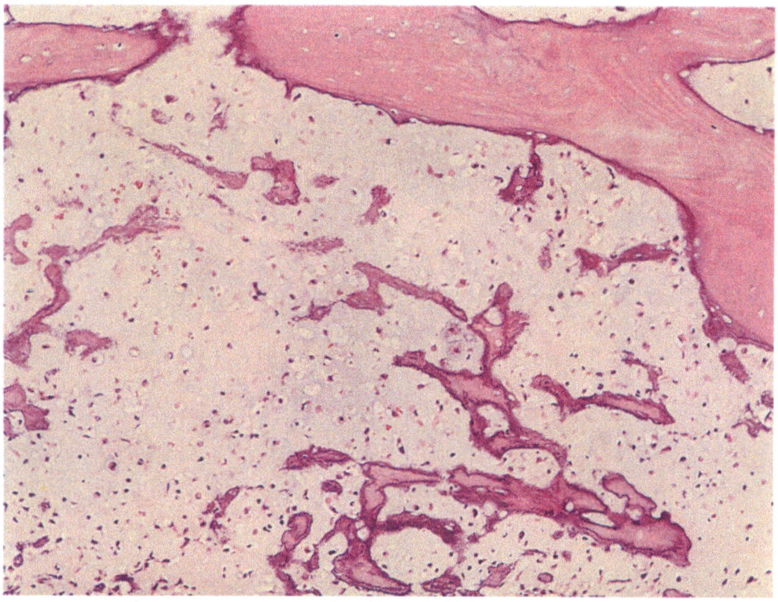

a

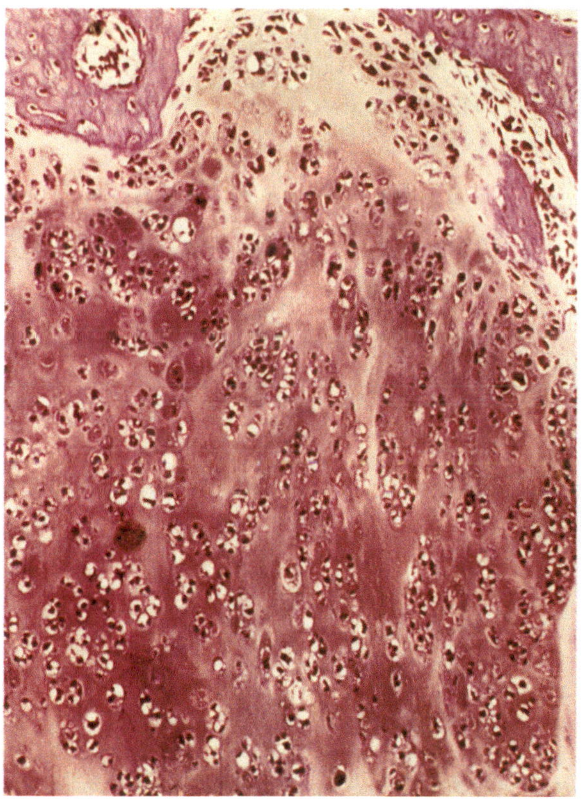

b

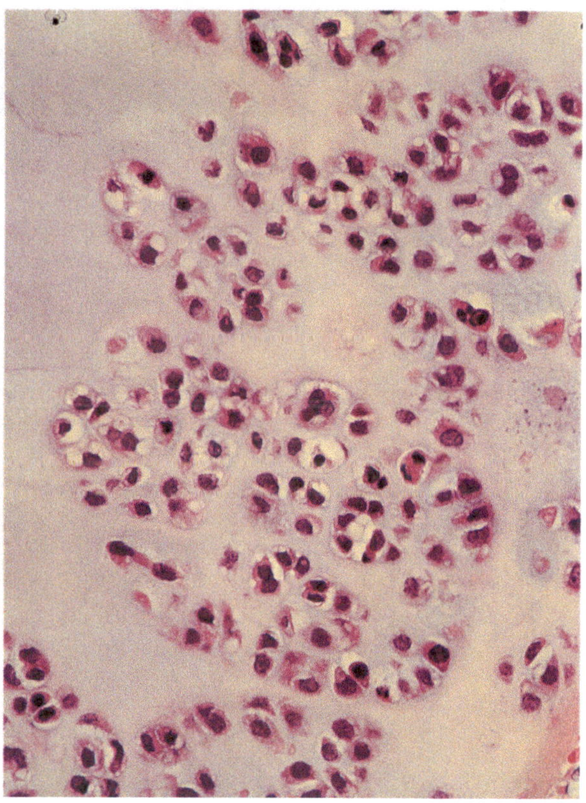

c

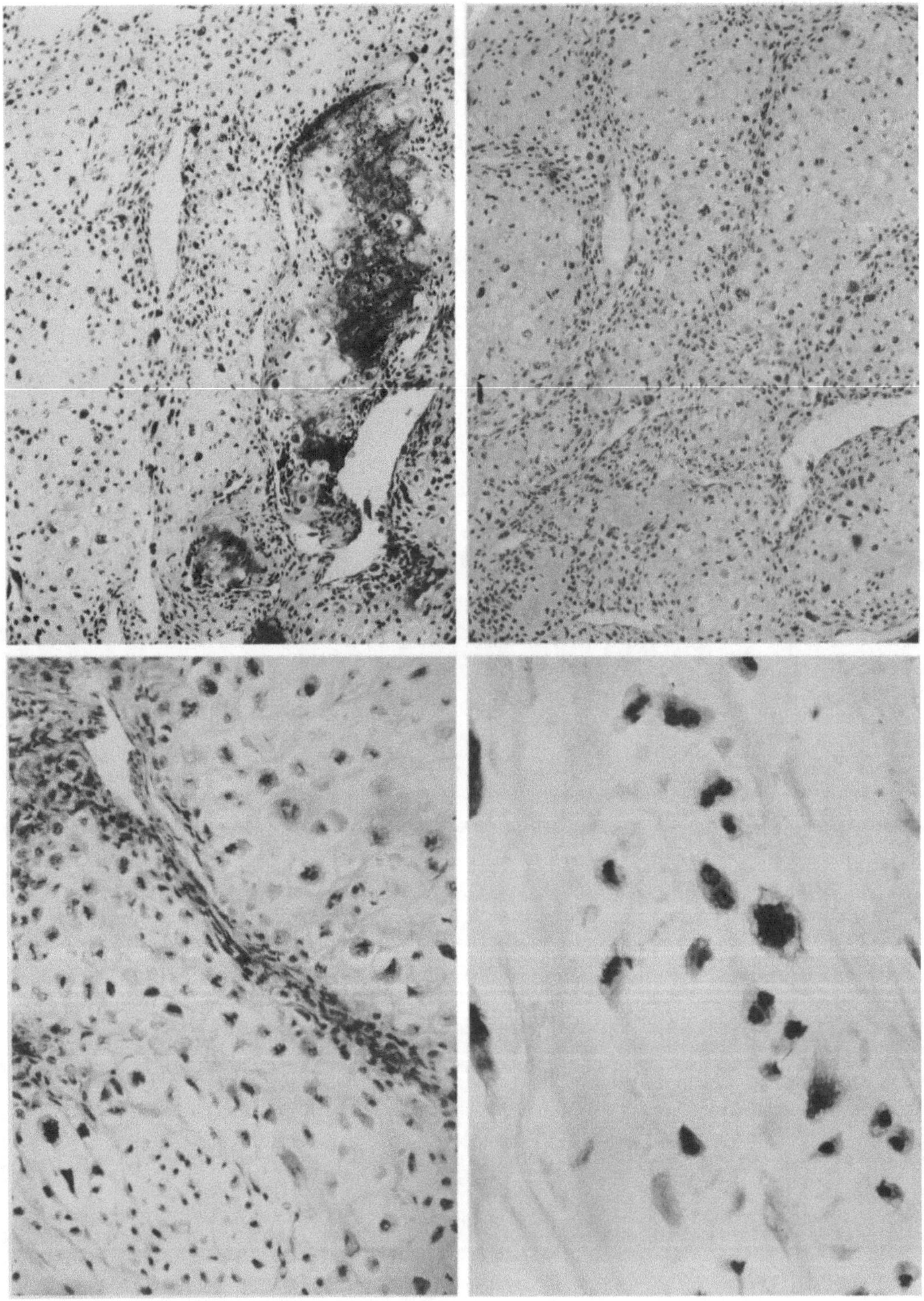

a b c d

Fig. II.87a–d. Photomicrographs of moderately well differentiated chondrosarcomas (grade II) at lower (**a,b**) and higher (**c,d**) magnification. Cartilage cells with plump, often double or some bizarre hyperchromatic nuclei are more frequently seen. **a,b** ×100; **c** ×250; **d** ×400

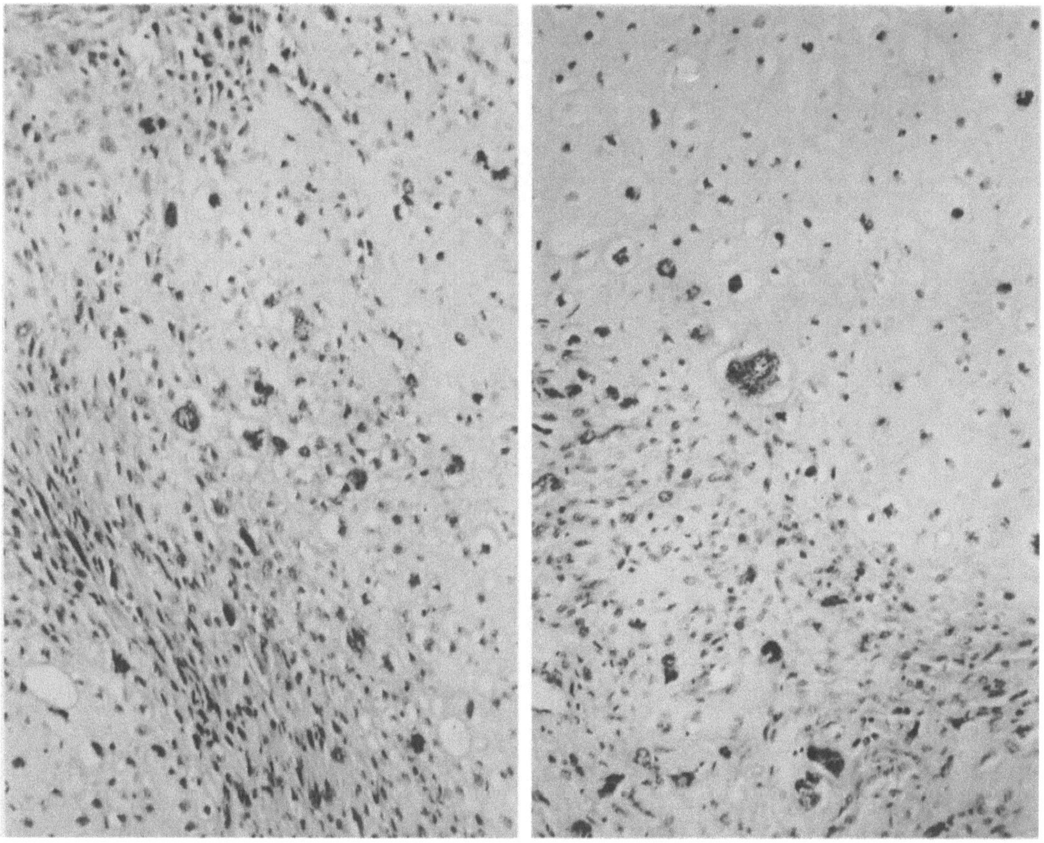

a b

Fig. II.88a,b. Photomicrographs of a high-grade malignant chondrosarcoma (grade III) showing a great number of cells with plump or bizarre, often double, nuclei. The septa between the tumor lobules are frequently rich in spindle-shaped cells. a,b ×120

nancy (Lichtenstein and Jaffe 1943; O'Neal and Ackerman 1952), as also do highly undifferentiated cells, especially fibroblastlike spindle cells in the periphery of or separating the tumor lobules (Evans et al. 1977) (see Fig. II.92c,d). The presence of such spindle-cell areas between more or less malignant cartilage nodules is distinct from the features of "dedifferentiated chondrosarcoma," in which the second, anaplastic element is clearly separated from the low-grade chondrosarcoma. The significance of myxomatous changes in relation to the prognosis of the tumor is still disputed. Some authors (Keiller 1925; Jaffe and Lichtenstein 1943; O'Neal and Ackerman 1952; and ourselves) disagree with the idea that myxomatous stromal change in itself is sinister, whereas others place importance on this finding (Henderson and Dahlin 1963; Copeland and Geschickter 1965; Dahlin and Unni 1986).

However, tumors with more or less conspicuous myxoid areas (Fig. II.90a) should not be confused with the so-called myxoid chondrosarcoma (Enzinger and Shiraki 1972) (Figs. II.90b, II.91), an entity not infrequently found primarily in the deep soft tissues of the extremities, especially the musculature. Examples of myxoid chondrosarcoma, which have been referred to also as "chordoid sarcoma" (Martin et al. 1973) because of their superficial resemblance to chordoma, are extremely rare arising within bone and we have only two such cases in our files. Therefore, the number of 61 cases reported by Huvos (1991) seems clearly too high compared with our and other authors' experience, and possibly includes conventional chondrosarcoma with a conspicuous myxoid component. However, the microscopic and ultrastructural features of "myxoid chondrosarcoma" are distinctive (Fig. II.91), revealing characteristic alignment of the tumor cells in strands and chords, separated by large amounts of mucoid material (Fig. II.90b). Ultrastructurally, the tumor cells show conspicuous, densely packed

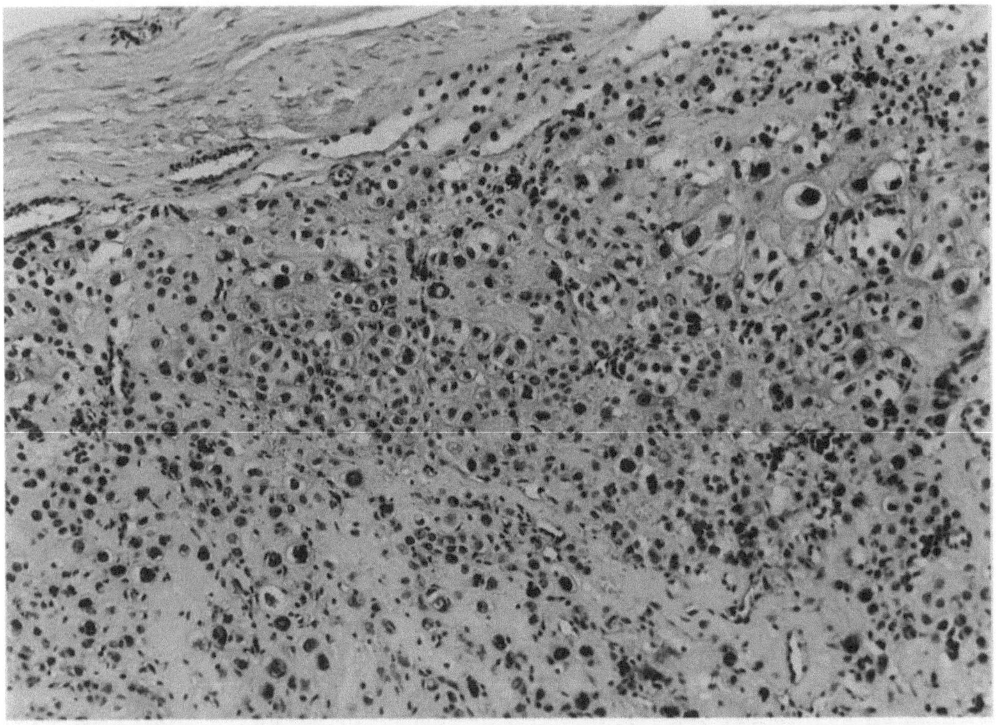

a

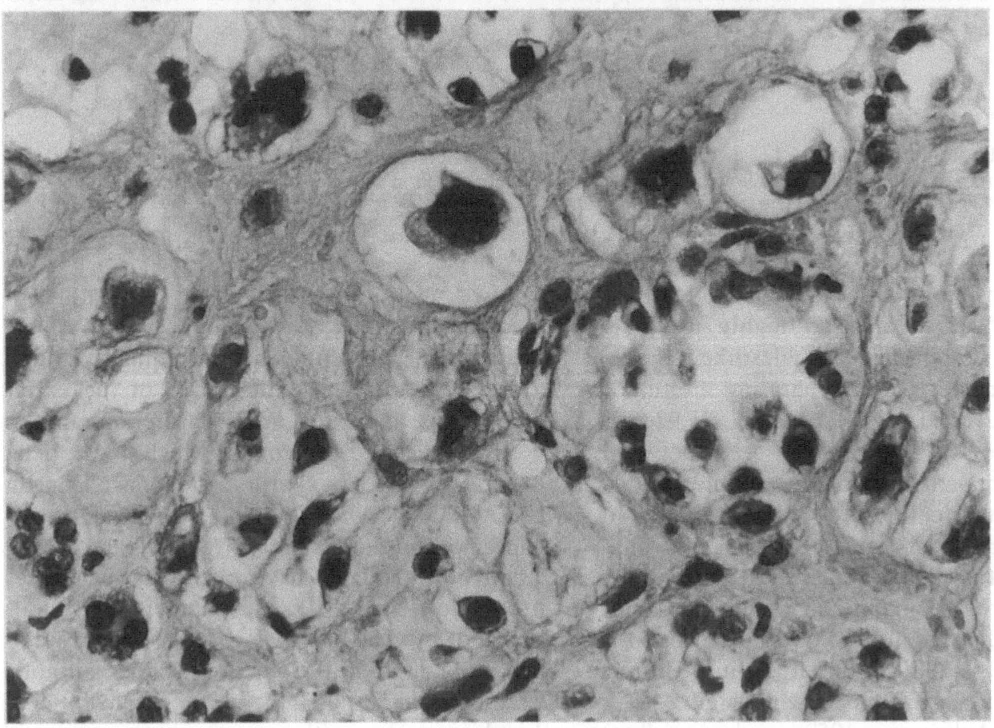

b

Fig. II.89a,b. Photomicrographs for grade III chondrosarcoma showing at lower and higher magnification the great number and pleomorphism of tumor cells. **a** ×200, **b** ×600

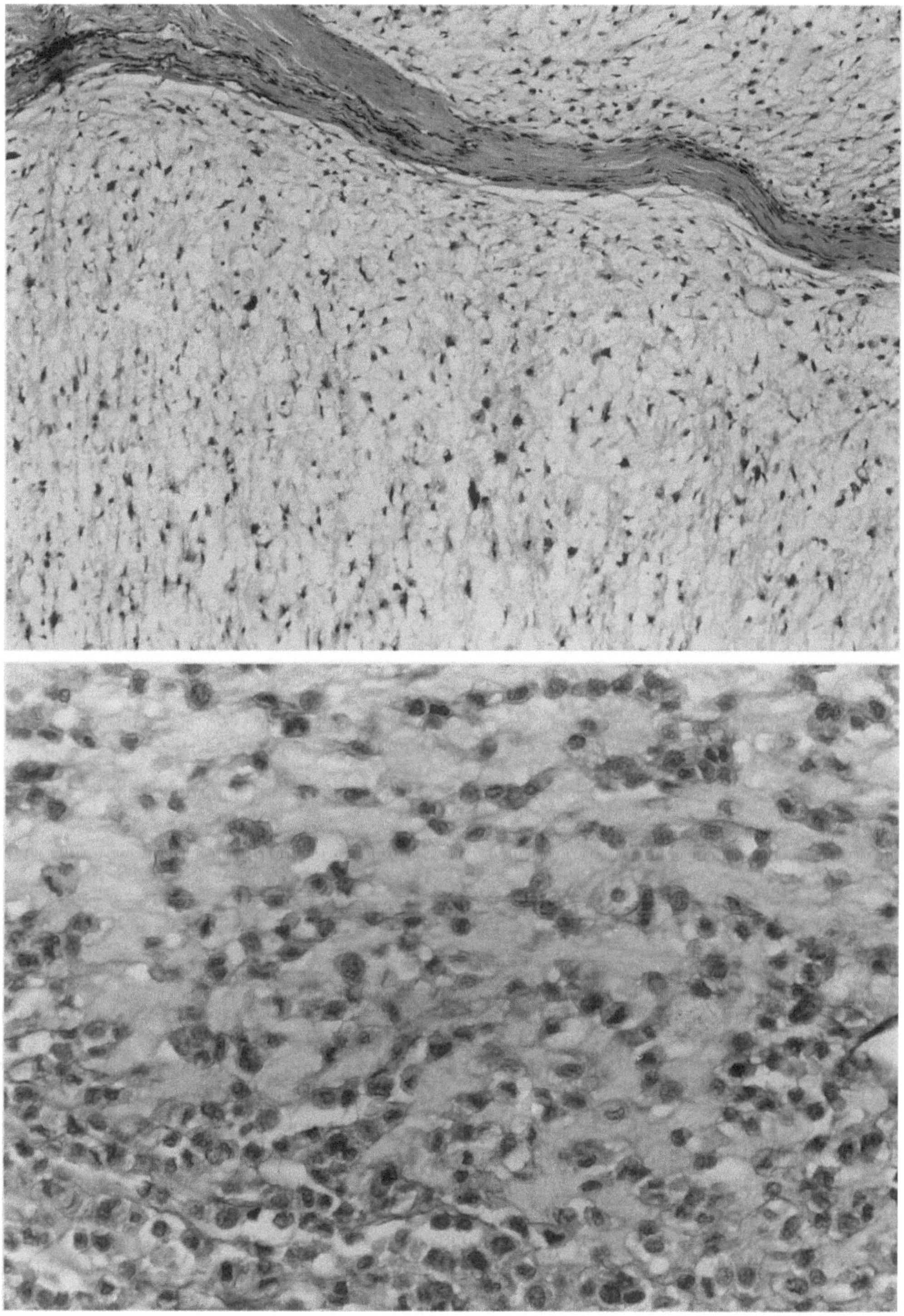

a

b

Fig. II.90a,b. Photomicrographs showing the different features of **a** conventional chondrosarcoma with myxoid area and **b** myxoid chondrosarcoma (chordoid sarcoma) with cords of epithelioidlike cells separated by a myxoid stroma. The differential diagnosis with myxoid angioblastoma and chordoma may be difficult. **a** ×150, **b** ×400

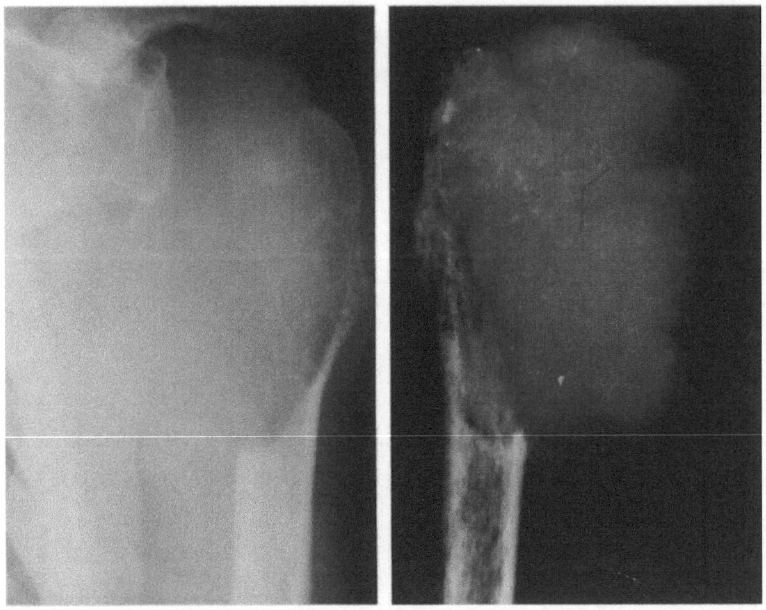

a b

Fig. II.91a,b. Male, 62 years old. Myxoid chondrosarcoma of humerus (same case as in Fig. II.90b; see that figure for histologic features). **a** Clinical radiograph and **b** radiograph of resected specimen show a large osteolytic lesion of the upper end, which has expanded and in great part destroyed the thinned cortex. Intraosseous myxoid chondrosarcoma is extremely rare and is also referred to as chordoid sarcoma

Table II.3. Grading of chondrosarcomas

Cytologic pattern	Low grade	Moderately malignant	Highly malignant
Variation in nuclear size	Slight Moderate number of plump nuclei	Moderate Many plump nuclei	Evident polymorphism Large number of plump nuclei
Double nuclei	Low incidence May be plump	Frequent plump double nuclei	Numerous
Multinucleate atypical giant cells	Absent	Absent or rare	Occasional to frequent
Calcification	Frequent conspicuous	Occasional	Absent or scarce

bundles or arrays of microtubules within the rough endoplasmic reticulum (Fu and Kay 1974; Wetzel and Reuhl 1980; Pardo-Mindan et al. 1981).

Myxoid chondrosarcoma is a tumor of relatively low grade malignancy, which nonetheless is capable of recurrence and metastasis; however, it may occur years after the initial diagnosis.

Applying the cytologic criteria of Lichtenstein and Jaffe (1943) and others, O'Neal and Ackerman (1952) divided chondrosarcomas into low-grade, moderately malignant, and highly malignant, using the patterns shown in Table II.3 (slightly modified by this author).

Although the preceding criteria are applied by most pathologists, they are highly subjective; therefore, the structural features of histopathologic appearance have been suggested as an aid to the differential diagnosis of enchondroma and low-grade chondrosarcoma. Sanerkin (1980), who recommended a combined cytologic study of smeared preparations and histopathologic study of the tissue structure, gave great importance to the invasiveness of the tumor in relation to the host bone. He considered a characteristic pattern of this feature to be the direct and intimate abutment of the tumor on eroded bone, where osteoclasts are no longer present on the bone surface, having been overtaken and killed by the tumor. This permeative pattern of chondrosarcoma characterized by a single confluent mass of cartilage replacing marrow and trapping or encasing the host bone's lamellar trabeculae on all sides is considered diagnostic by Mirra et al. (1985). Moreover, the scalloping and focal destruction of the cortex, spread of the tumor through haversian systems resulting in a secondary cortical thickening, and tumor lobules abutting the periosteum with formation of a soft tissue mass are characteristic indicators of malignancy.

Both the cytologic findings of plump and multinucleated cartilage cells and the permeation or invasiveness of the tumor through host cancellous bone are important diagnostic patterns for chondrosarcoma. The most important pathologic feature is the endosteal scalloping (see Figs. II.77, II.78) and/or focal cortical destruction that is often associated with cortical thickening and occasionally with invasion of soft tissues. The clinical presentation also determines whether or not a cartilage tumor in an adult is a low-grade chondrosarcoma or an old benign cartilage tumor. The presence of pain and the roentgenographic features of endosteal cortical resorption associated with cortical destruction and/or cortical thickening are almost always diagnostic of chondrosarcoma (see Figs. II.75–II.81).

However, cytologic and even histologic criteria, as we stated in the introduction to this chapter, cannot be applied to tumors of all sites, because some of them exhibit evident discrepancies between the histologic appearance and biologic behavior. Thus, tumors located in the tubular bones of hands and feet, in the synovial membrane, or subperiosteally (juxtacortically) behave generally as benign tumors, despite the fact that they often exhibit features which in other sites would be classified as low-grade chondrosarcoma.

Genuine chondrosarcomas of the hands and feet occur rarely. There are several reports on chondrosarcomas of the hands and feet; however, with the exception of a few publications (Dahlin and Salvador 1974; Roberts and Price 1977), only single or a few cases are reported, and the papers often include a review of the literature (Lansche and Spjut 1958, one case; Jacobson and Spjut 1960, three cases; Gottschalk and Smith 1963, one case; Pachter and Alpert 1964, two cases; Mangini 1967, one case among 153 chondromas of the hand; Salib 1967, three cases; Patel et al. 1977, one case). Schajowicz and Cambiaggi (1961) found one case among 153 chondromas of the hand. We have records of 14 cases of chondrosarcoma of the tubular bones of hands (9) and feet (5) from among 368 enchondromas of this location, that is, 4%.

The number of chondrosarcomas (30 cases, 20 seen in consultation) reported by Dahlin and Salvador (1974) among 62 chondromas of hands and feet treated at the Mayo Clinic, and the 19 cases reported by Roberts and Price (1977) from the Bristol Tumour Registry, are probably too high and do not correspond to the real incidence. Both institutions, being reference centers, collect more atypical and malignant cases than do other institutions. It is interesting that none of the 19 cases of Roberts and Price is known to have metastasized, possibly due to the more radical treatment of these tumors (amputation of the digit or ray) or to an overdiagnosis in some cases, that is, interpreting some cellular chondromas, with or without destruction of the cortex, as chondrosarcomas.

In our series, as in others, the well-differentiated low-grade chondrosarcoma accounts for a large majority (approximately 60%) of cases, the high-grade types being infrequent. It should be emphasized that the nuclear changes indicating malignancy may often be found in only a few fields; therefore, most authors prefer an ample open biopsy, avoiding degenerated and calcified areas and examining many sections. In our experience, percutaneous puncture (aspiration) biopsy and taking tissue from different areas and depths gave positive results in a great number of cases.

Performing a biopsy of a cartilaginous tumor always carries with it the great risk of implantation in neighboring soft tissues, even occasionally in the tract of a needle biopsy, with the increased danger of local recurrence. In order to avoid these complications, and in cases in which tumor resection is planned, the area where the biopsy was performed should be included in the excision field.

Electron Microscopy. In contrast to the numerous ultrastructural studies of normal cartilage, there are only a few reports of malignant cartilage tumors. Anderson et al. (1963) reported one case of chondrosarcoma of the scapula, and this writer in collaboration with others (1974) described the ultrastructure in seven cases of central chondrosarcoma, trying to establish a correlation between the ultrastructure and the histologic grade of malignancy. In cases of low-grade malignancy, a high density of organelles was observed, whereas a low density of organelles and more bizarre nuclei with prominent nucleoli were seen in the higher grades of malignancy.

In addition to other features different from those of normal chondrocytes, an inverse relationship between glycogen content and the histologic grade of malignancy was noted.

Although a systemic search was not performed, no viruslike particles, such as the A type viruslike intracisternal particles described by Morton et al. (1969) in a chondrosarcoma, were discovered. As we did, Spjut et al. (1971) noted evident alterations of the endoplasmic reticulum, but they also noted great similarities with normal immature cartilage cells.

Biochemistry and Flow Cytometry. The biochemical structure of chondrosarcoma has been studied extensively by Rosenberg and associates (1976) and in Mankin's laboratory (Mankin et al. 1979, 1980a,b). The first group isolated in pure form by dissociative density gradients, and then characterized, a proteoglycan subunit and proteoglycan aggregate. Proteoglycan subunits from sarcomas and immature cartilage were of approximately the same size, but sarcoma contained only chondroitin sulfate and essentially no keratan sulfate. Their data furthermore suggest that the malignant chondrocytes of human chondrosarcomas may lack galactosyltranferase essential for keratan sulfate synthesis. Mankin et al. (1979, 1980a,b), in a combined histologic and biochemical study of 72 cartilage tumors, tried to establish a valid relationship between histologic grade of malignancy and biochemical analysis. They classified the tumor histologically in six different groups and suggested that certain simple biochemical studies coupled with careful histologic observation could be of great value in assessment of malignancy of the lesions.

The introduction of newer diagnostic methods, such as the study of cellular DNA content, initially by Feulgen DNA absorption microfluorometry (Schajowicz et al. 1976) and more recently by laser-based flow cytofluorometric analysis by propidium iodide staining (Awtar 1975; Kreicbergs et al. 1982; Mankin et al. 1985), makes it possible to perform rapid determinations of DNA content per cell. However, ploidy determinations are meant not to replace but only to complement conventional histopathologic malignancy grading in chondrosarcoma. The main advantage of ploidy determination seems to be the recognition of highly malignant areas among grade I chondrosarcomas by virtue of the presence of cells with hyperploid DNA content. Further investigations, with longer follow-up periods, complemented by tissue cultures, are necessary to determine the real prognostic value of this method.

Treatment. The treatment of chondrosarcoma is preferably surgical, and the indication for the extent of the intervention depends not only on the histologic grade of malignancy but also on the local conditions, that is, involvement of the cortex with or without extension into the neighboring soft tissues (Campanacci et al. 1975; Barnes and Catto 1966). The type of treatment according to grading and local conditions is described in detail in Chap. X.

The prognostic factors, especially the relationship between histopathology and tumor behavior, were examined by Evans et al. (1977) in 71 cases seen at the M.D. Anderson Hospital in Houston, Texas. The tumors were grouped into grades I, II, and III on the basis of nuclear size, cellularity, and mitotic rate. The 5-year survival rates of patients with grade I, II, and III tumors were 90%, 81%, and 29%, respectively.

In other series, the 5-year survival rates were not so favorable, varying from 48.6% (McKenna et al. 1966) to 61% (Henderson and Dahlin 1963). In general, the 10-year survival rate is approximately 40% in the most important series (e.g., 41% in Henderson and Dahlin's series). The results presented in a review of 168 cases filed in our laboratory (Mondolfo 1968) were much less favorable (a 10-year survival rate of approximately 23%) because this series included many older cases that had already had local recurrences or were not treated radically enough, according to the criteria applied at present.

The majority of chondrosarcomas are well differentiated and have a great tendency to recur locally after incomplete excision. The tumor grows slowly, extending into neighboring tissues, but metastases are rare and late. They are more frequent in high-grade tumors, and vascular invasion with large thrombi was observed in two of our patients and in several reported cases.

The most common site of metastasis is the lung and more rarely brain (Clark and Maloney 1974), liver, kidney, and lymph nodes (Spjut et al. 1971); other bones were involved in four of our cases and in 18% of the cases reported by McKenna et al. (1966).

Radiotherapy has not been successful in the treatment of chondrosarcoma. In the few cases in our material in which radiotherapy was used for palliation in tumors not amenable to surgical removal, the results were disappointing. Some pain relief or reduction of the tumor mass was obtained only occasionally; this has also been the experience of other authors (see Chap. X). There seems to be little experience with chemotherapy.

"Dedifferentiated" Chondrosarcoma

Definition, WHO: *"A highly anaplastic sarcoma juxtaposed to a borderline or low-grade malignant chondrosarcoma. There is an abrupt transition between the two components."*

"Dedifferentiation" of a histologically borderline or low-grade and clinically indolent cartilaginous tumor, often present for years, into a highly anaplastic juxtaposed tumor with a uniformly poor prognosis, has been emphasized by Dahlin and Beabout (1971) as an important problem. Such conversion occurred in 33 of their 370 chondrosarcomas (10%). A more recent publication of the same institution (Mayo Clinic) (Dahlin and Unni 1986; Frassica et al. 1986) reported 78 cases out of 714 chondrosarcomas (11%). The same percentage was found in the files of the Rizzoli Institute (Capanna et al. 1988). The percentage was a little lower (6%) in the records of the M.D. Anderson Hospital and Tumor Institute of Houston, with only 26 of 430 chondrosarcomas (Johnson et al. 1986).

In contrast to the frequent recurrences of conventional, well-differentiated chondrosarcomas which show little or no change in histologic features, in the so-called dedifferentiated chondrosarcoma the second, additional element is highly anaplastic. This element was a spindle-cell sarcoma (fibrosarcoma) in 22 cases of Dahlin and Beabout (1971), and an osteosarcoma in the remaining 11 cases. In the more recent series of the Mayo Clinic (Dahlin and Unni 1986), the dedifferentiated portion had the histologic pattern of a fibrosarcoma in 33 cases and of an osteosarcoma in 43 cases; only two cases were judged to be malignant fibrous histiocytomas. The M.D. Anderson Institute researchers used the name "additional mesenchymal component" in reference to the dedifferentiated portion and classified this component histologically as malignant fibrous histiocytoma (16 cases), rhabdomyosarcoma (4), low-grade fibrosarcoma (3), osteosarcoma (2), or undifferentiated sarcoma (1).

There are several reports in the literature with a smaller number of cases, in which the most frequent dedifferentiated tumor was a spindle-cell tumor (fibrosarcoma) (Mirra and Marcove 1974; McFarland et al. 1977). However, Sanerkin and Woods (1979) reported on two cases in which the anaplastic area was composed of malignant fibrous histiocytoma. This tumor type was present in 14 of the 18 patients who had "dedifferentiated chondrosarcoma" in the series of McCarthy and Dorfman (1982). One-third of the lesions dedifferentiated into malignant fibrous histiocytoma in the Rizzoli series (Capanna 1988).

According to our present knowledge, most pathologists do not accept the concept of dedifferentiation of an already well differentiated cell. This problem has been discussed at a symposium on bone tumors by a group of specialized bone pathologists including Fechner, Huvos, Mirra, Spjut, and Dahlin (Fechner et al. 1984). Although they all questioned the accuracy of the concept of "dedifferentiation" in the pathogenesis of this tumor, they suggested continuing the use of the term "dedifferentiated chondrosarcoma" as a distinct, well-defined entity because it remains useful to indicate the tumor's more malignant behavior and poor prognosis.

However, what seems more probable in the opinion of several pathologists is that there are phenotypically distinct primitive cell clones present within a human chondrosarcoma and that these have the capability of differentiation into separate lines with different histologic characteristics, such as fibrosarcoma, osteosarcoma, malignant fibrous histiocytoma, and, more rarely, rhabdomyosarcoma. This hypothesis has been supported by an immunohistochemical and biochemical study of a cultured human chondrosarcoma, demonstrating the existence of four different clonal cell lines within the parent tumor (Gitelis et al. 1989).

Therefore, the term "progression," introduced by Foulds in 1949, was also proposed by us to characterize the phenomenon of increased malignancy exhibited by some cartilage tumors during their course, expressed by an increased growth rate, rapid metastatic spread, loss of histologic differentiation (anaplasia), and increased mitotic rate. This term would be a more logical and appropriate alternative to the term "chondrosarcoma with an additional mesenchymal component," proposed by the M.D. Anderson Institute (Johnson et al. 1986; Tetú et al. 1986). Huvos recently suggested (1991) the designation "spindle-cell chondrosarcoma," which, however, in our opinion does not express the prognostic significance of this tumor type.

In the writer's opinion, distinction from high-grade malignant (poorly differentiated) chondrosarcoma does not seem justified in many cases. Together with other authors (Barnes and Catto 1966; Evans et al. 1977), the author interprets the presence of extensive undifferentiated spindle-cell areas in the periphery or between the cartilage tumor lobules as being indicative of *progression* of a cartilaginous tumor to a high grade of malignancy (see Figs. II.88, II.92). Such progression (Van Rijssel 1973) can be found in many other malignant bone tumors, such as osteosarcomas or fibrosarcomas, and possibly depends on immunologic factors of the host.

There is no unequivocal proof that the dedifferentiated elements are really collagen-producing fibroblasts. In an ultramicroscopic study of one case of dedifferentiated chondrosarcoma, Kahn (1976), comparing the spindle-cell areas of this tumor with those of a poorly differentiated chondrosarcoma and a few mesenchymal chondrosarcomas reported in the literature (Fu and Kay 1974; Steiner et al. 1973), did not find fundamental differences in the three tumor types. He stated that the few isolated examples studied ultrastructurally did not permit one to arrive at definite conclusions.

Clinical and Radiologic Features. The tumor involves most frequently the pelvis and the long bones (Fig. II.93), particularly the femur and humerus (Figs. II.94, II.95). The average patient age is 40–50 years, most patients being over 20. There is no sex predilection, unlike the conventional central chondrosarcoma, in which there is a male predominance. Radiographically the lesions may appear similar to ordinary chondrosarcoma with typical calcification of the chondroid matrix. The presence, however, of a larger area of cortical lysis, particularly if associated with a large amount of unmineralized matrix, suggests a more aggressive lesion. The prognosis of "dedifferentiated chondrosarcoma" is generally poor, in spite of radical surgical treatment. The overall survival rate for 5 years is generally lower than 25%.

Secondary Chondrosarcoma

The development of a secondary chondrosarcoma in a proved benign enchondroma seems to be extremely rare; however, it is difficult to give any unequivocal estimate of the real frequency of this complication. In the Mayo Clinic series of 59 cases of secondary chondrosarcoma, none was observed in solitary enchondroma (Dahlin 1978). Most authors agree that is difficult or almost impossible to document histologically and/or radiologically the malignant degeneration of a solitary benign enchondroma. In retrospective revisions of the original histologic sections, many early cases demonstrated the misinterpretation of the surgical material as enchondroma, the tumors actually being low-grade malignancies from the beginning. This author does not believe that the demonstration of both benign and malignant tissue patterns signifies the diagnosis of secondary chondrosarcoma, because many malignant tumors may present both well-differentiated and clearly malignant areas. Malignant degeneration of previously benign cartilage tumor (enchondroma) seems to be less frequent than the 50% suggested by Mirra et al. (1985) and Wilner (1982).

In our files, we have no case of proved malignant transformation of an unquestionably benign solitary chondroma. On the other hand, chondrosarcomatous transformation (occurring in one or, rarely, more bones) is a frequent complication in *multiple enchondromatosis* with or without Ollier's disease or Maffucci's syndrome. We mentioned earlier that the incidence of malignant change varies from 20% to 50% in different series. In our series we found it in 8 of 40 cases of multiple enchondromatosis (20%) (see Figs. II.17, II.20, II.22).

There is no doubt that secondary chondrosarcoma may develop from the cartilage cap of a *solitary* or, more commonly, *multiple osteochondroma* (Figs. II.96–II.103). The frequency of this secondary chondrosarcoma, which is generally classified as peripheral or exostotic (eccentric) chondrosarcoma, has been the subject of considerable discussion. It has been estimated as less than 1% in solitary and as approximately 10% in multiple osteochondromatosis. These figures are speculative, because many adolescents are not followed into adult life and most statistics come

Fig. II.92. a,b Photomicrographs of so-called dedifferentiated chondrosarcoma showing more or less well-differentiated chondroid tissue adjacent to highly cellular areas rich in spindle cells with a fibrosarcomatous pattern. **c,d** The anaplastic and spindle-cell areas separate cartilage lobules, and there is no abrupt zone between the low-grade chondrosarcoma and the cellular anaplastic tumor. These features may be observed in conventional high-grade chondrosarcoma. **a,c** ×250; **b,d** ×400

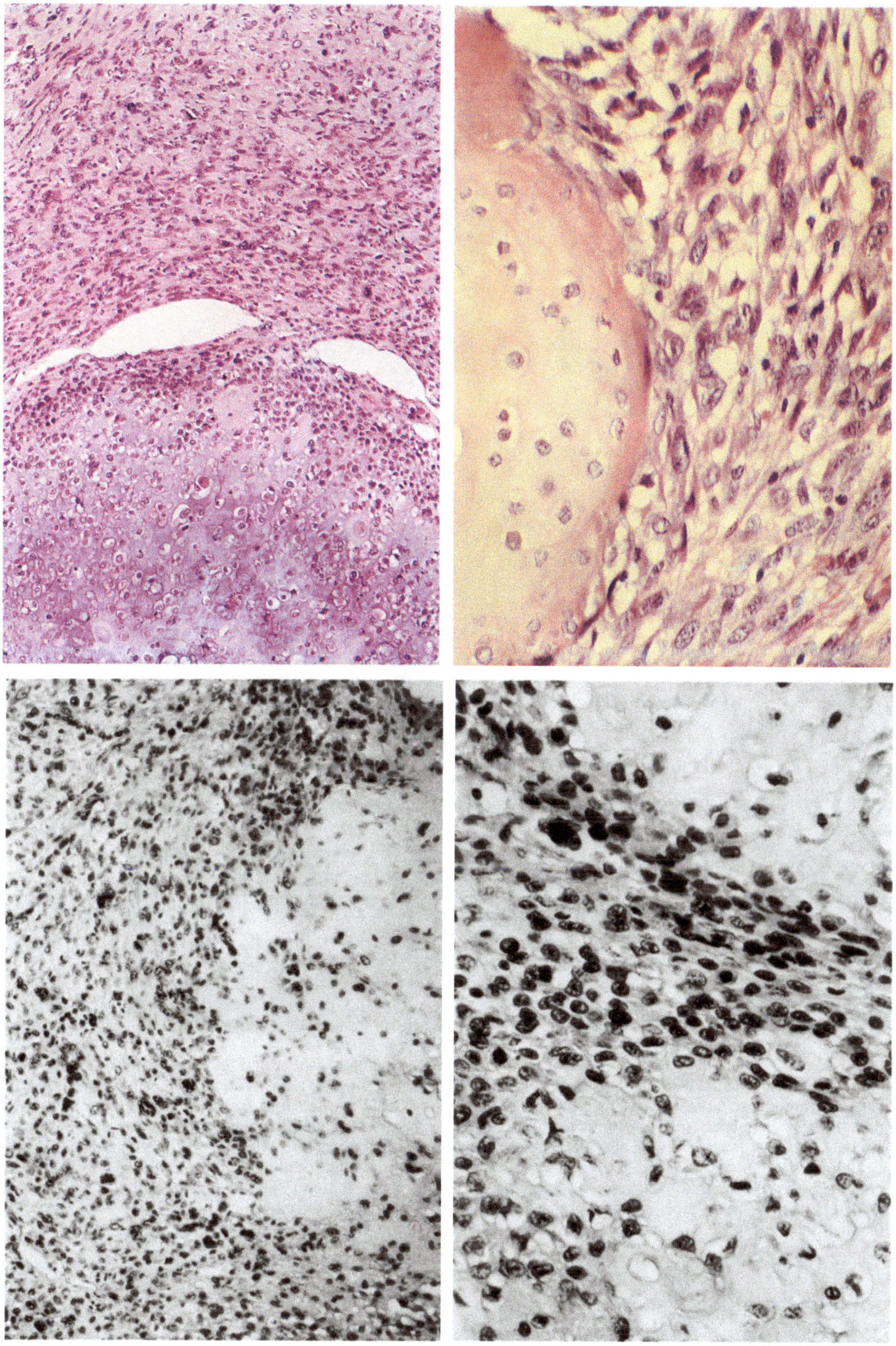

a b c d

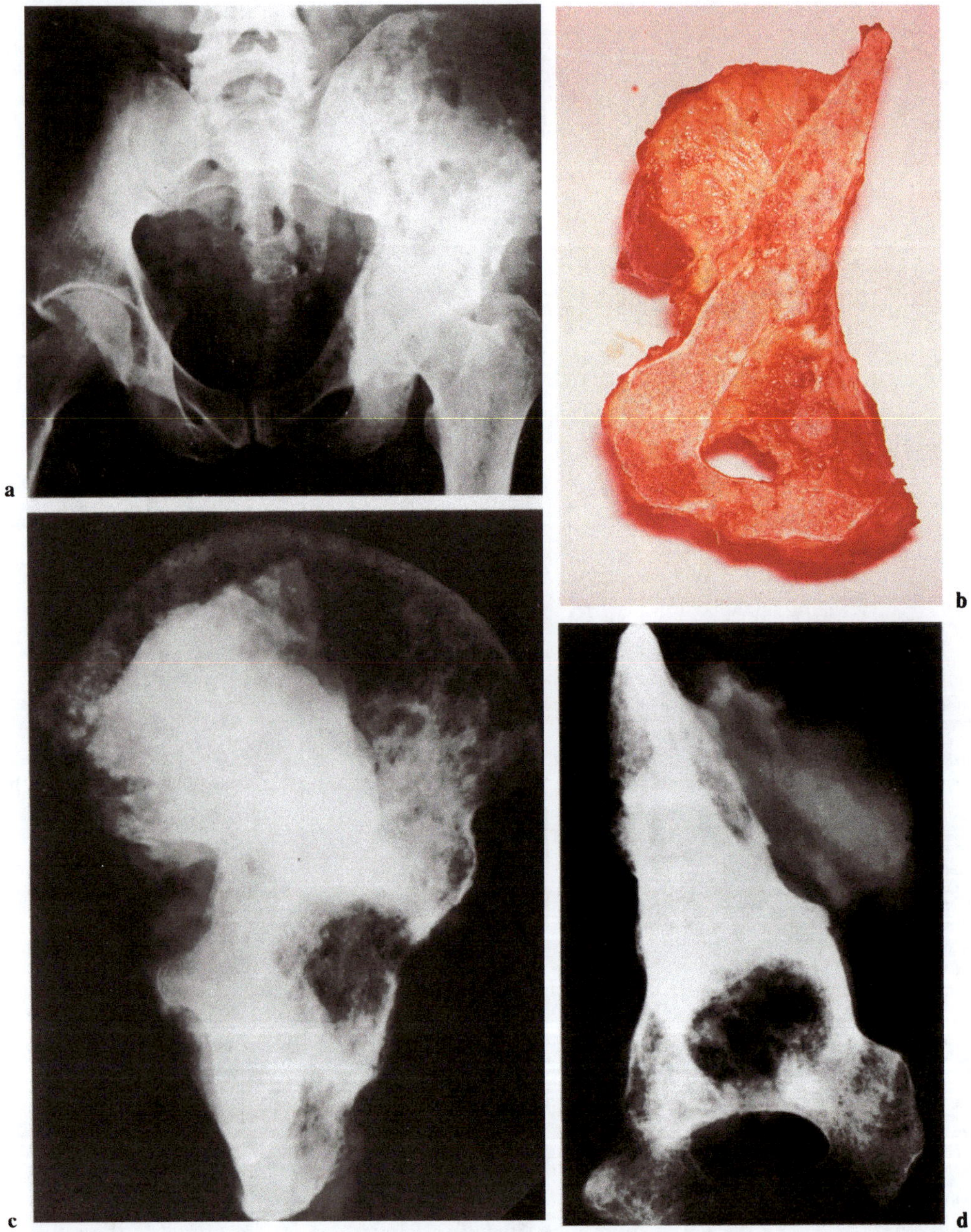

Fig. II.93a–d. Male, 39 years old. So-called dedifferentiated chondrosarcoma of ilium. **a** Radiograph showing irregular radiodense area, involving almost the entire ilium. Patient complained of pain for 3 years and sought help because of an increase in pain and the appearance of a swelling in the buttock. A hindquarter amputation was performed. **b** Radiograph showing the involvement of the iliac bone. **c** Photograph of the sectioned specimen demonstrates intraosseous tumor of characteristic cartilaginous aspect and an extraosseous fleshy, soft mass of grayish-pink color. The iliac veins were occupied by tumor tissue of the same aspect. **d** Radiograph of the specimen shown in **c**. Histologically, the tumor showed a central area of well or moderately differentiated chondrosarcoma, and a highly cellular spindle-cell tissue in the juxtaosseous mass. Patient died 6 months after operation with pulmonary and brain metastases

Fig. II.94a,b. Male, 48 years old with "dedifferentiated" chondrosarcoma of femur. **a** Radiograph shows irregular, radiodense and radiolucent lesion in the medullary cavity, with extraosseous soft tissue involvement. **b** Photograph of the specimen showing intraosseous lesion of cartilaginous aspect and extraosseous soft tumor mass at its medial aspect

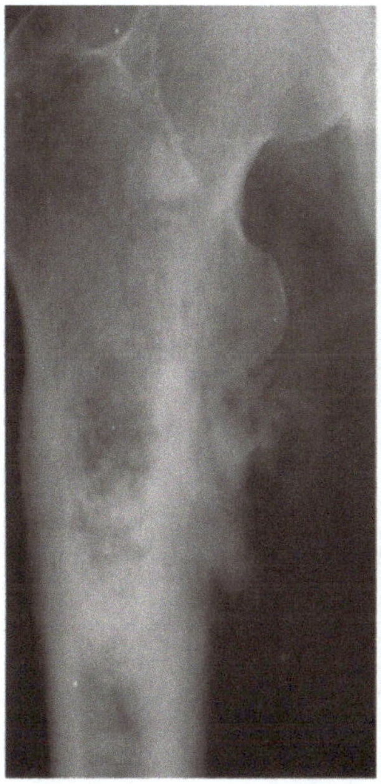

a

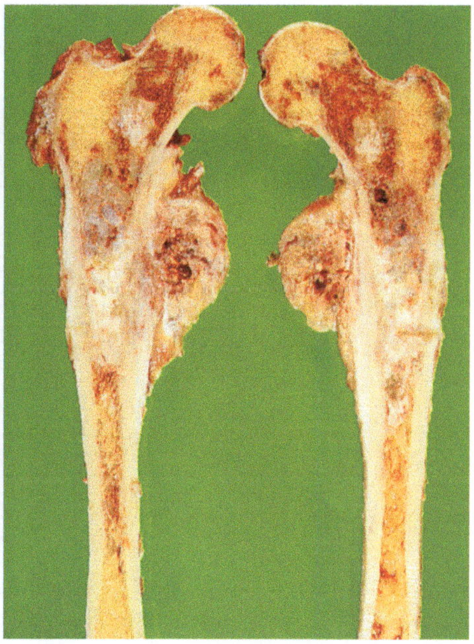

b

Fig. II.95a–c. Another case of "dedifferentiated" chondrosarcoma of femur. **a** Radiograph shows a predominantly radiolucent lesion of the upper third of the diaphysis with only slight calcification and a large soft tissue mass. **b** Photograph illustrates the cartilaginous features of the intraosseous tumor and the hemorrhagic aspect of the large fleshy extraosseous mass. **c** CT shows the intraosseous and extraosseous extension of the tumor

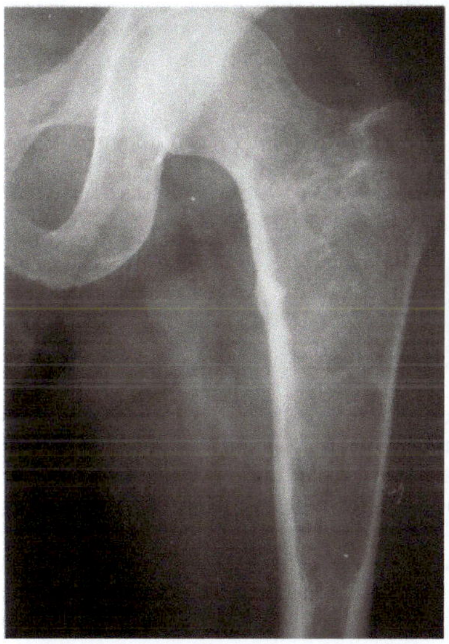

a

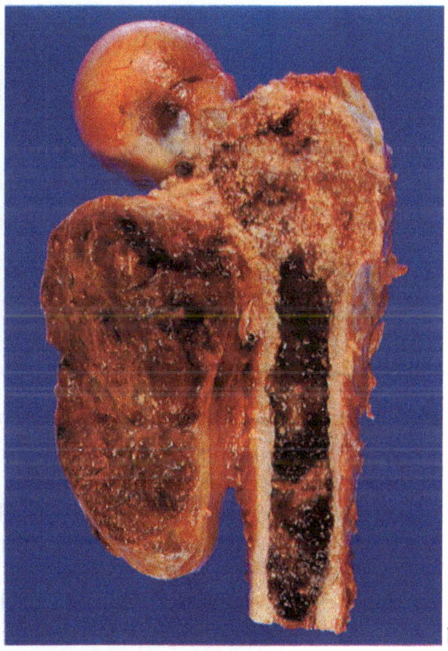

b

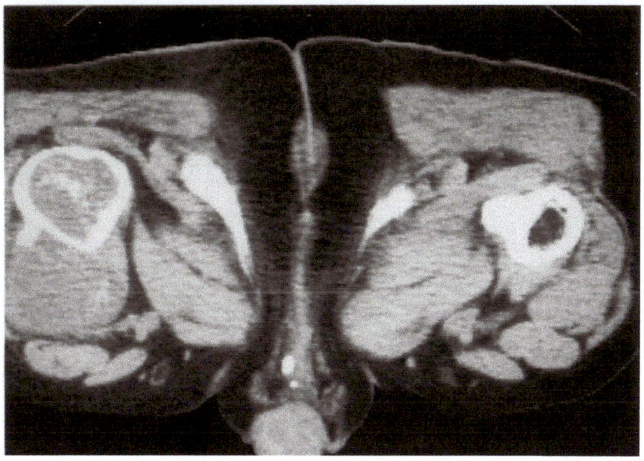

c

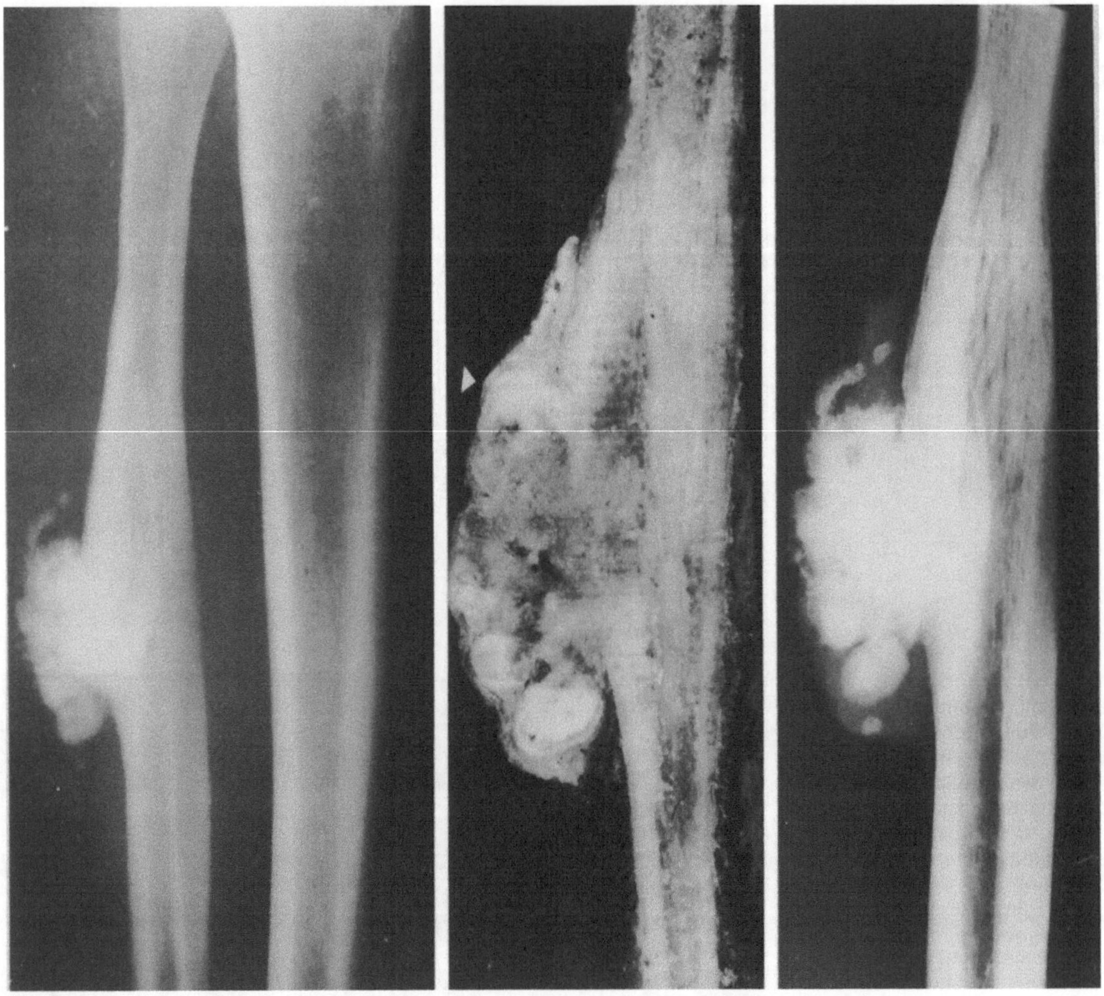

a, b c

Fig. II.96a–c. Female, 32 years old. Peripheral (exostotic) chondrosarcoma of fibula, secondary to solitary osteochondroma. **a** Radiograph shows a heavily calcified lesion with irregular contours and attached to the shaft by a broad base. A segmental resection was performed. **b** Photograph of the resected specimen shows an irregular cartilage cap in great part calcified and ossified. A juxtacortical osteosarcoma was excluded due to the continuity of the tumor spongiosa with that of the underlying fibula. **c** Radiograph of the specimen demonstrates the radiopacity and irregular lobulated surface of the lesion, suggesting juxtacortical osteosarcoma. Patient is living 6 years after resection

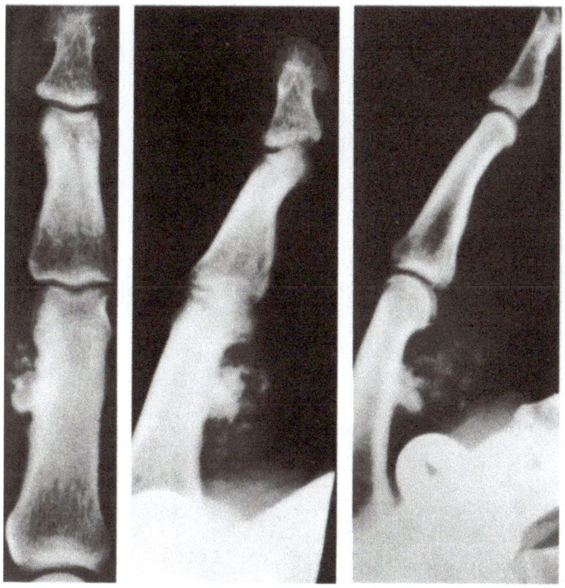

II.97
a b c

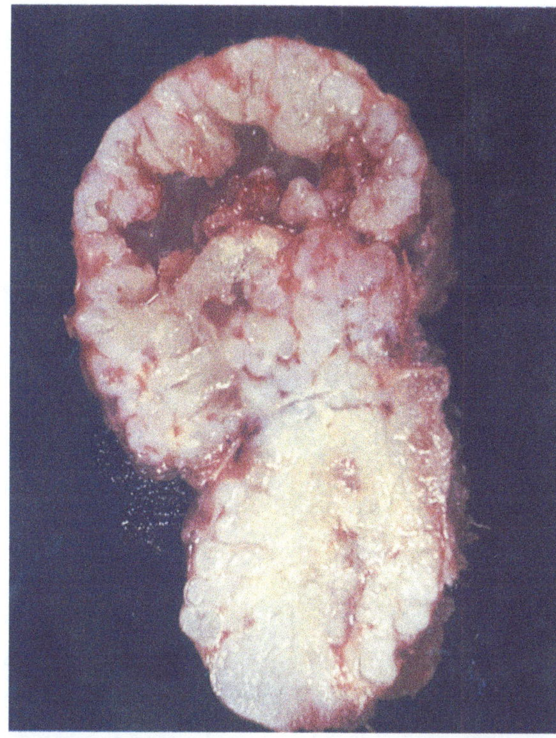

a II.98a

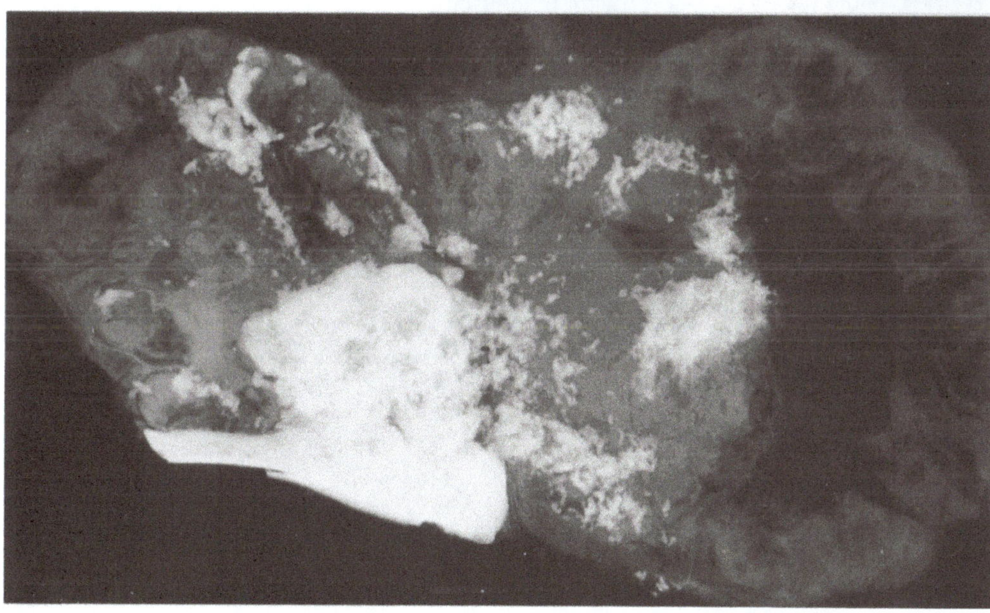

b

Fig. II.97a–c. Female, 36 years old. Peripheral chondrosarcoma of the phalanx secondary to osteochondroma. **a** Radiograph shows exostosis in great part sharply defined, with some spotty calcification. The lesion was excised and interpreted as osteochondroma, but recurred 1 year later; the radiologic aspect, revealing an irregular contour and coarse granular calcification, is shown in **b** and **c**. Reviewing the slides, a diagnosis of peripheral low-grade chondrosarcoma was made. (Courtesy of Dr. Stefani, Montivideo, Uruguay)

Fig. II.98a,b. Male, 40 years old. Peripheral chondrosarcoma of the ilium. **a** Photograph of a large chondrosarcoma (15 cm in its large diameter) showing the typical lobulated structure with areas of cystic degeneration, necrosis, and irregular foci of calcification. **b** Radiograph of a slab of the specimen showing irregular masses of coarse granular calcification and ossification. The tumor, which arose from the wing of the ilium, apparently originated in a previous osteochondroma

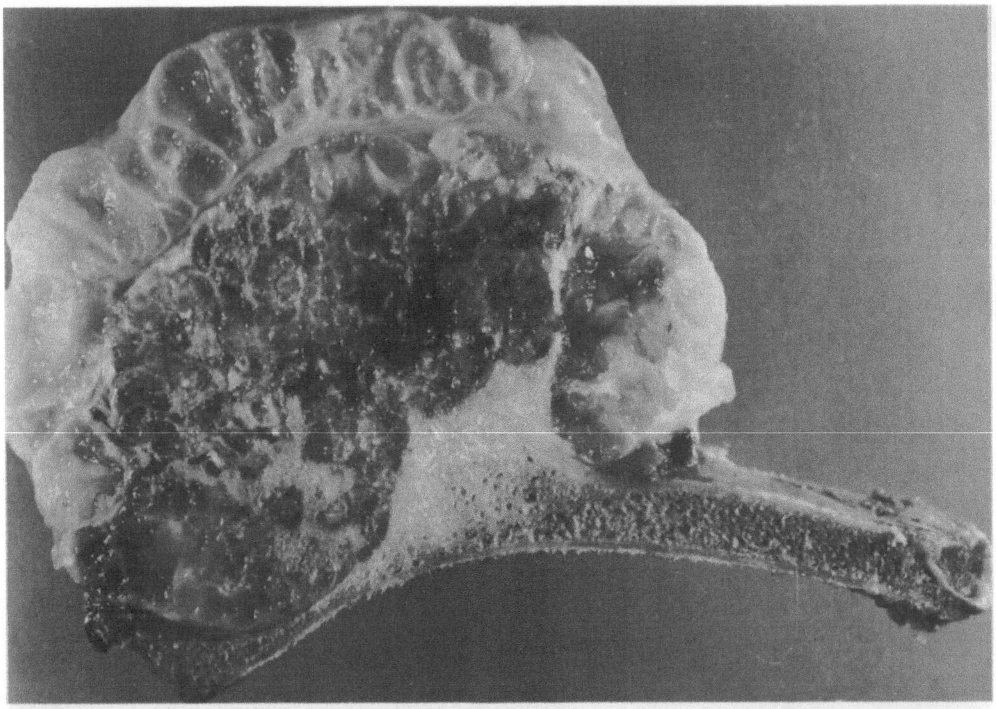

a

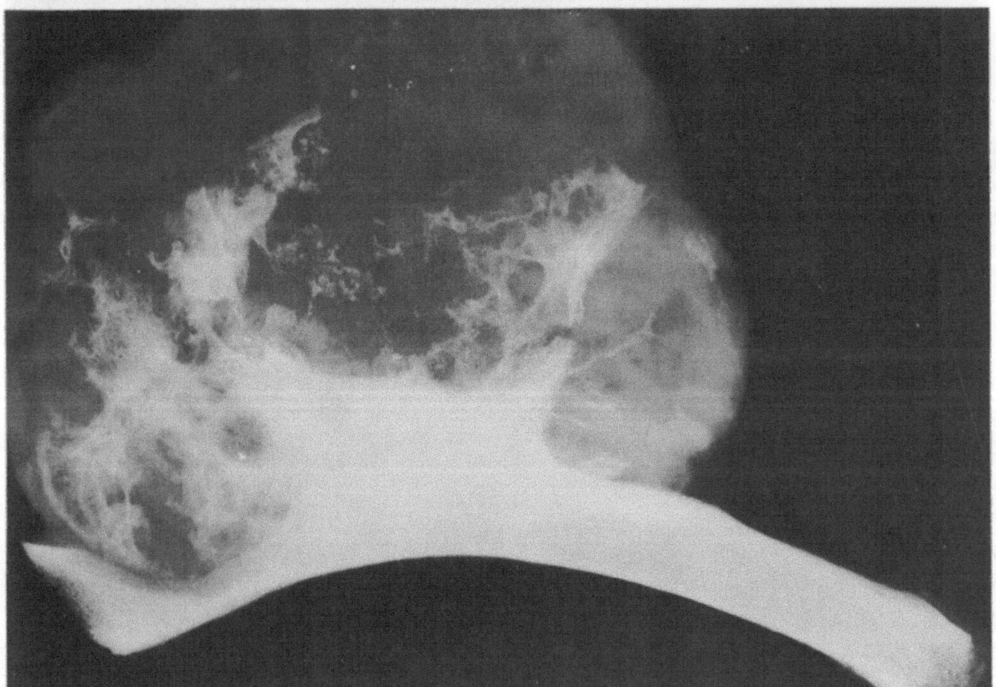

b

Fig. II.99a,b. Male, 20 years old. Chondrosarcoma of the ilium, secondary to osteochondroma. **a** Photograph and **b** radiograph of large chondrosarcoma secondary to previous osteochondroma. Extensive areas of cystic softening, necrosis, and hemorrhage may be seen

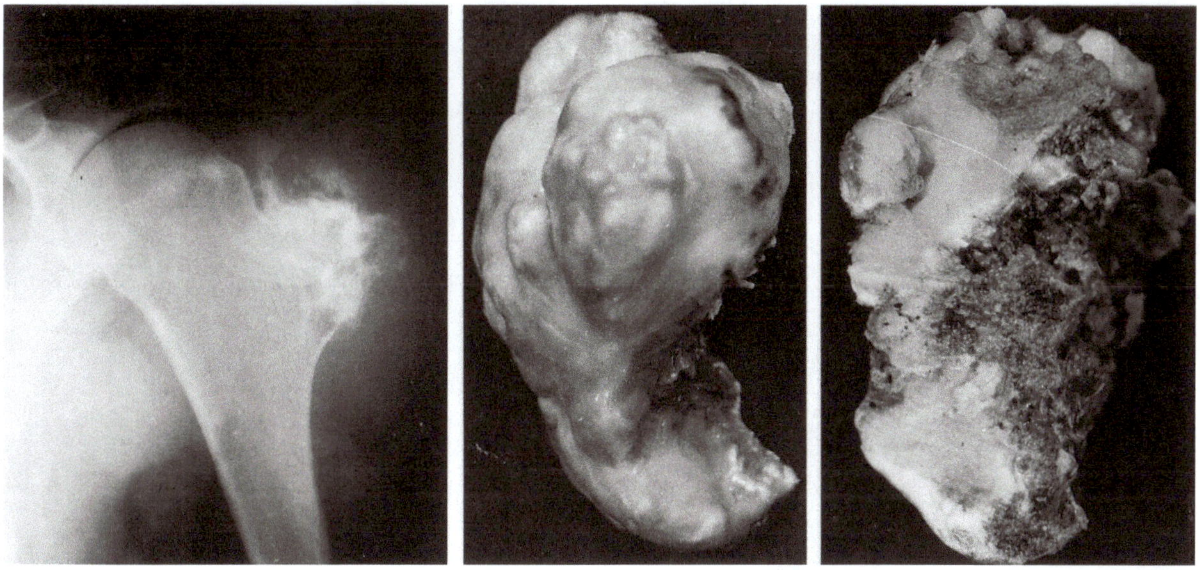

a b, c

Fig. II.100a–c. Male, 56 years old. Peripheral (exostotic) chondrosarcoma secondary to osteochondroma of humerus. **a** Radiograph shows the irregular borders of the surface of the lesion. **b,c** Photographs show the irregular lobulated surface and the thick cartilage cap with irregular borders in **c**

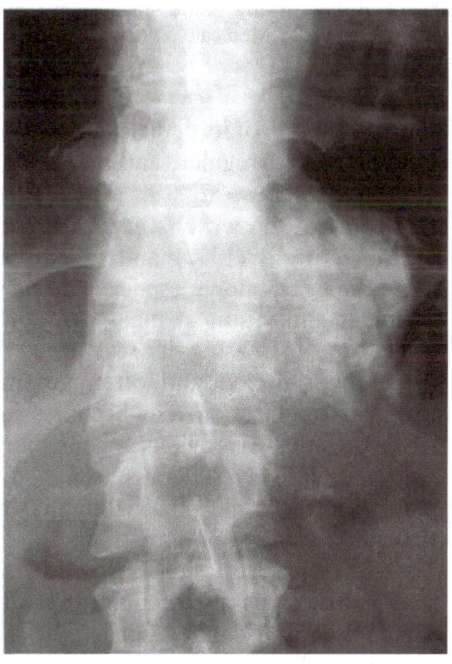

a

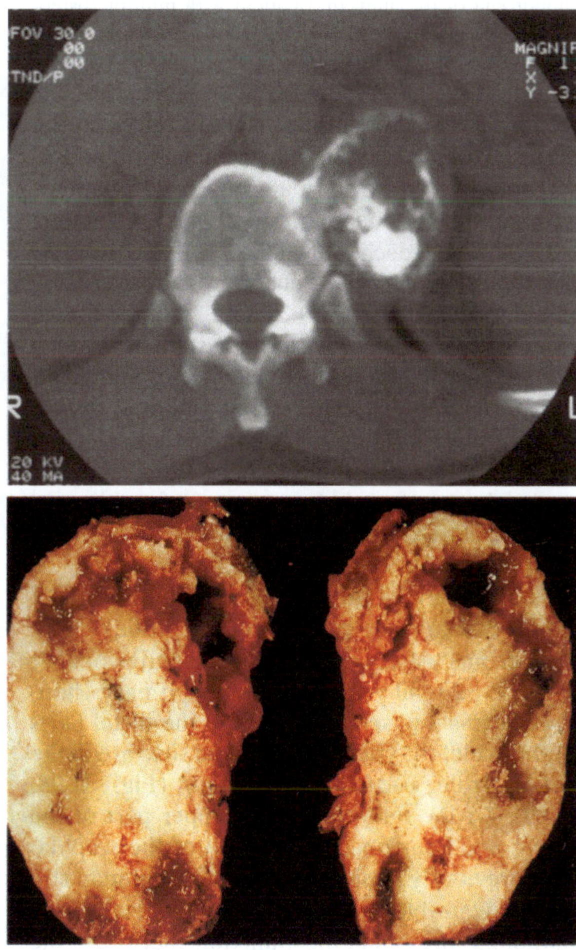

b c

Fig. II.101a–c. Male, 33 years old. Peripheral (exostotic) secondary low-grade chondrosarcoma of the 12th dorsal vertebra. **a** Radiograph shows large osteochondroma with irregular calcification in the upper portion, and an evident radiolucent area with ill-defined margins in the lower part. **b** CT scan reveals the origin of the tumor from the 12th vertebral body, with which it is united by an evident pedicle. **c** The cut surface of the resected specimen shows the thickness of the cartilage component. (St. Louis University Medical Center)

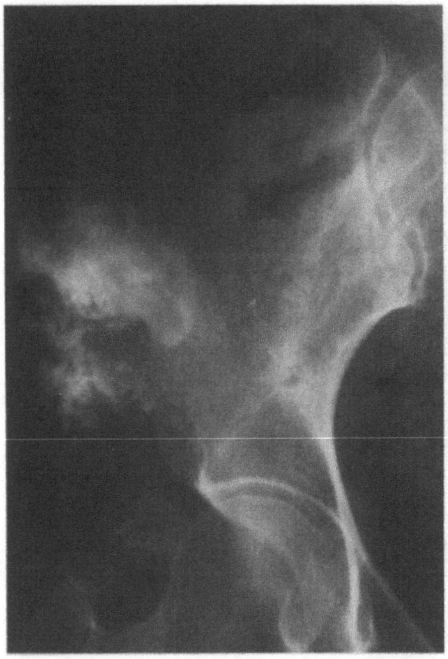

a

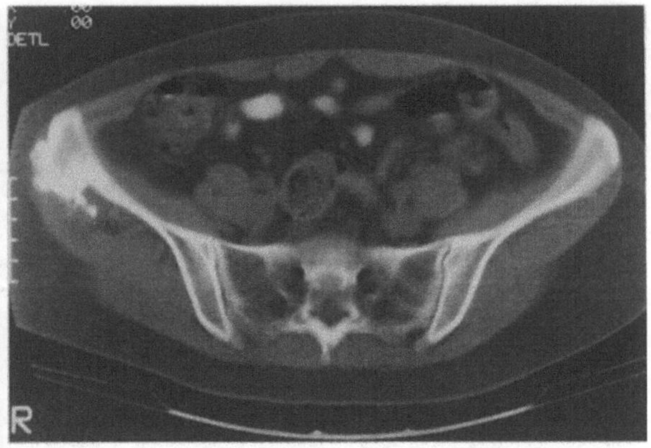

b

Fig. II.102a,b. Female, 35 years old. Peripheral (exostotic) chondrosarcoma secondary to an osteochondroma of the ilium in a patient with multiple osteochondromas. **a** Radiograph and **b** CT scan show the irregular margins of the lesion, which was in continuity with the underlying spongiosa of the ilium. The tumor was histologically of low-grade malignancy (grade I). (St. Louis University Medical Center)

from specialized or referral centers. Thus, in the Mayo Clinic series of 89 secondary chondrosarcomas, 28 occurred in a group of 115 patients with multiple osteochondromas (24%), 48 among 688 solitary osteochondromas (7%), and 13 in 59 patients with multiple enchondromatosis (22%) (Dahlin and Unni 1986). These findings are in evident disagreement with other statistics, which did not reveal such a high incidence of malignant transformation in solitary and multiple osteochondromas. Dahlin (1978) admits that selection factors make his figures unrealistic. In our material, we found four cases of malignant transformation among 1001 cases of solitary osteochondroma (0.4%), and ten cases among 63 patients with multiple osteochondromas (16%).

The secondary peripheral (exostotic) chondrosarcoma usually develops at a slightly younger age (i.e., 20–40 years) than does primary chondrosarcoma and seldom occurs in the distal parts of the skeleton. The most common sites are in the pelvic girdle, particularly the ilium (Figs. II.98, II.99, II.102), followed by the upper part of the femur and humerus (Fig. II.100), or the scapula. The previously benign osteochondroma may still be recognizable at its base radiologically and pathologically, but the junction between the spongious bone of its pedicle and the cartilage cap is much more irregular, and the width of the cap greatly increases in size (Figs. II.96–II.101). However, in the writer's experience, unlike that of Lichtenstein (1977) and others, a width of more than 1 cm alone, especially in pelvic lesions, is not an indication of malignancy. However, a large cap, increasing in size after the end of the growth period and often accompanied by irregular calcification that becomes indistinct or fuzzy beyond its previous regular borders or by pain of relatively sudden onset in a previously painless osteochondroma, is highly suspicious of malignant transformation.

In some large lesions, especially those localized in the pelvis or scapula and often heavily calcified with ill-defined borders, it is difficult to unequivocally determine the genesis, that is, primary and central or peripheral (secondary) (Figs. II.98, II.99).

The histologic criteria for the diagnosis of malignancy are the same as those applied for conventional central chondrosarcoma. Most peripheral chondrosarcomas are, in our and in others' experience, of low-grade malignancy, the prognosis being generally more favorable. In selected cases, particularly those localized in long

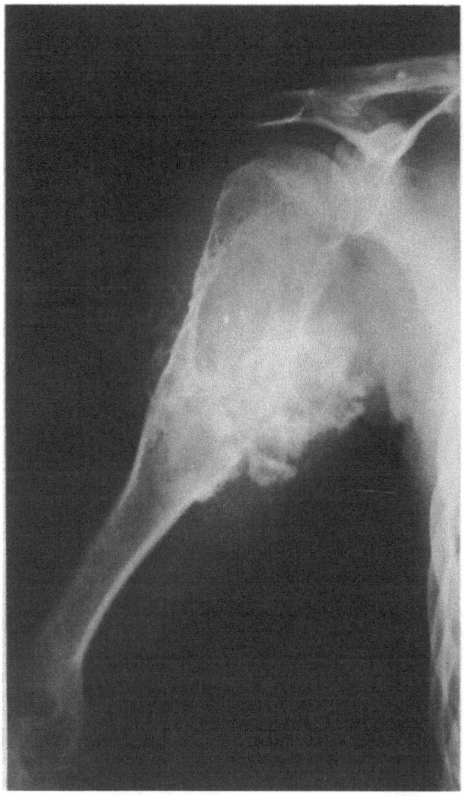

a

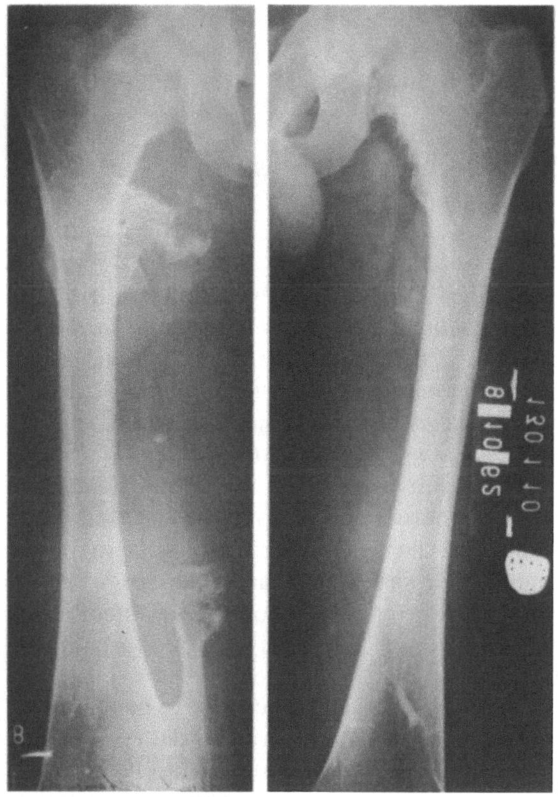

b, c

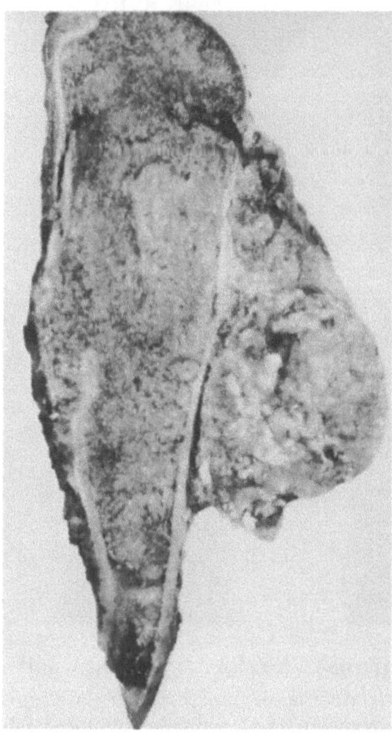

d

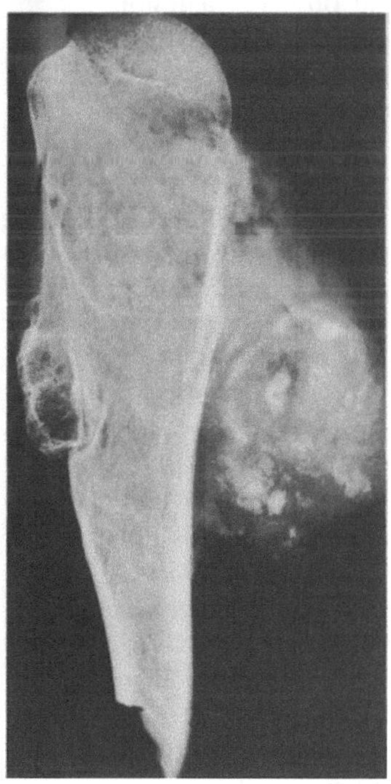

e

Fig. II.103a–e. Male, 19 years old. Multiple, hereditary osteochondromatosis with sarcomatous transformation in the humerus. Multiple osteochondromas in both extremities with sarcomatous change in one of the lesions of the humerus (**a**), which shows irregular, ill-defined borders. A resection of the upper third of the humerus was performed, but the tumor recurred locally 12 months later and forequarter amputation was performed. **d** Photograph and **e** radiograph of the resection specimens demonstrate the juxtaosseous tumor mass with foci of spotty calcification. Note the widening of the metaphyseal area, characteristic of multiple osteochondromatosis bones, a wide excision or en bloc resection may be curative.

2. Juxtacortical (Periosteal) Chondrosarcoma

Definition, WHO: *"A malignant cartilage-forming tumor arising from the external surface of a bone, usually characterized by well-differentiated lobulated cartilage with extensive areas of spotty calcification and enchondral ossification; however, tumor bone or osteoid is absent."*

This entity is rare and must be distinguished from chondrosarcoma arising as a result of malignant changes in the cartilage cap of an osteochondroma (secondary chondrosarcoma), which, in our opinion, should be termed "peripheral" or "exostotic" chondrosarcoma. Lichtenstein (1955) reported one case located in the upper shaft of the humerus of a young boy, as a distinct tumor type for which he used the term "periosteal" chondrosarcoma; in 1958, Jaffe stated that "occasionally one observes a lesion which represents the malignant counterpart of the juxtacortical chondroma," introducing the broader name "juxtacortical chondrosarcoma," emphasizing its relatively good prognosis even after local resection (Cooper 1965). The writer reported in 1977 the clinicopathologic features of seven cases of "juxtacortical chondrosarcoma" of probable periosteal origin, the term preferred by WHO to "periosteal chondrosarcoma"; that number had increased to 13 by the end of 1985.

In all cases, the lesion involved the shaft of a long bone, most often the femur, and in two cases two different long bones were affected. Six of the seven patients were male and all were in their twenties. The characteristic appearance was that of a small tumor adjacent to the cortex with areas of spotty calcification, often accompanied by radiating bone spicules perpendicular to the bone shaft and a typical Codman's triangle (Figs. II.104–II.108). Histologically, all tumors showed a cartilaginous lobular pattern, well delimited on the surface and seldom infiltrating the cortex; areas of spotty calcification and endochondral ossification were often present, but tumor osteoid and bone were conspicuously absent (Figs. II.109–II.112). Despite the occasionally ominous histologic aspect, the prognosis proved to be relatively favorable compared with that of the

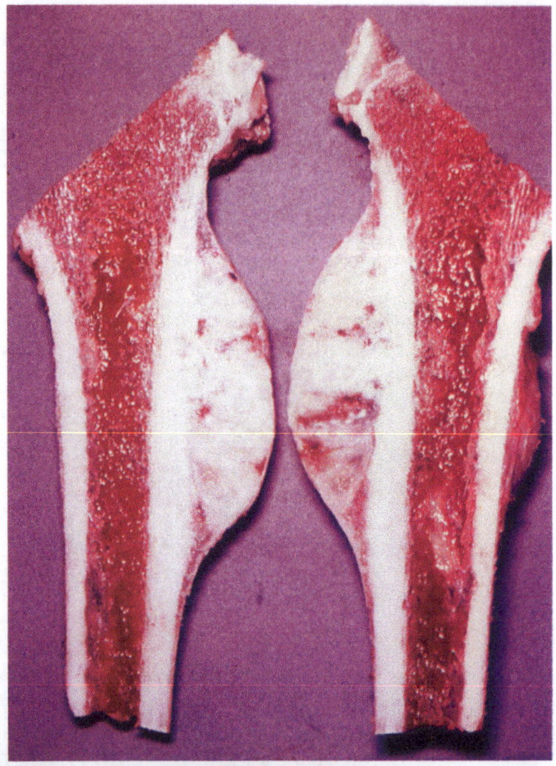

a

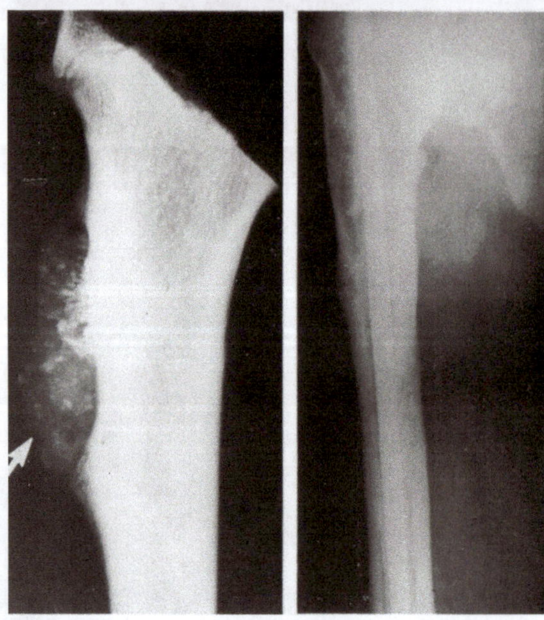

b, c

Fig. II.104a–c. Male, 17 years old. Juxtacortical chondrosarcoma of upper femur. **a** Photograph of the resected specimen showing a lobulated, sharply defined tumor of hard consistency; longitudinal section shows the tumor to be clearly extraosseous and juxtacortical, apparently of subperiosteal origin and of typical cartilaginous aspect. **b** Radiograph of the specimen showed the characteristic spotty calcification. **c** Radiograph shows the perfect consolidation of the bone graft. The patient was in good general health 12 years after en bloc resection. (Schajowicz 1978)

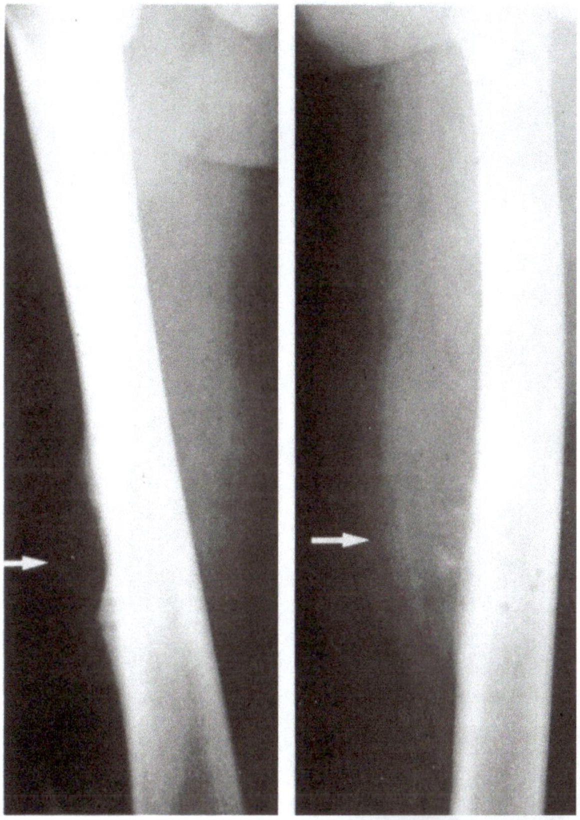

a

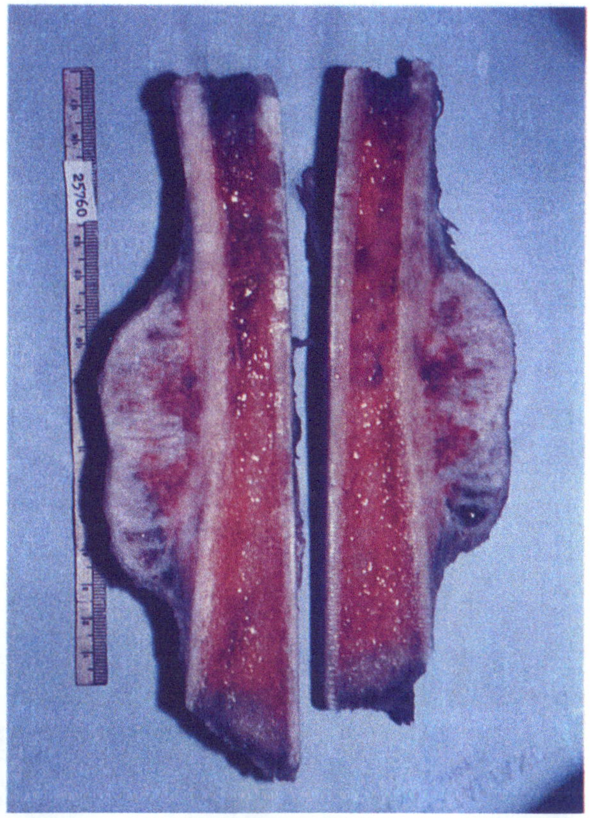

b

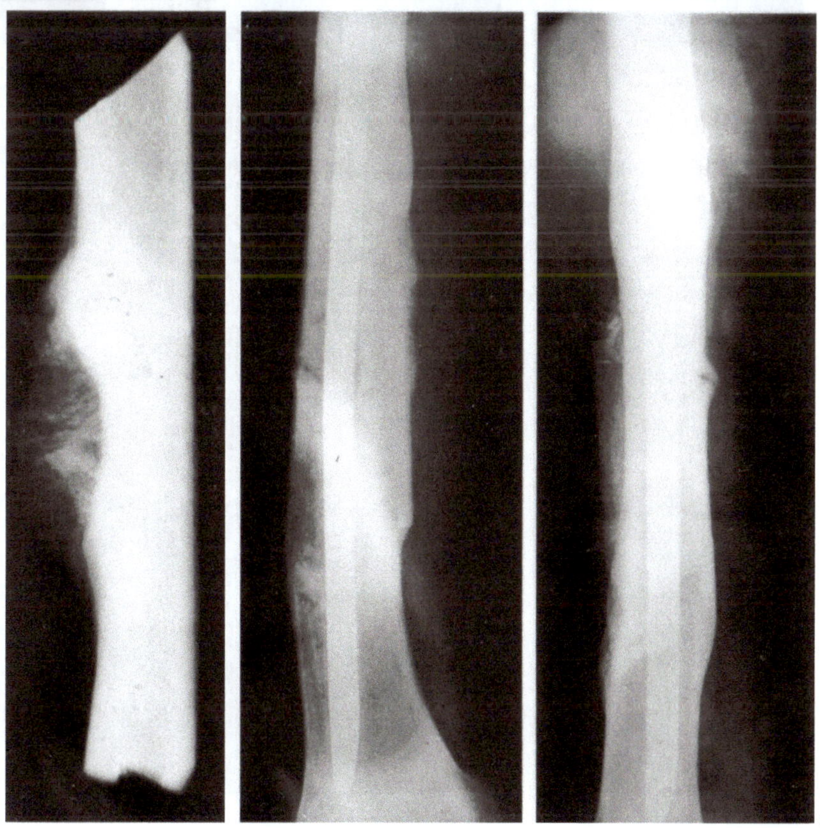

c, d

Fig. II.105a–d. Male, 17 years old. Juxtacortical chondrosarcoma of the femur. **a** Anteroposterior and lateral radiographs show a small juxtaosseous soft tissue mass with spotty calcification and radiating bone spicules producing a slight erosion of the subjacent cortex and typical Codman's triangles. **b** Photograph and **c** radiograph show the characteristic chondroid aspect of the tumor with zones of calcification and endochondral ossification near the underlying sclerotic cortex; radiating spicules are clearly seen in **c. d** Results 3½ years after wide block resection and allograft. (**b–d**, Schajowicz 1978)

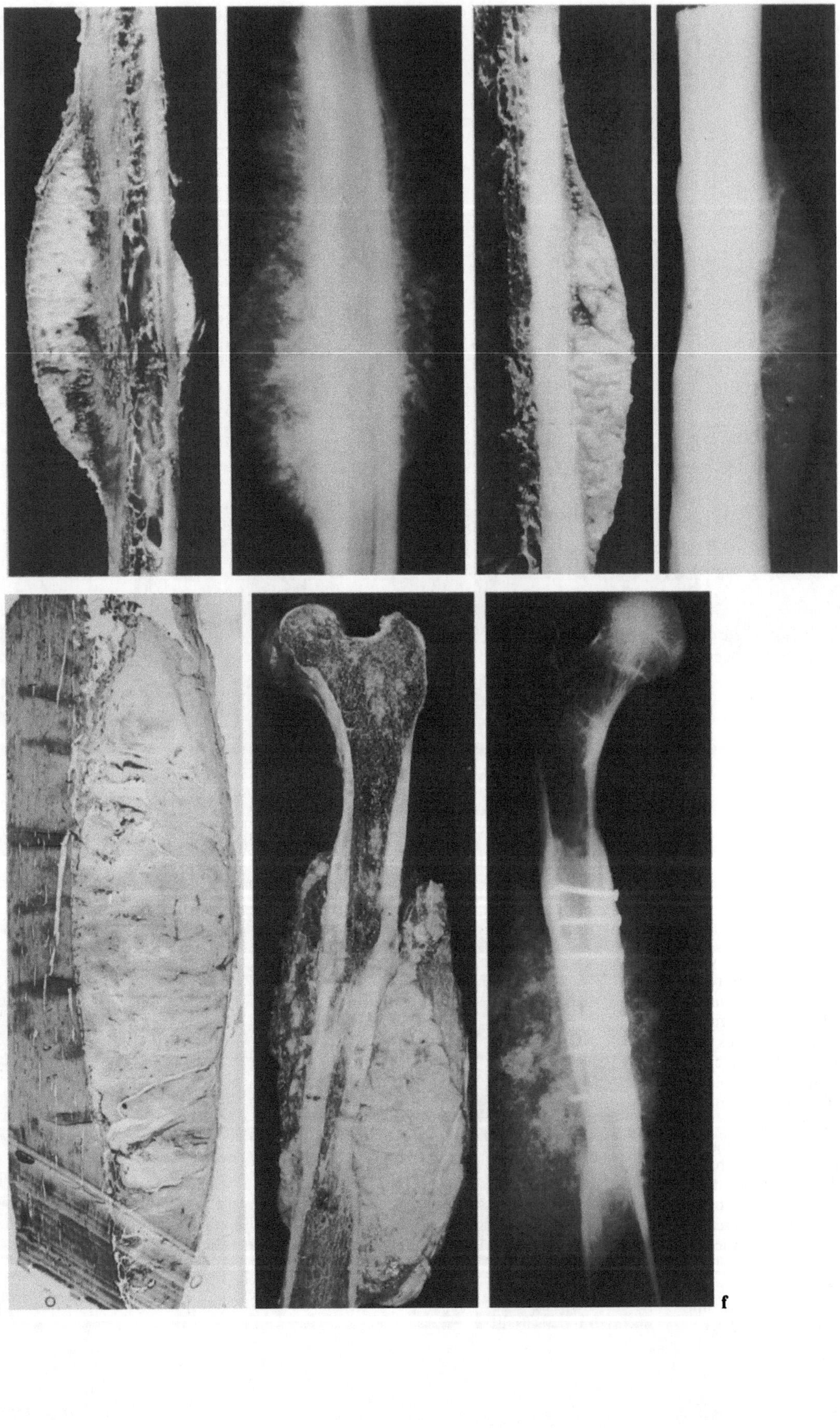

a, b c

d, e f

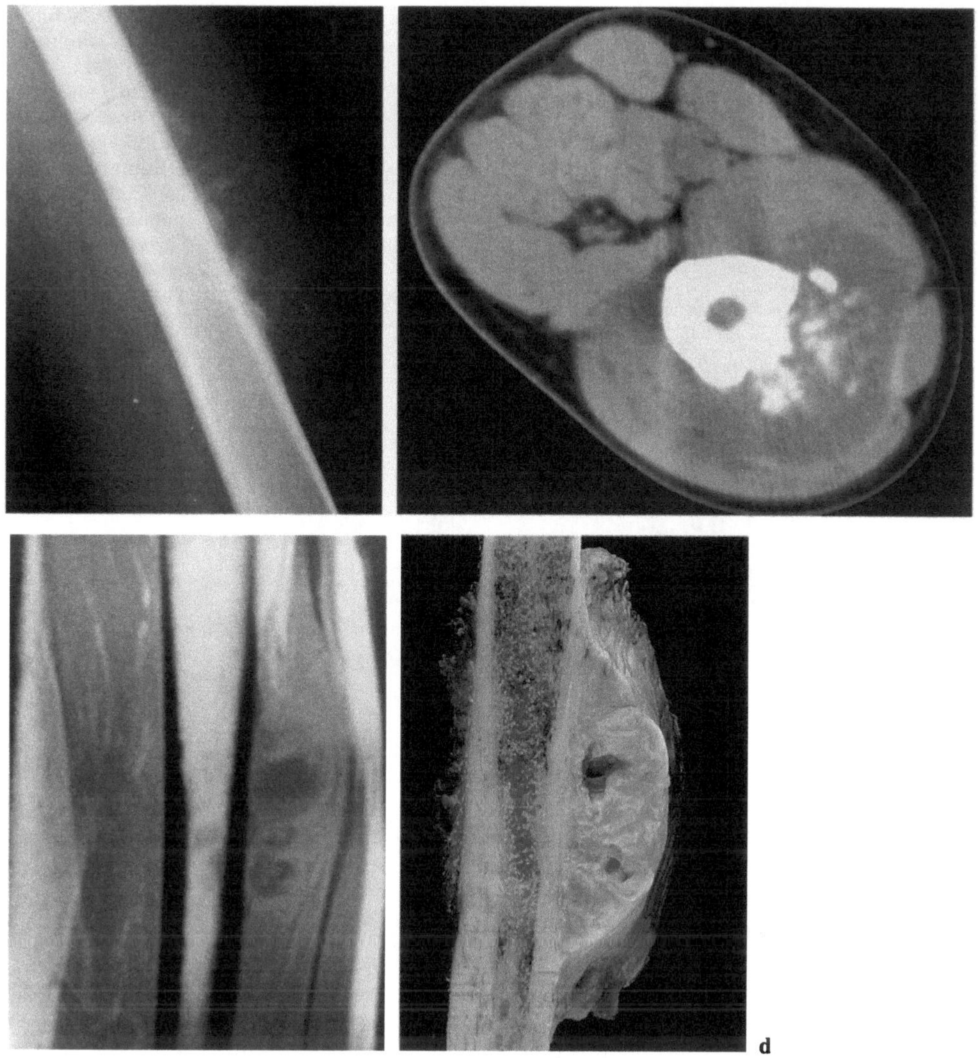

a b c d

◀ **Fig. II.106a–f.** Male, 16 years old (brother of patient illustrated in Fig. II.104). Juxtacortical (periosteal) chondrosarcoma of fibula and femur. **a,b** Photograph and radiograph of the resected specimen of the fibula, showing a lobulated juxtacortical tumor of cartilaginous aspect with a sharply defined surface. The tumor has partly destroyed the enlarged cortex on one side only, without invading the medulla. **c,d** Photograph, radiograph, and photomicrograph of resected metastatic tumor located in the femoral shaft that appeared 2½ years later. Histologically, the tumor was more malignant (grade III) than the fibular lesion. Three years later a large recurrence of the femoral tumor appeared and a disarticulation through the hip was performed. **e,f** Photograph and radiograph of the disarticulation specimen. The patient died with generalized metastases 15 years after onset of symptoms and 10 years after disarticulation. (Schajowicz 1978)

▲
Fig. II.107a–d. Female, 22 years old. Juxtacortical (periosteal) chondrosarcoma of femur. **a** Lateral radiograph shows a juxtaosseous soft tissue mass with irregular spotty calcification, producing only slight erosion of the subjacent cortex. **b** CT scan and **c** MRI illustrate the juxtaosseous location of the tumor, which has not penetrated the medullary cavity. **d** Photograph of the resected specimen shows the cartilaginous, partly cystic aspect of the lesion. (St. Louis University Medical Center)

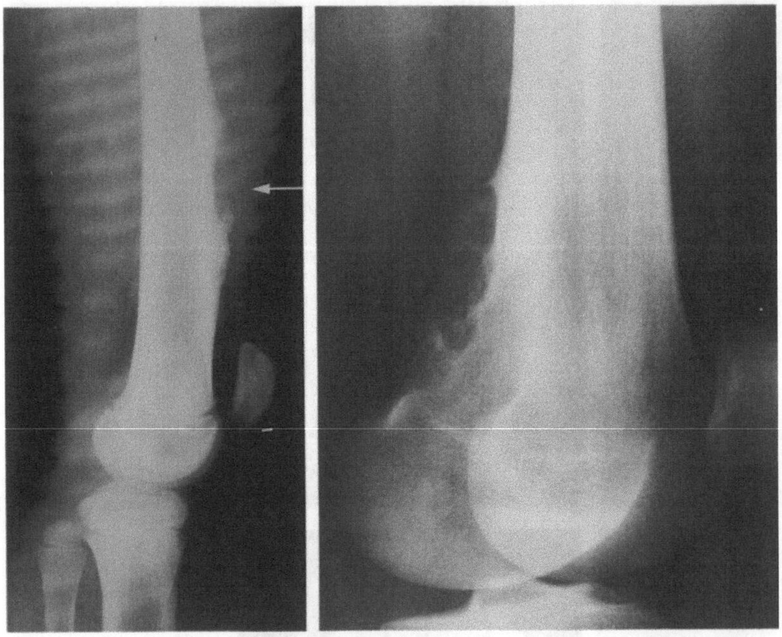

a b

Fig. II.108a,b. Juxtacortical (periosteal) chondrosarcoma of femoral diaphysis in a 14-year-old boy. **a** The lateral radiograph shows a small, juxtaosseous soft tissue mass (*arrow*) with only slight calcification and erosion of the adjacent cortex; typical Codman's triangles are seen on both edges of the lesion. **b** Periosteal (juxtacortical) chondroma of the lower metaphysis of the femur. Lateral radiograph shows a well-circumscribed, eccentric lesion with scalloping of the underlying cortex. Only a minimal amount of calcified cartilage was visible. (Schajowicz and McGuire 1989)

usual central chondrosarcoma of a similar grade of malignancy.

The problems in differential diagnosis arise with the periosteal (juxtacortical) chondroma, peripheral (exostotic or eccentric) chondrosarcoma, and particularly the so-called periosteal osteogenic sarcoma described by Unni et al. (1976) as a new and distinct entity with particular differences from "parosteal osteogenic sarcoma."

Periosteal (juxtacortical) chondroma is more common than juxtacortical (periosteal) chondrosarcoma. It involves the long bones of the hands and feet more frequently, but also the long limb bones. Although at times it may show some nuclear atypism and a higher cellularity, the cartilage cells are generally uninuclear and the nuclei are rarely plump. In the writer's opinion, some reported cases with a relatively high degree of cellular atypism and/or intramedullary penetration are really juxtacortical (periosteal) chondrosarcomas. The few cases of recurrences (Nosanchuk and Kaufer 1969) possibly stem from their incomplete excision or from failure to recognize malignancy.

Peripheral (exostotic or eccentric) chondrosarcoma is a relatively rare malignant change arising in the cartilage cap of an osteochondroma, a change more frequently associated with multiple osteochondromas. It is generally found in the metaphyseal region of a long bone or in a flat bone, especially the ilium, and it has in most cases a still recognizable pedicle of cancellous bone continuous with the spongiosa underlying the medullary cavity (see Figs. II.100–II.102).

However, the main problem of differential diagnosis is the so-called periosteal osteogenic sarcoma (Unni et al. 1976) or "periosteal" osteosarcoma (Dahlin 1978). Histologically, all reported cases of those series were "chondroblastic" osteosarcomas, with radiologic and pathologic features so similar to those of our juxtacortical chondrosarcomas that perhaps many of their cases were in fact juxtacortical (periosteal) chondrosarcomas. In our cases we have never seen clearly evident production of malignant osteoid, forming "fine lacelike osteoid" with or without mineralization characteristic of periosteal osteosarcoma. The only illustration in their article (Unni et al. 1976), which supposedly demonstrates this pattern, shows in our opinion some scant cartilage matrix and not tumor osteoid. With this comment we do not intend to deny the existence of rare cases of a "periosteal" osteogenic sarcoma or osteosarcoma of the chondroblastic type arising at the surface of bone with clinical and pathologic features different from the conventional "parosteal (juxtacortical) osteosarcoma." Indeed, we have observed nine cases of this type, as we discussed in Chap. I.

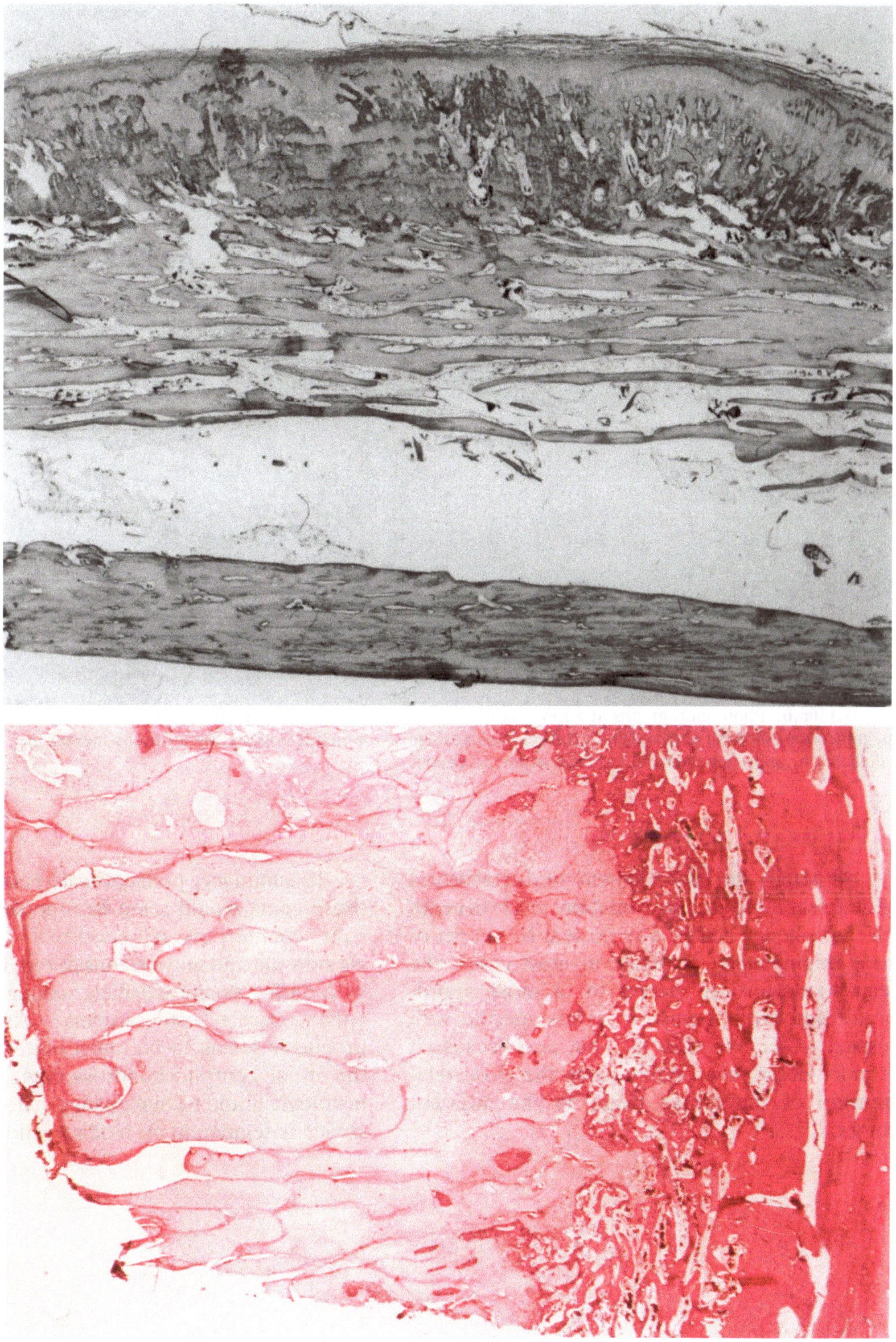

a

b

Fig. II.109a,b. Topographic photomicrograph shows the characteristic juxtacortical subperiosteal location of the tumor without penetration into the medullary cavity. ×10 a 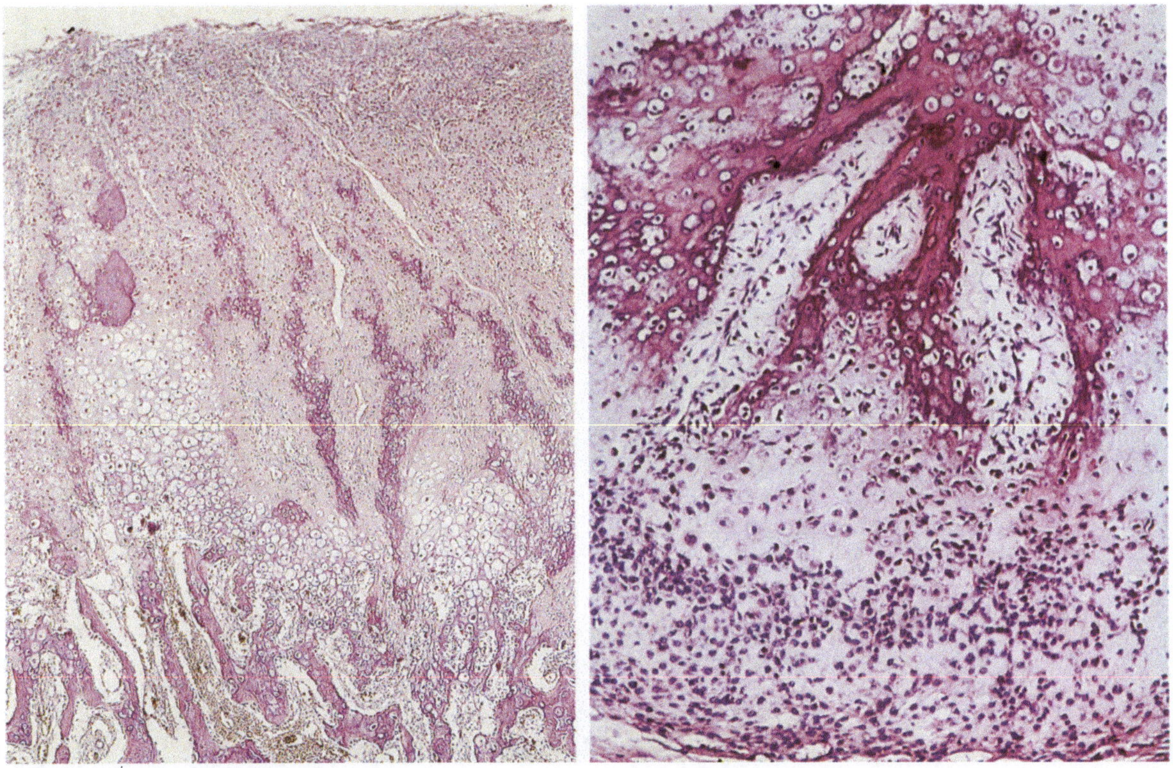 b

Fig. II.110a,b. Photomicrographs at **a** lower and **b** higher magnification, showing perpendicular trabeculae, cartilage calcification, and endochondral ossification in the deeper zone and a cellular undifferentiated area at the surface, which is covered by a fibrous membrane. **a** ×40, **b** ×100

Although the development of juxtacortical chondrosarcoma in close relation to or beneath the periosteum makes a periosteal or subperiosteal origin highly probable in most cases, the term "juxtacortical" seems to us more appropriate not only because it is less specific with respect to the site of origin, but also because it is more descriptive, emphasizing the close relationship of the tumor tissue to the adjacent cortex.

In summary, juxtacortical (periosteal) chondrosarcoma would seem to represent the malignant counterpart of periosteal (juxtacortical) chondroma and may be considered, in accordance with Jaffe, as the cartilage analog of parosteal (juxtacortical) osteosarcoma. As such, the prognosis seems to be much better than that of the usual central chondrosarcoma of a similar histologic grade of malignancy. The treatment of choice is segmental en bloc resection.

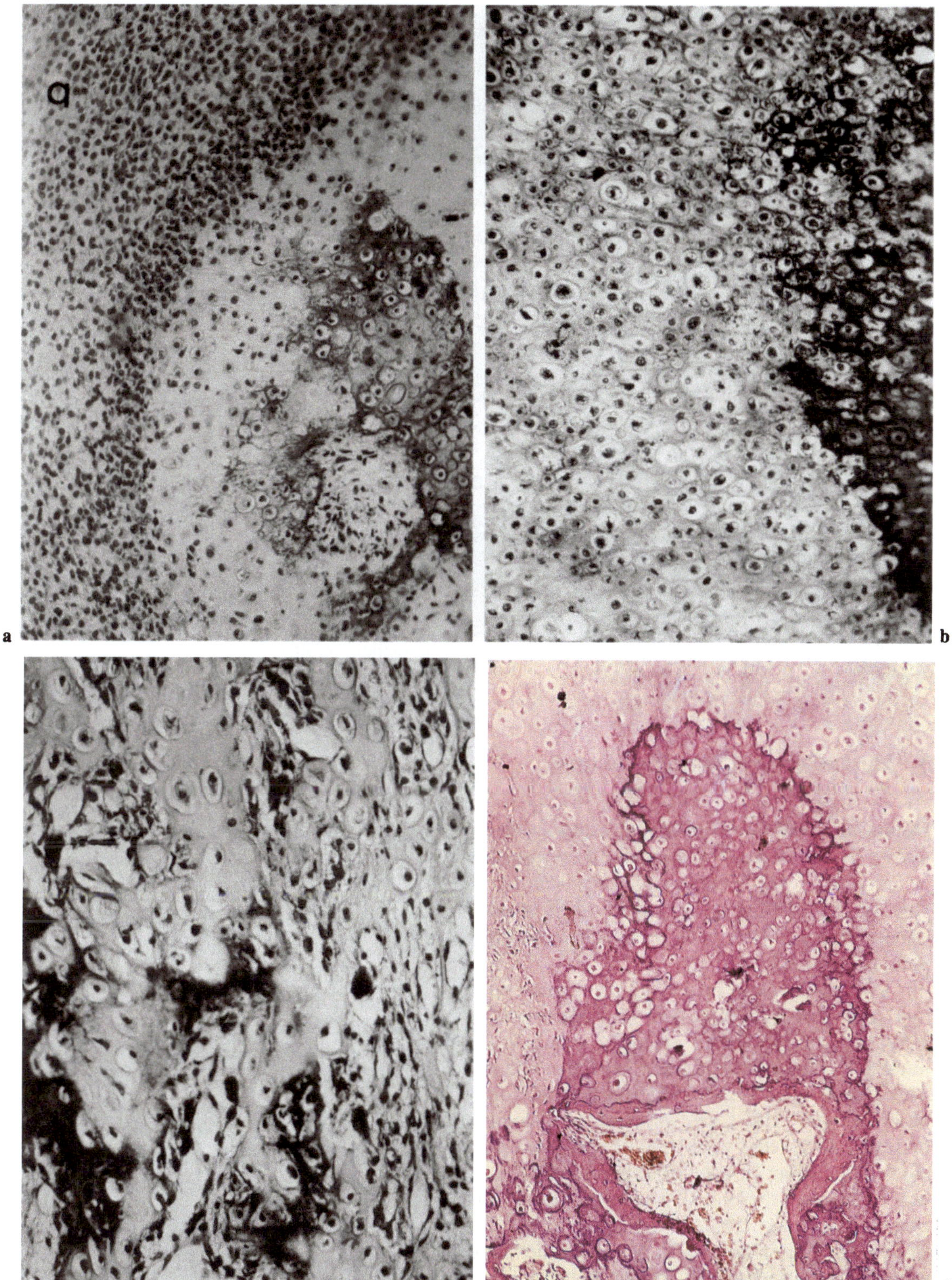

Fig. II.111a–d. Photomicrographs showing the typical histologic features of juxtacortical chondrosarcoma. **a** Peripheral cellular undifferentiated area on the *left* and a more differentiated, partially calcified zone on the *right*. **b** A moderately well differentiated cartilaginous area, in part showing conspicuous calcification. **c** Cartilage with beginning calcification, shown at a higher magnification. **d** Tumor cartilage with an advancing zone of endochondral ossification. (**d**, Schajowicz 1978) **a,b** ×100; **c** ×250; **d** ×100

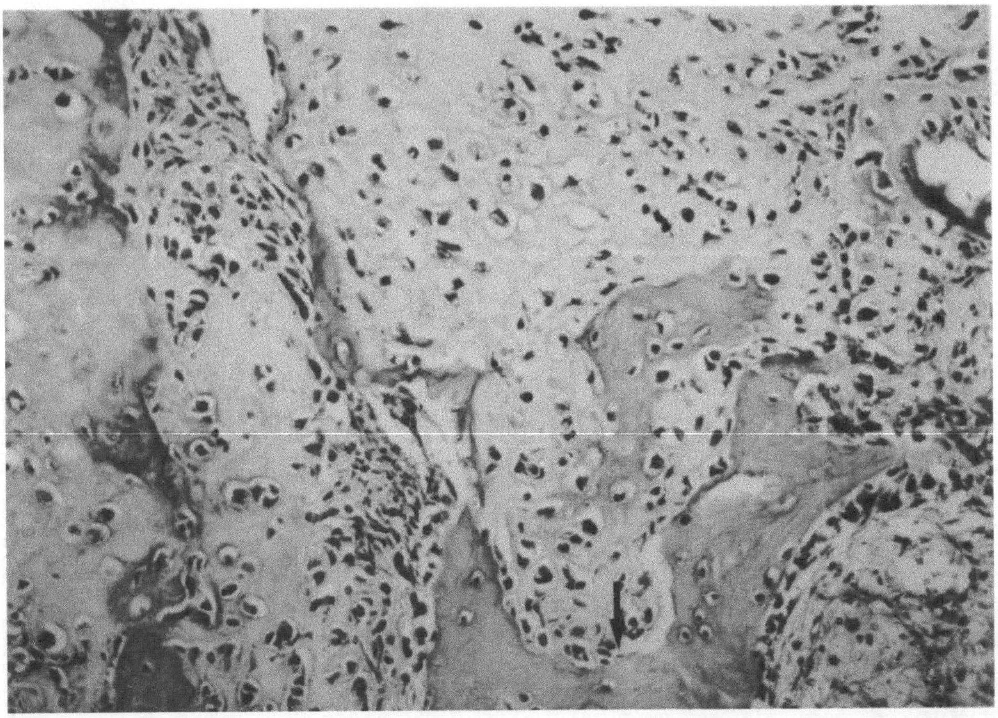

Fig. I.112. Photomicrograph showing at higher magnification the conspicuous cellular proliferation and pleomorphism, cartilage calcification, and reactive bone formation. ×250

3. Mesenchymal Chondrosarcoma

Definition, WHO: *"A malignant tumor, characterized by the presence of scattered areas of more or less differentiated cartilage together with highly vascular spindle-celled or round-celled mesenchymal tissue, often with a hemangiopericytomatous pattern."*

Two cases of this rare malignant tumor were first reported by Lichtenstein and Bernstein in 1959 as a distinct entity among a group of 25 unusual benign and malignant cartilage tumors. Three years later Dahlin and Henderson (1962) described ten more cases with similar histologic features, followed by reports of one or a few cases by Dowling (1964), Spjut et al. (1971), and others, some of these arising in extraskeletal soft tissues (Goldman 1967; Nezelof et al. 1965). Thirty new cases from the Mayo Clinic were reported by Salvador et al. (1971). The number of reported cases increased in later years as a result of contributions by Mazabraud (1974), Pepe et al. (1977), Harwood et al. (1981), Christiansen (1982), Dabska and Huvos (1983), Huvos et al. (1983), Bertoni et al. (1983), and Dahlin and Unni (1986). Approximately one-third of the lesions arose in extraskeletal soft tissues (Guccioni et al. 1973; Bertoni et al. 1983; Enzinger and Weiss 1988). More than 250 cases have been reported in the literature (Christiansen 1982). The lower extremities and the jaws were the most common sites of origin, but a wide variety of bones may be affected, including ribs and pelvic bones. There was a slight predominance in females, unlike conventional chondrosarcoma, and more than half the patients were in the second and third decades of life, ranging in age from 5 to 70 years, with an average age of 26 years (Huvos 1991). We have in our files 22 cases, four of which were referred to us from other countries. The tumors were located in the femur (six cases), tibia (three cases), vertebra (two cases), maxilla (three cases), scapula, and metatarsal bone (one case each). One case was multicentric, as were some other reported cases (Dahlin and Henderson 1962; Pepe et al. 1977; Lichtenstein and Bernstein 1959). Four cases arose in extraosseous soft tissue of the thigh (three cases) and leg (one case).

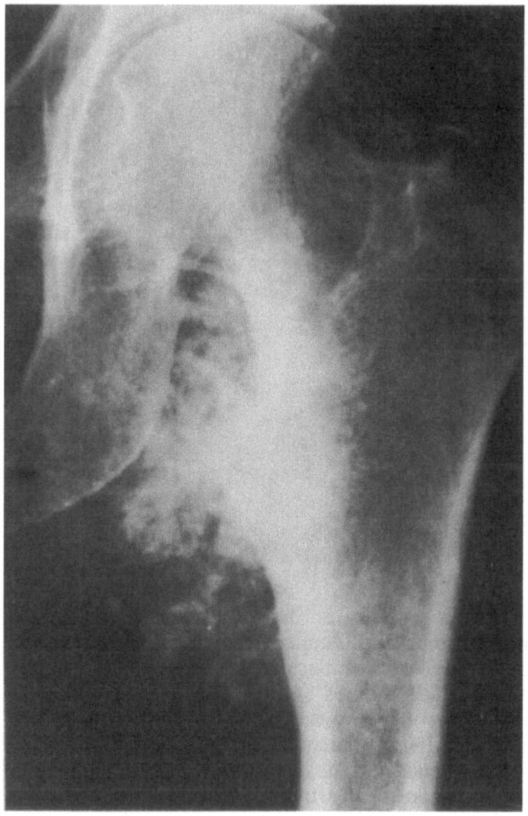

Clinical and Radiologic Features. The clinical symptoms were not characteristic, swelling and pain being the main symptoms in most cases. Pathologic fracture was found only exceptionally. The duration of symptoms prior to the histologic diagnosis was extremely variable, ranging from a few days to several years.

Most of the tumors arising in soft tissues could be visualized radiographically, showing stippled, relatively heavy calcifications (Fig. II.113). In bones, the lesions are predominantly osteolytic with ill-defined borders (Figs. II.114–

◀ **Fig. II.113.** Male, 70 years old. Mesenchymal chondrosarcoma of soft tissue origin. Radiograph shows a large juxtaosseous lesion, with conspicuous coarse spotty calcification and ill-defined contour in the region of the small trochanter. (Courtesy of Dr. Mazabraud, Paris)

Fig. II.114a–c. Male, 57 years old. Mesenchymal chondrosarcoma of scapula. **a** Radiograph shows an osteolytic lesion that has expanded and widely destroyed the lower half of the scapula. **b** Photograph and **c** radiograph of the resected scapula show the large size of the tumor of grayish-white color with central areas of hemorrhages and necrosis; the tumor has completely destroyed the body of the scapula
▼

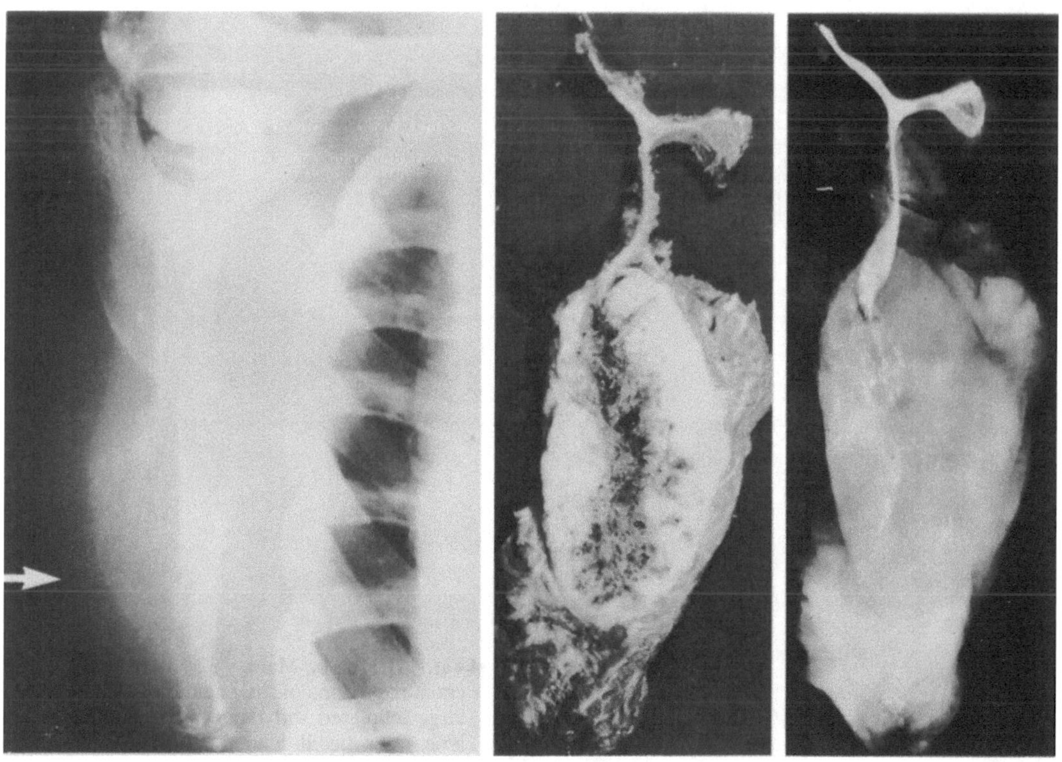

a **b, c**

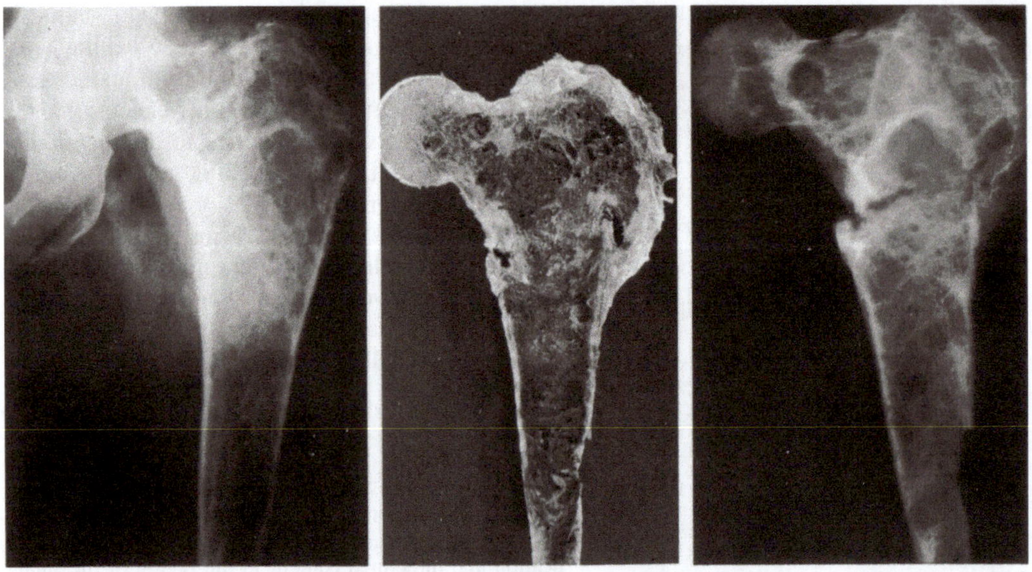

a, b c

▲ **Fig. II.115a–c.** Female, 38 years old. Mesenchymal chondrosarcoma of the upper femoral end. **a** Radiograph shows a radiolucent trabeculated lesion that has slightly expanded the thinned cortex. **b** Photograph and **c** radiograph of the resection specimen showing a soft hemorrhagic lesion that occupies the upper third of the shaft and extends into the femoral neck. The fracture seen in the specimen is an artifact. The patient was in good general health 6 years after resection followed by a prosthetic device

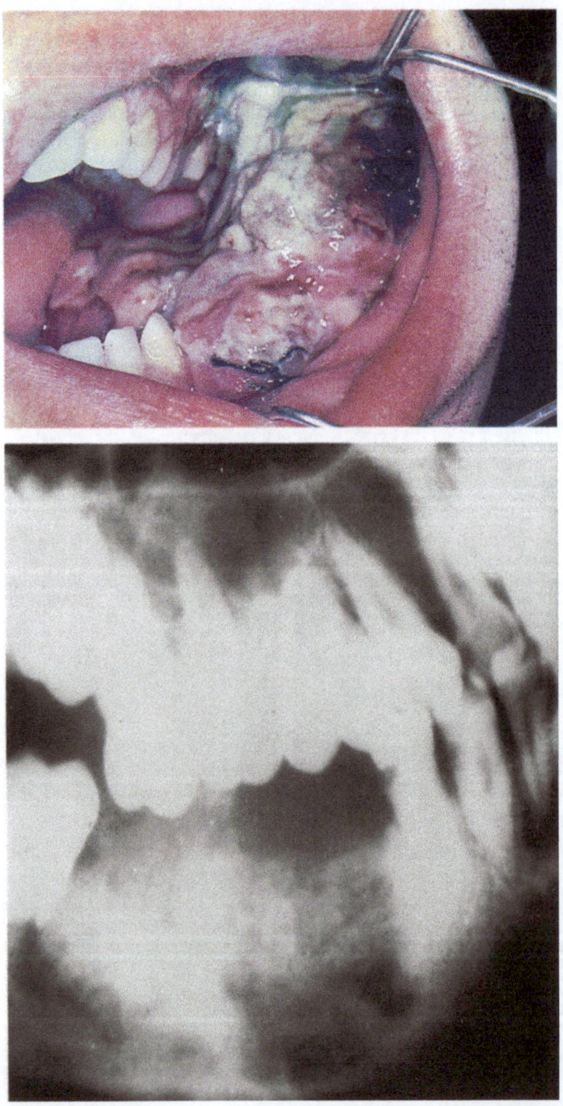

a

b

◀ **Fig. II.116a,b.** Male, 32 years old. Mesenchymal chondrosarcoma of the mandible. **a** Photograph shows the large lobulated soft tissue mass. **b** Radiograph reveals a lytic–sclerotic ill-defined lesion partially destroying the cortex

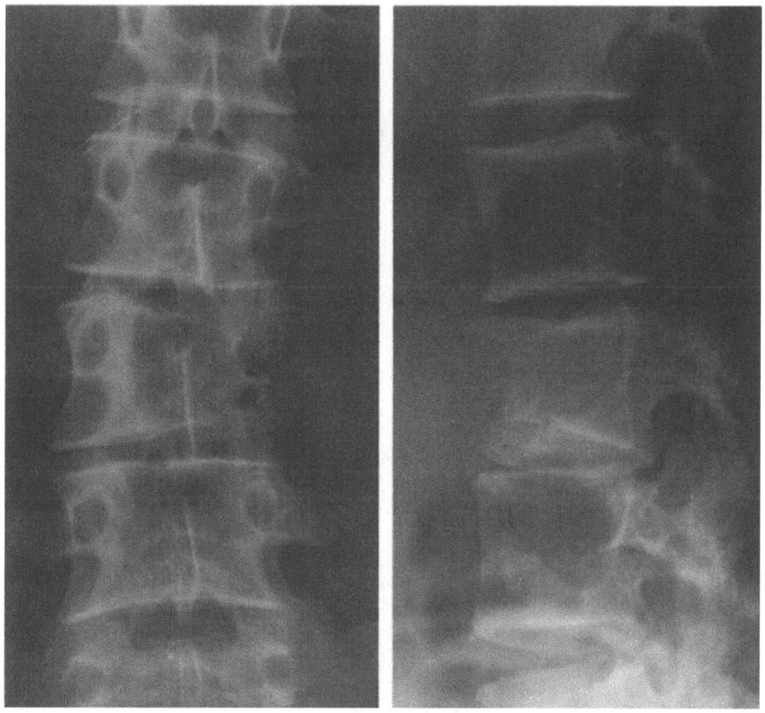

a b

Fig. II.117. Female, 14 years old. Mesenchymal chondrosarcoma of spine. Anteroposterior and lateral radiographs show an osteolytic, poorly delimited lesion which has destroyed the anterolateral aspect of the third lumbar vertebral body

II.118), exhibiting in most cases irregular calcification and sometimes distension or destruction of the thinned cortex.

In general, the characteristics were those of a malignant tumor, often indistinguishable from conventional chondrosarcoma.

Pathologic Findings. *Gross Pathology.* The macroscopic aspect is variable, showing areas of soft consistency, of grayish-white or yellowish color, alternating with firm or hard areas of frankly cartilaginous aspect with relatively extensive areas of calcification. In one of our cases, zones of necrosis and hemorrhage were conspicuous (Fig. II.114).

Histopathology. The histologic features are highly characteristic and are clearly distinct from those of conventional chondrosarcoma. Most of the tumor tissue is formed by a dense mass of round or spindle cells of uniform size with round or ovoid nuclei, without prominent nucleoli, alternating with scant or more conspicuous areas of cartilage that may be well differentiated or less mature, resembling the cartilage of conventional chondrosarcoma (Fig. II.119). Moderate to conspicuous mineralization of cartilage tissue, followed occasionally by endochondral ossification, is a frequent finding. The histologic pattern of the undifferentiated cellular areas resembles that observed in the round-cell sarcomas, particularly Ewing sarcoma or reticulum-cell sarcoma (malignant lymphoma), the reticulin fiber distribution being irregular and variable, surrounding individual or groups of cells.

In two cases we found abundant cytoplasmic glycogen granules, making confusion with Ewing sarcoma more likely, especially in tumors with scanty cartilage. *Electron microscopic studies* of single cases of mesenchymal chondrosarcoma (Steiner et al. 1973; Fu and Kay 1974; Mikata et al. 1977; Martínez-Tello and Navas-Palacios 1982) show the resemblance between the tumor cartilage and young hyaline or fetal cartilage. Steiner et al. suggest that the tumor originates from primitive cartilage-forming mesenchyme. In their case a large number of tumor cells remained in an early, undifferentiated state, whereas others had undergone cartilaginous differentiation; glycogen was scarce or lacking.

A frequent finding in our experience was a perivascular arrangement of the tumor cells, resulting in a characteristic *hemangiopericytomatous* pattern (Fig. II.119). This resemblance to hemangiopericytoma had already been emphasized by Dahlin and Henderson (1962), and it is mentioned in most reports. In fact, a tumor involving the orbit was reported as hemangio-

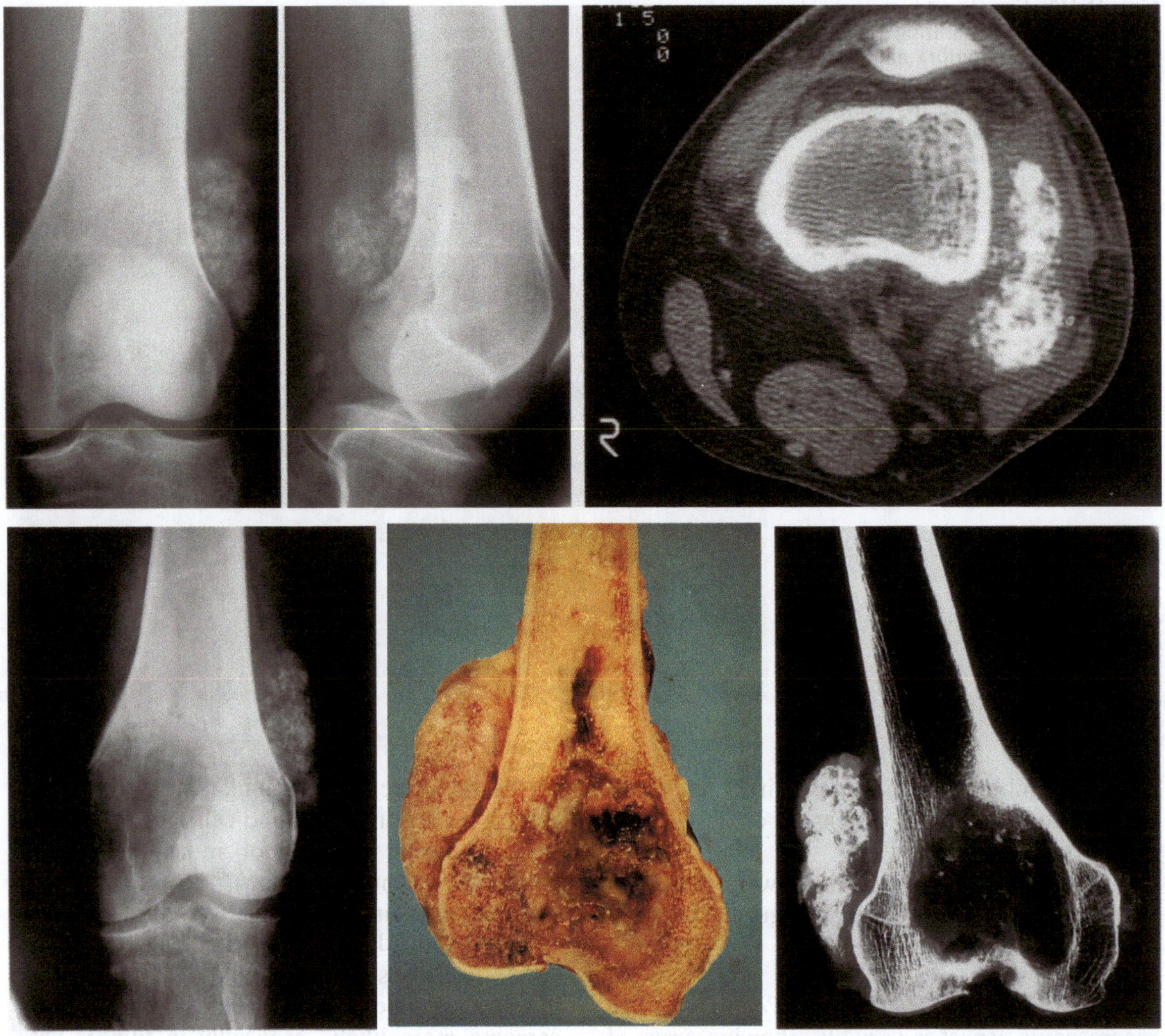

a b c, d e

Fig. II.118a–e. Male, 25 years old. Mesenchymal chondrosarcoma of femur. **a** Anteroposterior and lateral radiographs show a juxtaosseous soft tissue mass with spotty calcification. There was no clear evidence of medullary involvement. **b** Three months later an evident ill-defined osteolytic lesion was seen in the distal end of the femur, clearly shown on CT scan (**c**). **d** Photograph and **e** radiograph of the specimen demonstrate the intraosseous involvement and origin of the tumor

pericytoma with cartilaginous differentiation (Rech 1966). Huvos (1991) subdivided mesenchymal chondrosarcoma into two distinct groups, the better differentiated hemangiopericytomatoid variant, and the less differentiated small-cell type with zones of anaplastic round or spindle cells (small-cell type) dominating the microscopic picture.

This combination of vascular, cartilaginous, and structurally undifferentiated mesenchymal tissue induces us to believe that this entity could be a mixed mesenchymal tumor (malignant mesenchymoma). Several of the cases reported by Hutter et al. (1966) under the term "primitive multipotential primary sarcoma of bone" are, in our opinion, mesenchymal chondrosarcoma or Ewing sarcoma with reactive bone formation, the same as most of the cases published by Jacobson (1977) as "polyhistioma, a pluripotential small round-cell sarcoma of bone and soft tissue."

Treatment and Prognosis. The treatment was variable in our cases and in most cases from the literature; definite conclusions are not possible due to the limited number of reported cases. Radical surgical treatment seems to have given the best results.

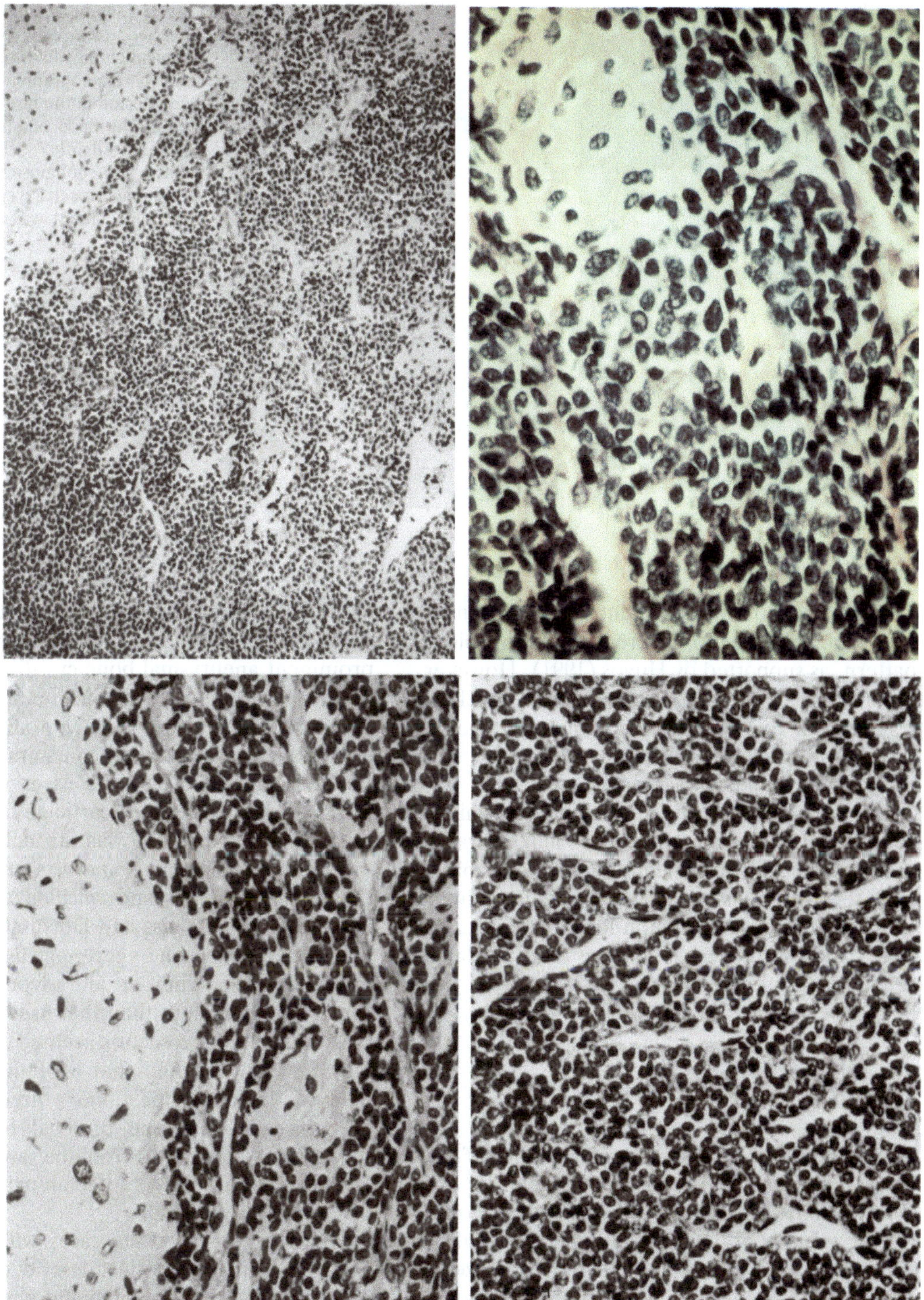

Fig. II.119a–d. Microphotographs of lower (**a**) and higher (**b–d**) magnification show a highly vascular round-celled "undifferentiated" tissue together with scattered areas of more or less differentiated cartilage. The hemangiopericytomatous structure is clearly seen. **a** ×100; **b–d** ×400 a 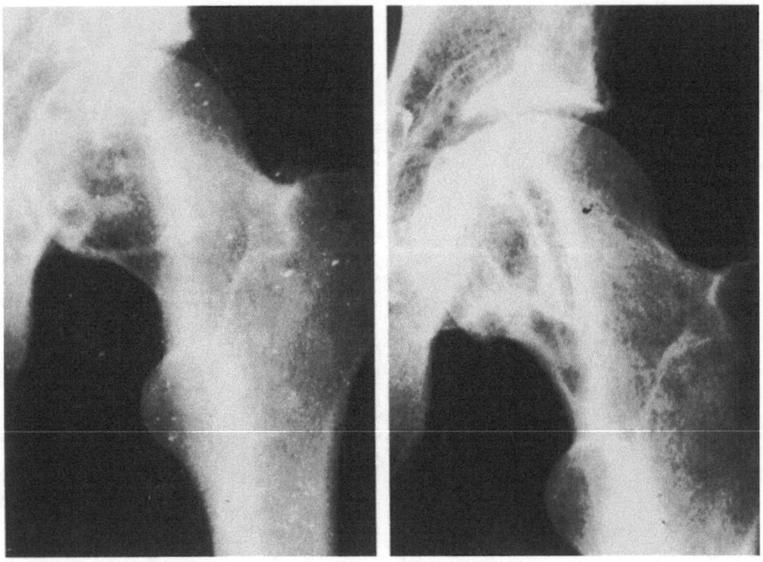 b

Fig. II.120a,b. Male, 26 years old. So-called clear-cell chondrosarcoma (atypical chondroblastoma) of femoral head. **a** Radiograph shows a radiolucent lesion in the non-weight-bearing area of the head of femur, with well-defined, slightly sclerotic border toward the spongiosa. **b** Radiograph shows the aspect 2 years after curettage. The patient was well 30 months later

We have not found evident differences in the evolution according to the predominant histologic pattern, as supported by Huvos (1991). However, according to Huvos, patients with a small-cell lesion seem to respond to combination chemotherapy and radiotherapy similarly to those with other small round-cell sarcomas.

It is possible that the predominance of highly cellular undifferentiated zones makes radiotherapy and adjuvant chemotherapy advisable.

Hematogenous metastases are frequent in the lungs and also in uncommon locations, including bones and soft tissues, sometimes after a delay of several years.

4. Clear-Cell Chondrosarcoma

Definition, WHO: *"A rare cartilage tumor of low-grade malignancy, characterized by rounded cells with conspicuous clear or vacuolated cytoplasm."*

In a survey of the bone tumors treated at the Mayo Clinic, Unni et al. (1976) recognized a group of 16 patients with destructive cartilaginous tumors of low-grade malignancy, which originally were considered benign. The tumor usually affected adults, involving most commonly the proximal femur, humerus, or tibia (Figs. II.120, II.122). Radiographically, it was generally well defined and often indistinguishable from chondroblastoma, although it occasionally exhibited progression of the process. Histologically, areas with benign giant cells and stromal cells similar to those seen in chondroblastoma, sometimes with prominent aneurysmal bone cyst-like areas, were observed. However, a distinctive finding was the presence of numerous cells with abundant, clear cytoplasm and of areas of conventional chondrosarcoma in about half the cases (Figs. II.121, II.122). As in normal cartilage and cartilage tumors, S-100 protein was strongly positive in most chondroblastomas and was most intense in the vacuolated cells and calcified areas (Monda and Wick 1985; Weiss and Dorfman 1986).

Because excision or curettage usually resulted in recurrence, Unni et al. advocated a more aggressive treatment than that used for chondroblastoma: en bloc resection seemed to be curative. However, they stated that 4 of the 16 patients died as a result of the tumor, three with metastatic disease, and one of local effects of the tumor. In a later report from the same institution, Bjornsson et al. (1984) noted an overall mortality of 15% in 47 patients.

We have observed six cases with the clinical and histologic features just described. Three were located in the femoral head and one in the upper tibial end, and they were interpreted by us primarily as "atypical" chondroblastoma (Fig. II.122). Two patients were well 3 years after conservative treatment (curettage); a third patient was lost to follow-up. En bloc resection of the tumor of the upper tibia was performed, and the patient was free of disease 5 years later.

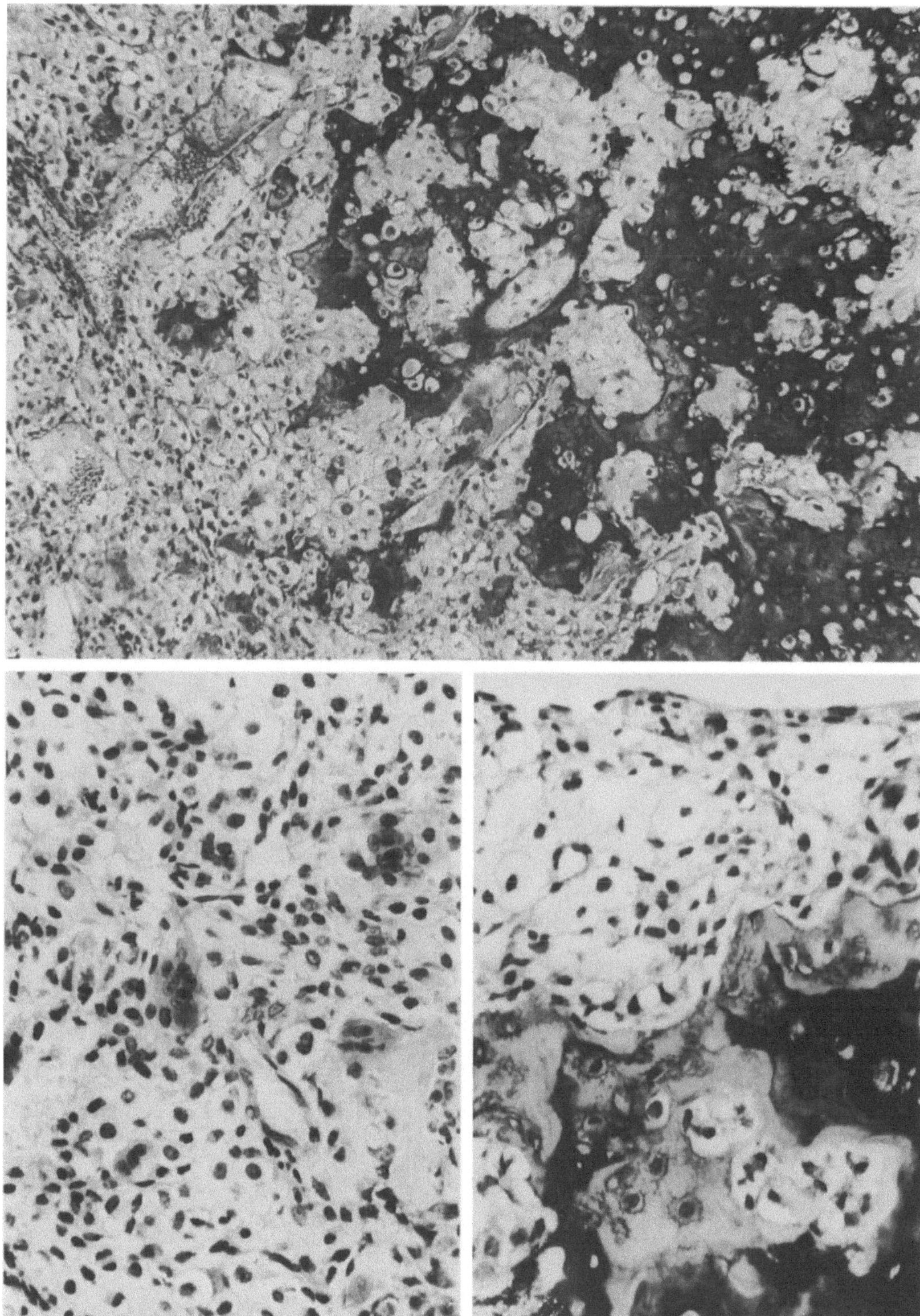

a

b c

Fig. II.121a–c. Photomicrographs of same case. **a** Extensive areas of calcified tumor cartilage. **b** Cells with abundant clear cytoplasm, intermingled with some multinucleated giant cells of osteoclast type. **c** Clear cells and calcified cartilage. **a** ×120; **b,c** ×300

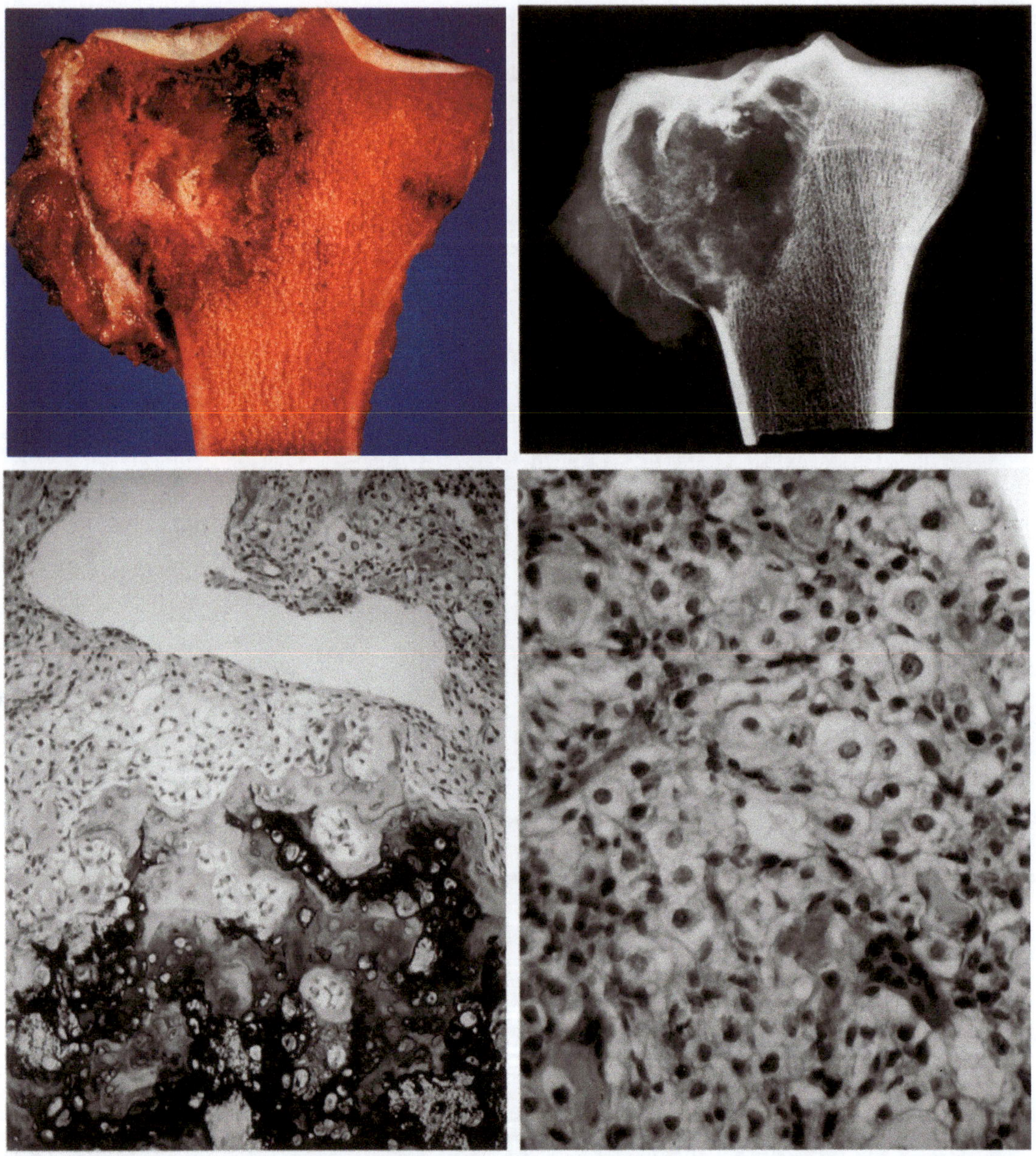

a b c d

Fig. II.122a–d. Female, 25 years old with clear-cell chondrosarcoma of the tibia. **a** Photograph and **b** radiograph of the resected specimen show a grayish and hemorrhagic, eccentric lesion in the upper metaepiphyseal region, expanding the thinned cortex. **c,d** Photomicrographs demonstrate the characteristic histologic features. **c** ×100, **d** ×400

We believe that the histologic features of the tumor cells should be investigated further, histochemically and ultrastructurally, in order to clarify the histogenesis of this rare type of tumor.

It cannot be denied that clear-cell chondrosarcoma could be an atypical, more aggressive chondroblastoma (Huvos et al. 1977) or the malignant transformation or counterpart of chondroblastoma, similar to "malignant (aggressive) osteoblastoma" reported by Schajowicz and Lemos (1976).

References

Chondroma and Osteochondroma

Aegerter E, Kirkpatrick JAJ (1975) Orthopedic diseases: physiology, pathology, radiology, 4th edn. W.B. Saunders, Philadelphia

Anastasi GW, Wertheimer HM, Brown JR (1963) Popliteal aneurysm with osteochondroma of the femur. Arch Surg 87:636–639

André L, Dymlin JF, Elner A, Hogeman KE (1963) Maffucci's syndrome. Report of four cases. Acta Chir Scan 126:397–405

Bauer TW, Dorfman HD, Latham JT Jr (1982) Periosteal chondroma: a clinicopathologic study of 23 cases. Am J Surg Pathol 6:631–637

Bean WB (1958) Dyschondroplasia and hemangiomata (Maffucci's syndrome). Arch Intern Med 102:544–550

Bethge JFJ (1963) Hereditäre multiple Exostosen und ihre pathogenetische Deutung. Arch Orthop Unfallchir 54:667–696

Borges AM, Huvos AG, Smith J (1981) Bursa formation and synovial chondrometaplasia associated with osteochondromas. Am J Clin Pathol 75:648

Boriani S, Bacchini P, Bertoni F et al. (1983) Periosteal chondroma: a review of twenty cases. J Bone Joint Surg [Am] 65:205–212

Campanacci M, Leonessa C, Boni A (1975) Cartilaginous tumors in the hand bones: report of 112 cases. Chir Organi Mov 62:483–490

Cannon SR, Sweetnam DR (1985) Multiple chondrosarcomas in dyschondroplasia (Ollier's disease). Cancer 55:836–840

Cary R (1965) Juxtacortical chondroma. J Bone Joint Surg [Am] 47:1405

Clark PM, Keokarn T (1965) Popliteal aneurysm complicating benign osteocartilaginous exostosis. Review of the literature and report of one case. J Bone Joint Surg [Am] 47:1386–1388

Crandall BF, Field LL, Sparkes RS et al. (1984) Hereditary multiple exostoses: report of a family. Clin Orthop 190:217–219

Dahlin DC (1978) Bone tumors, 3rd edn. Charles C. Thomas, Springfield, IL

Dahlin DC, Unni KK (1986) Bone tumors: general aspects and data on 8542 cases. Charles C. Thomas, Springfield, IL

D'Ambrosia R, Ferguson AB Jr (1968) The formation of osteochondroma by epiphyseal cartilage transplantation. Clin Orthop 61:103–115

Davies CWT (1985) Bizarre parosteal osteochondromatous proliferation in the hand: a case report. J Bone Joint Surg [Am] 67:648–650

DeSantos LA, Spjut HJ (1981) Periosteal chondroma: a radiographic spectrum. Skeletal Radiol 6:15–20

Ehrenfried A (1915) Multiple cartilaginous exostoses, hereditary deforming chondrodysplasia. JAMA 64:1642–1646

Ehrenfried A (1917) Hereditary deforming chondrodysplasia: more cases. Am J Orthop 15:463–478

El-Khoury GY, Bassett GS (1979) Symptomatic bursa formation with osteochondromas. AJR 130:331

Fairbank HAT (1948) Dyschondroplasia. Synonyms: Ollier's disease, multiple enchondroma. J Bone Joint Surg [Br] 30:689–708

Fairbank HAT (1949) Diaphyseal aclasis. J Bone Joint Surg [Br] 31:105–113

Fairbank HAT (1956) Dysplasia epiphysialis hemimelica (tarso-epiphyseal aclasis). J Bone Joint Surg [Br] 38:237–257

Ferguson AB Jr (1947) Calcified medullary defects in bone. J Bone Joint Surg 29:598

Ferriter P, Hirschy J, Kesseler H et al. (1983) Popliteal pseudoaneurysm: a case report. J Bone Joint Surg [Am] 65:695–697

Fischer MR, Hernandez RJ, Poznanski AK et al. (1984) Case report 262. Diagnosis: dysplasia epiphysealis hemimelica (DEH) – Trevor disease. Skeletal Radiol 11:147–150

Fornasier VL, McGonigal D (1977) Periosteal chondroma. Clin Orthop 124:233–236

Garrison RC, Unni KK, McLeod RA et al. (1982) Chondrosarcoma arising in osteochondroma. Cancer 49:1890–1897

Goodman SB, Bell RS, Fornasier VL et al. (1984) Ollier's disease with multiple sarcomatous transformations. Hum Pathol 15:91–93

Hershey SL, Lansden FT (1972) Osteochondromas as a cause of false popliteal aneurysms. Review of the literature and report of two cases. J Bone Joint Surg [Am] 54:1765–1768

Hudson TM, Springfield DS, Spanier SS et al. (1984) Benign exostoses and exostotic chondrosarcomas: evaluation of cartilage thickness by CT. Radiology 152:595–599

Huvos AG (1991) Bone tumors: diagnosis, treatment, prognosis W.B. Saunders, Philadelphia

Jaffe HL (1943) Hereditary multiple exostosis. Arch Pathol 36:335–357

Jaffe HL (1956) Juxtacortical chondroma. Bull Hosp Joint Dis 17:20–29

Jaffe HL (1958) Tumors and tumorous conditions of the bones and joints. Lea & Febiger, Philadelphia

Keats TE (1957) Dysplasia epiphysialis hemimelica (tarso-epiphyseal aclasis). Radiology 68:558–563

Keith A (1919–1920) Studies on the anatomical changes which accompany certain growth disorders of the human body. I. The nature of the structural alterations in the disorder known as multiple exostoses. J Anat 54:101–115

Kettlekamp DB, Campbell CJ, Bonfiglio M (1966) Dysplasia epiphysealis hemimelica. J Bone Joint Surg [Am] 48:746–766

Laurence W, Franklin EL (1953) Calcifying enchondroma of long bones. J Bone Joint Surg [Br] 35:225-228
Lewis MM, Kenan S, Yabut SM et al. (1990) Periosteal chondroma: a report of ten cases and review of the literature. Clin Orthop 256:185-192
Lewis RJ, Ketcham AS (1973) Maffucci's syndrome: functional and neoplastic significance. Case report and review of the literature. J Bone Joint Surg [Am] 55:1465-1479
Libshitz HI, Cohen MA (1982) Radiation-induced osteochondromas. Radiology 142:643-647
Lichtenstein L (1977) Bone tumors, 5th edn. C.V. Mosby, St. Louis
Lichtenstein L, Bernstein D (1959) Unusual benign and malignant chondroid tumors of bone. Cancer 12:1142-1157
Lichtenstein L, Hall JE (1952) Periostal chondroma. A distinctive benign cartilage tumor. J Bone Joint Surg [Am] 34:691-697
Maffucci A (1881) Di un caso di encondroma ed angioma multiplo. Mov Med Chir 13:399-412
Marcove RC, Huvos AG (1971) Cartilaginous tumors of the ribs. Cancer 27:794-801
Marcove RC, Stovell PB, Huvos AG, Bollough PG (1977) The use of cryosurgery in the treatment of low and medium grade chondrosarcoma. Clin Orthop 122:147-155
Marmor L (1964) Periosteal chondroma (juxtacortical chondroma). Clin Orthop 367:150-153
Merlino AF, Nixon JE (1964) Periosteal chondroma. Am J Surg 107:773-776
Milgram JW (1983) The origins of osteochondromas and enchondromas: a histopathologic study. Clin Orthop 174:264-294
Mirra JM, Picci P, Gold RH (1989) Bone tumors: clinical, radiologic and pathologic correlations. Lea & Febiger, Philadelphia
Moser RP (1990) Cartilaginous tumors of the skeleton. AFIP atlas of radiologic-pathologic correlations. Fasc II. Hanley & Belfus, Philadelphia
Murphy FD Jr, Blount WP (1962) Cartilaginous exostoses following irradiation. J Bone Joint Surg [Am] 44:662-668
Nojima T, Unni KK, McLeod RA et al. (1985) Periosteal chondroma and periosteal chondrosarcoma. Am J Surg Pathol 9:666-677
Nora FD, Dahlin DC, Beabout JW (1983) Bizarre parosteal osteochondromatous proliferation of the hands and feet. Am J Surg Pathol 7:245-250
Norman A, Sissons HA (1984) Radiographic hallmarks of peripheral chondromas. Radiology 151:589
Nosanchuk JK, Kaufer H (1969) Recurrent periosteal chondroma. Report of two cases and review of the literature. J Bone Joint Surg [Am] 51:375-380
Ollier L (1900) De la dyschondroplasie. Bull Soc Chir Lyon 3:22
Peterson HA (1989) Multiple hereditary osteochondromata. Clin Orthop 239:222
Rockwell MA, Saiter ET, Enneking WF (1972) Periosteal chondroma. J Bone Joint Surg [Am] 54:102-108
Sanerkin NG (1980) The diagnosis and grading of chondrosarcoma of bone. A combined cytologic and histologic approach. Cancer 45:582-594
Scaglietti O, Stringa G (1957) Periosteal myxoma of infancy and periosteal chondroma of adolescence, with local malignancy. Clin Orthop 9:147-157
Schajowicz F, Aiello CL, Slullitel JA (1970) Cystic and pseudocystic lesions of the terminal phalange with special reference to epidermoid cysts. Clin Orthop 68:84-92
Scherer E (1928) Exostosen, Enchondrome und ihre Beziehung zum Periost. Frankf Pathol 36:587
Schwartz HS, Zimmerman NB, Simon MA et al. (1987) The malignant potential of enchondromatosis. J Bone Joint Surg [Am] 69:269-274
Shapiro F, Simon S, Glincher MJ (1979) Hereditary multiple exostoses. J Bone Joint Surg [Am] 61:815
Shellito JG, Dockerty MB (1948) Cartilaginous tumors of the hand. Surg Gynecol Obstet 86:465-472
Slullitel I, Schajowicz F, Slullitel J (1954) Condromas e infartos isquémicos calcificados de los huesos largos. Bol Trab Soc Argent Ortop Traumatol 14:3-11
Slullitel JA, Schajowicz F, Slullitel J (1971) Osteochondrome solitair avec degenerscence maligne vers un sarcome osteogenique. Rev Clin Orthop 57:471-478
Solomon L (1963) Hereditary multiple exostosis. J Bone Joint Surg [Br] 45:292-304
Spjut HJ, Dorfman HD, Fechner RE, Ackerman LV (1971) Tumors of bone and cartilage. Atlas of tumor pathology, 2nd series, Fasc 5. Armed Forces Institute of Pathology, Washington DC
Sun TC, Swee RG (1985) Chondrosarcoma in Maffucci's syndrome. J Bone Joint Surg [Am] 67:1214-1219
Takigawa KMD (1971) Chondroma of the bones of the hand: a review of 110 cases. J Bone Joint Surg [Am] 53:1591-1600
Tiwisina T (1954) Dyschondroplasia (Ollier) mit multiplen Hämangiomen und örtlicher maligner Entartung (Chondrosarkom). Beitr Klin Chir 88:8-15
Trevor D (1950) Tarso-epiphyseal aclasis: a congenital error of epiphyseal development. J Bone Joint Surg [Br] 32:204
Twiston-Davies CW (1985) Bizarre parosteal osteochondromatous proliferation in the hand: a case report. J Bone Joint Surg [Am] 67:648-650
Vallance R, Hamblen DL, Kelly IG (1985) Vascular complications of osteochondromas. Clin Radiol 36:639
Virchow R (1891) Über multiple Exostosen. Berl Klin Wochenschr 28:1082
Wilner D (1982) Radiology of bone tumors and allied disorders. W.B. Saunders, Philadelphia

Chondroblastoma (Epiphyseal Chondroblastoma, Benign Chondroblastoma)

Abdul-Karim FW, Ayala AG, Spjut HJ (1985) Case report 321. Diagnosis: extraosseous chondroblastoma in the subcutaneous tissues of the right shoulder. Skeletal Radiol 14:73-75
Aronson RS, Hart WR, Martel W (1976) Metaphyseal chondroblastoma. AJR 127:686-688
Bertoni F, Unni KK, Beabout JW et al. (1987) Chondroblastoma of the skull and facial bones. Am J Clin Pathol 88:1-9
Bliss DG, Mann RJ (1985) Chondroblastoma of a metacarpal: report of a case and review of the literature. Clin Orthop 194:211-213

Bloem JL, Mulder JD (1985) Chondroblastoma: a clinical and radiological study of 104 cases. Skeletal Radiol 14:1–9

Bone Tumour Committee of the Japanese Orthopaedic Association National Cancer Center (1966) Collections of the registry of bone tumours in Japan, pp 93, 99

Brasse F, Schmitt M, Hoeffel JC et al. (1985) A case of vertebral chondroblastoma. Rev Chir Orthop 71:389–392

Brecher ME, Simon MA (1988) Chondroblastoma: an immunohistochemical study. Hum Pathol 19:1043–1047

Buraczewski J, Lysakowska J, Rudowski W (1957) Chondroblastoma (Codman's tumour) of the thoracic spine. J Bone Joint Surg [Br] 39:705–710

Campanacci M, Giunti A, Martucci E et al. (1977) Epiphyseal chondroblastoma: a study of 39 cases. Ital J Orthop Traumatol, English edn 3:67–74

Castleman B, McNeill JM (1966) Bone and joint clinicopathological conferences of the Massachusetts General Hospital. Little, Brown, Boston, p 220

Codman EA (1931) Epiphyseal chondromatous giant-cell tumors of the upper end of the humerus. Surg Gynecol Obstet 52:543–548

Coleman SS (1966) Benign chondroblastoma with recurrent soft-tissue and intra-articular lesions. J Bone Joint Surg [Am] 48:1554–1560

Coley BL (1960) Neoplasms of bone, 2nd edn. Harper (Hoeber), New York, p 131

Coley BL, Santoro AJ (1947) Benign central cartilaginous tumors of bone. Surgery 22:411–423

Copeland M, Geschickter CF (1949) Chondroblastic tumors of bone. Benign and malignant. Ann Surg 129:724–735

Copeland MM, Geschickter CF (1965) Cartilaginous tumors of bone. In: Tumors of bone and soft tissue. Papers presented at the University of Texas M.D. Anderson Hospital and Tumor Institute. Yearbook Medical, Chicago, p 279

Corsat J, Tomeno B, Forest M, Vinh TS (1989) Chondroblastomes bénins: une revue de 30 cas. Rev Chir Orthop 75:179–187

Dahlin DC (1956) Chondromyxoid fibroma of bone with emphasis on its morphological relationship to benign chondroblastoma. Cancer 9:195–203

Dahlin DC (1978) Bone tumors, 3rd edn. Charles C. Thomas, Springfield, IL

Dahlin DC, Ivins JC (1972) Benign chondroblastoma. A study of 125 cases. Cancer 30:401–413

Dahlin DC, Unni KK (1986) Bone tumors: general aspects and data on 8542 cases. Charles C. Thomas, Springfield, IL

Denko JV, Krauel LH (1955) Benign chondroblastoma of bone. An unusual localization in temporal bone. Arch Pathol 59:710–711

Ewing J (1928) Neoplastic diseases. A treatise of tumors, 3rd edn. W.B. Saunders, Philadelphia

Fechner RE, Wilde HD (1974) Chondroblastoma in the metaphysis of the femoral neck. A case report and review of the literature. J Bone Joint Surg [Am] 56:413–415

Feldman E (1977) Cartilaginous tumors and cartilage-forming tumor-like conditions of the bones and soft tissues. Encyclopedia of medical radiology, vol 6, Bone tumors. Springer, Berlin Heidelberg New York, pp 83–242

Flanning CV, Sneige NS, Carrasco CH et al. (1990) Fine needle aspiration cytology of chondroblastoma of bone. Cancer 65:1847–1863

Green P, Whittaker RP (1975) Benign chondroblastoma. Case report with pulmonary metastasis. J Bone Joint Surg [Am] 57:418–420

Hatcher CH (1945) The development of sarcoma in bone subjected to roentgen or radium irradiation. J Bone Joint Surg 27:179

Hull MT, Gonzalez-Crussi F, DeRosa GP et al. (1977) Aggressive chondroblastoma. Report of a case with multiple bone and soft tissue involvement. Clin Orthop 126:261–265

Huvos A, Marcove R, Erlandson R, Mike MD (1972) Chondroblastoma of bone. Cancer 29:760–771

Huvos AG, Higinbotham NL, Marcove RC et al. (1977) Aggressive behaviour and metastases with report of a new case. Clin Orthop 126:266–272

Jaffe HL (1958) Tumors and tumorous conditions of the bone and joints. Lea & Febiger, Philadelphia

Jaffe HL, Lichtenstein L (1942) Benign chondroblastoma of bone. A reinterpretation of the so-called calcifying or chondromatous giant cell tumor. Am J Pathol 18:969–983

Kahn LB, Wood FM, Ackerman LV (1969) Malignant chondroblastoma. Report of two cases and review of the literature. Arch Pathol 88:371–376

Kingsley TC, Markel SF (1971) Extraskeletal chondroblastoma: a report of the first reocrded case. Cancer 27:203–206

Kolodny A (1927) Bone sarcoma. The primary malignant tumors of bone and the giant cell tumor. Surg Gyencol Obstet 55:Suppl I

Kurt AM, Unni KK, Sim FH, McLeod RA (1989) Chondroblastoma of bone. Hum Pathol 20:965–976

Kyriakos M, Land VJ, Penning L et al. (1985) Metastatic chondroblastoma: report of a fatal case with a review of the literature on atypical, aggressive, and malignant chondroblastoma. Cancer 55:1770–1789

Levine GD, Bensch KMD (1972) Chondroblastoma. The nature of the basic cell. A study by means of histochemistry, tissue culture, electron microscopy and autoradiography. Cancer 29:1546–1562

Lichtenstein L (1952) Bone tumors, 2nd edn. C.V. Mosby, St. Louis

Lichtenstein L (1965) Bone tumors, 3rd edn. C.V. Mosby, St. Louis

Lichtenstein L, Bernstein D (1959) Unusual benign and malignant chondroid tumors of bone. Cancer 12: 1141–1157

Mayo-Smith W, Rosenberg AE, Khurana JS et al. (1990) Chondroblastoma of the rib: a case report and review of the literature. Clin Orthop 251:230–234

Mirra JM, Ulich TR, Eckardt JJ et al. (1983) "Aggressive" chondroblastoma. Light and ultra-microscopic findings after en bloc resection. Clin Orthop 178:276–284

Monda L, Wick MR (1985) S-100 protein immunostaining in the differential diagnosis of chondroblastoma. Hum Pathol 16:287–293

Moser RP (1990) Cartilaginous tumors of the skeleton. AFIP atlas of radiologic-pathologic correlations. Fasc II. Hanley & Belfus, Philadelphia

Ohno T, Park P, Oguro K et al. (1986) Ultrastructural study of clear-cell chondrosarcoma. Ultrastruct Pathol 10:321–330

Reyes CV, Kathuria S (1979) Recurrent and aggressive chondroblastoma of the pelvis with late malignant

neoplastic changes. Am J Surg Pathol (1979) 3:449–455
Riddell RD, Louis CJ, Bromberger H (1973) Pulmonary metastases from chondroblastoma of the tibia. Report of a case. J Bone Joint Surg [Br] 55:848–853
Salzer M, Salzer-Kuntschik M, Kretschmer G (1968) Das benigne Chondroblastom. Arch Orthop Unfallchir 64:229–244
Schajowicz F (1947) Epiphyseal chondroblastoma. Proc 4th International Cancer Research Congr, p 70
Schajowicz F, Gallardo H (1970) Epiphyseal chondroblastoma of bone. A clinico-pathological study of sixty-nine cases. J Bone Joint Surg [Br] 52:205–226
Schajowicz F, Cabrini RL, Simes RK et al. (1974) Ultrastructure of chondrosarcoma. Clin Orthop 100: 378–386
Schajowicz F, Donato de Próspero, Cosentino E (1990) Case report 641. Chondroblastoma-like osteosarcoma. Skeletal Radiol 19:603–606
Sherman RS, Uzel AR (1956) Benign chondroblastoma of bone. Its roentgen diagnosis. AJR 76:1132–1140
Sirsat MV, Doctor VM (1970) Benign chondroblastoma of bone. Report of a case of malignant transformation. J Bone Joint Surg [Br] 42:741–745
Sotelo-Avila C, Sundaram M, Kryriakos M et al. (1986) Case report 373. Skeletal Radiol 15:387
Springfield DS, Capanna R, Gherlinzoni F et al. (1985) Chondroblastoma: a review of seventy cases. J Bone Joint Surg [Am] 67:748–755
Sundaram M, McGuire MH, Naunheim K et al. (1988) Case report 467: cystic chondroblastoma left 4th rib. Skeletal Radiol 17:136–140
Sundaram TKS (1966) Benign chondroblastoma. J Bone Joint Surg [Br] 48:92–104
Valls J, Ottolenghi C, Schajowicz F (1951) Epiphyseal chondroblastoma of bone. J Bone Joint Surg [Am] 33:997–1009
Weiss APC, Dorfman HD (1986) S-100 protein in human cartilage lesions. J Bone Joint Surg [Am] 68:521–526
Wellman KF (1969) Chondroblastoma of the scapula. Cancer 24:408–416
Welsh RA, Meyer AT (1964) A histogenetic study of chondroblastoma. Cancer 17:578–589
Wirman JA, Crissman JD, Aron BF (1979) Metastatic chondroblastoma. Report of an unusual case treated with radiotherapy. Cancer 44:87–93
Wisniewski M, Toker C, Anderson PJ et al. (1973) Chondroblastoma of the cervical spine. Case report. J Neurosurg 38:763–766
Wright JL, Sherman MS (1964) An unusual chondroblastoma. J Bone Joint Surg [Am] 46:597–600

Chondromyxoid Fibroma (Fibromyxoid Chondroma)

Adler CP (1981) Fibromyxoma of the femoral neck. J Cancer Res Clin Oncol 101:183–189
Aegerter E, Kirkpatrick JA Jr (1975) Orthopedic diseases: physiology, pathology, radiology, 4th edn. W.B. Saunders, Philadelphia
Andrew T, Kenwright J, Woods C (1982) Periosteal chondromyxoid fibroma of the tibia: a case report. Acta Orthop Scand 53:467–470
Barros RE, Dominguez FV, Cabrini RL (1969) Myxoma of the jaws. Oral Surg 27:225–236
Bauer WH, Harell A (1954) Myxoma of bone. J Bone Joint Surg [Am] 36:263–266
Benedetti GB, Canepa G, Garcia M (1962) Il fibroma condromixoide dell'osso. Revisione critica della letteratura ed indagini istologiche ed istochemiche su 8 casi. Arch Putti Chir Organi Mov 17:44–72
Benson WR, Bass S (1975) Chondromyxoid fibroma. First report of occurrence of this tumor in vertebral column. Am J Clin Pathol 25:1290–1292
Bialik V, Kedar A, Ben-Arie Y et al. (1985) Case report 315. Diagnosis: parosteal (periosteal, juxtacortical) chondromyxoid fibroma of the upper end of the femur. Skeletal Radiol 13:323–326
Bloodgood JC (1924) Bone tumors. Myxoma. Ann Surg 80:817–833
Bone Tumour Committee of the Japanese Orthopaedic Association National Cancer Center (1966) Collections of the bone tumours in Japan, pp 98–99
Caballes RL (1979) Fibromyxoma of bone. Radiology 130:97–99
Chacha PB, Tan KK (1972) Periosteal myxoma of the femur: a case report. J Bone Joint Surg [Am] 54: 1091–1094
Coley BL, Santoro AJ (1947) Benign central cartilaginous tumours of bone. Surgery 22:411–423
Crabbé WA (1962) Chondromyxoid fibroma of bone. Proc R Soc Med 55:353
Dahlin DC (1956) Chondromyxoid fibroma of bone, with emphasis on its morphological relationship to benign chondroblastoma. Cancer 9:195–203
Dahlin DC (1967) Bone tumors, 2nd edn. Charles C. Thomas, Springfield, IL, pp 48–57
Dahlin DC (1978) Bone tumors, 3rd edn. Charles C. Thomas, Springfield, IL
Dahlin DC, Unni KK (1986) Bone tumors: general aspects and data on 8542 cases. Charles C. Thomas, Springfield, IL
Dahlin DC, Wells AH, Henderson ED (1953) Chondromyxoid fibroma of bone. J Bone Joint Surg [Am] 35:831–834
Feldman F (1977) Cartilaginous tumors and cartilage forming tumor like conditions of the bones and soft tissues. In: Ranniger K (ed) Bone tumors. Diseases of the skeletal system. Springer, Berlin Heidelberg New York
Feldman F, Hecht HL, Johnston AD (1970) Chondromyxoid fibroma of bone. Radiology 94:249–260
Gherlinzoni F, Rock M, Picci P (1983) Chondromyxoid fibroma. The experience at Istituto Ortopedico Rizzoli. J Bone Joint Surg [Am] 65:198–204
Gilmer WS, Highley GB, Kilgore WE (1963) Atlas of bone tumors, including tumor-like lesions. C.V. Mosby, St. Louis, pp 36–39
Goldman AB, Vigorita VJ (1983) Case report 245: fibromyxoma of the femur. Skeletal Radiol 10: 197–200
Goorwitch J (1951) Chondromyxoid fibroma of rib; report of an unusual benign primary tumor. Dis Chest 30:186–193
Hutchison J, Park WW (1960) Chondromyxoid fibroma of bone. J Bone Joint Surg [Br] 52:542–548
Iwata S, Coley BL (1958) Report of six cases of chondromyxoid fibroma of bone. Surg Gynecol Obstet 101:571–576

Jaffe HL (1958) Tumors and tumorous conditions of the bones and joints. Lea & Febiger, Philadelphia

Jaffe HL, Lichtenstein L (1948) Chondromyxoid fibroma of bone: a distinctive benign tumor likely to be mistaken especially for chondrosarcoma. Arch Pathol 45:541–551

Kangur TT, Dahlin DC, Turlington EG (1975) Myxomatous tumors of the jaws. J Oral Surg 33:523–528

Kreicbergs A, Lonnquist PA, Willems J (1985) Chondromyxoid fibroma: a review of the literature and a report on our own experience. Acta Pathol Microbiol Immunol Scand [A] 93:189–197

Kyriakos M (1979) Soft tissue implantation of chondromyxoid fibroma. Am J Surg Pathol 3:363–372

Lichtenstein L (1977) Bone tumors, 5th edn. C.V. Mosby, St. Louis

Lichtenstein L, Bernstein D (1959) Unusual benign and malignant chondroid tumors of bone. Cancer 12:1142–1157

Marcove RC, Kambolis C, Bullough PG, Jaffe HL (1964) Fibromyxoma of bone: a report of three cases. Cancer 17:1209–1213

Marcove RC, Lindeque BG, Huvos AG (1989) Fibromyxoma of the bone. Surg Gynecol Obstet 169:115–118

McLure DK, Dahlin DC (1977) Myxoma of bone: report of 3 cases. Mayo Clin Proc 52:249–253

Monda L, Wick MR (1985) S-100 protein immunostaining in the differential diagnosis of chondroblastoma. Hum Pathol 16:287–293

Netherlands Committee on Bone Tumours (1966) Radiological atlas of bone tumours, vol 1. Mouton, The Hague, p 6

Nunez C, Bennett T, Bohlman HH (1982) Chondromyxoid fibroma of the thoracic spine: case report and review of the literature. Spine 7:436–439

Ottolenghi CE, Petracchi LJ (1953) Chondromyxosarcoma of the calcaneus. J Bone Joint Surg [Am] 35:211–214

Perou ML, Kolis JA, Zaeske EV et al. (1967) Myxoma of the toe: case report. Cancer 20:1030–1034

Rahimi A, Beabout JW, Ivins JC et al. (1972) Chondromyxoid fibroma: a clinicopathologic study of 76 cases. Cancer 30:726–736

Ralph LL (1962) Chondromyxoid fibroma of bone. J Bone Joint Surg [Br] 44:7–24

Scaglietti O, Stringa G (1956) Mixoma periostale dell'infanzia e condroma periostale dell'adolescenza a malignita locale. Arch Putti Chir Organi Mov 7:13–28

Scaglietti O, Stringa G (1961) Myxoma of bone in childhood. J Bone Joint Surg [Am] 43:67–80

Schajowicz F (1987) Chondromyxoid fibroma: report of three cases with predominant cortical involvement. Radiology 164:783–786

Schajowicz F, Cabrini RL (1958a) Histochemical studies on glycogen in normal ossification and calcification. J Bone Joint Surg [Am] 40:1081

Schajowicz F, Cabrini RL (1958b) Histochemical localization of acid phosphatase in bone tissue. Science 127:1447

Schajowicz F, Gallardo H (1971) Chondromyxoid fibroma (fibromyxoid chondroma) of bone. Clinicopathological study of 32 cases. J Bone Joint Surg [Br] 53:198–216

Steiner GC (1979) Ultrastructure of benign cartilaginous tumors of intraosseous origin. Hum Pathol 10:71–86

Teitelbaum SL, Bessone L (1969) Resection of a large chondromyxoid fibroma of the sternum. Report of the first case and review of the literature. J Thorac Cardiovasc Surg 57:333–349

Turcotte B, Pugh DG, Dahlin DC (1962) The roentgenologic aspects of chondromyxoid fibroma of bone. Am J Roentgenol Radium Ther Nucl Med 87:1085–1095

Ushigome S, Takakuwa T, Shinagawa T et al. (1982) Chondromyxoid fibroma of bone: an electron microscopic observation. Acta Pathol Jpn 32:113–122

Ushigome S, Takakuwa T, Shinagawa T et al. (1984) Ultrastructure of cartilaginous tumors and S-100 protein in the tumors. With reference to the histogenesis of chondroblastoma, chondromyxoid fibroma and mesenchymal chondrosarcoma. Acta Pathol Jpn 34:1285–1300

Weiss APC, Dorfman HD (1986) S-100 protein in human cartilage lesions. J Bone Joint Surg [Am] 68:521–526

Zillmer DA, Dorfman HD (1989) Chondromyxoid fibroma of bone: thirty-six cases with clinicopathologic correlation. Hum Pathol 20:952–964

Chondrosarcoma

Alho A, Connor JF, Mankin HJ, Schiller AL, Campbell CJ (1983) Assessment of malignancy of cartilage tumors using flow cytometry: a preliminary report. J Bone Joint Surg [Am] 65:779–785

Anderson CE, Ludowieg J, Eyring EJ, Horowitz B (1963) Ultrastructure and chemical composition of chondrosarcoma: report of one case. J Bone Joint Surg [Am] 45:753

Angervall L, Kindblom LG (1980) Clear-cell chondrosarcoma: a light- and electron-microscopic and histochemical study of two cases. Virchows Arch [A] 389:27–41

Aprin H, Riseborough EJ, Hall JE (1982) Chondrosarcoma in children and adolescents. Clin Orthop 166:226–232

Awtar K (1975) Rapid flow cytofluorometric analysis of mammalian cell cycle by propidium iodide staining. J Cell Biol 66:188

Barnes R, Catto M (1966) Chondrosarcoma of bone. J Bone Joint Surg [Br] 48:729–764

Boström H, Friberg U, Larsson KS et al. (1968) In vitro incorporation of S^{35}-sulfate in chondrosarcomatous tissue. Acta Orthop Scand 39:58–72

Buckwalter JA (1983) The structure of human chondrosarcoma proteoglycans. J Bone Joint Surg [Am] 65:958–974

Campanacci M, Guernelli N, Leonessa C, Boni A (1975) Chondrosarcoma: a study of 133 cases, 80 with long-term follow-up. Ital J Orthop Traumatol 1:387–414

Cannon SR, Sweetnam DR (1985) Multiple chondrosarcomas in dyschondroplasia (Ollier's disease). Cancer 55:836–840

Chamber RG, Friedel W (1976) Chondrosarcoma of the larynx. Laryngoscope 86:713–717

Clark JV, Maloney AF (1974) Letter: chondrosarcoma. Arch Pathol 98:69

Coley BL, Higinbotham NL (1954) Secondary chondrosarcoma. Ann Surg 139:547–559

Coltrera MD, Googe PB, Harrist TJ et al. (1986) Chondrosarcoma of the temporal bone. Diagnosis and treatment of 13 cases and review of the literature. Cancer 58:2689–2696

Copeland MM, Geschickter CG (1965) Cartilaginous tumors of bone. In: Dybala LW, Freitag SB, Culhane DC (eds) Tumors of bone and soft tissue. Yearbook Medical, Chicago, pp 279–298

Dahlin DC (1976) Chondrosarcoma and its "variant." In: Ackerman LV, Spjut HJ, Abell MR (eds) Bone and joints. Williams & Wilkins, Baltimore, pp 300–311

Dahlin DC (1978) Bone tumors, 3rd edn. Charles C. Thomas, Springfield, IL

Dahlin DC, Henderson ED (1956) Chondrosarcoma, a surgical and pathological problem. Review of 212 cases. J Bone Joint Surg [Am] 38:1025–1038

Dahlin DC, Salvador AH (1974) Chondrosarcomas of bone of the hands and feet. A study of 30 cases. Cancer 34:755–760

Dahlin DC, Unni KK (1986) Bone tumors: general aspects and data on 8542 cases. Charles C. Thomas, Springfield, IL

Enzinger FM, Shiraki M (1972) Extraskeletal myxoid chondrosarcoma. An analysis of 36 cases. Hum Pathol 36:421–435

Erlandson RA, Huvos AG (1974) Chondrosarcoma: a light and electron-microscope study. Cancer 34:1642–1652

Evans HL, Ayala AG, Rohmsdahl MD (1977) Prognostic factors in chondrosarcoma of bone: a clinicopathologic analysis with emphasis on histologic grading. Cancer 40:808–837

Ewing JA (1939) A review of the classification of bone tumors. Bull Am Coll Surg 24:290–295

Faraggiana T, Sender B, Glicksman P (1981) Light- and electron-microscopic study of clear cell chondrosarcoma. Am J Clin Pathol 75:117–121

Fu YS, Kay S (1974) Comparative ultrastructural study of mesenchymal chondrosarcoma and myxoid chondrosarcoma. Cancer 33:1531–1542

Garrison RC, Unni KK, McLeod RA, Pritchard DJ, Dahlin DC (1982) Chondrosarcoma arising in osteochondroma. Cancer 49:1890–1897

Gilmer WS Jr, Kilgore W, Smith H (1963) Central cartilage tumors of bone. Clin Orthop 26:81–103

Gitelis S, Bertoni F, Picci P, Campanacci M (1981) Chondrosarcoma of bone: the experience at the Istituto Ortopedico Rizzoli. J Bone Joint Surg [Am] 63:1248–1257

Goethals PL, Dahlin DC, Devine KD (1963) Cartilaginous tumors of the larynx. Surg Gynecol Obstet 117:77–82

Gottschalk RG, Smith RT (1963) Chondrosarcoma of the hand. Report of a case with radioactive sulphur studies and review of literature. J Bone Joint Surg [Am] 45:141–150

Gottschalk RG, Alpert LK, Albert RE (1959) The use of large amounts of radioactive sulfur in patients with advanced chondrosarcomas. Cancer Res 19:1070–1077

Grabias S, Mankin HJ (1974) Chondrosarcoma arising in histologically proved unicameral bone cyst: a case report. J Bone Joint Surg [Am] 56:1501–1509

Harwood AR, Krajbich JI, Fornasier VL (1980) Radiotherapy of chondrosarcoma of bone. Cancer 45:2769–2777

Hatcher CH, Campbell JC (1951) Benign chondroblastoma of bone: its histologic variations and a report of late sarcoma in the site of bone. Bull Hosp Joint Dis 12:411–430

Healy JH, Lane JM (1986) Chondrosarcoma. Clin Orthop 204:119–129

Heffelfinger MJ, Dahlin DC, MacCarty CS et al. (1973) Chordomas and cartilaginous tumors at the skull base. Cancer 32:410–420

Henderson ED, Dahlin DC (1963) Chondrosarcoma of bone: a study of 288 cases. J Bone Joint Surg [Am] 45:1450–1458

Hudson TM, Springfield DS, Spanier SS et al. (1984) Benign exostoses and exostotic chondrosarcoma: evaluation of cartilage thickness by CT. Radiology 12:595–599

Huvos AG (1991) Bone tumors: diagnosis, treatment, prognosis. W.B. Saunders, Philadelphia

Huvos AG, Marcove RC (1987) Chondrosarcomas in the young. A clinicopathologic analysis of 79 patients younger than 21 years of age. Am J Surg Pathol 11:930–942

Huvos AG, Higinbotham NL, Miller TR (1972) Bone sarcomas arising in fibrous dysplasia. J Bone Joint Surg [Am] 54:1047–1056

Jacobson E, Spjut HJ (1960) Chondrosarcoma of the bones of the hand: report of three cases. Acta Radiol Scand 54:426–436

Jaffe HL (1958) Tumors and tumorous conditions of the bones and joints. Lea & Febiger, Philadelphia

Jaworski RC (1984) Intermitochondrial paracrystalline inclusions in chondrosarcoma. Pathology 16:172–173

Justis EJ Jr, Dart RC (1983) Chondrosarcoma of the hand with metastasis: a review of the literature and case report. J Hand Surg 8:320–324

Keiller VH (1925) Cartilaginous tumors of bone. Surg Gynecol Obstet 40:510–521

Kenney PJ, Gilula LA, Murphy WA (1981) The use of computed tomography to distinguish osteochondroma and chondrosarcoma. Radiology 139:129–137

Kragh LV, Dahlin DC, Erich JB (1960) Cartilaginous tumors of the jaws and facial regions. Am J Surg 99:852–856

Kreicbergs A, Boquist L, Borssén B, Larsson SE (1982) Prognostic factors in chondrosarcoma: a comparative study of cellular DNA content and clinicopathologic features. Cancer 50:577–583

Kreicbergs A, Silvferswärd C, Tribukait B (1984) Flow DNA analysis of primary bone tumors: relationship between cellular DNA content and histopathologic classification. Cancer 53:129–136

Lansche WE, Spjut HJ (1958) Chondrosarcoma of the small bones of the hands. J Bone Joint Surg [Am] 40:1139–1145

Larsson SE, Borssen R, Boquest L (1979) Chondrosarcoma: multifactorial clinical and histopathological study with particular regard to therapy and survival. Int Orthop 2:333–341

Lewis MM, Marcove RC, Bullough PG (1975) Chondrosarcoma of the foot: a case report and review of the literature. Cancer 36:586–589

Lichtenstein L (1977) Bone tumors, 5th edn. C.V. Mosby, St. Louis

Lichtenstein L, Jaffe HL (1943) Chondrosarcoma of bone. Am J Pathol 19:553–589

Lindbom A, Soderberg G, Spjut HJ (1961) Primary chondrosarcoma of bone. Acta Radiol 55:81–96

Lodwick GS (1965) A systemic approach to roentgen diagnosis of bone tumors. Tumors of bone and soft tissues. Yearbook Medical, Chicago

Lodwick GS (1984) The radiologist's role in the management of chondrosarcoma. Radiology 150:275

Mangini U (1967) Tumors of the skeleton of the hand. Bull Hosp Joint Dis 38:61–108

Mankin HJ, Cantley KP, Lippiello L, Schiller AL (1979) The biology of human chondrosarcoma. Histological and biochemical classification of 74 tumors. Trans 25th Annu Meet Orthop Res Soc 4:173

Mankin HJ, Cantley KP, Lippiello L, Schiller AL, Campbell CJ (1980a) The biology of human chondrosarcoma. I. Description of the cases, grading, and biochemical analyses. J Bone Joint Surg [Am] 62:160–176

Mankin HJ, Cantley KP, Schiller AL, Lippiello L (1980b) The biology of human chondrosarcoma. II. Variation in chemical composition among types and subtypes of benign and malignant cartilage tumors. J Bone Joint Surg [Am] 62:176–188

Mankin HJ, Conner JF, Schiller AL et al. (1985) Grading of bone tumors by analysis of nuclear DNA content using flow cytometry. J Bone Joint Surg [Am] 67: 404–413

Marcove RC (1977) Chondrosarcoma: diagnosis and treatment. Orthop Clin North Am 8:811–820

Marcove RC, Huvos AG (1971) Cartilaginous tumors of the ribs. Cancer 27:794–801

Marcove RC, Mike V, Hutter RVP, Huvos AG (1972) Chondrosarcoma of the pelvis and upper end of the femur. J Bone Joint Surg [Am] 54:561–572

Marcove RC, Stovell PB, Huvos AG, Bullough PG (1977) The use of cryosurgery in the treatment of low and medium grade chondrosarcoma. Clin Orthop 12:147 155

Martin RF, Melnick PJ, Warner NE et al. (1973) Chordoid sarcoma. Am J Clin Pathol 59:623–635

McCarthy EF, Dorfman HD (1982) Chondrosarcoma of bone with dedifferentiation: a study of eighteen cases. Hum Pathol 13:36–40

McKenna RJ, Schwinn CP, Soong KY, Higinbotham NL (1966) Sarcomata of the osteogenic series (osteosarcoma, fibrosarcoma, chondrosarcoma, periosteal osteogenic sarcoma and sarcomata arising in abnormal bone. An analysis of 552 cases. J Bone Joint Surg [Am] 48:1–26

Mirra JM, Gold R, Downs J et al. (1985) A new histologic approach to the differentiation of enchondroma from chondrosarcoma of bones. A clinico-pathologic analysis of 51 cases. Clin Orthop 201:214–237

Mondolfo S (1968) Chondrosarcomas. Rev Ortop Traumatol Lat-Am 13:159–170

Morton DL, Malmgren RA, Hall WT, Schidlowsky G (1969) Immunologic and virus studies with human sarcomas. Surgery 66:152

Neel HB III, Unni KK (1982) Cartilaginous tumors of the larynx: a series of 33 patients. Otolaryngol Head Neck Surg 90:201–207

O'Neal LW, Ackerman LV (1952) Chondrosarcoma of bone. Cancer 5:551–577

Pachter MR, Alpert M (1964) Chondrosarcoma of the foot skeleton. J Bone Joint Surg [Am] 46:601–607

Palmieri TJ (1984) Chondrosarcoma of the hand. J Hand Surg 9:332–338

Pardo-Mindan FJ, Guillen FJ, Villas C et al. (1981) A comparative ultrastructural study of chondrosarcoma, chordoid sarcoma, and chordoma. Cancer 47:2611–2619

Patel MR, Pearlman HS, Engler J, Wallowick BS (1977) Chondrosarcoma of the proximal phalanx of the finger. Review of the literature and report of a case. J Bone Joint Surg [Am] 59:401–403

Phemister DV (1930) Chondrosarcoma of bone. Surg Gynecol Obstet 50:216–233

Povýsil C, Matejovsky Z (1985) A comparative ultrastructural study of chondrosarcoma, chordoid sarcoma, chordoma and chordoma periphericum. Pathol Res Pract 179:546–559

Price CH, Goldie W (1969) Paget's sarcoma of bone. A study of 80 cases from the Bristol and the Leeds bone tumour registers. J Bone Joint Surg [Br] 51:205–224

Pritchard DJ, Lunke RJ, Taylor WF, Dahlin DC, Medley BE (1980) Chondrosarcoma: a clinicopathologic and statistical analysis. Cancer 45:149–157

Remberger K, Gay S (1977) Immunohistochemical demonstration of different collagen types in the normal epiphyseal plate and in benign and malignant tumors of bone and cartilage. Z Krebsforsch 90:95–106

Roberg OT (1935) Chondrosarcoma. The relation of structure and location to the clinical course. Surg Gynecol Obstet 61:68–82

Roberts PH, Price CHG (1977) Chondrosarcoma of the bones of the hands. J Bone Joint Surg [Br] 59:213–221

Rosenberg L, Francis K, Gallo G, Margolis R, Strider W, Pal S (1976) Isolation and characterization of proteoglycan subunit and proteoglycan aggregate from human chondrosarcoma. Trans 22nd Ann Meet Orthop Res Soc 1:32

Rosenthal DI, Schiller AL, Mankin HJ (1984) Chondrosarcoma: correlation of radiological and histological grade. Radiology 150:21–26

Salib PI (1967) Chondrosarcoma: a study of the cases treated at the Massachusetts General Hospital in 27 years (1937–1963). Am J Orthop 9:240–242

Sanerkin NG (1980) The diagnosis and grading of chondrosarcoma of bone: a combined cytologic and histologic approach. Cancer 45:582–594

Schajowicz F, Bessone JE (1967) Chondrosarcoma in three brothers. J Bone Joint Surg [Am] 49:129–141

Schajowicz F, Cambiaggi JE (1961) Chondrosarcoma de mano. Bol Trab Soc Argent Traumatol 25:191–198

Schajowicz F, Defilippi-Novoa CA, Firpo CA (1967) Thorotrast induced chondrosarcoma of the axilla. Am J Roentgenol Radium Ther Nucl Med 100:931–937

Schajowicz F, Cabrini RL, Simes RJ, Klein-Szanto AIP (1974) Ultrastructure of chondrosarcoma. Clin Orthop 100:378–386

Schajowicz F, Giménez IB, Conti CJ et al. (1976) Estudio microespectrofotométrico de ADN en condromas y condrosarcomas. Bol Trab Soc Argent Ortop Traumatol 41:147–154

Shives TC, McLeod RA, Unni KK, Schray MF (1990) Chondrosarcoma of the spine. J Bone Joint Surg [Am] 17:1158–1165

Slullitel JA, Schajowicz F, Slullitel J (1971) Ostéochondrome solitaire avec dégénerescence maligne vers un sarcome ostéogenique. Rev Chir Orthop 57:471–478

Spjut HJ, Dorfman HD, Fechner RE, Ackerman LV (1971) Tumors of bone and cartilage. Atlas of tumor pathology, 2nd series, Fasc 5. Armed Forces Institute of Pathology, Washington, DC

Suit HD, Goitein M, Munzenrider J et al. (1982) Definitive radiation therapy for chordoma and

chondrosarcoma of base of skull and cervical spine. J Neurosurg 56:377–385
Thomson AD, Turner-Warwick RT (1955) Skeletal sarcomata and giant-cell tumor. J Bone Joint Surg [Br] 37:266–303
Trias A, Basora J, Sánchez G et al. (1978) Chondrosarcoma of the hand. Clin Orthop 134:297–300
Weiss SW (1976) Ultrastructure of the so-called "chondroid sarcoma." Evidence supporting cartilaginous differentiation. Cancer 37:300–306
Wetzel WJ, Reuhl KR (1980) Microtubular aggregates in the rough endoplasmic reticulum of a myxoid chondrosarcoma. Ultrastruct Pathol 1:519–525
Wilner D (1982) Radiology of bone tumors and allied disorders. W.B. Saunders, Philadelphia
Wolford JF, Bedetti CD (1988) Skeletal myxoid chondrosarcoma with microtubular aggregates within rough endoplasmic reticulum. Arch Pathol Lab Med 112:77–81
Wu KK, Collon DJ, Guise ER (1980) Extra-osseous chondrosarcoma: report of five cases and review of the literature. J Bone Joint Surg [Am] 62:189–194
Yaghmai I (1978) Angiographic features of chondromas and chondrosarcomas. Skeletal Radiol 3:91–98

Dedifferentiated Chondrosarcoma

Abenoza P, Neumann MP, Manivel JC et al. (1986) Dedifferentiated chondrosarcoma: an ultrastructural study of two cases, with immunocytochemical correlations. Ultrastruct Pathol 10:529–538
Astorino RN, Tesluk H (1985) Dedifferentiated chondrosarcoma with a rhabdomyosarcomatous component. Hum Pathol 16:318–320
Barnes R, Catto M (1966) Chondrosarcoma of bone. J Bone Joint Surg [Br] 48:729–764
Bertoni F, Present D, Picci P et al. (1985) Case report 301. Diagnosis: dedifferentiated chondrosarcoma of the upper end of the humerus. Skeletal Radiol 13:228–232
Campanacci M, Bertoni F, Capanna R (1979) Dedifferentiated chondrosarcomas. Ital J Orthop Traumatol 5:331–341
Capanna R, Bertoni F, Betteli G et al. (1988) Dedifferentiated chondrosarcoma. J Bone Joint Surgery [Am] 70:60–69
Dahlin DC, Beabout JW (1971) Dedifferentiation of low-grade chondrosarcoma. Cancer 28:461–466
Dahlin DC, Unni KK (1986) Bone tumors: general aspects and data on 8542 cases. Charles C. Thomas, Springfield, IL
DeLange EE, Pope TL Jr, Fechner RE (1986) Dedifferentiated chondrosarcoma: radiographic features. Radiology 160:489–492
Evans HL, Ayala AG, Rohmsdahl MD (1977) Prognostic factors in chondrosarcoma of bone. A clinicopathologic analysis with emphasis on histologic grading. Cancer 40:808–837
Fechner RE, Huvos AG, Mirra JM et al. (1984) A symposium on the pathology of bone tumors. Pathology Annual. Part I. Appleton-Century-Crofts, Norwalk, CT
Foulds L (1949) Mammary tumors in hybrid mice; growth and progression of spontaneous tumors. Br J Cancer 3:345–375
Frassica FJ, Unni KK, Beabout JW et al. (1986) Dedifferentiated chondrosarcoma: a report of the clinicopathological features and treatment of seventy-eight cases. J Bone Joint Surg [Am] 68:1197–1205
Fu YS, Kay S (1974) Comparative ultrastructural study of mesenchymal chondrosarcoma and myxoid chondrosarcoma. Cancer 33:1531–1542
Gitelis S, Block JA, Inerot SE (1989) Clonal analysis of human chondrosarcoma. 35th Annual Meeting, Orthop Research Soc. Orthop Trans 13:443
Huvos AG (1991) Bone tumors: diagnosis, treatment, prognosis. W.B. Saunders, Philadelphia
Jaworski RC (1984) Dedifferentiated chondrosarcoma: an ultrastructural study. Cancer 53:2674–2678
Johnson S, Tetu B, Ayala AG et al. (1986) Chondrosarcoma with additional mesenchymal component (dedifferentiated chondrosarcoma). I. A clinicopathologic study of 26 cases. Cancer 58:278–286
Kahn LB (1976) Chondrosarcoma with dedifferentiated loci: a comparative and ultrastructural study. Cancer 37:1365–1375
McCarthy EF, Dorfman HD (1982) Chondrosarcoma of bone with dedifferentiation: a study of eighteen cases. Hum Pathol 13:36–40
McFarland GB, McKinley LM, Reed RJ (1977) Dedifferentiation of low-grade chondrosarcomas. Clin Orthop 122:157–164
Mirra JM, Marcove RC (1974) Fibrosarcomatous dedifferentiation of primary and secondary chondrosarcoma: review of five cases. J Bone Joint Surg [Am] 56:285–296
Steiner GC, Mirra JM, Bullough PG (1973) Mesenchymal chondrosarcoma. A study of the ultrastructure. Cancer 32:926–939
Tetú B, Ordóñez NG, Ayala AG et al. (1986) Chondrosarcoma with additional mesenchymal component (dedifferentiated chondrosarcoma). II. An immunohistochemical and electron microscopic study. Cancer 58:287–298
Van Rijssel TG (1973) Progression in bone tumors. Proc Symp Colston Res Soc 24:88–91

Juxtacortical (Periosteal) Chondrosarcoma

Cooper RR (1965) Juxtacortical chondrosarcoma. J Bone Joint Surg [Am] 57:524–528
Dahlin DC (1978) Bone tumors, 3rd edn. Charles C. Thomas, Springfield, IL
Jaffe HL (1958) Tumors and tumorous conditions of the bones and joints. Lea & Febiger, Philadelphia
Jokl P, Albright JA, Goodman AH (1971) Juxtacortical chondrosarcoma of the hand. J Bone Joint Surg [Am] 53:1370–1376
Lichtenstein L (1955) Tumors of periosteal origin. Cancer 8:1060–1069
Nojima T, Unni KK, McLeod RA et al. (1985) Periosteal chondroma and periosteal chondrosarcoma. Am J Surg Pathol 9:666–677

Norman A, Sissons HA (1984) Radiographic hallmarks of periosteal chondrosarcoma. Radiology 151:589–596
Nosanchuk JS, Kaufer H (1969) Recurrent periosteal chondroma. J Bone Joint Surg [Am] 51:375–380
Schajowicz F (1977) Juxtacortical chondrosarcoma. J Bone Joint Surg [Br] 59:473–480
Schajowicz F, Bessone JE (1967) Chondrosarcoma in three brothers. J Bone Joint Surg [Am] 49:129–141
Unni KK, Dahlin DC, Beabout JW (1976) Periosteal osteogenic sarcoma. Cancer 37:2476–2485
Wu KK, Kelly AP (1977) Periosteal (juxtacortical) chondrosarcoma: report of a case occurring in the hand. J Hand Surg 2:314–315

Mesenchymal Chondrosarcoma

Albores-Saavedra J, Angeles-Angeles A, Ridaura C et al. (1977) Embryonal chondrosarcoma in children. Patologia 15:153–162
Bertoni F, Picci P, Bacchini P et al. (1983) Mesenchymal chondrosarcoma of bone and soft tissue. Cancer 52:533–541
Christiansen RE Jr (1982) Mesenchymal chondrosarcoma of the jaws. Oral Surg 54:197–206
Dabska M, Huvos AG (1983) Mesenchymal chondrosarcoma in the young. Virchows Arch [A] 399:89–104
Dahlin DC, Henderson ED (1962) Mesenchymal chondrosarcoma. Further observations on a new entity. Cancer 15:410–417
Dahlin DC, Unni KK (1986) Bone tumors: general aspects and data on 8542 cases. Charles C. Thomas, Springfield, IL
Dardick I, Lagace R, Carlier MT et al. (1983) Chordoid sarcoma (extraskeletal myxoid chondrosarcoma). Virchows Arch [A] 399:61–78
Dowling EA (1964) Mesenchymal chondrosarcoma. J Bone Joint Surg [Am] 46:747–754
Enzinger FM, Weiss SW (1988) Soft tissue tumors, 2nd edn. C.V. Mosby, St. Louis
Fu YS, Kay S (1974) Comparative ultrastructural study of mesenchymal chondrosarcoma and myxoid chondrosarcoma. Cancer 33:1531–1542
Goldman RL (1967) Mesenchymal chondrosarcoma. A rare malignant chondroid tumor usually primary in bone. Report of a case arising in extraskeletal soft tissue. Cancer 20:1494–1498
Guccioni JG, Font RL, Enzinger FM, Zimmerman LE (1973) Extraskeletal mesenchymal chondrosarcoma. Arch Pathol 95:336–340
Harwood AR, Krajbich JI, Fornasier VL (1981) Mesenchymal chondrosarcoma: a report of 17 cases. Clin Orthop 158:144–148
Hutter RVP, Foote RW Jr, Francis KC, Sherman RS (1966) Primitive multipotential primary sarcoma of bone. Cancer 19:1–25
Huvos AG (1991) Bone tumors: diagnosis, treatment, prognosis. W.B. Saunders, Philadelphia
Huvos AG, Rosen G, Dabska M et al. (1983) Mesenchymal chondrosarcoma. A clinicopathologic analysis of 35 patients with emphasis on treatment. Cancer 51:1230–1237
Jacobson SA (1977) Polyhistioma. A malignant tumor of bone and extraskeletal tissues. Cancer 40:2116–2130
Lichtenstein L, Bernstein D (1959) Unusual benign and malignant chondroid tumors of bone. Cancer 12:1142–1157
Martínez-Tello FJ, Navas-Palacios JJ (1982) Ultrastructural study of conventional chondrosarcomas and myxoid and mesenchymal chondrosarcomas. Virchows Arch [A] 396:197–211
Mazabraud A (1974) Mesenchymal chondrosarcoma: six cases. Rev Chir Orthop 60:197–203
Mikata A, Iri H, Inuya MA (1977) Mesenchymal chondrosarcoma: a case report with an ultrastructural study and review of Japanese literature. Acta Pathol Jpn 27:93–109
Nakashima Y, Unni KK, Shives TC et al. (1986) Mesenchymal chondrosarcoma of bone and soft tissue: a review of 111 cases. Cancer 57:2444–2453
Nezelof C, Mazabraud A, Meary R (1965) Le chondrosarcome mesenchymateux: a propos d'un cas de localization parachidienne. Arch Anat Pathol 13:26–28
Pepe AJ, Kuhlman RF, Miller DB (1977) Mesenchymal chondrosarcoma: a case report. J Bone Joint Surg [Am] 59:256–258
Rech MJ (1966) Hemangiopericytoma with cartilaginous differentiation involving orbit. Arch Ophthalmol 75:82–83
Salvador AH, Beabout JW, Dahlin DC (1971) Mesenchymal chondrosarcoma: observations on 30 new cases. Cancer 28:605–615
Schajowicz F, Ceballos E, Gallardo M (1973) Condrosarcoma mesenquimático: Estudio clínico patológico. Bol Soc Argent Ortop Traumatol 38:223–228
Scheithauer BW, Rubinstein LJ (1978) Meningeal mesenchymal chondrosarcoma: report of 8 cases with review of the literature. Cancer 42:2744–2752
Spjut HJ, Dorfman HD, Fechner RE, Ackerman LV (1971) Tumors of bone and cartilage. Atlas of tumor pathology, 2nd series, Fasc 5. Armed Forces Institute of Pathology, Washington, DC
Steiner GC, Mirra JM, Bullough PG (1973) Mesenchymal chondrosarcoma: a study of the ultrastructure. Cancer 32:926–939

Clear-Cell Chondrosarcoma

Bjornsson J, Unni KK, Dahlin DC, Beabout JW, Sim FH (1984) Clear cell chondrosarcoma of bone: observations in 47 cases. Am J Surg Pathol 8:223–230
Campanacci M, Bertoni F, Laus M (1980) Clear-cell chondrosarcoma. Ital J Orthop Traumatol 6:365–372
Faraggiana T, Sender B, Glicksman P (1981) Light- and electron-microscopic study of clear-cell chondrosarcoma. Am J Clin Pathol 75:117–121
Foulds L (1949) Mammary tumors in hybrid mice; growth and progression of spontaneous tumors. Br J Cancer 3:345–375
Huvos AG, Higinbotham NL, Marcove RC et al. (1977) Aggressive chondroblastoma: review of the literature of aggressive behaviour and metastases with report of a new case. Clin Orthop 126:266–272
Kahn LB, Wood FM, Ackerman LV (1969) Malignant chondroblastoma: report of two cases and review of the literature. Arch Pathol 45:541–551

Kumar R, David R, Cierney G III (1985) Clear-cell chondrosarcoma. Radiology 154:45–48

Le Charpentier Y, Forest M, Postel M et al. (1979) Clear-cell chondrosarcoma: a report of five cases including ultrastructural study. Cancer 44:622–629

Monda L, Wick MR (1985) S-100 protein immunostaining in the differential diagnosis of chondroblastoma. Hum Pathol 16:287–293

Salzer-Kuntschik M (1981) Clear-cell chondrosarcoma. J Cancer Res Clin Oncol 101:171–176

Schajowicz F, Gallardo H (1970) Epiphyseal chondroblastoma of bone: a clinico-pathological study of sixty-nine cases. J Bone Joint Surg [Br] 52:205–226

Schajowicz F, Lemos C (1976) Malignant osteoblastoma. J Bone Joint Surg [Br] 58:202

Unni KK, Dahlin DC, Beabout JW, Sim JH (1976) Chondrosarcoma clear cell variant: a report of sixteen cases. J Bone Joint Surg [Am] 58:676–683

Van Rijssel TG (1973) Progression in bone tumors. Proc Symp Colston Res Soc 24:88–91

Vauzelle JL, Caille JP, Patricot LM et al. (1978) Clear-cell chondrosarcoma: a new case. Lyon Med 240:25

Weiss APC, Dorfman HD (1986) S-100 protein in human cartilage lesions. J Bone Joint Surg [Am] 68:521–526

CHAPTER III
Giant-Cell Tumor (Osteoclastoma)

Definition, WHO: "*An aggressive tumor, characterized by richly vascularized tissue consisting of rather plump spindle-shaped or ovoid cells and by the presence of numerous giant cells of osteoclast type, which are uniformly distributed throughout the tumor tissue. Relatively little collagen is present. Areas of hemorrhage and regressive changes, such as necrosis, fibrosis, and fibrohistiocytic reaction, are frequently present, especially in larger or longstanding tumors.*"

Giant-cell tumor is one of the most problematic bone neoplasms. Many important questions concerning the histogenesis, clinicopathologic diagnosis, and treatment still remain the subject of considerable controversy. Separation of the true giant-cell tumor of bone from the group of so-called variants (Ewing 1928) and from other dysplastic, metabolic, or granulomatous bone lesions, with which it has been confused in the past, is often difficult.

It has become evident that the view held by Nelaton (1860), Gross (1879), and Bloodgood (1923) that the giant-cell tumor is a uniformly benign lesion is no longer valid. True giant-cell tumors can no longer be considered innocent growths; on the contrary, they represent a *progressive, potentially malignant process* that can recur in about 20%–40% of patients, undergo sarcomatous transformation in about 5%–10%, and even produce metastases without apparent previous malignant changes. Mirra (1980) suggested the term "low-grade malignant neoplastic giant-cell tumor" as the most appropriate designation, which is similar to Uehlinger's denomination "semimalignant" (1976). The alleged variants (Table III.1), on the other hand, usually have a favorable evolution and can be cured with curettage or roentgenotherapy in low doses.

Many lesions are classified as giant-cell tumors merely because of their roentgenographic appearance or because of the presence of giant cells in the histologic preparations, when actually the lesions so classified are of minor importance (see variants in Table III.1). This procedure has contributed to the prevailing confusion and has prevented the establishment of uniform criteria for the treatment of giant-cell tumors. More than in any other bone tumor, the clinical features, particularly the patient's age, the radiographic appearance, and the gross and microscopic features, must be considered together in order to reach an accurate diagnosis. However, the histologic appearance must be considered to be most important.

Incidence. Giant-cell tumor of bone is infrequent. There are only a few recent publications of large series of more than 50 cases, most of them reporting material from registries. For example, the Bristol Tumour Registry recorded 52 cases over a 25-year period (McGrath 1972), which had increased by 1978 to 135 cases (McInerney and Middlemis 1978), and the Swedish Cancer Registry recorded 53 cases over 10 years (Larsson et al. 1975). The important series of Goldenberg et al. (1970) cites 218 cases collected from six different institutions, including 74 cases from Jaffe's collection. There are only a few institutions that have published their own series: Hutter et al. (1962), reporting 76 cases from the Memorial Hospital, New York; Campanacci et al. (1975), with 209 cases from the Rizzoli Institute,

Table III.1. Giant-cell tumor variants (Ewing 1928)

Former variant designation	Present classification and synonyms
Chondromatous	Benign chondroblastoma Codman's tumor Epiphyseal chondroblastoma Epiphyseal chondromatous giant-cell tumor Chondroblastoma
Myxomatous	Chondromyxoid fibroma Fibromyxoid chondroma
Xanthomatous	Nonosteogenic fibroma Nonossifying fibroma Fibrous cortical defect Metaphyseal fibrous defect Histiocytic xanthogranuloma Benign fibrous histiocytoma
Telangiectatic or subperiosteal	Aneurysmal bone cyst Multilocular hematic bone cyst

Bologna; and Merle D'Aubigné and Tomeno (1977), with an analysis of the treatment of 85 giant-cell tumors recorded over a 22-year period (1950–1972) at the Hospital Cochin (Paris). Giant-cell tumor seems to be frequent in China, Sung et al. (1981) reporting 208 cases. The last and largest series is that of the Mayo Clinic (Dahlin and Unni 1986), with 425 cases collected over 70 years (including 20 cases of the so-called malignant giant-cell tumor), representing 5% of the total number of bone tumors. The most recent publication of Huvos (1991) reported 265 cases treated at the Memorial Hospital, and Campanacci (1990) reported 539 cases from the Rizzoli Institute, Bologna.

In a previous paper (1961), the writer reviewed a series of 85 giant-cell tumors studied in his laboratory in the course of 20 years. As of December 1985, the number of cases of true giant-cell tumors had increased to 460. Other giant-cell lesions of bone, including the so-called variants and solitary bone cysts, had increased to 1095. The incidence of true giant-cell tumors represents 8.6% of all bone tumors.

Clinical Findings. *Age and Sex.* The age and sex distribution is shown in Scheme III.1.

Almost all patients were skeletally mature; only 15 were under the age of 15 years, and the occurrence of a true giant-cell tumor under the age of 10 is exceptional (four cases). In Dahlin's series of 425 cases only three patients were under 10 years of age (8 or 9 years old) and eight were in the age group of 10–14 years; in Goldenberg's series no patients were under 10 years of age. As in other statistics, the greatest number of giant-cell tumors in our series occurred in patients between 20 and 40 years of age (61%), with a peak incidence in the third decade. Thirty-six patients were more than 50 years old, the oldest being 68 years old.

It is noteworthy that some European authors (Goidanich 1956), and especially French authors (Trifaud et al. 1956), reported a large number of cases of giant-cell tumors in children. Of the 89 cases in the series of Trifaud and associates, ten were in children under 10 years of age, and 42 were in patients younger than 20 years. In a revision of older material of the Children's

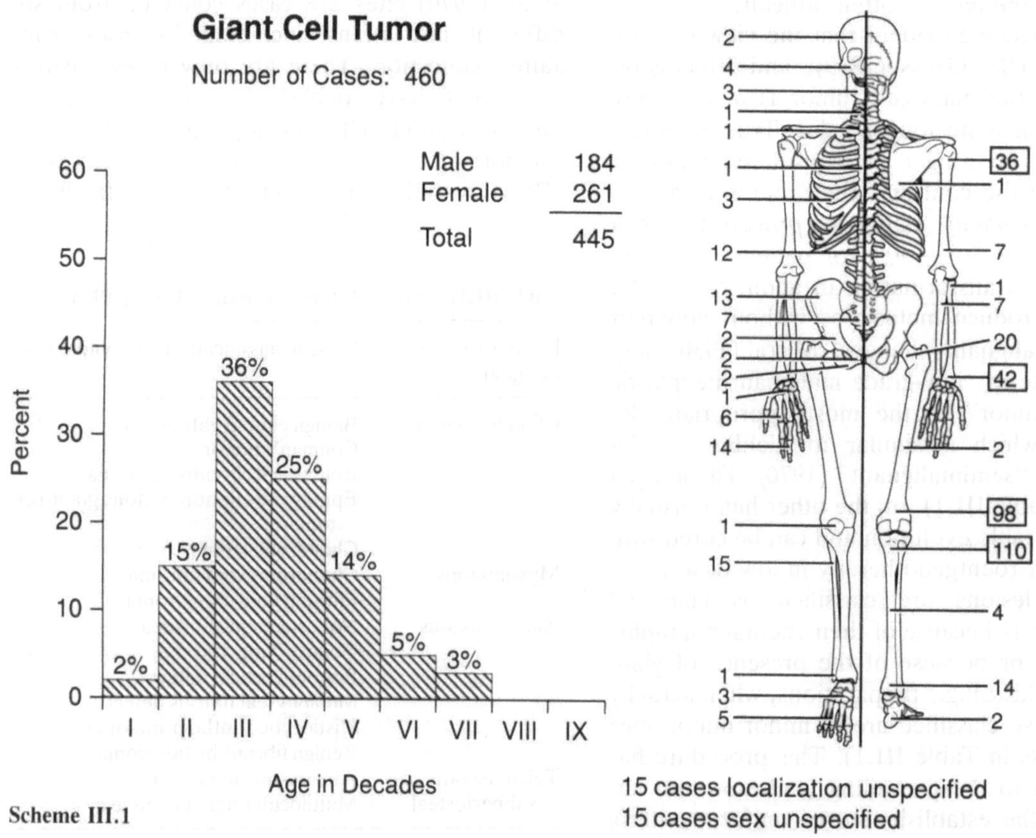

Scheme III.1

a b, c

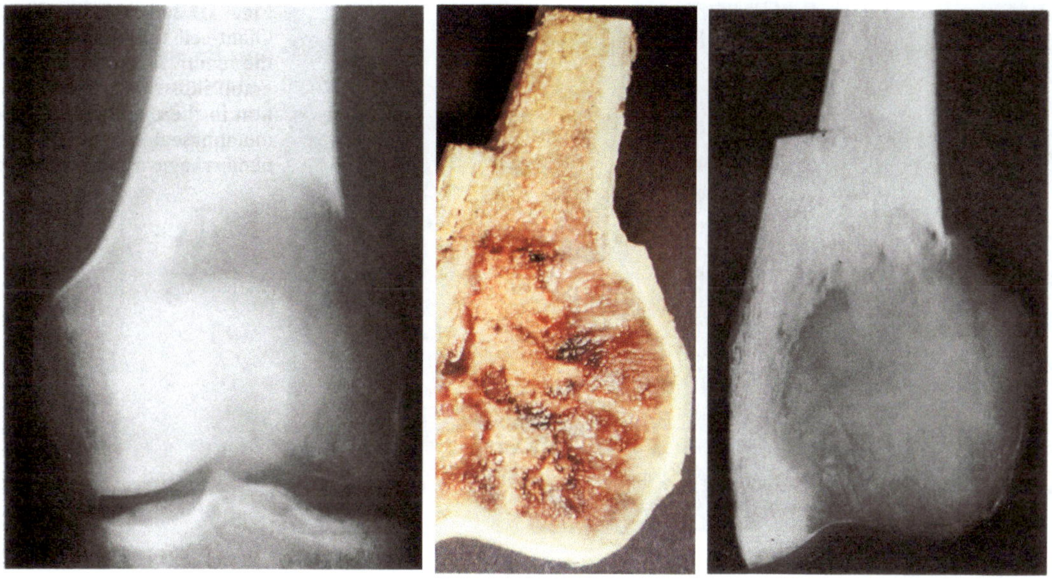

Fig. III.1a–c. Male, 56 years old. Giant-cell tumor of the lower end of the femur. **a** Radiograph illustrates a radiolucent lesion located eccentrically in the lateral femoral condyle and expanding the thinned cortex, which is destroyed in great part. Note the ill-defined borders toward the medullary cavity. **b** Photograph and **c** radiograph of a longitudinal section of the resection specimen

a b, c

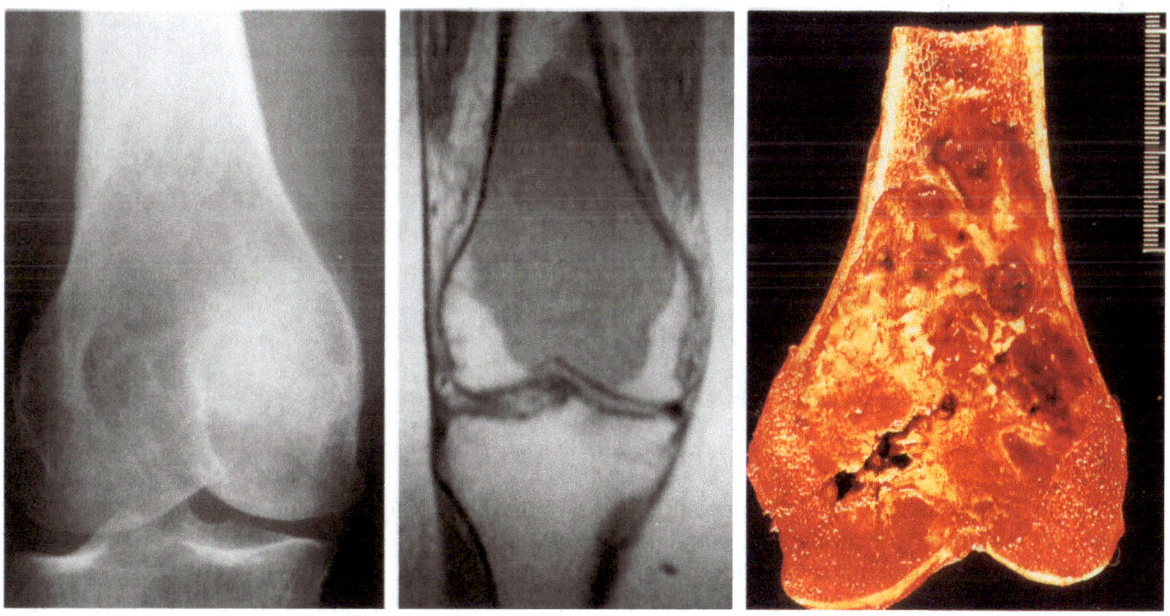

Fig. III.2a–c. Female, 33 years old. Giant-cell tumor of the lower end of the femur. **a** Radiograph shows the extension of the radiolucent lesion, which involves the whole width of the meta-epiphyseal region, as is better demonstrated on **b** T1-weighted coronal MRI scan and **c** a photograph of the resected specimen. This case, like the following figures, corresponds radiologically to the aggressive grade. (St. Louis University Medical Center)

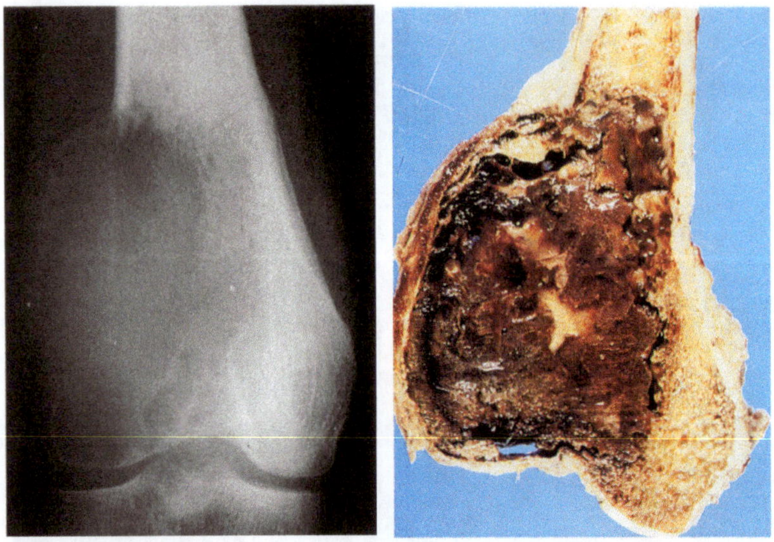

a b

Fig. III.3a,b. Male, 38 years old. Giant-cell tumor of the lower end of the femur. **a** Radiograph and **b** photograph illustrate the eccentric localization in the epiphysis and the adjacent metaphyseal region, and the reddish hemorrhagic aspect of this solid tumor

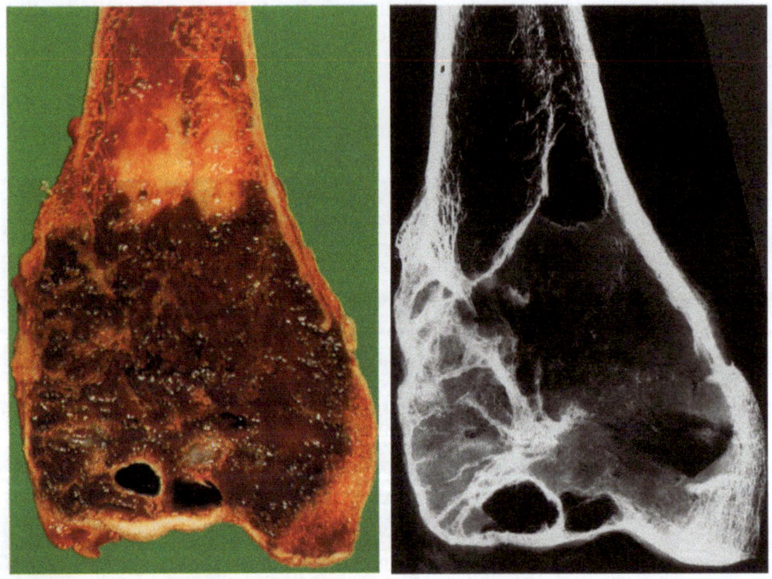

a b

Fig. III.4a,b. Female, 27 years old. Giant-cell tumor of the lower end of the femur. **a** Photograph and **b** radiograph of the resected specimen, showing the hemorrhagic aspect of the solid tumor, which occupies the whole width of the lower femur

Hospital in Buenos Aires, carried out with Dr. Derqui, 50 tumors or pseudotumors, simulating and classified as giant-cell tumor in children under 12 years of age, were reexamined; not one case of genuine giant-cell tumor was found (Schajowicz 1961).

In our series, the incidence in females was greater than in males by a ratio of 1.5 to 1. This agrees with the statistics of the majority of authors: Goldenberg et al. (1970) reported 125 females and 93 males; Dahlin and Unni (1986), 240 females and 185 males; and Huvos (1991), 147 females and 118 males. Campanacci (1990) found only a slight female predominance (52.5% to 47.5%).

Localization. As shown in Scheme III.1, the *most frequent anatomic sites* in our series were the lower end of the femur (98 cases) (Figs. III.1–III.5), upper end of the tibia (110 cases) (Figs. III.6–III.11), lower end of the radius (42 cases) (Figs. III.12b, III.13), and upper end of the humerus (36 cases) (Fig. III.14).

If we include the tumors at the upper fibular end (15 cases), approximately 50% occurred about the knee (Figs. III.15, III.16). The relative

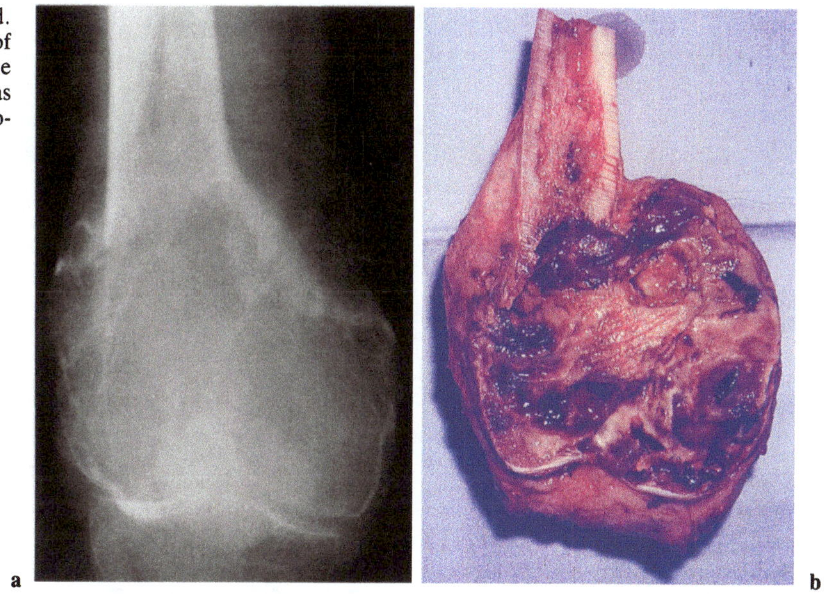

Fig. III.5a,b. Male, 36 years old. Giant-cell tumor of the lower end of the femur. **a** Radiograph showing the large size of the lesion, which has partly destroyed the cortex. **b** Photograph of the resected specimen

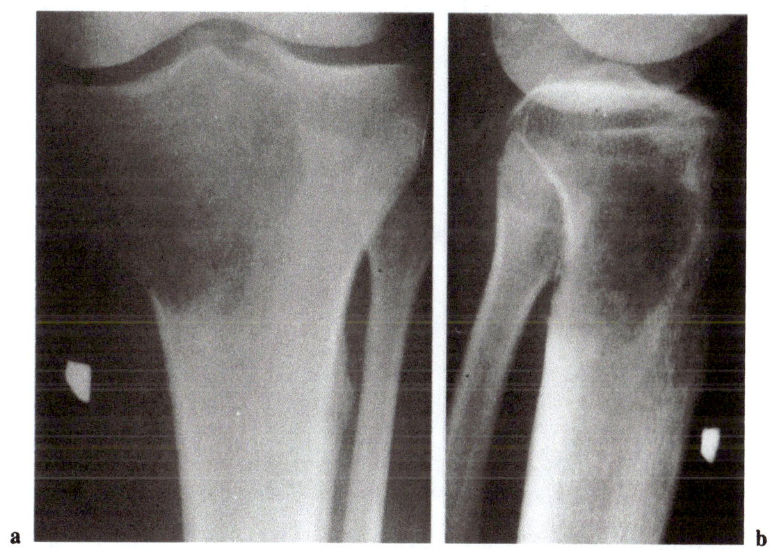

Fig. III.6a,b. Female, 48 years old. Giant-cell tumor of the upper end of the tibia. **a,b** Anteroposterior and lateral radiographs show a radiolucent, ill-defined lesion located eccentrically in the epiphysis of the tibia

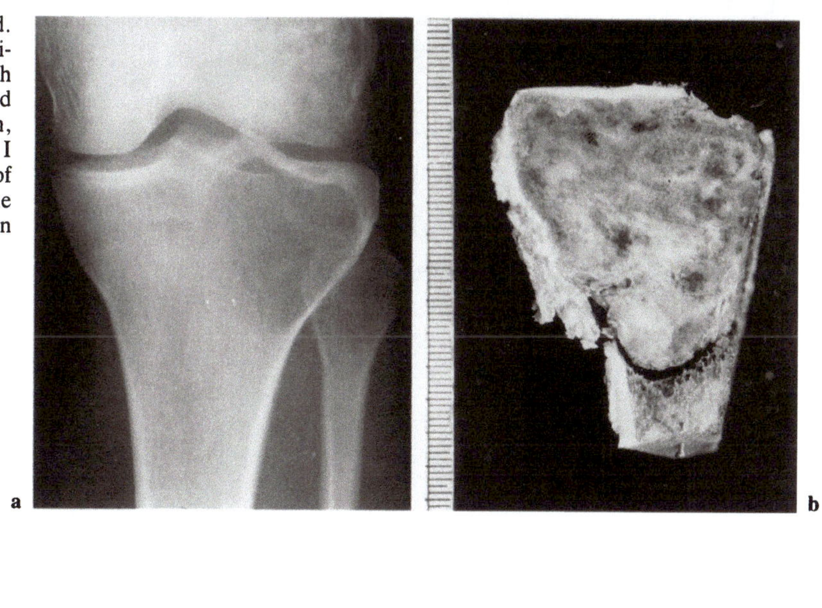

Fig. III.7a,b. Female, 25 years old. Giant-cell tumor of the upper epiphyseal end of the tibia. **a** Radiograph shows the small size of the tumor and its eccentric subchondral location, without expanding the cortex (grade I or quiescent type). **b** Photograph of the hemiresection demonstrates the solid aspect and juxta-articular location

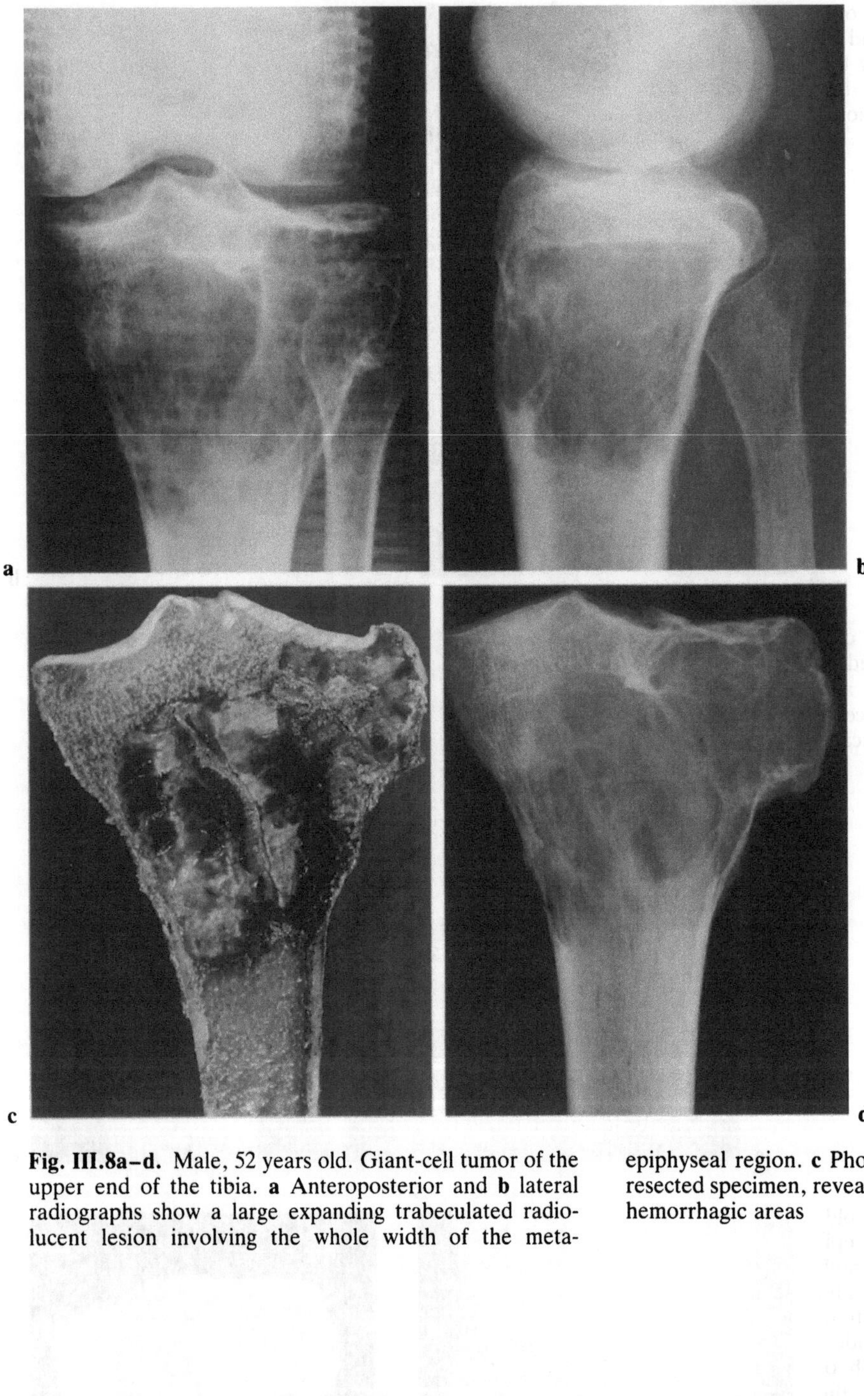

Fig. III.8a–d. Male, 52 years old. Giant-cell tumor of the upper end of the tibia. **a** Anteroposterior and **b** lateral radiographs show a large expanding trabeculated radiolucent lesion involving the whole width of the metaepiphyseal region. **c** Photograph and **d** radiograph of the resected specimen, revealing alternating grayish-white and hemorrhagic areas

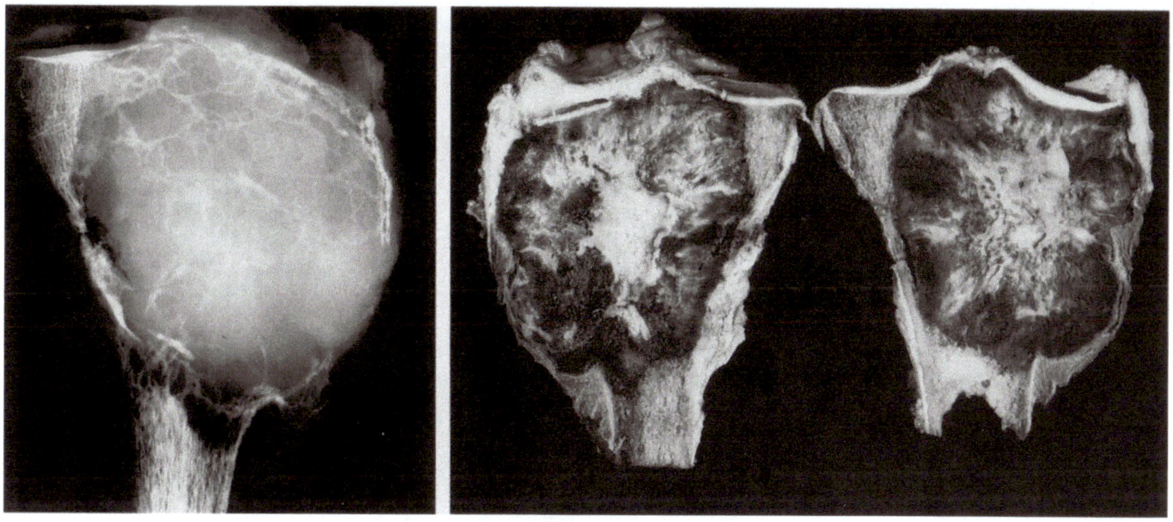

a b

Fig. III.9a,b. Female, 34 years old with giant-cell tumor of the upper end of the tibia. **a** Radiograph and **b** photograph show the large size of this trabeculated tumor, which has partly destroyed the extremely expanded and thinned cortex

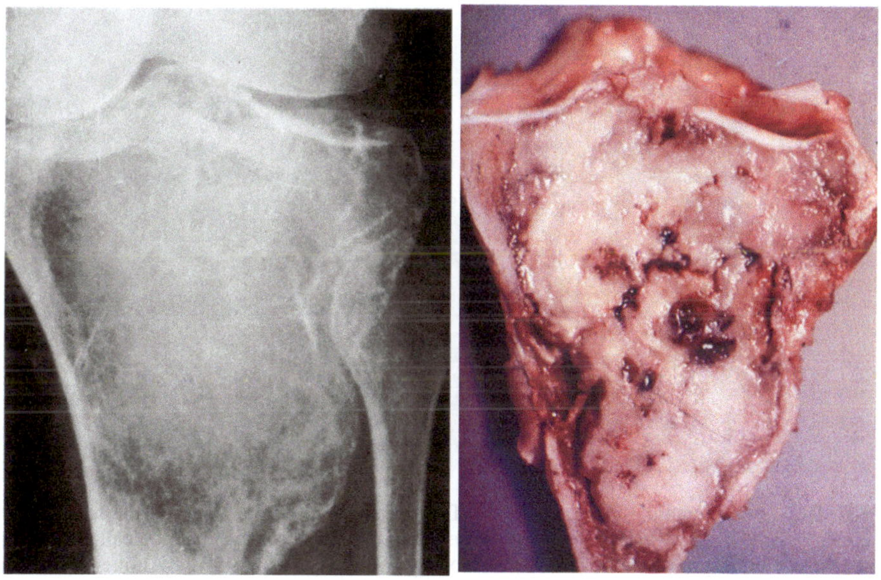

a b

Fig. III.10a,b. Female, 30 years old. Giant-cell tumor of the upper tibia. **a** Radiograph shows a large, osteolytic, expanding lesion involving the meta-epiphyseal region. **b** Photograph of the specimen reveals that most of the tumor is predominantly of grayish-white color with scarce hemorrhagic areas, and that it has expanded the cortex without perforating it

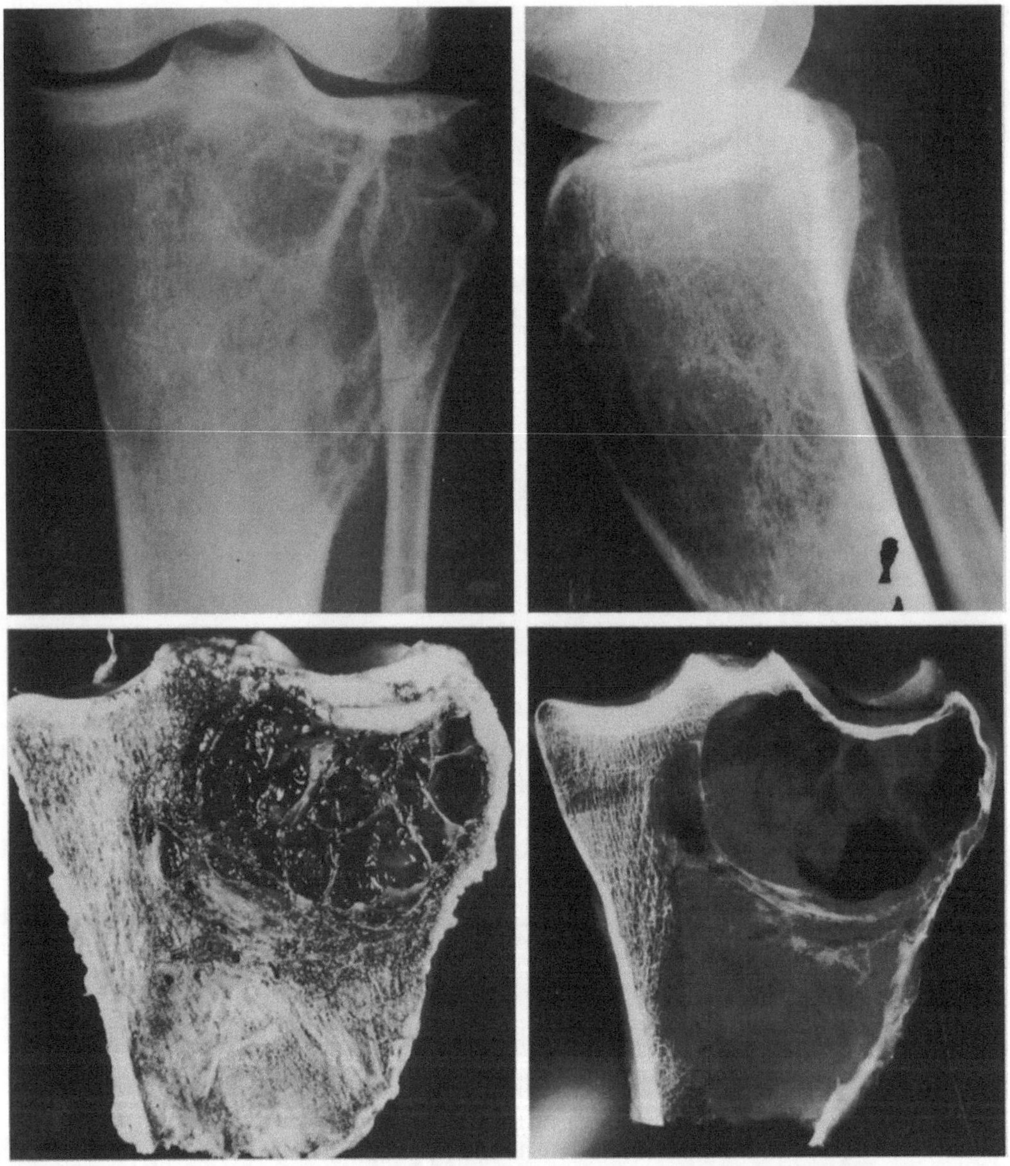

a b c

Fig. III.11a–c. Female, 26 years old. **a** Tumor of the upper end of tibia with features of giant-cell tumor and secondary aneurysmal bone cyst. **b** Photograph and **c** radiograph show the cystic, multiloculated aspect of the upper part of the lesion and the solid pattern of its lower part. Histologically, the cystic areas had the aspect of aneurysmal bone cyst. A segmental resection was performed, followed by cadaver bone graft

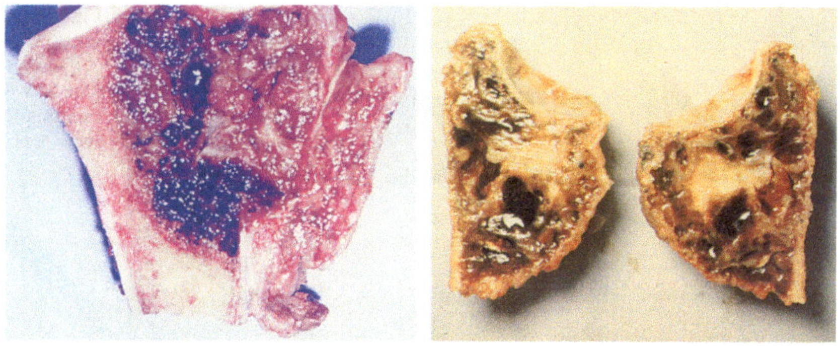

a b

Fig. III.12a,b. Photographs of two different cases of giant-cell tumor with secondary aneurysmal bone cyst-like changes located at **a** the proximal tibia and **b** the distal radius

Fig. III.13a–c. Female, 35 years old. Giant-cell tumor of the lower end of radius. **a** Anteroposterior and lateral radiographs reveal a large expansile lesion with extensive destruction of the thinned cortex and invasion of soft tissue. A malignant tumor was suspected, but no histologic signs of malignancy were observed. **b** Photograph and **c** radiograph of the resected specimen illustrate the solid aspect of most of the tumor, with large cystic, blood-filled spaces at its lower aspect, grossly and histologically similar to aneurysmal bone cyst

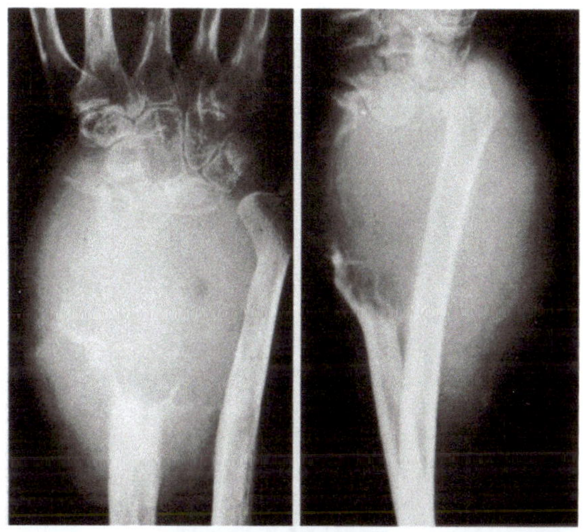

a

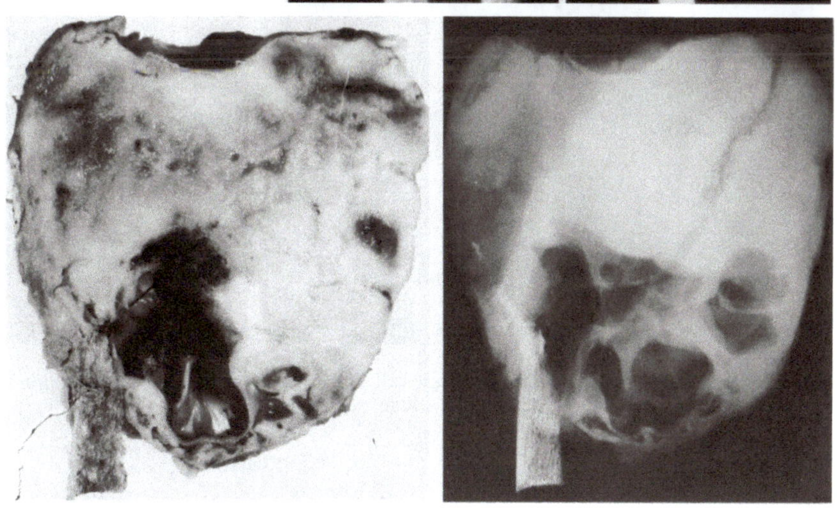

b c

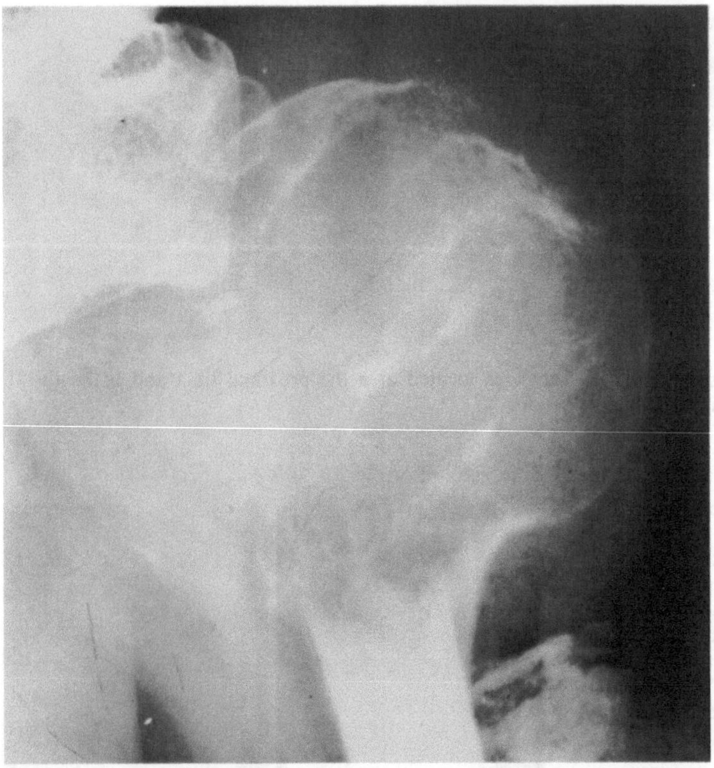

Fig. III.14. Female, 17 years old. Radiograph showing the enormous size of a giant-cell tumor of the upper end of the humerus, which was histologically without sign of malignancy; the patient is well and without recurrence 2 years after wide bloc resection

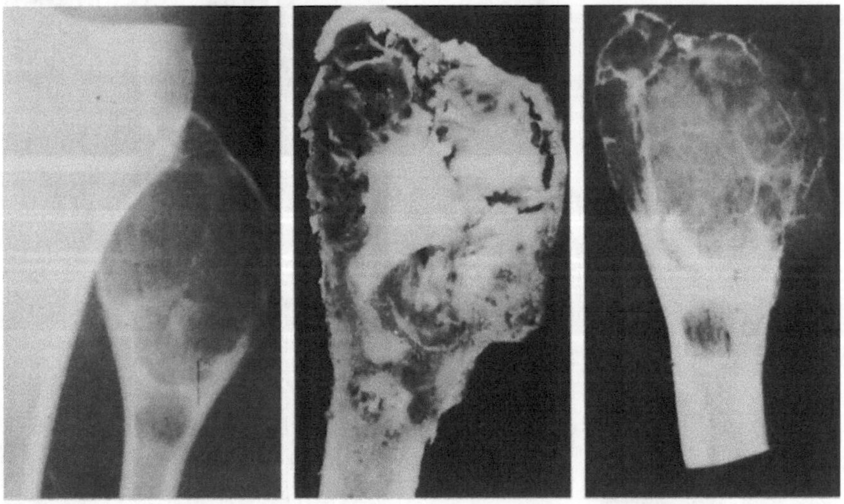

a, b c

Fig. III.15a–c. Female, 27 years old. Giant-cell tumor of upper end of fibula. **a** Radiograph shows a lytic expansile lesion. **b** Photograph and **c** radiograph of the resected specimen

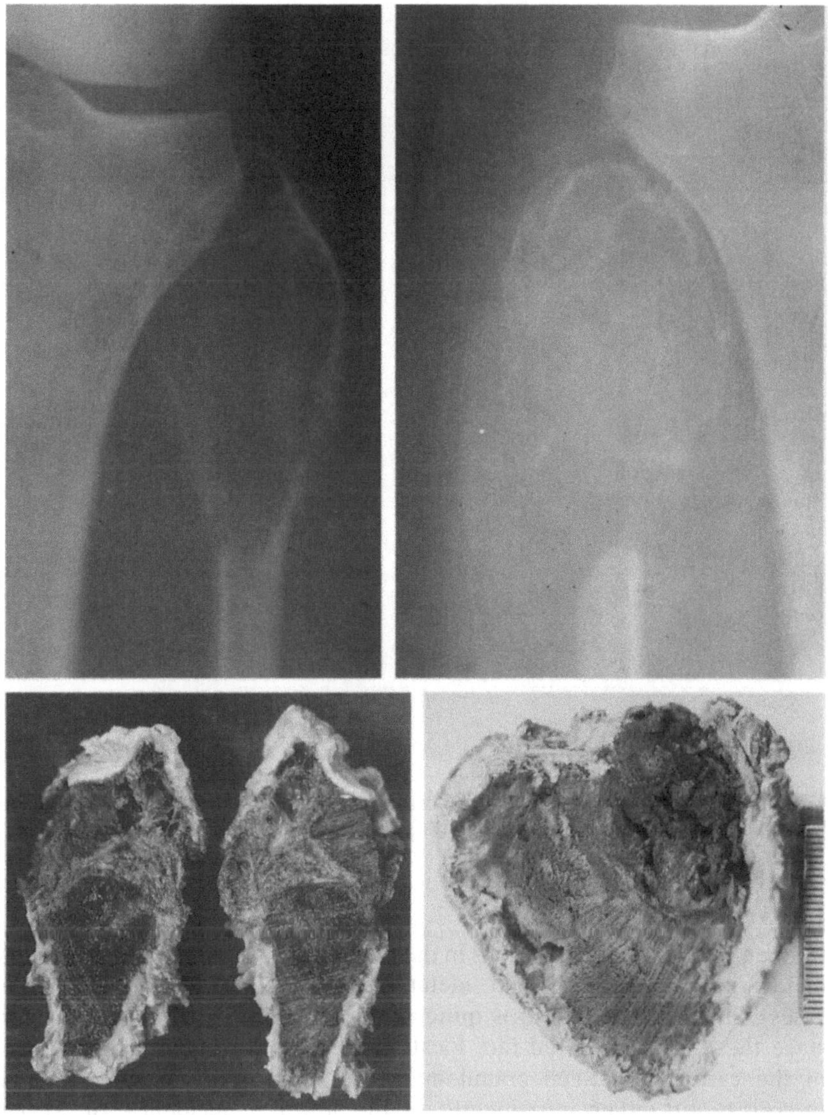

Fig. III.16a–d. Female, 41 years old. Recurrent giant-cell tumor of the upper end of the fibula. **a** Radiograph and **b** photograph of the resected specimen show an expansile, radiolucent, solid hemorrhagic lesion. **c** Radiograph and **d** photograph of the apparently subperiosteal recurrence at the same site, similar to the primary tumor, 10 months after the resection

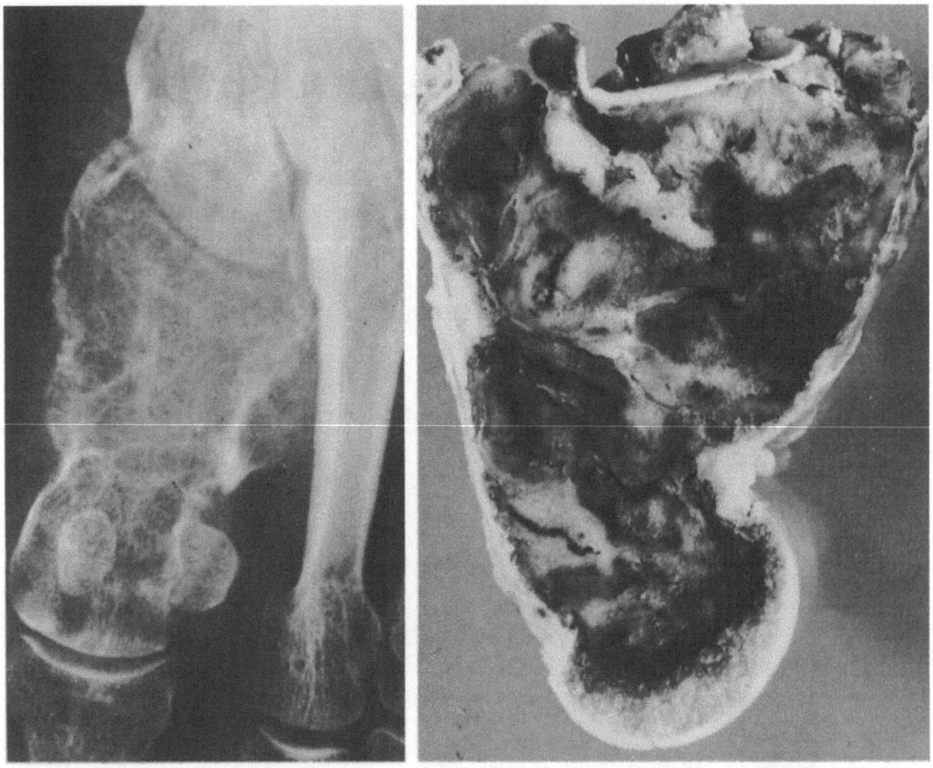

a b

Fig. III.17a,b. Male, 45 years old. Giant cell-tumor of the first metatarsal bone. **a** Radiograph and **b** photograph of the specimen reveal that the tumor occupies almost the whole length of the metatarsus

frequency in this series of lesions in the phalanges, metacarpals (20 cases), and metatarsals (five cases) (Figs. III.17, III.18) is quite remarkable, since these are considered rare locations, unlike in the case of giant-cell granuloma. Giant-cell tumors occur rather infrequently in the lower end of the tibia (Fig. III.19), upper end of the femur, the sacrum (Fig. III.20), and the spine (13 cases) (Figs. III.21–III.23). The involvement of patella, ribs, scapula, mandible (three cases), pelvic bones, and cranial bones was rare (Figs. III.24–III.26).

The occurrence of true giant-cell tumors in the jaw bones is still disputed, but, although extremely rare, is now accepted by several authors (Small and Rowe 1975) (Fig. III.27). Bhaskar et al. (1959), who reviewed 104 giant-cell lesions of the jaws, did not find a single case of genuine giant-cell tumor. It is true that most giant-cell lesions of the jaws are "reparative giant-cell granulomas" (Jaffe 1953a), classified as "giant-cell granulomas" by Pindborg and Kramer (1971); however, a few cases of genuine giant cell tumor have been observed by the writer (three cases) and by others, especially oral pathologists (Pindborg and Kramer 1971).

Our figures agree in general with those of other publications (Jaffe 1958; Lichtenstein 1977). One remarkable exception is the high incidence of 31 cases of giant-cell tumors of vertebrae above the sacrum published by Dahlin (1977), as compared with 13 cases in our series and none in the series of Campanacci (1981). In the writer's opinion this number should be taken with some reservation, because only 16 cases have been reported later from the Mayo Clinic files by Dahlin and Unni (1986).

In four of our patients, giant-cell tumors were found in multiple sites (multicentric): the first in three locations simultaneously, the iliac bone, femur, and tibia; the second in the lower radius and a metacarpal bone of the same site (Fig. III.28); the third, in the tibia and lower end of the femur, a new tumor appearing later in the upper femoral end; and the fourth in the upper tibia and lower femur. Only a few authors have reported multiple locations. Among others, McGrath (1972) reported one case among 52 with four loci;

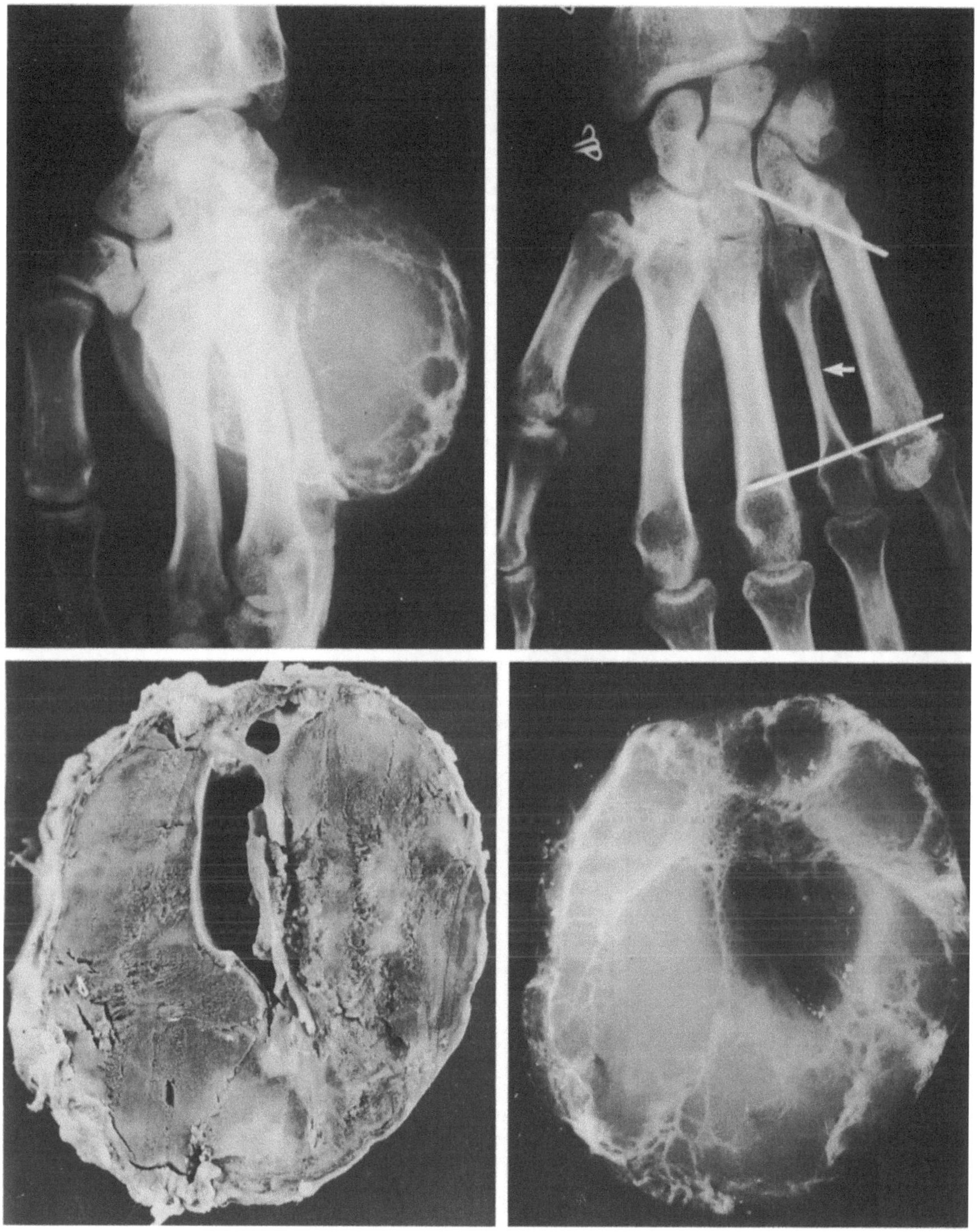

a b c d

Fig. III.18a–d. Female, 22 years old. Giant-cell tumor of fifth metacarpal bone. **a** Radiograph shows the widely distended bone contour of the tumor, which involves the whole extent of the bone and has caused compression atrophy of the adjacent fourth metacarpal, seen in **b**, a radiograph taken 10 months after resection and bone grafting. **c**,**d**, Solid aspect of the tumor that was previously diagnosed clinically as an aneurysmal bone cyst. (**c**,**d**, Schajowicz 1961)

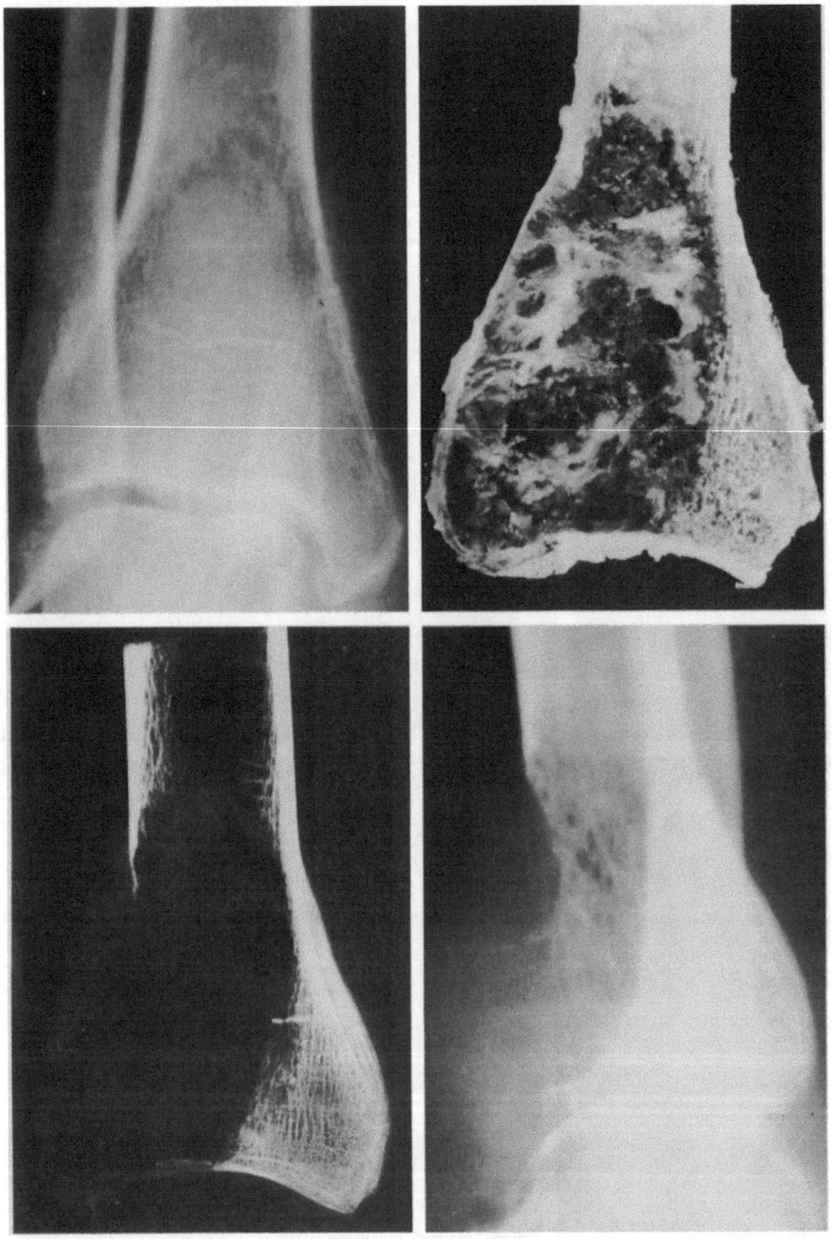

a b c

Fig. III.19a–c. Female, 24 years old. Giant-cell tumor of lower end of the tibia. **a** Radiographs show the extensive destruction of the posterior cortex. **b** Photograph shows the characteristic features of giant-cell tumor. **c** Radiograph of a thin slab reveals the osteolytic feature of the lesion

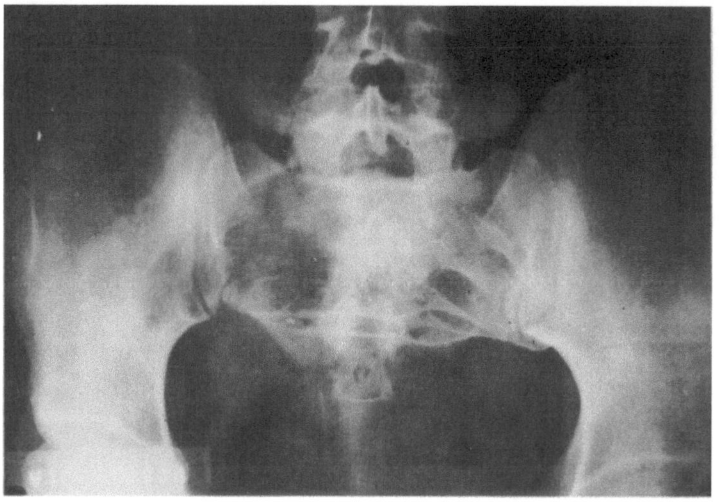

Fig. III.20. Female, 20 years. Giant-cell tumor of the sacrum

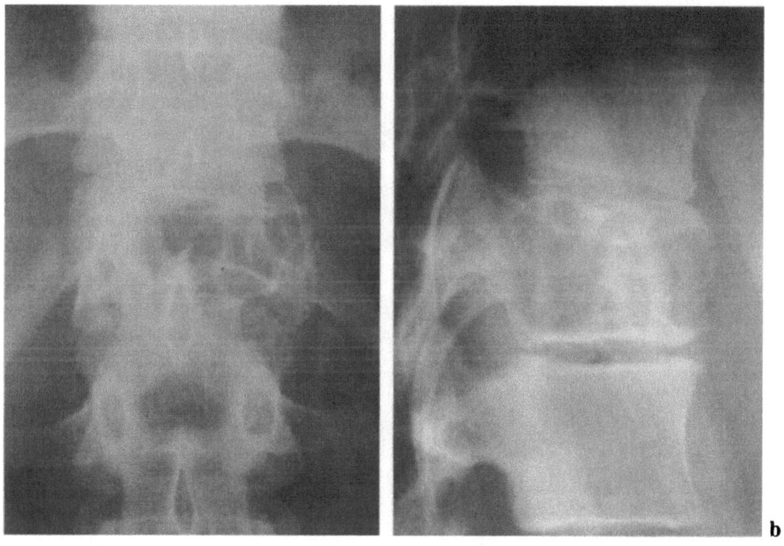

Fig. III.21a,b. Giant-cell tumor of the 12th thoracic vertebra. **a** Antero-posterior and **b** lateral radiographs show a radiolucent trabeculated and slightly expansile lesion of the vertebral body

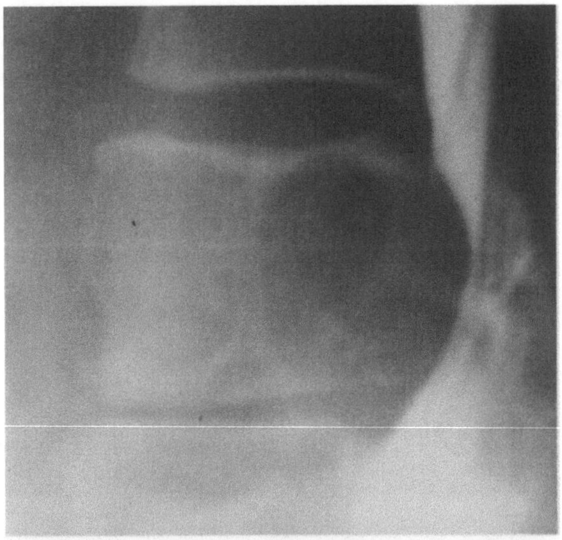

a

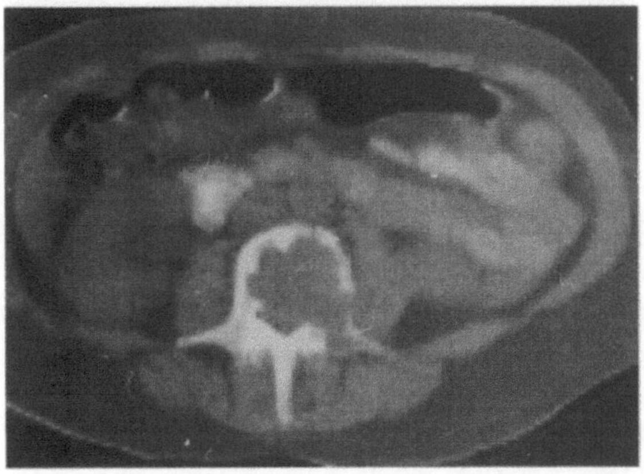

b

Fig. III.22a,b. Giant-cell tumor of the second lumbar vertebra. **a** Lateral radiograph shows a lytic expansile lesion in the posterior aspect of the vertebral body, protruding into the spinal canal. **b** CT scan revealing the extension of the tumor, which has partly destroyed the cortex

Fig. III.23a,b. Two advanced cases of vertebral giant-cell tumors. **a** Female, 26 years old, showing complete collapse of the body of L2 (vertebra plana). **b** Male, 29 years old, with extensive destruction of C7 and T1

▼

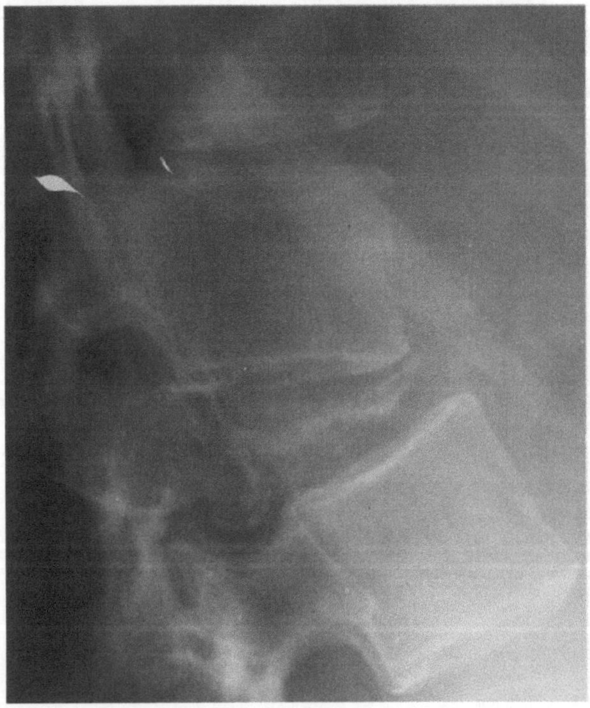

a

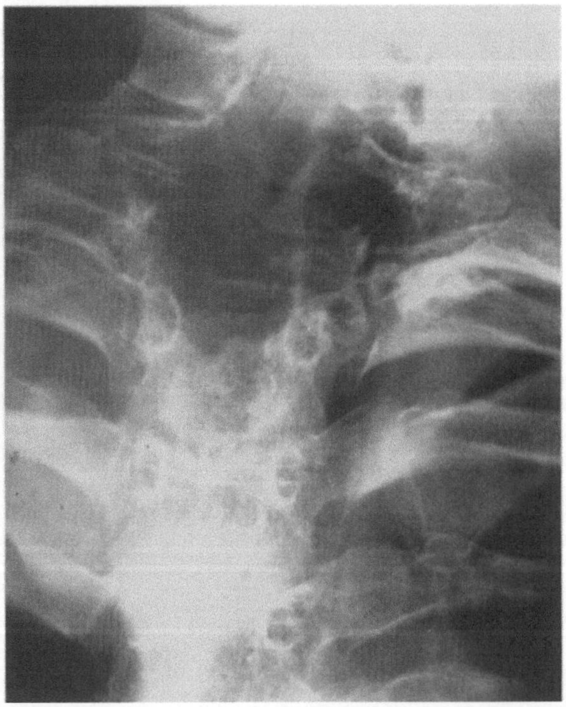

b

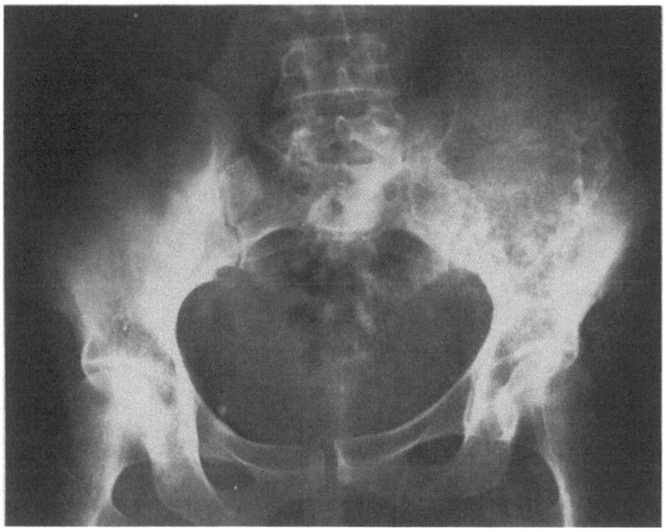

Fig. III.24. Female, 50 years old. Giant-cell tumor of the iliac wing

a
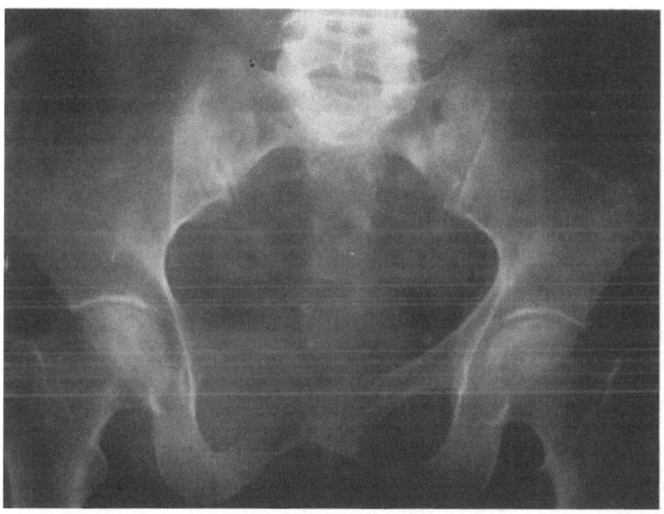

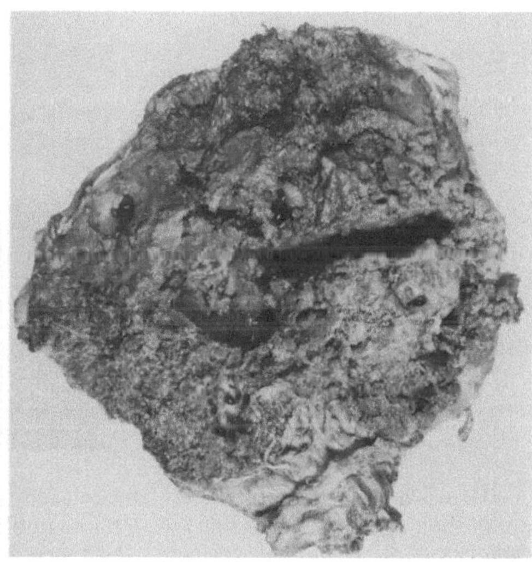
b

c
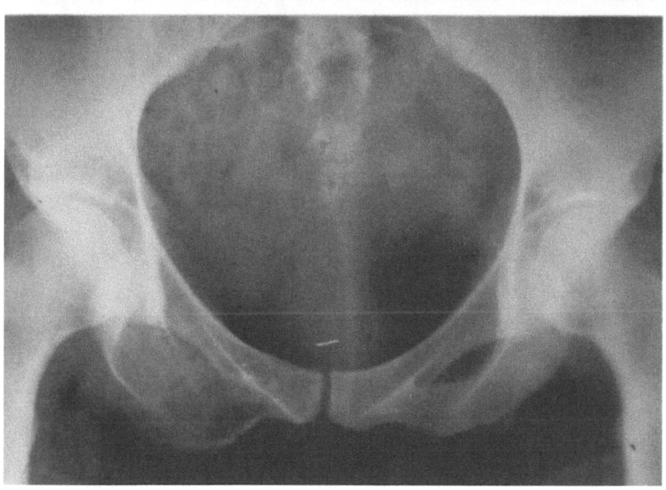

Fig. III.25a–c. Two different cases of pelvic giant-cell tumor. **a** Female, 59 years old. Radiograph shows a large osteolytic expansile lesion in the iliopubic ramus, suggesting a diagnosis of aneurysmal bone cyst. **b** Photograph of the resected tumor shows its solid hemorrhagic aspect. **c** Female, 34 years old, with a smaller radiolucent lesion in the ischium

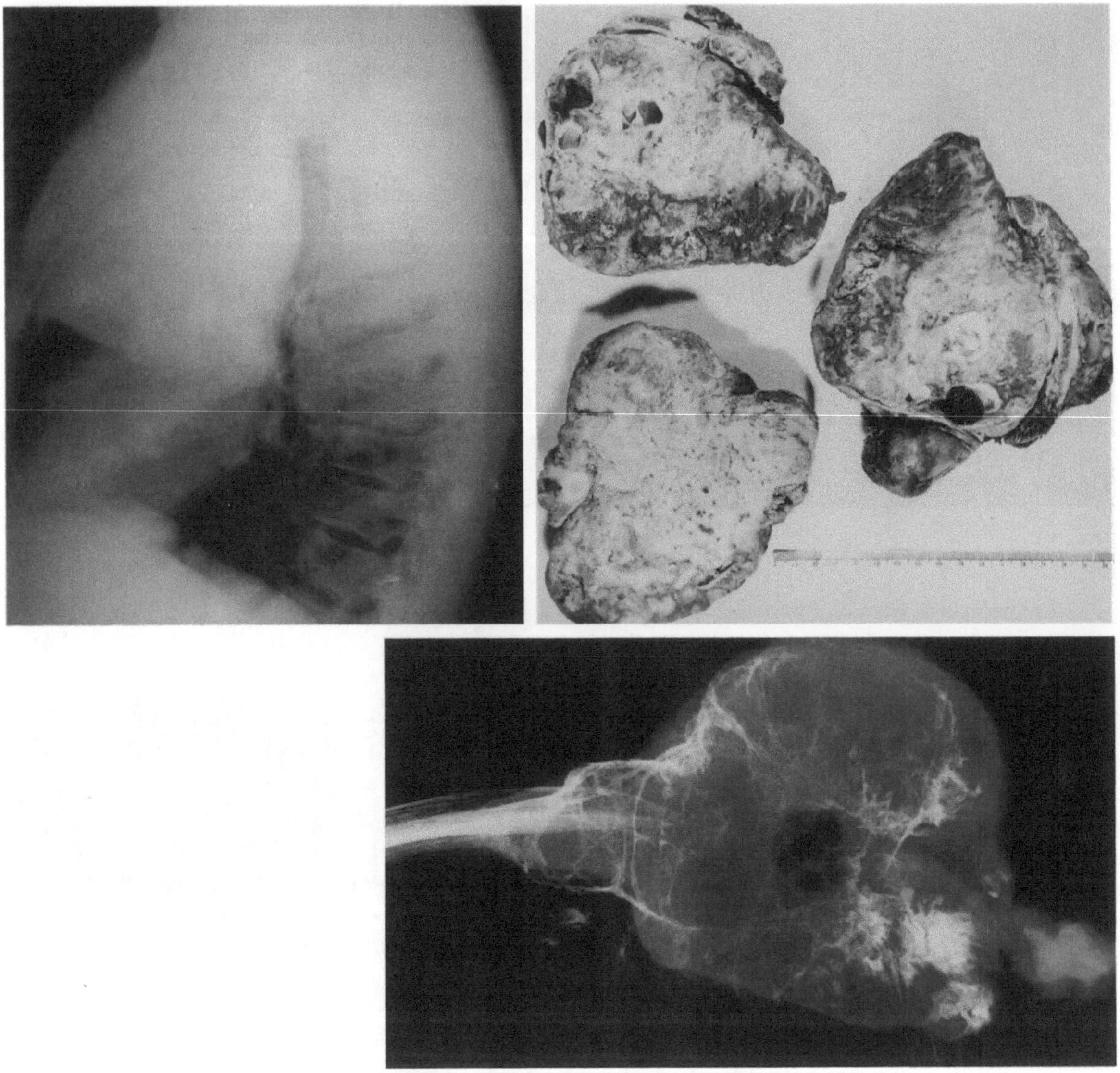

a b c

Fig. III.26a–c. Male, 42 years old. Giant-cell tumor in a rare location in the rib. **a** Radiograph, **b** photograph, and **c** radiograph of the resected specimen, which included the adjacent rib, show the solid aspect and large size of the widely expanded tumor

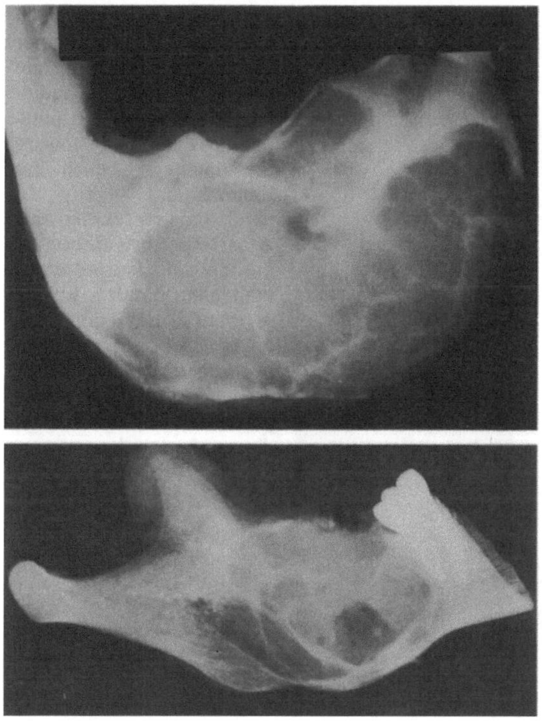

a

b

Fig. III.27a,b. Two cases of genuine giant-cell tumor of mandible, showing lytic expansile and trabeculated lesions, suggesting ameloblastoma

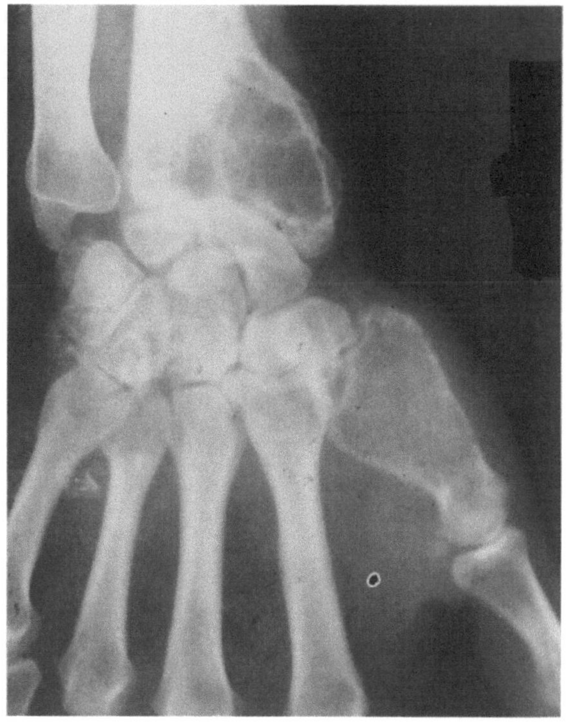

Fig. III.28. Male, 31 years old. Multicentric synchronous giant-cell tumor in the lower end of the radius and first metacarpal bone

Goldenberg et al. (1970), four cases with double lesions; and Dahlin (1978), two cases with two tumors each. The same author, in association with Sim and Beabout (Sim et al. 1977), reported 11 cases of multicentric giant-cell tumors with 35 individual tumors; three of them were treated at the Mayo Clinic between 1909 and 1976, and eight more were seen in consultation. They found seven other cases in the literature, including one of our cases and the cases of Tornberg (1975). We agree with these authors that it is sometimes difficult to distinguish a multicentric giant-cell tumor from a primary giant-cell tumor with metastatic spread, or from "brown tumors" in hyperparathyroidism. More recently, Peimer et al. (1980), Singson and Feldman (1983), and Ladanyi et al. (1989) have reported multicentric lesions.

Almost all giant-cell tumors were located at the epiphyseal end of a long tubular bone in a skeletally mature patient, most frequently abutting the articular cartilage and extending toward the metaphysis. In only three cases was the tumor located in the metaphysis and separated by a still-open cartilage plate from the epiphysis, and in three other cases the tumor was metadiaphyseal (Fig. III.29; cf. case of telangiectatic osteosarcoma in Fig. III.30).

Similar exceptional cases, limited to the metaphysis in skeletally immature patients, have been reported by Sherman and Fabricius (1961), Goldenberg et al. (1970; two cases), Peison and Feigenbaum (1976), Picci et al. (1983; 2%), and Dahlin and Unni (1986, three cases). Others, confined to the shaft or extending to the shaft from the metaphysis, were published by McGrath in 1972 (two cases) and by Campanacci et al. (1973), with one case in the shaft and two in the lower metaphysis of the femur; a similar case was reported by Huvos (1991) located in the distal femoral diaphysis in a 7-year-old child (Fig. 179). It is noticeable that all tumors located in the shaft, including the writer's cases, involved the femur, except one recent case sent in consultation from Sao Paulo, which was located in the humeral diaphysis (Fig. III.31).

Symptoms. The most frequent, and generally the first symptom, was pain of increasing intensity, associated with local swelling and tenderness of the affected area. Limitation of motion of the adjacent joint, most frequently the knee, was

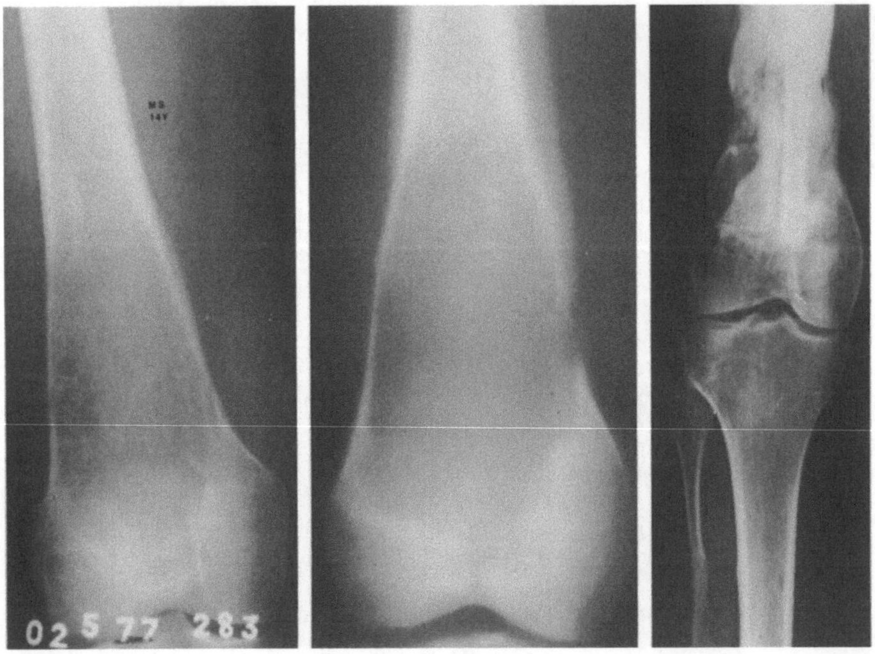

a, b c

Fig. III.29a–c. Female, 14 years old. Giant-cell tumor of femur. **a** Radiograph and **b** tomogram show a radiolucent lesion in the metaphysis extending toward the diaphysis, which has thinned and slightly expanded the cortex, showing a scarce periosteal reaction at one side, suggesting a malignant tumor. A wide segmental resection followed by bone grafts was performed. **c** Radiologic aspect 2 years later. The patient is well and without disease 8 years later

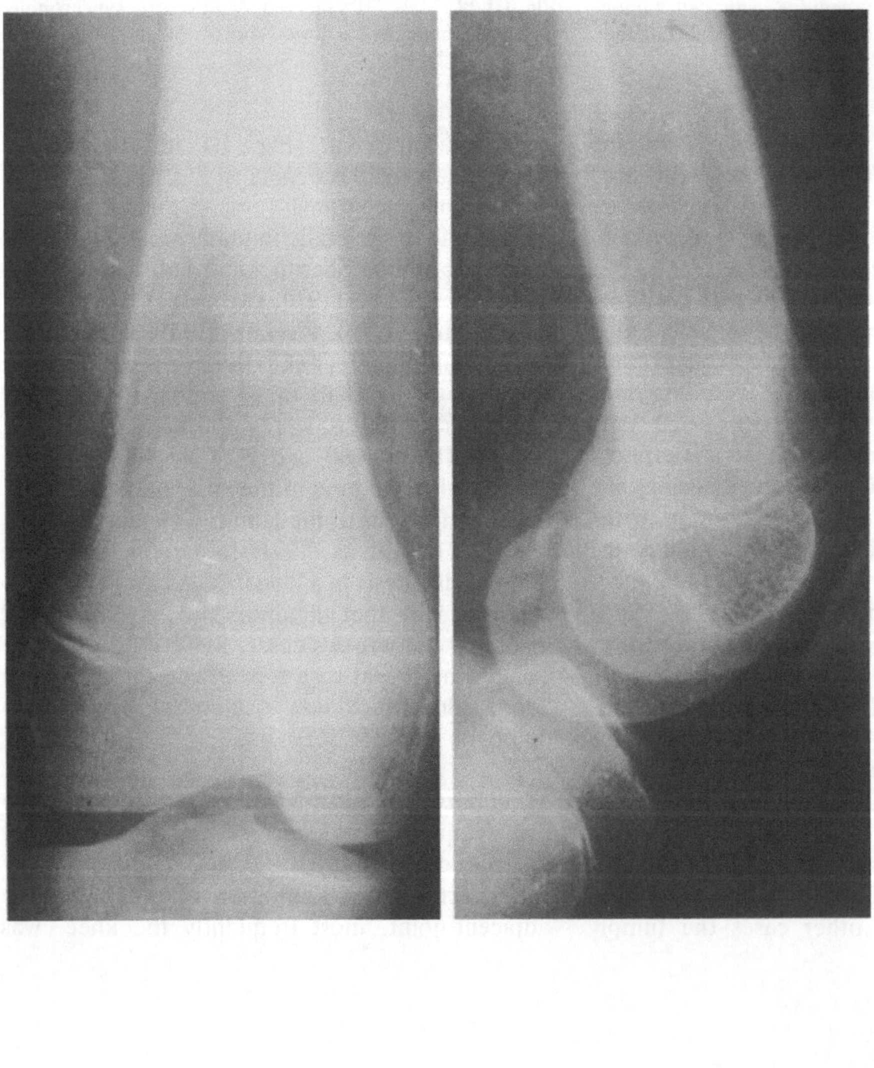

a b

Fig. III.30. Female, 14 years old, with similar radiologic features to the case in Fig. III.29, corresponding to a telangiectatic osteosarcoma

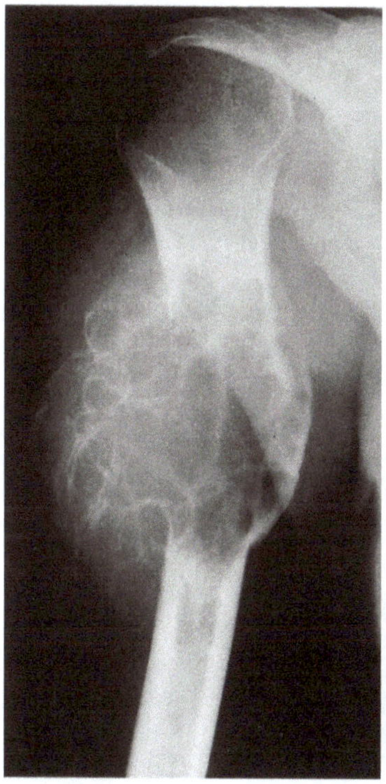

a

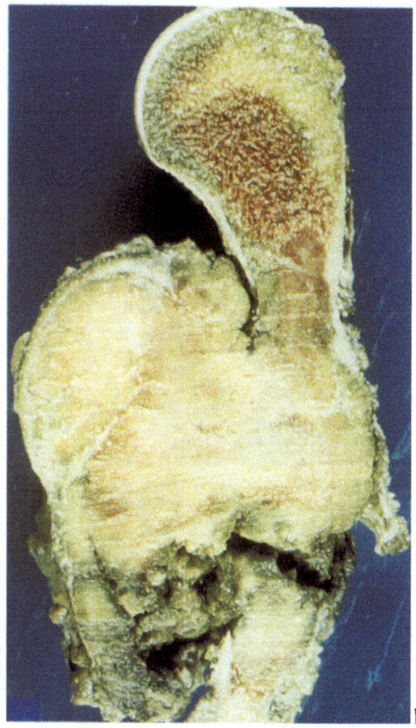

b

Fig. III.31a,b. Another exceptional case of giant-cell tumor of diaphyseal location in the humerus, showing in **a** a radiolucent, trabeculated, and widely expansile lesion. Radiologically, a metastatic tumor or hyperparathyroidism was suspected. **b** Photograph of the resected specimen shows a solid, predominantly grayish-white tumor which partly destroyed the cortex. (Courtesy of Dr. José Donato de Próspero, Sao Paulo, Brazil)

present in many patients. A pathologic fracture was infrequent and was occasionally the first symptom.

Radiographic Features. The most common appearance in a long bone was a radiolucent expanding zone, located eccentrically in the epiphyseal end, generally in a skeletally mature patient (Figs. III.1, III.7). The lesion extended both toward the articular cartilage and the metaphyseal region and occupied in more advanced cases the entire width of the bone (Figs. III.3–III.6, III.8). This was the most frequent finding in tumors of the lower end of the radius (Fig. III.13). The cortex was generally thinned, distended, and often partially destroyed, but a periosteal reaction was generally lacking. The limits between tumor and neighboring spongiosa were imprecise, and a sclerotic bone rim was generally not observed. Trabeculation in giant-cell tumor was infrequent in untreated lesions and appears to be a feature of nonaggressive tumors undergoing spontaneous regression (Jaffe 1958). Although at the present state of knowledge it is not possible to accurately predict clinical behavior on the basis of clinical and roentgenographic features, the division of giant-cell tumor into three categories, e.g., Campanacci's grades I, II, and III, which corresponds to Enneking's quiescent (latent), active, and aggressive stages, seems to be more helpful for prognosis and treatment than histologic grading. Of Campanacci's cases 20% were of grade I, 60% of grade II, and 20% of grade III. We have already mentioned the extreme rarity of metaphyseal or diaphyseal locations. In our series, we did not have a single lesion located primarily in a still-growing epiphysis and only one such case is mentioned by Dahlin and Unni (1986).

Pathologic Findings. *Gross Pathology.* The tumor presents, on section, a characteristic appearance. Although there is considerable variability, all specimens show extensive soft fleshy areas that alternate in color from gray to a light red or dark hemorrhagic hue. The gray zones are of a somewhat firmer consistency, but they are friable. The tumor is situated eccentrically in the epiphysis (Figs. III.1, III.7), extending toward the articular cartilage and toward the metaphysis. In the more advanced stages, these tumors may occupy the entire metaphyseal and epiphyseal region (Figs. III.2–III.4, III.8). These extensive tumors are usually observed in the upper extremity, especially in the lower end of the radius (Figs. III.12b, III.13). The explanation for the high incidence of extensive tumors in the upper extremity would appear to be that these tumors do not cause symptoms, or only with delay, when they are located in non-

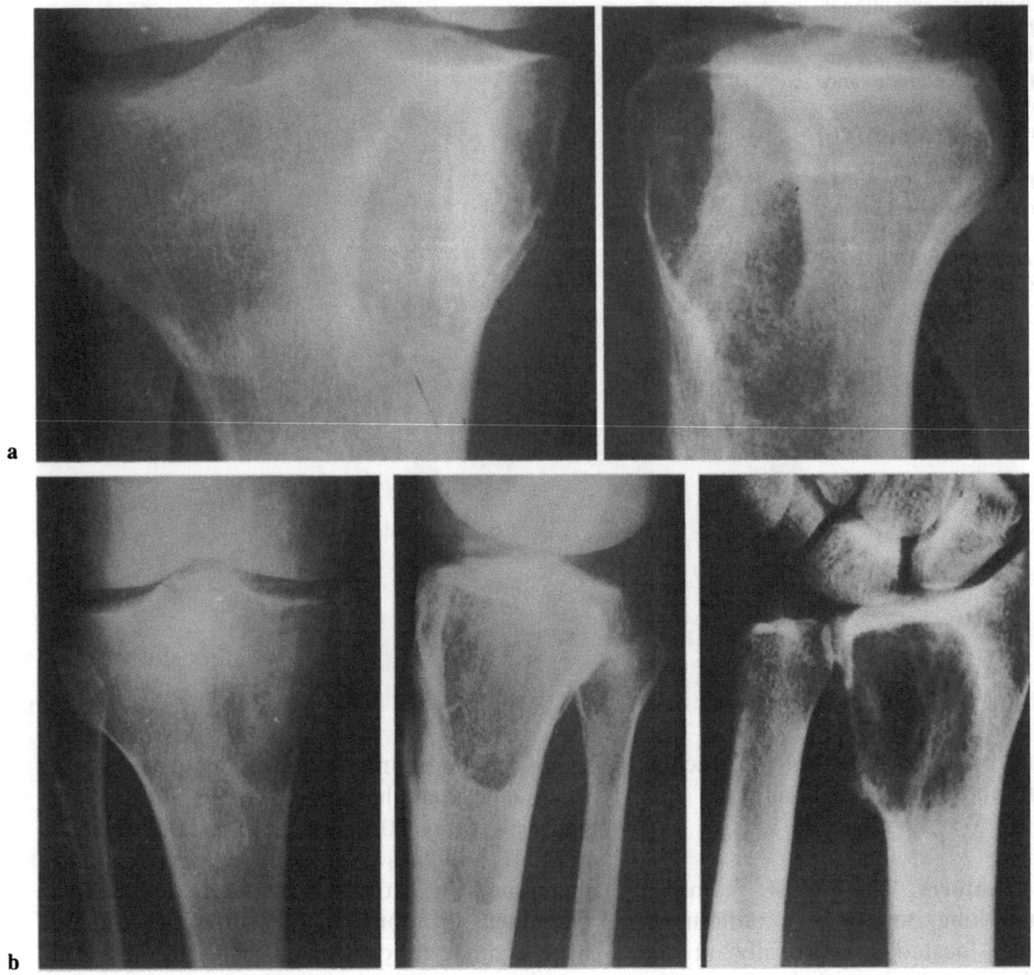

Fig. III.32a–c. Three different cases of xanthomatous type of giant-cell tumor. **a** Male, 36 years old. Anteroposterior and lateral radiographs show an eccentric lesion of the upper tibial end, with well-defined borders. **b** Male, 34 years old, with similar lesion. **c** Male, 43 years old, with radiolucent, well-limited lesion in the lower end of radius. The radiographic features correspond to Campanacci's grade I and Enneking's quiescent (latent) stage

weight-bearing bones (Fig. III.14). As a result, patients do not seek medical care until their tumors are far advanced. In the phalanges or metacarpals the tumor may occupy nearly all of the bone (Figs. III.17, III.18).

The tumor is traversed by thin septa of connective tissue and surrounded by a thin bone shell that in the more advanced cases is distended beyond the surfaces of the adjacent normal bone as if it were inflated (radiologic grade II or active). This thin shell of bone does not represent the expanded cortex. Rather, it is a new, displaced cortex formed by osteoclastic resorption of the endosteal surface and constant periosteal new-bone deposition, a mechanism well described by Virchow.

In advanced tumors, hemorrhage is more abundant, and small bright red or brownish cystic cavities are present (Figs. III.3, III.4). In some cases, part of the tumor is replaced by large cystic cavities filled with blood and traversed by thin septa, a pattern similar to that seen in aneurysmal

Fig. III.33a–d. Photomicrographs showing at lower and higher magnification different histologic features of the xanthomatous type of giant-cell tumor. Areas of this fibroxanthomatous aspect may predominate and are similar to those observed in non-ossifying fibroma (metaphyseal fibrous defect) or cases now referred to as fibrous histiocytoma: **a**,**b** spindle-celled fibrous tissue with a storiform pattern and a variable number of multinucleated giant cells of osteoclast type; **c**,**d** hemosiderin pigment and more or less numerous lipid-bearing histiocytes (xanthoma cells). **a**,**c** ×200, **b**,**d** ×400

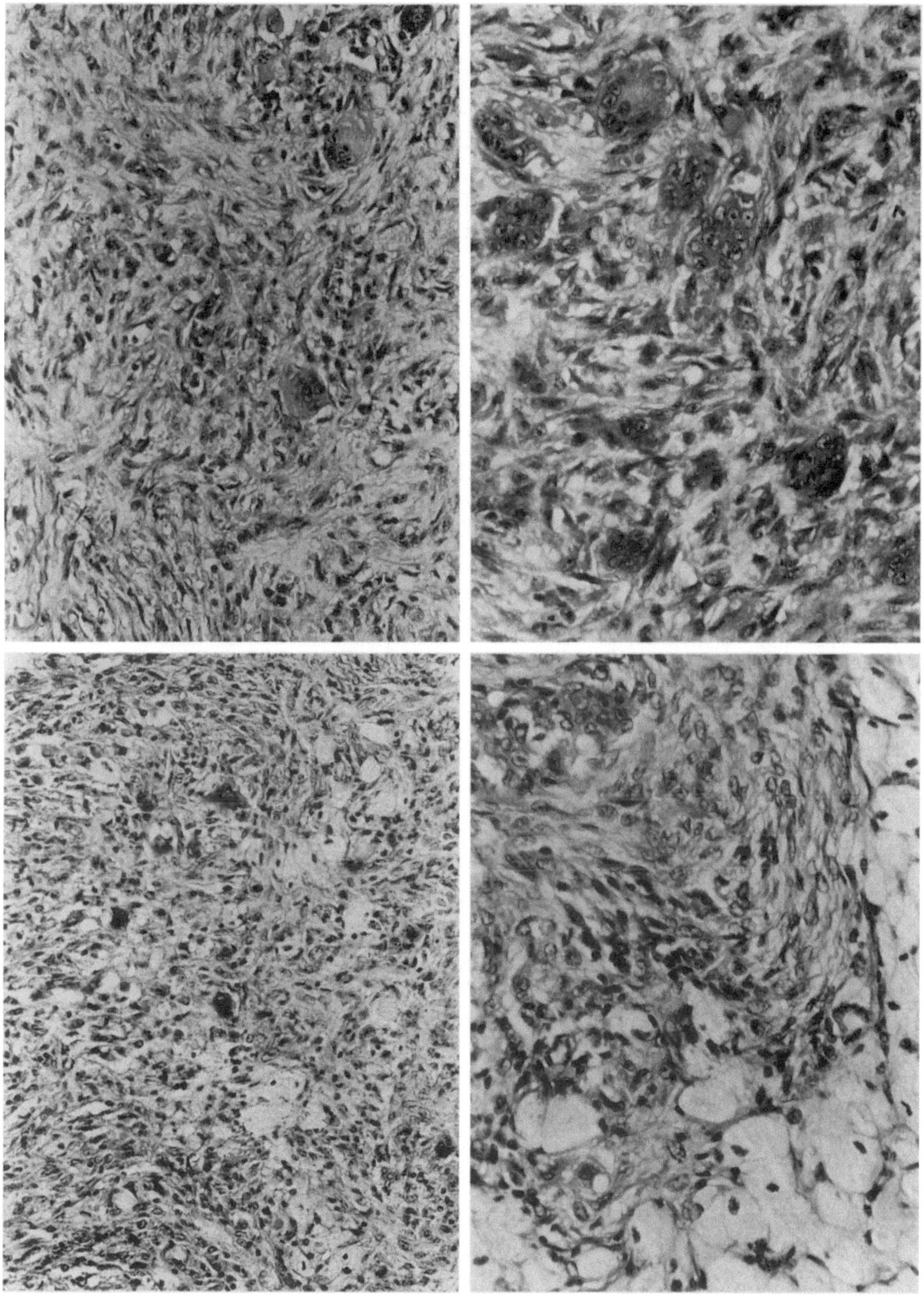

a b c d

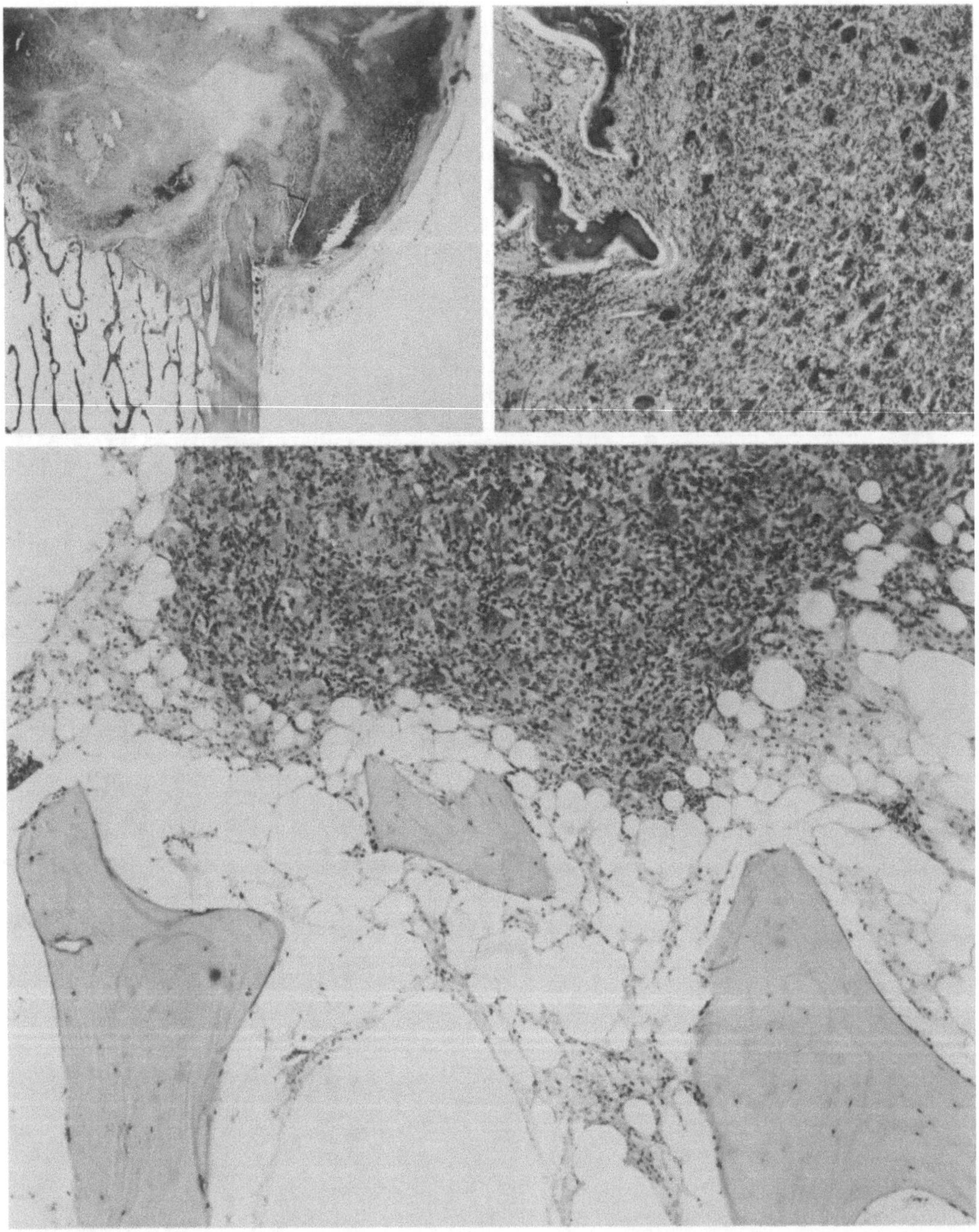

a b c

Fig. III.34a–c. Photomicrographs showing at low magnification (**a**) the destruction of the bone cortex and the extension of the tumor into the extraosseous soft tissue and marrow spaces, where there is no reactive bone formation or a fibrous membrane. This feature can be seen clearly in **c** and explains the frequency of recurrences after curettage. In **b** a fibrous septum, showing reactive new bone formation, is observed. **a** ×10, **b** ×40, **c** ×60

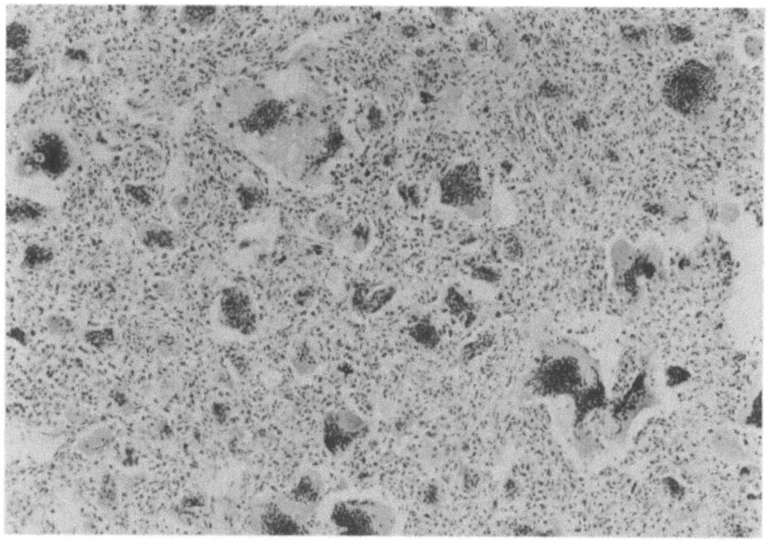

a

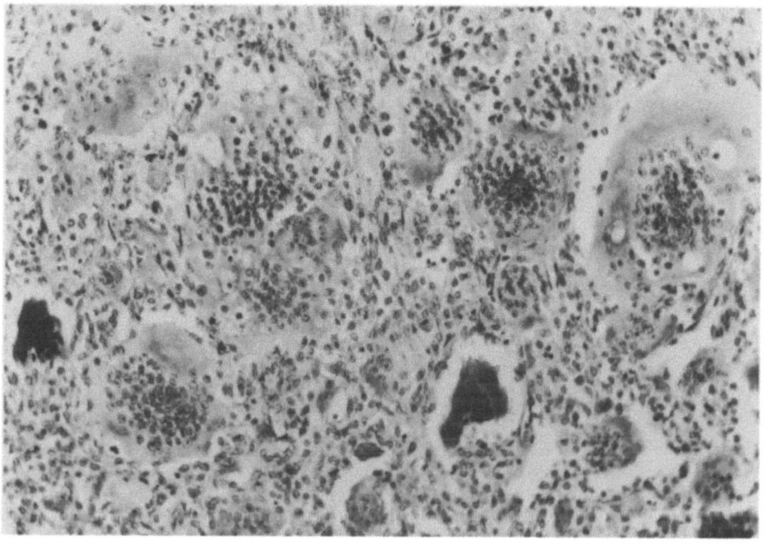

b

Fig. III.35a,b. Photomicrographs showing the characteristic histologic pattern of giant-cell tumor with numerous multinucleated giant cells that are uniformly distributed and separated by mononuclear stromal cells. Sometimes there are numerous vacuoles in the cytoplasm of the giant cells, and their nuclei are pyknotic. **a** ×100, **b** ×200

cyst (Figs. III.11, III.12). However, although the cystic areas may be extensive, they never occupy the major part of the tumor.

Yellowish-gray necrotic areas or zones of a sulfur-yellow color typical of xanthoma are often seen in limited areas, especially in advanced lesions. Occasionally, however, these xanthomatous or fibroxanthomatous areas constitute a major portion of the tumor (Figs. III.32, III.33).

A giant-cell tumor, even in its more advanced stages, respects the articular cartilage, which is only rarely perforated. Invasion of the joint space by the tumor is somewhat more frequent by way of the synovial and capsular tissues after the thin, newly formed bone cortex has been destroyed. Perforation or partial destruction of the thinned and widely expanded cortex (radiologically aggressive type) occurs often and does not indicate that the tumor is malignant. The margins of the tumor within the metaphyseal spongy tissue are not well defined; there is no delimiting fibrous or bone membrane. This explains the frequency of recurrences after curettage (Fig. III.34).

Microscopic Pathology. The histologic diagnosis should be based on a study of those areas that have not been modified by extensive hemorrhage and by such phenomena as necrosis or cicatricial fibrosis. In well-preserved areas, the histologic structure is characterized by a great number of multinucleated giant cells that are uniformly distributed in the tumor (Figs. III.34–III.37). These cells are irregularly delimited and have prolongations of their abundant cytoplasm, which is more or less basophilic and homogeneous or slightly granular. Sometimes, there are numerous

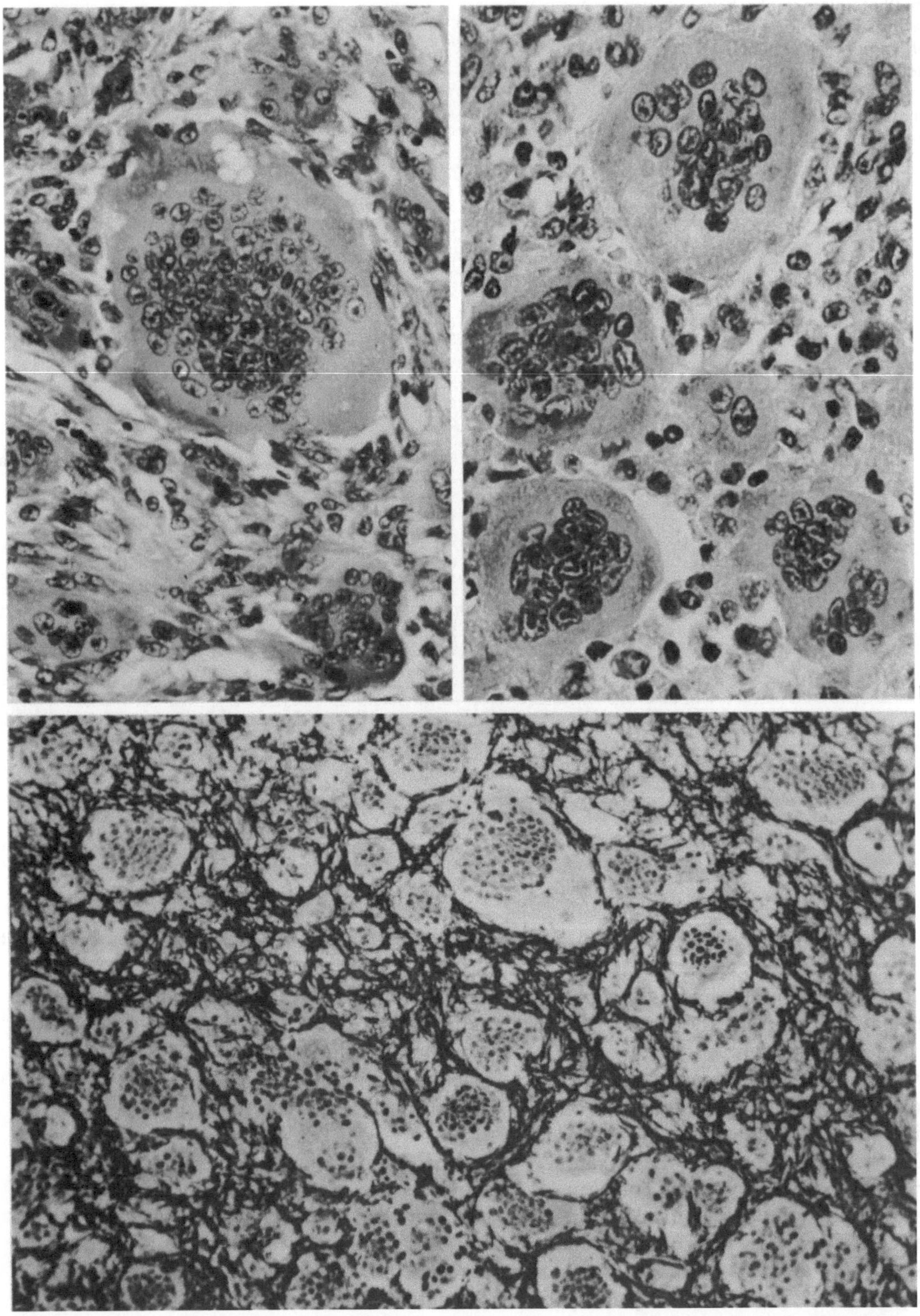

a b c

Fig. III.36a,b. Photomicrographs showing at high magnification the features of the multinucleated cells, the nuclei of which are identical to those of mononuclear stromal cells. These cells are round, oval, or fusiform in shape and generally have large nuclei with little chromatin and only one or two inconspicuous nucleoli. **c** Reticulin stained with Del Rio Hortega's silver impregnation technique. Numerous reticulin fibers, forming a dense network, surround individual cells and encircle the giant cells. **a,b** ×400, **c** ×120

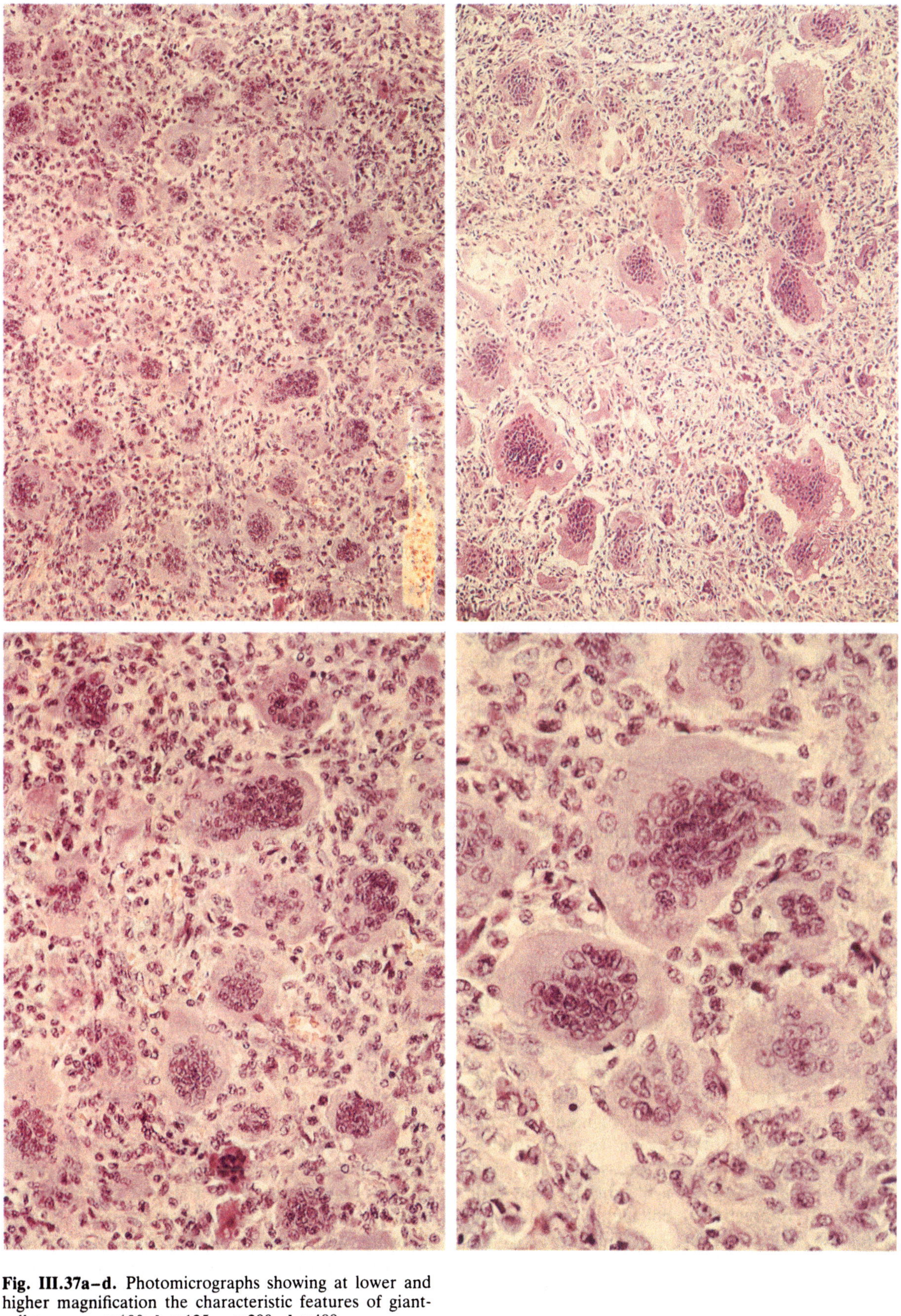

a b c d

Fig. III.37a–d. Photomicrographs showing at lower and higher magnification the characteristic features of giant-cell tumor. **a** ×100, **b** ×125, **c** ×200, **d** ×400

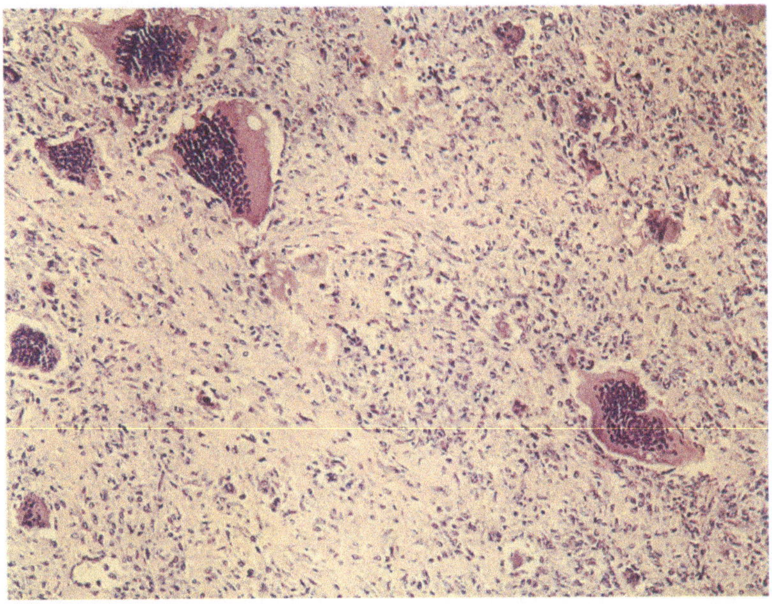

Fig. III.38. Photomicrograph showing an area with a predominantly fibrous stroma and scarce giant cells. This pattern may be seen occasionally in some older or larger tumors. ×120

vacuoles of different sizes in the cytoplasm. The size and number of nuclei are variable, but usually there are more than 15–20, and there may be hundreds (Figs. III.36, III.37). The appearance of the nuclei is identical to that of the nuclei of the mononuclear stromal cells, which constitute the other essential element of the tumor. These cells are ovoid or spindle shaped and generally have large nuclei with scarce chromatin and only one or two inconspicuous nucleoli; usually, there are only a few typical mitoses to be found (Fig. III.36).

With the usual staining techniques, the tumor shows little collagenous stroma in the zones of active growth; nevertheless, with silver stains, a dense network of reticulin fibrils is seen surrounding the individual cells without penetrating the giant cells (Fig. III.36c).

The tumor is rich in newly formed blood vessels with walls composed only of endothelial cells, and in vascular channels that are lined by tumor cells themselves or by an endothelial layer. This vascular pattern would explain the presence of abundant hemorrhages, both recent and old, with phagocytosis of blood pigment by the mononuclear cells of the stroma. In most tumors, there are generally limited areas that are composed of spindle cells of a fibroblastic type with abundant intercellular collagenous substance (Fig. III.38). However, predominance of the fibrous stroma is observed in the so-called reparative giant-cell granuloma of the mandible, as also in those of hands and feet (Fig. III.39). Occasionally, groups of lipoid-bearing foam cells (xanthomatous cells) are present, particularly in the vicinity of necrotic foci. In these areas, the giant cells are moderate in size and few in number, or there are none at all, being replaced by fibrous tissue. According to Jaffe, this pattern reflects spontaneous regression and healing of the tumor. In an occasional giant-cell tumor, this "healing reaction" may predominate over the characteristic tissue, a histologic pattern that seems to indicate a favorable prognosis, as proposed by Scaglietti and Mondolfo (1938) many years ago. Several epiphyseal lesions have been observed by this author in which almost the whole specimen showed this *fibroxanthomatous* pattern with only scattered giant cells (Fig. III.33). The histologic features of these cases were similar to those observed in histiocytic xanthogranulomas or nonossifying fibromas (metaphyseal fibrous defects), or cases now referred to as benign fibrous histiocytoma. Whether they constitute a healing reaction in a genuine giant-cell tumor, as suggested by Jaffe, or a less aggressive type of giant-cell tumor, is not yet completely clear. However, in our experience, it seems that this special pattern is associated with the roentgenographic features of grade I (latent or quiescent) tumors; that is, eccentric nonexpanding lesions showing well-defined, slightly sclerotic borders towards the spongiosa, which generally have a more favorable prognosis.

Fig. III.39a,b. Photomicrographs illustrating the histologic pattern of reparative giant-cell granuloma of the mandible. The giant cells are few in number and small in size, separated by an abundant loose connective stroma. **a** ×120, **b** ×300

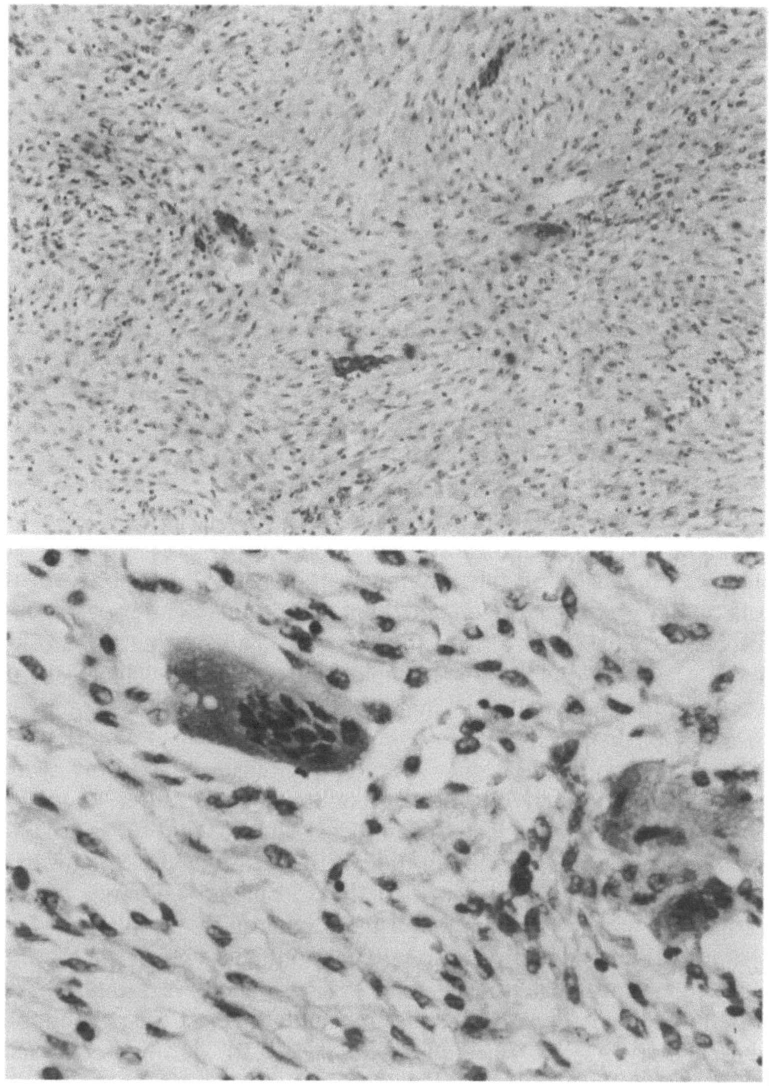

Some of the lesions with the above-mentioned radiologic and histologic features, that is, a predominant fibroxanthomatous pattern, have recently been misdiagnosed as "fibrous histiocytoma" of epiphyseal location (Bertoni et al. 1986; Matsuno 1990). It is noteworthy that in all but one of 43 patients reported by Goldenberg et al. (1970) in whom the tumor showed these histologic features, the lesion healed following the primary operation (either curettage with bone graft or excision combined with bone graft).

The collagenous septa of variable thickness that traverse the tumor frequently contain trabeculae of newly formed bone or osteoid, which may also be found in the vicinity of hemorrhagic and necrotic areas or after microfractures, and are generally reactive in nature. The possibility that the tumor cells can themselves form bone or osteoid cannot be completely excluded, but if that happens it is a rare finding involving limited areas, and should alert the pathologist to the possibility of a malignant bone-forming tumor. We did not find evidence of cartilage formation in genuine giant-cell tumor, except in areas of microfractures.

Johnston (1977) noted the presence of lymphocytic infiltration in stromal tissue, especially in areas of giant-cell activity, which he related to a possible cell-mediated immunity response from the host. He believes that the presence of lymphocytes together with giant cells, which he interprets as multinucleated macrophages, reflects a favorable prognosis in terms of local control of the lesion and long-term survival of the host.

A small number of osteolytic lesions, almost exclusively occurring in the tubular bones of the *hand*, have been reported under the term "giant-cell reaction of bone" (Ackerman and Spjut 1962; D'Alonzo et al. 1972; Jernstrom and Stark 1971; Schwinn 1976) or "giant-cell reparative granuloma." They are differentiated from true giant-cell tumors by the prominence of osteoid production and by a definitely fibrous stroma (see Chap. IX).

Histochemical Studies. The writer published in 1961 the results of an extensive histochemical study on a series of giant-cell tumors and the so-called variants, demonstrating that the histochemical behavior of the multinucleated giant cell of the giant-cell tumor and that of normal osteoclasts and chondroclasts are identical. This finding, in the writer's opinion, indicates a close relationship and similarity in the physiologic behavior of these cells.

Like Gomori (1941), the writer found intense acid phosphatase activity but no alkaline phosphatase in the multinucleated giant cells, and no alkaline or acid phosphatase in the stromal cells. Identical results were obtained in the so-called variants of giant-cell tumor and granulomatous lesions and foreign body reactions. These findings were confirmed by other authors (Pais and Barrufaldi 1958; Pepler 1958; Jeffree and Price 1965; Thiery et al. 1974; Kraievski et al. 1970). Therefore, histochemical methods are of no value in the differential diagnosis of these entities.

Our histochemical studies have also indicated the presence in all types of giant cells of the enzymes β-glucuronidase and succinate dehydrogenase and of nonglycogen carbohydrates, principally acid mucopolysaccharides and scarce complex lipids. It would seem that the metabolic and enzymatic activities of the multinucleated giant cells are related to the digestion, solution, and elimination of several classes of substances, i.e., there is evident macrophagic activity.

The stromal cells of giant-cell tumor do not generally show enzymatic reactions, possibly with the exception of *nonspecific esterase*, nor do they possess glycogen, mucopolysaccharides, or glycolipids in significant amounts.

In vitro cell cultures identified three major cell types based on morphologic characteristics, patterns of specific surface antigens, presence of receptors for hormones, and cell production (Goldring et al. 1986). One population consisted of mononuclear cells that expressed monocyte-macrophage (histiocyte) markers. These cells lacked receptors for skeletal hormones and did not persist in culture. A distinct population of mononuclear cells proliferated in culture, and these cells most likely represent the neoplastic elements of the tumors. The cells phenotypically resembled connective tissue stromal cells, i.e., they did not express macrophage surface antigens and they produced collagens (types I and III). They also possessed receptors for parathyroid hormones. The third population of tumor cells consisted of multinucleated giant cells. These cells lacked monocyte-macrophage surface antigens and possessed receptors for calcitonin, a phenotypic marker for osteoclasts. Goldring et al. (1986) also confirmed that the multinucleated giant cells present in early cultures do not persist after passage (Gallardo et al. 1970) and suggested that these cells are formed by fusion from mononuclear cell precursors which possibly lose their specific antigens, preventing their identification.

Electron Microscopy. The ultrastructural features of giant-cell tumors have been studied in different centers (Hanaoka et al. 1970; Ueno 1964; Kuwana 1967; Steiner et al. 1972; among others). All authors confirmed the ultrastructural similarity of osteoclasts and giant cells of giant-cell tumors, both of which are characterized by a large number of mitochondria, relatively sparse, rough endoplasmic reticulum, and a variable number of lysosomelike bodies in different cells (Fig. III.40). However, a characteristic brush border is generally lacking. According to Steiner et al., there was a discrepancy between the small number of lysosomelike bodies and the high acid phosphatase activity of giant cells found by the writer and other authors. Thiery et al. (1974) found abundant acid phosphatase activity in lysosomes concentrated around the Golgi apparatus.

The giant cells appear to arise by fusion of mononuclear tumor cells, but most investigators, including this author, could not demonstrate this mechanism with any certainty. On the other hand, Thiery et al. (1974) were more inclined to advocate the mechanism of amitotic nuclear division.

According to most authors, the stromal cells are undifferentiated mesenchymal or connective tissue cells with features suggestive of fibroblasts and histiocytes (Steiner et al. 1972; Spjut et al. 1971). However, the low number of cells of

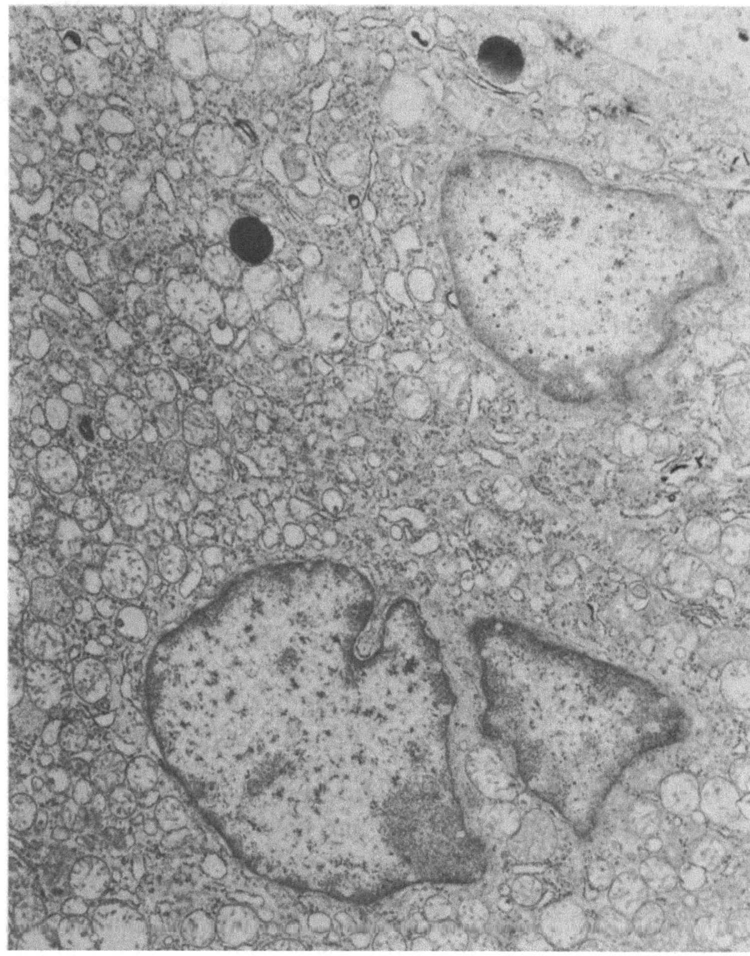

Fig. III.40. Electron micrograph of part of a giant cell showing three nuclei and the great number of mitochondria

histiocytic macrophage line does not seem to justify the classification of giant-cell tumor as a tumor of histiocytic derivation, as suggested by Huvos (1979).

In recent decades, viruslike intranuclear inclusions have been reported in the giant cells of some cases of giant-cell tumor, similar to those described in the osteoclasts of Paget disease by Welsh and Meyer (1970), Rebel et al. (1974), Mills and Singer (1976), Le Charpentier et al. (1977), Fornasier et al. (1985), Schajowicz et al. (1985), Vacher-Lavenu et al. (1981), and Abelanet et al. (1986).

Pathogenesis. The histogenesis of giant-cell tumor is still unclear. Almost all authors, including the writer, agree that the giant-cell tumor is a neoplastic process, and that the mononuclear stromal cell originates from the undifferentiated mesenchymal cells or cells of the supporting connective tissue of the bone marrow (Goldring et al. 1986), interpreted by some authors as reticulohistiocytic elements (Huvos 1979). The multinucleated giant cell is derived from these same immature cells, with their tendency toward histiocytic and fibroblastic differentiation, either by agglutination or conglomeration of the stromal cells, as held by the majority of authors, or by repeated division of the stromal-cell nucleus without the corresponding cytoplasmic division, as suspected by Virchow and reiterated by von Albertini (1928). After studying the cytologic details of smears from numerous giant-cell tumors and from cells in tissue culture, Lustig and the writer (1944) proved the existence of this last mechanism, at least in some giant cells in tissue culture, probably by amitotic division or nuclear segmentation. The majority of ultrastructural studies, however, are more inclined to support the conglomeration mechanism without offering definitive proof.

Microspectrophotometric studies performed by the writer (Schajowicz et al. 1977) in tumoral processes with giant cells also seem to favor this last histogenesis. Our studies and those of other authors (Thiery et al. 1974), however, could not completely resolve this problem. In addition to the more frequent conglomeration process, exceptional amitotic cellular division cannot be entirely denied.

Owing to the great resemblance between the histochemical and ultramicroscopic behavior of the osteoclast and the giant cell, the latter can be considered the neoplastic deviation of the osteoclast. This would explain certain morphologic differences between the two, such as the greater size and greater number of giant-cell nuclei and an abundance of these cells in a giant-cell tumor that far surpasses any functional requirement.

For these reasons, the term "osteoclastoma," which has been used by most British authors from Stewart (1914) to the present, is perfectly justified; it seems clear that the multinucleated giant cell of the giant-cell tumor belongs to the same family as the normal osteoclast and that, even though it is a neoplastic element, it would be expected to exhibit a bone-destroying function. Aegerter also prefers the term "osteoclastoma" (Aegerter and Kirkpatrick 1975). Until the histogenesis of this tumor is completely defined, the writer prefers, as in the WHO classification system, to continue using the neutral term "giant-cell tumor of bone," with "osteoclastoma" as a synonym. In addition to the preceding ultrastructural finding, the histiocytic nature of some of the stromal cells appears to be confirmed not only by immunohistochemical and ultramicroscopic studies, but also by the application of silver stains of Del Rio Hortega. These stains not only show abundant reticulin fibrils involving each stromal cell, but also stain specifically those cells that present ramified or ameboid prolongations, often providing contact between them and the giant cells. This is a feature that is characteristic of reticuloendothelial elements, according to Del Rio Hortega.

The giant cell appears to have a limited life span. In tissue culture, degenerative phenomena begin after 18–72 h, whereas the fundamental mononuclear cell is still actively growing. These regressive changes are also often seen in histologic sections of giant-cell tumors and consist of nuclear pyknosis and karyorrhexis or karyolysis, which are frequently combined with vacuolar degeneration of the cytoplasm.

Clinical-Histologic Correlation. An important question raised by nearly all authors concerns the reliability of grading giant-cell tumors as a guide to prognosis, that is, the possibility of predicting with any assurance the ultimate outcome of a given case based on the initial histology of the tumor.

Grading of these tumors was proposed many years ago by Stewart (1914) and Ewing (1922), and was especially emphasized by Jaffe, Lichtenstein, and Portis (1940), who defined three grades: benign, aggressive, and malignant. Meyerding (1941), the Bone Sarcoma Registry, and many others distinguished a benign and a malignant form (Murphy and Ackerman 1956; Hutter et al. 1962; Spjut et al. 1971; Dahlin 1978).

However, most authors (Spjut et al. 1971; Goldenberg et al. 1970; McGrath 1972; Larsson et al. 1975; Mclnerney and Middlemis 1978) since then have contended that giant-cell tumors that prove to be aggressive or frankly malignant are not initially distinguishable histologically from those with a benign course. In later publications, Jaffe (1953b, 1958) called the giant-cell tumor a treacherous lesion and mentioned four cases in which pulmonary metastases occurred without the original tumors or their metastases ever developing frankly malignant histologic characteristics. He stated that "unfortunately one really cannot predict from the histological pattern which cases will metastasize." A small but increasing number of similar cases have been reported by other authors (Finch and Gleave 1926; Dyke 1931; Murphy and Ackerman 1956; Jewell and Bush 1964; Spjut et al. 1971; Pan et al. 1964; Lasser and Tetewsky 1957; Gresen et al. 1973; Maloney et al. 1983; Vanel et al. 1983; Bertoni et al. 1985, 1988; Wray et al. 1990). The eight cases quoted by Dahlin and Unni in their monograph (1986) were published previously by Rock et al. (1984). It is noteworthy that almost all cases with metastases had been treated previously (Figs. III.41, III.42) (Schajowicz et al. 1972). Despite the conclusion that grading the primary tumor does not have prognostic value, several authors (Spjut et al. 1971; Goldenberg et al. 1970; Huvos 1991; and others) insist that grading giant-cell tumors is nonetheless worthwhile because it "emphasizes the unpredictable behavior of tumors and the need for prolonged and careful follow-up."

A careful histopathologic review of our material and correlation of these findings with the clinical features confirmed the almost generally accepted view that *grading is without practical*

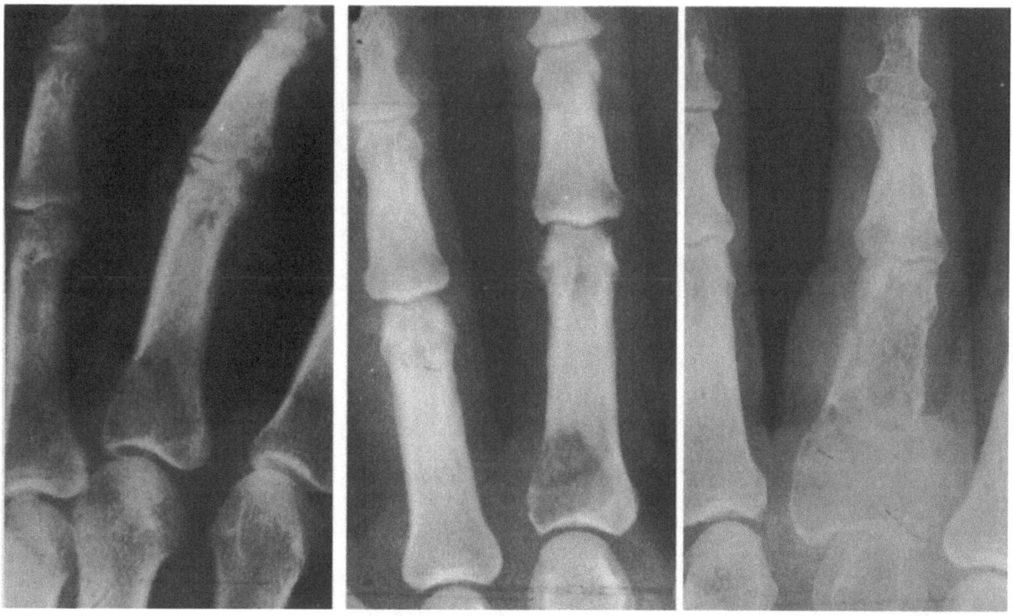

a b

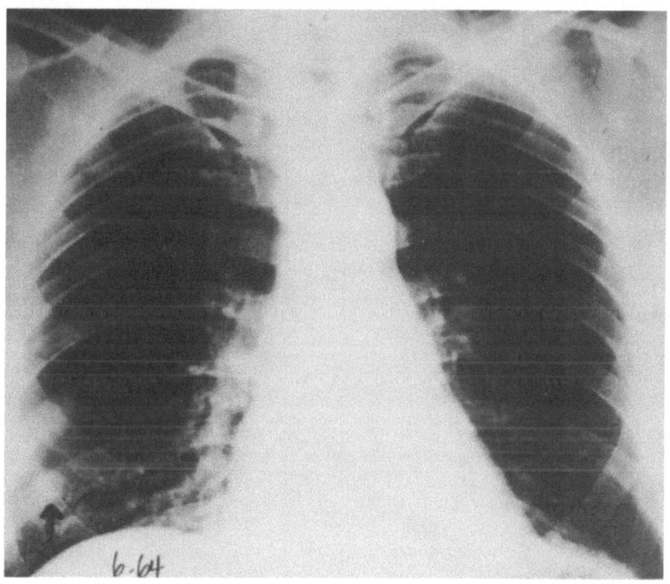

c

Fig. III.41a–c. Female, 46 years old. Giant-cell tumor of proximal phalanx of finger with pulmonary metastases. **a** Lateral and anteroposterior radiograph before operation. **b** Recurrence after curettage, showing extension of the tumor and destruction of the cortex with soft tissue invasion. **c** Radiograph of the lungs, showing a small metastatic nodule in the right lower lobe. (Schajowicz et al. 1972)

value, because prediction of the evolution of a giant-cell tumor based on its histologic features is impossible. It is doubtful that the not-infrequent finding of isolated giant cells or groups of tumor cells in blood vessels near the tumor has prognostic implications; further investigations are necessary to solve this important problem.

However, our experience confirms the statement of Goldenberg et al. that the predominance of *xanthomatous areas* associated with abundant fibrous tissue and scarce giant cells, often of smaller size, commonly associated with a quiescent (grade I) radiologic appearance, constitutes a histopathologic pattern of *prognostic value*, with a high cure rate after simple curettage and bone grafts. Analysis of this factor awaits a longer-term follow-up of our cases.

"Malignant" Giant-Cell Tumor. Considerable confusion exists concerning what constitutes a "malignant" giant-cell tumor based on histologic and/or clinical criteria; the relative incidence is extremely variable in the different larger series, ranging from 7% (Goldenberg et al. 1970) and 8% (Mnaymneh et al. 1964) up to 19% (McGrath 1972). McGrath divided malignant giant-cell

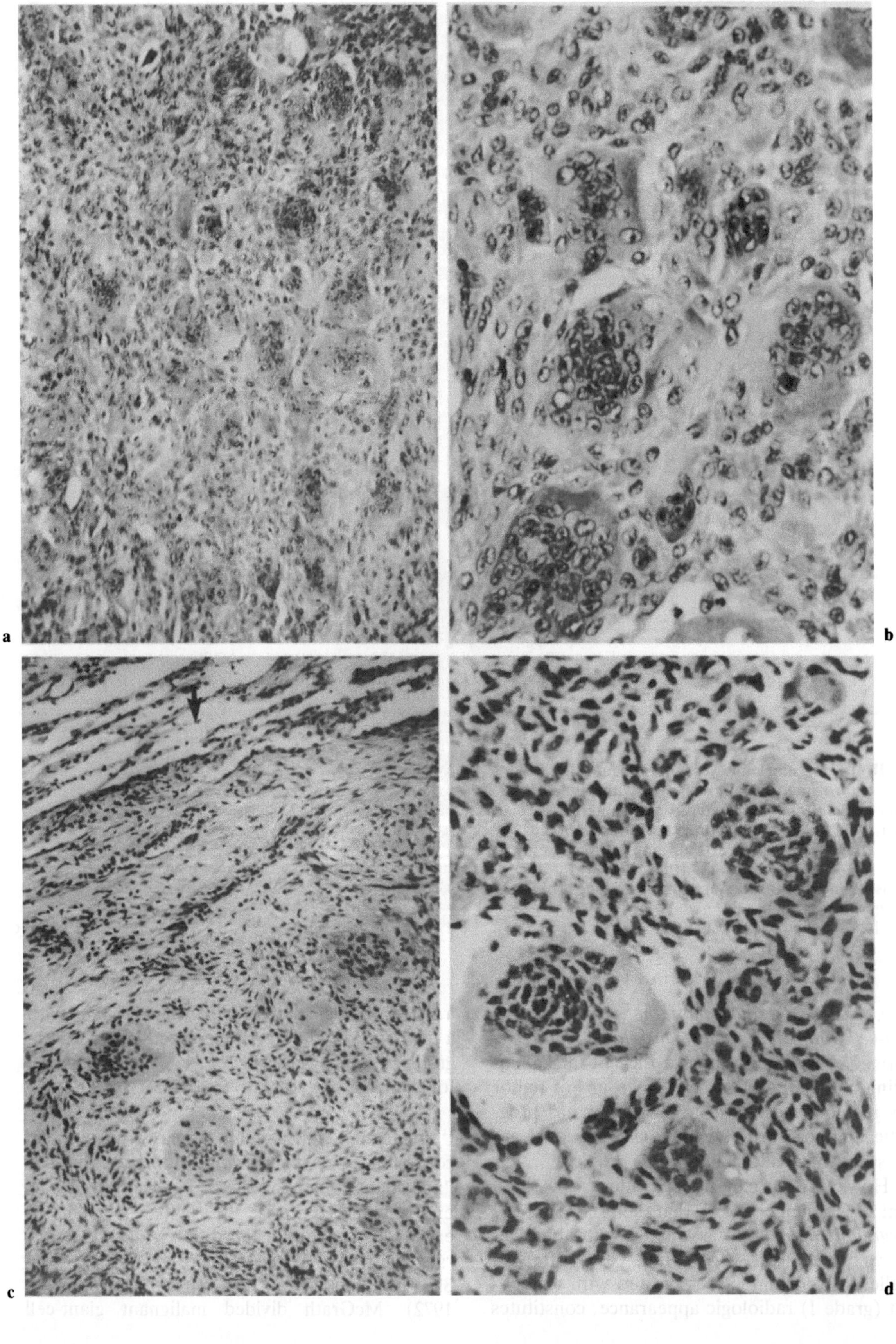
a
b
c
d

a 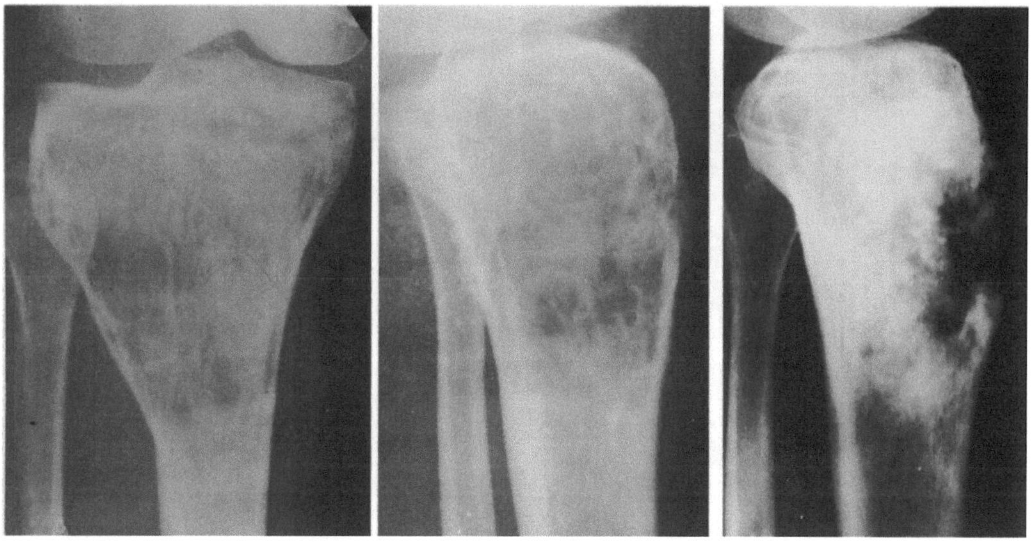 b

Fig. III.43a,b. Female, 21 years old. Giant-cell tumor of the upper end of tibia. **a** Anteroposterior and lateral radiographs. A curettage was performed after a previous biopsy and the remitted material showed the histologic features of giant-cell tumor without any sign of malignancy. **b** Radiograph 24 months after the curettage shows a sclerotic and osteolytic lesion that has destroyed the cortex with clear evidence of malignancy. A biopsy revealed an osteosarcoma. This was, in our experience, one of only two cases of sarcomatous transformation that occurred *without* irradiation

tumors into three types: (1) *primary*, in which the tumor was malignant from the onset (his two cases were located in the femoral shaft and were probably telangiectatic osteosarcomas); (2) *evolutionary*, in which a typical tumor progressed to a malignant form within a short period; and (3) *secondary*, in which a typical tumor underwent sarcomatous changes after a relatively long symptom-free period, usually after irradiation (four cases). It is noteworthy that the number of cases classified as malignant giant-cell tumor at the Memorial Hospital in New York during the period 1949–1977 decreased from 36 (Hutter et al. 1962) to only eight in the more recent report by Nascimento et al. (1979) from the same institution.

According to Dahlin (1978), who reported on 20 cases, "to be certain of the diagnosis of malignant giant-cell tumor, the pathologist must be able to demonstrate zones of typical benign giant-cell tumor in the malignant neoplasm under appraisal or in previous tissue obtained from the same neoplasm." According to this definition of malignant giant-cell tumor, 15 of the 20 tumors occurred *after treatment* for typical benign giant-cell tumors. Thirteen of the 15 "secondary" malignant tumors occurred subsequent to histologically verified benign giant-cell tumors at intervals that averaged 10.8 years from the time of treatment of the benign neoplasm, which included *irradiation* in each instance. The other two developed after bone grafting, without irradiation. Five patients had sarcomas present in portions of typical giant-cell tumors at the time of their first operations. With the exception of two patients, in whom sarcomatous transformation occurred 28 months (Schajowicz 1981) and 20 years (Gitelis et al. 1990), respectively, after previous curettage and bone grafting as treatment of a typical giant-cell tumor (Fig. III.43), all our cases occurred after radiation therapy, whether associated with conservative surgical intervention (seven cases) or not (three cases) (Fig. III.44).

The majority of the sarcomas were fibrosarcomas, and the remainder were osteosarcomas (two cases). This agrees with other published cases, which include only a few osteosarcomas (Cahan et al. 1948; Cruz et al. 1957; Sabanas et al. 1956). In general, postradiation sarcoma

Fig. III.42a–d. Same case as in Fig. III.41. **a,b** Photomicrographs illustrating the histologic appearance of the recurrent tumor of the phalanx, showing a typical giant-cell tumor without signs of malignancy. **c,d** Photomicrographs showing the histologic aspect of the excised pulmonary metastases without features of malignancy. **a** ×160; **b** ×320, **c** ×160, **d** ×250

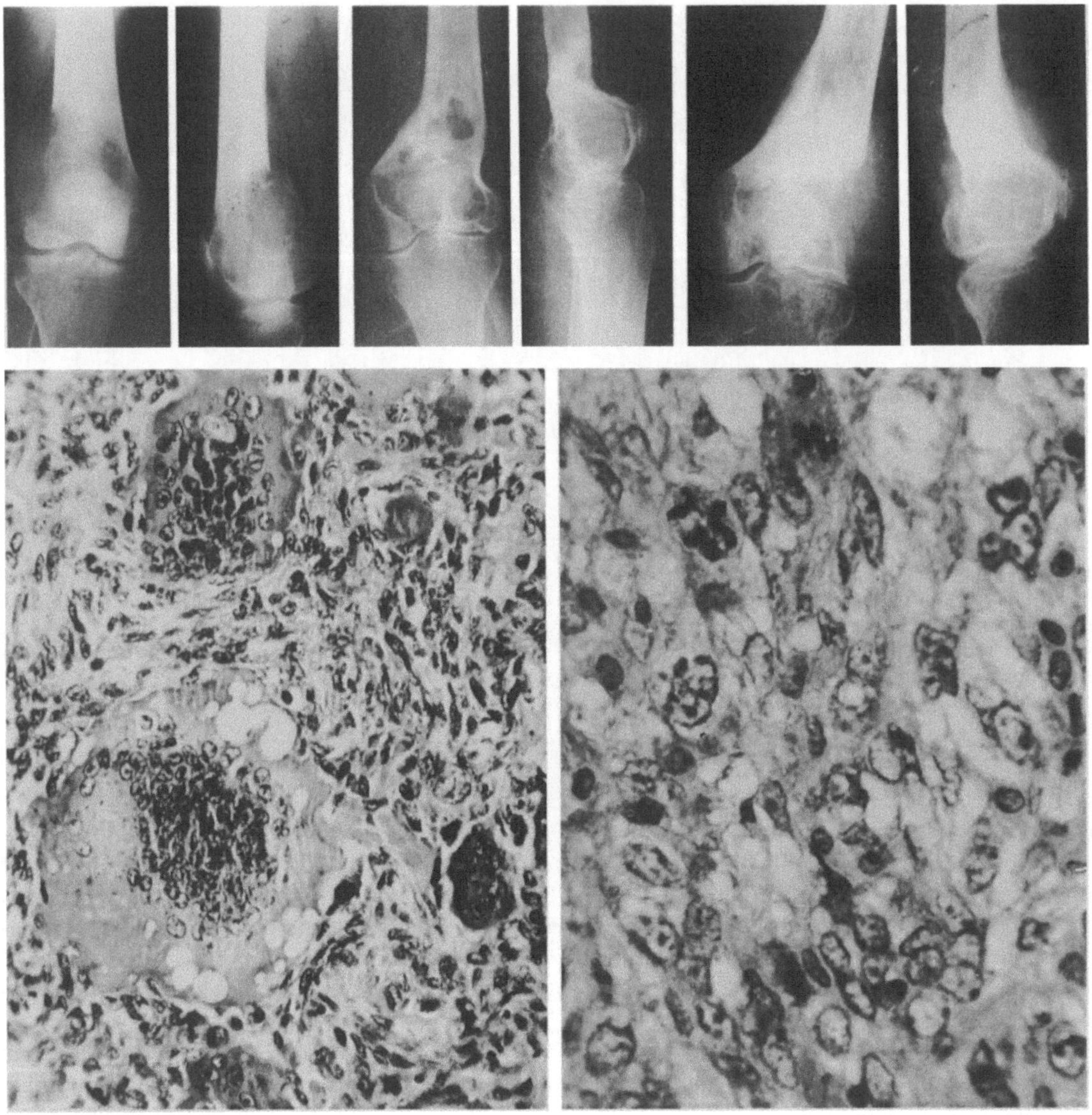

a, b c

d e

Fig. III.44a–e. Female, 20 years old. Sarcomatous transformation of benign giant-cell tumor of the lower end of femur, 18 years after curettage and radiotherapy. **a** Anteroposterior and lateral radiographs before treatment. **b** Radiograph 12 years later showing apparent recurrence of tumor. **c** Radiograph 18 years after initial treatment revealing a destructive osteolytic lesion, extending into soft tissue. An amputation was performed, and the patient died 6 months later with pulmonary metastases. **d,e** Photomicrographs of the original biopsy (giant-cell tumor) and of the amputation specimen showing spindle-cell sarcoma (fibrosarcoma). **d** ×180, **e** ×400

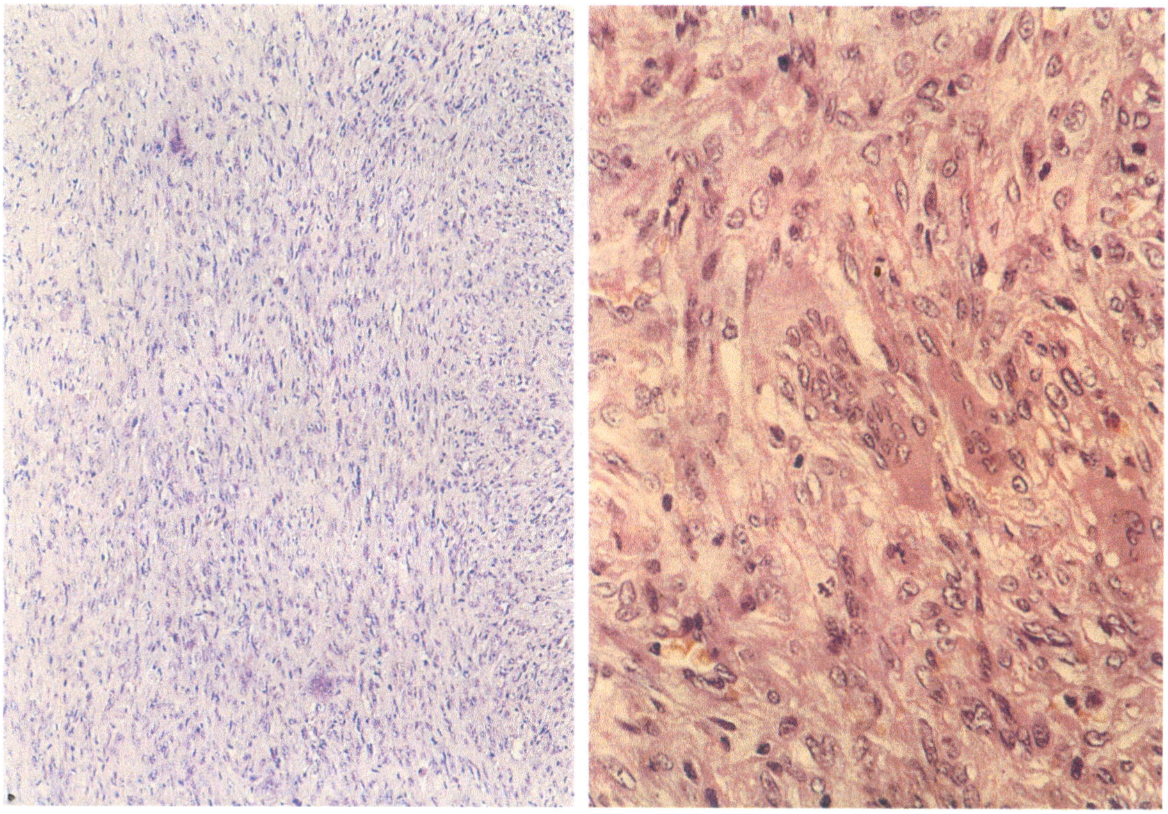

Fig. III.45a,b. Photomicrographs at **a** lower and **b** higher magnification of a fibrosarcoma containing a number of multinucleated giant cells. Such cases are occasionally interpreted as malignant giant-cell tumors. **a** ×120, **b** ×300

occurs in about 10% of cases (Cade 1949), although some statistics go as high as 15% (Jaffe 1958; Thomson and Turner-Warwick 1955).

The interval between commencement of radiation therapy and the appearance of sarcoma is generally 5–8 years. In our series it was between 3 and 18 years (Schajowicz and Slullitel 1966), but other authors (Cahan et al. 1948; Cruz et al. 1957; Jaffe 1958) mention cases in which the sarcoma appeared 22 and 23 years, or even 38 years (Dahlin 1978) after roentgenotherapy. Whether the action of the roentgen rays on the tumor cells is the cause of this late transformation, due to biologic changes in the stromal cells, demonstrable as cytologic changes, or whether it is the harmful effect of irradiation on neighboring healthy tissue (Hatcher 1945), is still an unsolved problem of only academic interest. The finding of fibrosarcomatous areas alongside areas showing the histologic pattern of typical giant-cell tumor appears to argue in favor of a true sarcomatous transformation of a preexistent, apparently benign giant-cell tumor.

In the writer's opinion, shared by Mirra (1980) and others, cases reported as "primary" malignant giant-cell tumors were really sarcomas rich in multinucleated giant cells of the osteoclast type, the majority being telangiectatic osteosarcomas, giant-cell rich osteosarcomas (Bathurst and Sanerkin 1986), fibrosarcomas (Fig. III.45; see also Chap. VI) or malignant fibrous histiocytomas.

Our experience supports Dahlin's statement that the entity *primary, diffusely malignant giant-cell tumor* with a roentgenogram consonant with the diagnosis of true giant-cell tumor *is extremely unusual*. No such case was found either in his or in our series. It is interesting that in the last editions of his book, Dahlin entitled the corresponding chapter "Malignancy in giant-cell tumors" (Dahlin and Unni 1986).

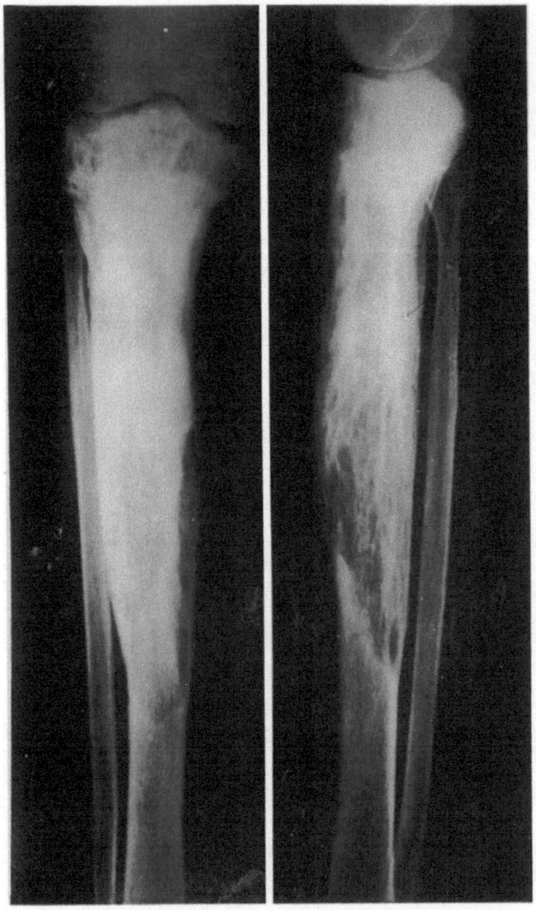

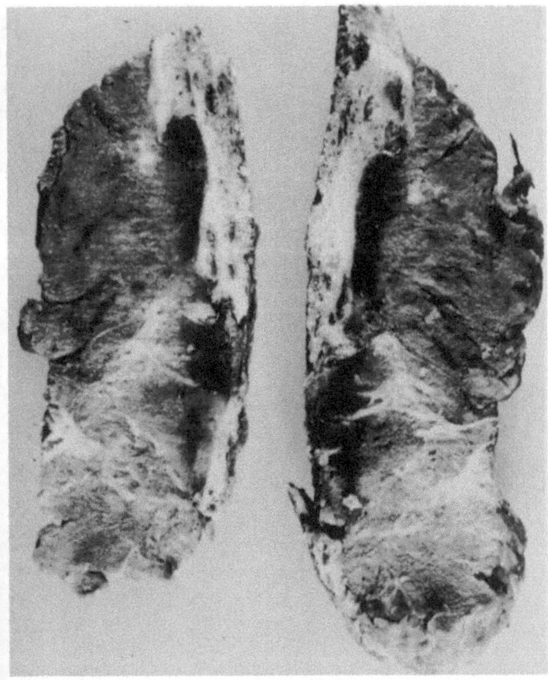

b

a

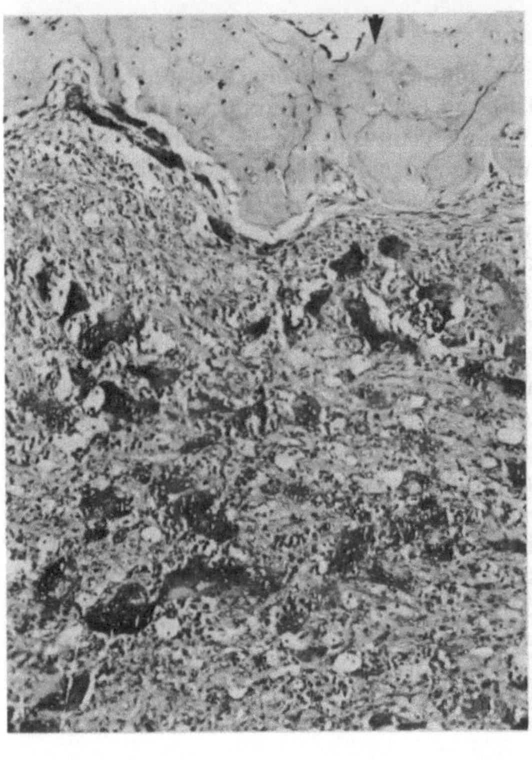

c

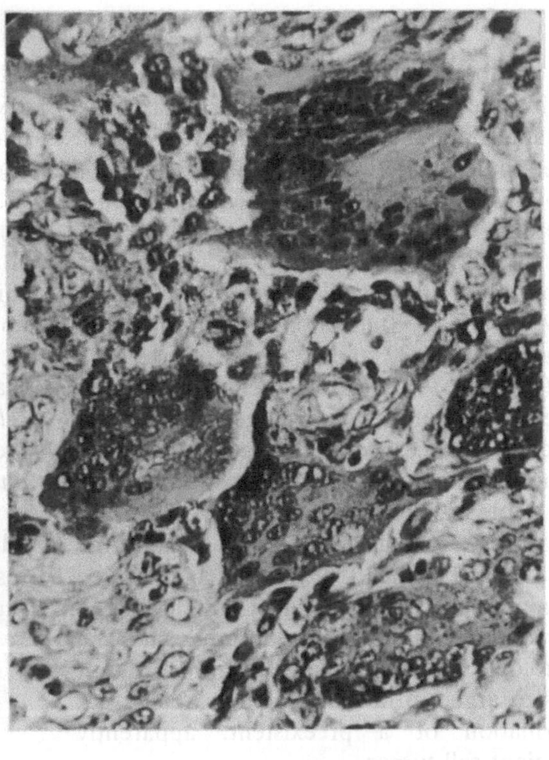

d

Giant-Cell Tumor in Paget Disease

The existence of a giant-cell tumor with no histologic signs of malignancy complicating Paget disease of bone is extremely rare. However, this possibility should be recognized, because sarcomas arising out of Paget disease always have a poor prognosis and with rare exceptions (Schatzki and Dudley 1961; Schajowicz et al. 1983) are rapidly fatal. Paradoxically, giant-cell tumors associated with Paget disease are not as aggressive as genuine giant-cell tumors originating in normal bones.

The fact that a fairly large number of giant cells of the osteoclastic type can be observed with some frequency in sarcomas arising in Paget disease (Schajowicz et al. 1983) shows that great care should be taken when making the diagnosis. One does not want to overestimate a benign tumor and therefore indicate radical treatment, or to underestimate a highly malignant tumor that is nearly always fatal.

In 1962, Hutter and associates reported five cases of benign giant-cell tumor sarcoma complicating Paget disease, observed at the Memorial Hospital, New York, and added an equal number of cases from the literature. These authors gave a detailed description of the clinical course and pathologic findings. One year later from the same center, McKenna et al. (1964) reported from the English literature, 12 cases (including five of their own) of benign giant-cell tumor as a complication in Paget disease. To those 12 cases, this writer has added another case in which the tumor was localized in the diaphysis of the tibia in a monostotic lesion in a 45-year-old patient who was followed for more than 4 years (Schajowicz and Slullitel 1966). This case recurred twice and finally an amputation was performed because of a secondary infection (Fig. III.46). More recently we observed another case, located in the clavicle (Schajowicz et al. 1983).

Goldenberg et al. (1970) reported four cases of giant-cell tumor in bones affected by polyostotic Paget disease (among a total of 218 giant-cell tumors; two of the four cases had already been reported) and collected 16 cases from the literature. It is noteworthy that most cases had a predilection for the bones of the skull and face (Jaffe 1958): three cases were found in the skull, three in the maxilla, and one in the mandible. The ilium was the next in order of frequency with four cases; only three cases were located in long bones, two in the tibia and one in the humerus. This is in direct contrast to the usual location of the genuine giant-cell tumor originating in bones unaffected by Paget disease.

One of the skull lesions, which corresponded to a multicentric giant-cell tumor, was mentioned by Jaffe (1958). From 1949 to 1967, it developed 21 foci of separate giant-cell tumors in various parts of the skull and face, as well as six lesions in the axial skeleton (Goldenberg et al. 1970). Mirra and Gold (1982) reported viruslike intranuclear inclusions, similar to those observed in the osteoclasts of Paget disease in a giant-cell tumor of the femur associated with Paget disease.

Fig. III.46a–d. Male, 45 years old. Giant-cell tumor of tibia associated with Paget disease of bone. **a** Anteroposterior and lateral radiographs showing a typical lesion of Paget disease involving the upper half of the tibia with an elongated osteolytic lesion of the anteromedial diaphysis, apparently destroying the thinned cortex. **b** Photograph of the resected specimen showing the extraosseous extension of the tumor, with its brown color. **c,d** Photomicrographs showing the histologic pattern of the giant-cell tumor; there is no sign of malignancy. At *top* in **c**, note a bone trabecula with the characteristic mosaic pattern of Paget disease. (Schajowicz and Slullitel 1966) **c** ×100, **d** ×400

References

Abelanet R, Daudet-Monsac M, Laoussadi S et al. (1986) Frequency and diagnostic value of the virus-like filamentous intranuclear inclusions in giant cell tumor of bone, not associated with Paget's disease: a study of 43 cases. Virchows Arch [A] 410:65–68

Ackerman LV, Spjut HJ (1962) Tumors of bone and cartilage. Atlas of tumor pathology, Fasc 4. Armed Forces Institute of Pathology, Washington, DC

Aegerter EE (1947) Giant cell tumors of bone: a critical survey. Am J Pathol 23:283–297

Aegerter EE, Kirkpatrick JA Jr (1975) Orthopedic diseases: physiology, pathology, radiology, 4th edn. W.B. Saunders, Philadelphia

Aoki J, Moser RP, Vinh TN (1989) Giant-cell tumor of the scapula: a review of 13 cases. Skeletal Radiol 18:427–434

Aparisi T, Arborgh B, Ericsson JLE (1977) Giant cell tumor of bone: detailed fine structural analysis of different cell components. Virchows Arch [A] 376:273–298

Aparisi T, Arborgh B, Ericsson JLE (1978) Giant cell tumor of bone: fine structural localization of alkaline phosphatase. Virchows Arch [A] 378:287–295

Athanasou NA, Bliss E, Gatter KC et al. (1985) An immunohistological study of giant-cell tumor of bone: evidence for an osteoclast origin of the giant cells. J Pathol 147:153–158

Bernstrom P, Stark HH (1971) Giant cell reaction of a metacarpal. Am J Clin Pathol 55:77–81

Bertheussen KJ, Holck S, Schiodt T (1983) Giant cell lesion of bone of the hand with particular emphasis on giant cell reparative granuloma. J Hand Surg [Am] 8:46–49

Bertoni F, Present D, Enneking WF (1985) Giant-cell tumor of bone with pulmonary metastases. J Bone Joint Surg [Am] 8:890–900

Bertoni F, Calderoni P, Bacchini P et al. (1986) Benign fibrous histiocytoma of bone. J Bone Joint Surg [Am] 68:1225–1230

Bertoni F, Present D, Sudanese A et al. (1988) Giant-cell tumor of bone with pulmonary metastases. Six case reports and a review of the literature. Clin Orthop 237:275–285

Bhaskar SN, Bernier JL, Godby F (1959) Aneurysmal bone cyst and other giant cell lesions of the jaws; report of 104 cases. J Oral Surg 17:30–41

Bloodgood JC (1923) Benign giant-cell tumor of bone: its diagnosis and conservative treatment. Am J Surg 37:105–116

Boquist L, Larsson SE, Lorentzon R (1976) Genuine giant-cell tumour of bone: a combined cytological, histopathological and ultrastructural study. Pathol Eur 11:117–127

Brecher ME, Franklin WA, Simon MA (1986) Immunohistochemical study of mononuclear phagocyte antigens in giant cell tumor of bone. Am J Pathol 125:252–257

Bridge JA, Neff JR, Bhatja PS, Singer WG, Murphy MD (1990) Cytogenetic findings and biologic behaviour of giant cell tumors of bone. Cancer 65:2697–2703

Burmester GR, Winchester RJ, Dimitriu-Bona A et al. (1983) Delineation of four cell types comprising the giant cell tumor of bone. Expression of IA and monocyte-macrophage lineage antigens. J Clin Invest 71:1633–1648

Caballes RL (1981) The mechanism of metastasis in the so-called "benign giant cell tumor of bone." Hum Pathol 12:762–767

Cade S (1949) Giant-cell tumour of bone (editorial). J Bone Joint Surg [Br] 31:158–160

Cahan GW, Woodard HQ, Higinbotham NL, Stewart JW, Coley BL (1948) Sarcoma arising in irradiated bone: report of eleven cases. Cancer 1:3–29

Campanacci M (1981) Tumori delle ossa e delle parti molli. 2 volumes. Aulo Gaggi Editore, Bologna, Italy

Campanacci M (1990) Bone and soft tissue tumors. Springer, Vienna New York

Campanacci M, Giunti A, Olmi R (1973) La localizazzione meta-diafisiaria del tumore a cellula giganti. Chir Organi Mov 62:29–38

Campanacci M, Giunti A, Olmi R (1975) Giant-cell tumors of bone: a study of 209 cases with long-term follow-up in 130. Ital J Orthop Traumatol 1:249–277

Campanacci M, Baldini N, Boriani S et al. (1987) Giant-cell tumor of bone. J Bone Joint Surg [Am] 69:106–114

Campbell CJ, Akbarnia BA (1975) Giant-cell tumor of the radius treated by massive resection and tibial bone graft. J Bone Joint Surg [Am] 57:982–986

Caskey PM, Wolf MD, Fechner RE (1985) Multicentric giant cell reparative granuloma of the small bones of the hand: a case report and review of the literature. Clin Orthop 193:199–205

Coley BL, Higinbotham NL, Kogure T (1958) Giant cell tumor of bone. Am J Surg 96:479–491

Cooper KL, Beabout JW, Dahlin DC (1984) Giant cell tumor: ossification in soft-tissue implants. Radiology 15:597–602

Cruz M, Coley BL, Stewart FW (1957) Post irradiation bone sarcoma: report of 11 cases. Cancer 10:72–88

Dahlin DC (1978) Bone tumors, 3rd edn. Charles C. Thomas, Springfield, IL

Dahlin DC (1977) Giant cell tumor of vertebrae above the sacrum: a review of 31 cases. Cancer 39:1350–1356

Dahlin DC, Unni KK (1986) Bone tumors: general aspects and data on 8542 cases. Charles C. Thomas, Springfield, IL

Dahlin DC, Cupps RE, Johnson EW Jr (1970) Giant-cell tumor: a study of 195 cases. Cancer 25:1061–1070

D'Alonzo RT, Pitcock JA, Milford LW (1972) Giant-cell reaction of bone: report of two cases. J Bone Joint Surg [Am] 54:1267–1271

De Santis E, Porfiri B, Simoni C et al. (1982) L'ultrastruttural del tumore a cellule giganti dell'osso. Arch Putti Chir Organi Mov 32:333–344

Duncan CP, Morton KS, Arthur JF (1983) Giant cell tumour of bone: its aggressiveness and potential for malignant changes. Can J Surg 26:475–477

Dyke SC (1931) Metastases of the "benign" giant cell tumor of bone (osteoclastoma). J Pathol Bacteriol 34:259–263

Eckhardt JJ, Grogan TJ (1986) Giant cell tumor of bone. Clin Orthop 204:45–58

Ewing J (1922) A review and classification of bone sarcomas. Arch Surg 4:485–533

Ewing J (1928) The classification and treatment of bone sarcomas. Cancer. Wood, New York, p 365

Finch GF, Gleave HH (1926) A case of osteoclastoma (myeloid sarcoma, benign giant tumor) with pulmonary metastases. J Pathol Bacteriol 29:339

Fitzpatrick DJ, Bullough PG (1977) Giant cell tumor of the lunate bone: a case report. J Hand Surg 2:269–270

Fornasier VL, Flores L, Hastings D et al. (1985) Virus-like filamentous intranuclear inclusions in a giant-cell tumor, not associated with Paget's disease of bone. J Bone Joint Surg [Am] 67:333–336

Gallardo H, Lustig ES, Schajowicz F (1970) Growth and maintenance of human giant cell bone tumors (osteoclastomas) in continuous culture. Oncology 24:146–159

Gilmer WS (1954) Histochemical studies in bone disease. I. Distribution of acid and alkaline phosphatase in bone tumors as a diagnostic acid. J Bone Joint Surg [Am] 36:182–183

Gitelis S, Wang J, Quast M, Schajowicz F, Templeton A (1990) Recurrence of a giant-cell tumor with malignant transformation to a fibrosarcoma 25 years after primary treatment. J Bone Joint Surg [Am] 71:757–761

Glass TA, Mills SE, Fechner RE et al. (1983) Giant-cell reparative granuloma of the hands and feet. Radiology 149:65–68

Goidanich IF (1956) I tumori primitivi dell'osso. Atti 41st Congr Soc Ital Ortop Traumatol

Goldenberg RR, Campbell CJ, Bonfiglio M (1970) Giant-cell tumor of bone: an analysis of 218 cases. J Bone Joint Surg [Am] 52:619–663

Goldring SR, Schiller AL, Mankin HJ et al. (1986) Characterization of cells from human giant cell tumors of bone. Clin Orthop 204:59–74

Goldring SR, Roelke MS, Petrison KK et al. (1987) Human giant cell tumors of bone: identification and characterization of cell types. J Clin Invest 79:483–491

Gomori G (1941) Distribution of acid phosphatase in tissues under normal and pathologic conditions. Arch Pathol 32:189–199

Gomori G (1956) Histochemical methods for acid phosphatase. Stain Technol 4:425–461

Gresen AA, Dahlin DC, Peterson LFA, Payne WS (1973) "Benign" giant cell tumor of bone metastasizing to lung: report of a case. Ann Thorac Surg 16:531–535

Gross SA (1879) Sarcoma of the long bone: based upon a study of 175 cases. Am J Med Sci 155:2–57

Hanaoka H, Friedman B, Mack RP (1970) Ultrastructure and histogenesis of giant cell tumors of bone. Cancer 25:1408

Hancox N (1956) The osteoclast. In: Bourne GH (ed) The biochemistry and physiology of bone. Academic, New York

Hatcher CH (1945) The pathogenesis of localized fibrous lesion in the metaphyses of long bones. Ann Surg 122:1016–1030

Hermann SD, Mesgarzadeh M, Bonakdarpour A et al. (1987) The role of magnetic resonance imaging in giant cell tumor of bone. Skeletal Radiol 16:635–643

Horton MA, Lewis D, McNulty K et al. (1985) Monoclonal antibodies to osteoclastomas (giant cell bone tumors): definition of osteoclast-specific cellular antigens. Cancer Res 45:5663–5669

Hutter RVP, Worcester JN Jr, Francis KC, Foote FW Jr, Stewart FW (1962) Benign and malignant giant cell tumors of bone: a clinicopathological analysis of the natural history of the disease. Cancer 15:653–690

Huvos AG (1979) Bone tumors: diagnosis, treatment and prognosis. W.B. Saunders, Philadelphia

Huvos AG (1991) Bone tumors: diagnosis, treatment, prognosis. W.B. Saunders, Philadelphia

Imura S, Takeda M (1968) Histochemical and electron microscopic studies on the giant cell tumors of bone (especially cultured cells). Springer, New York Berlin Heidelberg

Jacobs P (1972) The diagnosis of osteoclastoma (giant cell tumors): a radiological and pathological correlation. Br J Radiol 45:121–136

Jaffe HL (1953a) Giant cell reparative granuloma, traumatic bone cyst, and fibrous (fibro-osseous) dysplasia of the jaw bones. J Oral Surg 67:159–175

Jaffe HL (1953b) Giant cell tumour (osteoclastoma) of bones: its pathologic delimitation and the inherent clinical implications. Ann R Coll Surg Engl 13:343–355

Jaffe HL (1958) Tumors and tumorous conditions of the bones and joints. Lea & Febiger, Philadelphia

Jaffe JL, Lichtenstein L, Portis RB (1940) Giant cell tumor of bone: its pathologic appearance, grading, supposed variants and treatment. Arch Pathol 30:993–1031

Jeffree GM, Price CHG (1965) Bone tumors and their enzymes: a study of the phosphatases, non-specific esterases and betaglucuronidase of osteogenic and cartilaginous tumors, fibroblastic and giant cell lesions. J Bone Joint Surg [Br] 47:120

Jernstrom P, Stark HH (1971) Giant cell reaction of a metacarpal. Am J Clin Pathol 55:77–81

Jewell JH, Bush LF (1964) "Benign" giant cell tumor of bone with a solitary pulmonary metastasis: a case report. J Bone Joint Surg [Am] 56:848–852

Johnston J (1977) Giant cell tumor of bone: the role of the giant cell in orthopedic pathology. Orthop Clin North Am 8:751–770

Kraievski NA, Raikhlin NT, Soloviov JN (1970) Histochemical characteristics of giant cell bone tumors. Folia Histochem Cytochem (Krakow) 8:3–10

Kuwana K (1967) Electron microscopic study on giant cell tumor of bone. Nippon Geka Hokan 36:819

Ladanyi M, Traganos F, Huvos AG (1989) Benign metastasizing giant-cell tumors of bone: a DNA flow cytometric study. Cancer 64:1521–1526

Larsson SE, Lorentzon R, Boquist L (1975) Giant cell tumor of bone: a demographic, clinical and histopathological study of all cases recorded in the Swedish Cancer Registry for the years 1958 through 1968. J Bone Joint Surg [Am] 57:167–173

Lasser EC, Tetewsky H (1957) Metastasizing giant cell tumors: report of an unusual case with indolent bone and pulmonary metastases. Am J Roentgenol Radium Ther Nucl Med 78:804–811

Le Charpentier Y, Forest M, Daudet-Monsac M et al. (1975) Ultrastructure of giant cell tumors of bone. Rev Chir Orthop 61:387–390

Le Charpentier Y, Le Charpentier M, Forest M et al. (1977) Intranuclear inclusions in giant cell bone tumor. Demonstration by electron microscopy. Nouv Presse Med 6:259–262

Lichtenstein L (1977) Bone tumors, 5th edn. C.V. Mosby, St. Louis

Louis DS, Hankin FM, Braunstein EM (1986) Giant cell tumour of the triquetrum. J Hand Surg [Br] 11:279–280

Lustig ES, Schajowicz F (1944) Cultivo de tejido de tumor gigantocelular de los huesos. Contribución a la histogénesis de la célula gigante. Rev Ortop Traumatol 14:134–151

Maloney WG, Vaughan LM, Jones MH, Ross J (1983) Benign metastasizing giant-cell tumor of bone. Report of three cases and review of the literature. Clin Orthop 243:208–215

Mankin HJ, Fogelson FS, Trasher AZ, Jaffer F (1976) Massive resection and autograft transplantation in the treatment of malignant bone tumors. N Engl J Med 294:1247

Marcove RC, Weis LD, Vaghaiwalla MR, Pearson NR, Huvos AG (1978) Cryosurgey in the treatment of giant cell tumors of bone: a report of 52 consecutive cases. Cancer 41:957–969

Matsuno T (1990) Benign fibrous histiocytoma involving the ends of long bone. Skeletal Radiol 19:561–566

McCarthy EF (1980) Giant-cell tumor of bone: an historical perspective. Clin Orthop 153:14–25

McCarthy EF, Serrano JA, Wasserkrug HL et al. (1979) The ultrastructural localization of secretory acid phosphatase in giant cell tumor of bone. Clin Orthop 141:295–302

McGrath PM (1972) Giant cell tumours of bone: an analysis of 52 cases. J Bone Joint Surg [Br] 52:216–219

McInerney DP, Middlemis JH (1978) Giant cell tumors of bone. Skeletal Radiol 2:195–204

McKenna RJ, Schwinn CP, Soong KY, Higinbotham NL (1964) Osteogenic sarcoma arising in Paget's disease. Cancer 17:42–66

Merle d'Aubigné R, Tomeno B (1977) The treatment of giant cell tumors: an analysis of 85 consecutive cases. Int Orthop 1:159–164

Meyerding HW (1941) Benign and malignant giant cell tumor of bone: diagnosis and results of treatment. JAMA 117:1849–1855

Mills BG, Singer FR (1976) Nuclear inclusions in Paget's disease of bone. Science 194:201–202

Mirra JM (1980) Bone tumors: diagnosis and treatment. J.B. Lippincott, Philadelphia

Mirra JM, Gold RH (1982) Giant cell tumor containing viral-like intranuclear inclusions, in association with Paget disease. Skeletal Radiol 8:67–70

Mirra JM, Ulich T, Magidson J et al. (1982) A case of probable benign pulmonary "metastases" or implants arising from a giant cell tumor of bone. Clin Orthop 162:245–254

Mnaymneh WA, Dudley HR, Mnaymneh LG (1964) Giant cell tumor of bone. J Bone Joint Surg [Am] 46:63–75

Murphy WR, Ackerman LV (1956) Benign and malignant giant cell tumors of bone. Cancer 9:317–339

Nascimento AG, Huvos AG, Marcove RC (1979) Primary malignant giant cell tumor of bone: a study of eight cases and review of the literature. Cancer 44:1393–1402

Nelaton E (1860) D'une nouvelle espèce de tumeurs benignes des os, ou tumeurs a myeloplaxes. Delahaye, Paris

Ottolenghi CE (1972) Massive osteo- and osteoarticular bone grafts. Technic and results of 62 cases. Clin Orthop 87:156–164

Pais C, Barrufaldi O (1958) Richerche istochimiche sui tumori a mieloplassi (contributo allo studio istogenetico del tumore delle cellule giganti; significato dei reperti nella valutazione della malignita). Arch Putti Chir Organi Mov 9:12–46

Pan P, Dahlin DC, Lipscomb PR, Bernatz PE (1964) "Benign" giant cell tumor of the radius with pulmonary metastasis. Proc Staff Meet Mayo Clin 39:344–349

Parish FF (1973) Allograft replacement of all or part of a long bone following excision of a tumor: report of 21 cases. J Bone Joint Surg [Am] 55:1–22

Peimer CA, Schiller AL, Mankin HJ et al. (1980) Multicentric giant cell tumor. J Bone Joint Surg [Am] 62:652–656

Peison B, Feigenbaum J (1976) Metaphysial giant-cell tumor in a girl of 14. Radiology 118:145–146

Pepler WD (1958) The histochemistry of a giant cell tumour (osteoclastoma and giant cell epulis). J Pathol Bacteriol 76:505–510

Persson B, Wouters HW (1976) Curettage and acrylic cementation in surgery of giant cell tumors of bone. Clin Orthop 120:125–133

Picci P, Manfrini M, Zucchi V et al. (1983) Giant-cell tumor bone in skeletally immature patients. J Bone Joint Surg [Am] 65:486–490

Pindborg JJ, Kramer IR (1971) Histological typing of odontogenic tumors, jaw cysts and allied lesions, vol 5. World Health Organization, Geneva

Rebel A, Malkani K, Basle M (1974) Anomalies nucleaires des ostéoclastes de la maladie osseuse de Paget. Nouv Presse Med 3:1299–1301

Reddy CRRM, Rao PS, Rajakumari K (1974) Giant cell tumors of bone in South India. J Bone Joint Surg [Am] 56:617–619

Rock MG, Pritchard DJ, Unni KK (1984) Metastases from histologically benign giant-cell tumor of bone. J Bone Joint Surg [Am] 66:269–274

Rock MG, Sim FH, Unni KK et al. (1986) Secondary malignant giant-cell tumor of bone. Clinicopathological assessment of 19 patients. J Bone Joint Surg [Am] 68:1073–1079

Roessner A, von-Bassewitz DB, Schlake W et al. (1984) Biologic characterization of human bone tumors. III. Giant cell tumor of bone: a combined electron microscopical, histochemical, and autoradiographical study. Pathol Res Pract 178:431–440

Russell DS (1949) Malignant osteoclastoma and the association of malignant osteoclastoma with Paget's osteitis deformans. J Bone Joint Surg [Br] 31:281–290

Sabanas AO, Dahlin DC, Childs DS Jr et al. (1956) Postradiation sarcoma of bone. Cancer 9:528–542

Savini R, Gherlinzoni F, Morandi M et al. (1983) Surgical treatment of giant-cell tumor of the spine. The experience at the Istituto Ortopedico Rizzoli. J Bone Joint Surg [Am] 65:1283–1289

Scaglietti O, Mondolfo S (1938) Sulla varieta xantomatosa die tumori gigantocellulari. Chir Organi Mov 23:435–459

Schajowicz F (1961) Giant cell tumors of bone (osteoclastoma): a pathological and histochemical study. J Bone Joint Surg [Am] 43:1–29

Schajowicz F (1981) Tumors and tumorlike lesions of bone and joints. Springer, New York Berlin Heidelberg

Schajowicz F, Cabrini RL (1954) Histochemical studies of bone in normal and pathological conditions. With special reference to alkaline phosphatase, glycogen and mucopolysaccharides. J Bone Joint Surg [Br] 36:474–489

Schajowicz F, Cabrini RL (1958) Histochemical localization of acid phosphatase in bone tissue. Science 127:1447–1448

Schajowicz F, Oleaga Alarcon F (1945) La transformación sarcomatosa de la osteitis deformante de Paget. Bol Trab Soc Argent Cirug Ortop 10:116–130

Schajowicz F, Slullitel J (1966) Giant cell tumor associated with Paget's disease of bone. J Bone Joint Surg [Am] 48:1340–1349

Schajowicz F, Ackerman LV, Sissons HA (1972) Histological typing of bone tumors. International histological classification of tumors, No. 6. World Health Organization, Geneva

Schajowicz F, Giménez IB, Cabrini RL (1977) Estudio microespectrofotométrico del ADN de las células gigantes multinucleadas en el osteoclastoma y osteosarcoma. Bol Trab Soc Argent Ortop Traumatol 42:323–330

Schajowicz F, Cabrini RL, Gimenez I (1981) Microspectrophotometric quantitation of DNA in bone tumors with giant cells (osteoclastoma, osteosarcoma and chondroblastoma). Clin Orthop 156:91–97

Schajowicz F, Santini Araujo E, Berenstein M (1983) Sarcoma complicating Paget's disease of bone. A clinicopathological study of 62 cases. J Bone Joint Surg [Br] 65:299–307

Schajowicz F, Ubios AM, Santini Araujo E et al. (1985) Virus-like intranuclear inclusions in giant cell tumor of bone. Clin Orthop 201:247–250

Schatzki SC, Dudley HR (1961) Bone sarcoma complicating Paget's disease. A report of 3 cases with long survival. Cancer 14:517–523

Schwinn P (1976) Giant cell lesions of bone. In: Bones and joints, I.A.P. Monogr No. 17. Williams & Wilkins, Baltimore, pp 236–299

Sherman M, Fabricius R (1961) Giant cell tumor in metaphysis in a child. Report of an unusual case. J Bone Joint Surg [Am] 43:1225–1229
Shuffstall RM, Gregory JE (1953) Osteoid formation in giant cell tumors of bone. Am J Pathol 29:1123–1127
Sim FH, Dahlin DC, Beabout JW (1977) Multicentric giant cell tumors of bone. J Bone Joint Surg [Am] 59:1052–1060
Singson R, Feldman F (1983) Case report 229. Diagnosis: multiple (multicentric) giant cell tumors of bone. Skeletal Radiol 9:276–281
Slullitel I, Slullitel J, Schajowicz F (1959) Tumor de células gigantes con transformación sarcomatosa a los 18 años. Bol Trab Soc Argent Ortop Traumatol 24:85–93
Small S, Rowe NH (1975) A "true giant cell tumor" in the mandible? J Oral Surg 33:296–301
Spjut HJ, Dorfman HD, Fechner RE, Ackerman LV (1971) Tumors of bone and cartilage. Atlas of tumor pathology, 2nd series, Fasc 5. Armed Forces Institute of Pathology, Washington, DC
Steiner GC, Ghosh L, Dorfman HD (1972) Ultrastructure of giant cell tumors of bone. Hum Pathol 3:569–586
Stewart MJ (1914) Observations on myeloid sarcoma with an analysis of 50 cases. Lancet II:1236–1242
Sung HW, Kuo DP, Shu WP et al. (1981) Giant-cell tumor of bone: analysis of 280 cases in Chinese patients. J Bone Joint Surg [Am] 64:755–761
Sybrandy S, De la Fuente AA (1973) Multiple giant-cell tumor of bone: report of a case. J Bone Joint Surg [Br] 55:350–356
Thiery JP, Mazabraud A, Veisin MC, Lacroix G (1974) L'étude cytologique de la tumeur à cellules géantes. Rev Chir Orthop 61:337–386
Thomson AD, Turner-Warwick RT (1955) Skeletal sarcomata and giant cell tumours. J Bone Joint Surg [Br] 37:266–303
Tornberg DN, Dick HM, Johnston AD (1975) Multicentric giant-cell tumors in the long bones: a case report. J Bone Joint Surg [Am] 57:420–422
Trifaud A, Faysse R, Papillon J (1956) Les tumeurs à myéloplaxes des os ou tumeurs à cellules géantes. Rev Chir Orthop 43:413–513
Troup JB, Dahlin DC, Coventry MB (1960) The significance of giant cells in osteogenic sarcoma. Do they indicate a relationship between osteogenic sarcoma and giant cell tumors of bone? Proc Staff Meet Mayo Clin 35:170–186
Uehlinger E (1976) Primary malignancy, secondary malignancy and semimalignancy of bone tumors. In: Grundmann E (ed) Malignant bone tumors. Springer, New York Berlin Heidelberg, pp 109–119
Ueno K (1964) Electron microscopic observations of giant cell tumors of bone. J Jpn Orthop Assoc 38:724
Vacher-Lavenu MC, Louvel A, Daudet-Monsac M et al. (1981) Inclusions tubulofilamenteuses intranucleaired dans les cellules multinuclées des tumeurs à cellules géantes des os. Etude ultrastructurale d'une series de 31 tumeurs. CR Acad Sci Paris 293:639–644
Vanel D, Contesso G, Rebibo G et al. (1983) Benign giant-cell tumours of bone with pulmonary metastases and favourable prognosis. Report on two cases and review of the literature. Skeletal Radiol 10:221–226
Volkov M (1970) Allotransplantation of joints. J Bone Joint Surg [Am] 52:49
von Albertini A (1928) Gutartige Riesenzellengeschwülste. Thieme, Leipzig
Weinmann JP, Sicher H (1947) Bone and bones. Fundamentals of bone biology. C.V. Mosby, St. Louis
Welsh RA, Meyer AT (1970) Nuclear fragmentations and associated fibrils in giant cell tumor of bone. Lab Invest 22:63–72
Willis RA (1949) Pathology of osteoclastoma or giant cell tumour of bone. J Bone Joint Surg [Br] 31:236–240
Wilson PD, Lance EM (1965) Surgical reconstruction of the skeleton following segmental resection for bone tumors. J Bone Joint Surg [Am] 47:1629–1656
Windeyer BW, Woodyatt PB (1949) Osteoclastoma: a study of 38 cases. J Bone Joint Surg [Br] 31:252–267
Wold LE, Swee RG (1984) Giant cell tumor of the small bones of the hands and feet. Semin Diagn Pathol 1:173–184
Wold LE, Dobyns JH, Swee RG et al. (1986) Giant cell reaction (giant cell reparative granuloma) of small bones of the hands and feet. Am J Surg Pathol 10:491–496
Wray CC, MacDonald AW, Richardson RA (1990) Benign giant-cell tumor with metastases to bone and lung. J Bone Joint Surg [Br] 72:486–489
Xiang J, Spanier SS, Benson NA, Braylan RC (1987) Flow cytometric analysis of DNA in bone and soft tissue tumors using nuclear suspensions. Cancer 59:1951–1958
Yoshida H, Akeho M, Yumoto T (1982) Giant cell tumor of bone. Enzyme histochemical, biochemical and tissue culture studies. Virchows Arch [A] 395:319–330

CHAPTER IV

Marrow Tumors (Round-Cell Tumors)

Although some 70 years have elapsed since Ewing (1921) described as a distinct clinico-pathologic entity the "diffuse endothelioma of bone," which he later termed "endothelial myeloma" (1924), the precise histogenesis of this neoplasm remains unresolved – this despite the numerous ultrastructural, histochemical, immunohistochemical, and other more sophisticated studies published in recent years.

The difficulties of differential diagnosis within the group of malignant small (blue) round-cell tumors of bone and specifically Ewing sarcoma, malignant lymphoma [formerly termed "primary reticulum-cell sarcoma of bone" by Parker and Jackson (1939)], metastatic neuroblastoma (sympathicoblastoma), and small-cell carcinoma are well known and of considerable interest to the practicing surgical pathologist. Although certain cases may be distinguished by clinical and roentgenographic examination, the definite diagnosis must fundamentally be based on histopathologic study. But even the diagnosis performed exclusively with cytomorphologic and conventional histopathologic methods may present great problems, particularly in poorly differentiated neoplasms that occur in unusual anatomic locations or affect individuals outside the usual age groups.

Moreover, the specificity of Ewing sarcoma as a distinct entity has been disputed in the last decade by several authors (Cavazzana et al. 1987; Llombart-Bosch et al. 1988) who have advocated a neural origin of most, if not all, Ewing sarcomas. This view was already supported some time ago by several British authors who, under the influence of Willis (Willis 1940, 1967; Colville and Willis 1933), believed that most cases were really metastases of neuroblastoma or undifferentiated carcinoma. In 1984, Jaffe et al. distinguished a new entity under the denomination "primary neuroectodermal tumor of bone (PNET)," which resembles the peripheral neuroepithelioma of soft tissues. They based this diagnosis particularly on the positive immunohistochemical staining with neuron-specific enolase (NSE), a technique considered specific for tumors of neural origin, especially neuroblastoma (Triche and Askin 1983; Tsokos et al. 1984; Osborn et al. 1986), irrespective of the degree of histologic differentiation (see section on PNET).

1. Ewing Sarcoma

Definition, WHO: *"A malignant tumor with a rather uniform histological appearance composed of densely-packed small cells with round nuclei but without distinct cytoplasmic outlines or prominent nucleoli. The tumor tissue is typically divided into irregular strands or lobules by fibrous septa, but the intercellular network of reticulin fibers which is a feature of malignant lymphoma is not seen. Mitoses are infrequent. Hemorrhages and areas of necrosis are common."*

Incidence. Ewing sarcoma accounts for 272 cases or 11% of the malignant bone tumors in our files. This percentage is slightly higher than that in Dahlin and Unni's (1986) series of 402 cases, in which Ewing sarcoma accounted for 6% of the malignant bone tumors. Ewing sarcoma is rare in black populations of both the United States and Africa, who seem to be genetically resistant (Fraumeni and Glass 1970; Linden and Dunn 1970; Williams 1975), and uncommon in Chinese (Li et al. 1980).

Clinical Findings. *Sex and Age.* Scheme IV.1 shows the distribution according to sex and age. It coincides, with slight variations, with the findings of other authors. Males were affected slightly more often than females.

The predominant age was between 5 and 15 years, the tumor being exceedingly rare after the third decade and uncommon before the fifth year; 91% of tumors occured before 20 years of age.

Localization. The preferred anatomic sites were the diaphyseal or metadiaphyseal regions of long bones, the femur (81 cases), tibia (32 cases), and

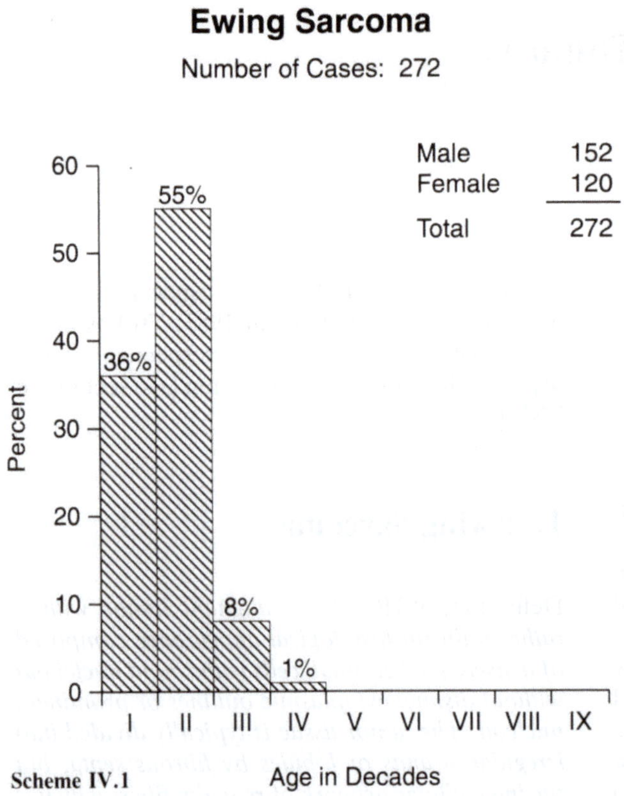

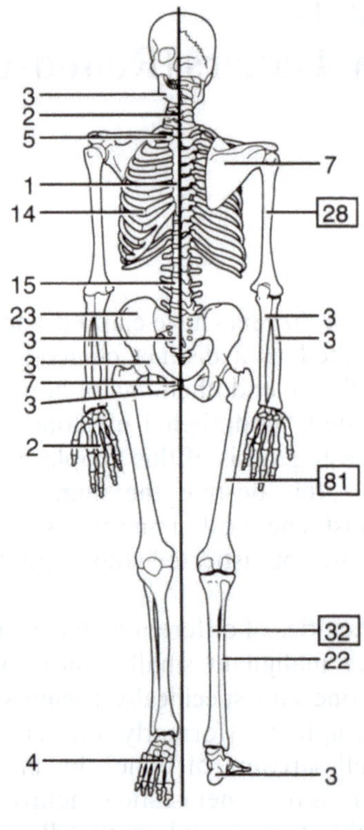

Scheme IV.1

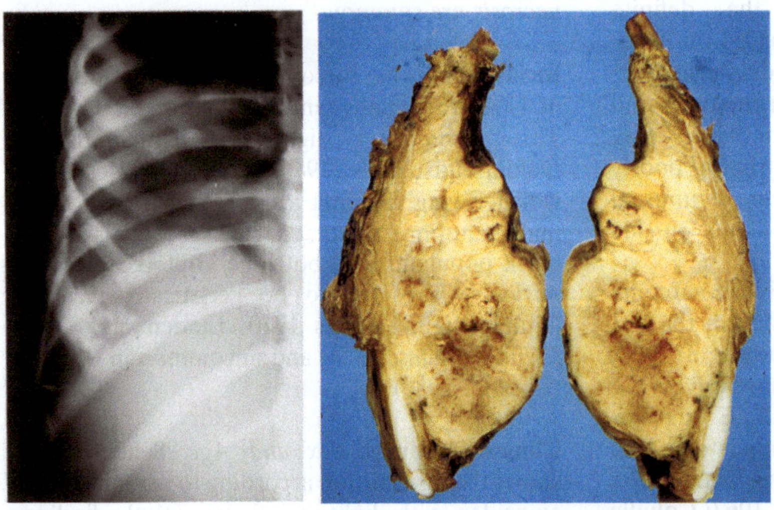

Fig. IV.1. a Destructive rib lesion in 11-year-old male. b Photograph of resected specimen showing obvious bony involvement with a large soft tissue component

humerus (28 cases) being the most commonly affected bones. Some flat and short bones are also frequently involved, especially the pelvis (ilium) (23 cases), spine (17 cases), and ribs (14 cases) (Fig. IV.1). Hands and feet and other sites were rarely involved. An epiphyseal location was exceptional in our material.

Symptoms. The most common complaint was pain and tenderness, accompanied in later stages by swelling or the presence of a palpable mass in the area of the tumor. The general health of the patients was frequently impaired – they often presented with fever, anemia, leukocytosis, and increased sedimentation rate. These symptoms,

Fig. IV.2. Male, 5 years old, Ewing sarcoma, shaft of ▶ femur. Radiograph shows a central irregular area of destruction surrounded by bone sclerosis. Note characteristic laminated "onion peel" periosteal reaction. (Schajowicz et al. 1972)

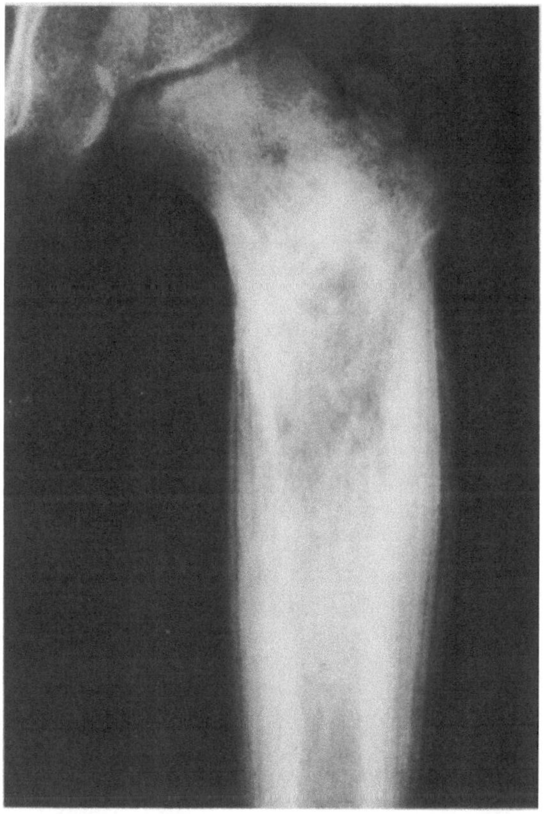

Fig. IV.3. Male, 13 years old. Ewing sarcoma of the shaft of fibula. Anteroposterior and lateral radiographs show a mottled area of bone destruction with laminated periosteal reaction of "onion-peel" appearance ▼

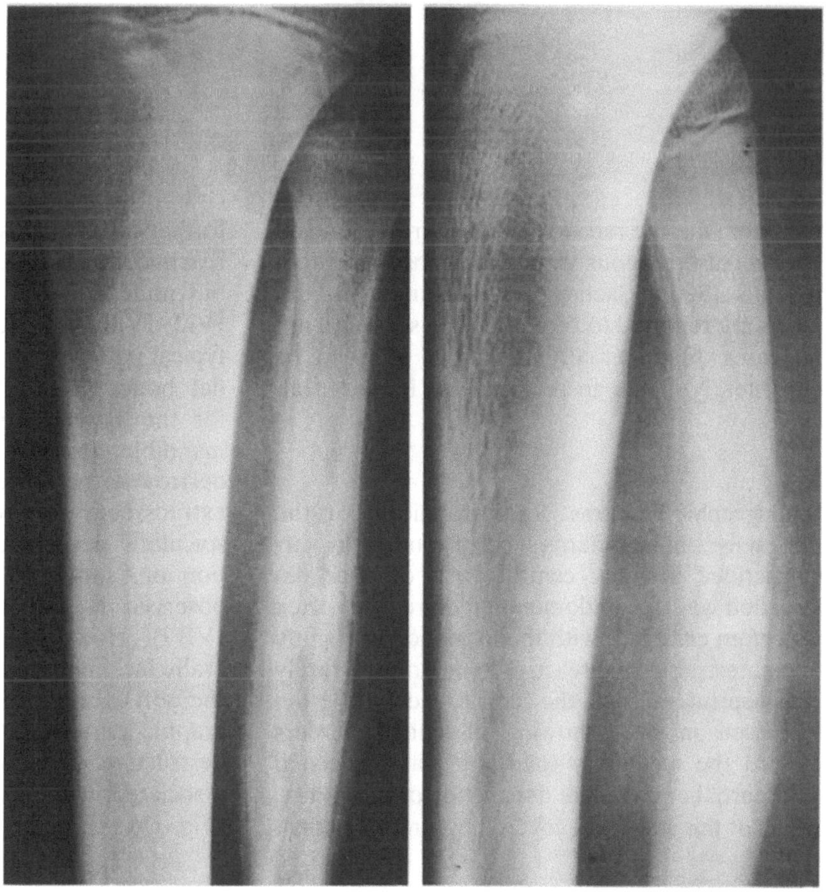

a b

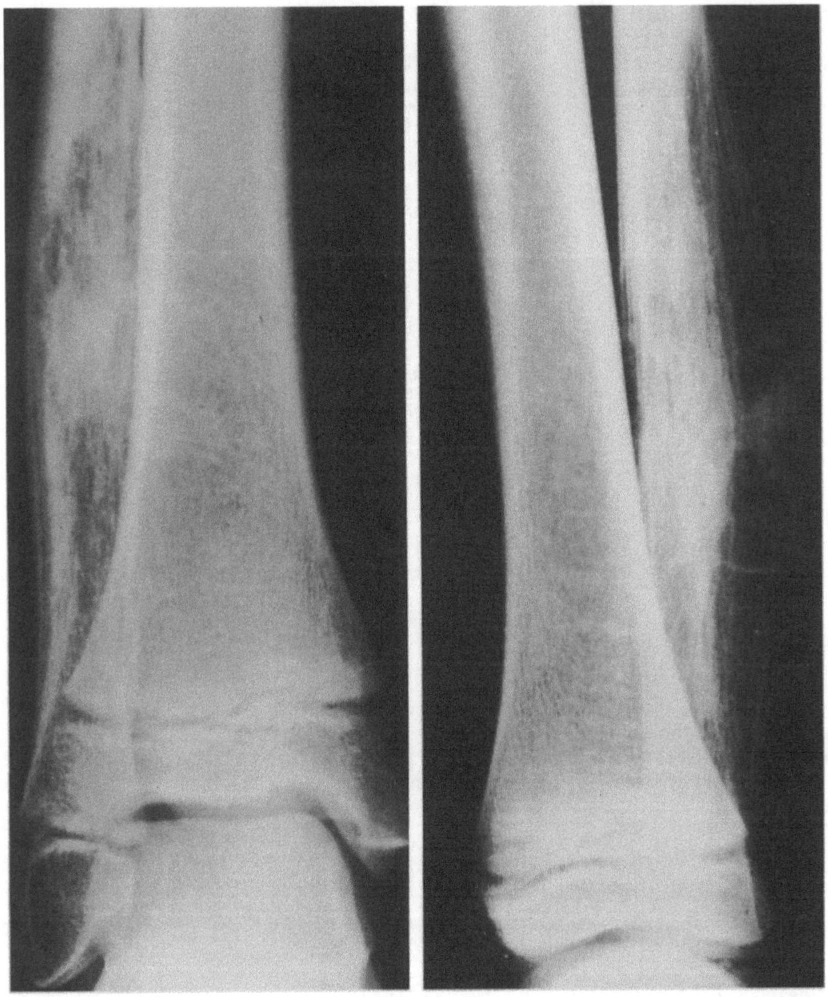

a b

Fig. IV.4. Male, 11 years old, Ewing sarcoma of fibula. Radiographs show radiolucent, irregular, ill-defined areas of osteolysis, periosteal lamellation, and perpendicular spicules

together with the radiographic features, led to an occasional erroneous clinical diagnosis of osteomyelitis. Serum lactate dehydrogenase (LDH) levels are reported to be elevated in some but not all cases (Bacci et al. 1985), but seem to be consistently higher in recurrences (Farley et al. 1987).

Radiographic Features. Radiographically, in the first stage, bone sclerosis accompanied by circumscribed irregular central areas of bone destruction was the predominant feature; the cortex was often enlarged, with the formation of slightly laminated periosteal reactive bone or more rarely radial spicules. Later, the central osteolytic lesion increased in size, showing ill-defined borders toward the medullary cavity. It was associated with partial or complete destruction of the cortex, which at this stage was covered by a more evident formation of periosteal laminated "onion peel" reactive bone. This pattern is a characteristic, but nondiagnostic, feature in long bones (Figs. IV.2–IV.8; however, cf. Figs. IV.9, IV.10); a typical pattern was generally lacking in short and flat bones (Figs. IV.11–IV.14; see Fig. IV.15 for the appearance in an unusual case in the mandible. In more advanced stages, the tumor destroyed the cortex, involving extensively the extraosseous soft tissues, sometimes provoking spicular, perpendicular reactive bone formation of "sunburst" appearance, similar to that observed in osteosarcoma (Figs. IV.5, IV.16, IV.17). However, Codman's triangle was generally lacking because of the rapid extension into the soft tissues. In the final stages, the radiographic pattern is often that of an extensive, destructive lesion, without any bone reaction and associated with an enormous soft tissue mass (Fig. IV.18).

Fig. IV.5. Female, 9 years old. Ewing sarcoma of femur. Anteroposterior and lateral radiographs show a radiolucent lesion at the anterolateral aspect of the metadiaphyseal region with periosteal reactive new-bone formation and Codman's triangles at its proximal end, suggestive of osteosarcoma

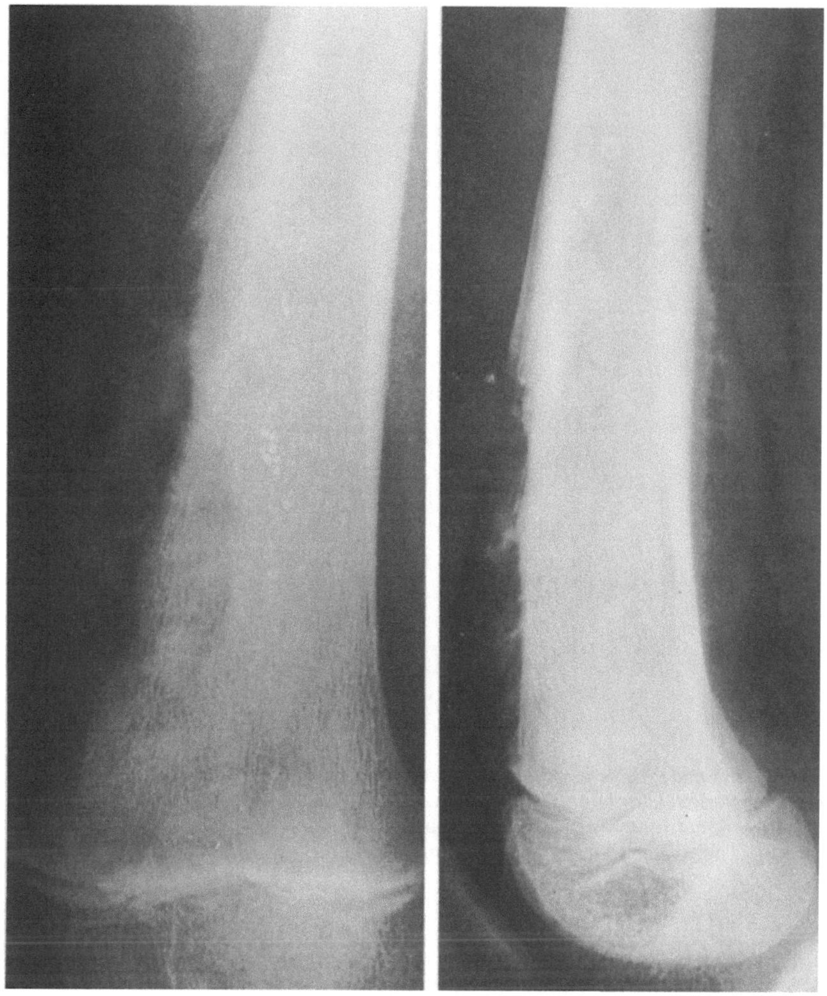

a b

Some benign lesions, especially osteomyelitis and eosinophilic granuloma, may simulate radiographically the appearance of Ewing sarcoma.

The malignant tumor that most commonly presents diagnostic problems is osteosarcoma, especially when localized in the diaphysis. Because of the striking tendency of Ewing sarcoma to involve other bones (Fig. IV.19), a bone scan is fundamental in detecting such lesions. Whether the presence of multiple bone lesions is a consequence of a metastatic spread or due to a multicentric origin is still disputed – the writer being more inclined to accept the former possibility.

Pathologic Findings. *Gross Pathology.* Like other pathologists, we have had only a few opportunities to examine entire specimens obtained from resection or amputation of untreated cases, because of the generalized primary type of treatment (chemotherapy and/or radiation therapy) used in Ewing sarcoma (Figs. IV.16–IV.18). In the nonmodified areas of the specimens, the medullary cavity was infiltrated by a tumor mass of soft consistency and grayish-white color, with numerous areas of hemorrhages and yellowish zones of extensive necrosis, often with cystic softening. This appearance suggests suppuration, which may lead to an erroneous impression of osteomyelitis. Frequently destruction of the cancellous bone trabeculae occurred, often accompanied by reactive new-bone formation and partial or complete infiltration of the marrow spaces to a degree greater than is apparent from the radiographic findings. This explains the necessity of irradiating the whole bone. The tumor permeated extensively the haversian channels of the cortex; in the earlier stages, there was little bone destruction, whereas

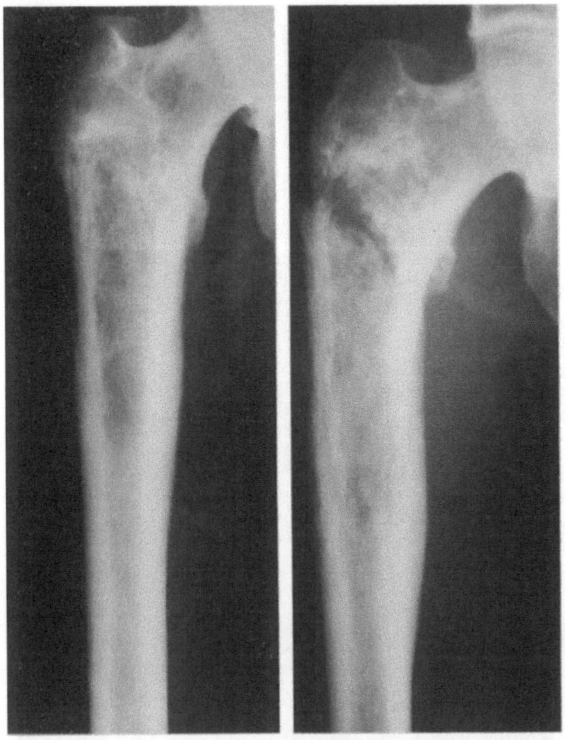

Fig. IV.6. Female, 18 years old. Ewing sarcoma of femur. Anteroposterior and lateral radiographs show an ill-defined permeative lesion in the upper third of the femur with slight periosteal reaction and pathologic fracture

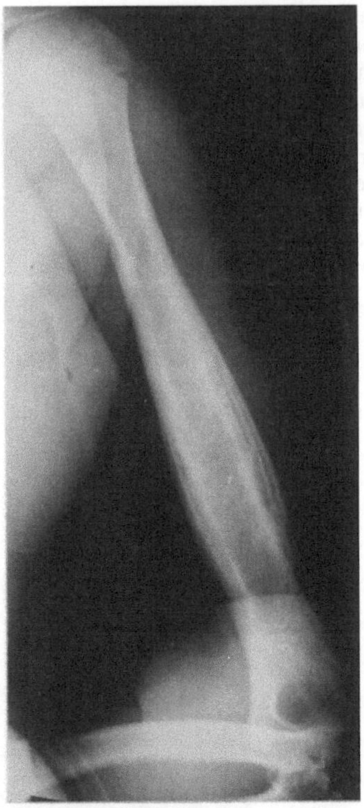

Fig. IV.7. Ten-year-old boy. Ewing sarcoma of the shaft of the humerus. Radiograph demonstrates a mottled area of bone destruction with an evident laminated periosteal reaction

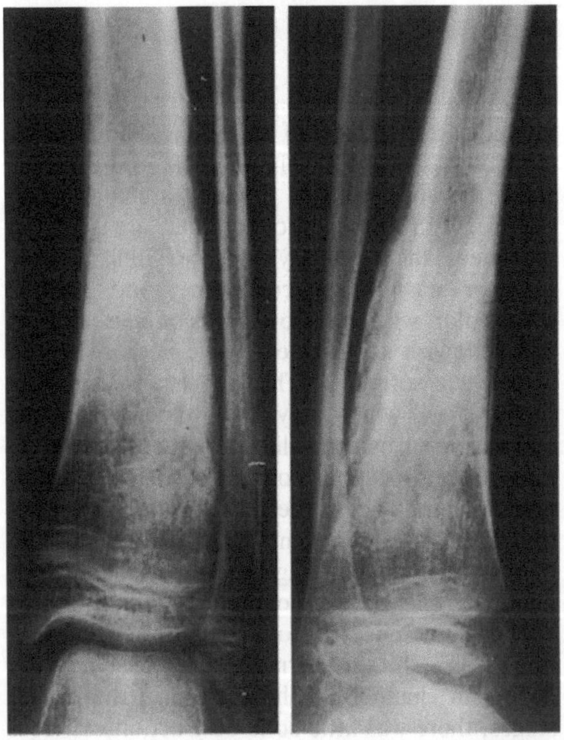

Fig. IV.8. Female, 5 years old. Ewing sarcoma of tibia. Anteroposterior and lateral radiographs show periosteal nonlaminated bone reaction at its lateral aspect and fine periosteal lamellae at the medial site

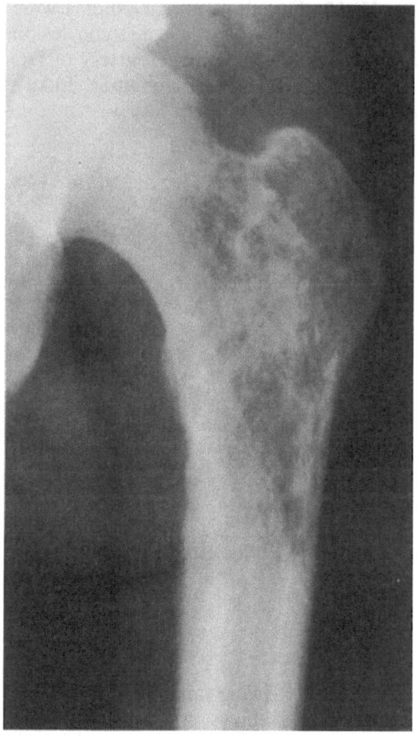

Fig. IV.9. Male, 19 years of age, Ewing sarcoma of the femur. Radiograph shows ill-defined permeative lesion in the upper third of the femur without evident periosteal reaction

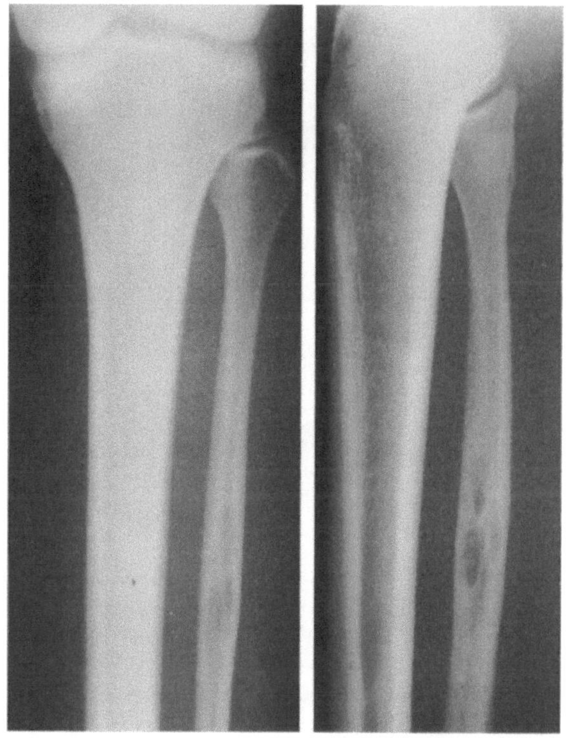

Fig. IV.10. Female, 18 years old. Ewing sarcoma of fibula. Anteroposterior and lateral radiographs show an osteolytic, apparently well-defined lesion in the midshaft without conspicuous periosteal reaction, suggesting a benign lesion

Fig. IV.11. Female, 19 years old. Ewing sarcoma of ilium. Radiograph illustrates destructive and sclerosing lesion in the ilium close to joint space, simulating an inflammatory process

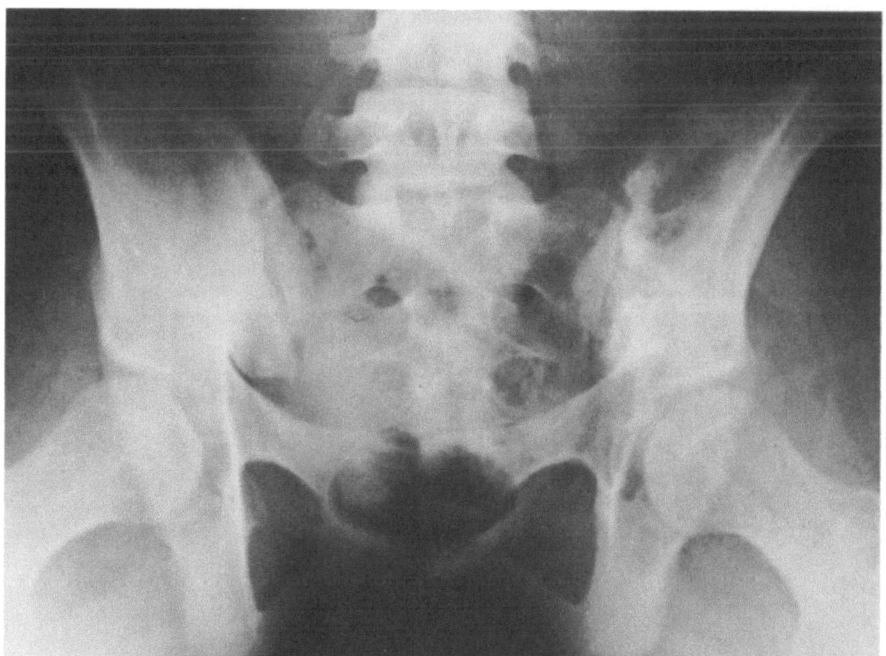

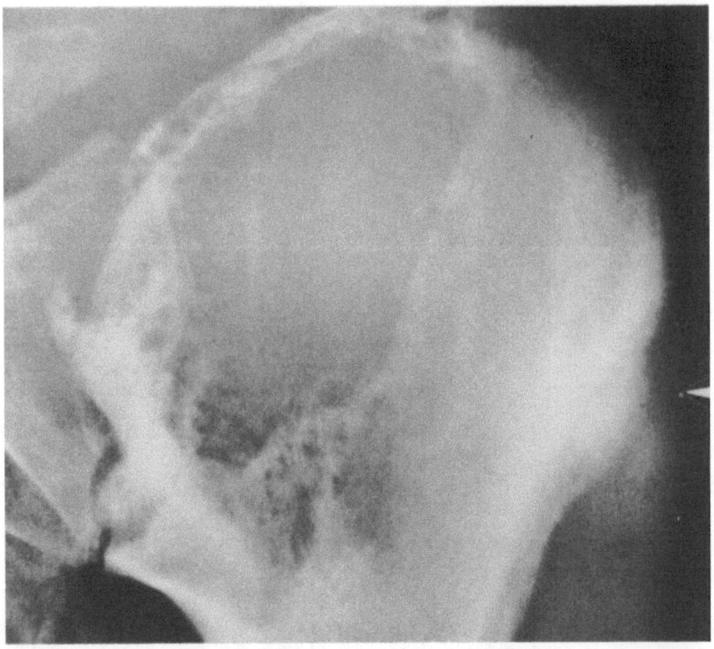

Fig. IV.12. Female, 18 years old. Ewing sarcoma of ilium. Large osteolytic lesion with permeative margins. (Courtesy of Dr. J. Petasnick, Rush-Presbyterian-St. Luke's Medical Center)

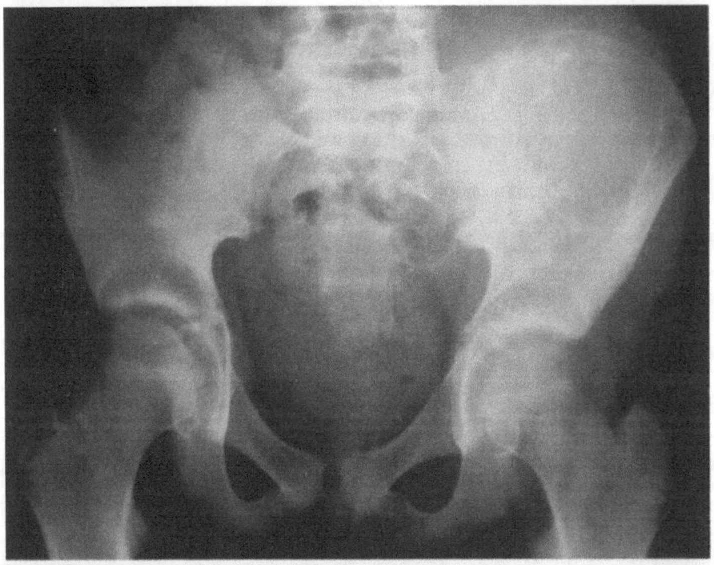

a

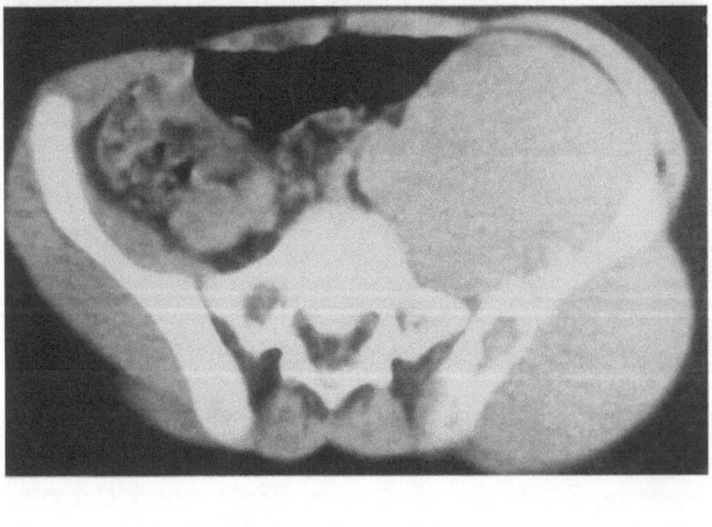

b

Fig. IV.13a,b. Ewing sarcoma of the ilium. **a** Radiograph shows a destructive and sclerotic poorly delimited lesion with soft tissue invasion at its upper aspect. **b** CT scan clearly reveals the bone involvement and the conspicuous penetration into the soft tissues

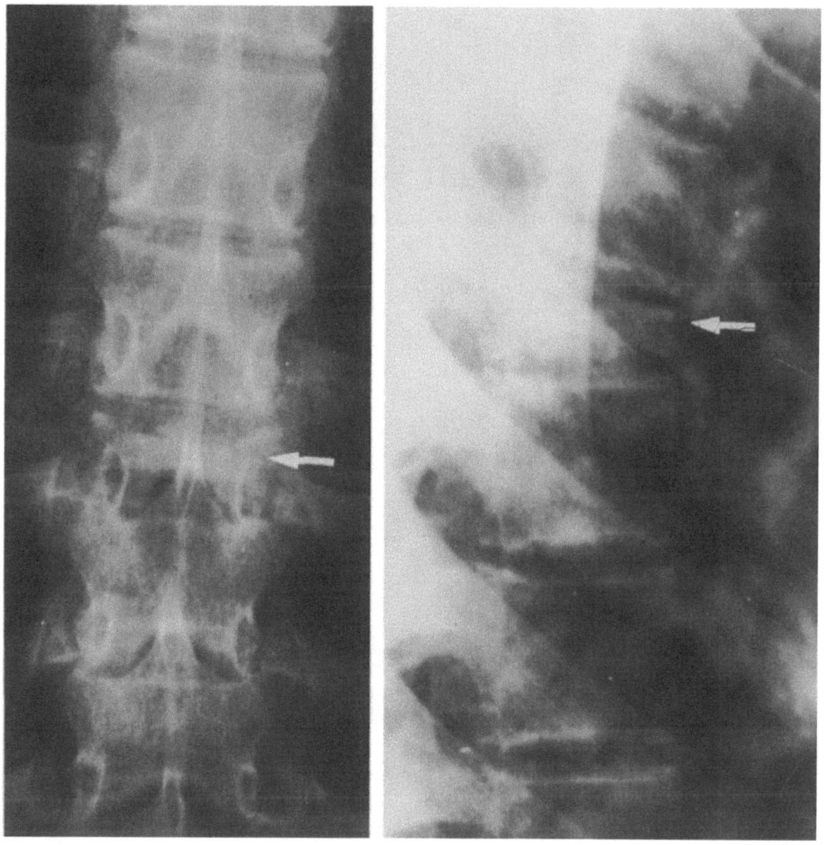

Fig. IV.14. Female, 15 years old. Ewing sarcoma of the ninth thoracic vertebra (*arrows*). Anteroposterior and lateral radiographs show compression of the vertebral body (vertebra plana). An identical appearance may be observed in eosinophilic granuloma

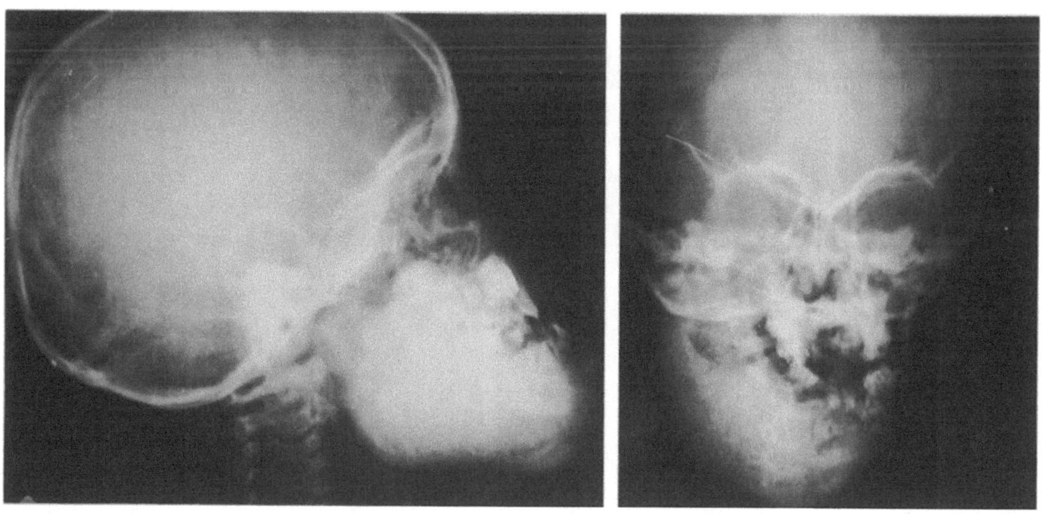

Fig. IV.15. Male, 5 years old. Ewing sarcoma of the mandible. Radiographs show an expanding sclerotic lesion with well-defined borders. This is an uncommon location and impossible to diagnose without biopsy

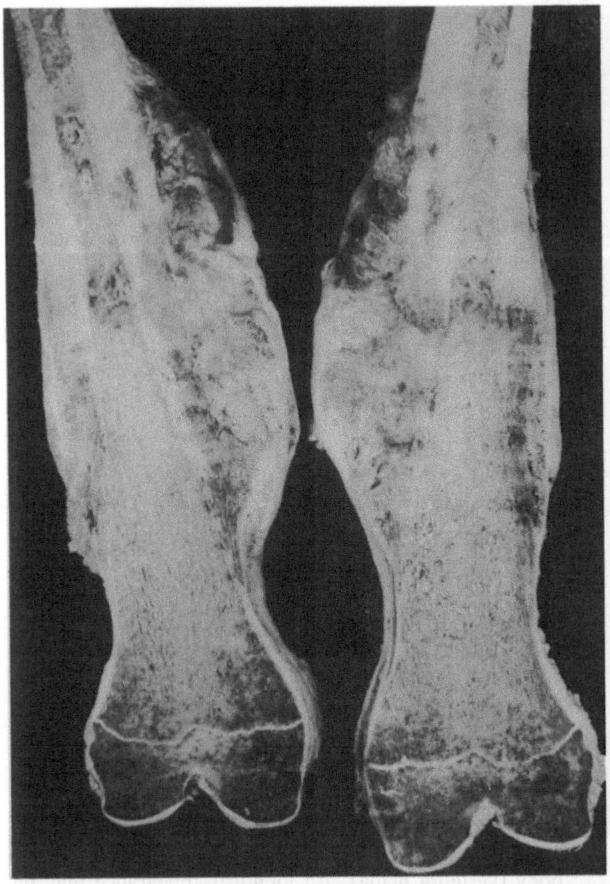
IV.16a

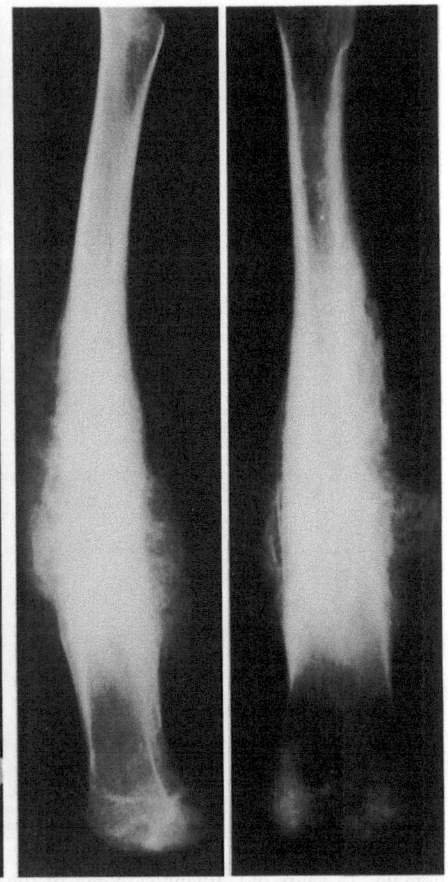
b

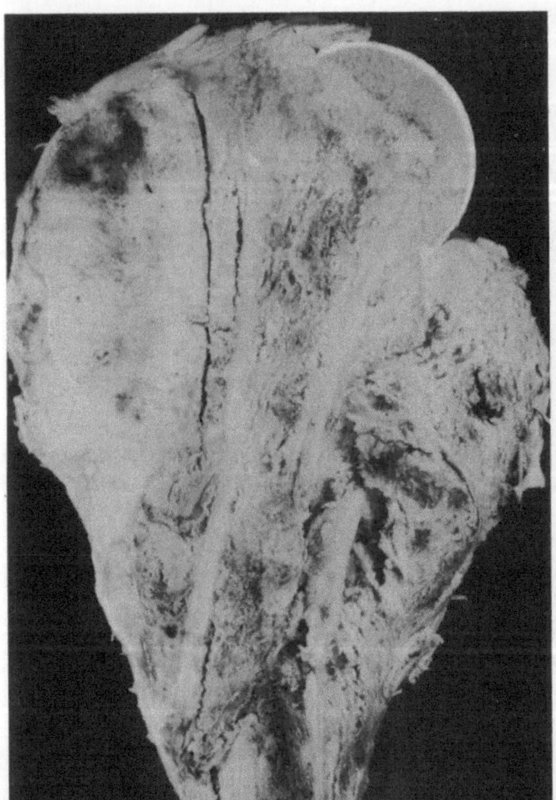
IV.17a

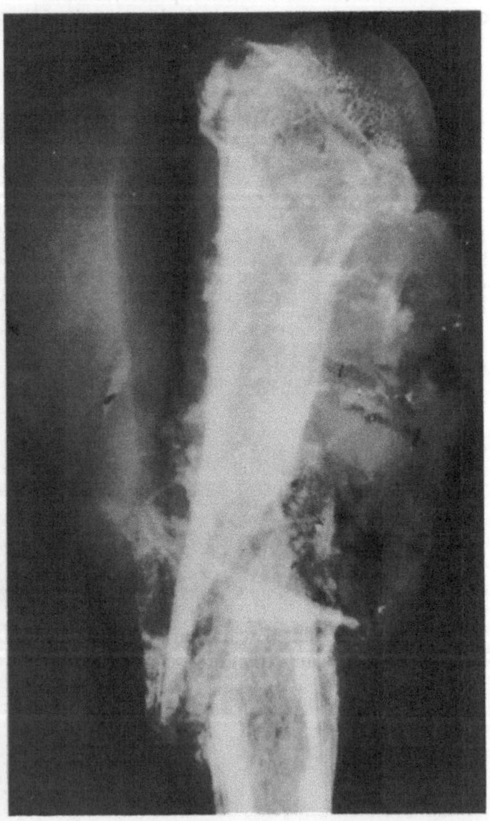
b

Fig. IV.16a,b. Female, 12 years old. Ewing sarcoma of the shaft of femur. Photograph and radiograph of the amputation specimen after radiation therapy, without chemotherapy, showing periosteal laminated and sunburst reactive bone formation

Fig. IV.17. Male, 16 years old. Ewing sarcoma of the humerus. Photograph and radiograph of amputation specimen show the enormous soft tissue and intramedullary extension of the tumor, with a pathologic fracture (**a**,**b**)

←

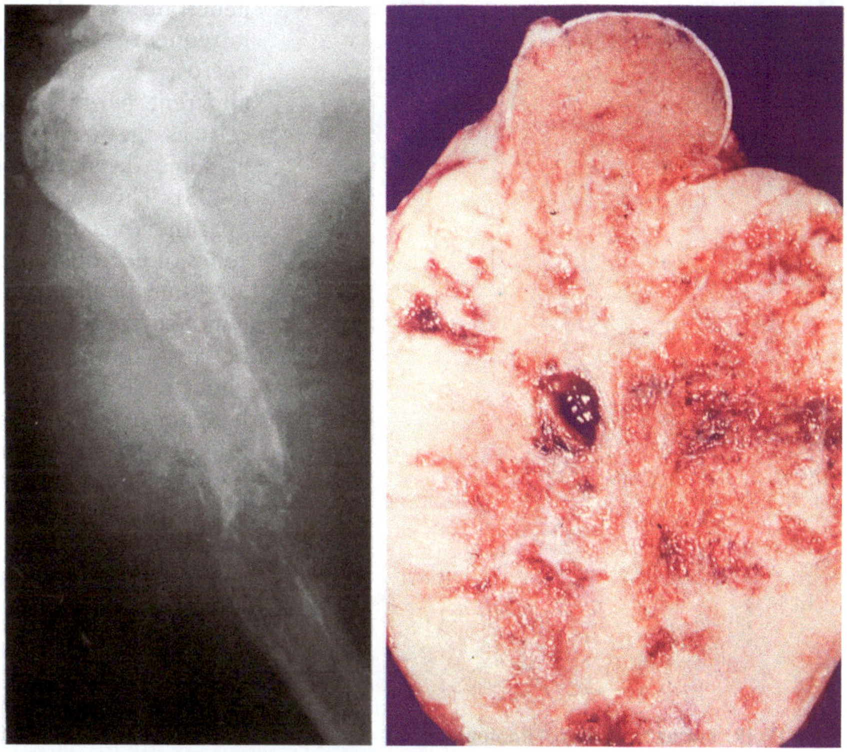

a

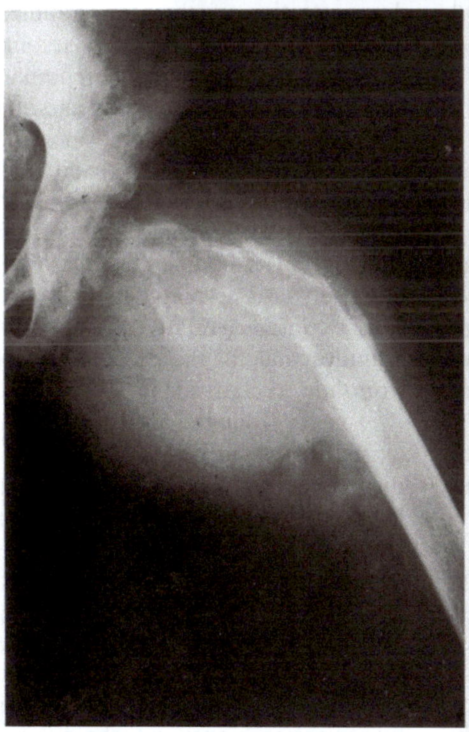

b

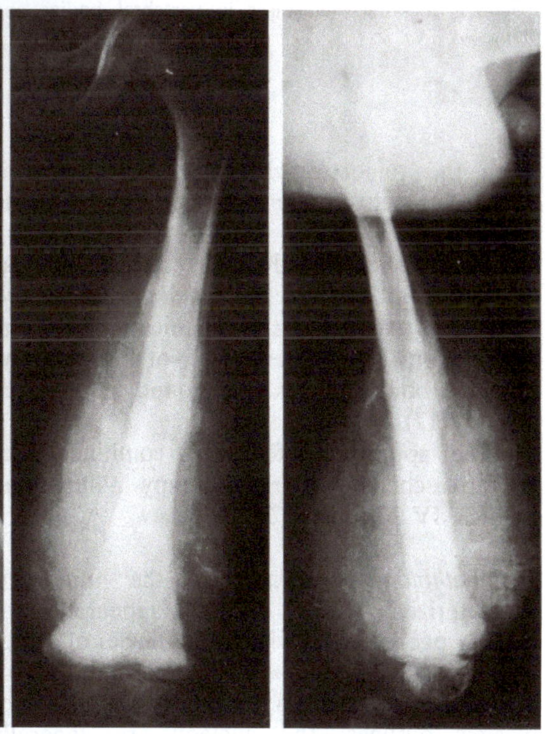

c

Fig. IV.18a–c. Three final stages of Ewing sarcoma, before the introduction of chemotherapy. **a** Male, 25 years old, with extensive destruction, pathologic fracture, and a large soft tissue mass, clearly visible in the photograph of the specimen. **b** Female, 15 years old, with extensive lesion, pathologic fracture, and large soft tissue mass in the upper femoral end. **c** Male, 4 years old, with an enormous tumor of bone and soft tissues that involves more than half of the femur

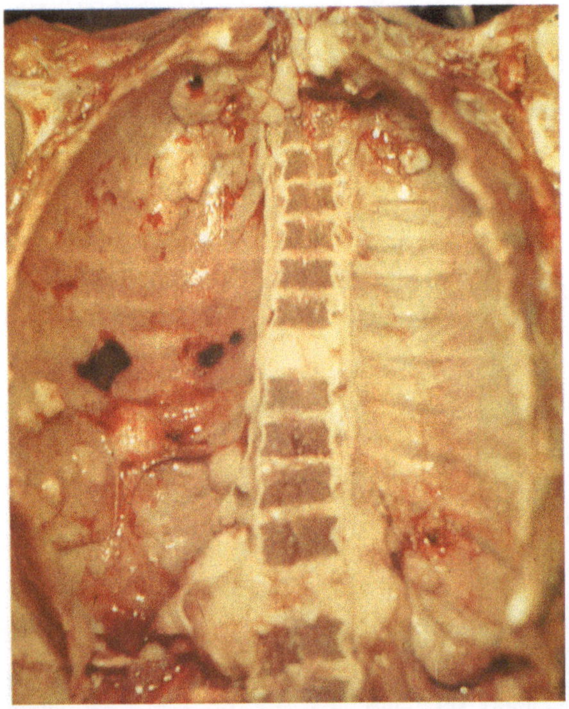

Fig. IV.19. Ewing sarcoma. Photograph of autopsy specimen showing metastases in vertebral bodies and pleura

when the tumor reached the periosteum, it produced reactive bone formation parallel to the bone surface.

In more advanced cases, the cortex was destroyed partly in several points, or completely, the central tumor mass communicating with the extraosseous soft tissue mass. Not infrequently, radiating bone spicules were found in this area (Fig. IV.17).

The appearance following combined preoperative chemo- and radiotherapy is illustrated by Figs. IV.20 and IV.21.

Histopathology. Histologically, the tumor is characterized by its uniform appearance of densely packed cells, with round nuclei of rather uniform size, about two or three times the size of a lymphocyte nucleus, without distinct cytoplasmic outlines; the nucleoli are generally inconspicuous (Figs. IV.22–IV.26).

Tumor bone or cartilage formation is absent. The tumor is divided into strands or lobules by conspicuous septa of fibrous tissue (Fig. IV.24). Silver stains demonstrate the lobular distribution of the reticulin fibers that surround large areas of tumor cells, into which few, if any, fibers penetrate (Fig. IV.27). Mitoses are present but infrequent. Hemorrhages and extensive areas of necrosis are common, sometimes producing an apparent perithelial arrangement of the viable cells as the necrosis of the tumor tissue occurs at some distance from the blood vessels (Fig. IV.23). This appearance gave origin to the term "perithelioma" in the older literature. In the zones of necrobiosis, the nuclei of the tumor cells are often small and pyknotic, about the size of a lymphocyte. These areas are particularly prone to be mistaken for malignant lymphoma of lymphocytic (lymphosarcoma) or mixed (histiocytic-lymphocytic lymphoma) type. Sometimes, the tumor cells are unusually large, surround small foci of necrosis, or yield alveolarlike or ganglionlike formations that resemble the rosettes of neuroblastoma (sympathicoblastoma) or PNET (Fig. IV.26). In some areas, the tumor cells directly surround blood-filled spaces, showing an endothelioid pattern (Fig. IV.28).

Histochemical Studies. In a paper published in 1959, the writer showed that the histochemical demonstration of glycogen granules in the cytoplasm of cells of Ewing sarcoma, and their absence in malignant lymphoma (reticulosarcoma), proved to be an easy and efficient method of differential diagnosis, provided that the specimens were properly fixed (alcohol 80% or Rossman's fluid, which is an alcoholic picric solution) and stained. The periodic acid-Schiff (PAS) stain as modified by McManus or Hotchkiss has been satisfactory. Part or most of the tumor cells contain relatively abundant glycogen granules that fill the cytoplasm and vary in size from fine to coarse (Fig. IV.29).

Apart from the necrotic zones, some areas existed in which glycogen was lacking. Previous digestion by ptyalin or Taka-diastase caused the PAS-positive granules to disappear, thus confirming that they were indeed glycogen. PAS staining with no or minimal nuclear counterstain is preferable because the glycogen granules are more clearly visible with this technique (Fig. IV.29b). The demonstration of glycogen is especially helpful in the small specimens obtained by aspiration biopsy, a technique used in many of our cases, and it could also be applied to the staining of smears prepared in these cases (see Introduction, Fig. 14). Fixation with 80% alcohol has the advantage of preserving alkaline phosphatase, and it gives more satisfactory results than Rossman's fluid. Formalin only inconstantly preserved glycogen, but in about half of the cases

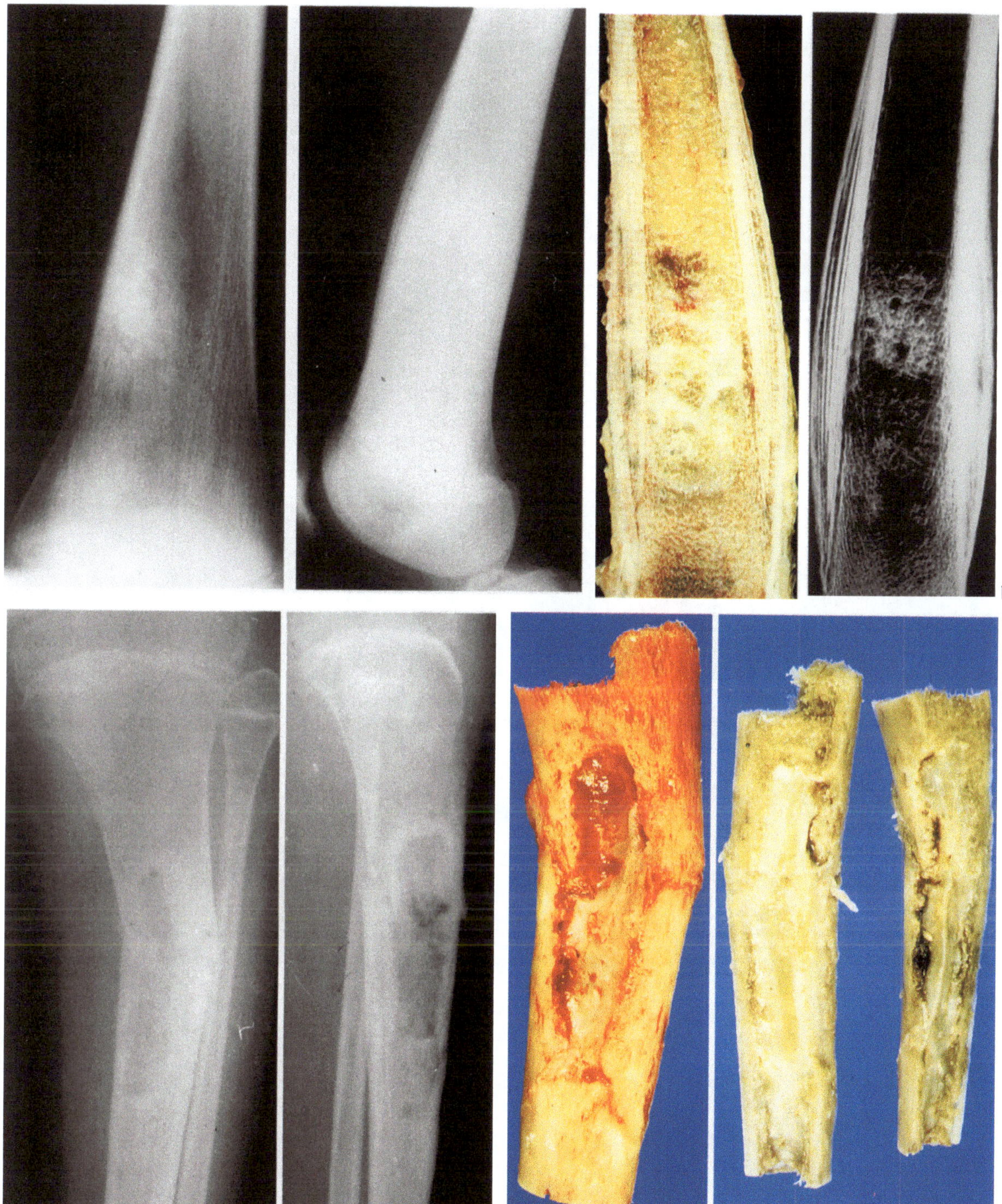

a b, c d e

Fig. IV.20a–e. Two cases of Ewing sarcoma showing the effect of combined preoperative chemo- and radiotherapy. **a** Male, 14 years old. Anteroposterior and lateral radiographs show a radiolucent permeative lesion in the lower third of the femur with coarse granular calcification and laminated periosteal reaction. **b** Photograph and **c** radiograph of the segmental resection showing the grayish-white necrotic and fibrotic tumor. The areas of calcification and laminated "onion-peel" periosteal reaction are clearly seen. **d,e** Female, 12 years old. **d** Anteroposterior and lateral radiographs showing an osteolytic lesion with a sclerotic border at its upper aspect, and pathologic fracture of the tibial diaphysis after chemo- and radiotherapy. **e** Photographs of the surface and section of the resected specimen show the complete necrosis and fibrosis of the tumor

a

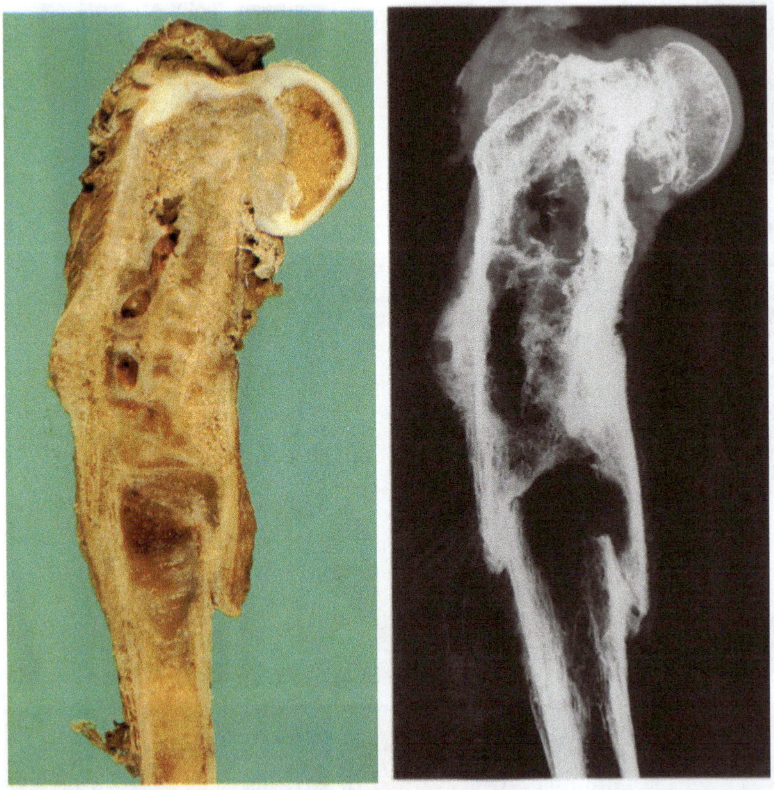

b

Fig. IV.21a,b. Twelve-year-old female. Ewing sarcoma of the upper third of the femur. **a** Photograph and **b** radiograph of the en bloc resected specimen after radio- and chemotherapy, showing the effect of treatment. In spite of the almost complete necrosis, histologically some scarce areas of viable tumor cells persist

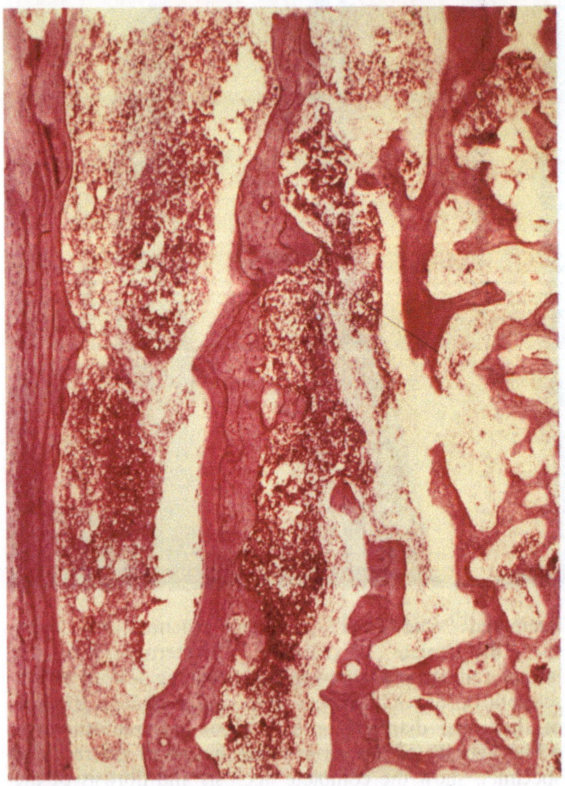

Fig. IV.22. Ewing sarcoma. Photomicrograph showing periosteal reactive bone formation. ×40

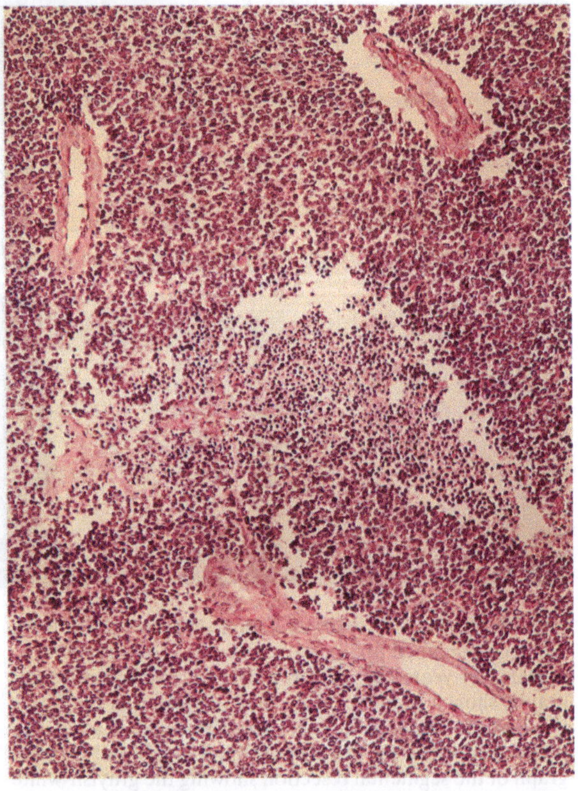

Fig. IV.23. Ewing sarcoma. Photomicrograph shows aspect of round nuclei of uniform size. In areas of necrosis at some distance from the blood vessels the nuclei are often small and pyknotic, about the size of lymphocytes. ×120

Fig. IV.24a,b. Photomicrographs showing at lower and higher magnification the densely packed small cells with round nuclei, forming compact masses or strands, separated by fibrous septa. **a** ×100, **b** ×400

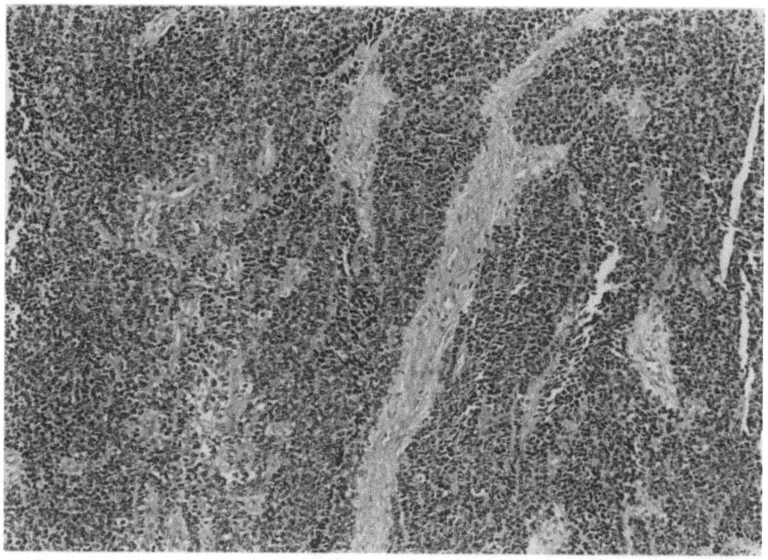

a

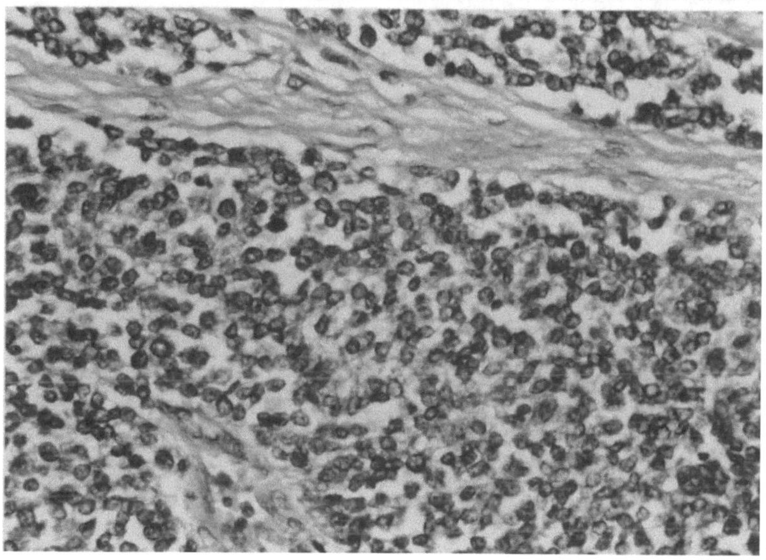

b

glycogen could still be demonstrated in material fixed in formalin for a long period. It is usually lacking in specimens decalcified with nitric or other strong acids. Therefore, the absence of glycogen in incorrectly treated material does not exclude the diagnosis of Ewing sarcoma.

Pomeroy and Johnson (1975) reported that glycogen was demonstrated in all their cases in which short fixation in neutral formalin was used. At the time of our first publication, we had studied only a few cases of metastatic neuroblastoma of bone in formalin-fixed material; despite the constant lack of glycogen in the tumor cells, we did not consider these results conclusive. In subsequent years, the material studied in our laboratory has increased notably, and the results obtained by us and by many others, with few exceptions, confirmed our previous findings with the routine light microscope. In a presentation at the 24th Symposium of the Colston Research Society held in Bristol we reported our results in 173 cases of Ewing sarcoma (Schajowicz 1973), 78 cases of malignant lymphoma, and 38 cases of metastatic neuroblastoma of bone, demonstrating the absence of glycogen not only in lymphoma but also in all cases of metastatic neuroblastoma investigated.

Several electron microscopic studies were reported, confirming the presence of varying amounts of glycogen in Ewing sarcoma (Friedman and Gold 1968; Kadin and Bensch 1971; Friedman and Hanaoka 1971; Hou-Jensen et al. 1972;

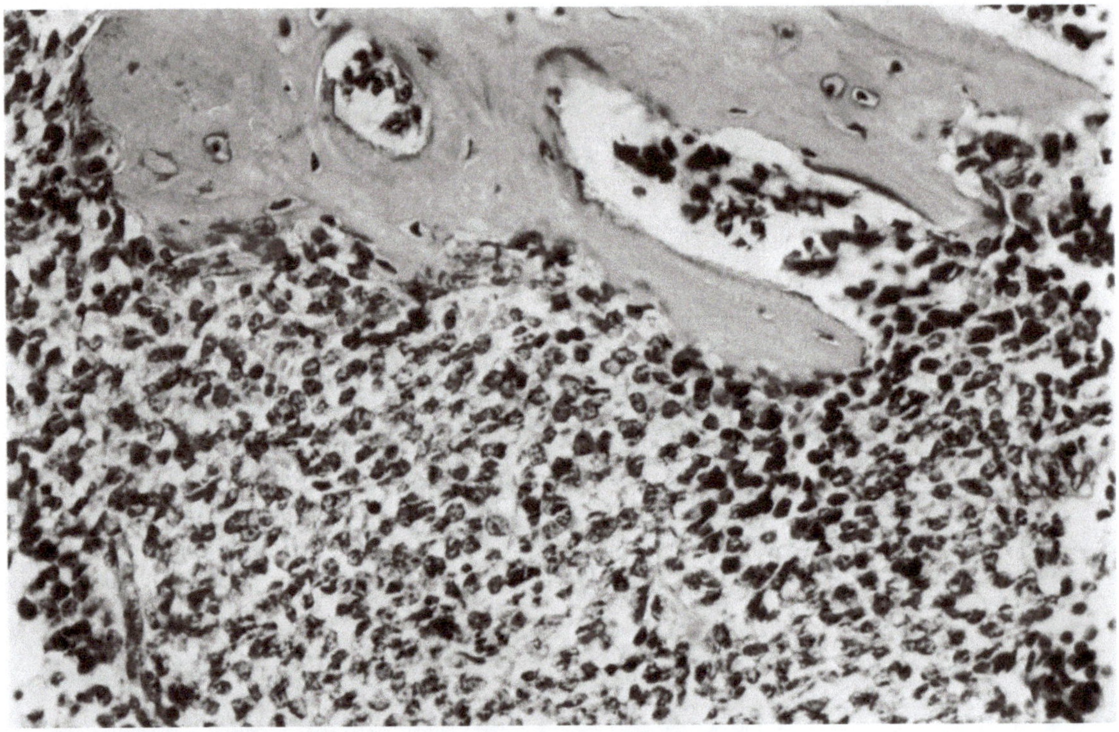

Fig. IV.25. Photomicrograph showing reactive bone formation. ×200

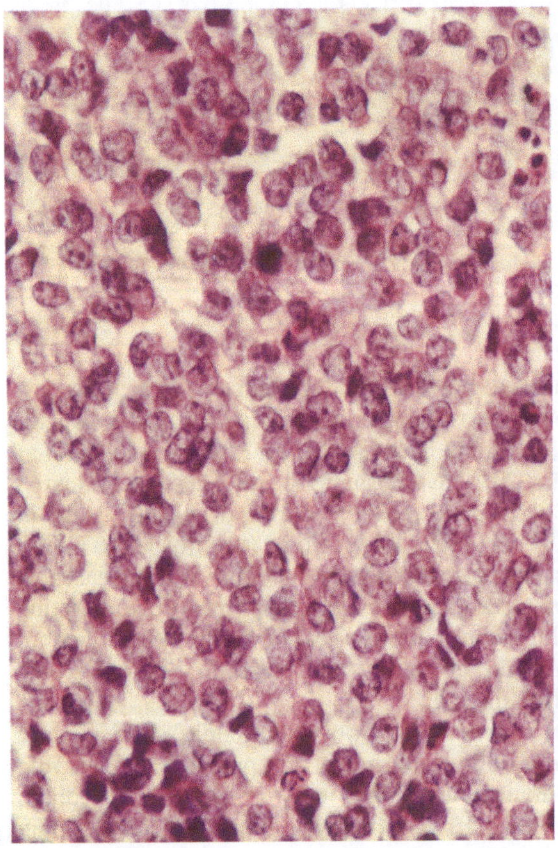

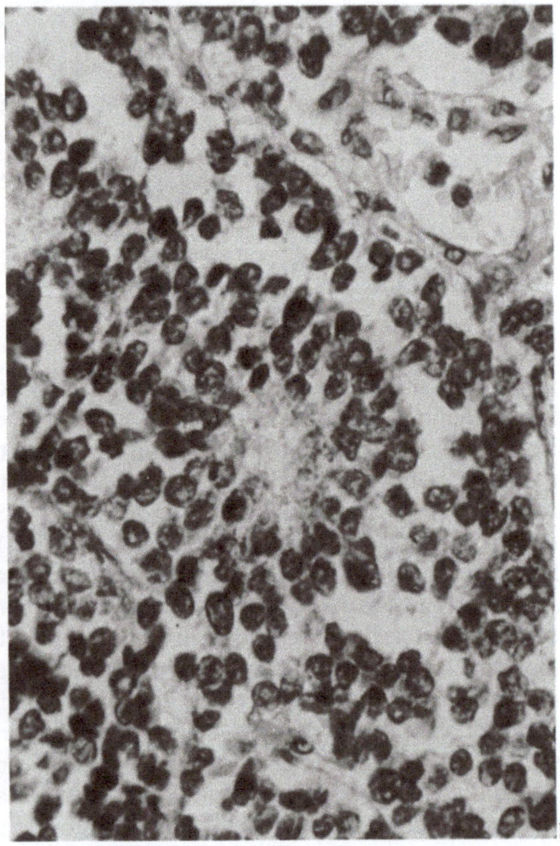

a b

Fig. IV.26a,b. Photomicrographs showing at high magnification the uniform aspect of the round nuclei without clear cytoplasmic outlines or prominent nucleoli. In **b**, pseudorosette pattern, resembling neuroblastoma. ×600

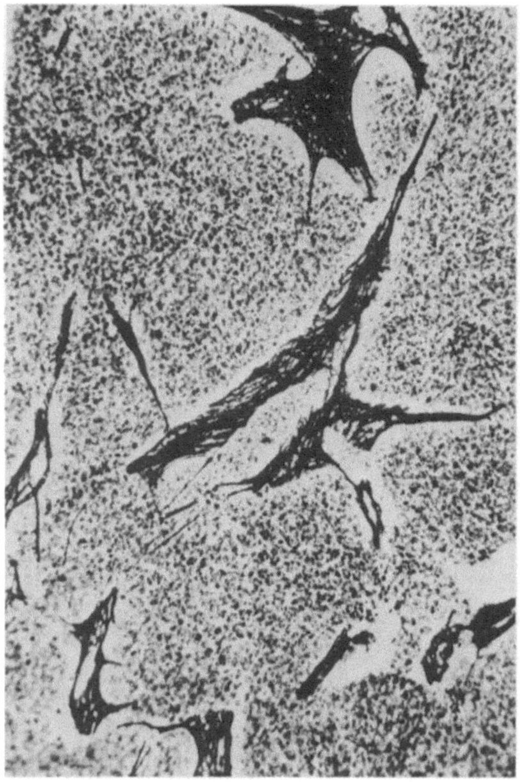

IV.27a

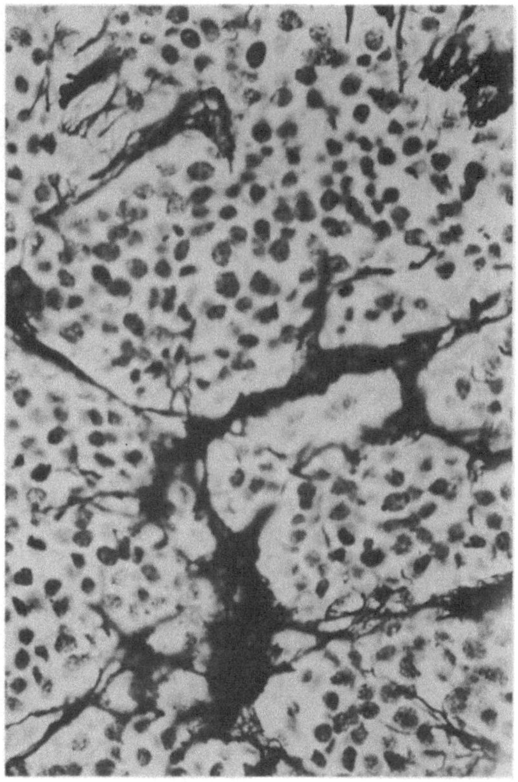

b

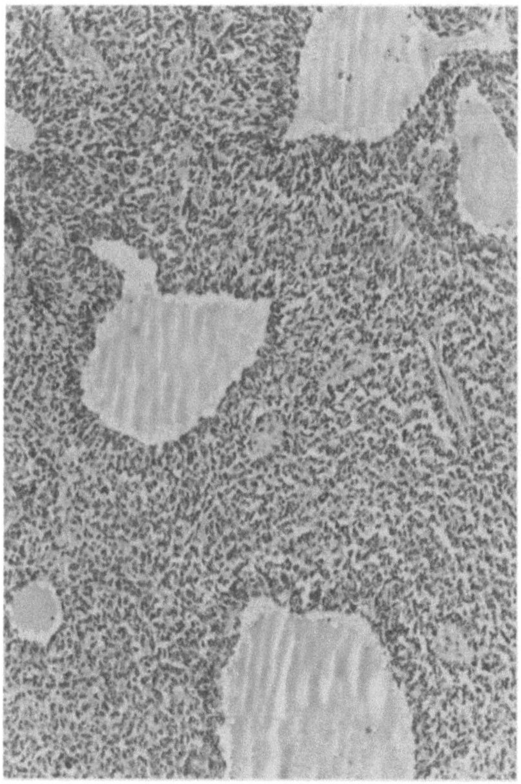

IV.28a

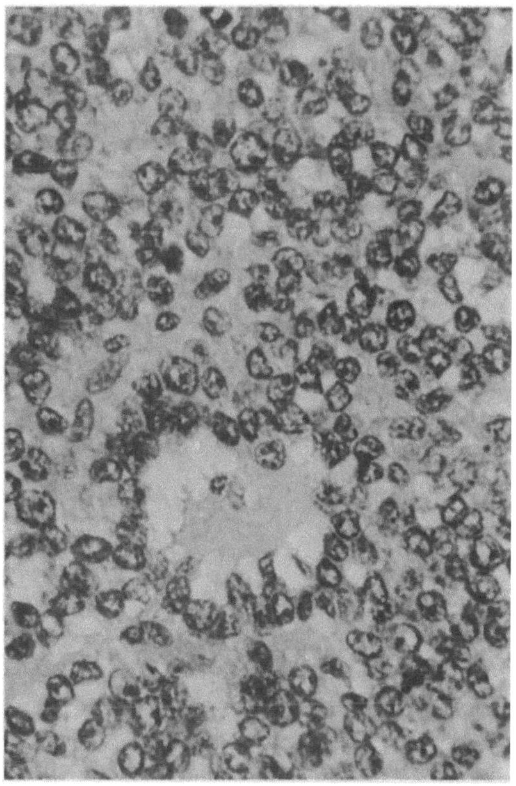

b

Fig. IV.27a,b. Photomicrographs showing at lower and higher magnification the reticulin fibers circumscribing large lobules of tumor cells (Del Rio Hortega's silver impregnation technique). **a** ×100, **b** ×400

Fig. IV.28a,b. Photomicrographs at lower and high magnification showing tumor cells, surrounding directly the lumen of vascular spaces. **a** ×160, **b** ×600 a 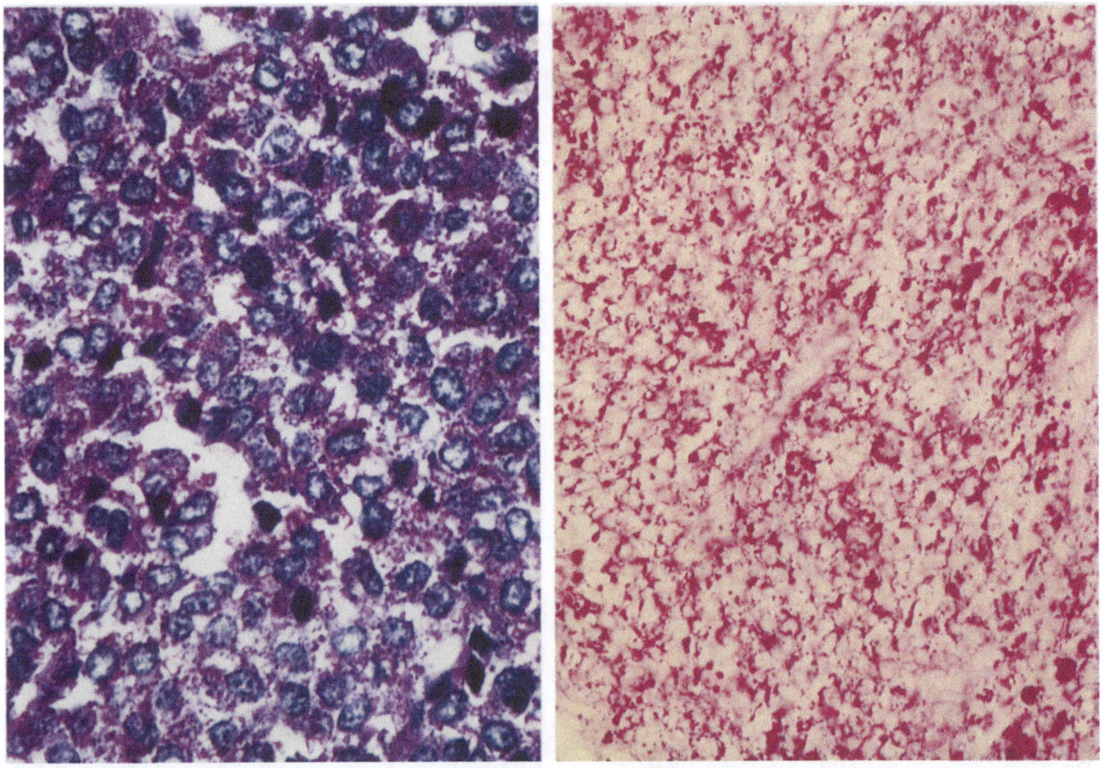 b

Fig. IV.29a,b. Photomicrographs showing stained glycogen granules in the cytoplasm of the tumor cells, more clearly visible in **b**, where the nuclei appear as clear disks, since no counterstain has been used (80% alcohol fixation, McMann's PAS stain). **a** ×400, **b** ×300

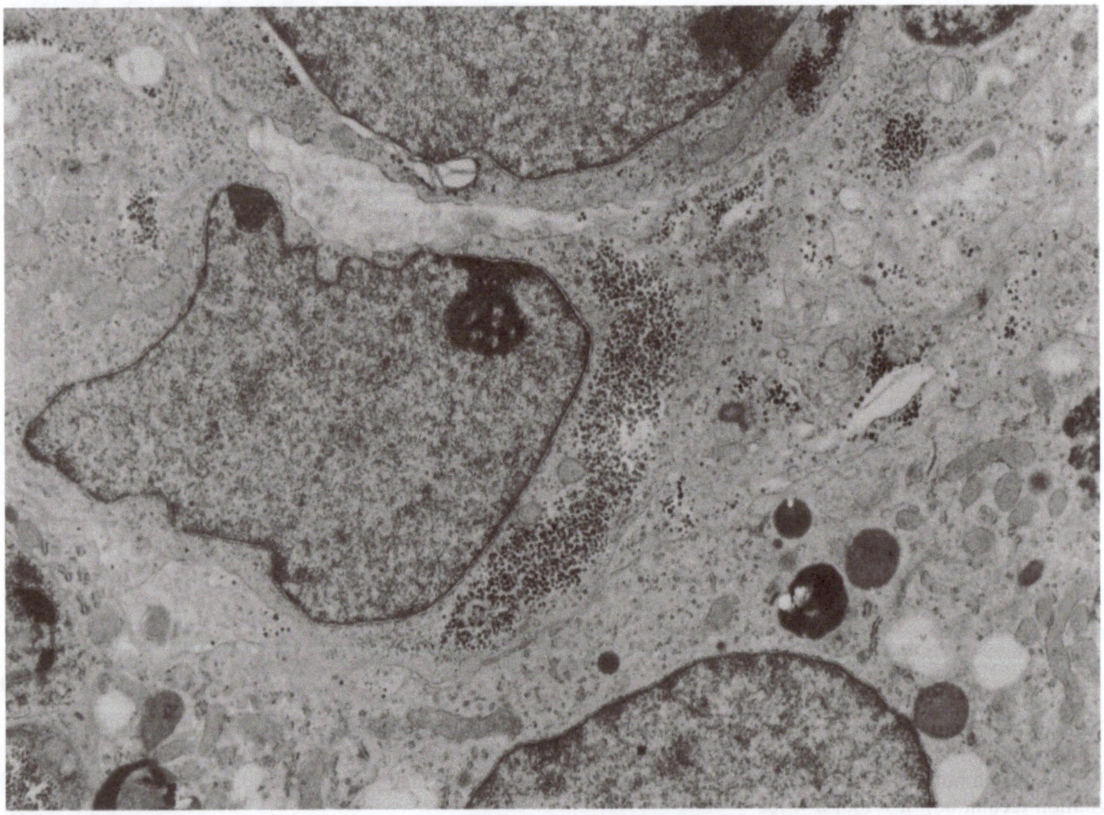

Fig. IV.30. Electron micrograph showing intracytoplasmic glycogen granules. ×15100

Ayala and Mackay 1977; Povysil and Matejovsky 1977) and its absence in malignant lymphoma (reticulo- and lymphosarcoma) and metastatic neuroblastoma (Friedman and Hanaoka 1971) (Fig. IV.30).

Ayala and Mackay (1977), who studied the ultrastructure of 40 well-documented cases of Ewing sarcoma seen at the M.D. Anderson Hospital, reported that glycogen was present in all tumors studied with the exception of two previously treated cases.

The findings of an important autopsy study at the National Cancer Institute (Bethesda) of 26 patients who received radiation therapy of the primary site plus adjuvant chemotherapy are extremely interesting (Telles et al. 1978). These authors showed that histologically the tumor at autopsy frequently had increased pleomorphism and increased numbers of bizarre giant cells; nevertheless, "these changes did not affect the presence of glycogen in tumor cells, thus reaffirming the importance of intracytoplasmic glycogen of Ewing's sarcoma." However, several authors (Price 1973; Triche and Ross 1978; Yunis et al. 1979) have reported the presence of variable amounts of glycogen in neuroblastoma, mostly by ultrastructural study and only rarely by light microscopy (Yunis et al. 1979). Therefore, the presence of glycogen alone is not advocated as sufficient to establish the diagnosis of Ewing sarcoma or to exclude neuroblastoma.

On the other hand, the recently described PNET (Jaffe et al. 1984) may also contain more or less abundant cytoplasmic granules of glycogen in about 10%–50% of cases (Llombart-Bosch et al. 1988).

Moreover, there are a few bone tumors that can present diagnostic difficulties due to an abundance of glycogen in their tumor cells. Cells in undifferentiated areas of osteosarcoma, particularly those present conspicuously in the so-called round-cell osteosarcoma (Sim et al. 1979), may contain glycogen (Schajowicz and Cabrini 1954). In these cases, the intense alkaline phosphatase activity of the osteosarcoma tumor cells and the presence of tumor osteoid trabeculae permit their differentiation from Ewing sarcoma, in which such activity or trabeculae are scarce or absent. Another tumoral process of bone or soft tissue origin, mesenchymal chondrosarcoma, frequently shows more or less abundant glycogen in the undifferentiated tumor cells; however, the presence of chondroid areas and the different clinical and radiologic features generally permit the correct diagnosis. Alveolar or embryonal rhabdomyosarcoma, which sometimes invades bone secondarily, may also show abundant cytoplasmic glycogen and other histologic features similar to those of Ewing sarcoma. Angervall and Enzinger reported a round-cell *soft tissue* tumor with cytologic and histochemical features, i.e., abundant cytoplasmic glycogen, resembling those of Ewing sarcoma. A few soft tissue tumors with the characteristics reported by the writer and others have been reported under the designation "extraskeletal Ewing sarcoma." One tumor examined under the electron microscope (Wigger et al. 1977) revealed many similarities with the ultrastructural features of classic Ewing sarcoma. The tumor described by Ewing as a distinct entity was of bone marrow (medullary) origin; it is therefore questionable whether a tumor of clearly soft tissue origin should be termed Ewing sarcoma, at least not until the histogenesis has been completely clarified.

Electron Microscopy. The ultrastructure of Ewing sarcoma has been the object of several studies (Friedman and Gold 1968; Nakayama et al. 1975; Takahashi et al. 1976; Llombart-Bosch et al. 1978; Ayala and Mackay 1977) using biopsy material and/or tissue culture material (Hou-Jensen et al. 1972; Kadin and Bensch 1971; Llombart-Bosch et al. 1990). With rare exceptions, all studies and our experience confirmed the presence of relatively abundant glycogen in the cytoplasm of many of the tumor cells, and its absence in malignant lymphoma and metastatic neuroblastoma. However, Triche and Ross (1978) reported an unusual case of a 13-year-old patient showing a glycogen-containing neuroblastoma upon electron microscopy that was PAS-negative in the initial bone marrow biopsies studied by light microscopy. As we stated above, several other authors (Price 1973; Triche and Ross 1978; Yunis et al. 1979) have also reported the presence of glycogen in neuroblastoma, mostly by ultrastructure.

The ultrastructural features described are essentially similar in all papers, that is, a predominant or *principal cell* type of polygonal size with cytoplasm poor in organelles and invariably with sparse endoplasmatic reticulum, few groups of mitochondria, and conspicuous Golgi complex. The nuclei are round or oval, the chromatin is typically fine and evenly distributed, and the single or multiple small nucleoli are clearly visible (Figs. IV.30, IV.31). Desmosomal intercellular connections or so-called atypical junction complexes have been described by several authors

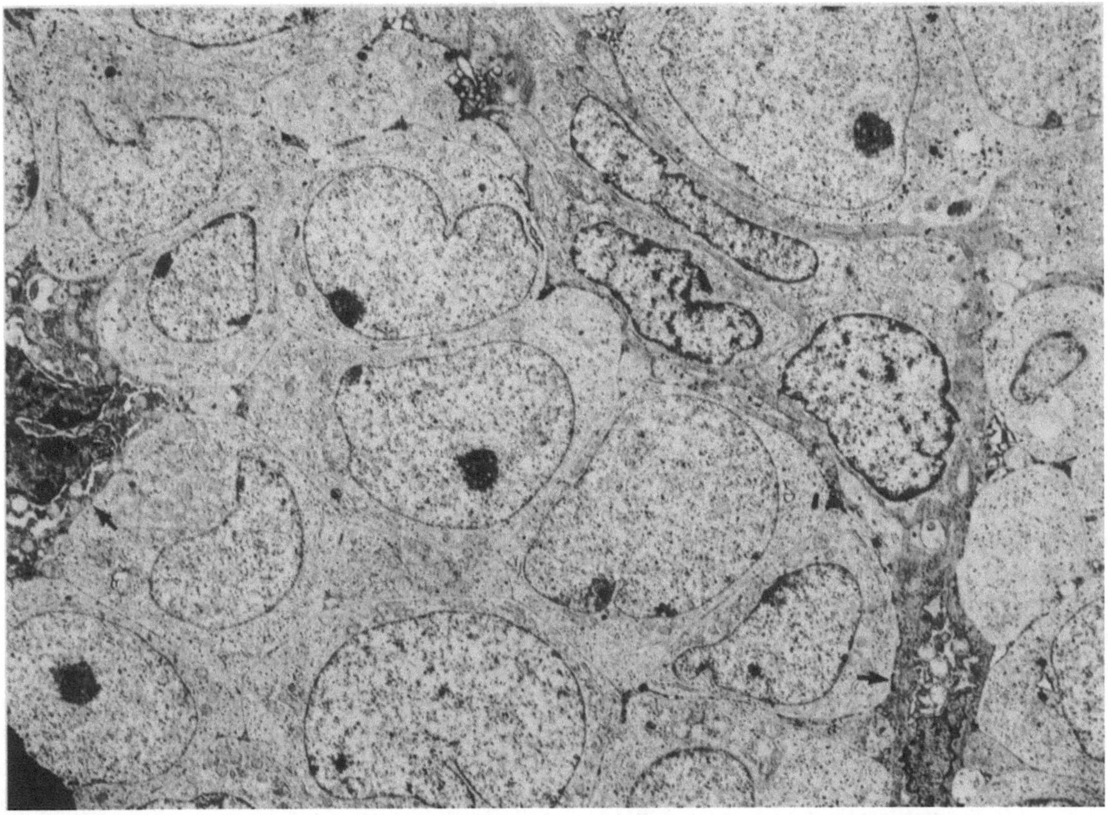

Fig. IV.31. Electron micrograph showing the characteristic principal cells of polygonal size with cytoplasm poor in organelles. The nuclei are round or oval with fine chromatin, the nucleoli contrast being clearly visible. Two dark cells, apparently degenerated tumor cells, are seen at the left (*arrow*) and lower borders. ×9000

(Hou-Jensen et al. 1972; Povysil and Matejovsky 1977; Llombart-Bosch et al. 1978) but were not found by others (Ayala and Mackay 1977). Besides the principal cell, a second type (secondary or *dark cell*) is usually present in small numbers (Fig. IV.31). The relationship of these cells to the prevailing principal cells is still disputed. They were thought to represent a local reaction of stroma cells to the surrounding sarcoma cells (Hou-Jensen et al. 1972) or principal cells in lymphoid maturation, thus suggesting that the tumor originated from immature reticulum cells (Friedman and Gold 1968). However, others (Kadin and Bensch 1971; Povysil and Matejovsky 1977; Llombart-Bosch et al. 1978), including the writer, believe that the dark cells probably represent degenerative tumor cells.

Cell-membrane-bound alkaline phosphatase activity of the principal cells has been demonstrated by Povysil and Matejovsky (1977) in the majority of their cases. Neurosecretory granules, intermediate filaments, and neurotubulelike structures are typically lacking in Ewing sarcoma.

Pathogenesis. Despite the extensive histologic, histochemical, immunohistochemical, tissue culture, and ultrastructural studies, the histogenesis of Ewing sarcoma remains obscure, and none of the findings presented to date can be regarded as unequivocal. Vascular endothelium (Ewing 1921, 1924) or perithelium, immature reticulum cells (Oberling 1928; Oberling and Raileanu 1932) undifferentiated mesenchymal cells (Melnick 1933; Jaffe 1958), and the myeloid cell (Kadin and Bensch 1971) have been considered to be the origin of the tumor cells.

A hemangiogenic origin, supported by Ewing, has been suggested due to the presence of desmosomal-type structures and basement membrane-like material or alkaline phosphatase positivity (Takahashi et al. 1976; Povysil and Matejovsky 1977; Llombart-Bosch et al. 1978), described in hemangiomatous neoplasms. The finding in some of the reported cases of areas resembling hemangiopericytoma, though infrequent, seems interesting because the presence of glycogen in the tumor cells of hemangiopericytoma (Battifora 1973) might indicate a relationship between the two tumors. However, there is no clear evidence that the vessels present are really part of the tumor. In conclusion, we agree with others that there is no definite proof of a vascular origin.

Since Oberling's work, the embryonic reticulum cell of the bone marrow has been considered the basic tumoral element. This view was supported by the ultrastructural interpretation of the dark cells as maturating reticulum cells by Friedman and Gold (1968). However, this maturative capacity is not accepted by other authors and the writer, who advocate that the dark cells represent degenerative regressive changes of the principal cell.

The myelogenous nature of the tumor cells, advocated by Kadin and Bensch and based fundamentally on the ultrastructure of the tumor cells in tissue culture, has not yet been confirmed by others.

In the writer's opinion, an origin from undifferentiated pluripotential supporting cells (stem cells) of bone marrow, as advocated by Jaffe (1958), with their limited potential for differentiation into various cell lines, appears most probable. However, the writer believes that the direction of this differentiation is not toward a histiocytic or lymphoid cell, but toward skeletogenic elements, without reaching the final goal, that is, reproducing osteoblasts (small-cell osteosarcoma) or chondroblasts (mesenchymal chondrosarcoma). The presence of abundant glycogen and membrane-bound alkaline phosphatase activity in the tumor cells of Ewing sarcoma, as observed in immature osteoblasts (Schajowicz and Cabrini 1954), appears to confirm this hypothesis.

Immunohistochemistry and Chromosomal Analysis. In recent years the introduction of new immunohistochemical methods applicable to formalin-fixed paraffin-embedded material, particularly using monoclonal antibodies, has helped to resolve the problem of distinguishing Ewing sarcoma from other round-cell tumors. An antibody that would be positive in all neuroblastomas and negative in all Ewing sarcomas – ideally sensitive and specific – would be of great value for the surgical pathologist. Thus, the reported presence of NSE in all neuroblastomas irrespective of histologic differentiation, and its absence in the other round-cell sarcomas, especially Ewing sarcoma and lymphoma of bone, attracted considerable attention (Triche and Askin 1983; Tsokos et al. 1984; Osborn et al. 1986; Llombart-Bosch et al. 1987). In the soft tissues, however, embryonal rhabdomyosarcoma was initially reported as negative for NSE, but later Osborn et al. (1986) reported two cases positive for NSE. These authors concluded that "NSE is not an appropriate marker to distinguish the different small round-cell tumors of children."

Unfortunately, neither of the two antibodies (monoclonal and polyclonal) against NSE comes close to achieving the desired outcome, as we found in a series of 30 Ewing sarcomas and 14 neuroblastomas studied at St. Louis University Medical Center in cooperation with Drs. Bedrossian and Sotelo. Both antibodies showed evident NSE positivity in several cases of Ewing sarcoma (30%) and were negative in four cases of histologically proven neuroblastoma, including two cases that also showed neurosecretory granules by electron microscopy.

Moreover, this same antibody was positive in a small proportion of nonneural tumors (Thomas et al. 1987), as also in 9 of 39 cases of Ewing sarcoma studied by Llombart-Bosch et al. (1987), in 3 of 11 Ewing sarcomas studied by Moll et al. (1987), and in 23 of 40 Ewing sarcomas (58%) studied by Pinto et al. (1989), again questioning the specificity of NSE immunoreactivity. Therefore, care should be exercised in not overinterpreting NSE positivity, particularly if polyclonal antibodies are used.

Recently a number of papers have been published supporting a neural differentiation or origin of Ewing sarcoma, mostly based on studies of tissue cultures with electron microscopy and/or scanning electron microscopy (Schmidt et al. 1982; Jaffe et al. 1984; Cavazzana et al. 1987, 1988; Llombart-Bosch et al. 1987, 1990) while others, based on keratin expression (Moll et al. 1987), have claimed heterogenetic pluripotential differentiation. This had already been suggested by Hutter et al. (1966) in their article on "primitive multipotential primary sarcoma of bone" and in Jacobson's report on "polyhistioma" (1977). According to the concept of Johnson (1953), the metabolic field or environment in which the tumor arises (diaphysis or metaphysis) is basic to its future differentiation. Keratin expression, however, is well documented in known neuroectodermal tumors (Cavazzana et al. 1987).

Significant controversy exists over whether Ewing sarcoma and PNET are closely related, if not the same tumor (Cavazzana et al. 1987; Llombart-Bosch et al. 1990). Both tumors share a

a, b

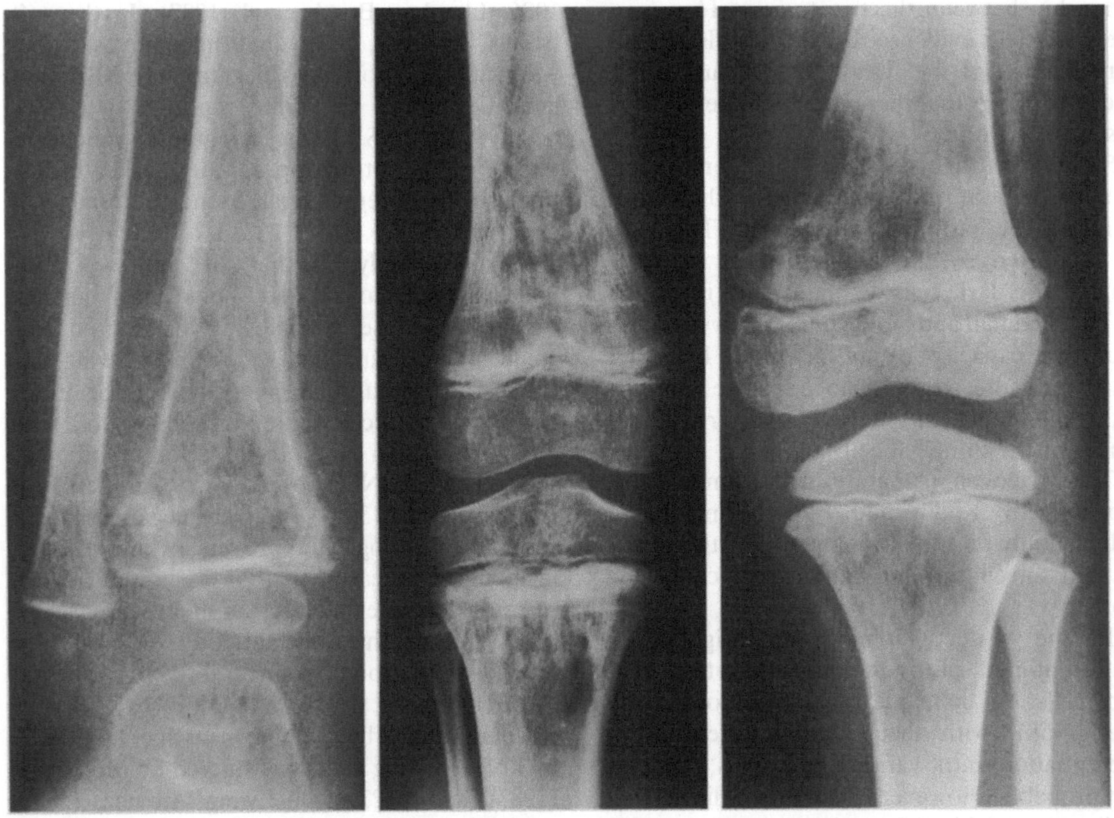

c

Fig. IV.32a–c. Patient, 4 years old, with metastatic neuroblastoma. **a** Radiograph shows irregular destructive lesion of the lower metaphysis of tibia with associated periosteal reaction. **b** Radiograph showing ill-defined areas of bone destruction with intervening sclerotic trabeculae in distal femur and proximal tibia. Radiolucent growth arrest lines are present in distal femur and proximal tibia. Similar lesions may be seen in acute leukemia. **c** 5-year-old patient with metastatic embryonal rhabdomyosarcoma. Radiograph shows ill-defined osteolytic lesions with cortical destruction in distal femoral and proximal tibial metaphyses. (Cases courtesy of Dr. J.P. Petasnick, Rush-Presbyterian-St. Luke's Medical Center)

positive reactivity with some neural markers, such as Leu-7 (HNK-1) HBA-7/1 (Fellinger et al. 1988), and a common cytogenetic abnormality (the chromosome 11;22 reciprocal translocation) (Aurias et al. 1984; Turc-Carell et al. 1984; Whang-Peng et al. 1984), which is lacking in neuroblastoma and other small round-cell tumors.

Therefore, the question arises whether all Ewing sarcomas represent a less differentiated form of neuroectodermal tumors of bone (PNET), or whether this diagnosis should be restricted only to atypical Ewing sarcomas and to those tumors presenting cytomorphologic neural features, such as Homer-Wright rosettes or pseudorosettes, among others.

Differential Diagnosis. Ewing sarcoma may present diagnostic difficulties, clinically and radiologically, with several nontumoral processes such as osteomyelitis, syphilis of bone, eosinophilic granuloma, or tumoral lesions, especially osteosarcoma. However, there are generally no major problems involved in distinguishing these processes histopathologically.

The clinical and, above all, histologic distinction of Ewing sarcoma from metastatic neuroblastoma (sympathicoblastoma) in its more immature form (sympathicogonioma of Del Rio Hortega), in which rosette-like structures are often lacking, may be extremely difficult (Fig. IV.34b). Neuroblastoma is more common in children under 5 years of age and rarely occurs in adults. Metastases in the skull, often accompanied by exophthalmos and radiolucent permeative lesions located preferentially in the metaphysis of long bones (humerus, femur), are frequent (Figs. IV.32, IV.33).

No glycogen was found in any of our cases that were correctly fixed (Fig. IV.34; cf. Fig.

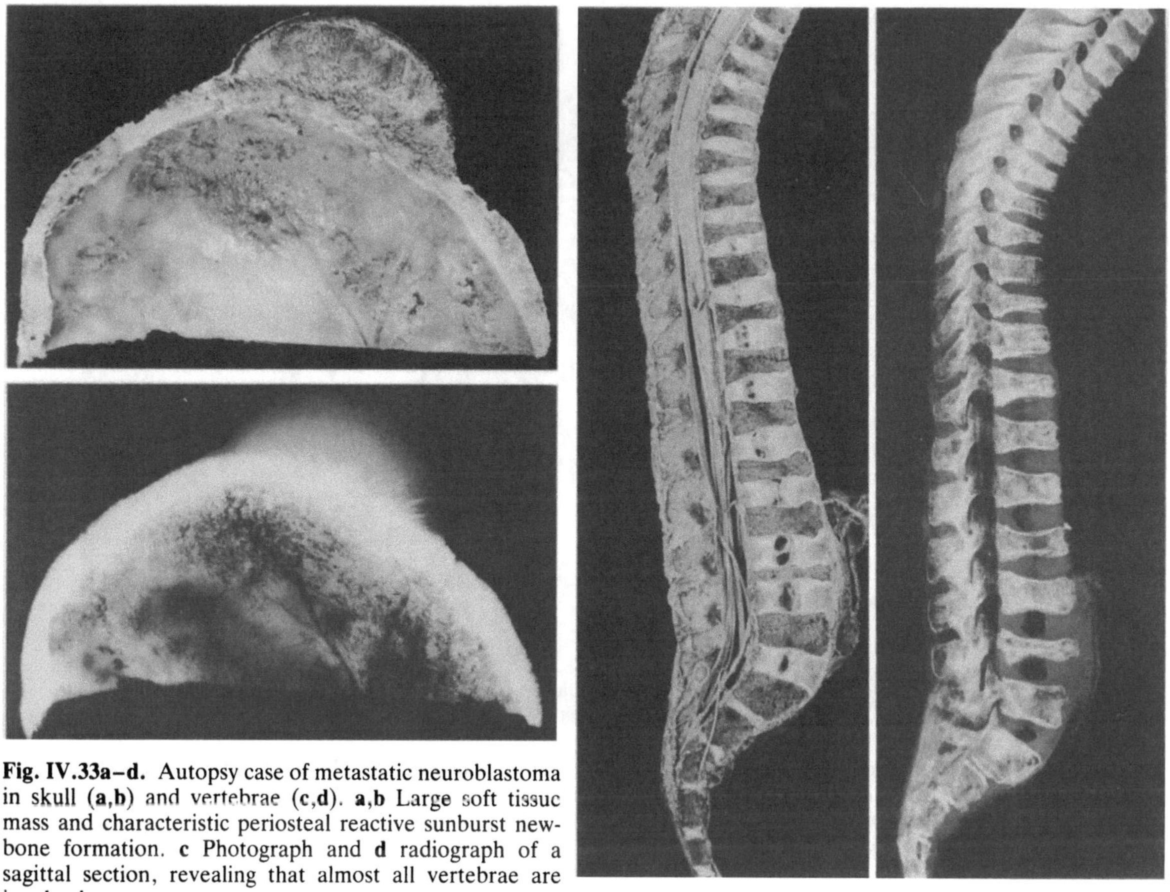

a

b

c, d

Fig. IV.33a–d. Autopsy case of metastatic neuroblastoma in skull (**a**,**b**) and vertebrae (**c**,**d**). **a**,**b** Large soft tissue mass and characteristic periosteal reactive sunburst new-bone formation. **c** Photograph and **d** radiograph of a sagittal section, revealing that almost all vertebrae are involved

IV.35) (Schajowicz 1973). Also, with special silver stains, nerve fibrils can often be demonstrated, particularly in the rosette-like structures. The biochemical tests for urinary catecholamine excretion (norepinephrine, epinephrine, and 3-methoxy-4-hydroxymandelic acid, VMA), have been positive in about 80% of our cases. Pretreatment levels appear to correlate with the extent of disease; however, the level does not seem to correlate with prognosis. Serial urinary catecholamine levels are helpful in predicting the clinical course of patients with neuroblastoma. Those patients who show a rapid return to normal urinary levels have a significantly better prognosis than those who do not. Finally, the most specific and definitive features of neuroblastoma can be observed with the electron microscope. Friedman and Hanaoka (1971) and subsequently other workers demonstrated the presence of neurosecretory granules and neural processes containing neurofibrils, which permit a definite distinction from other round-cell sarcomas of nonneural origin (Fig. IV.36).

Other malignant bone tumors containing extensive undifferentiated round-cell areas, such as some osteosarcomas ("round-cell osteosarcoma") (Sim et al. 1979) or mesenchymal chondrosarcoma, may present diagnostic problems for the pathologist because of the possible presence of cytoplasmic glycogen in some of these cases. The formation of tumor bone or cartilage, associated with the clinical features, often permits a definitive diagnosis. The differential diagnosis with PNET and malignant lymphoma (reticulo- and lymphosarcoma) is described in the following sections.

Whether the separation of classic Ewing sarcoma from PNET is only of academic importance or whether it is justified because of a different biologic behavior and more serious prognosis of PNET, associated with a different treatment, will only be resolved in future investigations involving a significant number of cases. It must be emphasized that great care should be exercised to arrive at a definite diagnosis of Ewing sarcoma, necessitating an ex-

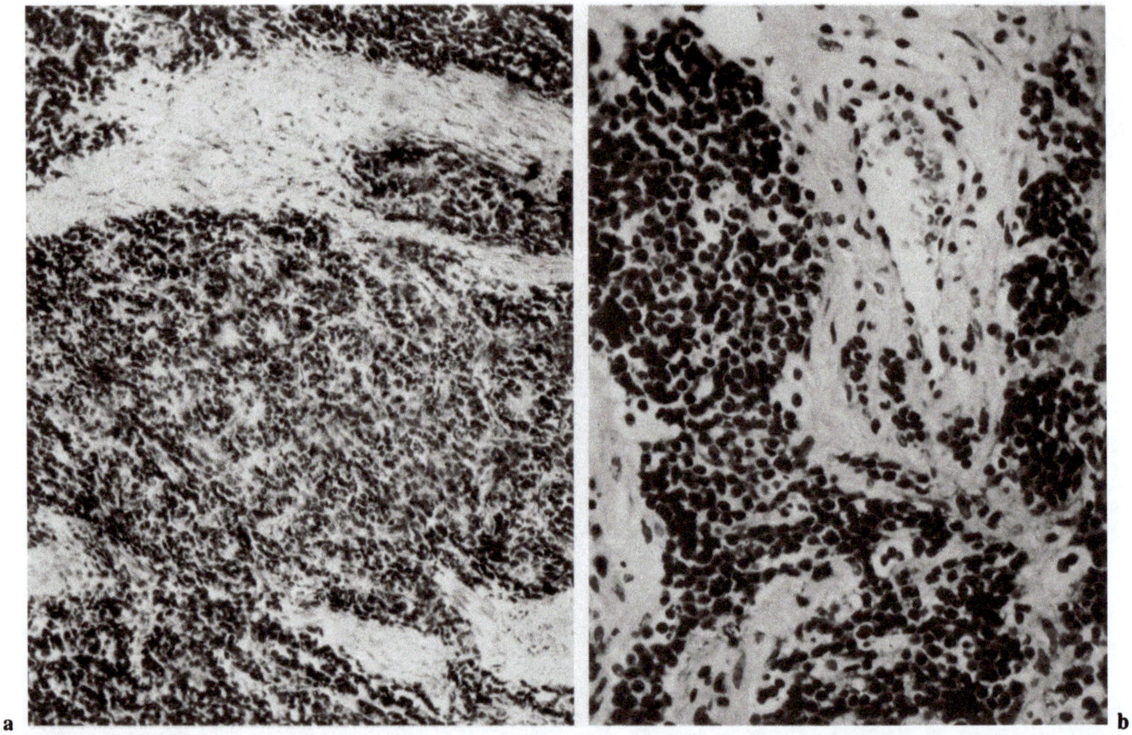

Fig. IV.34a,b. Photomicrographs of metastatic neuroblastoma. **a** Numerous rosettelike structures. Large tumor lobules are separated by conspicuous fibrous septa. **b** The tumor cells show small dark nuclei the size of a lymphocyte and form nodules or lobules of different sizes, separated by thick fibrous septa. Rosettelike structures are lacking in this more undifferentiated type (sympathogonioma of Del Rio Hortega). **a** ×100, **b** ×180

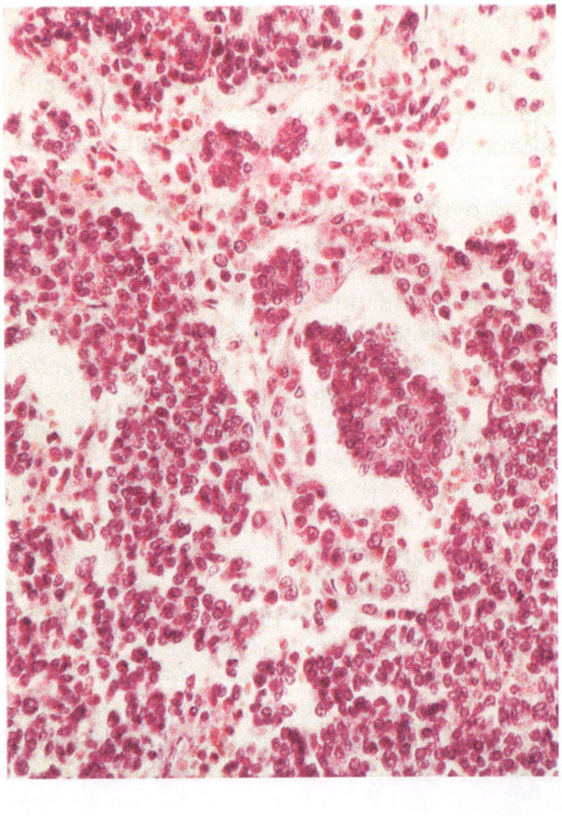

Fig. IV.35. Photomicrograph of Ewing sarcoma showing scanty rosettelike structures. Autopsy confirmed the diagnosis and revealed the presence of abundant glycogen. (Schajowicz 1973)

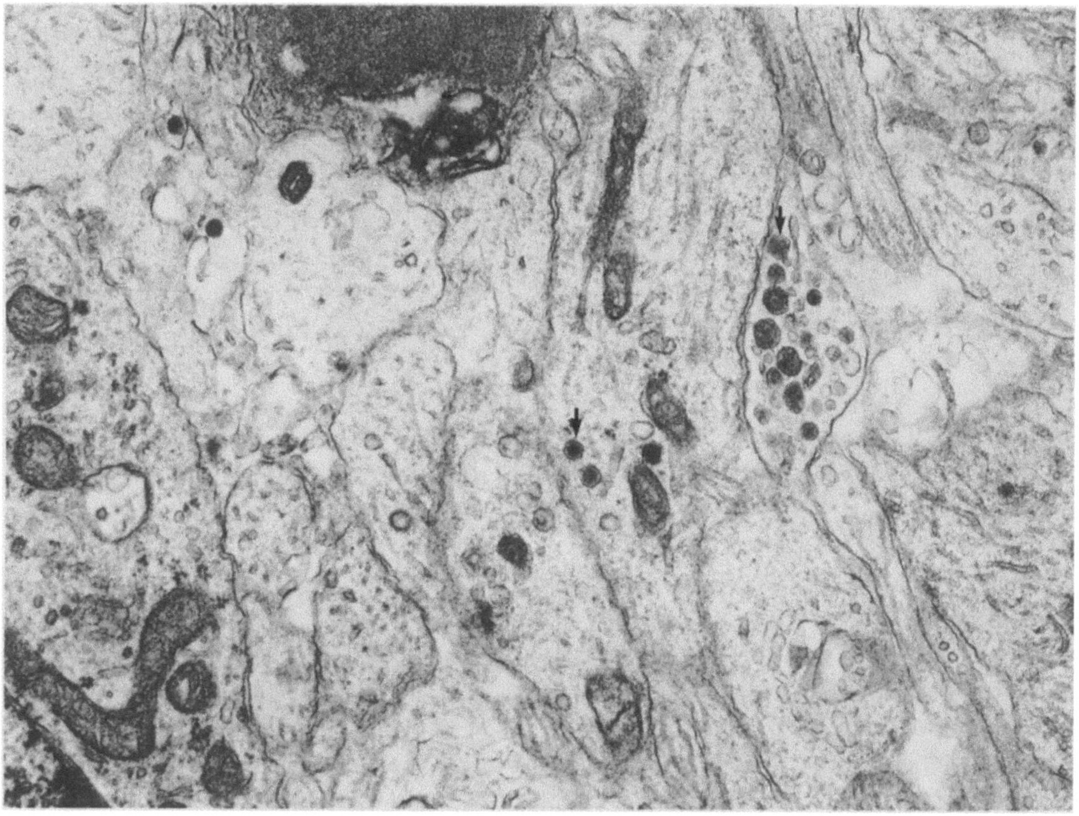

Fig. IV.36. Electron micrograph of neuroblastoma showing the presence of neurosecretory granules and neural processes containing neurofibrils. (Courtesy of Dr. H. Battifora, Northwestern University, Chicago, Illinois) ×43 000

haustive histochemical, immunohistochemical, and electron microscopic study, especially to rule out a tumor of neural origin.

2. Primary Neuroectodermal Tumor of Bone

Definition, WHO: *"A rare and highly malignant tumor that morphologically resembles the peripheral neuroepithelioma of soft tissues. Its distinction from Ewing sarcoma, when based solely on routine microscopy, is extremely difficult and uncertain."*

In 1984 Jaffe et al. reported four malignant small round-cell tumors of bone in children, which they called "neuroectodermal tumors of bone" and which resembled the peripheral neuroepithelioma of soft tissues. In spite of only scarce amounts of glycogen in both imprints and tissue sections, the initial diagnosis of the cases based on the clinical, roentgenographic, and histologic findings had been Ewing sarcoma. However, the demonstration of a lobular pattern, Homer-Wright rosettes, and NSE in tissue sections and in long-term tissue cultures resulted in the diagnosis of neuroectodermal tumor of bone, despite the lack of catecholamine secretion and of neurosecretory granules on ultrastructural study, except in one case.

As mentioned above, several authors later questioned the specificity of Ewing sarcoma and affirmed that most, if not all, Ewing sarcomas are actually neural neoplasms, that is, PNETs, based principally on immunohistochemical studies and in vitro cultures with electron microscopy and/or scanning electron microscopy (Cavazzana et al. 1987).

In 1988, Llombart-Bosch et al., reporting 14 cases of PNET, established the following clinical-pathologic criteria for its diagnosis:

The age and sex in this tumor group are quite similar to those observed in Ewing sarcoma, with a clear male predominance (11:3) and a median age of 14.4 years. The only outstanding clinical

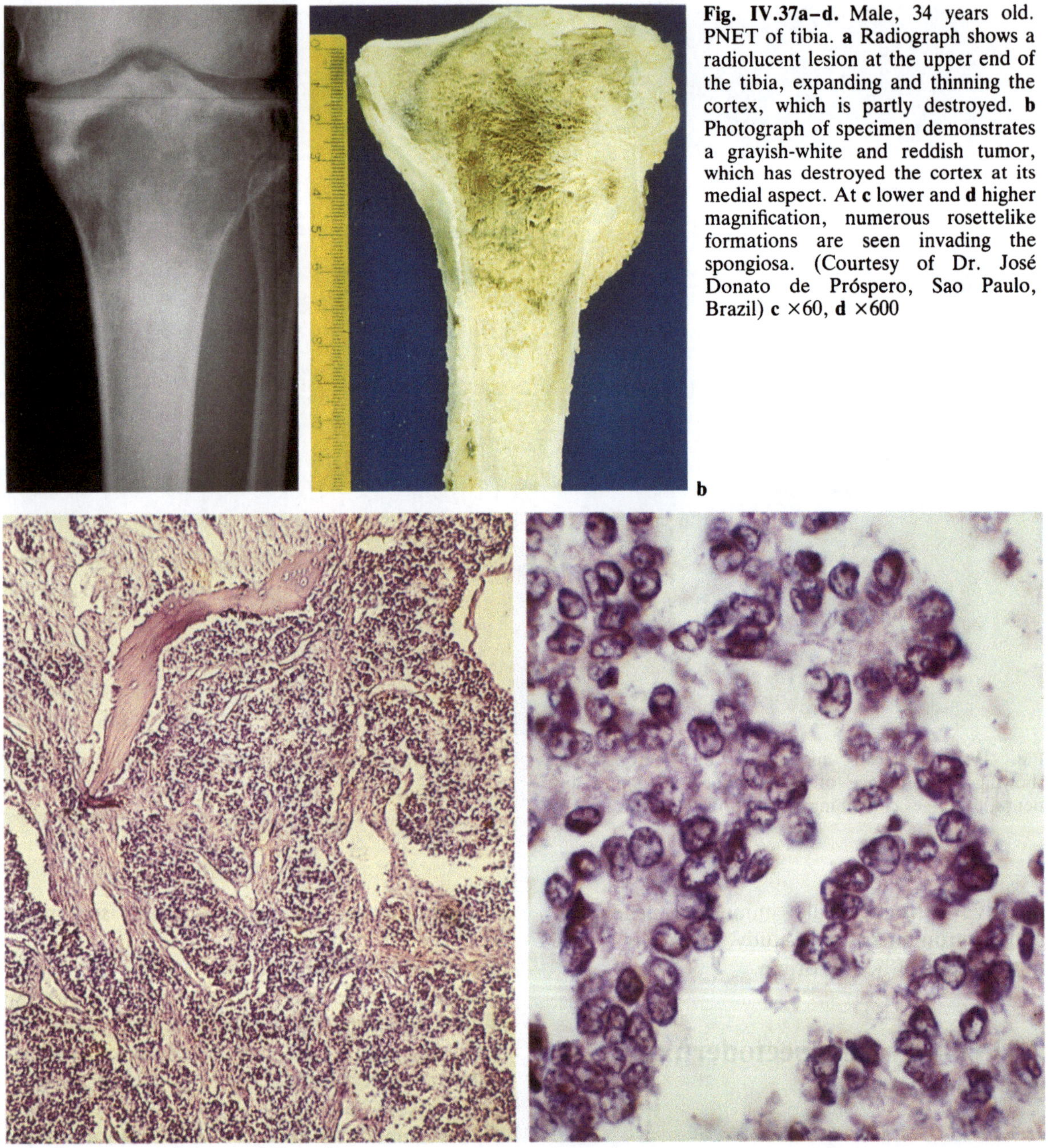

Fig. IV.37a–d. Male, 34 years old. PNET of tibia. **a** Radiograph shows a radiolucent lesion at the upper end of the tibia, expanding and thinning the cortex, which is partly destroyed. **b** Photograph of specimen demonstrates a grayish-white and reddish tumor, which has destroyed the cortex at its medial aspect. At **c** lower and **d** higher magnification, numerous rosettelike formations are seen invading the spongiosa. (Courtesy of Dr. José Donato de Próspero, Sao Paulo, Brazil) **c** ×60, **d** ×600

difference is the high malignancy displayed by PNET, which resembles the behavior observed in the peripheral neuroepithelioma group of soft tissue tumors (Miser et al. 1987).

Histologically the main features of this tumor which distinguish it from Ewing sarcoma, are: (1) the presence of numerous Homer-Wright rosettes or pseudorosettes, in clusters, distributed in a haphazard fashion; (2) cell and nuclear variation, showing more heterogeneity than is present in conventional Ewing sarcoma, but with similar glycogen deposits in approximately half of the cases (in 9 of 14 cases of Llombart-Bosch et al. 1988); and (3) a lobular pattern with faintly fibrillar interstitial stroma (Figs. IV.37, IV.38).

Electron microscopy shows neurosecretory granules, intermediate filaments, and neurotubulelike structures within the cytoplasm and in the cell processes. However, unlike in metastatic neuroblastoma, urinary catecholamine excretion is normal in PNET, and this helps to distinguish the two lesions (Table IV.1).

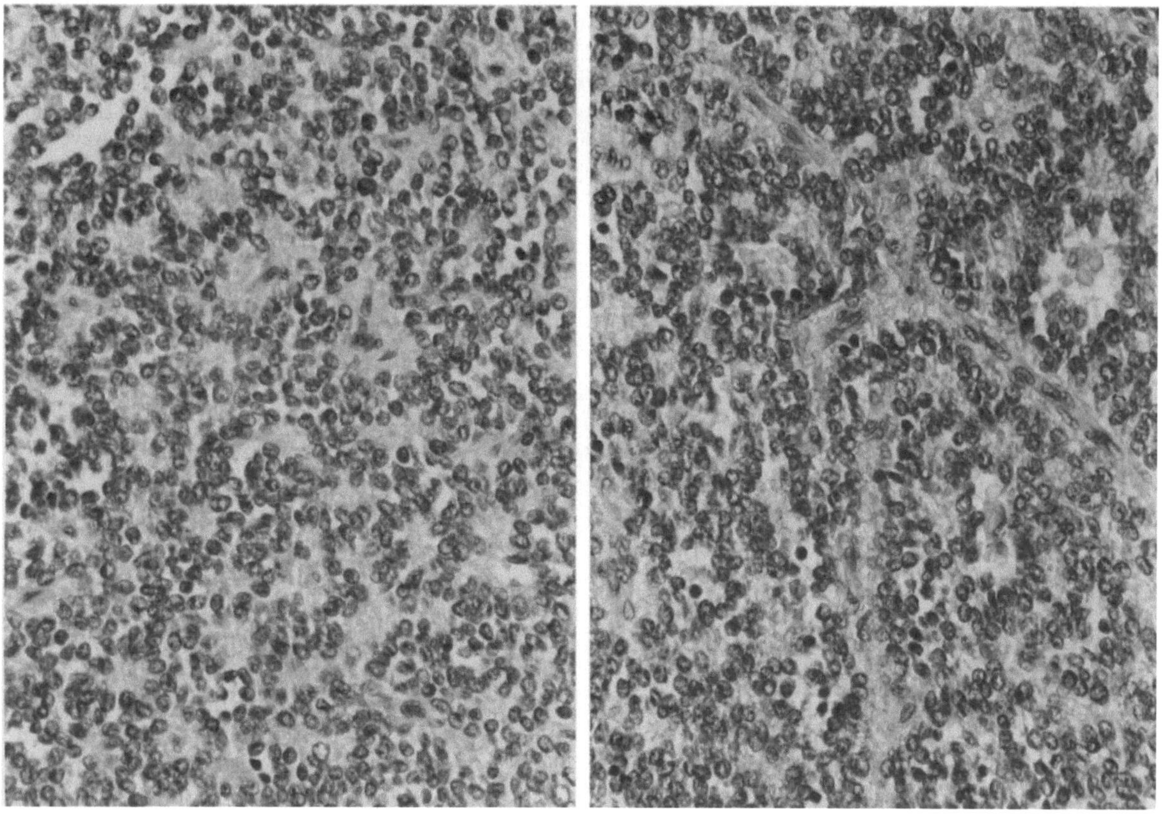

a b

Fig. IV.38a,b. Photomicrographs of other areas of the same case as in Fig. IV.37, revealing the conspicuous rosettoid formations and the uniform aspect of the round nuclei without clear cytoplasmic outlines, very similar to those of Ewing sarcoma. ×400

Table IV.1. Differential diagnosis of Ewing sarcoma and neural tumors

	Ewing sarcoma	Neuroectodermal tumor of bone	Metastatic neuroblastoma
Age	5–20 years	Median age 11 years	Under 5 years
Glycogen	+	(50%)	–
Ultrastructure	Undifferentiated (principal) cells Glycogen +	Neural processes Neurosecretory granules Glycogen	Neural Processes Neurosecretory granules Glycogen –
Neuron-specific enolase (NSE)	–	+	+
Urinary catecholamine	Normal	Normal	Elevated
Chromosomal translocation	Present	Present	Absent

The distinction between Ewing sarcoma, PNET, and other small round-cell tumors has been based particularly on the results of immunohistochemical staining with NSE and other neural markers (HNK-1, HBA-7/1, and others). However, these are positive not only in PNET, but also in a number of cases in which the histologic features are those of Ewing sarcoma. Moreover, the presence of a reciprocal 11;22 chromosome translocation is shared by both tumors, suggesting a close histogenetic relationship (Table IV.1).

As stated above in the section on Ewing sarcoma, this author believes that the diagnosis of PNET should be restricted to atypical Ewing sarcomas displaying morphologic evidence of neural differentiation by light and electron microscopy, accompanied by immunohistochemical studies (Figs. IV.37, IV.39).

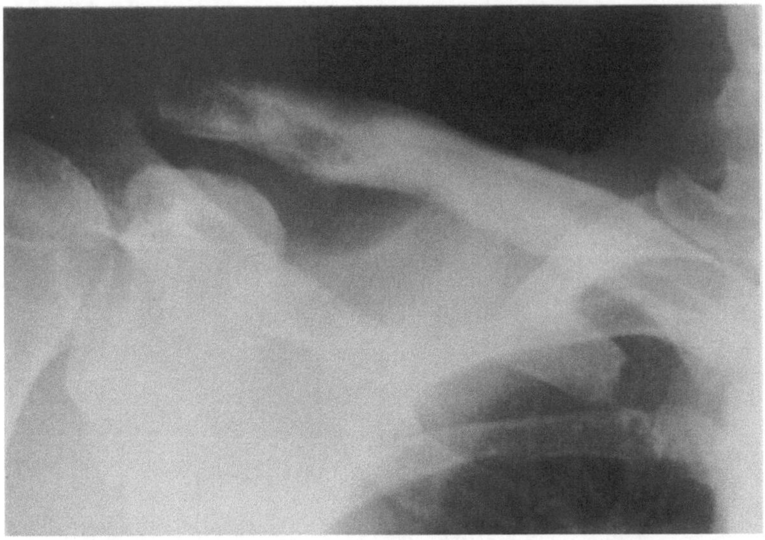

Fig. IV.39. Male, 20 years old. PNET of clavicle. Radiograph shows a mixed lytic–sclerotic permeative lesion at the external end of the clavicle, which was diagnosed as a small round-cell tumor, possibly Ewing sarcoma. However, the electron microscopic and immunohistochemical studies, revealing positivity for NSE and neurofilaments, inclined the diagnosis towards PNET. (Case from Rush-Presbyterian-St. Luke's Medical Center)

3. Malignant Lymphoma of Bone (Non-Hodgkin Lymphoma)

Definition, WHO: *Lymphoma of bone, formerly referred to as reticulum-cell sarcoma, has been defined as "a malignant lymphoid tumor with a rather varied histologic structure, considered to be primary in bone. The tumor cells are usually rounded and rather pleomorphic and may have well-defined cytoplasmic outlines; many of their nuclei are indented (cleaved) or horseshoe-shaped and have prominent nucleoli. In most cases numerous reticulin fibers are present and are distributed uniformly between the tumor cells."*

Non-Hodgkin lymphomas constitute a large group of neoplasms, the pathologic classification of which has long been controversial. The classification of Rappaport, proposed 25 years ago and subsequently widely used, was also previously employed in the first edition of this book. In more recent years new classifications have been proposed, including two which are based in part upon modern concepts of the immune system and lymphoid physiology (Lukes and Collins 1975; Lennert 1975). The Rappaport system has undergone considerable revision with the recognition of new clinicopathologic entities, but no consensus exists as to which system is most satisfactory with regard to clinical relevance and scientific accuracy.

In an attempt to resolve this problem, an international multi-institutional clinicopathologic study of 1177 cases of non-Hodgkin lymphoma was sponsored by the National Cancer Institute (Rosenberg et al. 1982). The reproducibility and clinical relevance of the six major classifications were tested. Immunologic methods were not employed. A working formulation of non-Hodgkin lymphoma was described which separated the disease into three groups (low grade, intermediate, and high grade), with ten major types, utilizing *morphologic* criteria only, giving equivalent terms for each type in the six major classifications. This formulation permits translation among the various systems and greatly facilitates clinical comparison of different reports and results of therapeutic trials.

It is not the purpose of this book to consider in detail this working formulation, and we will employ it only as far as current knowledge permits it to be applied to the rare "primary lymphomas" in bone.

Following Parker and Jackson's publication in 1939 of the "primary reticulum-cell sarcoma of bone," its separation from Ewing sarcoma as a distinct entity with characteristic clinical and pathologic features was generally accepted. Parker and Jackson collected 17 cases and noted the discrepancy that often existed between the size of the destructive bony lesion and the good general condition of the patient; they also pointed out that the clinical evolution seemed to be more favorable than that of Ewing sarcoma, 7 of 17 patients having survived longer than 10 years.

The term "reticulum-cell sarcoma" was used to describe tumors composed of reticulum-producing cells considered of histiocytic (monocytic-macrophage) origin. However, since the advent of newer classifications of non-Hodgkin lymphomas, it has been shown that the majority of the histiocytic lymphomas were in fact B- or T-cell lymphomas, and that true "histiocytic" or "reticulohistiocytic" lymphomas are rare (Isaacson et al. 1983).

This author and also others have not found nodular (follicular) lymphomas in bone (Dosoretz et al. 1982; Clayton et al. 1987; Ostrowski et al. 1986). "Primary" lymphoma of bone is defined as a solitary osseous lesion without involvement of other osseous or nonosseous sites within 6 months of the onset of symptoms. The involvement of regional lymph nodes does not exclude the diagnosis of primary lymphoma of bone. Adopting this definition, it becomes evident that many of the lymphomas reported in the older literature as "primary in bone" cannot be accepted as such by present standards because they were not adequately staged. Furthermore, the authors did not have the benefit of the new staging procedures such as radionuclide scanning, computed tomography, and magnetic resonance imaging. A great number of these cases were probably secondary deposits derived from tumors of lymph nodes or from other extranodal lesions. Although morphologically indistinguishable, they have a different clinical behavior and a worse prognosis, and are almost always fatal within 2 years, in contrast with the favorable prognosis of primary lymphomas in bone.

Primary osseous lesions in Hodgkin disease, in contrast to the secondary involvement of bone, seem to be extremely rare, and we did not observe any unequivocal case in our files. Of 13 cases of Hodgkin disease in bone found in the Mayo Clinic (Ostrowski et al. 1986), none had a single bone involvement.

Incidence. In our previous series (1981), 102 cases were classified as malignant non-Hodgkin lymphoma (63 primary and 39 secondary) and three as lymphosarcoma (well-differentiated lymphocytic lymphoma) primary in bone.

Huvos (1991), however, includes in his series of 158 "primary" lymphomas of bone studied at the Memorial Hospital from 1949 to 1983, 18 examples of multifocal osseous involvement in the absence of lymph node disease. At the Mayo Clinic (Dahlin and Unni 1986) 469 cases of malignant lymphoma of bone (primary and

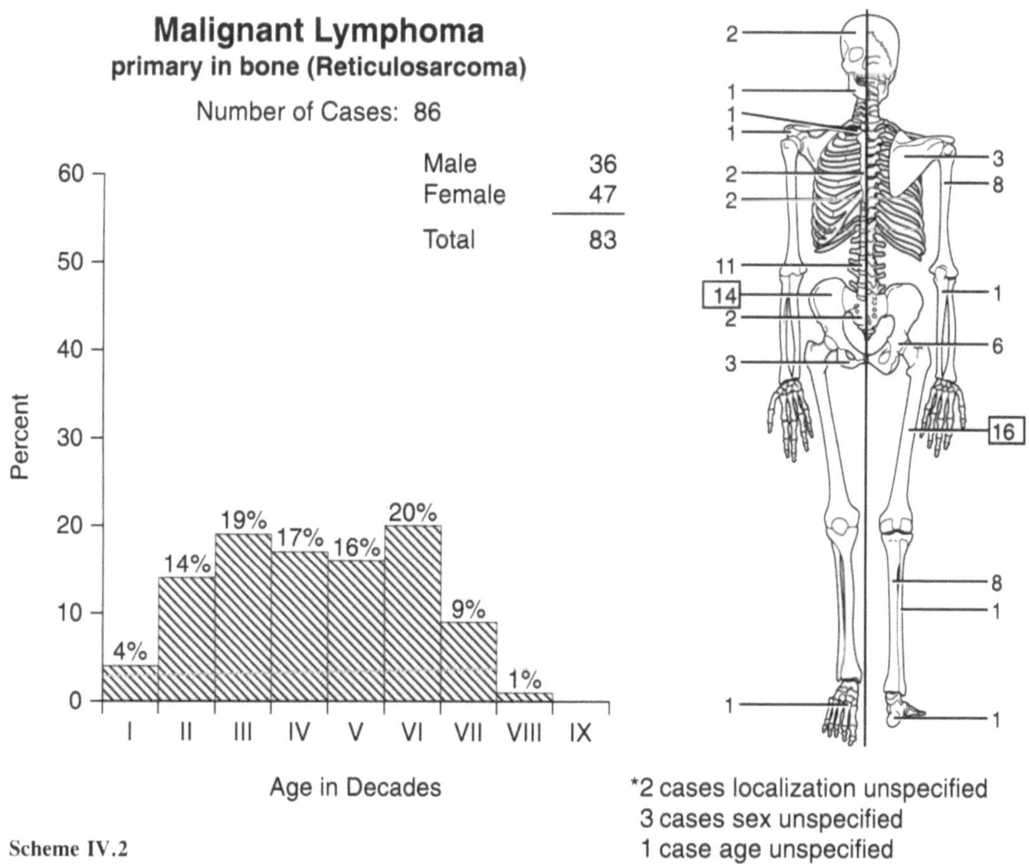

Scheme IV.2

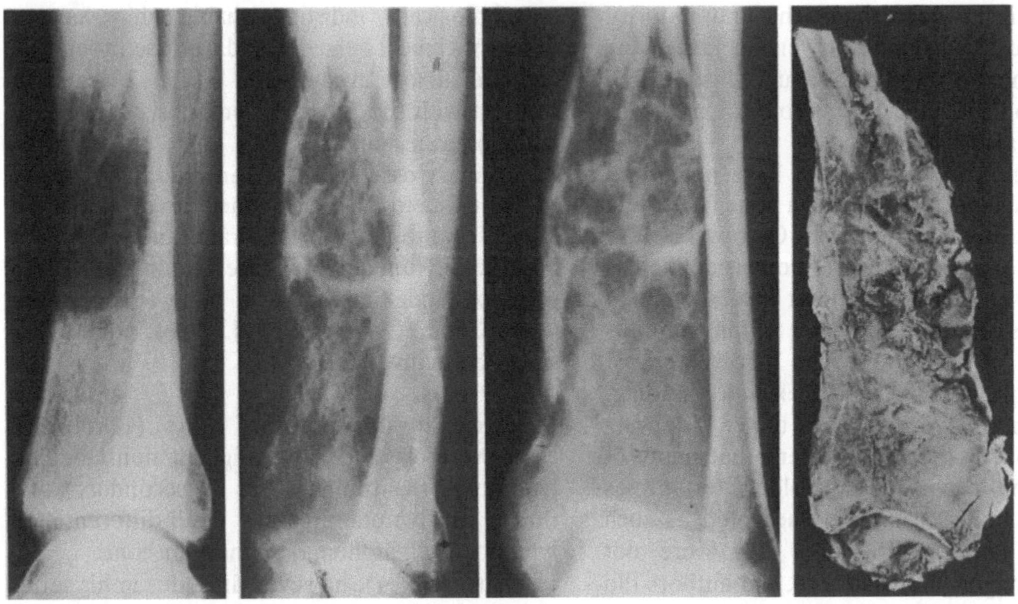

a b, c

Fig. IV.40a–c. Male, 26 years old. Primary lymphoma of tibia. **a** Radiograph of osteolytic lesion of the shaft of the tibia with ill-defined, permeative margins and destruction of the cortex. **b** Lateral and anteroposterior radiographs 6 months after radiotherapy showing extension of the lesion toward the distal end of the tibia. An en bloc resection followed by bone grafts was performed. The patient was in good health 6 years later. **c** Photograph of the resected specimen showing extension of the tumor into the soft tissues

secondary) were diagnosed, representing 7.2% of malignant bone tumors. In 202 cases (3.1%), the osseous involvement seemed to be the unique lesion.

Clinical Findings. *Sex and Age.* The sex, age, and skeletal distribution of 86 cases of non-Hodgkin lymphoma, primary in bone, are shown in Scheme IV.2; this lesion accounted for 4% of malignant bone tumors. Females predominated in our series (1.4:1), but males appear to be affected more frequently in other series, with a 2:1 or 3:2 ratio (Dahlin and Unni 1986; Huvos 1991).

Primary lymphoma (reticulosarcoma) can occur at any age. However, it was more common after the second decade, with a peak in the third decade. It was rare under 10 years of age, thus differing from Ewing sarcoma, which occurred most commonly in the first two decades, and from secondary lymphoma, which was more common after the fourth or fifth decade.

Localization. Primary lymphoma (reticulosarcoma) may involve any bone, but most commonly it is situated in short bones, especially the ilium (14 cases), vertebrae (11 cases), and scapula, and long tubular bones, particularly the femur (16 cases) and tibia (8 cases). This finding agrees with those of other large series (Francis et al. 1954; Wilson and Pugh 1955; Huvos 1991). In contrast to Dahlin and Unni's series (1986), in which there was a relatively high incidence of skull and mandibular tumors, cranial and mandibular involvement was rare in our series.

Symptoms. One of the most striking clinical features of primary lymphoma of bone is the remarkable contrast between the general well-being of the patient and the extensive painful, destructive lesion (Parker and Jackson 1939). The situation is very different in the secondary, disseminated form of lymphoma, which is almost always associated with a poor general condition and/or subfebrile temperature. Pain of variable intensity and duration, generally accompanied by swelling of the involved bone and local tenderness, is the most common complaint. The onset is often insidious and slow; several patients sought consultation months after symptoms started. Neurologic symptoms occurred in several cases localized in the vertebrae. Pathologic fracture was rare in our cases, but it occurred frequently (about 20%) in other series (Parker and Jackson 1939; Bethge 1955). Sometimes, it was the initial symptom.

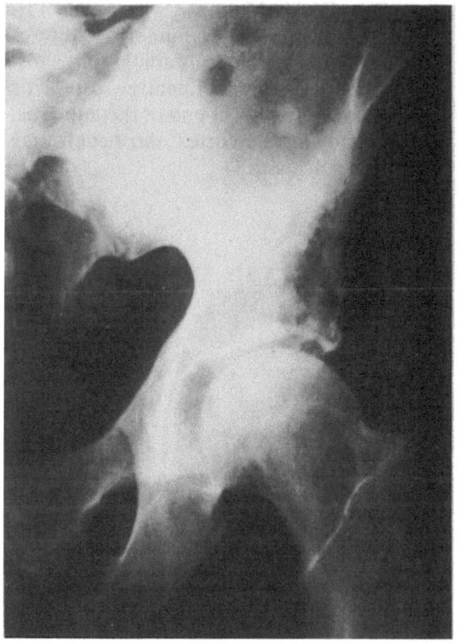

Fig. IV.41. Female, 60 years old. Primary lymphoma of ilium. Radiograph shows an osteolytic, ill-defined lesion with some reactive sclerosis

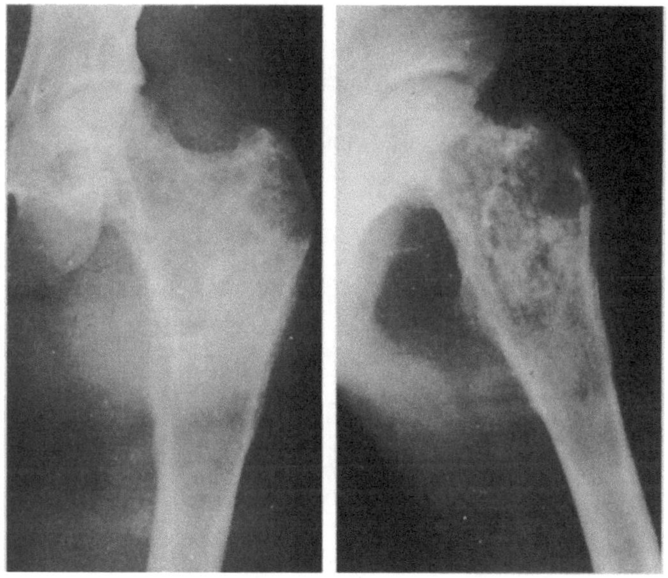

Fig. IV.42. Male, 19 years old. Primary lymphoma of femur. Anteroposterior and lateral radiographs show permeative lesion with ill-defined margins and periosteal reaction in the femoral neck extending toward the marrow cavity of the diaphysis

a

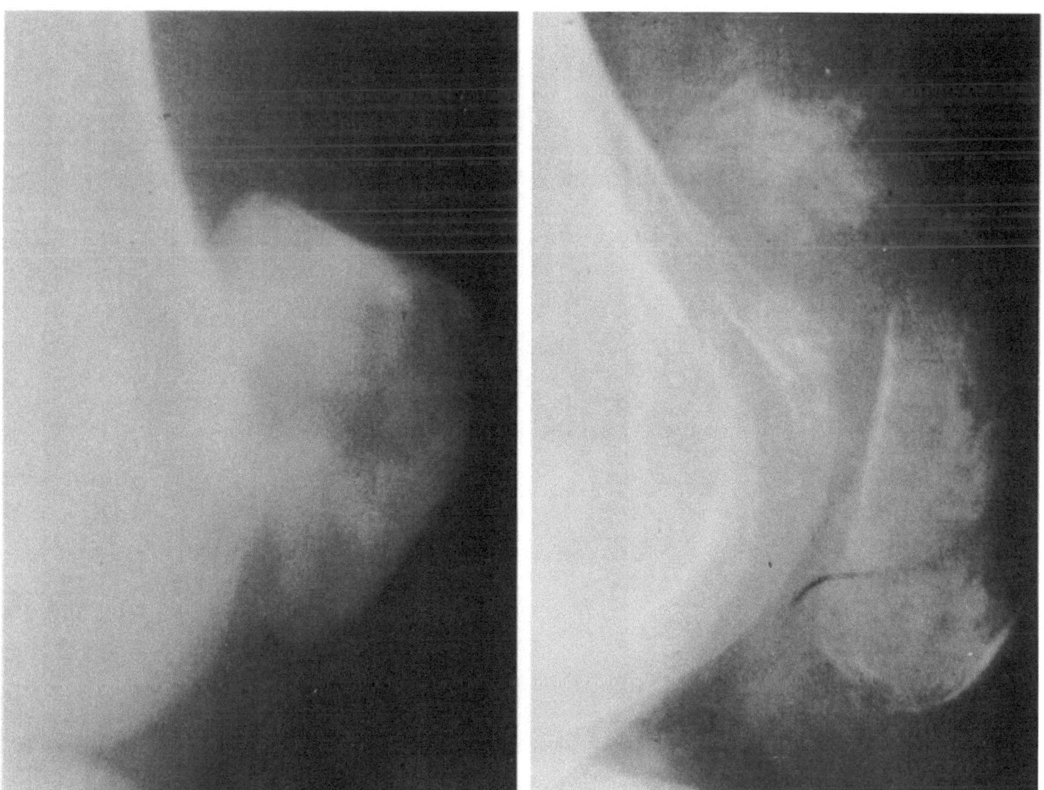

b

Fig. IV.43a,b. Male, 38 years old. Primary lymphoma of patella. **a** Radiograph shows radiolucent, ill-defined lesion. **b** Radiograph after a pathologic fracture illustrates the increase in size

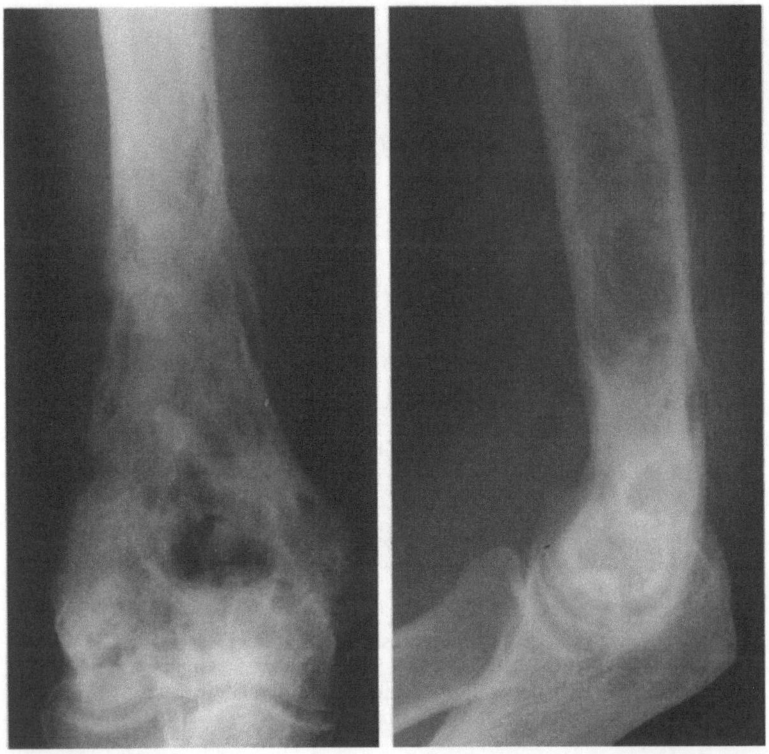

Fig. IV.44. Male, 43 years old. Primary lymphoma of humerus. Anteroposterior and lateral radiographs show a large, predominantly osteolytic lesion of the lower end of the humerus, destroying the cortex and penetrating into soft tissues

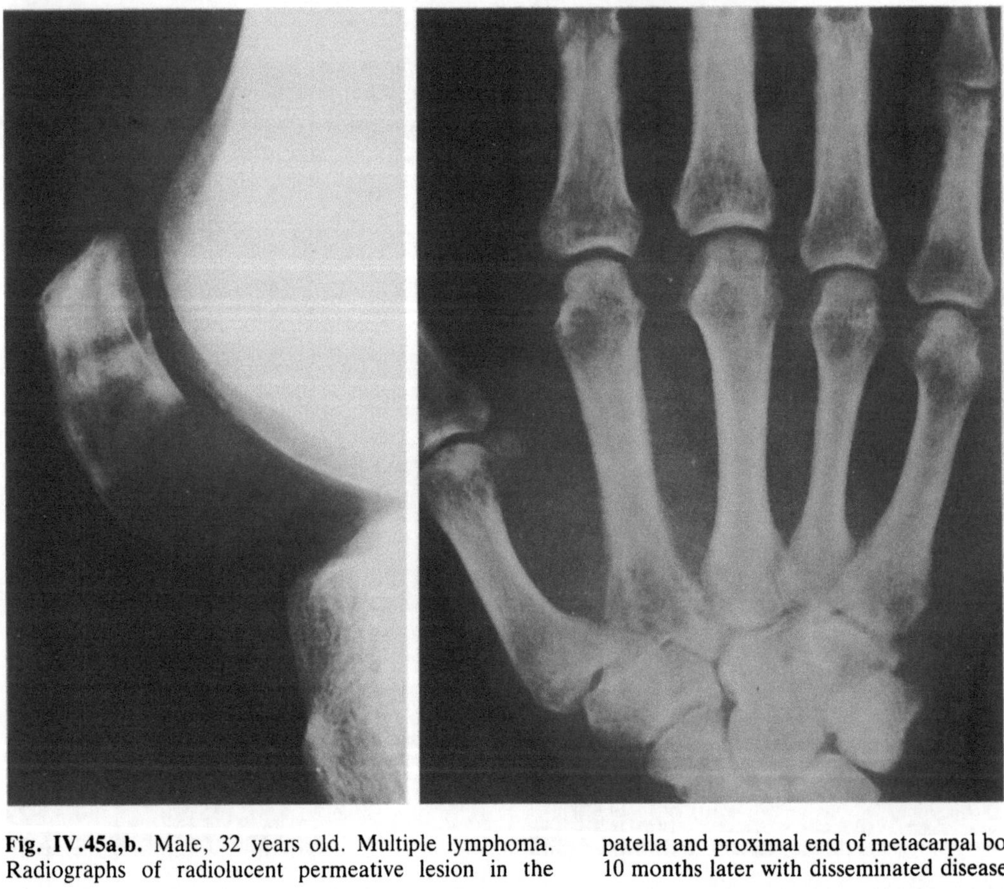

a b

Fig. IV.45a,b. Male, 32 years old. Multiple lymphoma. Radiographs of radiolucent permeative lesion in the patella and proximal end of metacarpal bone. Patient died 10 months later with disseminated disease

Fig. IV.46a–e. Female, 25 years old. Primary lymphoma of tibia, B-cell type. **a** Radiograph shows a poorly delimited, predominantly sclerotic lesion in the upper third of the tibia without soft tissue involvement. The hole (*arrow*) corresponds to a previous biopsy. **b** CT scan and **c** T1-weighted MRI show the compact sclerosis and the extension of the lesion in the medullary canal without penetration into soft tissues. The first biopsy was inclusive (chronic osteomyelitis? malignant histiocytic tumor?). **d** Photomicrograph of the second biopsy shows spindle-celled fibrous tissue with infiltration of round tumor cells, apparently malignant histiocytes and lymphocytes, and areas of necrosis including necrotic bony fragments. Both the large, obviously neoplastic cells and the smaller round cells exhibit leukocyte common antigen (**e**), and stained positive for B-cell marker L26. **d** ×100, **e** ×200

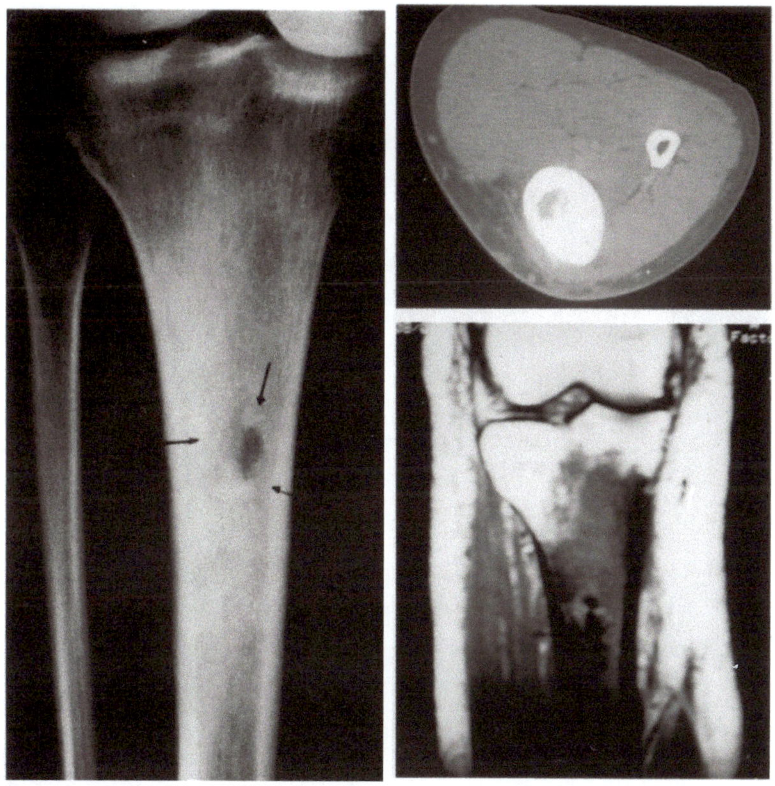

a b c

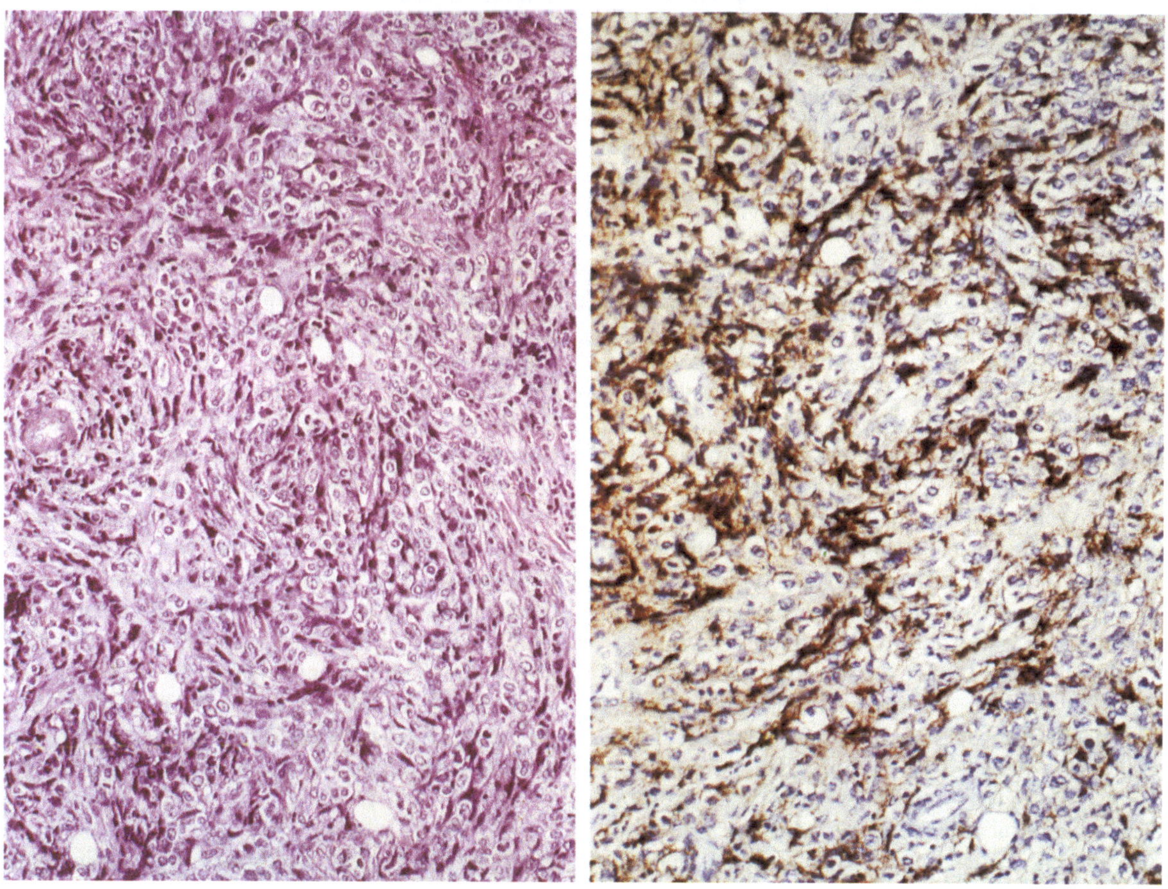

d e

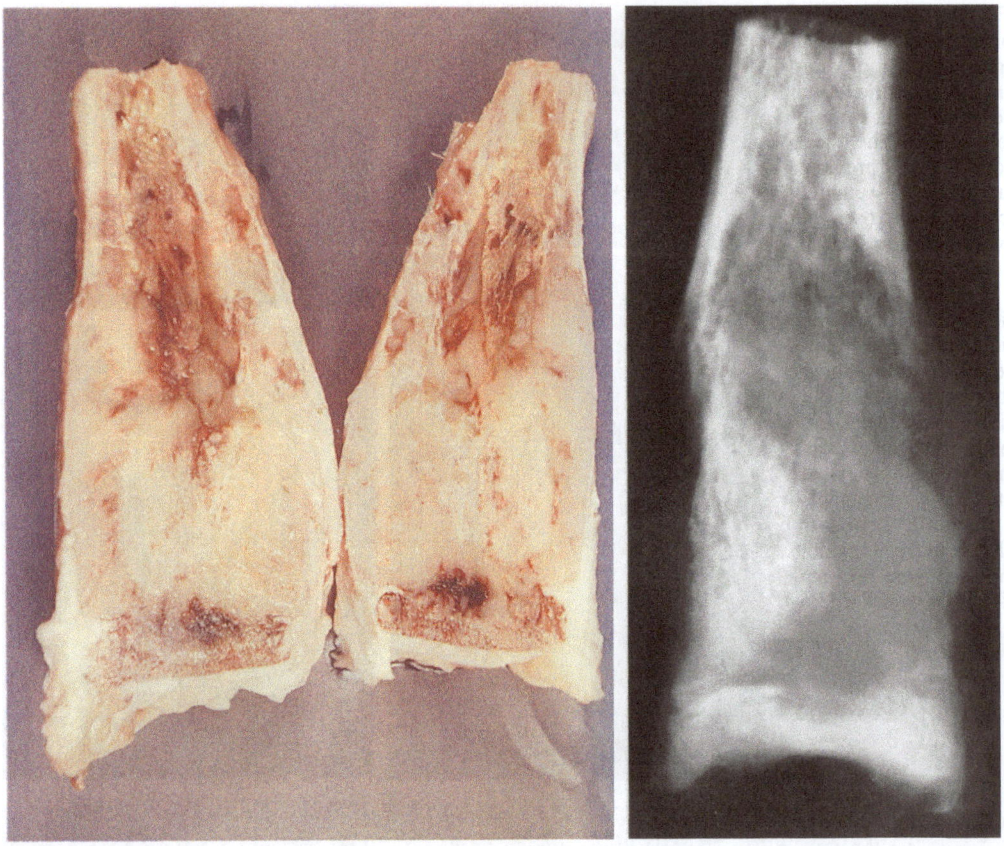

a b

Fig. IV.47a,b. Male, 10 years old. Primary lymphoma of tibia. **a** Photograph and **b** radiograph of the amputation specimen showing destruction of the cancellous and cortical bone and extension into the epiphysis and soft tissues. Some reactive sclerosis in the spongiosa is seen

Radiographic Features. The first changes are usually one or more small permeative areas of bone destruction arising in the medullary cavity of the metaphysis or diaphysis, or rarely in the epiphysis of a long or flat bone (Figs. IV.40–IV.44). The radiolucent lesions later become confluent, forming more extensive areas that reach the cortex, which is soon penetrated by the tumor and partially or completely destroyed, producing periosteal new-bone formation, which in our cases was not striking. A typical "onion peel" reaction was not found in our cases, and a "sunburst" pattern was infrequent. Total destruction of the cortex is invariably accompanied by a large soft tissue mass. Although the most characteristic and predominant feature is a mottled, permeative lesion with extensive bone destruction, sometimes foci of moderate or, rarely, conspicuous reactive bone formation in the medullary cavity or of the cortex may be observed; however, this was rather infrequent in our material (Figs. IV.45, IV.46).

Pathologic Findings. *Gross Pathology.* In cases in which we studied the anatomic specimen before and after treatment (radiotherapy and/or chemotherapy), the tumor had destroyed the cancellous bone in a wide area of the meta- or diaphyseal region, without sharp delimitation toward the surrounding bone. The cortical bone was thinned and distended or, more commonly, destroyed and perforated at several points, extending the tumor into the soft tissues. The periosteum commonly had not reacted or produced new bone, although this did occur on a small scale in the cancellous tissue surrounding the tumor. The tumor was grayish-white, and the consistency varied between firm and friable. Areas of necrosis were much less common and extensive than in Ewing sarcoma (Figs. IV.40, IV.47).

Histopathology. In former publications (Schajowicz 1973, 1981) this author tried to classify the malignant lymphomas of bone according to the criteria of Rappaport's (1966) classification of lymph node lymphomas. The great majority of our cases of primary lymphomas were classified as histiocytic (15) and histiocytic-lymphocytic (35), and only four as undifferentiated malignant lymphoma (reticulosarcoma). Three were classified as well-differentiated lymphocytic lymphomas (lymphosarcomas). In the last decade all lymphomas, when possible, were classified according to the Working Formulation (1982). In several of our older cases, adequate staging procedures had not been performed and a certain number of lesions then classified as "primary" in bone would probably be diagnosed at present as secondary or doubtful.

The histologic structure was variable and the tumor cells could be separated into various subgroups in most cases, the most important criteria being the predominance of large cells, the presence or absence of nuclear clefts (cleaved and noncleaved cells), and the degree of pleomorphism or anaplasia. The tumor cell was usually rounded, ovoid, or pleomorphic and had a slightly basophilic cytoplasm, often with well-defined outlines. The nuclei were commonly larger than in Ewing sarcoma, poor in chromatin, and oval to indented (cleaved) or horseshoe in shape; they often contained one or two prominent nucleoli (Figs. IV.48–IV.50). Only occasionally were more than one nucleus and an evident pleomorphic pattern observed. Tumors composed predominantly of histiocytic cells (monocytes-macrophages) were infrequent, and it was common to find among the tumor cells a conspicuous number of poorly and well-differentiated lymphocytes. To distinguish true histiocytic tumors (according to Rappaport's classification), immunohistochemistry is of great value and has the added advantage that it can be used in routine formalin-fixed paraffin-embedded tissue. Isaacson et al. (1983) found that α_1-antitrypsin is a more reliable marker than lysozyme for malignant histiocytes.

Furthermore, most histiocytic tumors showed a rich reticular framework and a characteristic distribution of the fibrils surrounding individual cells. However, this pattern also may be found in many of the large-cell lymphomas (Fig. IV.48c,d).

On the other hand, the Del Rio Hortega specific technique, used in our older cases, showed the wealth of predominantly ramified reticuloendothelial elements and their even distribution among the differentiated "histiocytic" elements in the tumors which we had previously classified as "histiocytic" or "histiocytic-lymphocytic" lymphomas; they corresponded to the original reticulosarcoma of Parker and Jackson.

The rare cases (three) of well-differentiated lymphocytic lymphoma (lymphosarcoma) and the few undifferentiated or anaplastic ("stem-cell") lymphomas were often difficult to distinguish from Ewing sarcoma. Both entities generally lack reticulin fibers and, more importantly, always lack glycogen, like all the other varieties of lymphoma. The possible prognostic significance of the morphologic cell pattern is described later.

We want to emphasize that the three cases of well-differentiated lymphoma, initially primary in bone, terminated with leukemic changes in peripheral blood (Figs. IV.51–IV.53).

In our few cases of Hodgkin disease (Figs. IV.54, IV.55) it was impossible to determine with absolute certainty whether the lesion was primarily intraosseous. Therefore, these cases have not been included in our statistical figures.

Finally, we want to stress that the cytologic investigation of smears in material obtained by needle biopsy or imprint preparation from the tumor tissue was extremely useful in all varieties of round-cell tumors of bone, especially in the precise diagnosis of the different types of malignant lymphoma. Differential diagnosis is sometimes difficult with undifferentiated metastatic carcinoma and with cases of poorly differentiated myelomas. In such cases, the immunologic and/or biochemical findings (urinary and serum protein) facilitate the diagnosis.

Electron Microscopy. Ultrastructural studies may be helpful in distinguishing Ewing sarcoma from malignant lymphoma (Friedman and Hanaoka 1971; Rice et al. 1973). The cells of the "reticulum-cell" type of malignant lymphoma appeared in Friedman and Hanaoka's study with considerable variation in size and shape, the cell membranes being convoluted with some villouslike projections. The nuclei were irregular, moderately electronlucent, but showed marginal chromatin condensation and often prominent nucleoli. A moderate number of mitochondria and ribosomes and an evident Golgi apparatus were present. Histiocytic propensity is shown by lysosomes and phagocytized material in the cytoplasm.

Between the cellular elements, there were two types of fibrils, unbanded, possibly reticulin, and others showing the typical banding of collagen. Cells of lymphomas of the well-differentiated lymphocytic type did not show constant

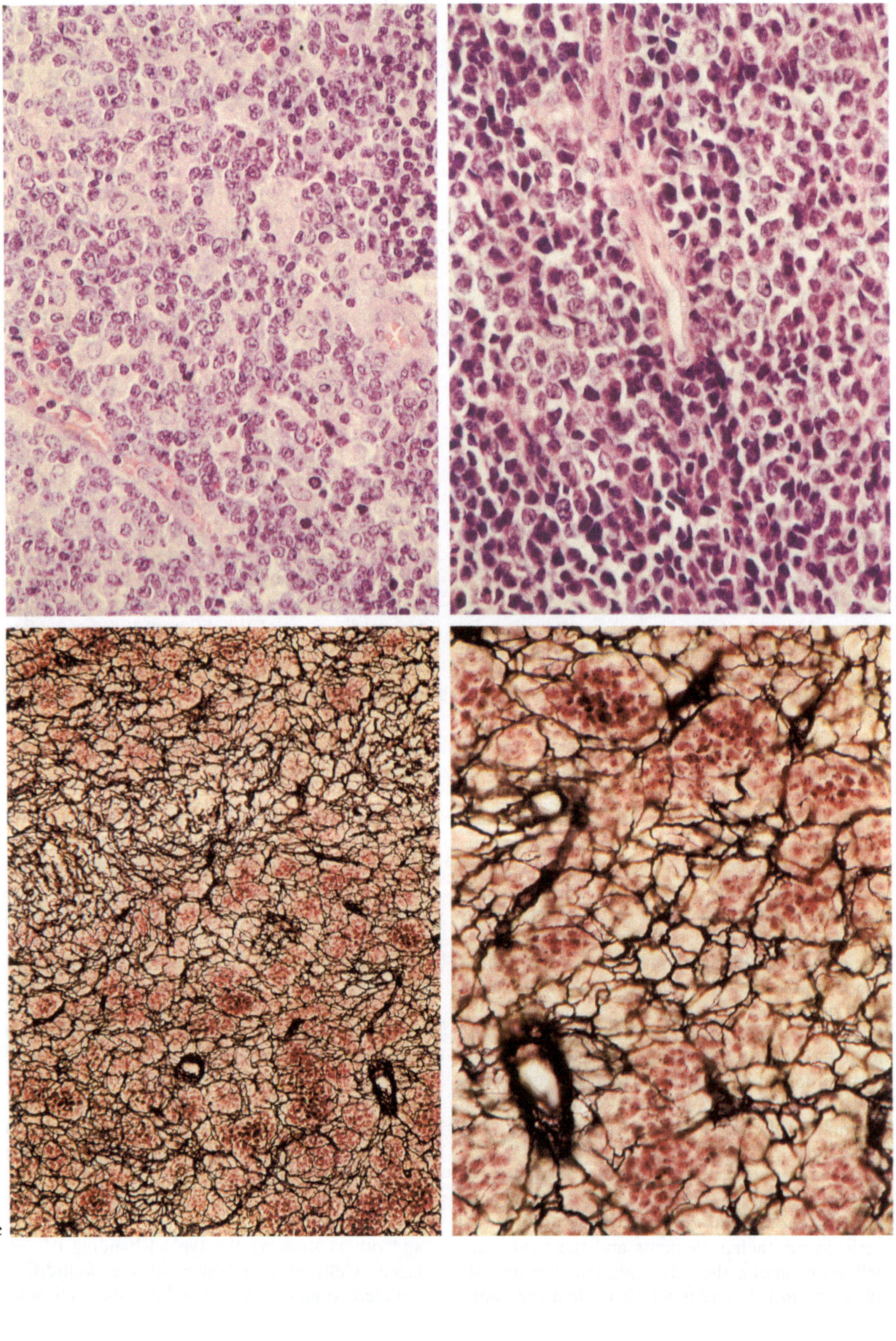

a b c d

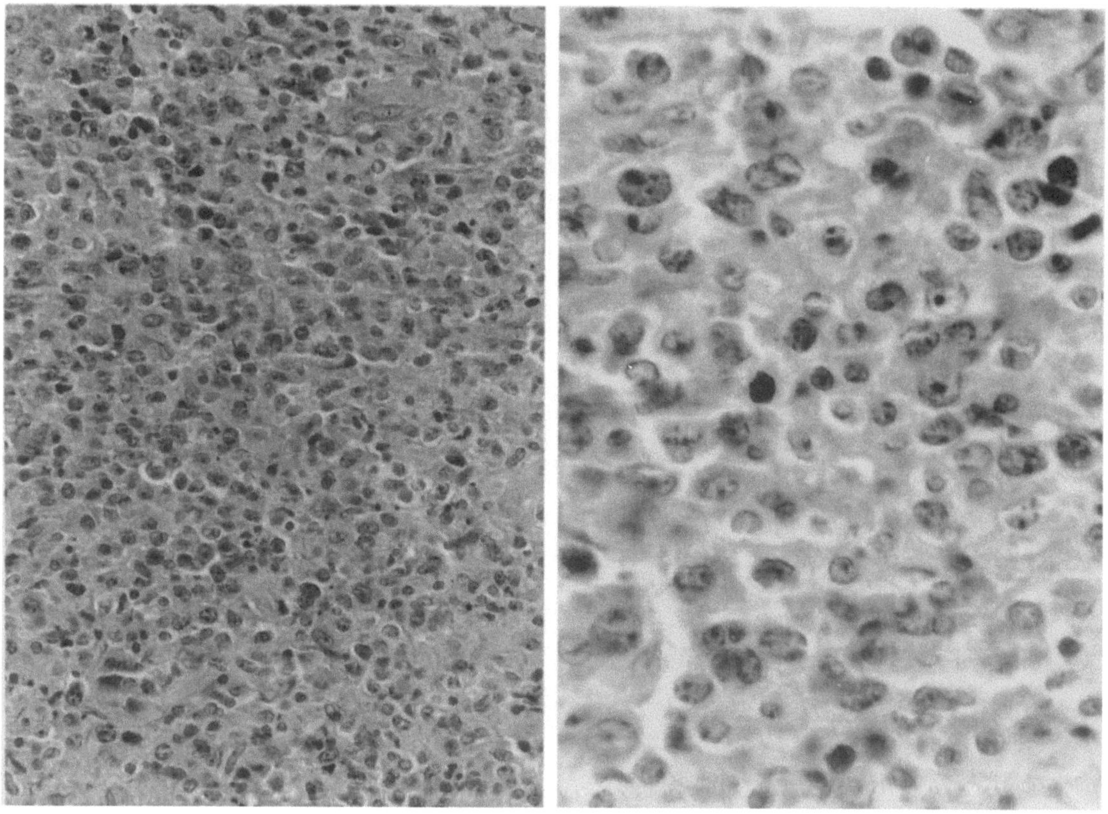

a b

Fig. IV.49a,b. Photomicrographs of primary lymphoma of bone showing at **a** lower and **b** higher magnification the histologic features of this predominantly cleaved large-cell lymphoma. The prominent nuclei of the tumor cell are well seen in **b**. **a** ×300, **b** ×600

Fig. IV.48a–d. Photomicrographs of primary lymphoma of bone. **a,b** The more pleomorphic aspect of the round cells, which frequently have well-defined cytoplasmic outlines and indented nuclei. Lymphocytic differentiation can be seen in **a** (*upper left corner*). **c,d** Del Rio Hortega's silver stain demonstrating abundant reticulin fibers forming a dense network surrounding individual (**c**) or small groups (**d**) of tumor cells. **a** ×300, **b** ×320, **c** ×180, **d** ×350

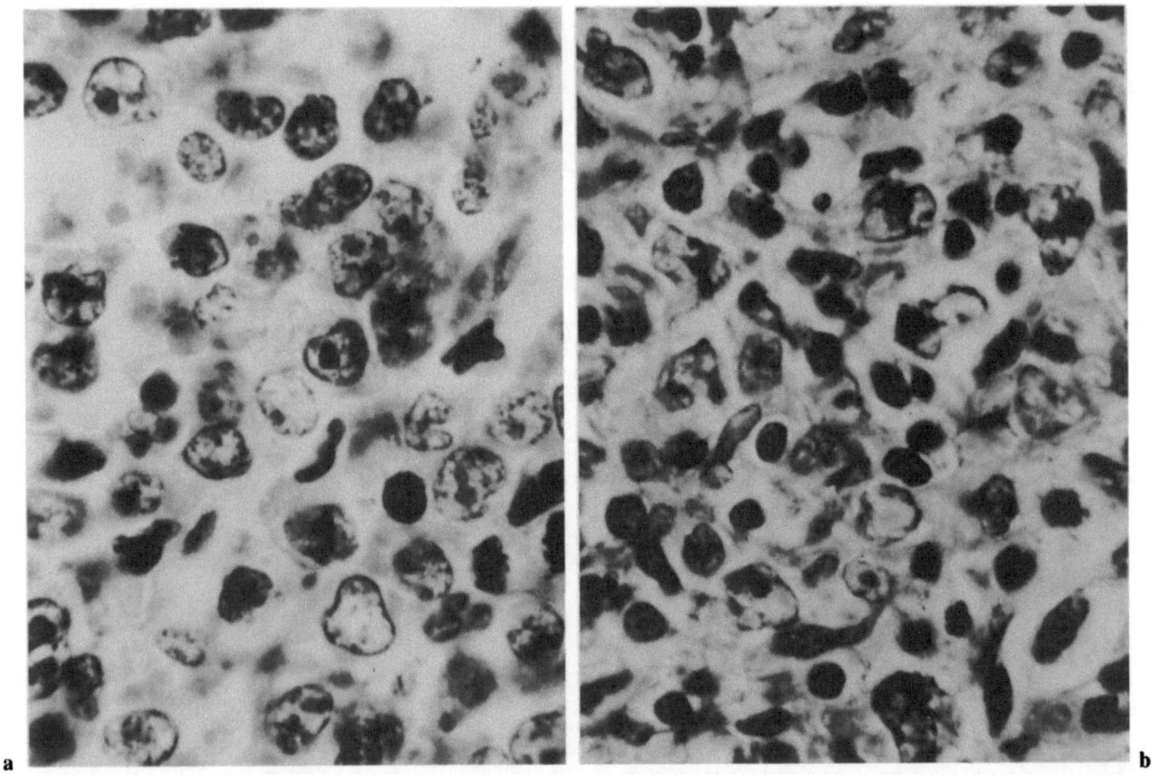

Fig. IV.50a,b. Photomicrographs of cleaved large-cell lymphoma showing the nuclear details at higher magnification. ×600

Fig. IV.51a,b. Male, 9 years old. Lymphosarcoma of humerus. a Radiograph shows an extensive osteolytic lesion of the upper end of the humerus. b Radiograph 6 months after radiotherapy ▼

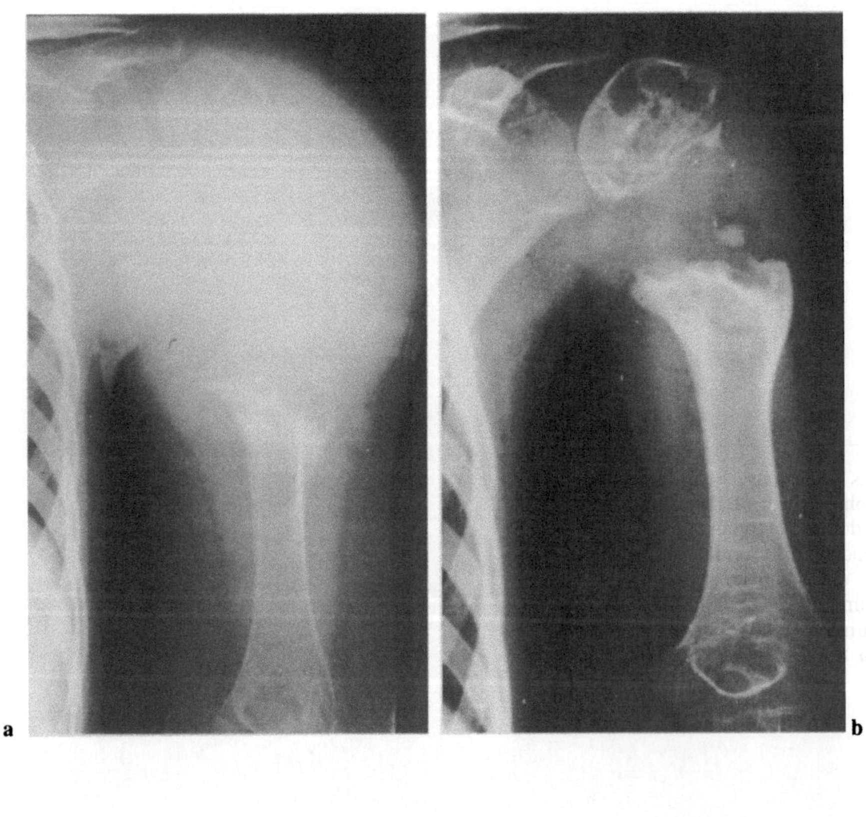

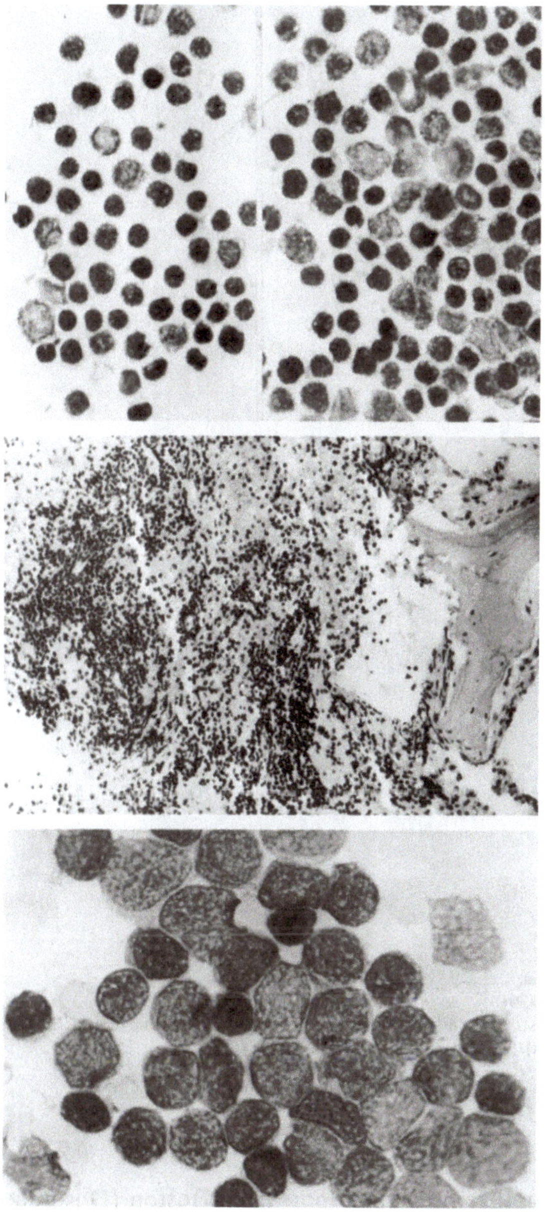

a

b

c

◀ **Fig. IV.52a–c.** Photomicrographs of lymphosarcoma of the upper end of humerus. **a** Smear and **b** histologic section of the aspirated material, showing predominantly well-differentiated lymphocyte. **c** Cytologic features of a lymph node biopsy (supraclavicular region) performed 1 year later showing a poorly differentiated lymphocytic lymphoma. **a** ×400, **b** ×100, **c** ×800

Fig. IV.53. Photomicrograph of lymphocytic lymphoma (lymphosarcoma) of calcaneus. ×100
▼

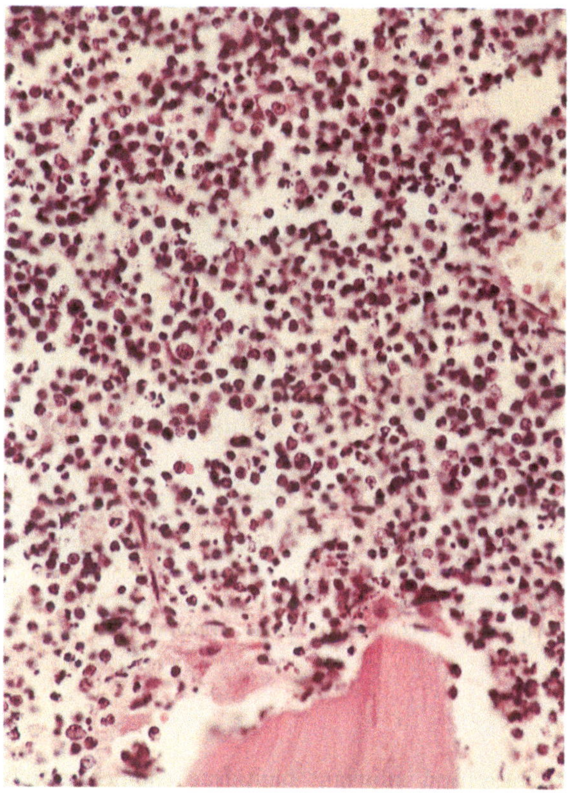

findings, but in general the size and shape of the nuclei were more uniform, and the cytoplasmic borders were more regular without evidence of phagocytic activity.

Treatment and Prognosis. The treatment of "reticulosarcoma" has changed over the years and varies in different institutions. Parker and Jackson (1939) advised early amputation followed by radiotherapy of the regional lymph nodes, one of the frequent sites of metastasis. Coley (1960) believed that the best treatment is radiotherapy, combined with the administration of Coley's toxins. All authors agree that the malignant lymphoma primary in bone is radiosensitive, but it is evident that even supervoltage radiotherapy in high doses (45–60 Gy), delivered to the entire bone, does not constitute a guarantee against recurrence.

The preferred treatment in our institution was wide excision (en bloc resection) of expendable bones (fibula, ribs) and also of other long or short bones when feasible, and only exceptionally amputation. This was accompanied by irradiation of the remaining bone and the regional lymph nodes. In recent years a combination of radio-

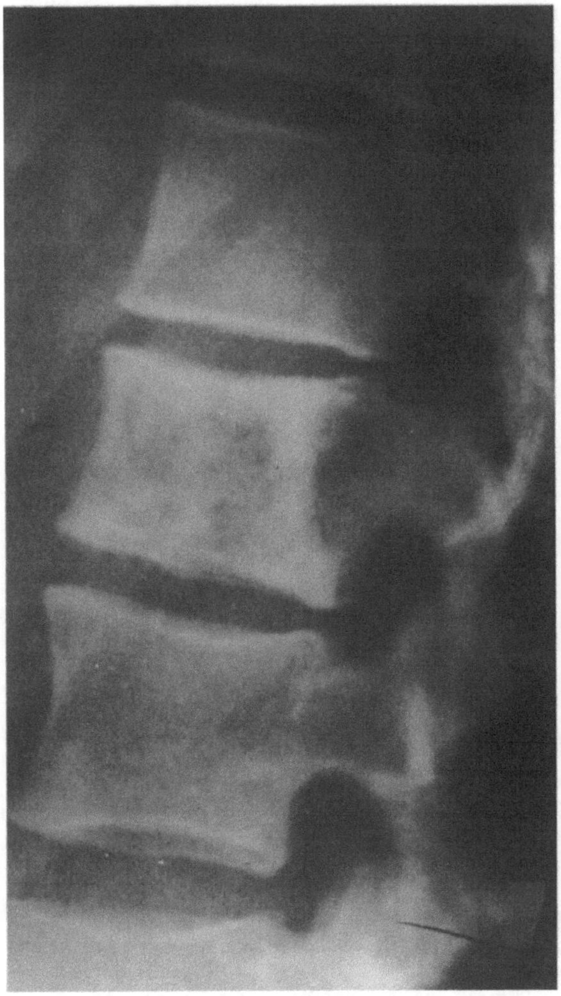
a

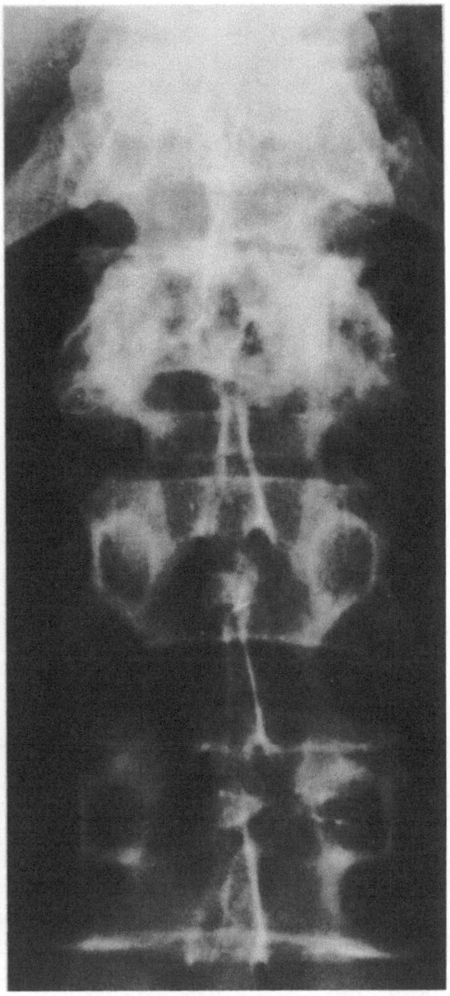
b

Fig. IV.54a,b. Female, 27 years old, with Hodgkin lymphoma, secondary in bone. Lateral and anteroposterior radiographs of osteolytic–sclerotic lesion of the first lumbar vertebra

therapy and adjuvant multidrug chemotherapy was given, including essentially the same drugs as are used in Ewing sarcoma, associated with surgery for local-regional disease. In disseminated disease and in surgically inaccessible lesions, aggressive chemotherapy is applied, together with irradiation of some focal lesions.

The histologic pattern of lymphoma significantly correlates with the *prognosis* of the disease, according to some authors (Dosoretz et al. 1982; Clayton et al. 1987). Of the 26 patients with large-cell lymphoma studied at the M.D. Anderson Hospital in Houston (Clayton et al. 1987), 17 were long-term survivors. Of those with large cleaved-cell lymphomas, 67% were long-term survivors, but only 20% of the patients with large non-cleaved cell lymphomas survived. Another previous report from Boston (Dosoretz et al. 1982) also emphasized the value of the morphology of the tumor cell, arriving at similar conclusions. However, extensive study of 22 patients with malignant lymphoma of bone from the Mayo Clinic (Ostrowski et al. 1986) failed to demonstrate a significant prognostic value of histologic typing of the lymphomas as assessed by either the Working Formulation or the Kiel system. Similarly, whether the lymphoma exhibited T-cell features or was of the cleaved-cell type was not found to be of prognostic relevance. However, the site and clinical stage of the disease (local vs disseminated lesions) and soft tissue invasion evidently affect the prognosis; thus, patients with primary osseous lymphoma were found to have a 55% 5-year survival rate by

Fig. IV.55. Autopsy specimen of a case of generalized Hodgkin lymphoma showing involvement of several vertebrae. Despite the infiltration of four vertebrae, radiologic osteolytic and sclerotic changes can be seen only in the two middle, completely involved vertebral bodies and not in the adjacent vertebrae, even in this 5-mm thick slab

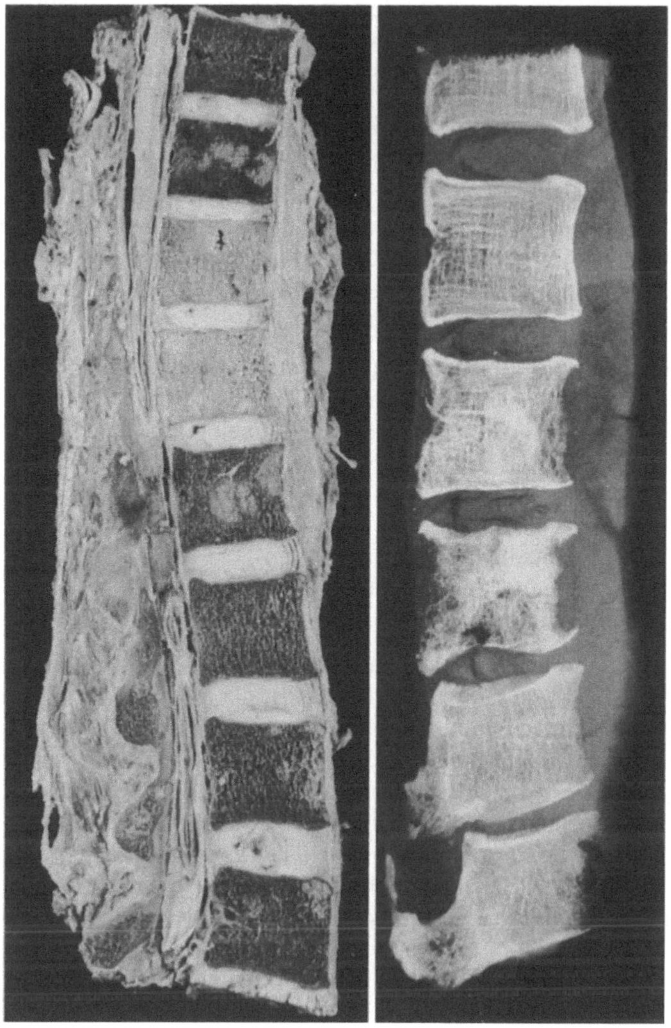
a b

Ostrowski et al. (1986), as against a rate of only 9% in those with disseminated disease. On the other hand, involvement of the pelvis and the vertebrae signifies a poor prognosis, with a high rate of recurrence and dissemination.

The prognosis in primary lymphosarcoma (well-differentiated lymphocytic lymphoma) seems to be poor. The few cases in our series died after 1 or 2 years with lymphatic leukemia.

Metastases in other organs occur in about 50% of cases, with a 20% frequency in lymph nodes and less common occurrence in bone and lungs, which is in contrast to the high frequency of their involvement in Ewing sarcoma.

4. Myeloma

Definition, WHO: "*A malignant tumor, usually showing multiple or diffuse bone involvement by neoplastic plasma cells with varying degrees of immaturity, including atypical forms. The lesions are often associated with the presence of abnormal proteins in the blood and urine, and occasionally with the presence of amyloid or para-amyloid in the tumor tissue or other organs.*"

Myeloma, or plasmacytic myelomatosis, and other immunoglobulin-producing monoclonal gammopathies have, in recent decades, been the object of several excellent monographs (Waldenström 1970; Snapper and Kahn 1971) and numerous papers covering clinical, therapeutic, biochemical, and immunologic aspects. However, the pathologic features have been less extensively treated, despite the excellent monograph edited by Azar and Potter (1973) and several other publications.

Since the historic papers of Dalrymple (1846) on "mollities ossium" and of Rustizky (1873) on "multiples Myelom," and Kahler's striking case (1889), the plasmacytic growths have been classified in several categories based on their gross and microscopic appearance.

1. Multiple myeloma (multiple plasma-cell myeloma, myelomatosis or Kahler's disease)
2. Disseminated nonosteolytic myelomatosis (diffuse decalcifying myelomatosis)
3. "Solitary" myeloma
4. Extraskeletal plasmacytoma
5. Plasma-cell leukemia
6. Malignant lymphomas with plasmacytic differentiation

Multiple myeloma is usually associated with IgG, IgA, or light-chain (Bence Jones) monoclonal immunoglobulin production by the tumor cells, and the appropriate M protein or polypeptide is detectable in the serum and/or urine by immunochemical techniques. The anomalous immunoglobulin is occasionally IgD or more rarely IgE. Myeloma with IgM has also been reported, but usually this form of monoclonal immunoglobulin production is associated with a lymphoplasmacytoid disease (Waldenström's disease or primary macroglobulinemia).

Incidence. If the cases diagnosed by hematologists through bone marrow aspiration are included, myeloma is the most common primary malignant bone tumor. In the Mayo Clinic series (Dahlin 1978) about half of the malignant tumors were myelomas. Kyle (1975), also from the Mayo Clinic, found 869 cases in a 12-year period. In our laboratory only material obtained directly by surgical or, more frequently, by needle biopsy of the radiologically visible lesion was studied. Our findings are based on the histologic study together with the cytologic observation of smears.

Myeloma, with 495 cases, accounted for 21% of the malignant tumors in our series. In recent years the number of cases has been increasing due to advances in diagnostic methods, especially biochemical and immunologic studies, including immunoelectrophoresis and immunofluorescence. In a review of multiple myeloma in the United States from 1950 to 1975, Blattner et al. (1981) found an incidence of 2 to 3 myeloma cases per 100000 people, with a higher incidence among black Americans, who also had a mortality twice as high as that of whites (Leech et al. 1983). The incidence rate is high in the Scandinavian countries (Waldenström 1970) but rare in Japan.

Clinical Findings. *Sex and Age.* In most series, as in ours, the tumor occurred predominantly in males: 61% in Kyle's series (1975) and 59% in ours. An exception was Griffiths' series (1966): among 243 cases he found a female predominance. Myeloma generally occurs in patients over 40 years of age (98% in Kyle's series), most frequently between 50 and 70 years; there was a peak in the sixth decade in our material, and myeloma was definitely rare under 30 years of age. Isolated cases have been reported in children (Gordon and Schneider 1940; Schmaus 1950; Porter 1963; Hewell and Alexanian 1976; Lazarus et al. 1980; Bernstein et al. 1985). Jaffe (1958) reported on a case in a 13-year-old child who died at 18 years of age. Maeda et al. (1973) reported a case of IgA monoclonal gammapathy in a 13-year-old child and reviewed ten cases of multiple myeloma previously reported in childhood.

In the cases of "solitary" myeloma, the age of onset seems to be lower; in four of our cases, it was under 40 and in two, under 30 years of age.

Localization. Myeloma involves primarily those bones that in adulthood contain red marrow and is therefore found mainly in vertebrae, ribs, skull, pelvis, and sternum; long bones, scapula, and mandible are also often affected. A single focus was initially found in several cases, but disseminated disease developed within 2 years. Only three cases remained solitary for more than 10 years and may be considered a "solitary" myeloma. They were located in dorsal and lumbar vertebrae (one case each) and in the upper end of the femur (one case).

Symptoms. The most frequent clinical manifestation was bone pain, of varying intensity and duration, generally referred to the thoracic region and spine. A common initial symptom was low back or sciatic pain, sometimes accompanied by neurologic symptoms, usually a consequence of spinal cord or nerve root compression after a pathologic fracture of a vertebral body or penetration of the tumor into the spinal canal. Pathologic fracture of other bones such as ribs or a long bone (femur, humerus) was common. Anemia, sometimes associated with abnormal hemorrhagic tendency, and signs of renal insufficiency were found in more than 50% of our cases. Loss of weight, fever, and general weakness were also frequently found. The presence of a palpable swelling was not uncommon, especially in lesions of the ribs, clavicle, sternum, cranial bones, and more rarely in long bones.

The laboratory findings in disseminated lesions are of utmost importance. Anemia, often severe, a high sedimentation rate, frequently above 100 mm in the first hours, and azotemia reflecting kidney involvement were common features. Hypercalcemia was a frequent finding, the degree being generally but not always related to the extent of bone destruction by the myelomatous tissue; it was found in approximately one-third of our patients and in 30% of Kyle's. In contrast to hyperparathyroidism, the serum alkaline phosphatase was normal except in cases of pathologic fracture, and the serum inorganic phosphate is generally normal or increased when renal complication develops in terminal stages of the disease. Smears of peripheral blood may show "rouleau" formation of red cells and the presence of occasional plasma cells. Cases with a large number of white cells and a high percentage of plasma cells are rare and are referred to as plasma-cell leukemia. The real incidence of this entity is disputed because of the different criteria used to classify it (Kyle et al. 1974). Kyle et al. arbitrarily define plasma-cell leukemia as a condition in which more than 20% of cells present in the peripheral blood are plasma cells, with an absolute plasmacytosis of more than 20000 plasma cells per cubic millimeter in conjunction with marrow plasma cell proliferation. Seventeen of the patients (1.6%) in the Kyle et al. series fulfilled these criteria. In 12 patients, the leukemia appeared before myeloma was diagnosed. Patients with plasma-cell leukemia had a much higher incidence of hepatosplenomegaly than did a group of patients with myeloma without leukemia. Serum protein electrophoresis was performed in 12 patients, and eight had an M component. In all patients, bone marrow examinations were positive for myeloma.

The study of the bone marrow by sternal or iliac marrow puncture is of fundamental diagnostic importance, especially in cases of diffuse lesions, when the radiologic findings are not characteristic. A 5%–10% increase in the number of *typical* plasma cells in itself does not permit the diagnosis of myeloma because this sign may be found in other diseases. Moreover, in some instances with involvement of the marrow by multiple medullary foci, separated by normal marrow, needle aspiration may yield no or only a few myeloma cells. On the other hand, the presence of numerous large cells, with one or more atypical, often bizarre nuclei, is conclusive.

The study of the serum and urinary proteins is of great diagnostic importance. In the majority of patients, the total serum protein is elevated due to an increase in the globulin fraction. Bence Jones proteinuria has been observed by Jaffe in about 40% of patients, and it was identified in

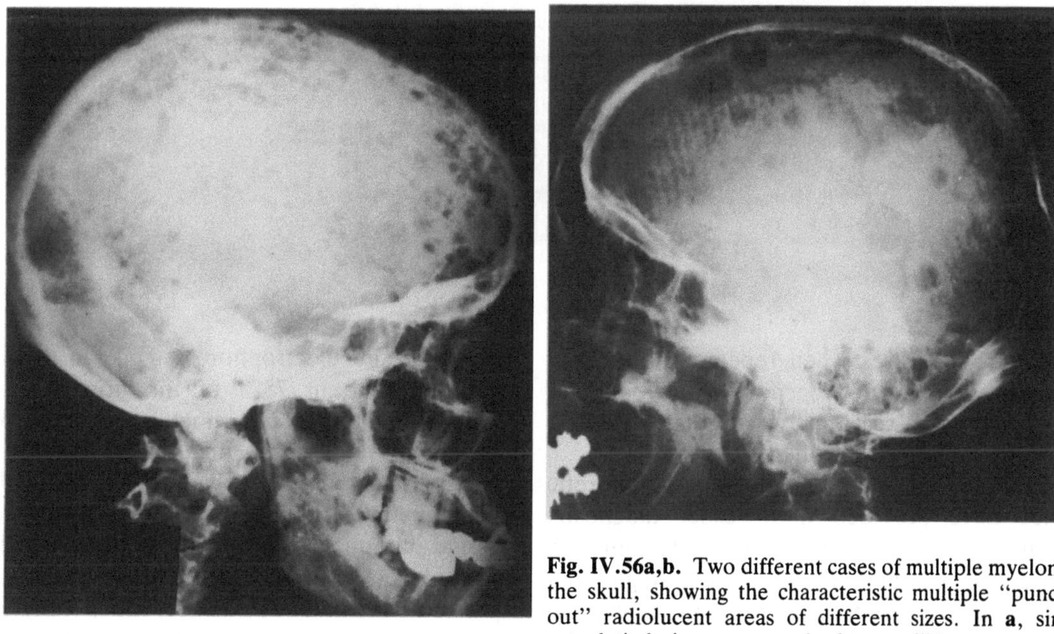

a b

Fig. IV.56a,b. Two different cases of multiple myeloma in the skull, showing the characteristic multiple "punched-out" radiolucent areas of different sizes. In **a**, similar osteolytic lesions are seen in the mandible

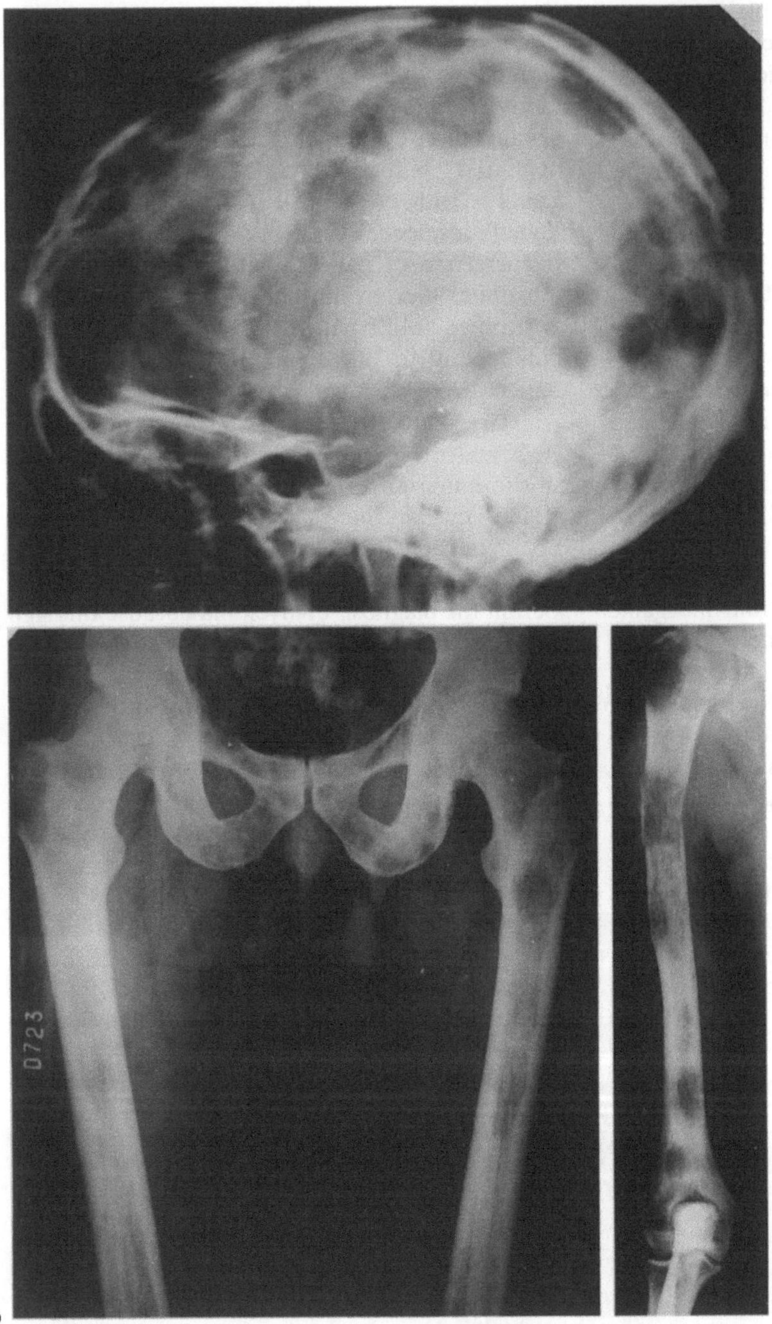

a b c

Fig. IV.57a–c. Multiple myeloma with numerous osteolytic "punched out" areas in **a** skull, **b** both femora, and **c** humerus

49% of Kyle's cases when repeatedly searched for. However, it is not specific for myeloma and may be found occasionally in other diseases, especially metastatic carcinoma.

Electrophoretic and immunoelectrophoretic studies have provided more exact diagnostic information and a more exact determination of the various globulin and immunoglobulin fractions and their possible prognostic implications. In a review of 869 cases, Kyle found upon serum protein electrophoresis a pike in 76% and a globulin pike in 75% of the urinary electrophoretic patterns. Immunoelectrophoresis of the serum showed a monoclonal heavy chain in 83% and a monoclonal light chain in 8% (Bence Jones proteinemia). Three cases failed to reveal monoclonal immunoglobulin in the serum or a Bence Jones protein in the urine; these cases are at present classified as "*nonsecretory*" myeloma; several observations of this type have been

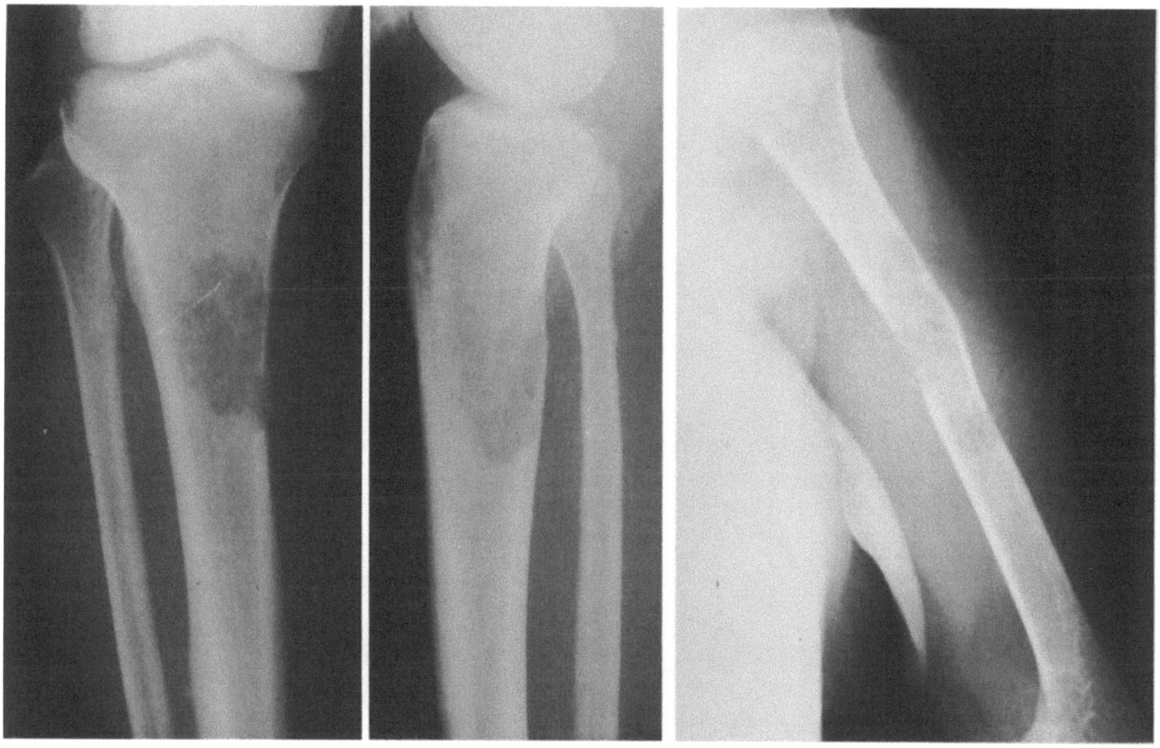

a b

Fig. IV.58a,b. Female, 70 years old. Multiple myeloma. **a** Anteroposterior and lateral radiographs show osteolytic lesion with permeative margins in the upper tibia. **b** Ill-defined permeative lesion of the humeral shaft with pathologic fracture. (Courtesy of Dr. J.P. Petasnick, Rush-Presbyterian-St. Luke's Medical Center)

reported (Azar et al. 1972). The incidence of such cases is reported to be 1%–2% of all myeloma patients.

Radiographic Features. The radiographic appearance is variable and depends on the clinical type. In the most common classic multiple myeloma, numerous round or oval osteolytic lesions with a characteristic punched-out aspect are seen (Figs. IV.56, IV.57, cf. Fig. IV.58; Fig. IV.59 illustrates simulation of multiple myeloma by metastases to the skull). The initially small radiolucent foci, which are clearly delimited without sclerotic margins, increase in size and may coalesce until much of the affected bone and/or the overlying cortex is destroyed (Fig. IV.60). Periosteal reaction or sclerosis of the margin of the lesion is infrequent, but it may be found after chemo- or radiotherapy. In some lesions, especially those located in a rib, in the sternum, or sometimes in a long bone, the tumor may expand the thinned cortex (Fig. IV.61). This ballooned appearance is more common in the slowly growing solitary or initially solitary lesion (Fig. IV.62). Linear residual bone trabeculae often produce a trabeculated or soap-bubble appearance (Figs. IV.61, IV.62) (Schajowicz et al. 1972).

Diffuse myelomatosis, which is characterized by extensive plasma-cell infiltration of bone marrow without formation of distinct tumor nodules and localized bone destruction, has the radiographic aspect of generalized bone rarefaction (osteoporosis). This pattern has been described by French authors (Lièvre 1955; Weissenbach and Lievre 1958) as "myelomatose diffuse decalcificante" (Fig. IV.63).

Pathologic fracture, especially of the vertebrae and ribs with collapse of the vertebral bodies, and also of long bones, is common in both types of myeloma (i.e., multiple myeloma and diffuse myelomatosis) (Figs. IV.64, IV.65).

Rarely, the bone lesions show evident *bone sclerosis* with the appearance of osteoblastic metastasis, showing a nodular or diffuse pattern, and they may be limited to one region of the skeleton. A small number of such sclerotic cases have been reported in the literature (Engels et al. 1960; Lowbeer 1969; Clarisse and Staple 1971; Waldenström 1970) and almost all monographs

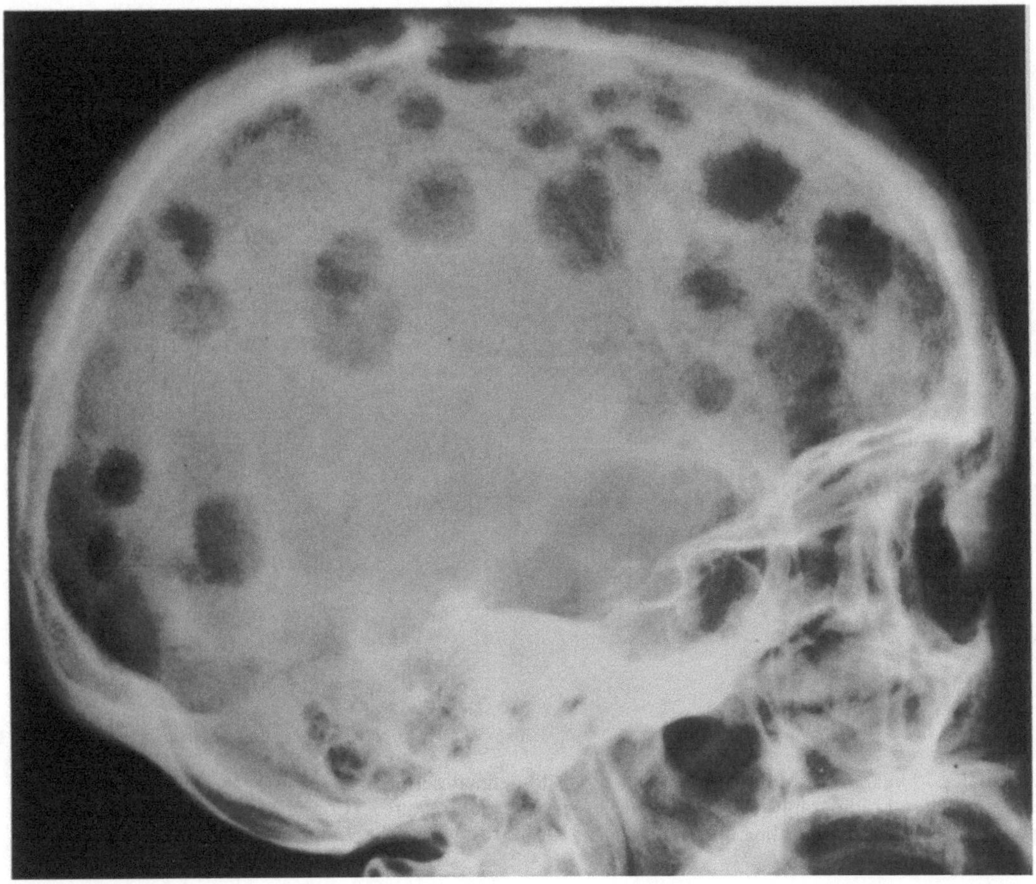

Fig. IV.59. Female, 45 years old. Metastases of breast carcinoma in skull. Radiograph shows multiple large osteolytic lesions similar to those observed in multiple myeloma. (Courtesy of J.P. Petasnick, Rush-Presbyterian-St. Luke's Medical Center)

illustrate single cases (Edeiken and Hodes 1977; Spjut et al. 1971; Lichtenstein 1977; Resnick and Niwayama 1988). The writer has observed two such cases and published one of them, which was associated with progressive polyneuropathy (Gravano et al. 1970) (Fig. IV.66). The incidence of polyneuropathy in sclerotic myeloma is about 30%–50%; Morley and Schweiger (1967), for example, found this association in 13 patients among a total of 33 examples of sclerotic myeloma recorded in the literature. Patients with sclerotic myeloma are on average younger than those with conventional myeloma. The clinical and laboratory findings that often characterize this syndrome, i.e., polyneuropathy, organomegaly, endocrinopathy, M protein, and skin changes (Bardwick et al. 1980; Takatsuki and Sanada 1983), have given rise to the acronymic designation "POEMS syndrome."

Pathologic Findings. The *gross* pattern of the skeletal lesions varies widely according to the different clinicoradiologic types (Figs. IV.67–IV.69). In the classic multiple myeloma, the red marrow, preferentially of short and flat bones, is replaced by small nodules, generally not larger than 1 cm, with intervening normal bone marrow. They often coalesce, forming large nodules that may occasionally occupy a major portion of a short bone (vertebra or rib), destroying the cancellous bone and part of the cortex, with penetration into the neighboring soft tissues (Figs. IV.70, IV.71). The tumor nodules are grayish-pink and of soft consistency. The often considerable bone destruction causes frequent fractures and collapse of vertebral bodies, leading to compression of spinal cord nerve roots or spinal nerves. Exceptionally, the plasma-cell nodules are accompanied by local deposits of a grayish-white tissue of firmer consistency, corresponding to amyloid.

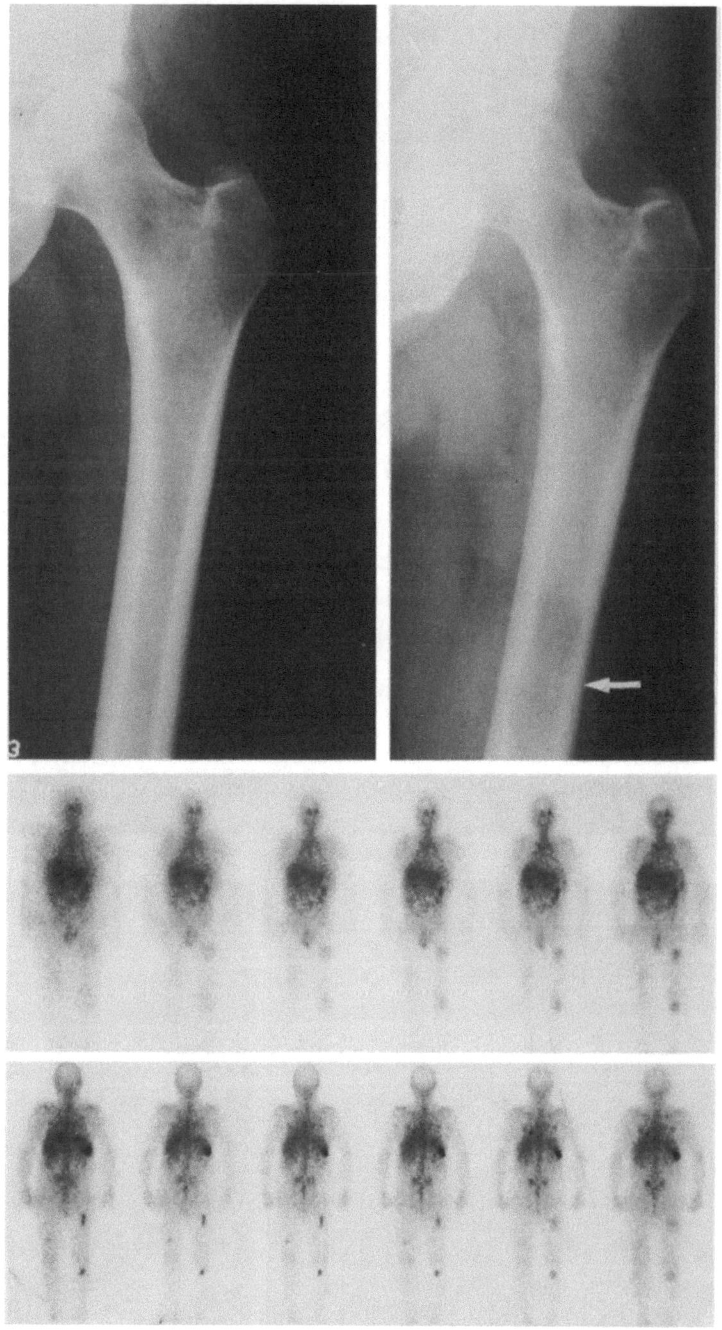

a b c

Fig. IV.60a–c. Male, 60 years old. Multiple myeloma. **a** Initial radiograph of femur (June 1977) shows no radiologic changes. However, the bone scan (**b**) with ^{99m}Tc-EHDP demonstrates uptake in the upper femur, tibia, and rib. **c** Radiograph taken in September 1977 revealed the osteolytic lesion in the femoral shaft. (Courtesy of Dr. W. Fordham, Rush-Presbyterian-St. Luke's Medical Center)

The process of intense bone destruction in multiple myeloma is the cause of the relatively conspicuous hypercalcemia with ensuing metastatic calcium deposits, especially in lungs and kidneys. Increased bone resorption results from the production of osteoclast-activating factor (OAF) by the neoplastic cells. The activation of osteoclasts by OAF can be blocked by prednisone (Mundy et al. 1974).

In the diffuse type of myelomatosis, the bone marrow is replaced entirely or in great part by a grayish-pink tissue, often hemorrhagic, which infiltrates diffusely the cancellous bone, accompanied by small tumor nodules, without producing evident bone destruction (Fig. IV.63). The radiographic expression of this pattern comprises diffuse, often generalized bone rarefaction (osteoporosis).

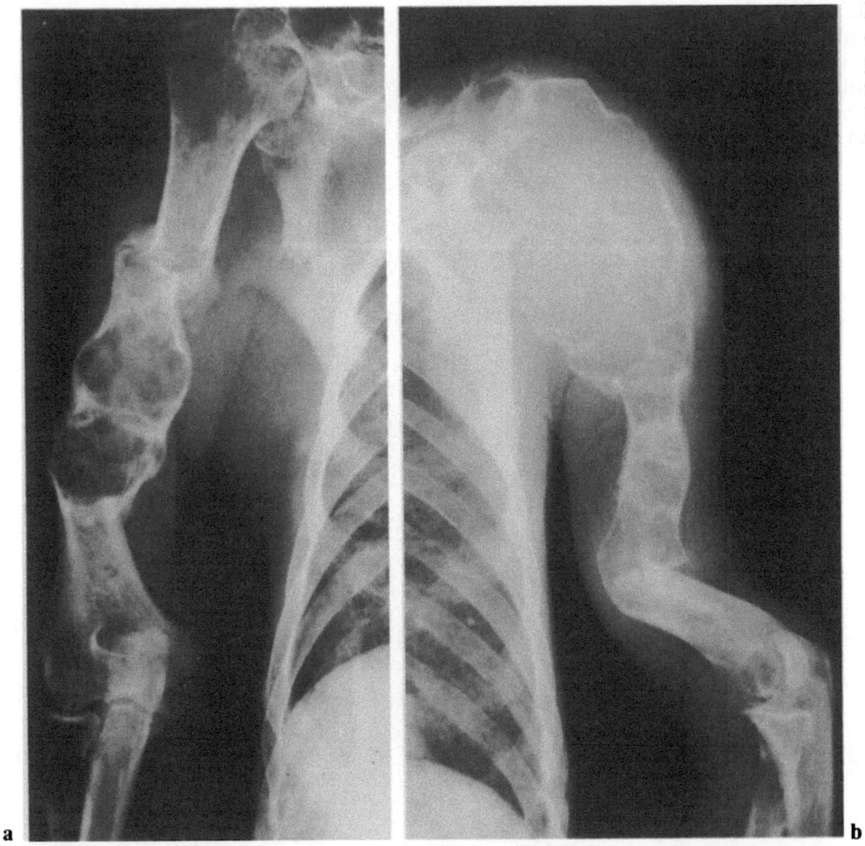

Fig. IV.61a,b. Male, 60 years old. Multiple myeloma. Radiographs showing widely disseminated large, expanding osteolytic lesions with pathologic fractures

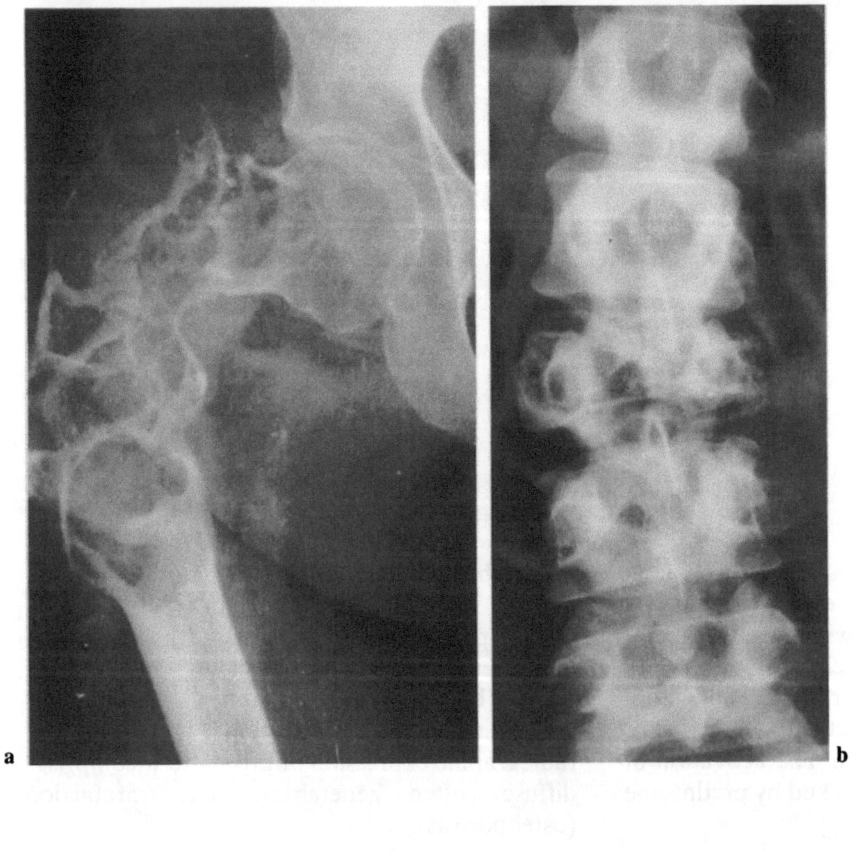

Fig. IV.62a,b. Female, 44 years old. Myeloma of the upper femur. **a** Radiograph at time of presentation shows an osteolytic, expanding, and trabeculated lesion suggestive of giant-cell tumor. **b** Two years later multiple lesions are seen in the spine; lesions subsequently appeared in the skull. (Schajowicz et al. 1972)

Fig. IV.63. Photograph and radiograph of a longitudinal, 5-mm-thick section of the spine showing predominantly diffuse infiltration of the cancellous bone with only scattered small areas of bone destruction. (Courtesy of Dr. Donato De Prospero, São Paulo, Brasil)

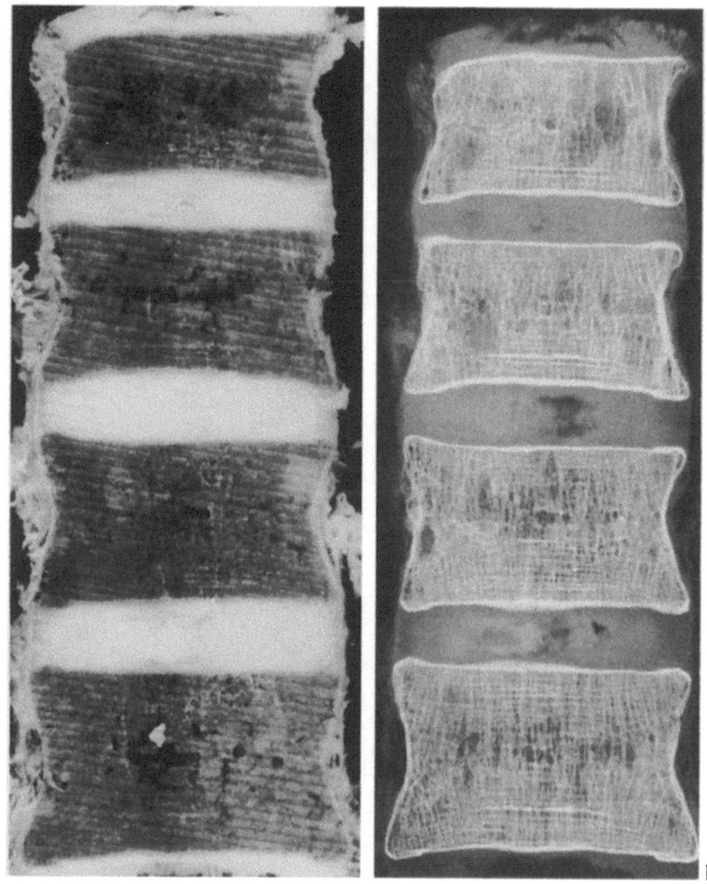

a b

Fig. IV.64a,b. Two cases of "solitary" myeloma of humerus (**a**) and fourth lumbar vertebra (**b**) in patients 47 years and 50 years old, respectively. Radiographs show purely osteolytic lesions. The humerus lesion was resected en bloc and the vertebral lesion was irradiated. Both patients were well and without dissemination after 6 years

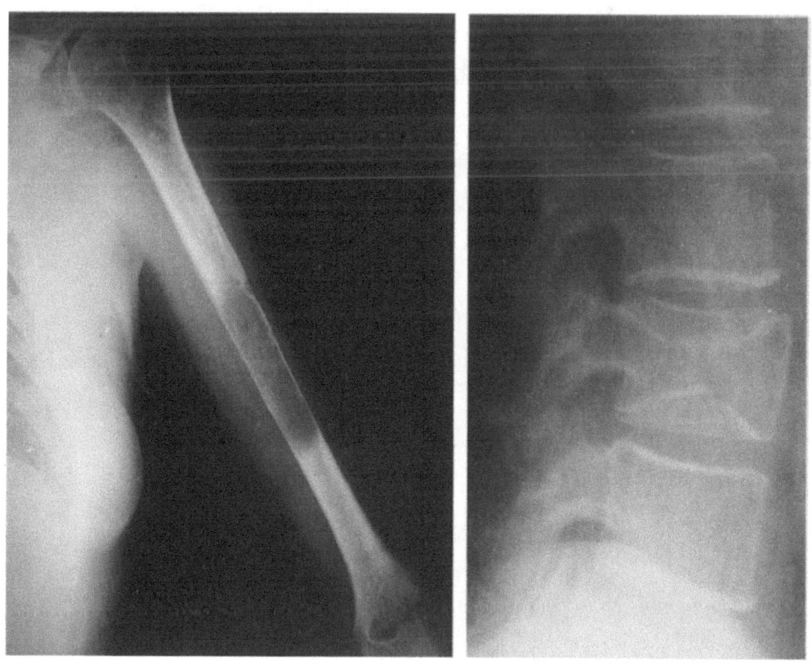

a b

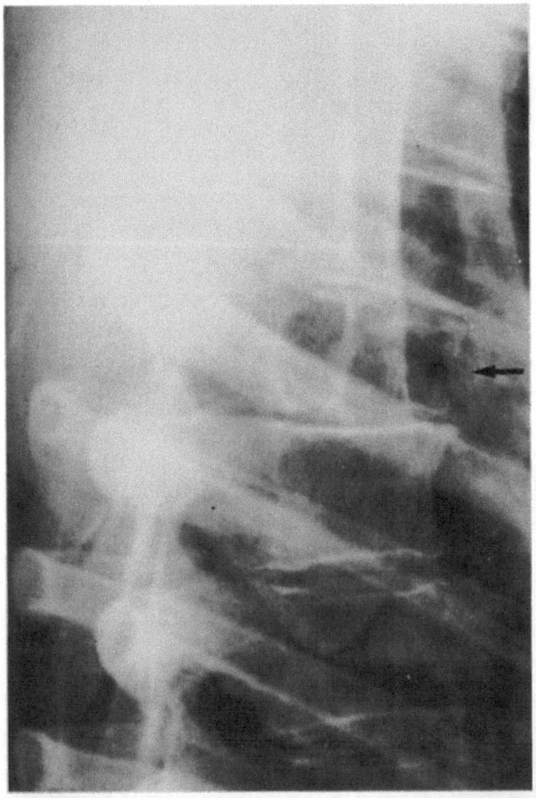

a

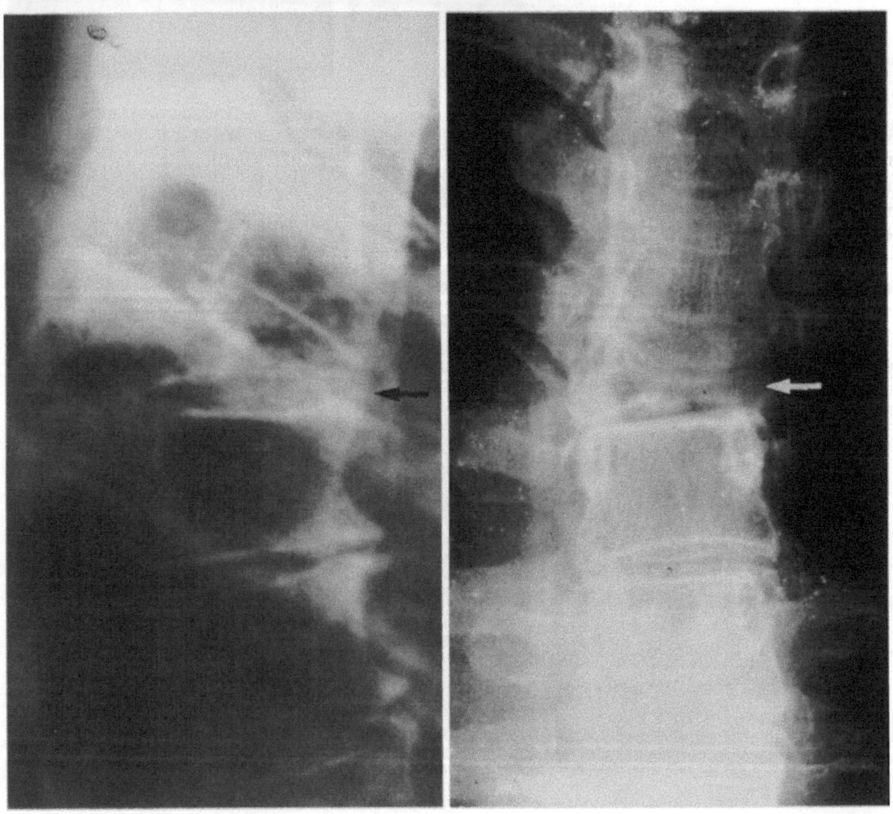

b

Fig. IV.65a,b. Male, 24 years old. "Solitary" myeloma of dorsal vertebra. **a** Radiograph of the initial osteolytic lesion of the vertebral body (*arrow*). A decompression due to neurologic syndrome was performed. The histologic study revealed a well-differentiated myeloma. The lesion was irradiated. **b** The lateral and anteroposterior radiographs 15 years later show the collapsed vertebral body. The patient was well and without symptoms 23 years after onset

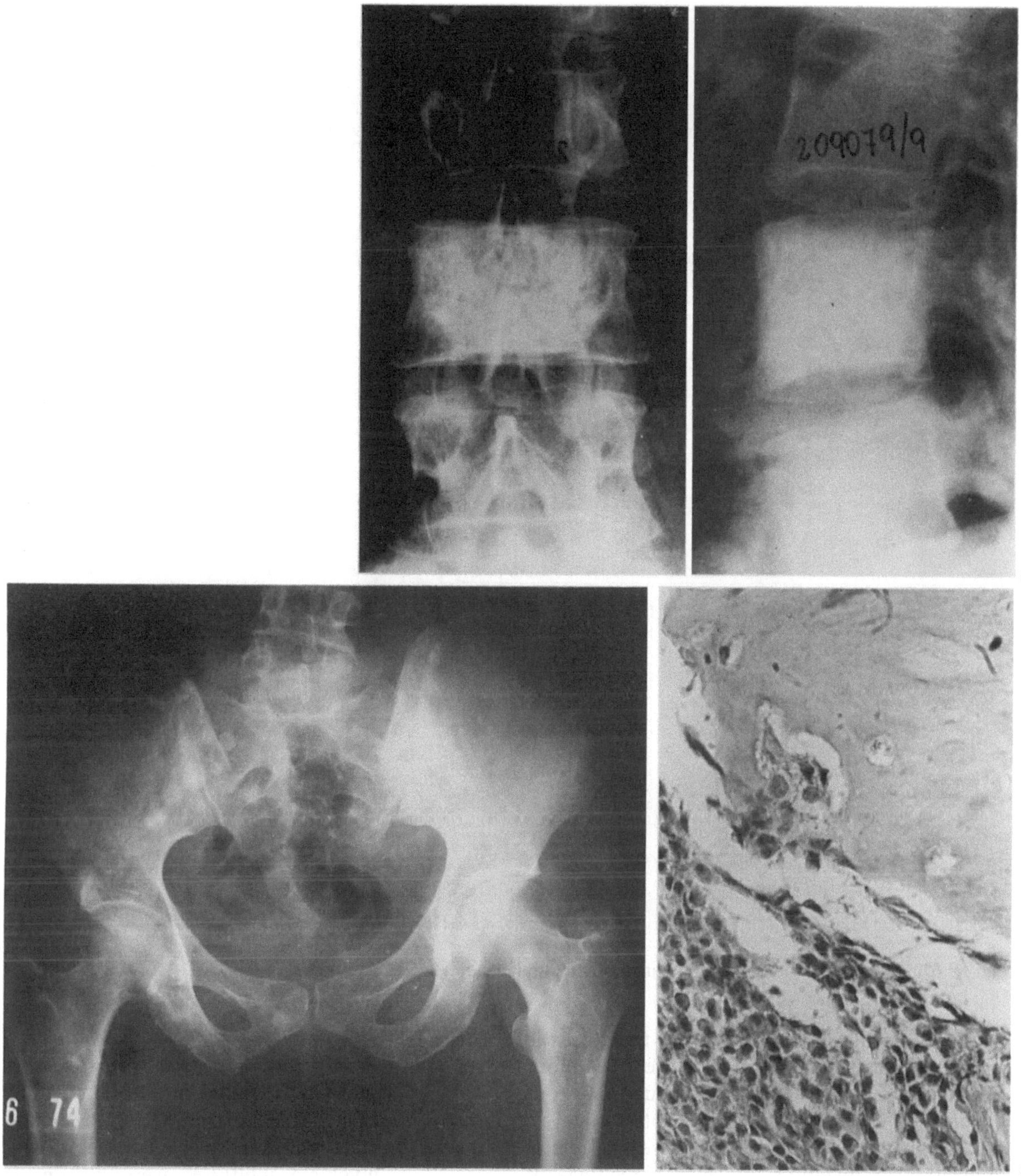

a b c

Fig. IV.66a–c. Female 56 years of age. Sclerotic type of multiple myeloma. **a** Anteroposterior and lateral radiographs of third lumbar vertebra show diffuse sclerosis of vertebral body with the appearance of an osteoblastic metastasis. **b** Nodular foci of sclerosis are seen in the ilium and sacrum. **c** Photomicrograph demonstrates the histologic pattern of a well-differentiated myeloma. At the *right upper corner* an enlarged laminar bone trabecula is seen. **c** ×250

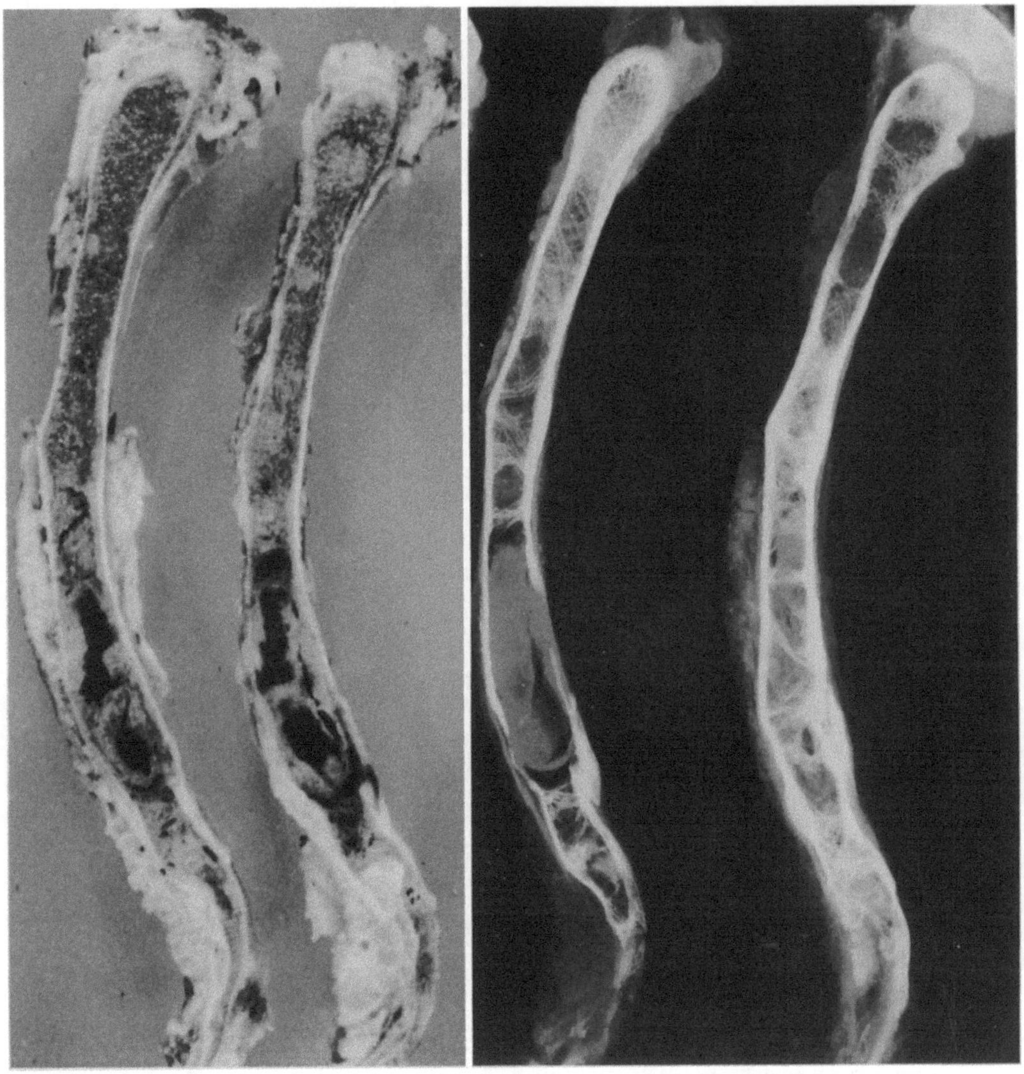

Fig. IV.67. Photograph and radiograph illustrating multiple osteolytic lesions of rib

In the localized (solitary) form, the cortex is sometimes destroyed over a wide area, but more frequently it is thinned and expanded, without penetration of the tumor into the soft tissue.

Autopsy studies have shown extraskeletal infiltration by myeloma in a high percentage of cases. Pasmantier and Azar (1969) analyzed 57 consecutive autopsies during a 15-year period. Depending on the presence or absence of grossly identifiable tumor outside the skeleton, they divided myeloma into three stages:

Stage I. *Intraskeletal*:
Grossly confined to the skeleton

Stage II. *Paraskeletal*:
Confined to the skeleton and by direct extension to immediate paraskeletal areas, as in paracostal, epidural, and subdural extensions

Stage III. *Extraskeletal*:
Presumably metastatic spread to sites such as regional or distant lymph nodes, spleen, liver, kidney, adrenals, etc.; extraskeletal gross or microscopic myeloma infiltrates were present in 65% of Pasmantier and Azar's series

According to Pasmantier and Azar, it was apparent that the vast majority of stage I myelomas are associated with well-differentiated or moderately differentiated histologic grade, whereas poorly differentiated growths are more prevalent in stage III myeloma.

Histologically, the tumor nodules are formed by a compact mass of round cells, of relatively uniform size, with no or scarce intercellular connective vascular stroma (Fig. IV.72). The fat

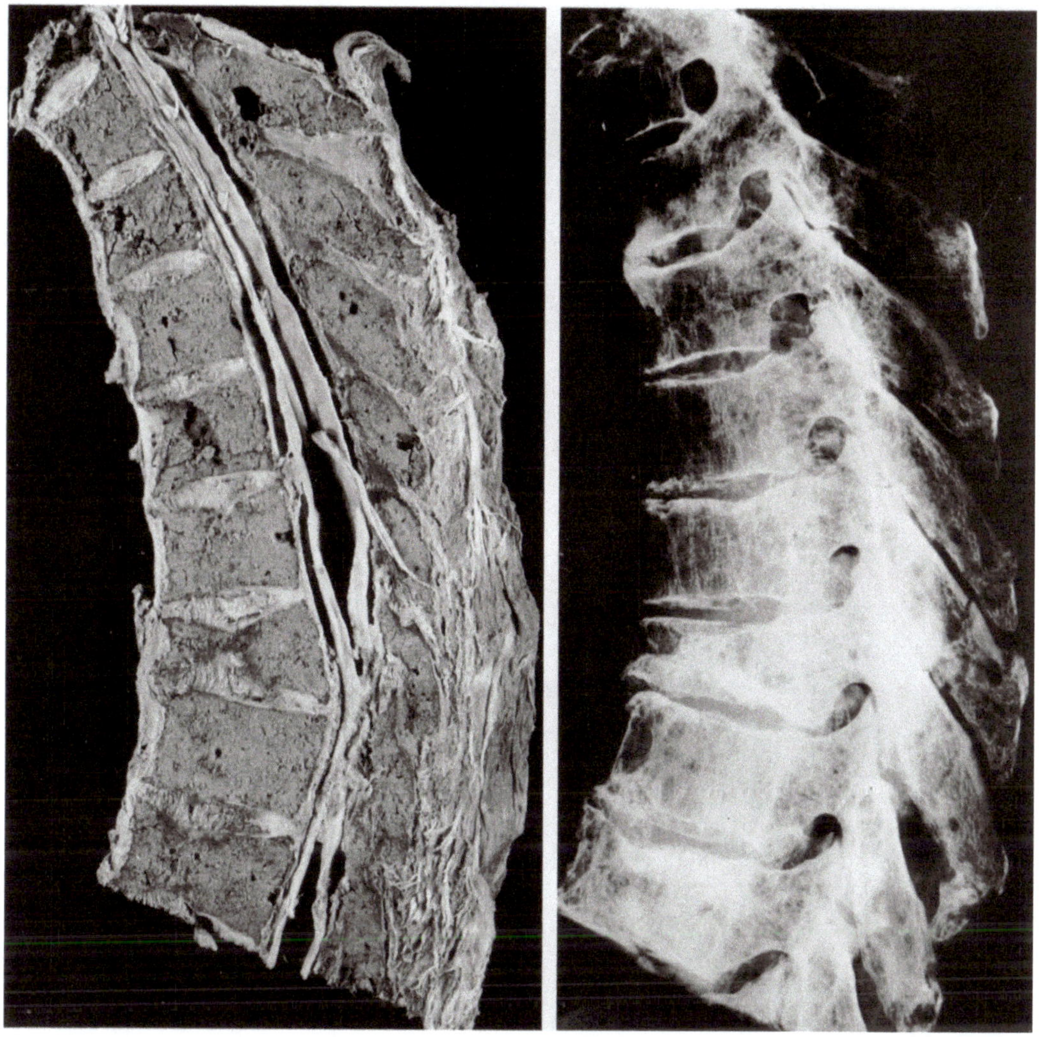

Fig. IV.68. Photograph and radiograph of the dorsal spine showing diffuse infiltration and disseminated osteolytic areas of vertebral bodies and spinal processes

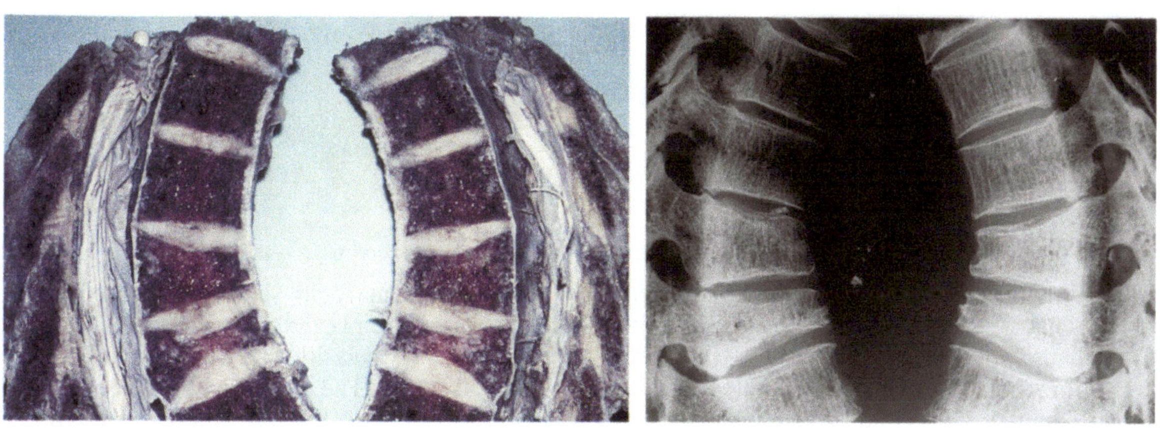

a b

Fig. IV.69a,b. Multiple myeloma. Photograph and radiograph of sagittal section autopsy specimen, showing compression fracture of two lumbar vertebrae

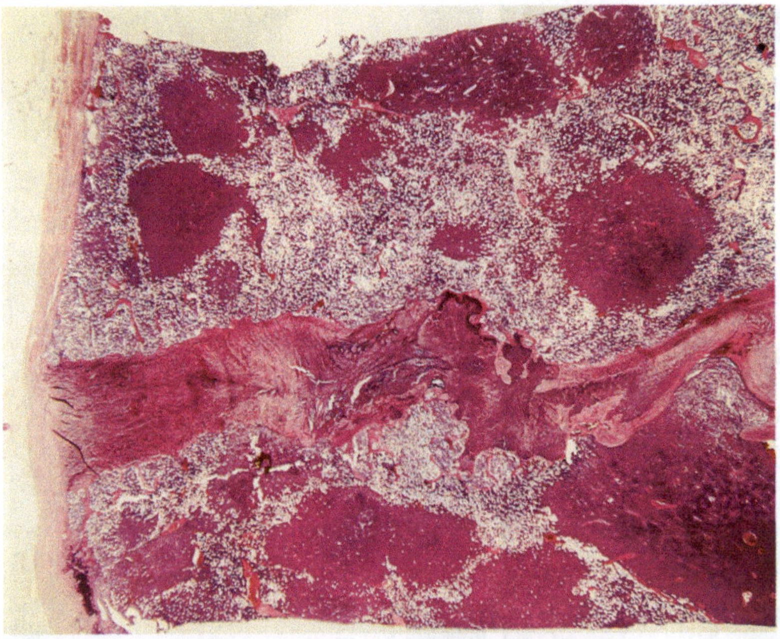

Fig. IV.70. Topographic photomicrograph illustrating multiple, in part confluent tumor nodules in the spongiosa of two adjacent vertebral bodies. ×8

Fig. IV.71a–c. Topographic photomicrographs illustrate large osteolytic lesions in the skull (**a**) and in the ribs (**b**,**c**). ×8
▼

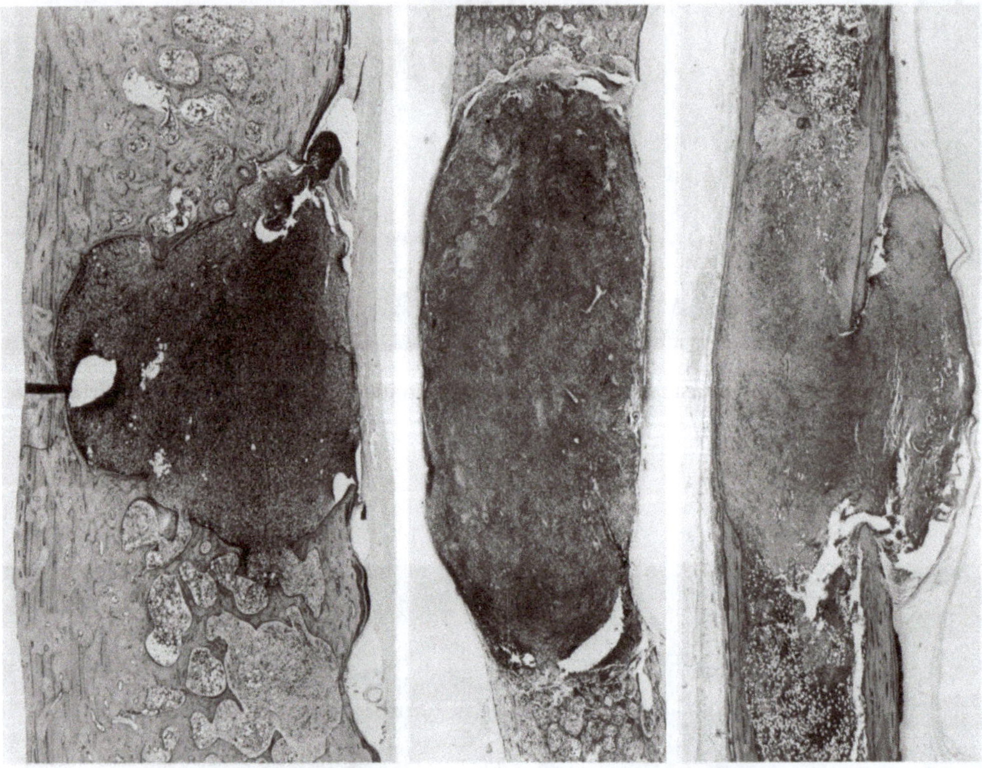

a **b, c**

cells normally present in the red marrow disappear almost completely due to the infiltrative and expansive growth of the tumor. The tumor cells form strands and lobules, separated by thin-walled capillary vessels and reticulin fibers that are abundant in the poorly differentiated tumors and scarce in the well-differentiated lesions.

The myeloma cells show a striking resemblance to mature plasma cells or their immediate precursors, a similarity that was emphasized in 1900 by Wright. The reactive plasma cells were first described by Ramón y Cajal (1906) as "céllulas cianófilas" due to their deep cytoplasmic basophilia. Marschalkó gave the first detailed

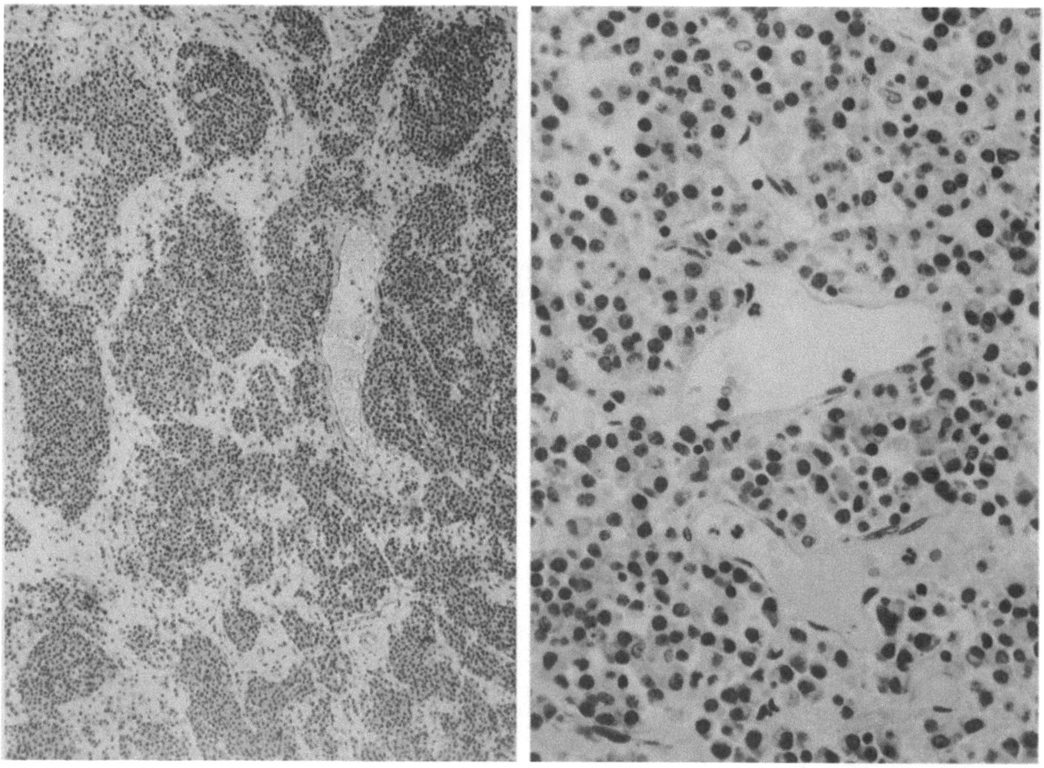

a b

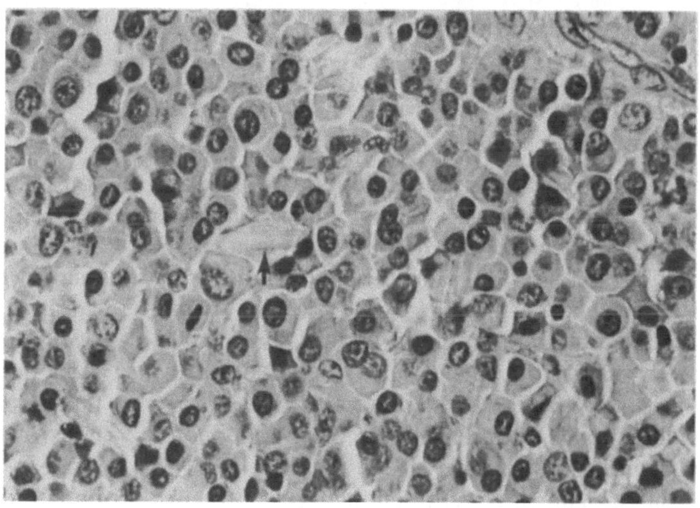

c

Fig. IV.72a–c. Photomicrographs of the histologic pattern of a well-differentiated myeloma. The tumor cells are mostly of uniform size showing distinct cytoplasmic outlines and only a few double nuclei resembling plasma cells. However, the nuclei are generally larger, the chromatin is irregularly dispersed, and the juxtanuclear halo is generally lacking. The tumor lobules are separated by capillary vessels. In **c** some crystals are seen (*arrow*). **a** ×60, **b** ×200, **c** ×600

description of the morphologic characteristics, emphasizing the distinctive features of the nucleus – its typical "cartwheel" pattern, its eccentric position, and the presence of a light-staining juxtanuclear area, which later came to be known as the Golgi apparatus.

Histochemically, the cytoplasm of plasma cells is rich in ribonucleoprotein, which is responsible for its intense basophilia and, particularly, for its pyroninophilia, which is regarded as an index of RNA contents of the cytoplasm and of the necleolus. The cytoplasm shows a variable degree of PAS staining that appears to reflect the presence or lack of stored immunoglobulin, particularly IgA. Lipoids are usually absent, as are alkaline phosphatase and NSE activity. Several morphologic variants of plasma cells appear to be related to the mode of secretion and antibody production, including Russell bodies, Mott cells, and "flaming" cells of Undritz. A more detailed description of these elements may be found in Azar and Potter's monograph (1973).

Malignant lymphomas with M component and plasmacytic differentiation may be observed,

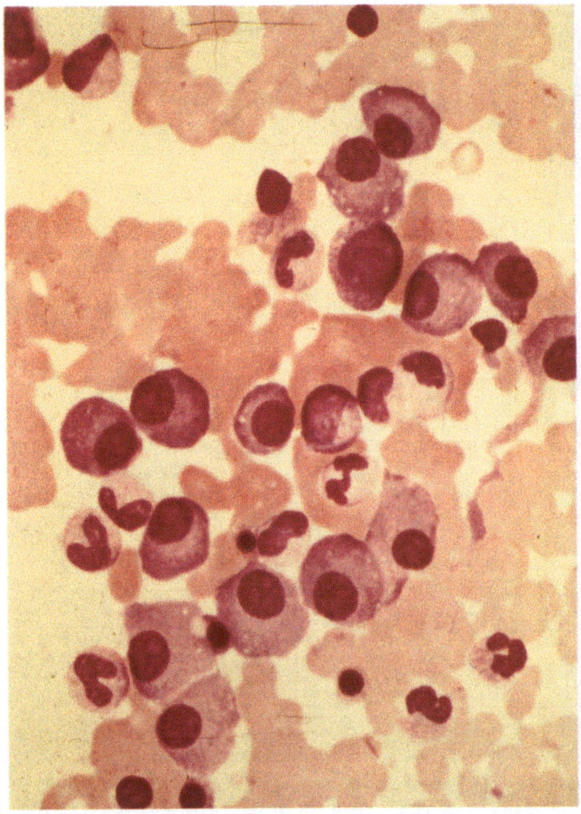
a

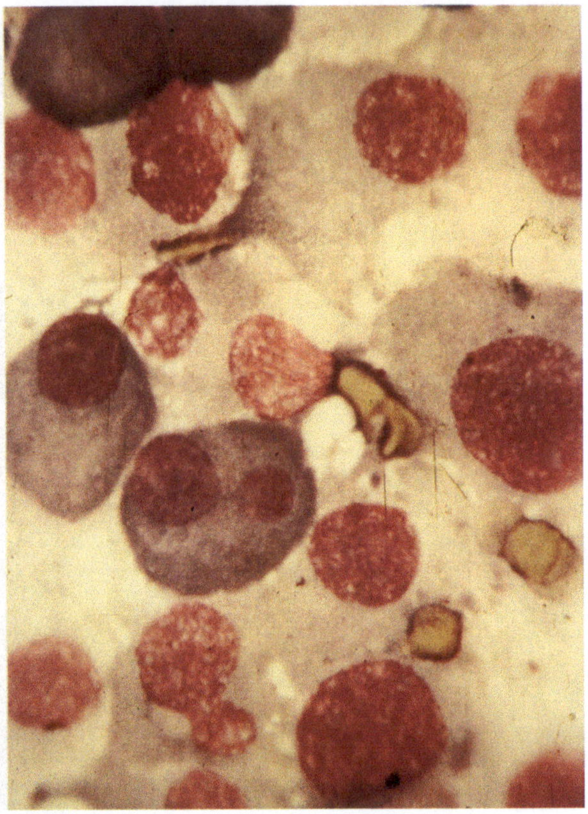
b

Fig. IV.73a,b. Multiple myeloma. Photomicrographs of smears from needle biopsy stained with May-Grünwald-Giemsa show plasma cells in different stages of evolution. **a** ×500, **b** ×800

one of the most common types of this association being Waldenström's macroglobulinemia. This syndrome is characterized by a striking increase in monoclonal IgM, accompanied by a number of hemorrhagic, hemolytic, and viscosity disturbances. The proliferating cells, usually found in the bone marrow, spleen, and lymph nodes, have the same features as plasma cells. The macroglobulin may be evident in the cytoplasm and/or nuclei of some of these cells in the form of PAS-positive globules representing glycoproteins. Occasionally, the histologic picture is pleomorphic. Some patients develop reticulosarcomas that are probably lymphoid tumors with pyroninophilic cytoplasm representing in vivo "immunoblastic" transformation of their original small lymphoid or lymphoplasmacytoid cells.

Although there may be variability in the tumor cells (myeloma cells), the general structure is uniform, showing different grades of cellular differentiation, with one or the other grade predominating in a particular tumor.

A well-differentiated type showing an evident resemblance to reactive plasma cells (Figs. IV.71, IV.73) and a poorly differentiated myeloma, with considerable pleomorphism and relatively large atypical, multinucleated cells, are described by all authors and have been related to the prognosis of the process (Figs. IV.74c, IV.75a).

It is sometimes difficult to assign the tumor to one of these two grades; an intermediate or moderately differentiated type was introduced that approaches the morphologic appearance of non-Hodgkin lymphoma. Under the light microscope, several features permit one to differentiate myeloma cells from reactive plasma cells: myeloma cells are often slightly larger; the nuclear chromatin is more abundant and dispersed, so that there is no "cartwheel" pattern; and the perinuclear halo (Golgi complex) is less evident in conventional histologic sections. This last feature, however, is clearly seen under the electron microscope; the same is true for Russell bodies, which are rarely seen under the light microscope.

Among the cells closely resembling plasmacytes, a variable number of tumor cells are seen showing large nuclei of irregular shape with scarce chromatin and prominent nucleoli, i.e., with the features of lymphoid cells or histiocytes (Fig. IV.74c). These elements may be numerous

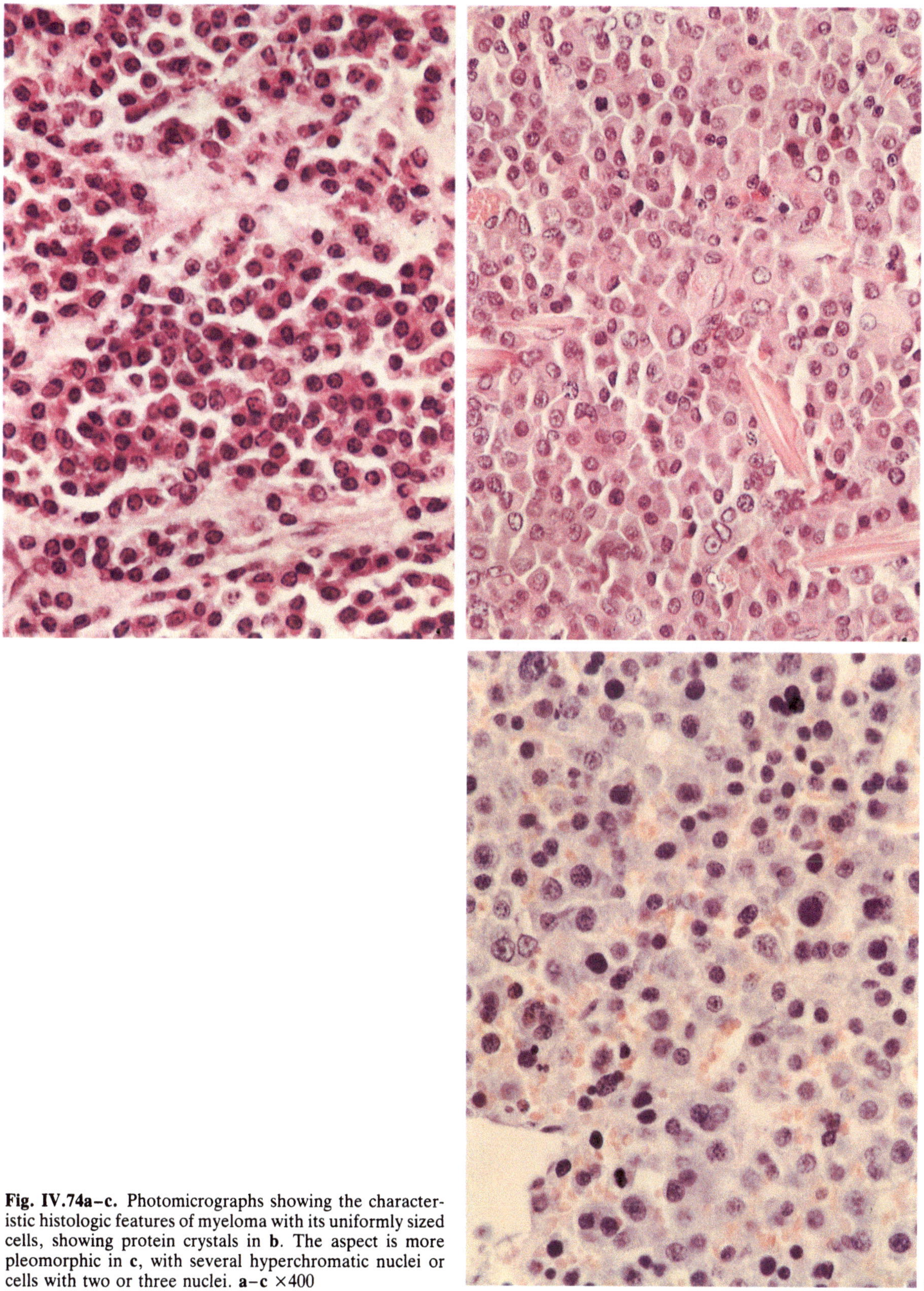

a b c

Fig. IV.74a–c. Photomicrographs showing the characteristic histologic features of myeloma with its uniformly sized cells, showing protein crystals in **b**. The aspect is more pleomorphic in **c**, with several hyperchromatic nuclei or cells with two or three nuclei. **a–c** ×400

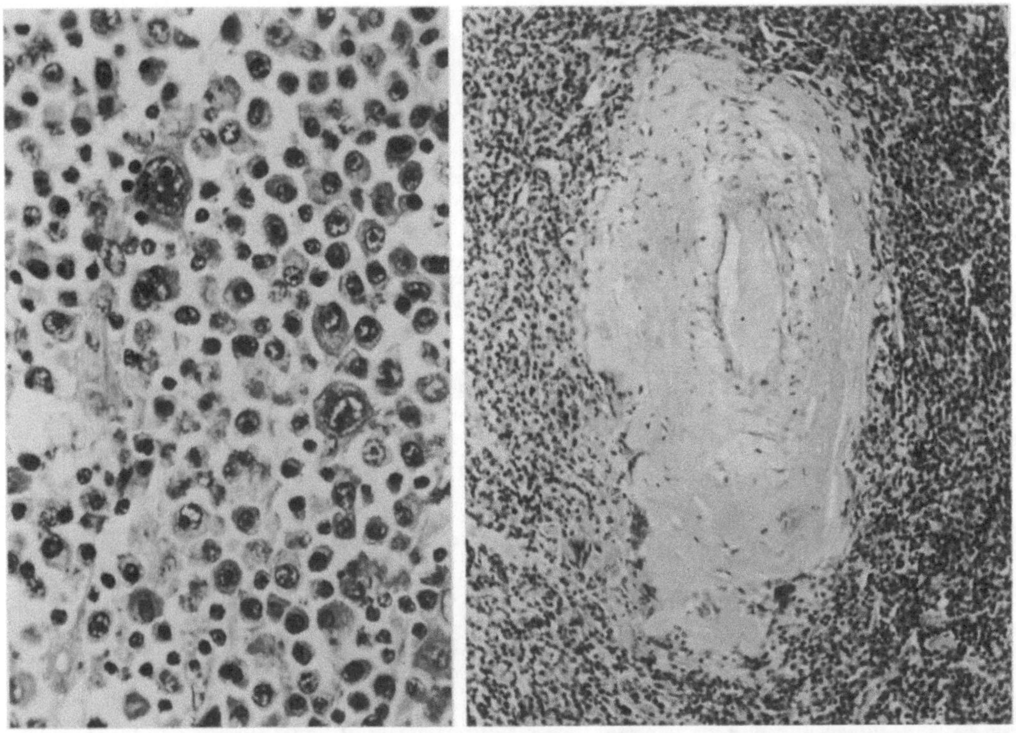

a b

Fig. IV.75. **a** Photomicrograph of the pleomorphic histologic pattern of a poorly differentiated anaplastic myeloma, revealing the presence of numerous cells with two or three hyperchromatic or large bizarre nuclei. **b** Perivascular deposit of amyloid is seen. **a** ×400, **b** ×100

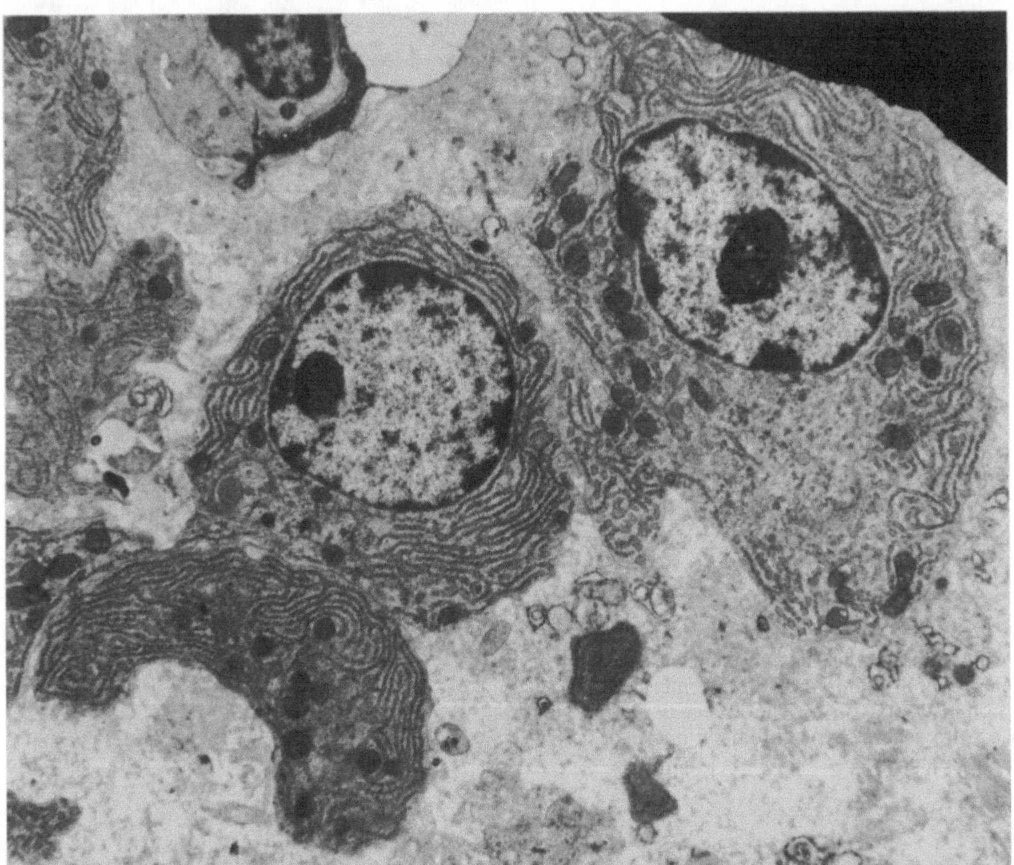

in some areas, causing problems in the differential diagnosis with lymphoma. In fact, for many years, an origin of the myeloma cells from immature reticulum cells was advocated. However, a number of experimental observations, especially in vitro, have demonstrated an origin in small lymphocytes, which are regarded as embryonal cells capable of different lines of differentiation, including plasmacytic.

Electron Microscopy. The ultrastructure of reactive plasmacytes and myeloma cells has been investigated extensively in recent decades (Maldonado et al. 1966), starting with the studies of Braunsteiner et al. (1953). In general, the fine structure of the myeloma cell is so similar to that observed in the parent reactive plasma or preplasma cell that it is often difficult to distinguish between the two.

Without going into detail, we shall mention some of the most characteristic features, which may be helpful in establishing a firm diagnosis of myeloma. The most typical feature is the presence of an abundant rough or granular endoplasmic reticulum closely folded in a lamellar fashion, involving a vast proportion of the cytoplasm but not the Golgi complex, which is well developed in most myeloma cells, suggesting a high degree of activity in protein storage and secretion (Fig. IV.76). It is well known that other specialized protein-synthesizing cells, especially osteoblasts, show identical structures. In addition to the most common lamellar pattern, the endoplasmic reticulum may present different features, preferentially different grades of a variable number of dilated cisternae, probably related to protein storage or to prolonged chemotherapy (Maldonado et al. 1966).

In addition, a great variety of cytoplasmic inclusions (dense bodies, Russell bodies, lysosomal granules, or crystals) may be found in myeloma cells. Crystalloid structures of different shapes are occasionally found in ordinary histologic sections and probably correspond to protein crystals (Fig. IV.74). Cytoplasmic crystalline inclusions are frequently found in the rare IgD myeloma (Ford et al. 1980; Jennette et al. 1981).

◄

Fig. IV.76. Electron micrograph shows the lamellated endoplasmic reticulum characteristic of myeloma cells. (Courtesy of Dr. H. Battifora, Northwestern University, Chicago) ×18500

Myeloma and Amyloidosis

The association of amyloidosis, i.e., the extracellular deposit of a protein-carbohydrate, partly fibrillar, with certain distinctive histochemical and optical properties, and multiple myeloma has been known since the last century. The distribution and staining reactions of amyloid deposits often resemble those of primary amyloidosis, except when the deposits occur in muscles and around joints in myeloma, resulting in arthritic manifestations (Kavanaugh 1978). No other neoplasm appears to have the same disposition toward amyloidosis that myeloma has; this alteration occurs in 10%–25% of cases (Bayrd and Bennett 1950; Kyle and Bayrd 1961; Lowell 1967). In the autopsy material of Pasmantier and Azar (1969), 15% had generalized amyloidosis with deposits in kidneys (6), spleen (3), adrenal gland (5), and liver (2), in contrast to the general opinion that it is more common in other organs (heart and alimentary tract, muscular tissue, peripheral nerves) and rare in parenchymatous organs. There is occasionally a localized deposition in the form of "amyloidomas" that originated at the site of skeletal or extraskeletal individual myeloma nodules.

Histologically, amyloid deposits are (a) characterized by small, often confluent nodules or perivascular deposits of homogeneous structure, (b) eosinophilic, and (c) often surrounded by foreign-body giant cells; Congo red and metachromatic staining may be negative, but special fluorescence techniques and polarization microscopy are usually conclusive (Azar and Potter 1973) (Fig. IV.75b).

In addition to generalized involvement of small vessels, granular or lumpy aggregates of amyloid may be found in intimate relation to myeloma cells (Dahlin and Dockerty 1950).

"Solitary" (Localized) Myeloma

The precise definition of "solitary" myeloma, a relatively uncommon lesion, has been a source of dispute. The long evolution and unpredictable behavior of this tumor is at present generally accepted, in contrast to the sometimes relatively short and invariably fatal course of multiple myeloma. The single focus, located more commonly in a long bone or in a vertebral body (Fig. IV.77; see also Figs. IV.64, IV.65), may remain

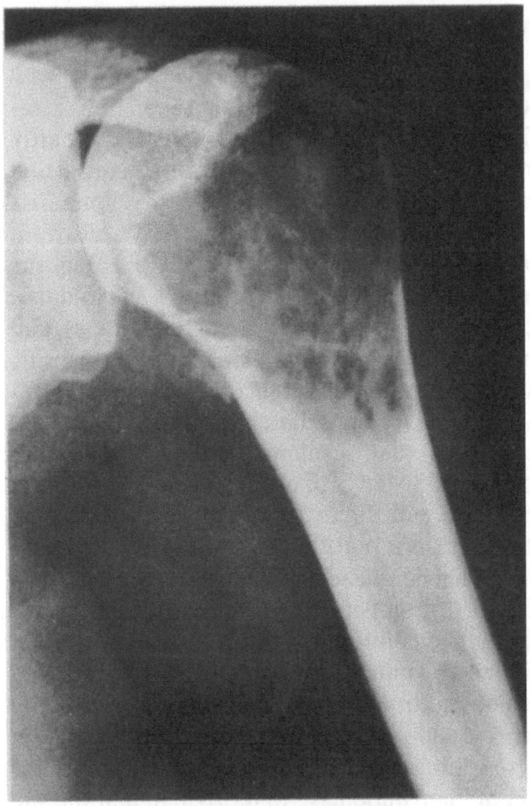

Fig. IV.77. Female, 40 years old. "Solitary" myeloma of humerus. Radiograph shows a large osteolytic lesion with ill-defined margins in the upper end of the humerus. The patient is well and without dissemination 9 years after segmental resection

localized for several years, and finally may disseminate (Gootnick 1945; McLauchlan 1973; Meyer and Schulz 1974; Bataille and Sany 1981; Bacci et al. 1982).

The prognosis is much better than that of multiple myeloma. There are exceptional cases that are free of disease after more than 10 years, because of proper treatment by excision and/or radiotherapy. The criteria for accepting a case as "solitary" are the absence of other radiologically proven lesions, negative sternal marrow biopsy, and the lack of dysproteinemia and urine protein alterations (Bichel and Kirketerp 1938). However, the necessary period of observation is still disputed; some authors accept an interval of 3 years (Christopherson and Miller 1950; Lichtenstein 1977) and others one of 5 years. Valderrama and Bullough (1968), in a review of 47 patients with myeloma of the spine, found apparently solitary lesions in 14. Five of the patients were alive and well without signs of dissemination 4–14 years later, with an average survival period of 10 years (Fig. IV.62). However, in five cases, dissemination occurred 2–14 years after the clinical diagnosis. Our experience is similar. We observed several patients in whom dissemination occurred after 3–10 years. Only three patients who could be followed were still living 10 years later: two after 11 and 12 years, in whom the tumor was localized in the femur and fifth lumbar vertebra, respectively, and one after 25 years with a tumor in the fifth dorsal vertebra, treated by radiotherapy (Fig. IV.65). It is interesting that the average age of the patients with "solitary" myeloma was lower than that of patients with disseminated lesions, and that patients are frequently below age 40. On the other hand, it is not possible to distinguish histologically the solitary from the multiple lesions – all stages of cytologic differentiation may be observed in both types.

In conclusion, there is clear evidence that "solitary" myeloma is only a clinical variant of myeloma, with stages of transition existing between the localized and disseminated types (Bataille and Sany 1981). Although some solitary lesions may show temporary electrophoretic changes, there are rare lesions with few foci and slow evolution with a normal electrophoretic pattern, although this occurs only in 1%–3% of cases.

Occasionally, a lesion with the histologic features of a myeloma may be found in an *extraskeletal location*, but as in intramedullary "solitary" myeloma, many cases reported in the literature as localized processes represent an extension or metastasis from an underlying skeletal plasmacytoma, or may long precede clinically occult but already disseminated myelomatosis. On the other hand, sometimes a plasma-cell *granuloma* is confused with a plasmacytoma. However, there is evidence that legitimate and primary extraskeletal plasmacytomas do exist, the most frequent locations being the air passages or in the conjunctiva (Hellwig 1943), and less common locations, the gastrointestinal tract and other organs. One of the earliest and best examples of a true plasmacytoma of lymph nodes was reported by Nelson and Lyons in 1957. It is important that the prognosis of localized extraskeletal plasmacytoma is favorable, like that of the solitary intramedullary lesions.

Myeloma Kidney. Several morphologic changes in patients with myelomatosis may lead to severe impairment of renal function. These lesions may be found alone or in combination and are as follows (Azar and Potter 1973):

1. Bence Jones lamellated protein casts with evidence of epithelial destruction or hypertrophy and with occasional formation of syncytial giant cells
2. Chronic and acute pyelonephritis
3. Calcium and urate casts, with or without metastatic calcinosis
4. Amyloidosis, primarily involving glomeruli and walls of small vessels
5. Infiltration by myeloma cells

Treatment and Prognosis. In localized lesions, surgical treatment, consisting of wide excision or en bloc resection with or without previous irradiation, may be applied to bones that can be removed without appreciable loss of function, such as rib, fibula, mandible, and scapula. Radiotherapy with a dosage of 30–40 Gy is another alternative in localized lesions, and it is the preferred treatment in tumors not amenable to surgery, especially those located in vertebral bodies. Even in this location, complete excision of one or two vertebral bodies has been attempted (Stener 1974). In patients with neurologic symptoms due to collapse of a vertebral body or penetration of the tumor into the spinal canal, decompression prior to irradiation is indicated. When a pathologic fracture occurs in a long bone, some kind of internal fixation should be performed, followed by radiotherapy.

When there is some doubt about possible dissemination or a second focus appears in a different bone, chemotherapy in association with irradiation is indicated. Although the effects of chemotherapy in multiple myelomas seem to be only temporary in many cases, in others, chemotherapy with one or preferably multiple drugs has produced long-term survival.

Various drugs have proved effective, and good results have been reported with phenylalanine mustard (Alkeran or melphalan) and cyclophosphamide (Cytoxan or Endoxan), with or without corticosteroids or other drugs. Several protocols with different combinations of agents are under trial. The Memorial Hospital, New York, uses the M-2 protocol, consisting of melphalan, cyclophosphamide, vincristine, prednisone, and BLNU, and conceived by Lee et al. (1974); this protocol produced an 80% objective response rate, with a median survival rate of 36 months. The Mayo Clinic's treatment preference (Kyle 1975, 1984) includes a combination of melphalan (0.15 mg/kg body weight, taken orally once a day) and prednisone (155 mg taken four times daily) for a 7-day period every 6 weeks.

The prognosis of multiple or diffuse myelomatosis is unfavorable; about 50% of patients die within 2 years after diagnosis, often due to renal insufficiency, infections, severe anemia, or generalized amyloidosis. Certain factors seem to affect the prognosis of individual cases. Patients with disseminated bone lesions associated with extraskeletal involvement (stages II and III) and histologically poor differentiation (Nordenson 1966) and patients with IgA myeloma were found to have a noticeably shorter survival time than those with IgG myeloma (Cooperative Study by Acute Leukemia Group B 1975).

We have already mentioned the better prognosis of the so-called solitary myeloma and emphasized the unpredictable nature of this variant of myeloma. Although dissemination may develop after a long, disease-free interval (2–10 years) following treatment, in rare cases it never occurs (Bataille and Sany 1981). Of 34 patients with solitary myeloma treated before 1960 in the Mayo Clinic, 18 were alive 5 years later. Seven of the latter group died at intervals that ranged from 7 to 24 years. Three of our patients with solitary lesions were living 11–25 years after local therapy (irradiation or decompression followed by irradiation in the vertebral lesions). Like Cohen et al. (1964), we did not find that the degree of differentiation affects the chance of prolonged survival with localized lesions, contrary to the apparently unfavorable prognosis of poorly differentiated tumors in disseminated disease.

References

Ewing Sarcoma, Primary Neuroectodermal Tumor and Malignant Lymphoma of Bone

Akhtar M, Ashraf M, Sabbah R (1985) Aspiration cytology of Ewing's sarcoma. Light and electron microscopic correlations. Cancer 56:2051–2060

Angervall L, Enzinger FM (1975) Extraskeletal neoplasm resembling Ewing's sarcoma. Cancer 36:240–251

Aurias A, Rimbaut C, Buffe D, Dubousset J, Mazabraud A (1983) Chromosomal translocation in Ewing's sarcoma. N Engl J Med 309:496

Aurias A, Rimbaut C, Buffe D, Zucker JM, Mazabraud A (1984) Translocation involving chromosome 22 in Ewing's sarcoma: a cytogenetic study of four fresh tumors. Cancer Genet Cytogenet 12:21

Ayala AG, Mackay B (1977) Ewing's sarcoma: an ultrastructural study. In: Dybala LW, Freitag SB, Culhane

DC (eds) Management of primary bone and soft tissue tumors, vol 10. Yearbook Medical, Chicago, pp 179–185

Bacci G, Capanna R, Orlandi M et al. (1985) Prognostic significance of serum lactic acid dehydrogenase in Ewing's tumor of bone. Ric Clin Lab 15:89–96

Bacci G, Jaffe N, Emiliani E et al. (1986) Therapy for primary non-Hodgkin's lymphoma of bone and a comparison of results with Ewing's sarcoma. Ten years' experience at the Istituto Ortopedico Rizzoli. Cancer 57:1468–1472

Baird RJ, Krause VW (1963) Ewing's tumor: a review of 33 cases. Can J Surg 6:136–140

Bator SM, Bauer TW, Marks KE et al. (1986) Periosteal Ewing's sarcoma. Cancer 58:1781–1784

Battifora J (1973) Hemangiopericytoma: ultrastructural study of five cases. Cancer 31:1418–1432

Bethge JFJ (1955) Die Ewingtumoren oder Omoblastome des Knochens. Differential-diagnostische und Kritische Erörterungen. Ergeb Chir Orthop 39:327–425

Bhansali SK, Desai PB (1963) Ewing's sarcoma: observations on 107 cases. J Bone Joint Surg [Am] 45:541–553

Callen DF, Smith RD, Bourne AJ (1987) Chromosomal analysis in Ewing sarcoma. Pathology 19:64–66

Cavazzana A, Miser JS, Jefferson HTL, Triche TJ (1987) Experimental evidence for a neural origin of Ewing's sarcoma. Am J Pathol 127:507

Cavazzana AO, Magnani JL, Ross RA et al. (1988) Ewing's sarcoma is an undifferentiated neuroectodermal tumor. Prog Clin Biol Res 271:487–498

Chan KW, Rosen G, Miller D et al. (1982) Hodgkin's disease in adolescents presenting as a primary bone lesion. Am J Pediatr Hematol Oncol 4:11–17

Clayton F, Butler JJ, Ayala AG et al. (1987) Non-Hodgkin's lymphoma in bone: pathologic and radiologic features with clinical correlates. Cancer 60:2494–2501

Coley BL (1960) Neoplasms of bone and related conditions: their etiology, pathogenesis, diagnosis and treatment, 2nd edn. Harper (Hoeber), New York

Coley BL, Higinbotham NL, Bowden L (1948) Endothelioma of bone (Ewing's sarcoma). Ann Surg 128:533–560

Coley BL, Higinbotham NL, Groesbeck HP (1950) Primary reticulum-cell sarcoma of bone. Summary of 37 cases. Radiology 55:641–658

Colville HC, Willis RA (1933) Neuroblastoma metastases in bone with a criticism of Ewing's endothelioma. Am J Pathol 9:421–430

Connor CL (1926) Endothelial myeloma, Ewing. Report of fifty-four cases. Arch Surg 12:789–829

Cossman J, Schnitzer B, Deegan MJ (1977) Immunologic surface markers in non-Hodgkin's lymphomas. Am J Pathol 87:19–32

Dahlin DC, Unni KK (1986) Bone tumors: general aspects and data on 8542 cases. Charles C. Thomas, Springfield, IL

Dahlin DC, Coventry MB, Scanlon PW (1961) Ewing's sarcoma: a critical analysis of 165 cases. J Bone Joint Surg [Am] 43:185–192

Dickman PS, Liotta LA, Triche TJ (1982) Ewing's sarcoma: characterization in established cultures and evidence of its histogenesis. Lab Invest 47:375–382

Dinshaw KA, Advani SH, Nair CN et al. (1984) Primary non-Hodgkin's lymphoma of bone. Indian J Cancer 20:275–282

Dosoretz DE, Raymond AK, Murphy GF et al. (1982) Primary lymphoma of bone. The relationship of morphologic diversity to clinical behavior. Cancer 50:1009–1014

Dosoretz DE, Murphy GF, Raymond AK et al. (1983) Radiation therapy for primary lymphoma of bone. Cancer 51:44–46

Dranoff G, Bigner DD (1984) A word of caution in the use of neuron-specific enolase expression in tumor diagnosis. Editorial. Arch Pathol Lab Med 108:535

Edwards JE (1940) Primary reticulum cell sarcoma of the spine: report of a case with autopsy. Am J Pathol 16:835–844

Ewing J (1921) Diffuse endothelioma of bone. Proc NY Pathol Soc 21:17–24

Ewing J (1924) Further report on endothelial myeloma. Proc NY Pathol Soc 24:93–101

Ewing J (1939) A review of the classification of bone tumors. Surg Gynecol Obstet 68:971–976

Falini B, Binazzi R, Pileri S et al. (1988) Large cell lymphoma of bone: a report of three cases of B-cell origin. Histopathology 12:177–190

Farley FA, Healey JH, Caparros-Sison B et al. (1987) Lactate dehydrogenase as a tumor marker for recurrent disease in Ewing's sarcoma. Cancer 59:1245–1248

Fellinger EF, Hamilton G, Salzer-Kuntschik M (1988) A new monoclonal antibody against a subgroup of malignant small round cell tumors. Proceedings of the First Meeting of the European Musculoskeletal Oncology Society (EMSOS), Vienna

Francis KC, Higinbotham NL, Coley BL (1954) Primary reticulum cell sarcoma of bone. Report of 44 cases. Surg Gynecol Obstet 99:142–146

Fraumeni JF Jr, Glass AG (1970) Rarity of Ewing's sarcoma among US Negro children. Letter to the editor. Lancet I:366–367

Friedman B, Gold H (1968) Ultrastructure of Ewing's sarcoma. Cancer 22:307–322

Friedman B, Hanaoka H (1971) Round cell sarcoma of bone. J Bone Joint Surg [Am] 53:1118–1136

Frouge C, Vanel D, Coffre C, Covaner D, Contesso G, Sarrazin D (1988) The role of magnetic resonance in the evaluation of Ewing's sarcoma. A report of 27 cases. Skeletal Radiol 17:387–392

Gall EA, Mallory TB (1942) Malignant lymphoma: a clinicopathologic survey of 618 cases. Am J Pathol 13:381–416

Greco MA, Steiner GC, Fazzini E (1988) Ewing's sarcoma with epithelial differentiation: fine structural and immunocytochemical study. Ultrastruct Pathol 12: 317–325

Hou-Jensen K, Priori E, Dmochowski L (1972) Studies on ultrastructure of Ewing's sarcoma of bone. Cancer 29:280–286

Howart JA, Thomas H, Waters KD et al. (1987) Malignant lymphoma of bone in children. Cancer 59:335–339

Hutter RVP, Foot FW Jr, Francis KC, Sherman RS (1966) Primitive multipotential primary sarcoma of bone. Cancer 99:1–25

Huvos AG (1991) Bone tumors: diagnosis, treatment, prognosis. W.B. Saunders, Philadelphia

Isayama T, Iwasaki H, Kikuchi M, Yoh S, Takagishi N (1990) Neuroectodermal tumor of bone. Evidence for neural differentiation in a cultured cell line. Cancer 65:1771–1781

Isaacson P, Wright DH, Jones DB (1983) Malignant lymphoma of true histiocytic (monocyte/macrophage) origin. Cancer 51:80–91

Ivins JC, Dahlin DC (1953) Reticulum-cell sarcoma of bone. J Bone Joint Surg [Am] 35:835–847

Jacobson SA (1977) Polyhistioma: a malignant tumor of bone and extra-skeletal tissues. Cancer 40:2116–2130

Jaffe N (1958) Tumors and tumorous conditions of the bones and joints. Lea & Febiger, Philadelphia

Jaffe N (ed) (1979) Progress in pediatric hematology oncology, vol II. Bone tumors in children. Publishing Science Group, Acton, Massachusetts

Jaffe R, Santamaria M, Yunis EJ et al. (1984) The neuroectodermal tumor of bone. Am J Surg Pathol 8:885–898

Jeffree GH (1973) Enzymes of round cell tumours in bone and soft tissue. A histochemical survey. J Pathol 113:101–105

Johnson LC (1953) A general theory of bone tumors. Bull NY Acad Med 29:164

Johnson RE, Pomeroy TC (1975) Evaluation of therapeutic results in Ewing's sarcoma. AJR 123:583–587

Joyce MJ, Harmon DC, Mankin HJ et al. (1984) Ewing sarcoma in female siblings: a clinical report and review of the literature. Cancer 53:1959–1962

Jurgens H, Exner V, Gadner H et al. (1988) Multidisciplinary treatment of primary Ewing's sarcoma of bone: a 6-year experience of a European cooperative trial. Cancer 61:23–32

Kadin ME, Bensch KG (1971) On the origin of Ewing's tumor. Cancer 27:257–273

Khanolkar VR (1948) Reticulum cell sarcoma of bone. Arch Pathol 46:467–476

Kissane JM, Askin FB, Foulkes M et al. (1983) Ewing's sarcoma of bone: clinicopathologic aspects of 303 cases from the Intergroup Ewing's Sarcoma Study. Hum Pathol 14:773–779

Larsson SE, Boquist L, Bergdahl L (1973) Ewing's sarcoma: a consecutive series of 64 cases diagnosed in Sweden, 1958–1967. Clin Orthop 94:263–272

Lennert K (1975) Morphology and classification of malignant lymphomas and so-called reticuloses. Acta Neuropathol (Suppl) 6:1–16

Lewis RJ, Marcove RC, Rosen G (1977) Ewing's sarcoma – functional effects of radiation therapy. J Bone Joint Surg [Am] 59:325–331

Li FP, Tu JT, Liu FS et al. (1980) Rarity of Ewing's sarcoma in China. Lancet I:1255

Lichtenstein L, Jaffe HL (1947) Ewing's sarcoma of bone. Am J Pathol 23:43–78

Linden G, Dunn JE (1970) Ewing's sarcoma in Negroes. Lancet I:1171

Llombart-Bosch A, Blache R, Peydro-Olaya A (1978) Ultrastructural study of 28 cases of Ewing's sarcoma. Typical and atypical forms. Cancer 41:1362–1373

Llombart-Bosch A, Blache R, Peydro-Olaya A (1982) Round-cell sarcomas of bone and their differential diagnosis with particular emphasis on Ewing's sarcoma and reticulosarcoma. A study of 233 tumors with optical and electron microscopic techniques. Pathol Annu 17:113–145

Llombart-Bosch A, Lacombe MJ, Contesso G et al. (1987) Small round blue cell sarcoma of bone mimicking atypical Ewing's sarcoma with neuroectodermal features. Cancer 60:1570–1582

Llombart-Bosch A, Lacombe MJ, Peydro-Olaya A et al. (1988) Malignant peripheral neuroectodermal tumors of bone other than Askin's neoplasm: characterization of 14 new cases with immunohistochemistry and electron microscopy. Virchows Arch [A] 412:421

Llombart-Bosch A, Carda C, Peydro-Olaya A et al. (1990) Soft tissue Ewing's sarcoma. Characterization in established cultures and xenografts with evidence of a neuroectodermic phenotype. Cancer 66:2589–2601

Loeffler JS, Tarbell NJ, Kozakewich H et al. (1986) Primary lymphoma of bone in children: analysis of treatment results with adriamycin, prednisone, Oncovin (APO), and local radiation therapy. J Clin Oncol 4:496–501

Lukes RJ, Butler JJ (1966) The pathology and nomenclature of Hodgkin's disease. Cancer Res 26: 1063–1081

Lukes RJ, Collins RD (1975) New approaches to the classification of the lymphomata. Br J Cancer (Suppl) 2:1–28

Lukes RJ, Craver L, Hall T, Rappaport H, Rubin P (1966) Report on nomenclature committee. Cancer Res 26 (Part I): 1311

Lumb G, Mackenzie DH (1956) Round cell tumours of bone. Br J Surg 43:380–389

MacIntosh DJ, Price CHG, Jeffree GM (1975) Ewing's tumor: a study of behavior and treatment in forty-seven cases. J Bone Joint Surg [Br] 57:331–340

MacIntosh DJ, Price CHG, Jeffree GM (1977) Malignant lymphoma (reticulosarcoma) in bone. Clin Oncol 3: 287–300

Magnus HA, Wood HL-C (1956) Primary reticulosarcoma of bone. J Bone Joint Surg [Br] 38:258–278

Mahoney JP, Alexander RW (1978) Ewing's sarcoma: a light- and electron-microscopic study of 21 cases. Am J Surg Pathol 2:283–298

Mahoney JP, Alexander RW (1980) Primary histiocytic lymphoma of bone: a light and ultrastructural study of four cases. Am J Surg Pathol 4:149–161

Maletz N, McMarrow LE, Greco A et al. (1986) Ewing's sarcoma. Pathology, tissue culture, and cytogenetics. Cancer 58:252–257

Martin SE, Dwyer A, Kissane JM et al. (1982) Small-cell osteosarcoma. Cancer 50:990–996

Mathé G, Rappaport H (1976) Histological and cytological typing of neoplastic diseases of haematopoietic and lymphoid tissues, No. 14. World Health Organization, Geneva

McCormack LJ, Dockerty MB, Ghormley RK (1952) Ewing's sarcoma. Cancer 5:85–99

McDonald I (1981) Malignant lymphoma associated with internal fixation of a fractured tibia. Cancer 48:1009–1011

Melnick PJ (1933) Histogenesis of Ewing's sarcoma with postmortem of a case. Am J Pathol 19:353

Miettinen M, Lehto VP, Virtanen I (1982) Histogenesis of Ewing's sarcoma: an evaluation of intermediate filaments and endothelial cell markers. Virchows Arch [B] 41:277–284

Miser JS, Kinsella TJ, Triche TJ et al. (1987) Treatment of peripheral neuroepithelioma in children and young adults. J Clin Oncol 5:1752–1758

Moll R, Lee I, Gould VE et al. (1987) Immunocytochemical analysis of Ewing's tumors. Patterns of expression of intermediate filaments and desmosomal proteins indicate cell type heterogeneity and pluripotential differentiation. Am J Pathol 127:288–304

Morris MW, Davey RF (1975) Immunologic and cytochemical properties of histiocytic and mixed histiocytic-lymphocytic lymphomas. Am J Clin Pathol 63:403–414

Nakayama I, Tsuda N, Muta H et al. (1975) Fine structure comparison of Ewing's sarcoma with neuroblastoma. Acta Pathol Jpn 25:251–268

Nascimento AG, Unni KK, Pritchard DJ et al. (1980) A clinicopathologic study of 20 cases of large-cell (atypical) Ewing sarcoma of bone. Am J Surg Pathol 4:29–36

Navas-Palacios JJ, Aparicio-Duque R, Valdés MD (1984) On the histogenesis of Ewing's sarcoma. An ultrastructural immunohistochemical and cytochemical study. Cancer 53:1882–1901

Neff JR (1986) Nonmetastatic Ewing's sarcoma of bone: the role of surgical therapy. Clin Orthop 204:111–117

Oberling C (1928) Les reticulosarcomes et les reticuloendotheliosarcomes de la moelle osseuse (sarcomes d'Ewing). Bull Assoc Fr Etude Cancer 17:259–296

Oberling CP, Raileanu C (1932) Nouvelles recherches sur les reticulosarcomes de la moelle osseuse (sarcomes d'Ewing). Bull Assoc Fr Etude Cancer 21:333–345

Osborn M, Dirk TH, Kaser H et al. (1986) Immunohistochemical localization of neurofilaments and neuron-specific enolase in 29 cases of neuroblastoma. Am J Pathol 122:433

Ostrowski ML, Unni KK, Banks PM et al. (1986) Malignant lymphoma of bone. Cancer 58:2646–2655

Parker F Jr, Jackson H Jr (1939) Primary reticulum cell sarcoma of bone. Surg Gynecol Obstet 68:45–53

Pinto A, Grant LH, Hayes FA et al. (1989) Immunohistochemical expression of neuron-specific enolase and Leu 7 in Ewing's sarcoma of bone. Cancer 64:1266

Polak M, Schajowicz F (1949) Patología e histogénesis del reticulosarcoma de los huesos. Rev Asoc Med Argent 63:162–170

Pomeroy TC, Johnson RE (1975) Combined modality therapy of Ewing's sarcoma. Cancer 35:36–47

Povysil C, Matejovsky Z (1977) Ultrastructure of Ewing's tumor. Virchows Arch [A] 374:303–316

Price CHG (1973) Discussion. In: Price CHG, Ross FGM (eds) Bone: certain aspects of neoplasia. F.A. Davis, Philadelphia

Price CHG, Jeffree GM (1977) Incidence of bone sarcoma in SW England, 1946–74, in relation to age, sex, tumour site and histology. Br J Cancer 36:511–522

Prieto F, Badia L, Montalar J et al. (1985) Translocation (11;22) in Ewing's sarcoma. Cancer Genet Cytogenet 17:87–89

Pritchard DJ, Dahlin DC, Dauphine RT, Taylor WR, Beabout JW (1975) Ewing's sarcoma: a clinicopathological and statistical analysis of patients surviving five years or longer. J Bone Joint Surg [Am] 57:10–16

Rappaport H (1966) Tumors of the hematopoietic system. In: Atlas of tumor pathology, Sect III, Fasc 8. Armed Forces of Pathology, Washington, DC

Reimer RR, Chabner BA, Young RC et al. (1977) Lymphoma presenting in bone: results of histopathology, staging, and therapy. Ann Intern Med 87:50–55

Rice RW, Cabot A, Johnston A (1973) The application of electron microscopy to the diagnostic differentiation of Ewing's sarcoma and reticulum cell sarcoma of bone. Clin Orthop 97:174–184

Rosenberg SA, Berard CW, Brown BW (1982) National Cancer Institute sponsored study of classifications of non-Hodgkin's lymphomas. Cancer 49:2112–2135

Salzer-Kuntschik M (1976) Cytologic and cytochemical behavior of primary malignant bone tumors. In: Grundmann E (ed) Malignant bone tumors. Springer, New York Berlin Heidelberg, pp 145–156

Schajowicz F (1959) Ewing's sarcoma and reticulum cell sarcoma of bone. With special reference to the histochemcal demonstration of glycogen as an aid to differential diagnosis. J Bone Joint Surg [Am] 41: 185–192

Schajowicz F (1973) Differential diagnosis of Ewing's sarcoma. Proc Symp Colston Res Soc 24:189–205

Schajowicz F (1981) Tumors and tumorlike lesions of bone and joints. Springer, New York Berlin Heidelberg

Schajowicz F, Cabrini RL (1954) Histochemical studies of bone in normal and pathological conditions. With special reference to alkaline phosphatase, glycogen and mucopolysaccharides. J Bone Joint Surg [Br] 36:474–489

Schajowicz F, McGuire MH (1989) Diagnostic difficulties in skeletal pathology. Clin Orthop 240:281

Schajowicz F, Ackerman LV, Sissons HA (1972) Histological typing of bone tumours. World Health Organization, Geneva

Schmidt D, Mackay B, Ayala AG (1982) Ewing's sarcoma with neuroblastoma-like features. Ultrastruct Pathol 3:143–151

Shoji H, Miller TR (1971) Primary reticulum cell sarcoma of bone. Significance of clinical features upon the prognosis. Cancer 28:1234–1244

Sim FH, Unni KK, Beabout JW, Dahin DD (1979) Osteosarcoma with small cells simulating Ewing's tumor of bone. J Bone Joint Surg [Am] 61:207

Steiner GC, Graham S, Lewis MM (1988) Malignant round cell tumor of bone with neural differentiation (neuroectodermal tumor). Ultrastruct Pathol 12: 505–512

Stout AP (1943) A discussion of the pathogenesis and histogenesis of Ewing's tumor of bone marrow. AJR 50:334–342

Strege DW, Manel DP, Vogler C, Schajowicz F (1990) Ewing's sarcoma in a phalanx of an infant's finger. J Bone Joint Surg [Am] 71:1262–1265

Sundaram M, Merenda G, McGuire M (1990) A skip lesion in association with Ewing's sarcoma. Report of a case. J Bone Joint Surg [Am] 71:764–768

Takahashi K, Sato T, Kojima M (1976) Cytological characterization and histogenesis of Ewing's sarcoma. Acta Pathol Jpn 26:167–190

Tayton KJJ (1980) Ewing's sarcoma at the site of a metal plate. Cancer 45:413–415

Telles NC, Rabson AS, Pomeroy TC (1978) Ewing's sarcoma: an autopsy study. Cancer 41:2321–2329

Thomas P, Battifora H, Maderino GL, Patrick J (1987) A monoclonal antibody against neuron-specific enolase: immunohistochemical comparison with a polyclonal antiserum. Am J Clin Pathol 88:146

Triche TJ, Askin FB (1983) Neuroblastoma and the differential diagnosis of small round blue cell tumors. Hum Pathol 14:569

Triche TJ, Ross WE (1978) Glycogen-containing neuroblastoma with clinical and histopathologic features of Ewing's sarcoma. Cancer 41:1425–1432

Tsokos M, Linnoilo RI, Chandra RS, Triche TJ (1984) Neuron-specific enolase in the diagnosis of neuroblastoma and other small round-cell tumors in children. Hum Pathol 15:575

Turc-Carel C, Phillip I, Berger MP et al. (1983) Chromosomal translocation in Ewing's sarcoma. N Engl J Med 309:497

Turc-Carel C, Phillip I, Berger MP et al. (1984) Chromosome study of Ewing's sarcoma (ES) cell lines. Consistency of a reciprocal translocation t(11;22) (q24;q12). Cancer Genet Cytogenet 12:1–19
Turc-Carel C, Aurias A, Mugneret F et al. (1988) Chromosomes in Ewing's sarcoma. I. An evaluation of 85 cases of remarkable consistency of t(11;22) (q24;q12). Cancer Genet Cytogenet 32:229–238
Ueda T, Aozasa K, Ohsawa M et al. (1989) Malignant lymphomas of bone in Japan. Cancer 64:2387–2392
Uehlinger E, Botstejn C, Schinz HR (1948) Ewingsarkom und Knochenretikulosarkom. Klinik, Diagnose und Differential-diagnose. Oncologia 1:193–245
Valls J, Muscolo D, Schajowicz F (1952) Reticulum-cell sarcoma of bone. J Bone Joint Surg [Br] 34:588–598
Whang-Peng J, Triche TJ, Knutsen T et al. (1984) Chromosome translocation in peripheral neuroepithelioma. N Engl J Med 311:584
Wick MR, Abenoza P, Manivel JC (1988) Diagnostic immunohistopathology. In: Gnepp DR (ed) Pathology of the head and neck. Churchill Livingstone, New York, pp 216–217
Wick R, Scheithauer BN, Hovasc H (1983) Neuron-specific enolase in neuroendocrine tumor, thymus, bronchus and skin. Am J Clin Pathol 29:703
Wigger HJ, Salazar GH, Blanc WA (1977) Extra-skeletal Ewing's sarcoma. An ultrastructural study. Arch Pathol Lab Med 101:446–449
Wilkins RM, Pritchard DJ, Burgert EO Jr et al. (1986) Ewing's sarcoma of bone. Experience with 140 patients. Cancer 58:2552–2555
Williams AO (1975) Tumors of childhood in Ibadan, Nigeria. Cancer 36:370–378
Willis RA (1940) Metastatic neuroblastoma in bone presenting the Ewing's syndrome with a discussion of "Ewing's sarcoma." Am J Pathol 16:317–329
Willis RA (1967) Ewing's tumor. In: Pathology of tumors, 4th edn. Butterworth, London
Wilson RW, Pugh DG (1955) Primary reticulum-cell sarcoma of bone, with emphasis on roentgen aspects. Radiology 65:343–351
Yunis EJ (1986) Ewing's sarcoma and related small round cell neoplasms of children. In: Arthur Purdy Stout Symposium. Am J Surg Pathol 10[Suppl]:54–62
Yunis EJ, Walpusk JA, Agostini RM et al. (1979) Glycogen in neuroblastomas. A light- and electron-microscopic study of 40 cases. Am J Surg Pathol 3:313–323

Myeloma

Alexanian R, Salmon S, Bonnet J et al. (1977) Combination therapy for multiple myeloma. Cancer 40: 2765–2771
Azar HA (1977) Plasma cell myelomatosis and other monoclonal gammapathies. In: Sheldon C (ed) Animal pathology. Appleton-Century-Crofts, New York, pp 463–489
Azar HA, Potter M (1973) Multiple myeloma and related disorders, vol 1. Harper & Row, New York
Azar HA, Zaino EC, Pham TD, Yannopoulos K (1972) "Nonsecretory" plasma cell myeloma. Observations on seven cases with electron microscope studies. Am J Clin Pathol 58:618
Bacci G, Calderoni P, Cervellati C et al. (1982) Solitary plasmacytoma of bone: a report on 19 cases. Ital J Orthop Traumatol 8:469–478
Bardwick PA, Zwaifler NJ, Grill GN et al. (1980) Plasma cell dyscrasia with polyneuropathy, organomegaly, endocrinopathy, M protein, and skin changes: the POEMS syndrome. Medicine 59:311–322
Bataille R, Sany J (1981) Solitary myeloma: clinical and prognostic features of a review of 114 cases. Cancer 48:845–851
Bataille R, Chevalier J, Rossi M et al. (1982) Bone scintigraphy in plasma-cell myeloma: a prospective study of 70 patients. Radiology 145:801–804
Bayrd ED, Bennett WA (1950) Amyloidosis complicating myeloma. Med Clin North Am 34:1151–1164
Berard CW, Dorfman F (1974) Histopathology of malignant lymphoma. Clin Haematol 3:39
Bernstein SC, Perez-Atayde AR, Weinstein HJ (1985) Multiple myeloma in a child. Cancer 56:2143–2147
Bichel J, Kirketerp P (1938) Notes on myeloma. Acta Radiol 19:487–503
Blattner WA, Blair A, Mason TJ (1981) Multiple myeloma in the United States, 1950–1975. Cancer 48:2547–2554
Braunsteiner H, Fellinger K, Pakesch F (1953) Demonstration of a cytoplasmic structure in plasma cells. Blood 8:916–922
Braylan RC, Jaffe ES, Berard CW (1975) Malignant lymphomas. Current classification and new observations. Pathol Annu 10:213–270
Christopherson WM, Miller HJ (1950) Reevaluation of solitary plasma-cell myeloma of bone. Cancer 3:240–252
Clarisse PDT, Staple TW (1971) Diffuse bone sclerosis in multiple myeloma. Radiology 99:327–328
Cohen DM, Svien HJ, Dahlin DC (1964) Long-term survival of patients with myeloma of the vertebral column. JAMA 187:914–917
Cooperative Study by Acute Leukemia Group B (1975) Correlation of abnormal immunoglobulin with clinical features of myeloma. Arch Intern Med 135:46–52
Costa G, Engle RL Jr, Schilling A et al. (1973) Melphalan and prednisone: an effective combination for the treatment of multiple myeloma. Am J Med 54:589–599
Dahlin DC (1978) Bone tumors, 3rd edn. Charles C. Thomas, Springfield, IL
Dahlin DC, Dockerty MB (1950) Amyloid and myeloma. Am J Pathol 26:581–593
Dalrymple J (1846) On the microscopical character of mollities ossium. Dublin QJ Med Sci 2:85–145
Edeiken J, Hodes PJ (1977) Roentgen diagnosis of disease of bone. Williams & Wilkins, Baltimore
Engels EP, Smith RC, Krantz S (1960) Bone sclerosis in multiple myeloma. Radiology 75:242–247
Ford HC, Casey BR, Walker S et al. (1980) Multiple myeloma with an IgD kappa monoclonal protein. Am J Clin Pathol 74:105–107
Gootnick LT (1945) Solitary myeloma: review of sixty-one cases. Radiology 45:385–391
Gordon J, Schneider B (1940) Plasma-cell myeloma in a child. Report of a case. Int Clin 4:173–181
Gravano L, Schajowicz F, Menzani A, Vaccaro A (1970) Mieloma múltiple de forma osteoblástica. Prensa Med Argent 57:1654–1663
Griffiths DLL (1966) Orthopaedic aspects of myelomatosis. J Bone Joint Surg [Br] 48:703–728

Hellwig CA (1943) Extramedullary plasma cell tumors as observed in various locations. Arch Pathol 36:95–111
Hewell GM, Alexanian R (1976) Multiple myeloma in young persons. Ann Intern Med 84:441–443
Jaffe HL (1958) Tumors and tumorous conditions of the bones and joints. Lea & Febiger, Philadelphia
Jennette JC, Wilkman AS, Benson JD (1981) IgD myeloma with intracytoplasmic crystalline inclusions. Am J Clin Pathol 74:231–235
Kahler O (1889) Zur Symptomatologie des multiplen Myeloms. Wien Med Presse 30:209–213, 253–255
Kavanaugh JH (1978) Multiple myeloma, amyloid arthropathy, and pathological fracture of the femur. A case report. J Bone Joint Surg [Am] 60:135–137
Kobayashi H, Ii K, Sano T et al. (1985) Plasma-cell dyscrasia with polyneuropathy and endocrine disorders associated with dysfunction of salivary glands. Am J Surg Pathol 9:759–763
Kyle RA (1975) Multiple myeloma: review of 869 cases. Mayo Clin Proc 50:29–40
Kyle RA (1984) Treatment of multiple myeloma: a small step forward? N Engl J Med 310:1382–1383
Kyle RA, Bayrd ED (1961) "Primary" systemic amyloidosis and myeloma: discussion of relationship and review of 81 cases. Arch Intern Med 107:344–353
Kyle RA, Maldonado JE, Bayrd ED (1974) Plasma cell leukemia. Report of 17 cases. Arch Intern Med 133: 813
Lazarus HM, Kellermeyer RW, Masamichi A et al. (1980) Multiple myeloma in young men: clinical course and electron microscopic studies of bone marrow plasma cells. Cancer 46:1397–1400
Lee BJ, Sahakian G, Clarkson BD et al. (1974) Combination chemotherapy of multiple myeloma with Alkeran, Cytoxan, vincristine, prednisone, and BCNU. Cancer 33:533–538
Leech SH, Bryan CF, Elston RC et al. (1983) Genetic studies in multiple myeloma. 1. Association with HLA-CW5. Cancer 51:1408–1411
Lichtenstein L (1977) Bone tumors, 5th edn. C.V. Mosby, St. Louis
Lièvre AJ (1955) Myelome multiple et myelomatose decalcificant diffuse. Presse Med 65:577
Lowbeer L (1969) Occurrence of osteosclerosis in multiple myeloma. Lab Med 10:396–397
Lowell DM (1967) Amyloid-producing plasmacytoma of the pelvis: case report and review of the literature. Arch Surg 94:899–903
MacIntyre W (1850) Case of mollities and fragilitas ossium accompanied with urine strongly charged with animal matter. Med Chir Soc Trans 33:211–232
Maeda K, Abesamis CM, Kuhn LM, Hyun BH (1973) Multiple myeloma in childhood: report of a case with breast tumors as a presenting manifestation. Am J Clin Pathol 60:552
Maldonado JE (1965) The ultrastructure of the myeloma cell. Thesis submitted to the Faculty of the Graduate School of the University of Minnesota
Maldonado JE, Brown AL Jr, Bayrd ED et al. (1966) Ultrastructure of the myeloma cell. Cancer 19:1613–1627
Mangalik A, Veliath AJ (1971) Osteosclerotic myeloma and peripheral neuropathy: a case report. Cancer 28:1040–1045
Mathe G, Rappaport H (1976) Histological and cytological typing of neoplastic disease of haematopoietic and lymphoid tissues. International classification of tumours, No 14. World Health Organization, Geneva
McLauchlan J (1973) Solitary myeloma of the clavicle with long survival after total excision: report of a case. J Bone Joint Surg [Br] 55:357–358
Meis JM, Butler JJ, Osborne BM et al. (1987) Solitary plasmacytomas of bone and extramedullary plasmacytomas. A clinicopathologic and immunohistochemical study. Cancer 59:1475–1485
Meyer JE, Schulz MD (1974) "Solitary" myeloma of bone: a review of 12 cases. Cancer 34:438–440
Mill WB, Griffith R (1980) The role of radiation therapy in the management of plasma cell tumors. Cancer 45: 647–652
Morley JB, Schweiger AC (1967) The relation between chronic polyneuropathy and osteosclerotic myeloma. J Neurol Neurosurg Psychiatry 30:432–442
Mundy GR, Raisz LG, Cooper RA, Schechter GP, Salmon SE (1974) Evidence for the secretion of an osteoclast stimulating factor in myeloma. N Engl J Med 291:1041–1046
Nelson MG, Lyons AR (1957) Plasmacytoma of lymph glands. Cancer 10:1275–1280
Nordenson NG (1966) Myelomatosis, a clinical review of 310 cases. Acta Med Scand [Suppl] 179:178–183
Okano H, Azar HA, Osserman EF (1966) Plasmacytic reticulum cell sarcoma: case report with electron microscopic studies. Am J Clin Pathol 46:546–555
Osserman EF, Takasuki K (1963) Plasma cell myeloma. Gamma globulin synthesis and structure. A review of biochemical and clinical data, with the description of a newly-recognized and related syndrome, "H_γ-2-chain (Franklin's) disease." Am J Med 42:357–384
Pasmantier MW, Azar HA (1969) Extraskeletal spread in multiple plasma cell myeloma: a review of 57 autopsied cases. Cancer 23:167–174
Porter FS Jr (1963) Multiple myeloma in a child. J Pediatr 62:602–604
Ramón y Cajal S (1906) Quelques antecedents histioriques ignorés sur les Plasmazellen. Anat Anz 29:666–673
Rappaport H (1966) Tumors of the hematopoietic system. In: Atlas of tumor pathology, Sect III, Fasc 8. Armed Forces Institute of Pathology, Washington, DC
Resnick D, Niwayama G (1988) Diagnosis of bone and joint disorders, 2nd edn, vol 6. W.B. Saunders, Philadelphia
Rustizky JV (1873) Multiples myelom. Dtsch Z Chir 3: 162–172
Schajowicz F, Ackerman LV, Sissons HA (1972) Histological typing of bone tumours. World Health Organization, Geneva
Schmaus KA (1950) Multiples Myeloma (Plasmacytom) bei einem Jugendichlen. Chirurg 21:48–50
Slavens JJ (1934) Multiple myeloma in a child. Am J Dis Child 47:821–835
Smetana K, Györkey F, Györkey P, Busch H (1973) Ultrastructural studies on human myeloma plasmacytes. Cancer Res 33:2300–2309
Snapper I, Kahn A (1971) Myelomatosis. Fundamentals and clinical features. University Park Press, Baltimore, Maryland
Spjut HJ, Dorfman HD, Fechner RE, Ackerman LV (1971) Tumors of bone and cartilage. Atlas of tumor pathology, 2nd series, Fasc 5. Armed Forces Institute of Pathology, Washington, DC
Stener B (1974) Resección de columna en el tratamiento de los tumores vertebrales. Arch Ortop Lat Am 1:189

Takatsuki K, Sanada I (1983) Plasma cell dyscrasia with polyneuropathy and endocrine disorders (clinical aspects). Pathol Clin Med 12:1663–1668

Tompkins EH (1960) The conversion of lymphocytes with "atypical nuclei" into plasma cells of the Marschalko type. Am J Pathol 37:175–189

Valderrama JAF, Bullough PG (1968) Solitary myeloma of the spine. J Bone Joint Surg [Br] 50:82–90

Valenzuela R, Govindarajan S, Tubbs R et al. (1979) IgD myeloma: report of a case with unusual clinical and immunologic features. Am J Clin Pathol 72:246–250

Waldenström J (1970) Diagnosis and treatment of multiple myeloma. Grune & Stratton, New York

Weissenbach P, Lièvre JA (1958) Myelomatose decalcificante diffuse. Bull Mem Hosp Paris, pp 1127, 1851

Wright JH (1900) A case of multiple myeloma. Trans Assoc Am Physicians 15:137–145

CHAPTER V
Vascular Tumors

The existing nomenclature of vascular tumors of bone, especially that of the malignant types, is confusing and far from uniform. Vascular tumors show a wide range of histologic appearances, varying from well-differentiated vasoformative lesions to highly anaplastic tumors. Different terms – such as hemangiosarcoma (angiosarcoma), hemangioendothelioma, and hemangioendotheliosarcoma – have been used as synonyms or have been divided into different grades, from well differentiated (grade I hemangioendothelioma) to poorly differentiated (grade III hemangioendothelioma). On the other hand, it is sometimes difficult to make a clear distinction between the relatively common hemangiomas and the rare angiosarcomas. Therefore the WHO classification includes an intermediate group of essentially low-grade tumors, comprising hemangioendothelioma (epithelioid hemangioendothelioma) and the extremely rare hemangiopericytoma, originating in bone (Table V.1). This last tumor type is considered in all reports as a distinct entity, and exceptionally may present frankly malignant histologic features and a metastatic potential.

A. Benign

1. Hemangioma

Definition, WHO: *"A benign lesion consisting of newly formed blood vessels, either of capillary or cavernous type."*

In contrast to the high incidence in soft tissues, hemangiomas are infrequent in bone when only the cases with clinical and radiologic evidence are considered.

However, hemangiomas, especially of the vertebral bodies, have been found with great frequency in the autopsy studies of German and Austrian pathologists, especially those performed in Schmorl's (Dresden) and Erdheim's (Vienna) institutes, because of the special interest of these workers in vertebral pathology. Thus Makrycostas (1927) reported 41 angiomas in 12 vertebral columns in patients without clinical symptoms. Töpfer (1928) found 257 vertebral angiomas in 2154 autopsies (11.92%), 34 of them multiple; and Junghanns (1932), of Schmorl's laboratory, mentioned 409 cases with 579 lesions found in 3829 vertebral columns. In none of these cases did the lesion provoke any clinical symptoms.

On the other hand, most spinal lesions are occasional radiologic findings or are discovered after consultation for back pain. These are the reasons why some pathologists consider hemangioma a developmental abnormality (hamartomatous malformation) or the result of localized venous stasis rather than a true neoplasm (Lichtenstein 1977; Aegerter and Kirkpatrick 1975).

Incidence. Hemangioma is infrequently diagnosed by the clinician and surgical pathologist. It accounted for only 1.2% of all bone tumors in our series (63 cases being identified) and for approximately 1% of the tumors of the Mayo Clinic series

Table V.1. Vascular tumors (WHO classification)

Benign	Intermediate	Malignant
Hemangioma	Hemangioendothelioma (epithelioid hemangioendothelioma, histiocytoid hemangioma)	Angiosarcoma
Lymphangioma Glomus tumor	Hemangiopericytoma	Hemangiopericytoma

(Dahlin and Unni 1986). Dorfman et al. (1971) reported 27 cases of hemangioma studied at the Hospital for Joint Diseases (New York) over a period of 40 years.

Clinical Findings. There was no sex predominance in most statistics, including ours, but in Dahlin's series (1978) the lesion was more frequent in females (3:2). It can be found in all age groups, but was more common in adults.

The most common anatomic sites were the spine and cranium; more rarely, long or other short bones were affected. Sherman and Wilner (1961) surveyed 60 hemangiomas of bone recorded in the literature and found that two-thirds were located in the vertebral column and skull, which agrees with Dahlin's and our figures. Wyke (1946), who surveyed the literature through 1949, found 40 cases of hemangioma located in the skull, most frequently in the parietal (20 cases) and frontal (10 cases) bones, and with an evident female predominance (3:1). Four of our patients had multiple disseminated lesions, which will be discussed later.

Symptoms. Many hemangiomas were asymptomatic or gave rise to moderate pain or swelling if located in a cranial or long bone. Vertebral lesions may produce back pain and, rarely, neurologic symptoms due to compression of the spinal cord or nerve roots, especially after a fracture.

Radiographic Features. The radiographic aspect of hemangioma may be uncharacteristic, consisting of a radiolucent defect with little or no periosteal reaction in a long or cranial bone. However, in vertebral lesions, the radiographic appearance is often characteristic, showing rarefaction with prominent parallel vertical striations or a honeycomb appearance (Figs. V.1–V.3). Nonvertebral lesions may also show coarse, irregular, or mostly longitudinal trabeculation (Figs. V.4, V.5). In cranial bones and occasionally in long bones and ribs, a circumscribed, round or oval, often honeycombed radiolucent area, tending to bulge the outer and sometimes the inner table of the cranium, is observed. In tangential views, the characteristic "sunburst" or "sun-ray" pattern ("sun-ray skull") is seen; this is produced by fine spicules of reactive new bone radiating from the center or perpendicularly toward the surface (Figs. V.6–V.8). A similar appearance may be found occasionally in osteosarcoma (Fig. V.9) and in an underlying meningioma penetrating into the calvarium (Fig. V.10).

Fig. V.1. Male, 38 years old. Hemangioma of second lumbar vertebra. Anteroposterior and lateral radiographs illustrate the normal contour of the vertebra, which shows rarefaction and thickened longitudinal trabeculae, producing a honeycomb aspect. Patient complained of pain for several months

Fig. V.2. Male, 45 years old. Paget disease of the third lumbar vertebra. Anteroposterior and lateral radiographs show similar exaggerated vertical striation

We observed one exceptional case of intracortical hemangioma located in the tibia in a woman 54 years of age, which caused marked pain and bone sclerosis, simulating an "osteoid osteoma" (Schajowicz et al. 1979) radiologically and macroscopically. Dorfman et al. (1971) reported another case with almost identical characteristics. In some other cases, published by Loxley et al. (1972), Sugiura (1975), Guerra et al. (1984), Pena et al. (1985), and Kenan et al. (1988) under the term "periosteal hemangioma," the lesion was extraosseous and subperiosteal, giving rise to a shallow cup-shaped depression in the cortex with marked local sclerosis of the underlying bone. Three similar lesions were seen in our series.

Pathologic Findings. The *gross appearance* is that of a dark red, predominantly friable and hemorrhagic tissue, often traversed by irregularly distributed or radiating bony spicules. The cortex is sometimes thinned and expanded, but rarely disrupted.

Histologically, hemangioma consists of a conglomerate of newly formed thin-walled vascular channels. In the majority of cases, most of the blood vessels were more or less dilated, being of the cavernous type that is more common in the cranial lesions. Others are predominantly of the less frequent capillary type, which was more common in long bones (Fig. V.11). In our experience, most of the vertebral lesions were of the mixed type. The vessels are usually filled with red blood cells, but occasionally the cavernous channels are empty. In that case it is difficult to be certain whether this is an artifact or actually lymphatic vessels, which would suggest the diagnosis of lymphangioma. In cases of "cystic angiomatosis," both types of vessels may coexist.

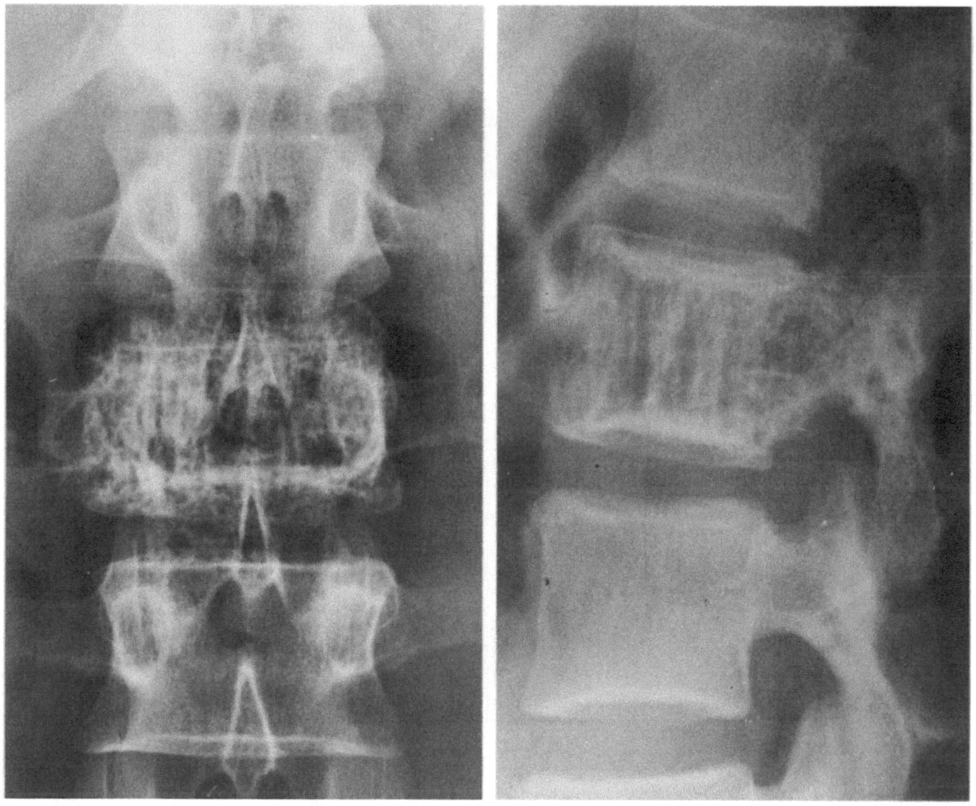

V.1a b

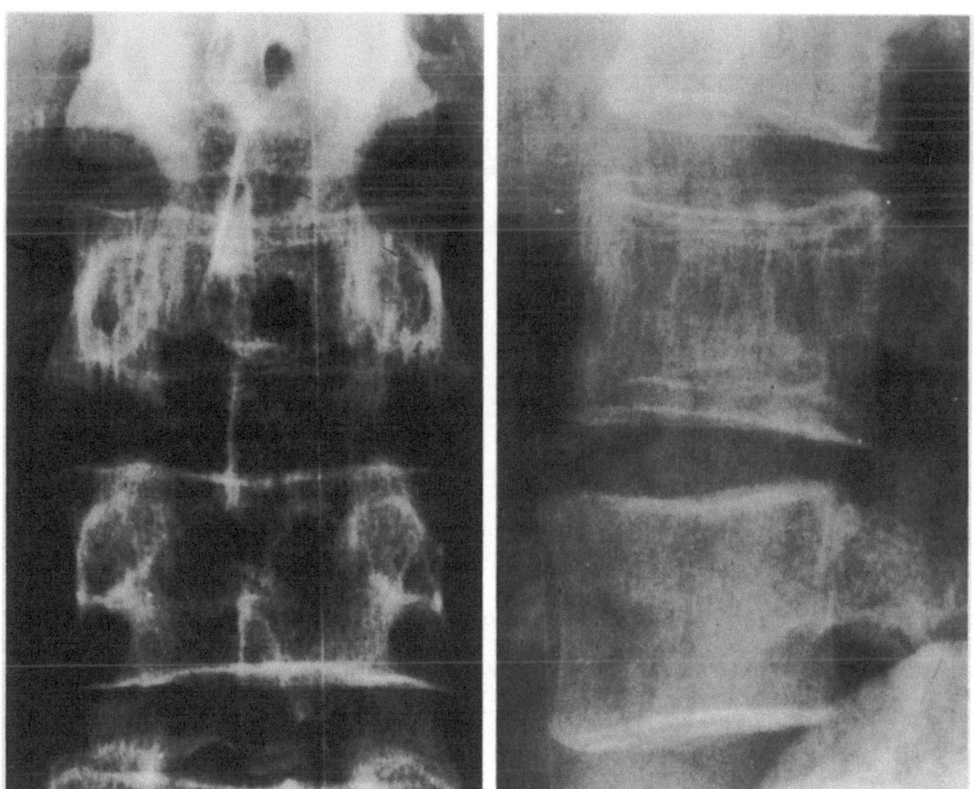

V.2a b

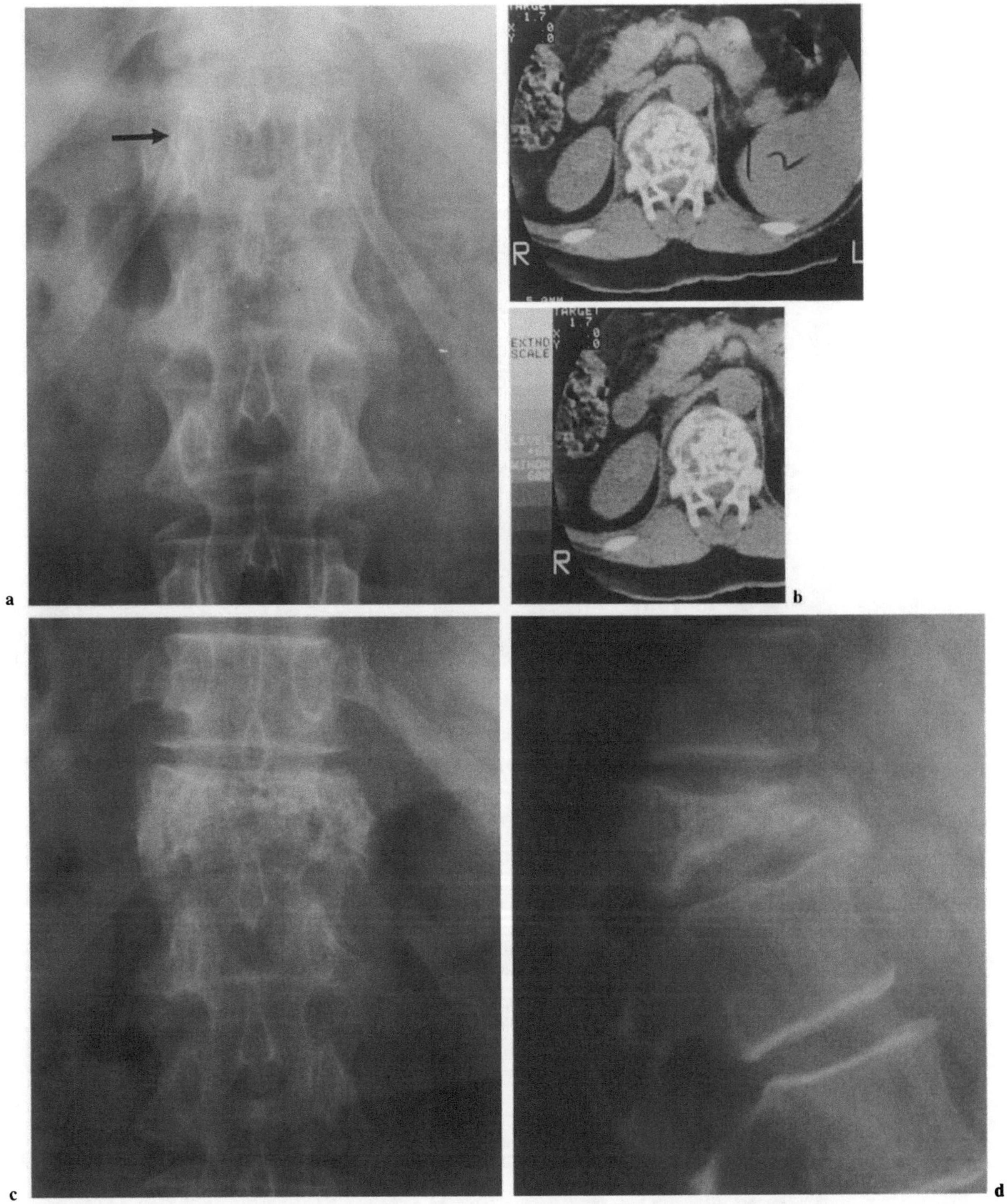

Fig. V.3a–d. Female, 45 years old. Hemangioma of twelfth dorsal vertebra. **a** Radiograph showing the typical longitudinal striation. **b** CT scan through the body of T12 reveals the characteristic punctate trabecular pattern. **c,d** Compression fracture causing pain and neurologic symptoms

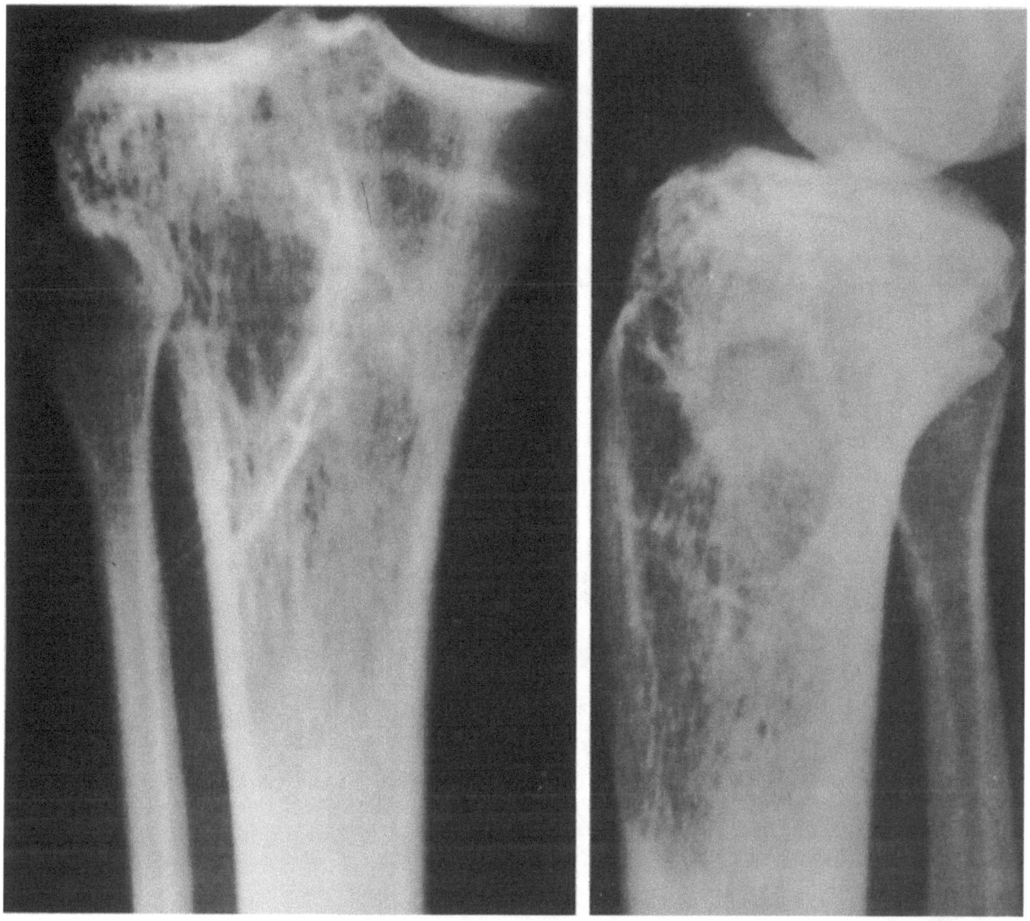

▲

Fig. V.4. Female, 51 years old. Hemangioma of the upper end of the tibia. Anteroposterior and lateral radiographs reveal a radiolucent ill-defined lesion, with coarse, mostly longitudinal trabeculation

Fig. V.5. Female, 20 years old. Hemangioma of the calcaneus. Radiograph shows osteolytic ill-defined multilocular lesion with coarse irregular trabeculation. (St. Louis University Medical Center) ▶

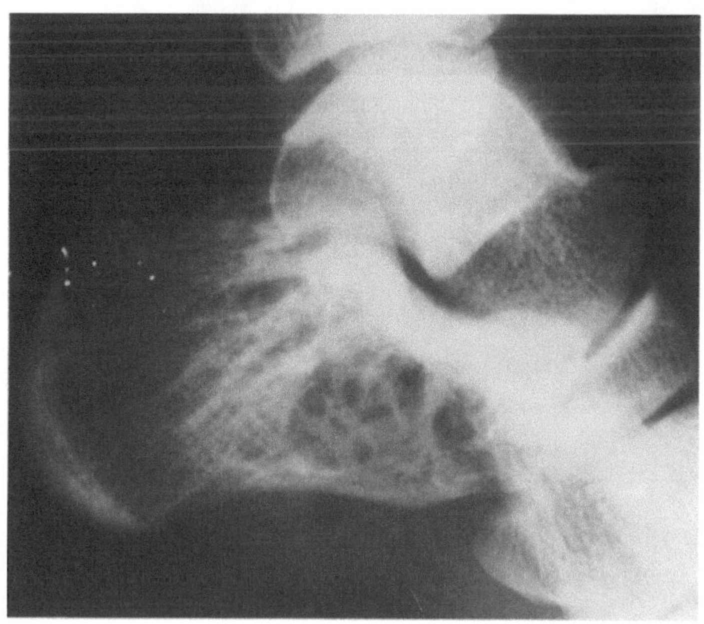

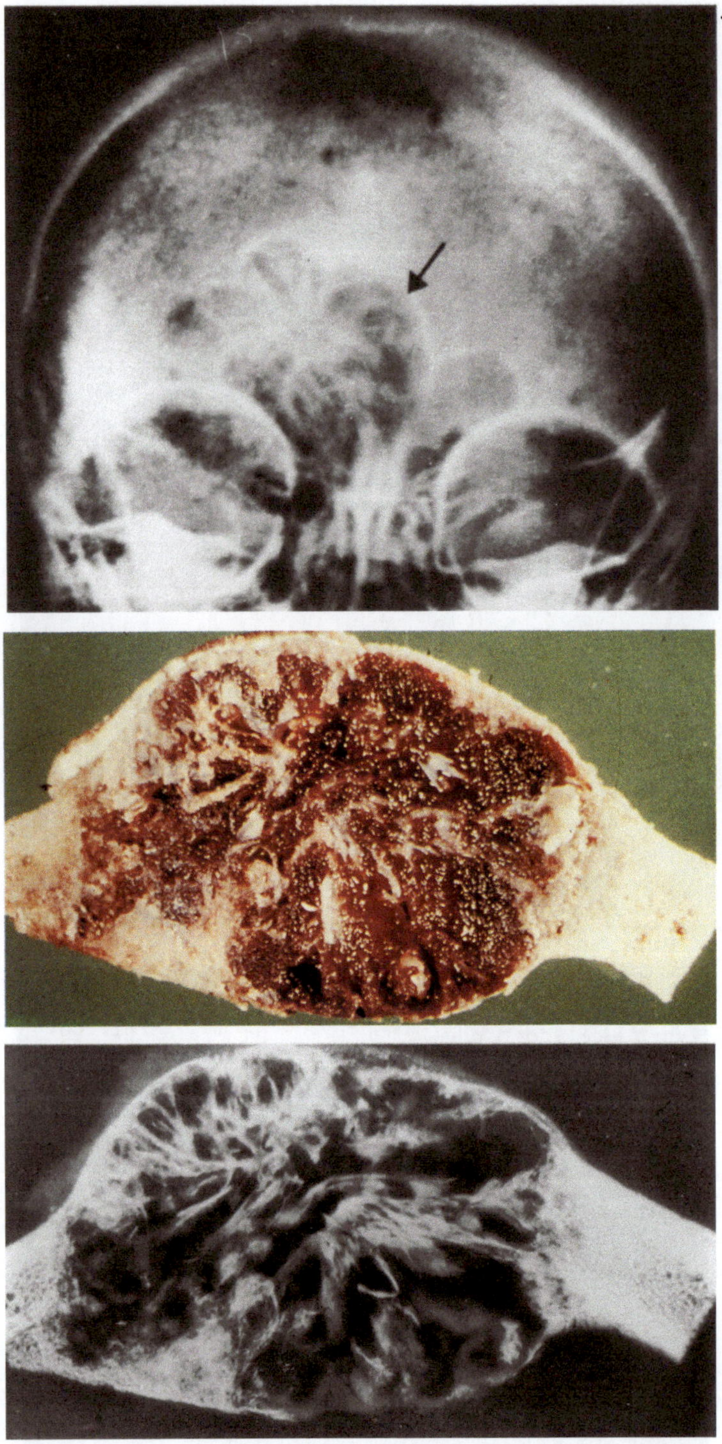

a

b

c

◀ **Fig. V.6a–c.** Female, 63 years old. Hemangioma of frontal bone. **a** Radiograph shows the sun-ray appearance of the lesion. **b** Photograph and **c** radiograph of the specimen demonstrate the highly vascular pattern of the lesion and the sun-ray appearance of the bony septa

Fig. V.7a,b. Female, 45 years old. Hemangioma of the skull. **a** Lateral radiograph reveals a lytic lesion of the frontal bone, expanding and thinning the outer table; radiating spicules are difficult to see in this radiograph, but are clearly noted in the radiographs of the specimen (**b**), which show the characteristic sunburst appearance ("sun-ray skull") ▶

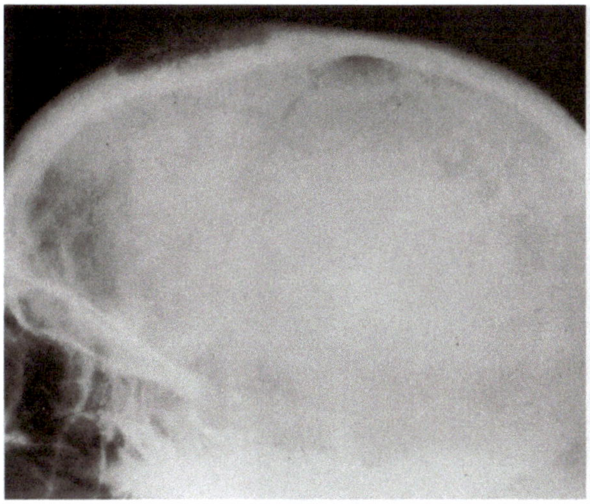

V.7a

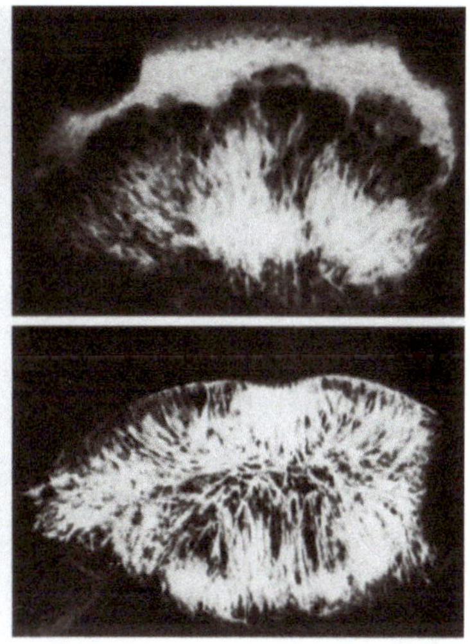

b

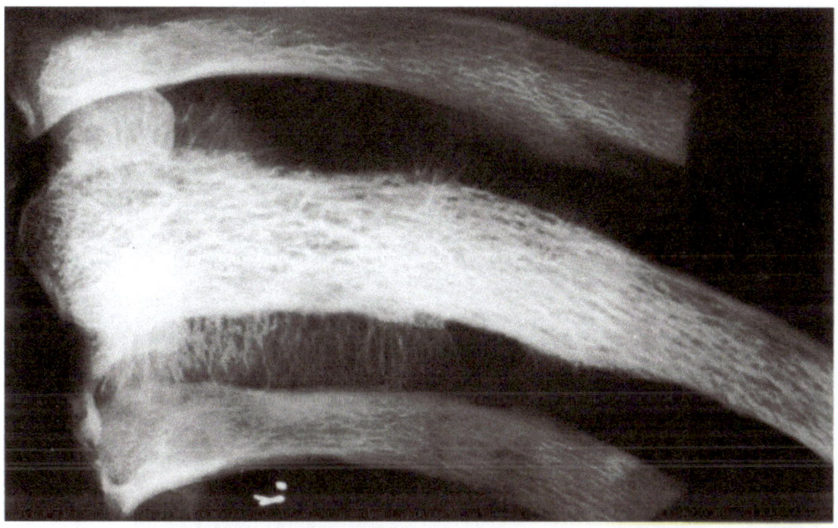

a

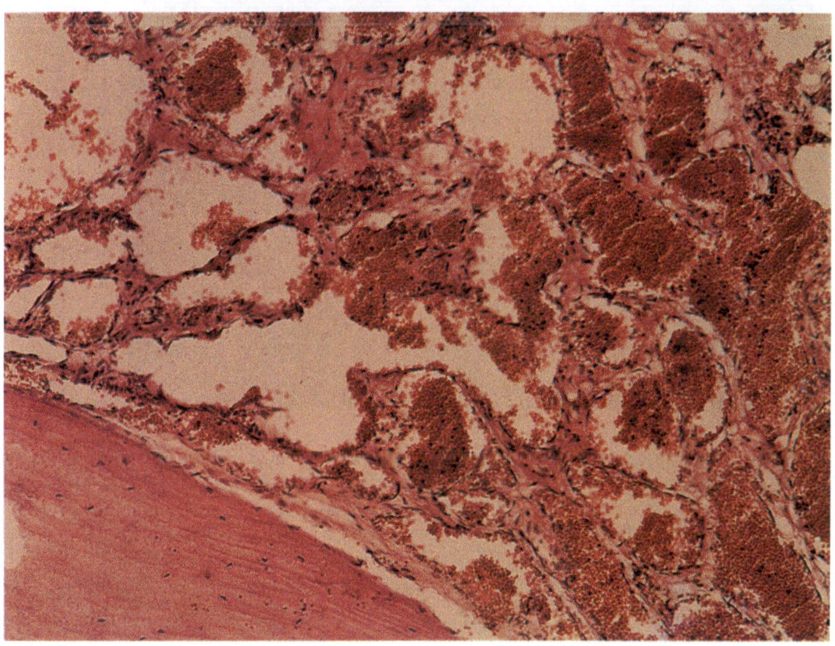

b

Fig. V.8a,b. Male, 25 years old. Hemangioma of rib. **a** Radiograph of the surgical specimen illustrates the characteristic thin bone spicules, perpendicular to the bone surface, and the honeycomb appearance of the spongiosa. **b** Photomicrograph showing dilated, blood-filled capillary vessels

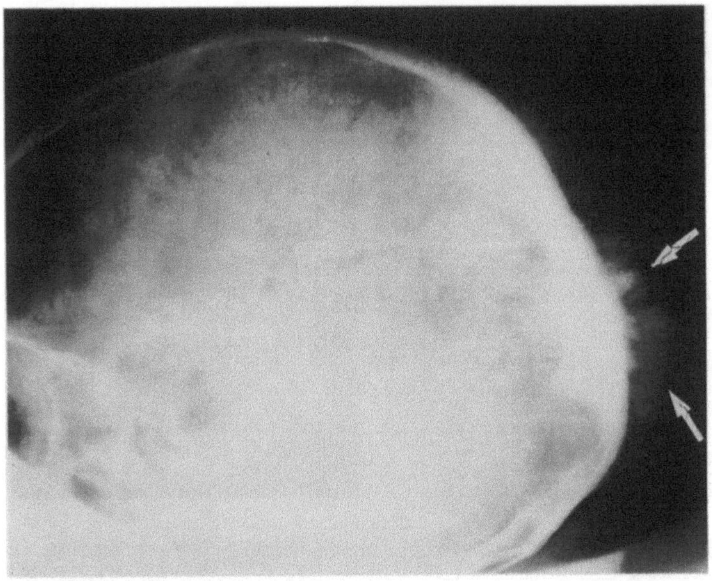

Fig. V.9. Male, 18 years old. Osteosarcoma of the skull. Radiograph illustrates perpendicular bone spicules in the occipital region, producing a similar sunburst appearance

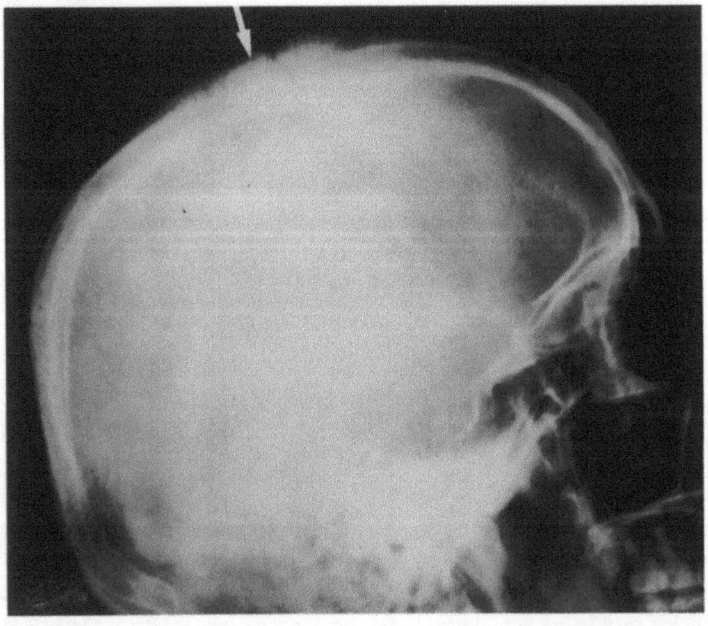

V.10a

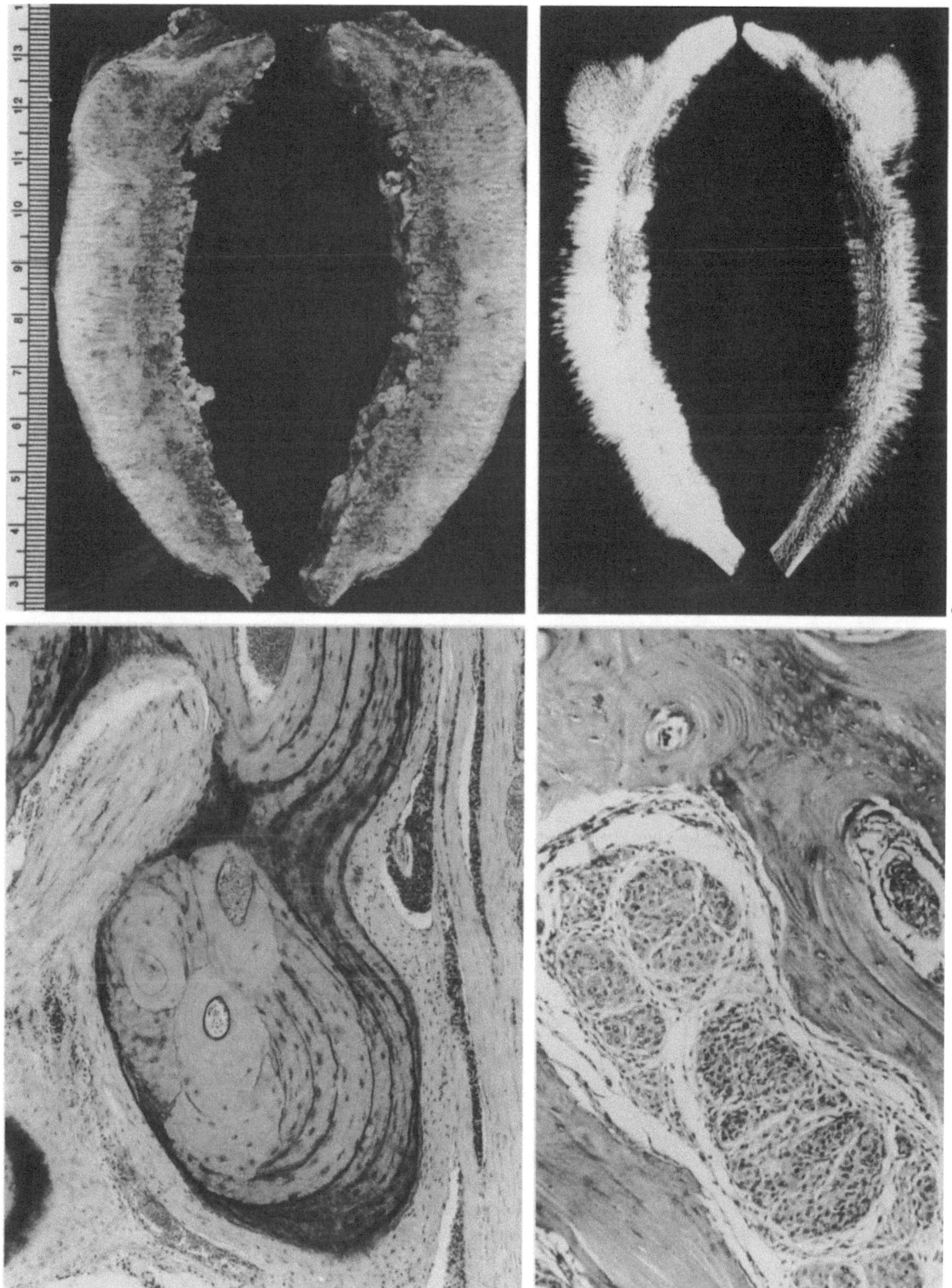

Fig. V.10a–e. Male, 52 years old. Meningioma with skull involvement. **a** Lateral radiograph shows bone spicules, with a sunburst pattern. **b** Photograph and **c** radiograph of the resected specimen show the enlarged and partially sclerotic skull with the evident sunburst appearance. **d**,**e** Photomicrographs at lower and higher magnification showing infiltration of the tumor between the enlarged bone trabeculae. **d** ×100, **e** ×200

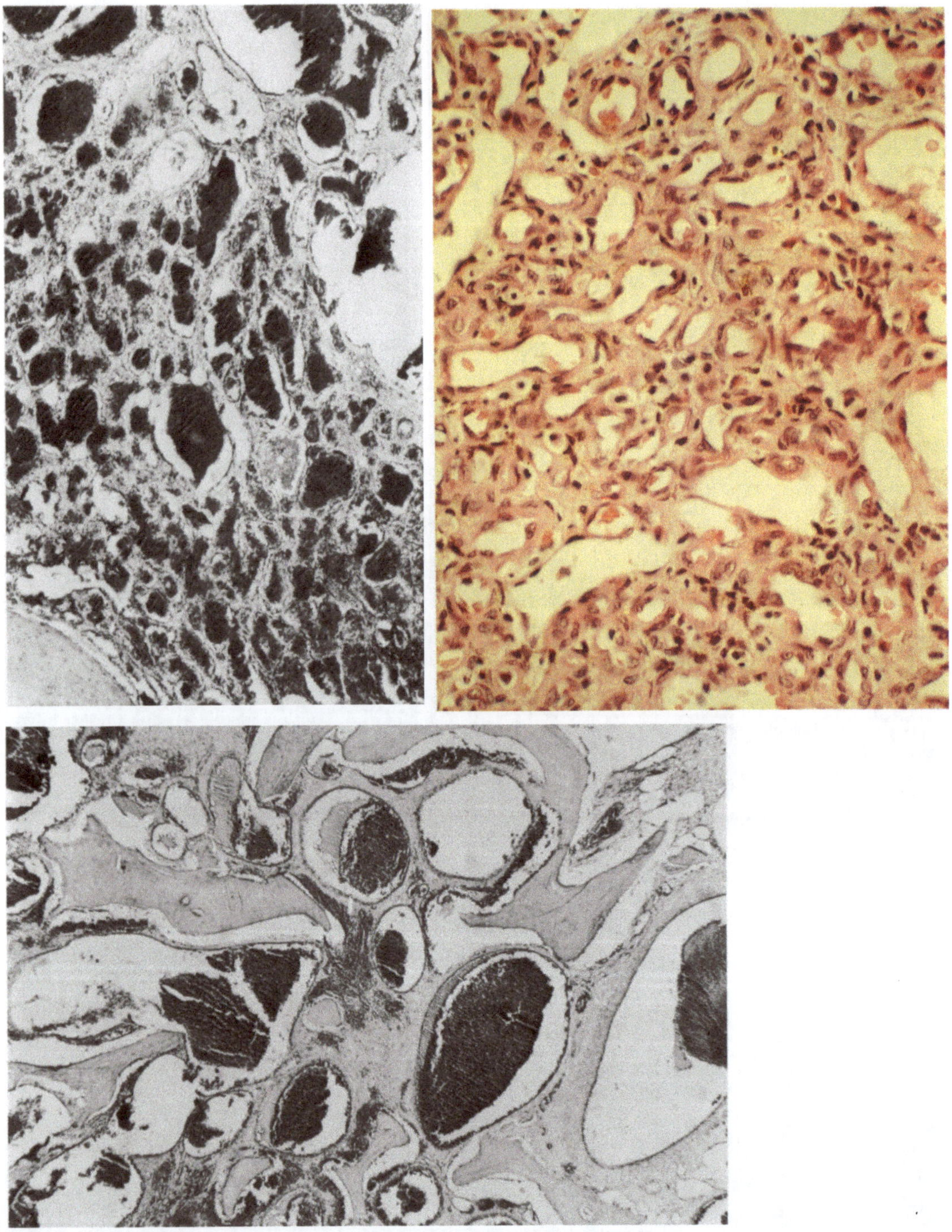

Fig. V.11a–c. Photomicrographs at lower (**a**,**b**) and higher (**c**) magnification showing the numerous thin-walled engorged blood vessels between the bone trabeculae. **a** and **b** are from the rib lesion and **c** from a calvarial hemangioma, which are generally of the cavernous type. **a**,**b** ×100, **c** ×250

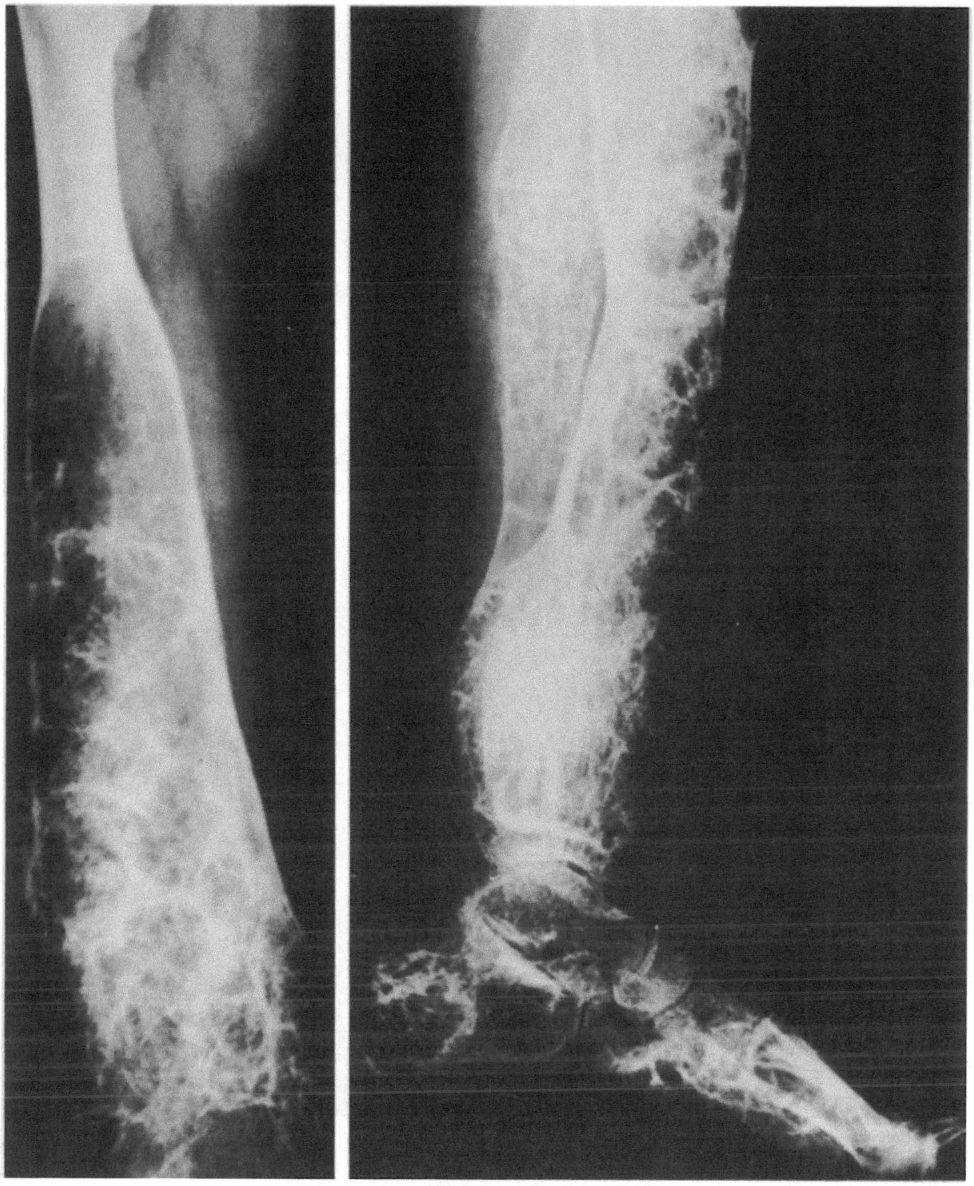

Fig. V.12. Hemangiomatosis of bone. Anteroposterior and lateral radiographs show extensive involvement of the entire shaft of the tibia and fibula, tarsal bones, and a great part of the femur with expansion of the bone, thinning of the cortices, and multiple radiolucent areas producing a honeycomb appearance

Hemangiomas may involve diffusely two or more bones of a single extremity or, rarely, several long, short, and flat bones, in which case it is classified as "diffuse skeletal hemangiomatosis" (Fig. V.12) (Singh et al. 1974; Ferretti et al. 1981). Patients with diffuse skeletal hemangiomatosis may develop intravascular coagulation (Kasabach-Merritt syndrome) (Lozman and Holmblad 1976). In our opinion, diffuse hemangiomatosis should be distinguished from "cystic angiomatosis" of bone because of their different radiologic and macroscopic aspects, and the better prognosis of the latter entity. Complete regression without any treatment is possible, although intermediate stages between both may exist.

Treatment. Hemangiomas of the vertebrae are often asymptomatic and do not require any treatment; some may undergo spontaneous regression with sclerotic reaction. In cases that cause pain or neurologic symptoms, surgical intervention (decompression and/or curettage) may be necessary, followed or not by radiotherapy.

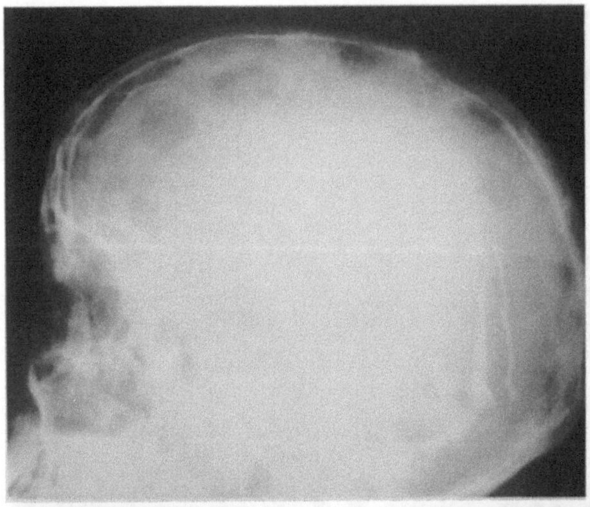
a

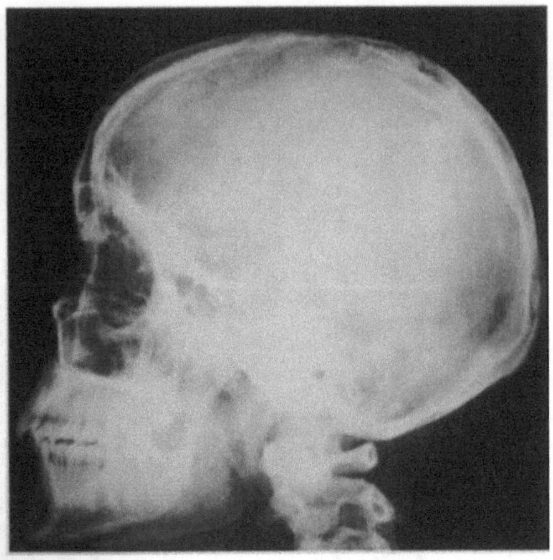
b

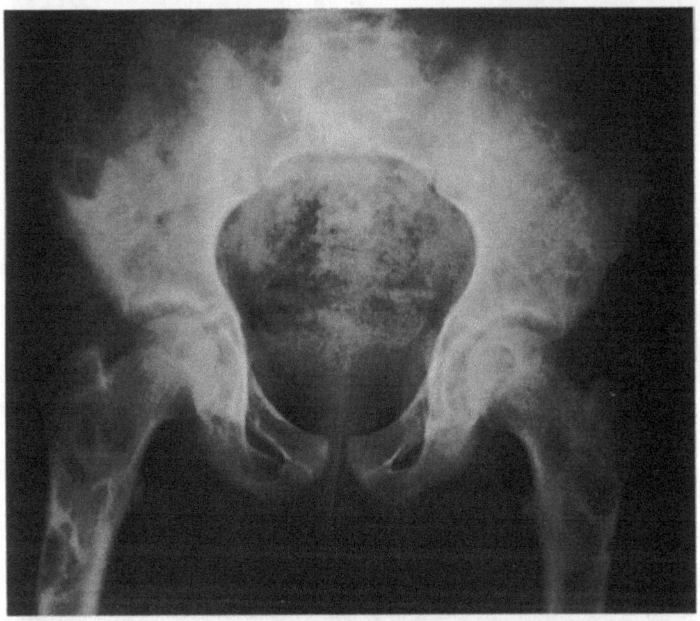
c

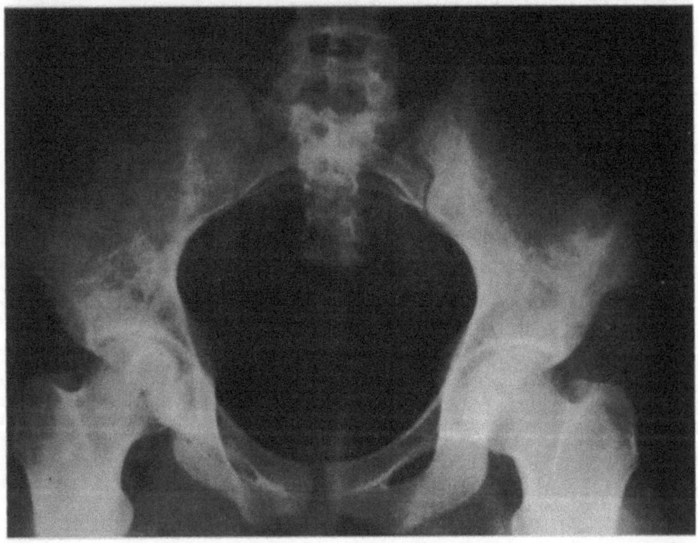
d

Fig. V.13a–g. Female, 15 years old. Cystic angiomatosis of bone. **a** Radiograph of the skull showing multiple cystic lesions of various sizes. **b** Seven years later, the cystic areas have almost completely disappeared without any treatment. **c** Initial radiograph showing numerous cystic lesions in the pelvis, femoral head, and uppermost third of the femur. **d** Seven years later, there has been regression with reduction or disappearance of almost all cysts. **e** Radiograph showing multiple cysts in several ribs, several of them slightly expanded. **f** Seven years later there was spontaneous regression of lesions. **g** Photograph and radiographs of a longitudinal section of the resected rib segment showing multiple confluent cystic lesions, in great part filled with blood. (Schajowicz et al. 1978)

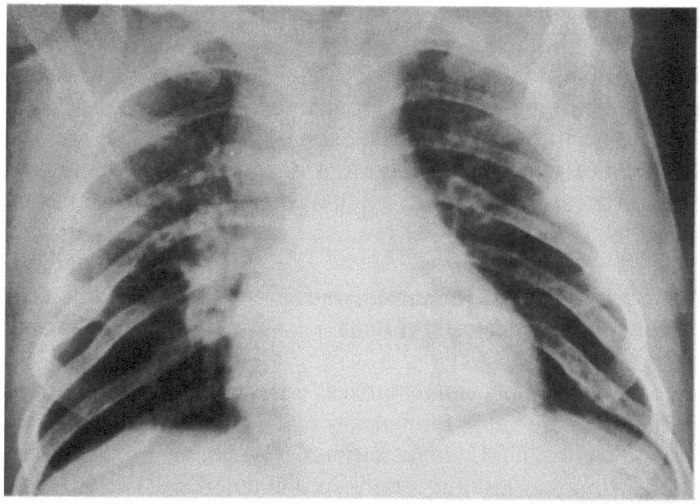
e

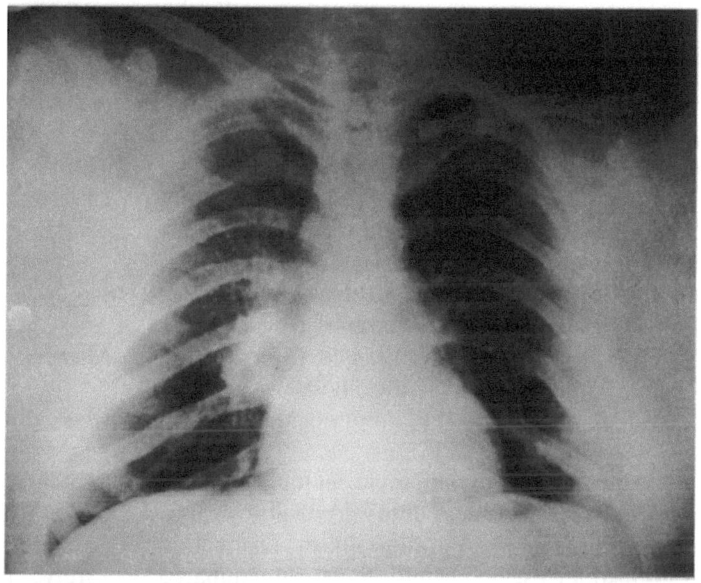
f

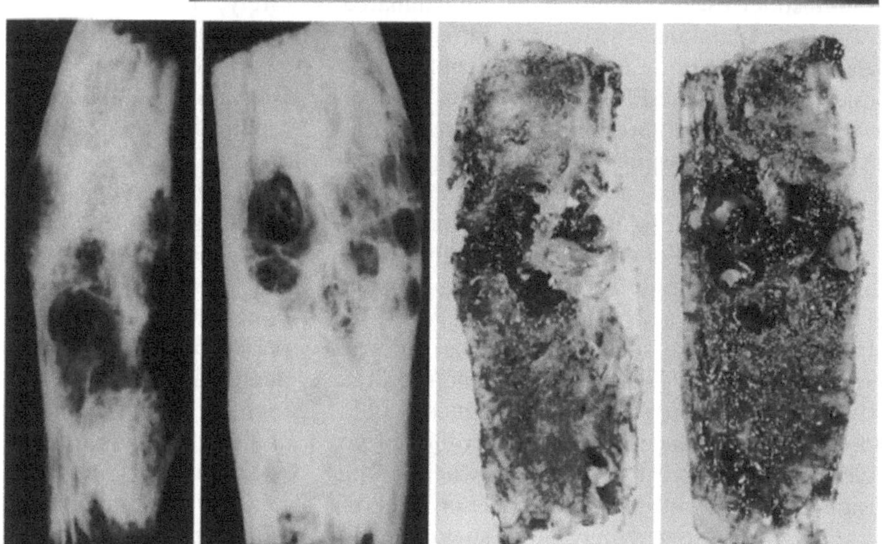
g

In some cases, roentgenotherapy may relieve pain and produce sclerosis of the lesion. Hemangiomas of the skull or long and short bones are best managed with en bloc resection of the lesions. In most of these locations, a biopsy may be necessary because it is often impossible to establish a correct diagnosis by other means.

Cystic Angiomatosis (Hamartomatous Hemolymphangiomatosis) of Bone

The name "cystic angiomatosis" of bone is applied to a rare but pathologically distinct entity, probably congenital, characterized by disseminated osteolytic lesions, often accompanied by angiomatous lesions of soft tissues, especially the spleen.

The process is more frequent in infants or young children during the first decade of life and tends to involve ribs, pelvis, femora, and skull, but only exceptionally the hands and feet. The radiologic features are characteristic, consisting in multiple roundish or ovoid cystic areas of different sizes, which are either sharply defined, often with slightly sclerotic borders, or confluent, giving a honeycombed appearance (this is especially common in the pelvis). In certain cases the cortex of some ribs or of the fibula was slightly expanded and thinned, but no periosteal reaction was observed (Fig. V.13).

The clinical and radiologic features make it possible to separate this entity from fibrous dysplasia and from hyperparathyroidism. Distinction from histiocytosis X (multiple or disseminated histiocytic granuloma with or without Hand-Schüller-Christian or Letterer-Siwe syndrome) is difficult (Parsons and Ebbs 1940). In fact, in all of our five cases, the presumptive diagnosis was histiocytosis X. Despite some radiographic differences, such as the lack of periosteal reaction in the long bone lesions (a frequent finding in histiocytosis X), the diagnosis must always be confirmed by histologic examination of a segment of affected bone, a rib (Figs. V.13g, V.14) or fibula being most convenient for this purpose (Schajowicz et al. 1978). With a puncture or a simple surgical biopsy, a definite diagnosis could not be made in the great majority of reported cases. It is important to establish whether the lesion involves only the skeleton, as in three of our five cases, or whether soft tissues are also involved, especially viscera; in the reported cases, the spleen has been most affected. Contrary to the often fatal evolution of these lesions, the prognosis is more favorable when the skeleton alone is affected or when there is only an associated subcutaneous soft tissue tumor (lymphangioma or hemangioma). In these cases, spontaneous regression of the cystic bone lesion may occur, as happened in some reported cases (Boyle 1972; Spjut and Lindbom 1962) and in two of our patients. For this reason, it is important to be familiar with the clinical, radiologic, and pathologic features of "cystic angiomatosis" in order to avoid unnecessary treatment. Splenectomy is, however, of value if the spleen alone among the viscera is affected (Ritchie and Zier 1956).

The term "cystic angiomatosis of bone" is preferred by us and most authors (Gramiak et al. 1957; Jacobs and Kimmelstiel 1953; Moseley and Starobin 1964) because in some cases a lymphangioma of the subcutaneous tissue and a hemangioma of the rib and tibia may coexist – as in one of our cases – or because blood vessels and lymphatics may be seen in the same lesion. The pathogenesis of this entity is still under discussion; we believe that the hypothesis of a multicentric congenital malformation – that is, a vascular hamartoma – is the most acceptable one.

Massive Osteolysis

Massive osteolysis, also called "disappearing bone," "phantom bone," or "Gorham's disease," is a rare progressive destructive disease of bone, probably caused by multiple or diffuse cavernous hemangiomas or lymphangiomas in bones, or rarely, by a combination of both. In 1954, Gorham et al. established massive osteolysis as a distinct clinical symptom, and 1 year later, Gorham and Stout (1955), in a summary of 24 reported cases, several of them histologically proven (Johnson and McClure 1958), showed that the histologic basis of the syndrome was angiomatosis of bone.

Massive osteolysis begins insidiously and is characterized by a progressive regional loss of bone with resultant deformity. After a variable period of activity, it generally undergoes spontaneous arrest, but exceptionally may progress rapidly, terminating fatally less than 2 years after clinical onset (Gorham et al. 1954; Hambach et al. 1958).

The great majority of patients are children or young adults. There is no evidence of genetic transmission or sex predilection.

The disease has a propensity for involvement of the shoulder girdle and the pelvis, with resorp-

Fig. V.14a–c. Photomicrographs showing at lower and higher magnification bone trabeculae separated by multiple large cystic spaces with a flattened endothelial layer, partly empty and partly occupied by red blood cells (Schajowicz et al. 1978). **a** ×55, **b** ×100, **c** ×100

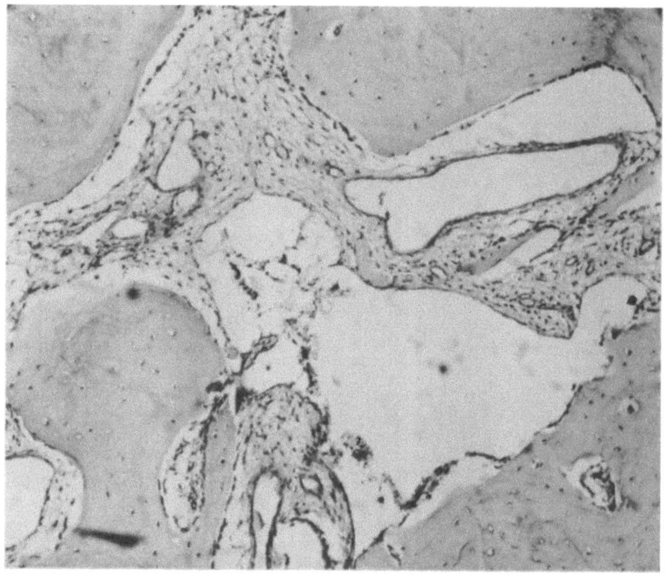

a

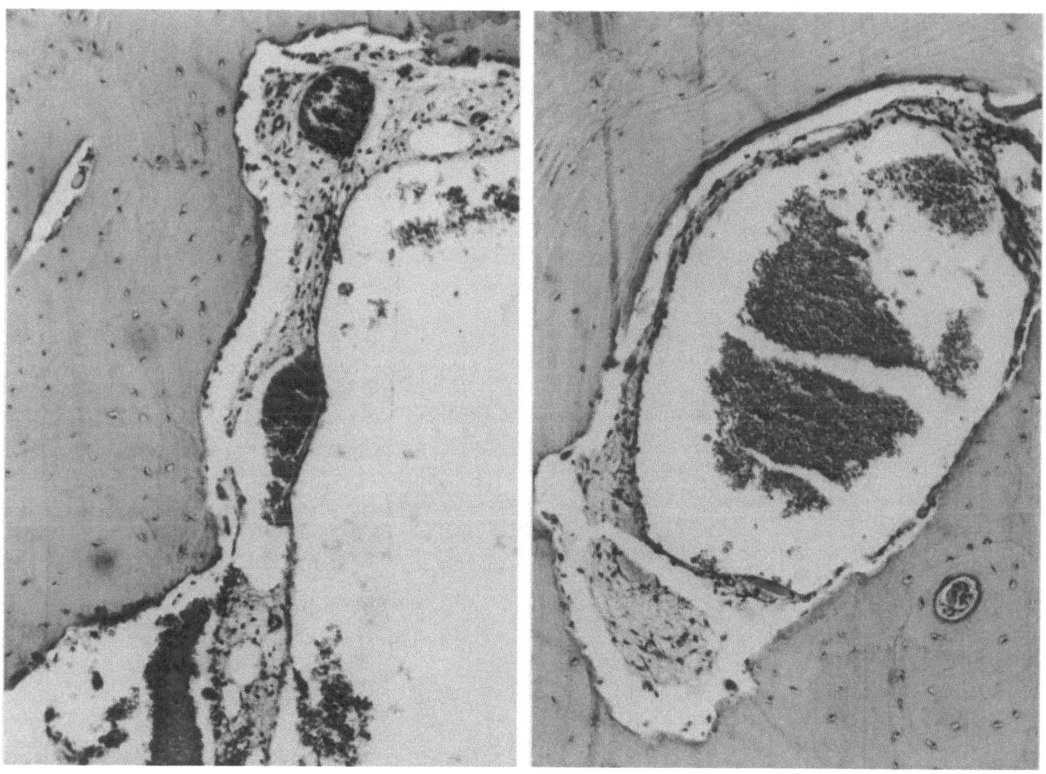

b c

tion of the proximal part of the humerus, clavicle, and scapula, or dissolution of the ilium, ischium, and part of the sacrum or upper femoral end (Sage and Allen 1974; Thompson and Schurman 1974; Heyden et al. 1977; Edwards et al. 1983; Cannon 1986; Choma et al. 1987).

The pathologic findings in the relatively few cases studied histologically include a marked increase in intraosseous capillaries, forming an anastomosing network of endothelium-lined channels, usually filled with red blood cells or serum; if they are empty, it is possible that these channels are lymphangiomas rather than hemangiomas. The case reported by Bickel and Broders (1947) as "primary lymphangioma of the ilium," in which there was progressive dissolution of the ilium, ischium, and parts of the vertebra, is evidently an example of "massive osteolysis."

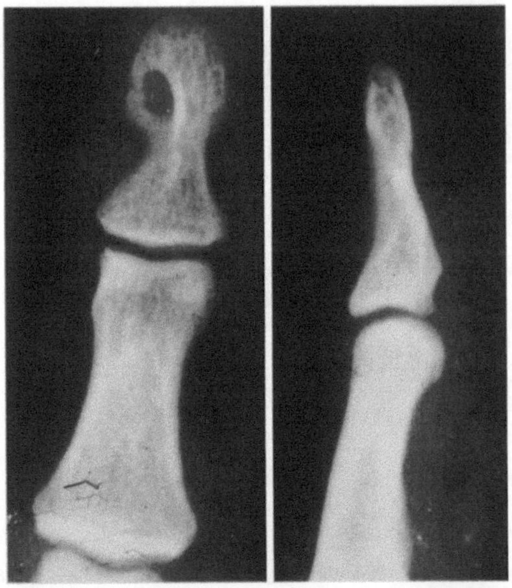

a

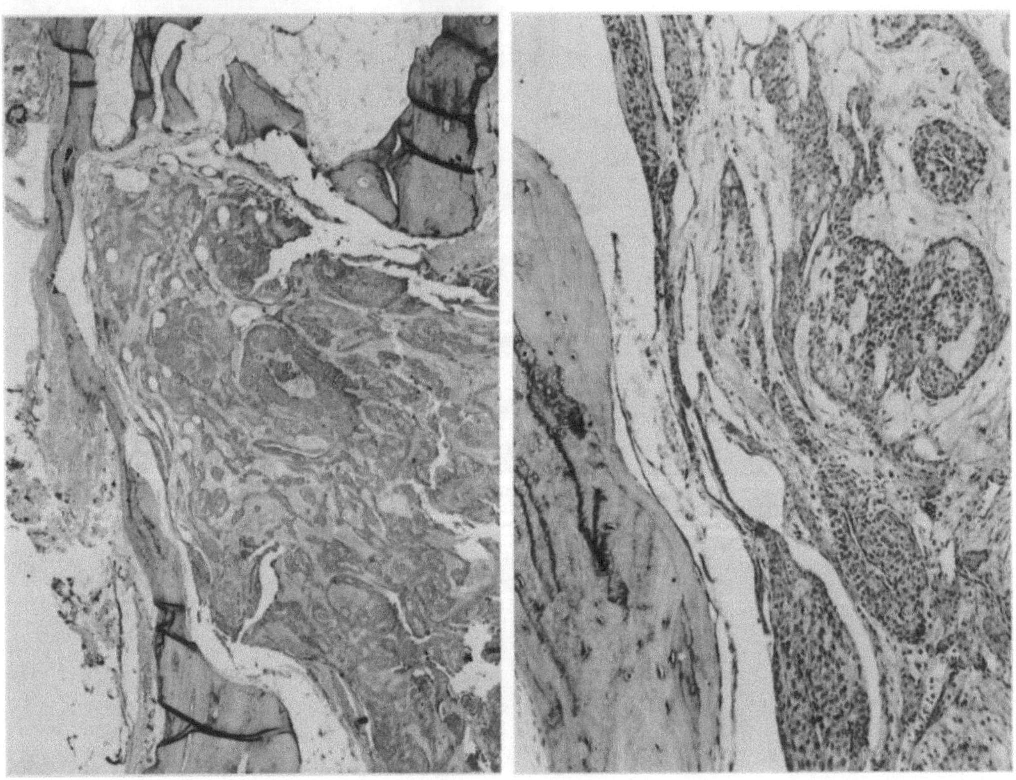

b c

Fig. V.15a–c. Male, 30 years old. Glomus tumor of terminal phalanx. **a** Anteroposterior and lateral radiographs show a cystic lesion, with a well-defined border, within the medullary cavity. **b,c** Photomicrographs illustrate at lower and higher magnification the intraosseous location of the tumor, which has thinned the cortex in **a** and is characterized by lobules and strands of cells showing a conspicuous perithelial pattern. **b** ×100, **c** ×200

2. Lymphangioma

Definition, WHO: *"A benign lesion consisting of newly formed lymph vessels, usually in the form of dilated cystic spaces."*

The presence of intraosseous lymphatics was denied in the past, but is now generally accepted. Their presence was demonstrated after the introduction of lymphangiography (Nixon 1970).

Proliferations of lymphatic vessels arising inside bone are extremely rare and are more frequently diffuse or multiple (Rosenquist and Wolfe 1958; Cohen and Craig 1955). Only exceptional solitary lymphangiomas have been reported (Falkner and Tilling 1956; Bullough and Goodfellow 1976; Jumbelic et al. 1984). Lichtenstein (1977) illustrated another case located on the tibial shaft. Some of the multiple lymphangiomas have been reported under the term "cystic angiomatosis," and as we mentioned previously, a combination of lymphatic and blood vessels may coexist in this entity (Schajowicz et al. 1978). Multiple or solitary lymphangiomas are probably not true neoplasms but rather vascular malformations (hamartomas).

3. Glomus Tumor (Glomangioma)

Definition, WHO: *"A benign lesion consisting of lobules and strands of rounded uniform cells intimately associated with vascular structures showing a perithelial pattern, and probably derived from the neuromyoarterial glomus"* (Masson 1935).

Glomus tumors arising within bone are extremely rare. Only isolated cases have been reported, almost all located in a terminal phalanx (Lattes and Bull 1948; Lehman and Kraissl 1949; Mackenzie 1962; Siegel 1967; Sugiura 1976; Chan 1981; Vetrani et al. 1982). Lichtenstein mentioned two cases in his book (1977) and Dahlin (1978) reported another similar case. Exceptionally the lesion was located in the pubis (Tang et al. 1976), middle phalanx (Bjorkengren et al. 1986), and coccyx (Pambakian and Smith 1981).

The writer has also studied two such cases (Schajowicz et al. 1970) (Fig. V.15). It is sometimes difficult to exclude the possibility of secondary erosion of bone by a glomus tumor originating in the adjacent soft tissues, which is more common.

Glomus tumors are always associated with severe pain; the primary intraosseous lesions have the radiologic appearance of an osteolytic well-delineated lesion, which may expand the thinned cortex slightly, without periosteal reaction, and which is invariably located in a terminal phalanx. Excision of the lesion is curative.

B. Intermediate or Indeterminate

Malignant bone tumors of unquestionable vascular origin are rare, and no center dedicated to the treatment of bone lesions has in its files an appreciable number of cases. In contrast, poorly differentiated, especially telangiectatic osteosarcomas are not infrequently classified as hemangiosarcomas. The nomenclature and definitions of malignant vascular tumors used in textbooks and other publications are confusing; the terms hemangiosarcoma, angiosarcoma, hemangioendothelioma, and malignant hemangioendothelioma have been used as synonyms (Jaffe 1958; Dahlin 1978) and only exceptionally to indicate separate pathologic entities with different clinical behaviors (Thomas 1942). Most authors have followed the criteria of Stout, who in 1943 described hemangioendothelioma as a tumor of blood vessels that exhibits (a) formation of atypical endothelial cells in greater numbers than are required to line the vessels with a simple endothelial membrane and (b) formation of vascular tubes with a delicate framework of reticulin fibers and a tendency for their lumens to anastomose. Most authors prefer to call all malignant vascular tumors "hemangioendothelioma" (Unni et al. 1971; Lichtenstein 1977; Dahlin 1978), using the term "angiosarcoma" as a synonym (Jaffe 1958; Spjut et al. 1971; Dahlin and Unni 1986). However, Unni et al. (1971) divided hemangioendothelioma into three different histologic grades, which seem to be related to prognosis, although they agree that grading is not easy and is "at best an approximation." A similar approach is followed by Campanacci et al. (1980). On the other hand, Dorfman et al. (1971) applied the term "hemangioendothelial sarcoma" to all malignant vascular tumors, which they divided into poorly differentiated (angiosarcoma) and well-differentiated types (hemangioendothelioma) with different clinical behavior, the latter having a better prognosis. Wold (1982a), in collaboration with his associates of the Mayo Clinic (see Dahlin and Unni 1986), likewise used the term "hemangioendothelial sarcoma" for all malignant vascular tumors, clearly illustrating the confusion in the literature. However, hemangiopericytoma originating in bone, which is extremely rare, is considered a distinct entity in all reports.

In view of the still-prevailing confusion in the nomenclature of vascular tumors, in its recent revision the WHO classification system continues to separate these lesions into *benign*, *intermediate or indeterminate* (which includes *hemangioendothelioma* and the rare *hemangiopericytoma*), and the *clearly malignant*, more anaplastic type, *angiosarcoma*. However, a clear distinction between these different vascular tumors may sometimes be difficult, especially between some capillary hemangiomas and well-differentiated hemangioendotheliomas. An indisputable case of primary lymphangiosarcoma in bone has not yet been reported.

1. Hemangioendothelioma

Definition, WHO: *"An aggressive, but virtually non-metastasizing tumor characterized by the presence of solid cell cords and vascular endothelial structures. The cells are often prominent and plump, but the frankly malignant features of angiosarcoma are lacking."*

Incidence. Hemangioendothelioma as defined by the WHO corresponds to the well-differentiated type of hemangioendothelial sarcoma of Dorfman et al. (1971) and to grade I and some grade II hemangioendotheliomas (angiosarcomas) of Unni et al. (1971) and Dahlin and Unni (1986). It was referred to as "histiocytoid hemangioma" by Rosai et al. in 1979, but more recently the term "epithelioid hemangioendothelioma" has been preferred by most authors (Weiss and Enzinger 1982; Maruyama et al. 1985; Tsuneyoshi et al. 1986; Martínez-Tello et al. 1989).

Hemangioendothelioma is a rare tumor: Only 15 cases have been recorded in our files, accounting for 0.63% of all primary malignant tumors. Dorfman et al. (1971) observed ten cases among 15 malignant vascular tumors of bone over a 40-year period.

It is difficult to determine the exact incidence of what we classify as "hemangioendothelioma," because in most publications all malignant vascular tumors, except hemangiopericytoma, are grouped together under the heading "hemangioendothelioma" (Otis et al. 1968; Dahlin 1978; Campanacci et al. 1980; Volpe and Mazabraud 1982; Dahlin and Unni 1986) or angiosarcoma (Jaffe 1958; Spjut et al. 1971).

Otis et al. (1968) found only 12 cases in the files of the Memorial Cancer Center (New York), including four previously published by Hartmann and Stewart (1962). In a later publication, 39 hemangioendotheliomas with unifocal (solitary) and ten with multifocal bone involvement were reported from the Memorial Hospital (Huvos 1991). Dahlin and Unni (1986) reported 60 cases, which represent less than 1% of malignant bone tumors in the Mayo Clinic series. In the series of 626 malignant primary bone lesions reported by the Netherlands Committee on Bone Tumors, there were seven cases of malignant vascular tumors (1%), and among 696 malignant bone tumors diagnosed during an 11-year period by the Swedish Cancer Registry, six were classified as malignant hemangioendothelioma (Larsson et al. 1975). In a review of the literature, Srinivasan et al. (1978) found 87 cases, adding two new ones.

Clinical Findings. About 65% of patients have been males, and no predilection for a particular

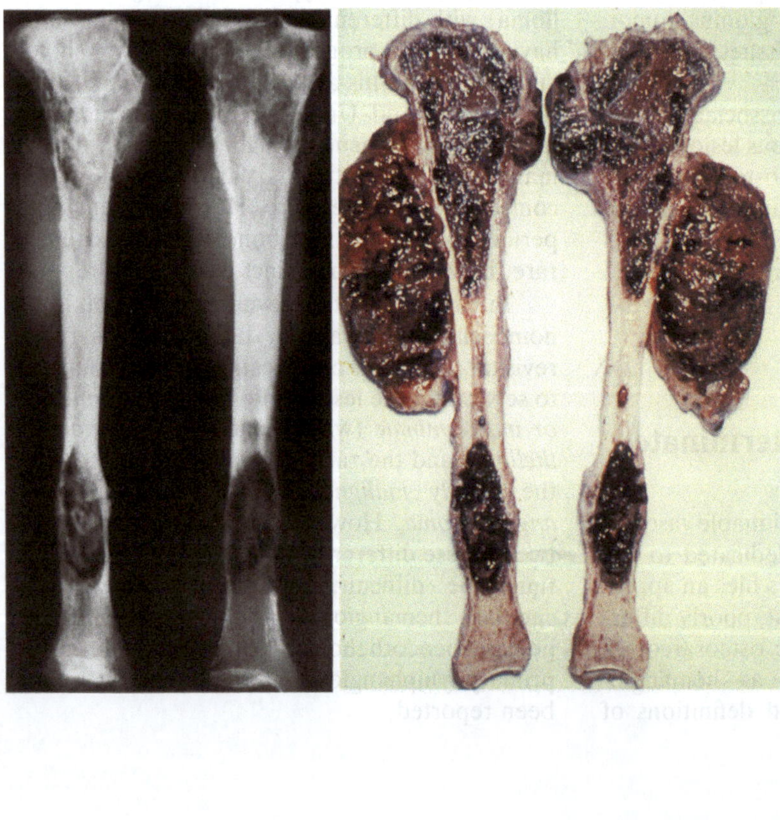

a b

Fig. V.16a,b. Male, 63 years old. Hemangioendothelioma with multiple lesions in the tibia and femur of the same limb. **a** Photograph and **b** radiograph of the amputation specimen. The histologic features of this case are shown in Fig. V.23 and correspond to the type referred to as "myxoid angioblastoma" by Mirra. (Schajowicz et al. 1972)

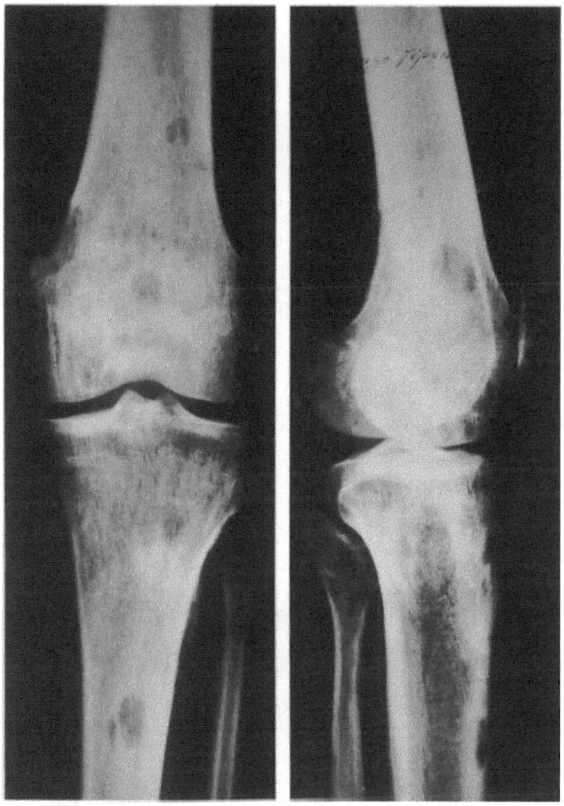

Fig. V.17. Male, 66 years old. Hemangioendothelioma with multiple lesions. Anteroposterior and lateral radiographs illustrate multiple cystic lesions of different sizes in tibia and femur

age group has been reported, which agrees with our experience. Due to the rarity of this group of well-differentiated tumors, it is difficult to give figures of statistical value about preferred localization or age. However, it seems that, as with age, any skeletal region may be affected, though with a preference for long tubular and pelvic bones. In our files, 15 cases were classified as hemangioendothelioma: seven were located in the tibia, two in the femur, one in the fibula, and one in the humerus. The remaining cases were located in different short bones, including one in the patella.

Like other vascular tumors, hemangioendothelioma may be multifocal (pluricentric). Multifocality was observed in four of our cases and in three of the ten cases of Dorfman's et al. series (1971). Dahlin (1978) mentioned that multifocality occurred in one-third of his cases; multiple foci were often limited to a single or several bones of the same extremity (Figs. V.16, V.17), as was also true in the ten multifocal cases in the series of Huvos.

Symptoms. Most patients complained of pain and/or swelling, sometimes accompanied by hemorrhagic joint effusion, which was the initial symptom in one of our cases located in the patella (Fig. V.18). Radiographically, the lesions were osteolytic, sometimes well delineated and sometimes permeative. In some cases, a trabeculated or honeycombed pattern was observed (Fig. V.19), and the cortex was expanded or partially destroyed, without evident periosteal reaction in most cases. In several cases, it was difficult to establish radiographically whether the tumor was benign or malignant. In one case the tumor was of apparently periosteal origin (Fig. V.20).

Pathologic Findings. The lesion has a typical *gross appearance* characterized by a dark red, hemorrhagic soft mass that is often well circumscribed or shows irregular margins. Other smaller foci may occasionally be observed in the medullary cavity of the same bone, but they are only sometimes visible radiographically. The tumor tissue, which may be traversed by some septa of reactive bone trabeculae, in some cases destroyed the cortex, penetrating extensively into the surrounding soft tissues (Fig. V.16). In the case located in the patella, the whole bone was involved with slight expansion and partial erosion of the cortex, penetrating into the synovial membrane and producing a hypertrophic, hemorrhagic synovitis (Fig. V.18).

Histologically, the vasoformative character of the tumor is clearly visible, showing all stages of evolution from solid cell cords to the formation of small, capillary-type blood vessels with prominent endothelial cells, commonly pleomorphic or of cubical to cylindrical shape (Figs. V.21, V.22). The prominent endothelial cells frequently show papillary intravascular projections, often with epithelial-like or histiocytelike features, exhibiting eosinophilic, sometimes vacuolated cytoplasm ("histiocytoid hemangioma" or "epithelioid endothelioma"). These areas may alternate with numerous, often dilated cavernous capillaries with flattened endothelia (Fig. V.23). Silver stains for reticulin fibers are of utmost importance in determining whether the cells are proliferating inside the vessel wall, as in hemangioendothelioma, or outside the vessel wall, which is characteristic of hemangiopericytoma (Fig. V.24). The stromal cells between the newly formed vessels are spindle shaped and usually do not show the atypical features of angiosarcoma, i.e., nuclear hyperchromatism,

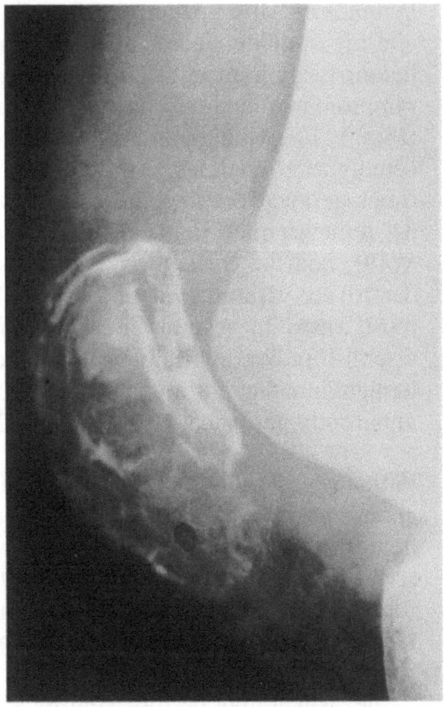

a

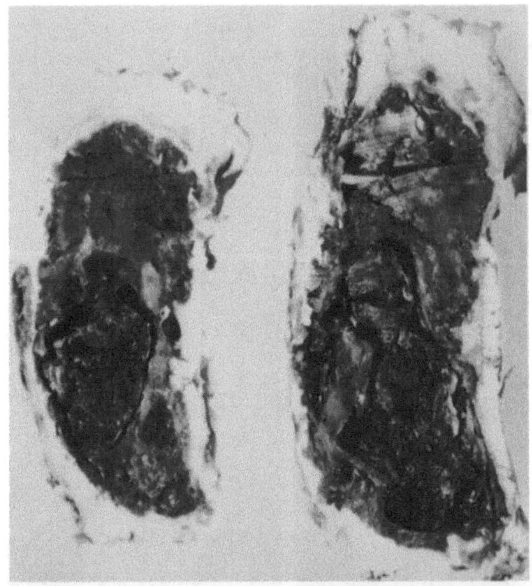

b

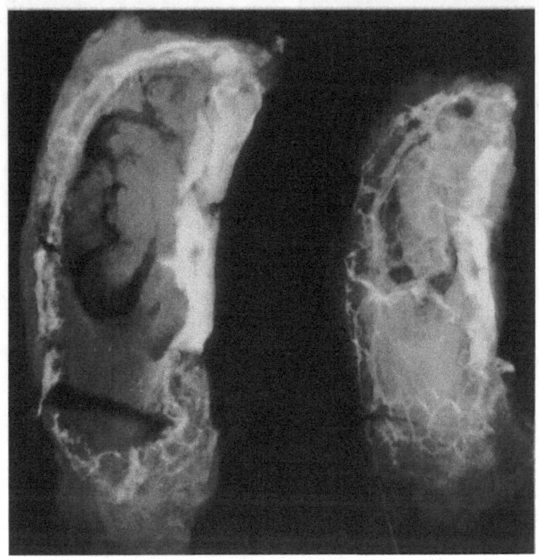

c

Fig. V.18a–c. Female, 13 years old. Hemangioendothelioma of patella. **a** Radiograph illustrates an osteolytic honeycombed lesion involving almost the entire patella. **b** Photograph and **c** radiograph of the excised patella show the dark red, hemorrhagic appearance of this osteolytic trabeculated lesion. The patient was well 5 years after excision of the patella and part of the synovial membrane, which was involved by the tumor

pleomorphism, and evident mitotic activity. The stroma may show an evident inflammatory reaction with prominent eosinophilia. A conspicuous myxoid stroma may be present; these cases have been referred to as "myxoid angioblastoma" (Mirra and Kameda 1985) and can be mistaken for "myxoid chondrosarcoma" (Fig. V.23). However, we want to emphasize that occasionally in some areas transitional stages between clearly well-differentiated types and highly anaplastic lesions may be found, making the exact categorization of some tumors difficult.

In cases in which the proliferation and hypertrophy and/or intravascular tufting of the endothelial cells are not conspicuous in part of the tumor, it may be difficult to distinguish capillary hemangioma from well-differentiated hemangioendothelioma. It is therefore important for the pathologist to examine as many tissue fragments of different areas as possible, in order to discover the characteristic histologic features.

Vascular tumors are characteristically bone-destroying lesions, and only scarce reactive bone formation is found in malignant tumors. Direct bone or osteoid formation by the tumor cells is never observed, nor are a conspicuous number of giant cells of osteoclast type associated with predominant vascular spaces. In the presence of such findings, the diagnosis is telangiectatic osteosarcoma or aneurysmal bone cyst, respectively,

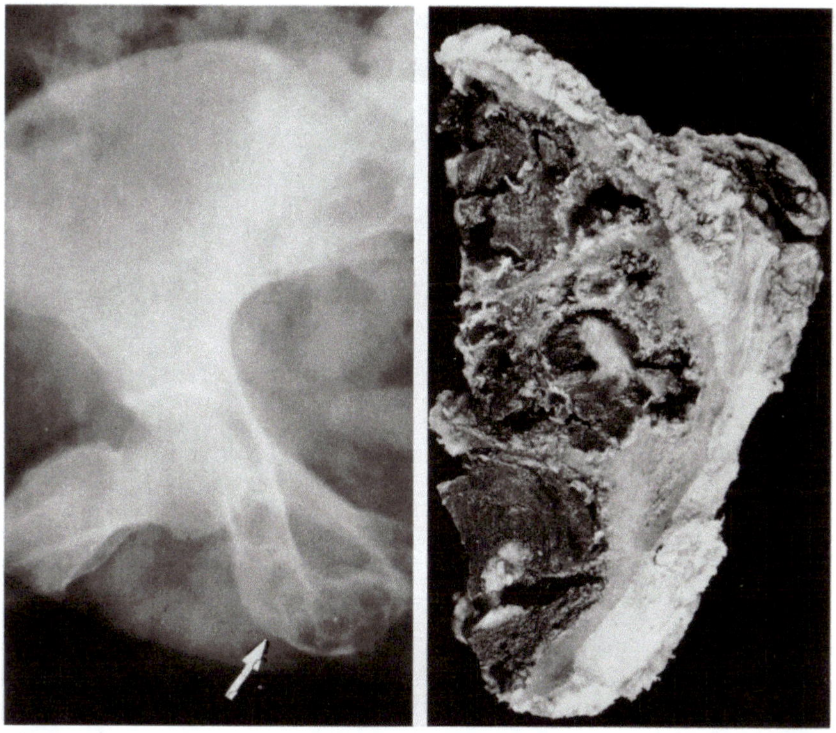

a b

Fig. V.19a,b. Female, 59 years old. Hemangioendothelioma of the ischium. **a** Radiograph shows a radiolucent, slightly expanding, multilocular lesion. **b** Photograph of the resected specimen reveals the vascular-hemorrhagic aspect

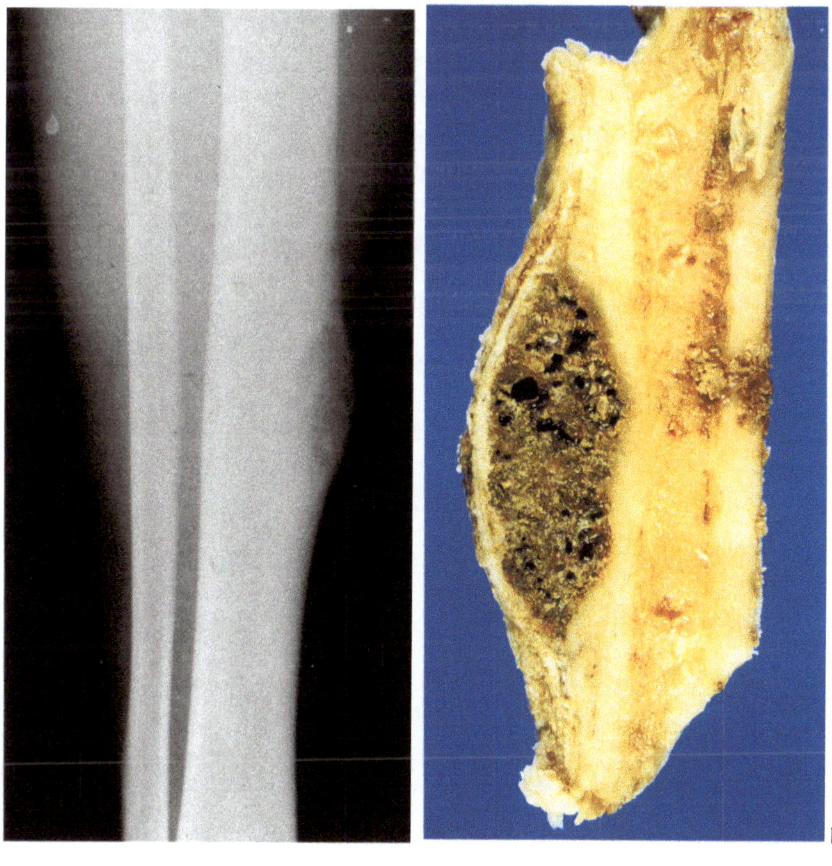

a b

Fig. V.20a,b. Female, 30 years old. Hemangioendothelioma of the tibia of probable periosteal origin. **a** Radiograph showing a radiolucent lesion of the diaphysis, which has expanded the thinned cortex and is covered by a thin shell of newly formed bone by the periosteum, as is seen in **b** a photograph of the specimen resected en bloc. The hemorrhagic tumor erodes the cortex, but does not penetrate into the medullary canal

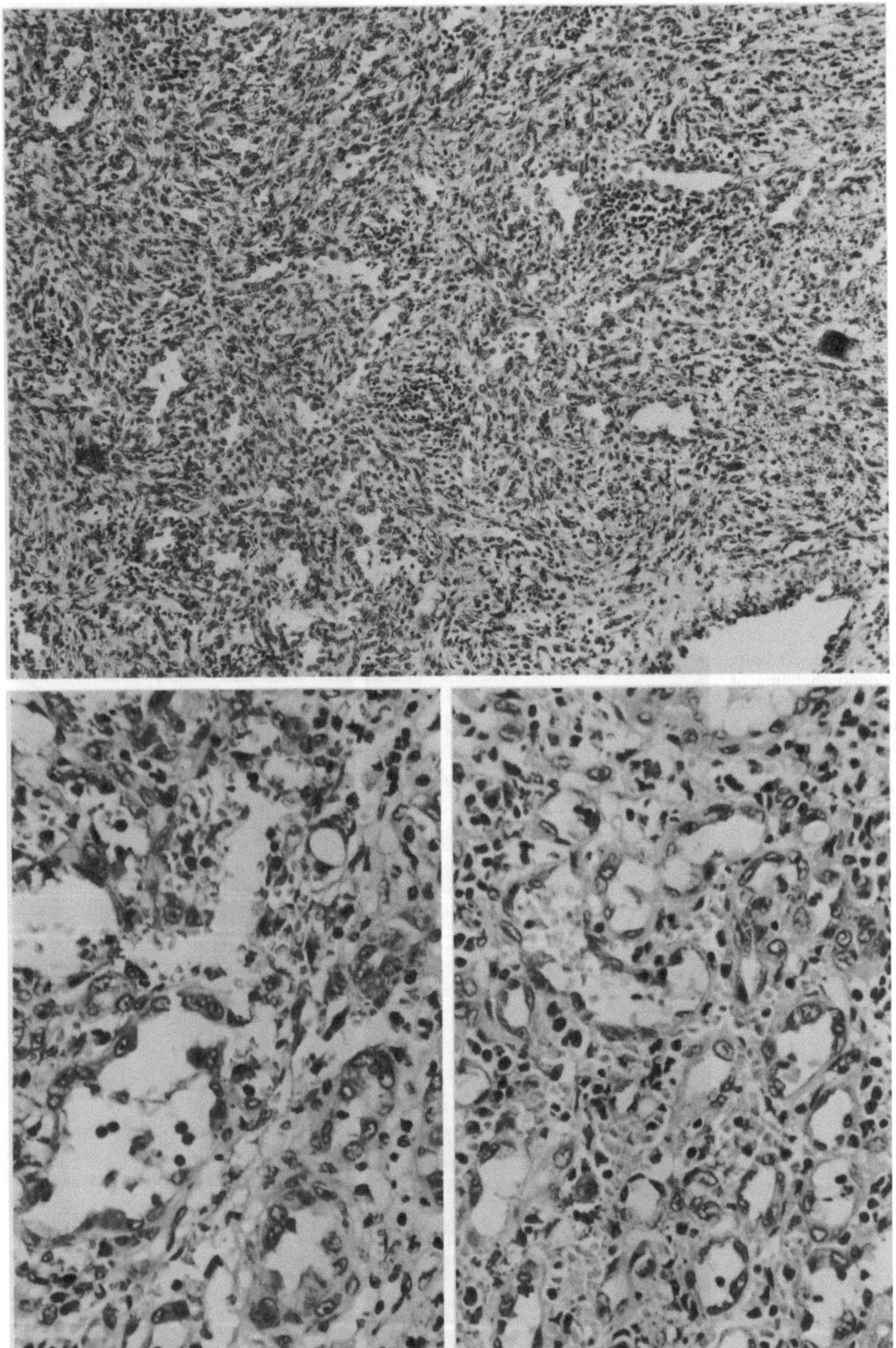

a

b

c

Fig. V.21a–c. Photomicrographs of hemangioendothelioma showing at lower and higher magnification the obvious vascular pattern with capillary spaces lined by prominent and plump endothelial cells. Note at the *left* more solid areas, but without revealing conspicuous cellular pleomorphism. **a** ×150, **b**,**c** ×400

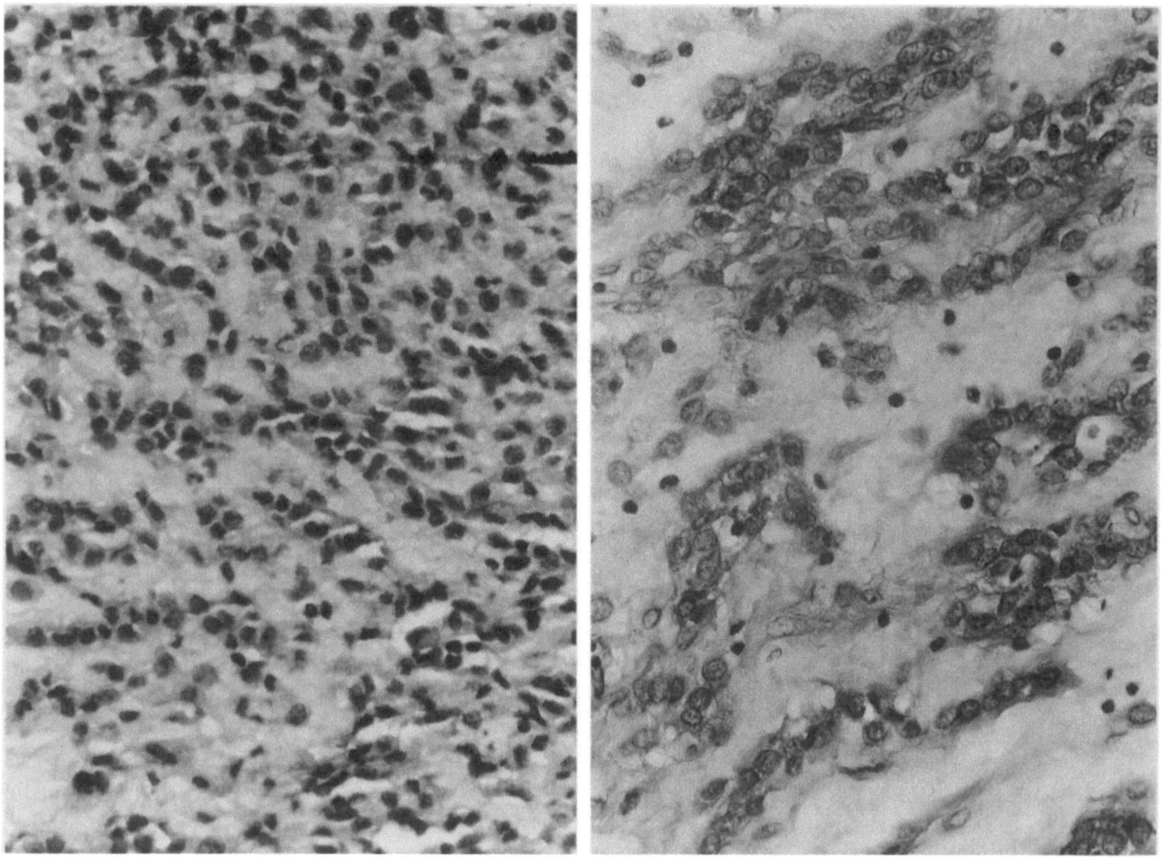

a b

Fig. V.22a,b. Photomicrographs of hemangioendothelioma showing, at lower and higher magnification, its characteristic features. **a** ×100, **b** ×400

according to the presence or lack of cellular atypism and pleomorphism. The differential diagnosis of malignant hemangioendothelioma (epithelioid hemangioendothelioma; histiocytoid hemangioma) with metastatic carcinoma or melanoma may be difficult. Monoclonal antibodies directed against keratins of various molecular weights are negative in vascular tumors, which are, on the other hand, positive for factor VIII-related antigen and *Ulex europaeus* immunoperoxidase staining.

Treatment and Prognosis. In localized single lesions, a wide resection was effective in several of our cases localized in the patella, ischium, and tibia. In multiple lesions located in one or in different bones of the same extremity, amputation seems to be the most appropriate treatment. According to Otis et al. (1968), patients with multiple lesions in the same extremity have a better prognosis than those with solitary ones. In their series, only one of four patients with multicentric lesions died, whereas six of seven patients with solitary lesions died. This apparent paradox of good prognosis in multifocal involvement is confirmed by Huvos (1991), with a greater number cases from the same institution (Memorial Hospital). It is explained by the fact that most multifocal bony presentations occur in patients with low-grade malignant hemangioendotheliomas (grade I hemangioendothelioma or epithelioid hemangioepithelioma). Eight of ten patients survived 5 years and only one died of disease within 2 years. Patients with a single hemangioendothelioma of bone had a much worse prognosis, with only 18% surviving 5 years. However, the experience of the Mayo Clinic does not agree with this finding (Unni et al. 1971).

The value of radiation therapy alone or in association with surgery as adjuvant treatment has not yet been established. Isolated examples of long-term survival in patients treated solely with radiotherapy have been reported (Morgenstern and Westing 1969; Larsson et al. 1975).

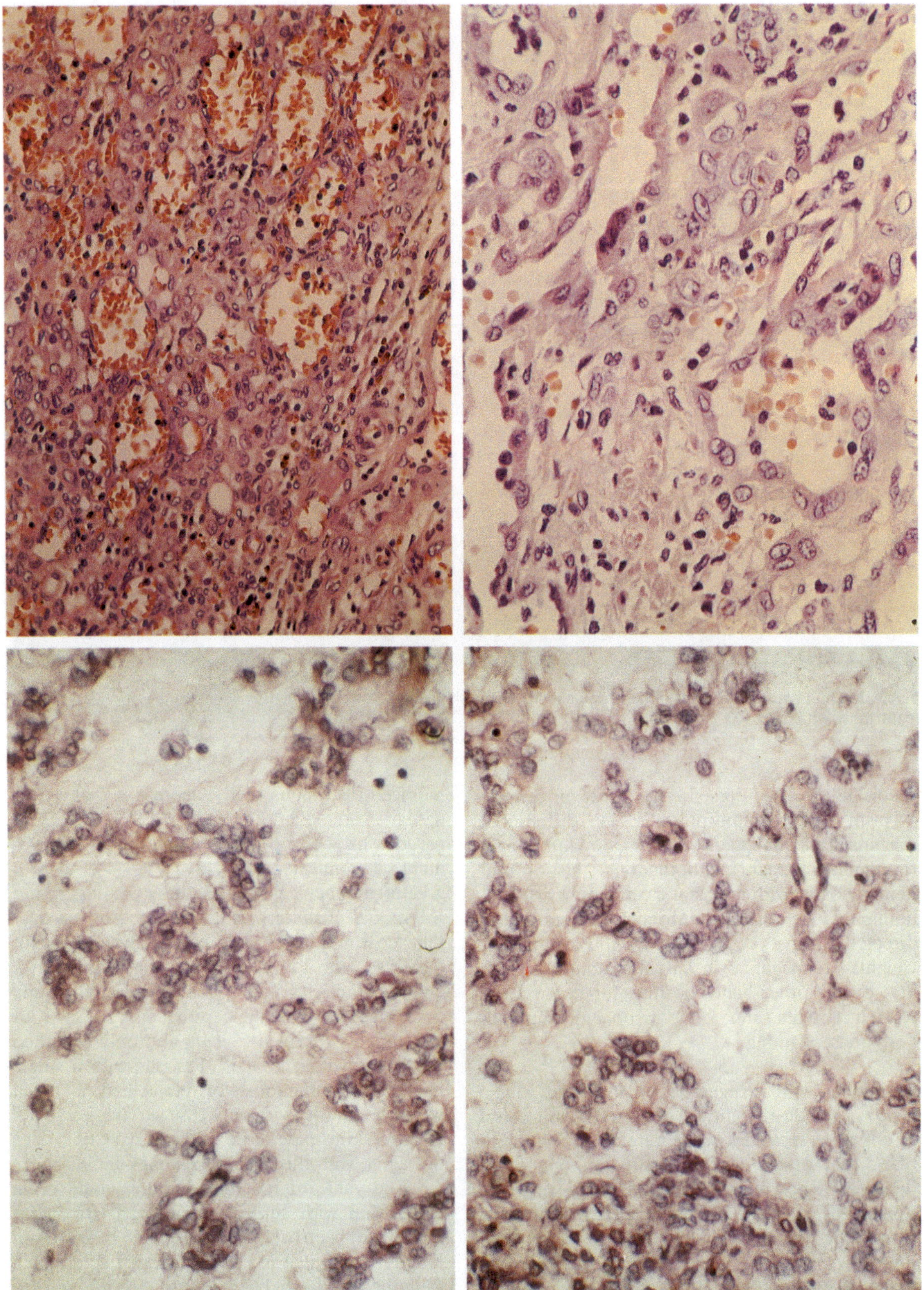

a b c d

Fig. V.24a,b. Photomicrographs illustrating more clearly the hypertrophied endothelial cells inside the basal membrane with a reticulin stain (Del Rio Hortega's silver impregnation technique for reticulin fibers). **a** ×150, **b** ×400

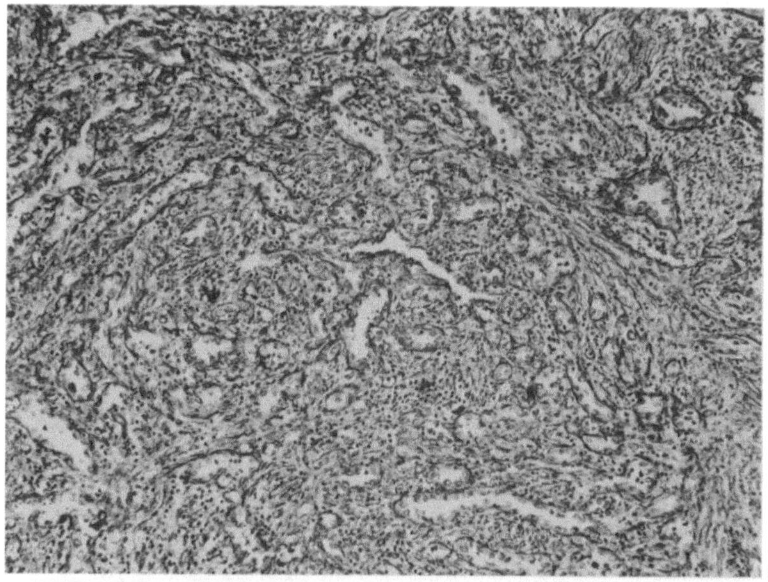

a

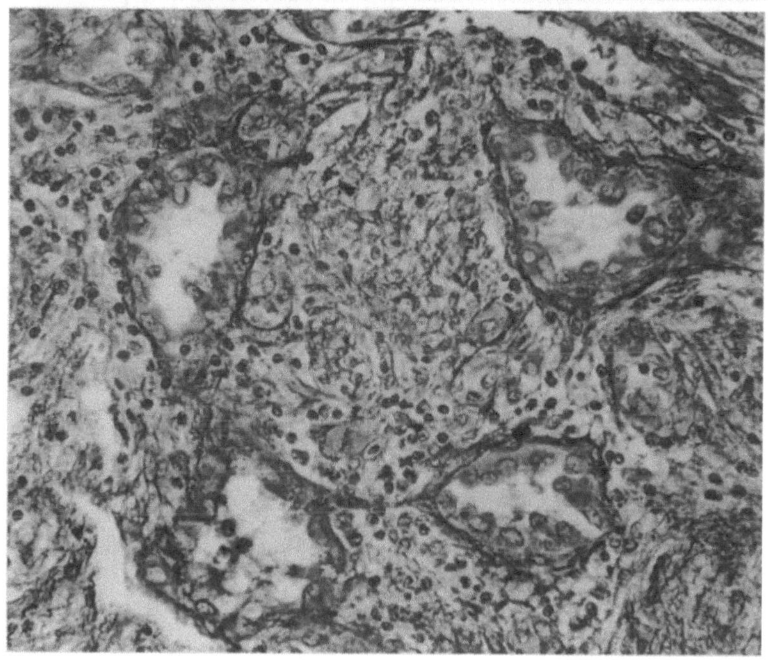

b

◀ **Fig. V.23a–d.** Photomicrographs of **a** lower and **b–d** higher magnification of "myxoid angioblastoma," showing individual nests and cords of epithelial-like cells, separated by a more or less abundant myxoid stroma. Intracytoplasmic vacuolization (blisters), a precursor to the development of vascular formation, is a characteristic finding, resembling "signet ring" cells of carcinoma. The differential diagnosis with chordoma and myxoid chondrosarcoma is difficult. **a** ×200, **b** ×400, **c,d** ×300

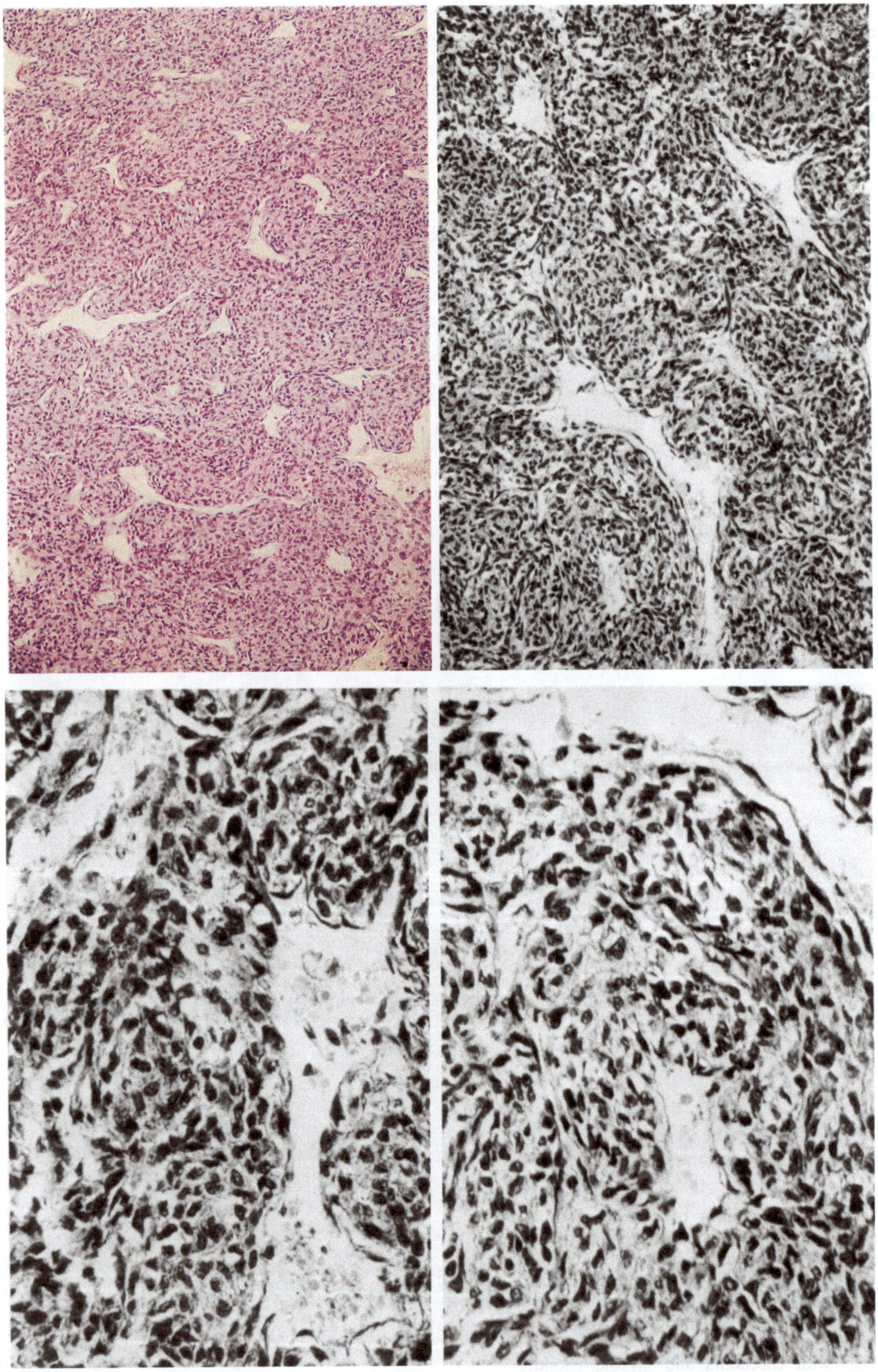

a b c d

Fig. V.25a–d. Photomicrographs of hemangiopericytoma showing vascular spaces lined by a single layer of flattened endothelial cells surrounded by proliferating tumor cells, without the frankly malignant features of angiosarcoma. **a**,**b** ×100, **c**,**d** ×250

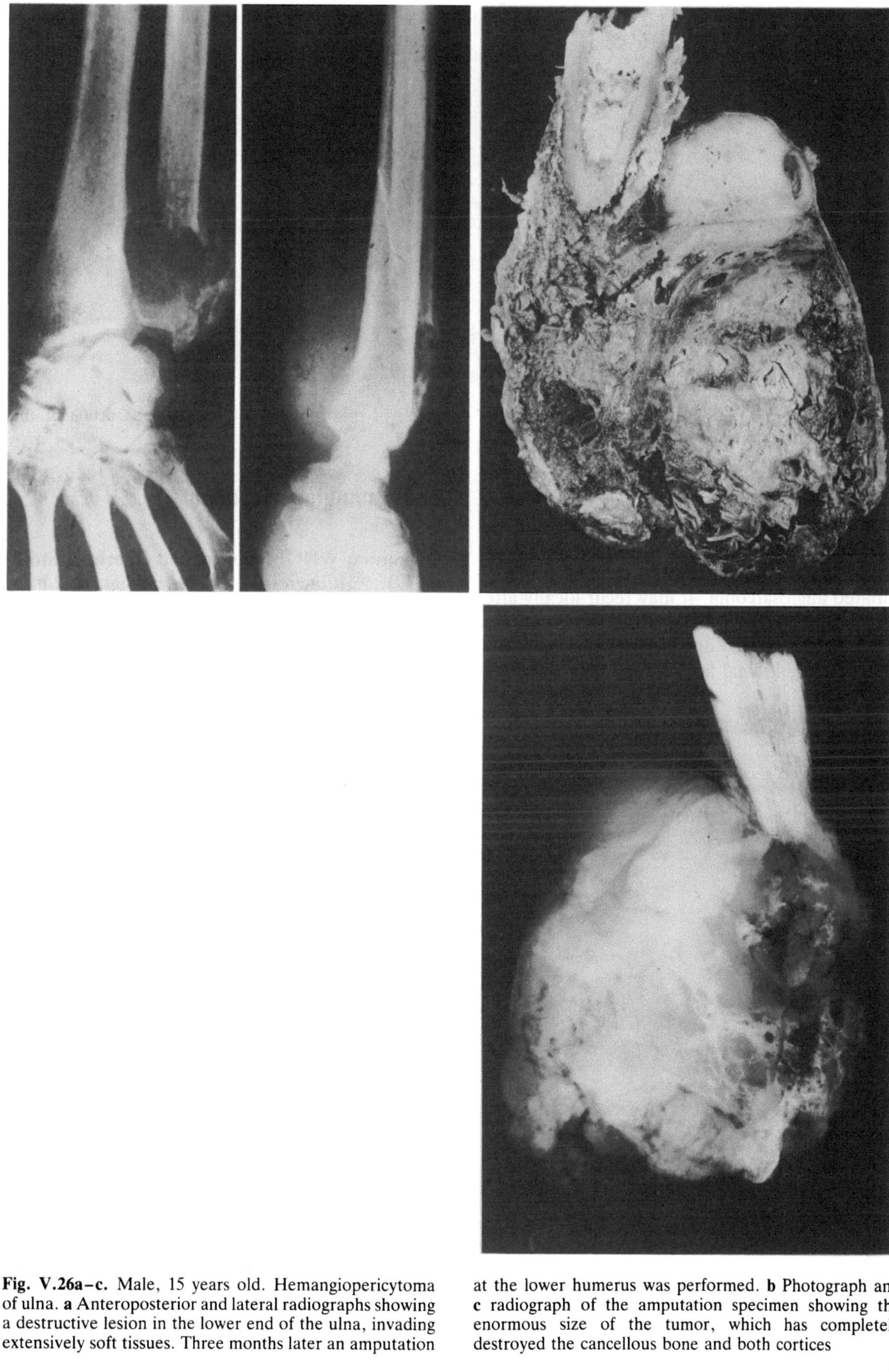

a b c

Fig. V.26a–c. Male, 15 years old. Hemangiopericytoma of ulna. **a** Anteroposterior and lateral radiographs showing a destructive lesion in the lower end of the ulna, invading extensively soft tissues. Three months later an amputation at the lower humerus was performed. **b** Photograph and **c** radiograph of the amputation specimen showing the enormous size of the tumor, which has completely destroyed the cancellous bone and both cortices

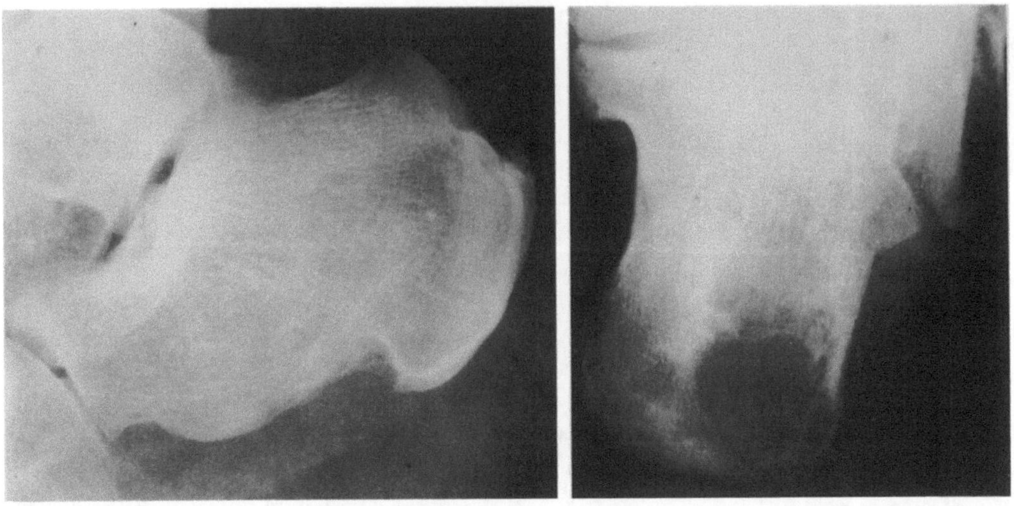

Fig. V.27. Male, 47 years old. Hemangiopericytoma of calcaneus. Radiograph shows an ill-defined radiolucent lesion of the calcaneus with partial destruction of the cortex

The evolution of hemangioendothelioma is unpredictable (Volpe and Mazabraud 1982), but according to our experience, it appears that the survival rate is higher than in the poorly differentiated angiosarcoma. It may recur locally after excision but it rarely metastasizes, although new foci may occasionally appear after treatment of a solitary or multifocal lesion.

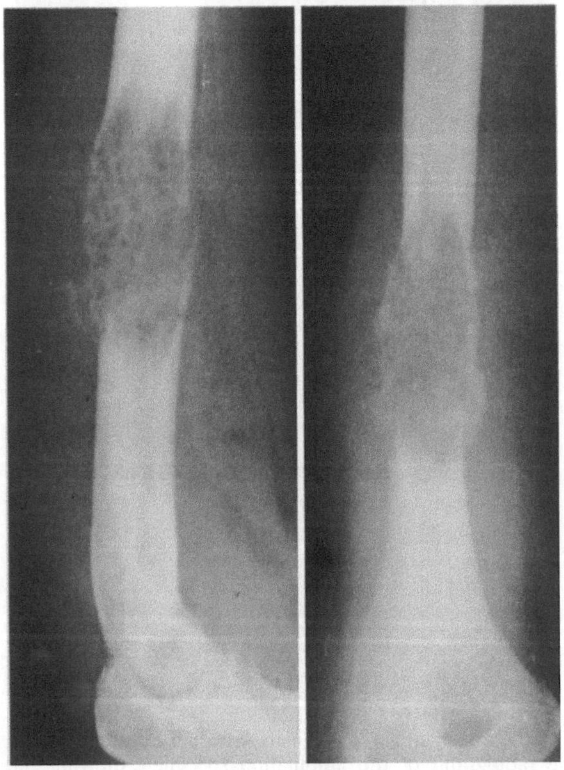

2. Hemangiopericytoma

Definition, WHO, following the criteria of Stout (1949): *"An aggressive or even malignant tumor characterized by a pattern of vascular spaces lined by a single layer of endothelial cells surrounded by zones of proliferating cells."*

As in the case of soft tissue tumors with an essentially similar histologic structure, the behavior of hemangiopericytoma originating in bone is unpredictable. The exact histologic criteria for the separation of low-grade and malignant variants have not yet been satisfactorily defined. However, some cases of hemangioperictyoma show evident features of malignancy, frank anaplasia and metastatic potential, associated with a bad prognosis. The perivascular pattern of these tumors can best be recognized in reticulin preparations. This rare tumor type has been accepted as an entity distinct from other malignant vascular tumors (Fig. V.25). Only a few cases have been reported in the literature (Marcial-Rojas 1960; Legré et al. 1966; Unni et al. 1971; Dunlop 1973; Lichtenstein 1977). We observed five cases involving the ulna (Fig. V.26), calcaneus (Fig. V.27), fibula, radius (Fig. V.28),

Fig. V.29. Female, 40 years old. Hemangiopericytoma of humerus with another focus in the sacrum. Anteroposterior and lateral radiographs reveal an osteolytic lesion that presents a finely honeycomblike pattern and that destroyed the cortices. (Courtesy of Dr. C. Lemos, Rio de Janeiro, Brasil)

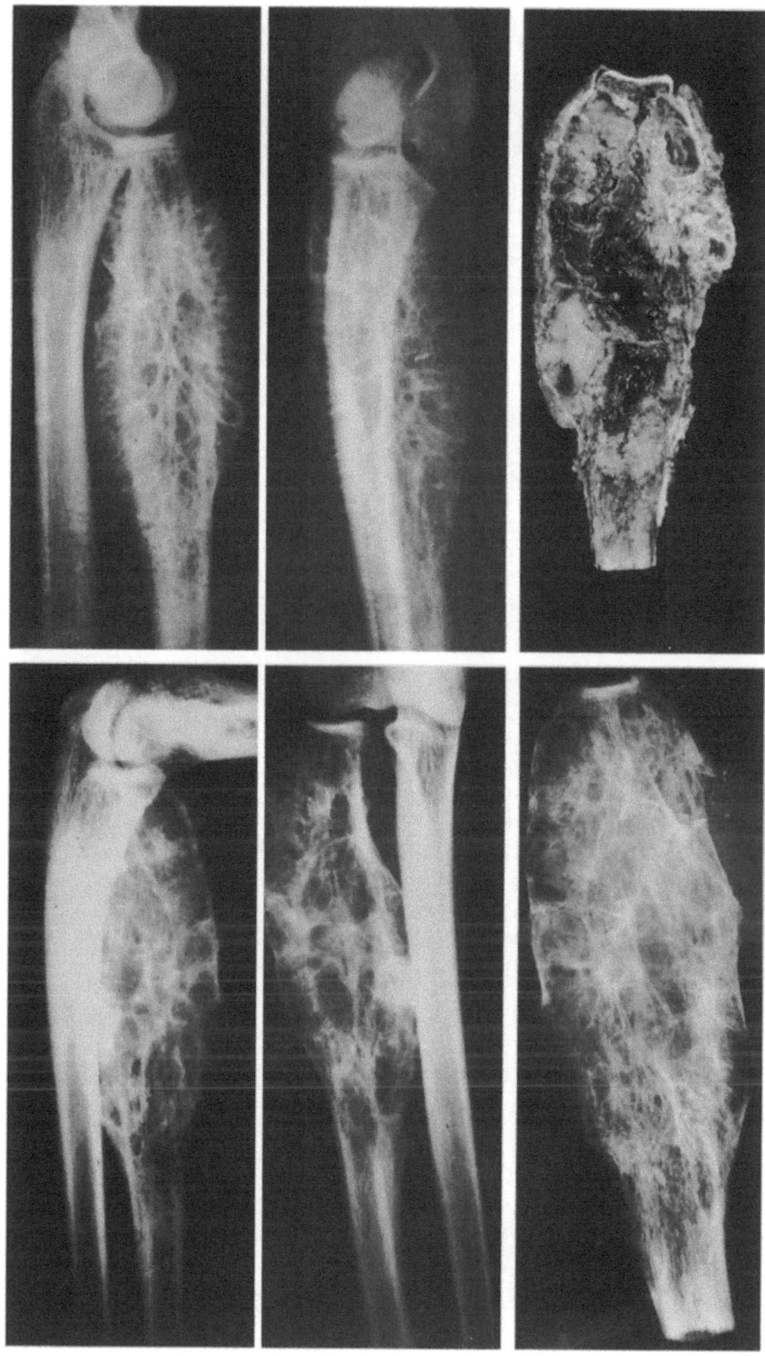

Fig. V.28a–d. Male, 16 years old. Hemangiopericytoma of radius. **a** Lateral and anteroposterior radiographs show a radiolucent lesion with a honeycomblike pattern and sunburst periosteal reaction. **b** Radiographs 4 months after irradiation showing regression of the lesion, which now has more regular contours. An amputation through the lower third of the humerus was carried out. **c** Photograph and **d** radiograph of the specimen show the hemorrhagic and honeycombed aspect of the tumor

and scapula. Other typical cases located in the humerus (Fig. V.29), radius, cervical spine, and mandible were seen in consultation. The seven cases reported by Dahlin and Unni were located in the ischium, the ilium, a dorsal vertebra, a rib, and the mandible. Six patients were studied at the Memorial Hospital (Huvos 1991). Most of the cases were in adults. Areas with hemangiopericytoma structures may be observed in several other tumors, i.e., osteosarcomas, fibrosarcomas, and more frequently in mesenchymal chondrosarcomas and synovial sarcomas.

Resection or amputation is the treatment indicated; the tumor may recur locally after resection, but the prognosis, although unpredictable, seems to be more favorable than that of the poorly differentiated angiosarcoma. The vascular pattern with characteristic perithelial proliferation of tumor cells can best be recognized using special reticulin stains.

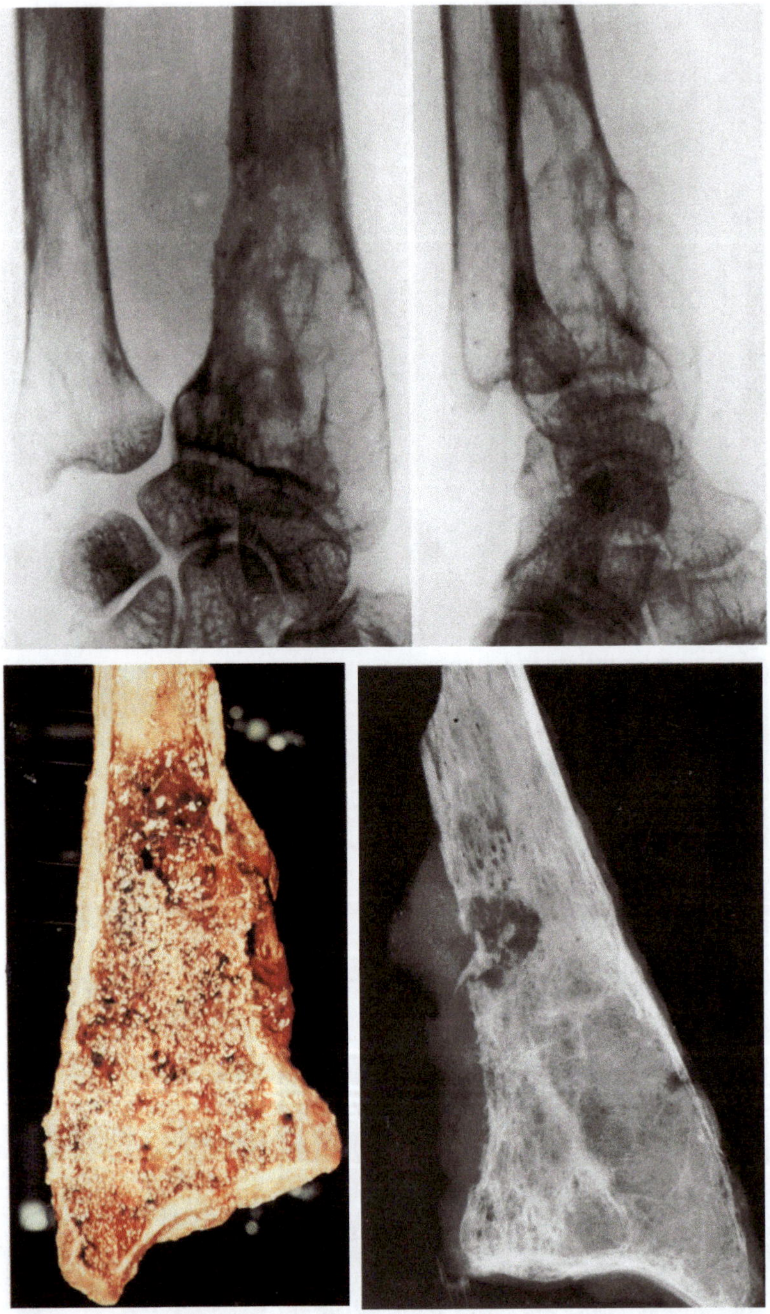

a

b

c

Fig. V.30a–c. Female, 30 years old. Angiosarcoma of radius. **a** Anteroposterior and lateral radiographs illustrate a radiolucent trabeculated lesion, expanding and partly destroying the thinned cortex at one side. A giant-cell tumor was ruled out by biopsy. An amputation was performed and another similar small lesion was found in the upper third of the radius. The patient died 1 year later with pulmonary metastasis. **b** Photograph and **c** radiograph of the specimen showing the dark, hemorrhagic tumor and the destruction of the cancellous bone and part of the thinned cortex

C. Malignant

1. Angiosarcoma

Definition, WHO: *"A malignant tumor characterized by the formation of irregular vascular channels, lined by one or more layers of atypical endothelial cells, often of immature appearance, and accompanied by solid masses of poorly differentiated or anaplastic tissue."*

This tumor type corresponds to the poorly differentiated hemangioendothelial sarcoma of Dorfman et al. (1971) and to grades II and III of hemangioendothelioma of Unni et al. (1971) and Dahlin and Unni (1986), that is, the high-grade malignant anaplastic types. Angiosarcoma appears to be even rarer than the better differentiated vascular tumors. Our series included 12 cases of angiosarcoma (0.43% of malignant tumors) and 15 cases of hemangioendothelioma. Dorfman et al. reported a lower

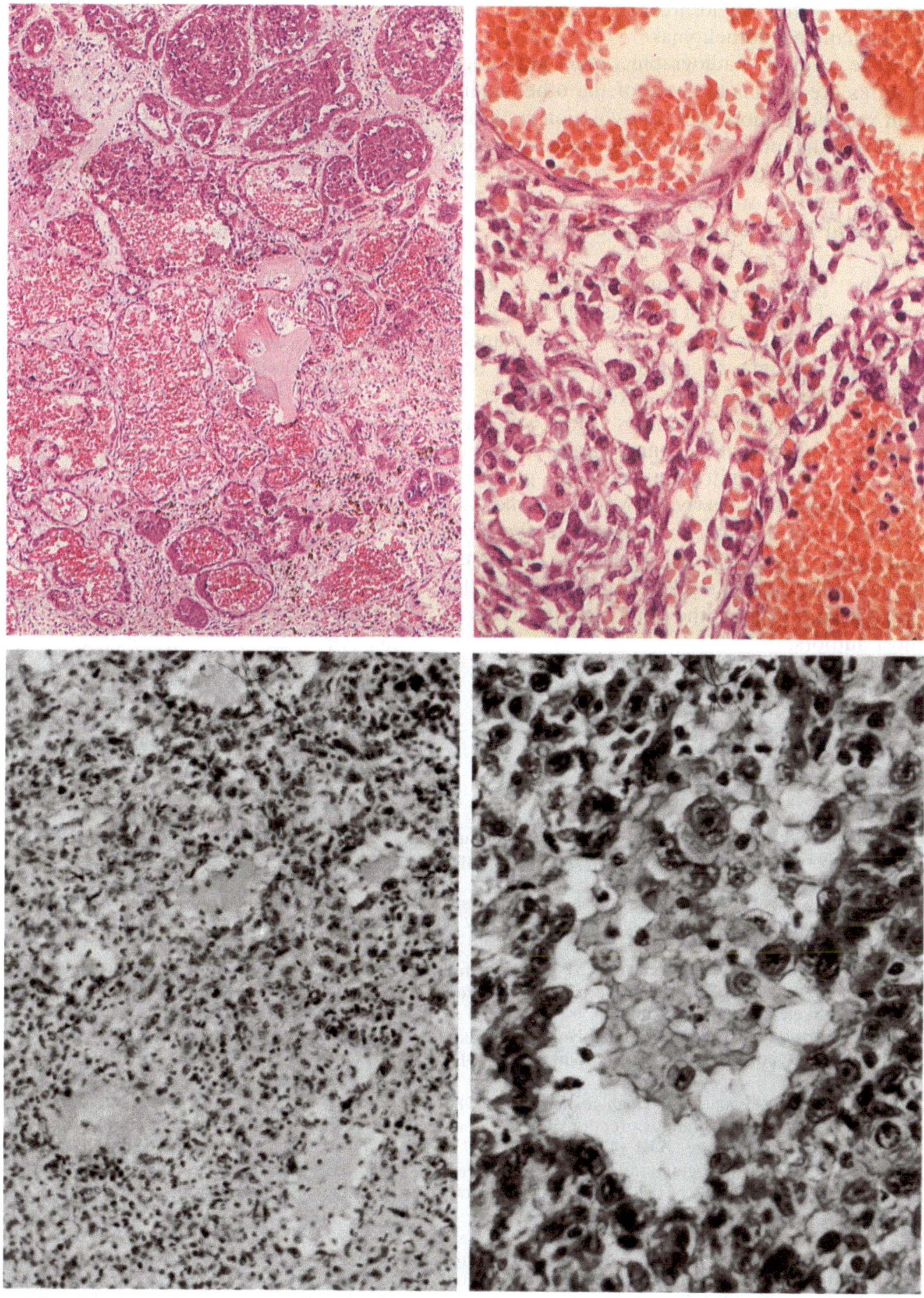

Fig. V.31a–d. Photomicrographs of angiosarcoma showing besides dilated blood-filled capillary vessels, irregular vascular spaces lined with one or more layers of atypical endothelial cells, frequently of immature appearance and accompanied by solid masses of poorly differentiated or anaplastic tissue. **a** ×125, **b** ×320, **c** ×100, **d** ×40 incidence – five angiosarcomas compared with ten hemangioendotheliomas.

The clinical, radiographic, and pathologic features are similar to those of the other malignant vascular tumors, but the evolution is usually more rapidly progressive, with more extensive erosion and destruction of the cortex and wide penetration into soft tissues (Figs. V.30, V.31). Multifocal bone lesions occurred in two of our cases.

The prognosis of angiosarcoma is more ominous. The survival of patients with high-grade malignant vascular tumors of bone (hemangioendotheliosarcoma or angiosarcoma) was only 20% in the Mayo Clinic series (Wold et al. 1982a). In contrast, patients with low-grade hemangioendothelial sarcomas (grade I tumors) had an almost uniformly excellent prognosis (95% disease-free survival). Most patients with angiosarcoma died with metastases in the lungs and other organs, including bones, less than 2 years after radical surgery (amputation or disarticulation), which is the treatment advocated by most authors.

References

Benign Vascular Tumors

Ackerman AJ, Hart MS (1942) Multiple primary hemangioma of the bones of the extremity. Am J Roentgenol Radium Ther 48:47

Aegerter E, Kirkpatrick JA Jr (1975) Orthopedic diseases: physiology, pathology, radiology, 4th edn. W.B. Saunders, Philadelphia

Baker ND, Greenspan A, Neuwirth M (1986) Symptomatic vertebral hemangiomas: a report of four cases. Skeletal Radiol 15:458–463

Bickel WH, Broders AC (1947) Primary lymphangioma of the ilium: report of a case. J Bone Joint Surg 29:517–522

Bjorkengren AG, Resnick D, Haghighi P et al. (1986) Intraosseous glomus tumor: report of a case and review of the literature. AJR 147:739–741

Boyle WJ (1972) Cystic angiomatosis of bone: a report of three cases and review of the literature. J Bone Joint Surg [Br] 54:626–636

Brower AC, Culver JE Jr, Keats TE (1973) Diffuse cystic angiomatosis of bone: report of two cases. Am J Roentgenol Radium Ther Nucl Med 118:456–463

Bucy PC, Capp CC (1930) Primary hemangioma of bone. With special reference to roentgenologic diagnosis. Am J Roentgenol Radium Ther Nucl Med 23:1–33

Bullough PG, Goodfellow JW (1976) Solitary lymphangioma of bone: a case report. J Bone Joint Surg [Am] 58:418–419

Cannon SR (1986) Massive osteolysis. A review of seven cases. J Bone Joint Surg [Br] 68:24–28

Chan CW (1981) Intraossoeus glomus tumor: case report. J Hand Surg 6:368–369

Choma ND, Biscotti CV, Bauer TW et al. (1987) Gorham's syndrome: a case report and review of the literature. Am J Med 83:1151–1156

Cohen J, Craig JM (1955) Multiple lymphangiectasis with involvement of bone. Am J Roentgenol Radium Ther Nucl Med 74:299

Cone RO, Hudkins P, Nguyen V et al. (1983) Histiocytoid hemangioma of bone: a benign lesion which may mimic angiosarcoma. Report of a case and review of literature. Skeletal Radiol 10:165–169

Dahlin DC (1978) Bone tumors, 3rd edn. Charles C. Thomas, Springfield, IL

Dahlin DC, Unni KK (1986) Bone tumors: general aspects and data on 8542 cases. Charles C. Thomas, Springfield, IL

Daniels RA, Weisenfeld I (1979) Tumorous phosphaturic osteomalacia: report of a case associated with multiple hemangiomas of bone. Am J Med 67:155–159

Dorfman HD, Steiner GC, Jaffe HL (1971) Vascular tumors of bone. Hum Pathol 2:349–376

Edwards WH Jr, Thompson RC Jr, Varsa EW (1983) Lymphangiomatosis and massive osteolysis of the cervical spine. A case report and review of the literature. Clin Orthop 177:222–229

Falkner S, Tilling G (1956) Primary lymphangioma of bone. Acta Orthop Scand 26:99–110

Ferretti A, Sadun F, Gherardi G (1981) Diffuse skeletal angiomatosis. Ital J Orthop Traumatol 7:353–358

Geschickter CF, Maseritz IH (1938) Primary hemangioma involving bones of the extremities. J Bone Joint Surg 20:888–900

Goidanich IF, Campanacci M (1962) Vascular hamartomata and infantile angioectatic osteohyperplasia. J Bone Joint Surg [Am] 44:815

Gorham LW, Stout AP (1955) Massive osteolysis (acute spontaneous absorption of bone): its relation to hemangiomatosis. J Bone Joint Surg [Am] 37:985–1004

Gorham LW, Wright AW, Schultz HH et al. (1954) Disappearing bones: a form of massive osteolysis. Report of two cases, one with autopsy findings. Am J Med 17:674–682

Graham JJ, Yang WC (1984) Vertebral hemangioma with compression fracture and paraparesis treated with preoperative embolization and vertebral resection. Spine 9:97–101

Gramiak R, Ruiz G, Campetti FL (1957) Cystic angiomatosis of bone. Radiology 69:347–353

Guerra J Jr, Resnick D, Cone R et al. (1984) Case report 273. Diagnosis: periosteal (parosteal, juxtacortical) vascular malformation. Skeletal Radiol 11:303–306

Hambach R, Pujman J, Maly V (1958) Massive osteolysis due to hemangiomatosis. Report of a case of Gorham's disease with autopsy. Radiology 71:43–47

Hayes JT, Brody GL (1961) Cystic lymphangiectasis of bone: a case report. J Bone Joint Surg [Am] 43:107–117

Heyden G, Kindblom LG, Nielsen JM (1977) Disappearing bone disease: a clinical and histological study. J Bone Joint Surg [Am] 59:57–61

Iglesias de la Torre L, Gomez Camajo M, Palacios GT (1939) Consideraciones clínicas, anatómicas y quirúrgicas del glomus tumoral de Masson. Cirug Ortop Traumatol 7:11–20

Jacobs JE, Kimmelstiel P (1953) Cystic angiomatosis of the skeletal system. J Bone Joint Surg [Am] 35:409–420

Johnson PM, McClure G (1958) Observations on massive osteolysis: a review of the literature and report of a case. Radiology 71:28–42

Jumbelic M, Feuerstein IM, Dorfman HD (1984) Solitary intraosseous lymphangioma: a case report. J Bone Joint Surg [Am] 66:1479–1481

Junghanns H (1932) Über die Haüfigkeit gutariger Geschwülste in den Wirbelkörpern (Angiome, Lipome, Osteoma). Arch Klin Chir 169:204–212

Kenan S, Bonar S, Jones C et al. (1988) Subperiosteal hemangioma: a case report and review of the literature. Clin Orthop 232:279–283

Koblenzer PJ, Bukowski MJ (1961) Angiomatosis (hamartomatous hemolymphangiomatosis). Pediatrics 28:65–76

Lattes R, Bull DC (1948) A case of glomus tumor with primary involvement of bone. Am Surg 127:187–191

Lehman W, Kraissl C (1949) Glomus tumor within bone. Surgery 28:218

Lichtenstein L (1977) Bone tumors, 5th edn. C.V. Mosby, St. Louis

Loxley SS, Thiemeyer JS Jr, Ellasser JC (1972) Periosteal hemangioma: a report of two cases. Clin Orthop 85:151–154

Lozman J, Holmblad J (1976) Cavernous hemangiomas associated with scoliosis and a localized consumptive coagulopathy: a case report. J Bone Joint Surg [Am] 58:1021–1024

Mackenzie DH (1962) Intraosseus glomus tumors: report of two cases. J Bone Joint Surg [Br] 44:648–651

Makrycostas K (1927) Über das Wirbelangiom-lipom und osteom. Virchows Arch [A] 265:259–303

Manning HJ (1951) Symptomatic hemangioma of the spine. Radiology 56:58–65

Masson P (1935) Les glomus cutanés de l'homme. Bull Soc Fr Dermatol Syphiligr 42:1174–1245

Mohan V, Gupta SK, Tuli SM et al. (1980) Symptomatic vertebral haemangiomas. Clin Radiol 31:575–579

Moseley LE, Starobin SG (1964) Cystic angiomatosis of bone: manifestations of a hamartomatous disease entity. Am J Roentgenol Radium Ther Nucl Med 91:1114–1120

Nixon GW (1970) Lymphangiomatosis of bone demonstrated by lymphangiography. Am J Roentgenol Radium Ther Nucl Med 110:582

Pambakian H, Smith MA (1981) Glomus tumours of the coccygeal body associated with coccydynia: a preliminary report. J Bone Joint Surg [Br] 63:424–426

Parsons LG, Ebbs JH (1940) Generalized angiomatosis presenting the clinical characteristics of storage reticulosis. Arch Dis Child 15:129

Pena JM, Calone JA, Ortega F (1985) Periosteal hemangioma of left fibula: case report 324. Skeletal Radiol 14:133–135

Ritchie G, Zier FG (1956) Hemangiomatosis of the skeleton and the spleen. J Bone Joint Surg [Am] 38:115–122

Rosai J, Gold J, Landy R (1979) The histiocytoid hemangiomas: a unifying concept embracing several previously described entities of skin, soft tissue, large vessels, bone and heart. Hum Pathol 10:707–730

Rosenquist CJ, Wolfe DC (1958) Lymphangioma of bone. J Bone Joint Surg [Am] 50:158–162

Ross JS, Masaryk TJ, Modic MT et al. (1987) Vertebral hemangiomas: MR imaging. Radiology 165:165–169

Sage MR, Allen PW (1974) Massive osteolysis. Report of a case. J Bone Joint Surg [Br] 56:130–135

Schajowicz F, Aiello CL, Slullitel I (1970) Cystic and pseudocystic lesions of the terminal phalange with special reference to epidermoid cysts. Clin Orthop 58:84–92

Schajowicz F, Aiello CL, Francone MV, Giannini GE (1978) Cystic angiomatosis (hamartous haemolymphangiomatosis) of bone: a clinicopathological study of three cases. J Bone Joint Surg [Br] 60:100–106

Schajowicz F, Rebecchini AC, Bosch-Mayol G (1979) Intracortical hemangioma simulating osteoid osteoma. J Bone Joint Surg [Br] 61:94–95

Schnyder P, Fankhauser H, Mansouri B (1986) Computed tomography in spinal hemangioma with cord compression: report of two cases. Skeletal Radiol 15:372–375

Seckler SG, Rubin H, Rabinowitz JG (1964) Systemic cystic angiomatosis. Am J Med 37:976–986

Sherman RS, Wilner D (1961) The roentgen diagnosis of hemangioma of bone. Am J Roentgenol Radium Ther Nucl Med 86:1146–1159

Siegel MW (1967) Intraosseous glomus tumor: a case report. Am J Orthop 9:68–69

Singh R, Grewal DS, Bannerjee AK et al. (1974) Haemangiomatosis of the skeleton: report of a case. J Bone Joint Surg [Br] 56:136–138

Spjut HJ, Lindbom A (1962) Skeletal angiomatosis: report of two cases. Acta Pathol Microbiol Scand 55:49–58

Sugiura I (1975) Tibial periosteal hemangioma. Clin Orthop 104:242–244

Sugiura I (1976) Intra-osseous glomus tumour: a case report. J Bone Joint Surg [Br] 58:245–247

Tang TT, Zuege RC, Babbitt DP et al. (1976) Angioglomoid tumor of bone. J Bone Joint Surg [Am] 58:873–876

Thompson JS, Schurman DJ (1974) Massive osteolysis: case report and review of literature. Clin Orthop 103:206–211

Töpfer D (1928) Zur Kenntnis der Wirbelangiome. Frankf Z Pathol 36:537–545

Tsuneyoshi M, Dorfman HD, Bauer TW (1986) Epithelioid hemangioendothelioma of bone. Am J Surg Pathol 10:754–764

Vetrani A, Milano C, Palombini L et al. (1982) Tumore glomico dell'osso (presentazione di un caso). Arch Putti Chir Organi Mov 32:329–332

Wallis LA, Asch T, Maisel BW (1964) Diffuse skeletal hemangiomatosis. Report of two cases and review of literature. Am J Med 37:545

Wold LE, Swee G, Sim FH (1985) Vascular lesions of bone. Pathol Annu (Pt 2):101–137

Wyke BD (1946) Primary hemangioma of the skull: a rare cranial tumor. Am J Roentgenol Radium Ther 61: 302–316

Yang ZY, Zhang LJ, Chen ZX et al. (1985) Hemangioma of the vertebral column: a report on 23 patients with special reference to functional recovery after radiation therapy. Acta Radiol [Oncol] 24:129–132

Intermediate and Malignant Vascular Tumors

Angervall L, Kindblom LG, Karlsson K et al. (1985) Atypical hemangioendothelioma of venous origin: a clinicopathologic, angiographic, immunohistochemical and ultrastructural study of two endothelial tumors within the concept of histiocytoid hemangioma. Am J Surg Pathol 9:504–516

Bohn LE, Dehner LP, Walker C Jr (1982) Case report 204: multicentric angiosarcoma of bone involving the right lower extremity. Skeletal Radiol 8:303–305

Bundens WD Jr, Brighton CT (1965) Malignant hemangioendothelioma of bone: report of two cases and review of the literature. J Bone Joint Surg [Am] 47:762–772

Campanacci M, Boriani S, Giunti A (1980) Hemangioendothelioma of bone: a study of 29 cases. Cancer 46:804–814

Chen KT, Hoffman KD, Hendricks EJ (1979) Angiosarcoma following therapeutic irradiation. Cancer 44:2044–2048

Chow RW, Wilson CB, Olsen ER (1970) Angiosarcoma of the skull: report of a case and review of the literature. Cancer 25:902–906

Craver WL, Brown BS (1979) Hemangioendothelioma of bone with pulmonary metastases: a 25-year course. Report of a case. Cancer 43:1917–1923

Dahlin DC (1978) Bone tumors, 3rd edn. Charles C. Thomas, Springfield, IL

Dahlin DC, Unni KK (1986) Bone tumors: general aspects and data on 8542 cases. Charles C. Thomas, Springfield, IL

DeSmet AA, Inscore D, Neff JR (1989) Case report 521: histiocytoid hemangioma of the distal end of the right humerus. Skeletal Radiol 18:60–65

Dorfman HD, Steiner GC, Jaffe HL (1971) Vascular tumors of bone. Hum Pathol 2:349–376

Dube VE, Fisher DE (1972) Hemangioendothelioma of the leg following fixation of the tibia. Cancer 30: 1260–1266

Dunlop J (1973) Primary haemangiopericytoma of bone: report of two cases. J Bone Joint Surg [Br] 55:854–857

Fulling KH, Gersell DJ (1983) Neoplastic angioendotheliomatosis: histological, immunohistochemical, and ultrastructural findings in two cases. Cancer 51:1107–1118

Garcia-Moral CA (1972) Malignant hemangioendothelioma of bone: review of world literature and report of two cases. Clin Orthop 82:70–79

Hartmann WH, Stewart FW (1962) Hemangioendothelioma of bone: unusual tumor characterized by indolent course. Cancer 15:846–854

Huvos AG (1991) Bone tumors: diagnosis, treatment, prognosis. W.B. Saunders, Philadelphia

Jaffe HL (1958) Tumors and tumorous conditions of the bones and joints. Lea & Febiger, Philadelphia

Khanna SD, Saigal RK (1974) Malignant haemangioendothelioma of bone: clinical-pathological report of 15 cases and review of literature. Indian J Surg 36: 144–146

Larsson SE, Lorentzon R, Boquist L (1975) Malignant hemangioendothelioma of bone. J Bone Joint Surg [Am] 57:84–89

Legré G, Payan H, Aubert M (1966) Osseous hemangiopericytoma. Rev Chir Orthop 52:551–559

Lichtenstein L (1977) Bone tumors, 5th edn. C.V. Mosby, St. Louis

Marcial-Rojas RA (1960) Primary hemangiopericytoma of bone: review of the literature and report of the first case with metastases. Cancer 13:308–311

Martínez-Tello FJ, Marcos-Robles J, Blanco-Lorenzo F (1989) Case report 520: primary epithelioid hemangioendothelioma of bone (polyostotic). Skeletal Radiol 18:55–59

Maruyama N, Kumagai Y, Ishida Y et al. (1985) Epithelioid haemangioendothelioma of the bone tissue. Virchows Arch [A] 407:159–165

Mirra JM, Kameda N (1985) Myxoid angioblastomatosis of bone: a case report of a rare multifocal entity with light, ultramicroscopic and immunopathologic correlation. Am J Surg Pathol 9:450

Morgenstern P, Westing SW (1969) Malignant hemangioendothelioma of bone. Cancer 23:221–224

Otis J, Hunter RVP, Foote FW, Marcove RC, Stewart W (1968) Haemangioendothelioma of bone. Surg Gynecol Obstet 127:295–305

Pearlman AW (1972) Hemangioendothelial sarcoma of bone: the role of irradiation and tumor growth studies. Bull Hosp Joint Dis 33:135–149

Rosai J, Gold J, Landy R (1979) The histiocytoid hemangiomas. Hum Pathol 10:707–730

Schajowicz F, Ackerman CV, Sissons HA (1972) Histological typing of bone tumours. Intermediate and histological classification of tumours, No. 6. WHO, Geneva

Spjut HJ, Dorfman HD, Fechner RE, Ackerman LV (1971) Tumors of bone and cartilage. Atlas of tumor pathology, 2nd series, Fasc 5. Armed Forces Institute of Pathology, Washington, DC

Srinivasan CK, Patel MR, Pearlman HS, Silver JW (1978) Malignant hemangioendothelioma of bone. Review of the literature and report of two cases. J Bone Joint Surg [Am] 60:696–700

Steiner GC, Dorfman HR (1972) Ultrastructure of hemangioendothelial sarcoma of bone. Cancer 29: 122–135

Stout AP (1943) Hemangioendothelioma: a tumor of blood vessels featuring vascular endothelial cells. Ann Surg 118:445–464

Stout AP (1949) Hemangiopericytoma: a study of 25 new cases. Cancer 2:1027–1054

Stout AP (1956) Tumors featuring pericytes: glomus tumor and hemangiopericytoma. Lab Invest 5:217–223

Thomas A (1942) Vascular tumors of bone: pathological and clinical study of 27 cases. Surg Gynecol Obstet 74:777–795

Tsuneyoshi M, Dorfman HD, Bauer TW (1986) Epithelioid hemangioendothelioma of bone: a clinicopathologic, ultrastructural and immunohistochemical study. Am J Surg Pathol 10:754–764

Unni KK, Ivins JC, Beabout JW, Dahlin DC (1971) Hemangioma, hemangiopericytoma and hemangioendothelioma (angiosarcoma) of bone. Cancer 27: 1403–1414

Volpe R, Mazabraud A (1982) Hemangioendothelioma (angiosarcoma) of bone: a distinct pathologic entity with an unpredictable course? Cancer 49:727–736

Weiss SW, Enzinger FM (1982) Epithelioid hemangioendothelioma: a vascular tumor often mistaken for a carcinoma. Cancer 50:970–981

Wold LE, Unni KK, Beabout JW et al. (1982a) Hemangioendothelial sarcoma of bone. Am J Surg Pathol 6:59–70

Wold LE, Unni KK, Cooper KL et al. (1982b) Hemangiopericytoma of bone. Am J Surg Pathol 6:53–58

CHAPTER VI

Other Connective Tissue Tumors

A. Benign

1. Benign Fibrous Histiocytoma

Definition, WHO: *"A benign lesion characterized by the presence of spindle-celled fibrous tissue with a storiform pattern and containing a variable number of multinucleated giant cells, hemosiderin pigment and lipid-bearing histiocytes (xanthoma cells)."*

The term "benign fibrous histiocytoma" implies a true tumor, although its histologic features are identical to those of metaphyseal fibrous defect (fibrous cortical defect and nonossifying fibroma), considered by all authorities to be a nonneoplastic lesion (possibly a developmental anomaly) since it is often self-limited or may become ossified and disappear.

The existence of benign fibrous histiocytoma as a separate entity is based exclusively on clinical differences from metaphyseal fibrous defect. These clinical differences include an older age group of patients and the lesion being confined, in contrast to metaphyseal fibrous defect, to the diaphysis or epiphysis of long bones, to the pelvis or ribs, or exceptionally to other bones (clavicle, spine, skull, patella) generally not involved by nonossifying fibroma. Moreover, the lesion is generally painful, even in the absence of fracture. In this author's opinion it is debatable whether histologically identical lesions should be classified as distinct entities – as a true tumor (benign fibrous histiocytoma) or as a nonneoplastic developmental anomaly (metaphyseal fibrous defect). The nomenclature of this group of lesions is confusing and various synonyms are used in the literature, such as xanthoma, fibroxanthoma, xanthogranuloma, and histiocytic xanthogranuloma (see section on metaphyseal fibrous defect in Chap. IX). The term "xanthoma" was used in the older literature (Bahls 1936; Burman and Sinberg 1938), and more recently xanthoma has been considered a specific tumor of bone (Dahlin and Unni 1986; Bertoni et al. 1988). Some xanthomas have been described in association with hyperproteinemia (Yagmai 1978). This author does not believe that separation of so-called primary xanthoma of bone as a distinct entity is justified; it corresponds, most authors agree, to unusually heavily "lipidized" (xanthomatous) variants of benign fibrous histiocytoma, in generally late stages.

Benign fibrous histiocytoma of bone is a rare lesion. Only a few single case reports (Bertoni et al. 1983; Destouet et al. 1980; Roessner et al. 1981) and some series with a small number of cases have appeared in the literature. Dahlin's textbook (1978) included a chapter "Benign and atypical fibrous histiocytomas," in which he reported seven cases from the Mayo Clinic series of more than 6000 cases. Dahlin mentioned that the histopathology of these lesions, which he considered true tumors, was similar to that of nonossifying fibroma, but he apparently distinguished them because of their atypical radiologic appearance, location, and the older age of the patients. In the later Mayo Clinic series (Dahlin and Unni 1986), the number of cases increased to ten tumors out of 8542. A few other series with a small number of cases have appeared in the recent literature (Fechner 1984, seven cases; Clarke et al. 1985, eight cases; Bertoni et al. 1986, seven cases from the Rizzoli Institute in Bologna). The diagnostic term "atypical fibrous histiocytoma," introduced by Dahlin, is ambiguous and its histologic features are not yet clearly defined. It tacitly admits the difficulties of classifying these lesions. It is probable that some exceptional reported cases (Saito and Caines 1977; Dahlin 1978) are actually low-grade malignant fibrous histiocytoma.

Age and Localization. Unlike in the case of nonossifying fibroma, most patients were adults, ranging from 15 to 60 years. Almost all the patients had pain, without evidence of a fracture. As mentioned above, benign fibrous histiocytoma involves most commonly the diaphysis or epiphysis of long bones, the pelvis, and ribs; however, other bones such as the clavicle, spine, and skull may rarely be involved. Two of our cases

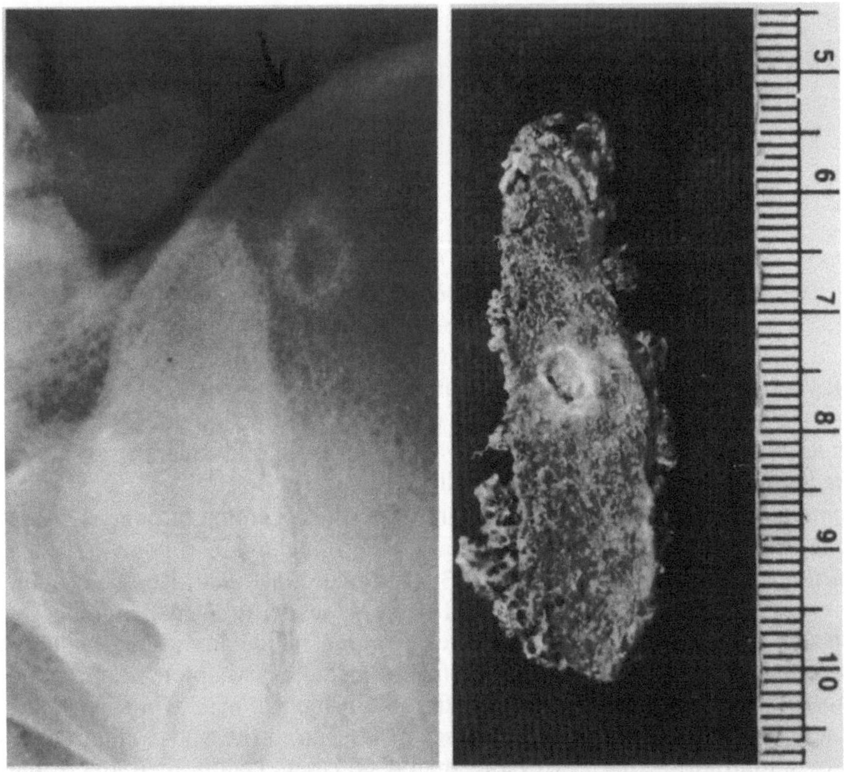

a b

Fig. VI.1a,b. Male, 19 years old. Benign fibrous histiocytoma in the ilium. **a** Radiograph shows a small radiolucent lesion surrounded by a sclerotic rim. **b** Photograph of the resected specimen shows the size of the lesion, which was yellowish in color

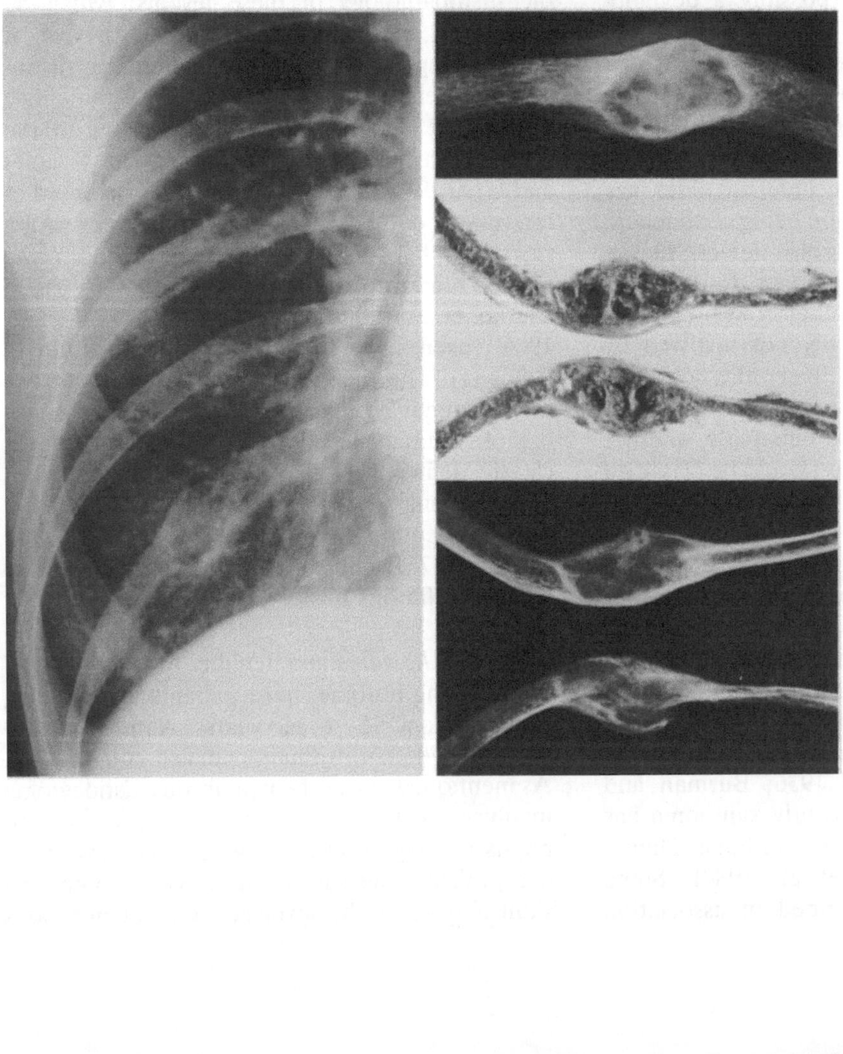

a b, c, d

Fig. VI.2a–d. Male, 51 years old. Fibrous histiocytoma in a rib. **a** Radiograph shows a radiolucent, slightly expanding lesion, suggesting fibrous dysplasia. **b** Radiograph of the resected rib segment illustrates clearly the well-defined sclerotic border of this radiolucent lesion. **c** Photograph and **d** radiograph of a longitudinal section demonstrating the dark-brownish color with some cystic areas of the lesion, its aspect being considerably different from that of fibrous dysplasia or "aneurysmal bone cyst" a 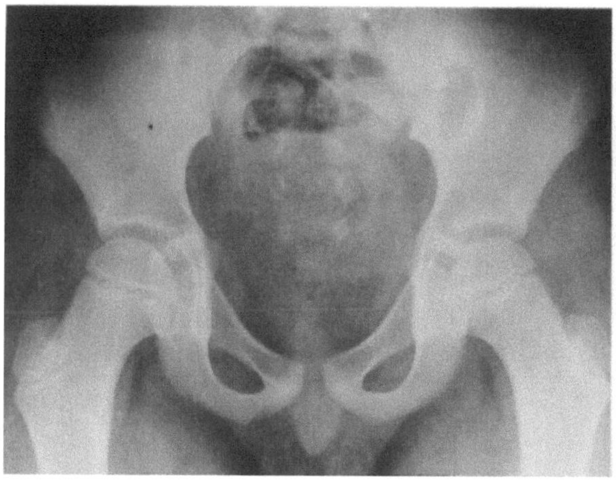 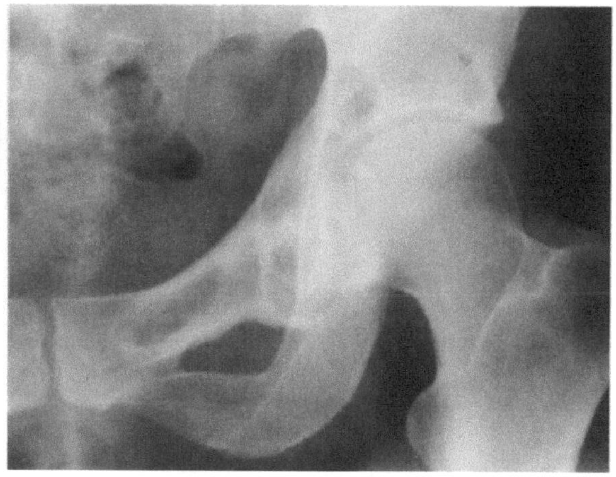 b

Fig. VI.3. a Male, 14 years old. Benign fibrous histiocytoma of the ilium, showing radiolucent lesion surrounded by a sclerotic border. **b** Female, 35 years old, with benign fibrous histiocytoma of the acetabular region. Radiograph demonstrates a radiolucent, trabeculated lesion, well delineated by sclerotic borders

Fig. VI.4a,b. Two cases of benign fibrous histiocytoma of epiphyseal location with radiologic features suggesting a diagnosis of giant-cell tumor. **a** Female, 19 years old. Radiograph shows a radiolucent trabeculated lesion, well defined by sclerotic borders, located centrally in the upper epiphysis of the tibia. **b** Female, 23 years old. Radiograph demonstrates an eccentric, radiolucent, well-delineated lesion in the distal epiphysis of the radius. Histologically in both cases the pattern was that of a purely fibrohistiocytic lesion without features of genuine giant-cell tumor

a 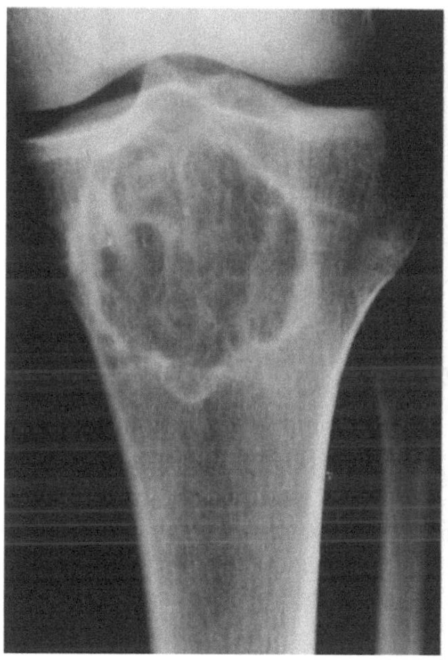 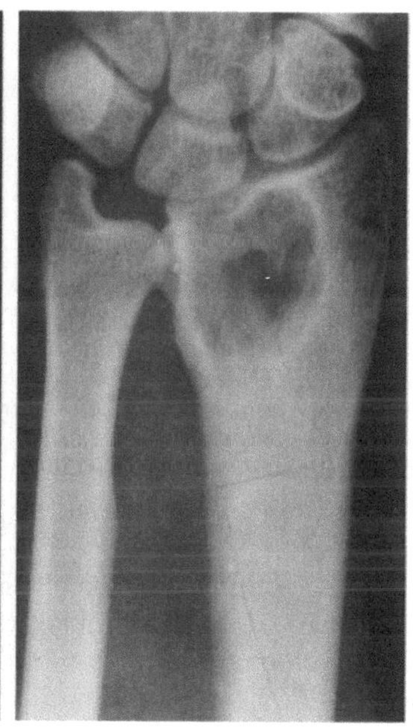 b

published in the first edition (Figs. IX.39, IX.40) as "metaphyseal fibrous defect," adopting the above criteria, would be classified now as benign fibrous histiocytoma. The first case is a lesion in the ilium of a 19-year-old male (Fig. VI.1) and the second is a rib lesion in a 51-year-old male (Fig. VI.2).

The radiographic features show a well-defined, radiolucent, sometimes slightly expanding lesion with sclerotic borders (Fig. VI.3). In long bones the lesion is situated centrally or eccentrically; the latter presentation is particularly common when it is located in an epiphysis. In this site the radiographic aspect is indistinguishable from the grade I (quiescent type) of giant-cell tumor (Fig. VI.4). As was stated in Chap. III, several such giant-cell tumors presented histologically focal or extensive areas of a fibrohistiocytic type similar to that seen in benign fibrous histiocytoma. When insufficient tumor material is studied, these histologic features, which are interpreted as secondary regressive or degenerative phenomena in an otherwise histologically typical giant-cell tumor, along with the adult age of the patient, may suggest the erroneous diagnosis of benign fibrous histiocytoma. Bertoni et al. (1986) therefore reviewed 350 cases of giant-cell tumor at the

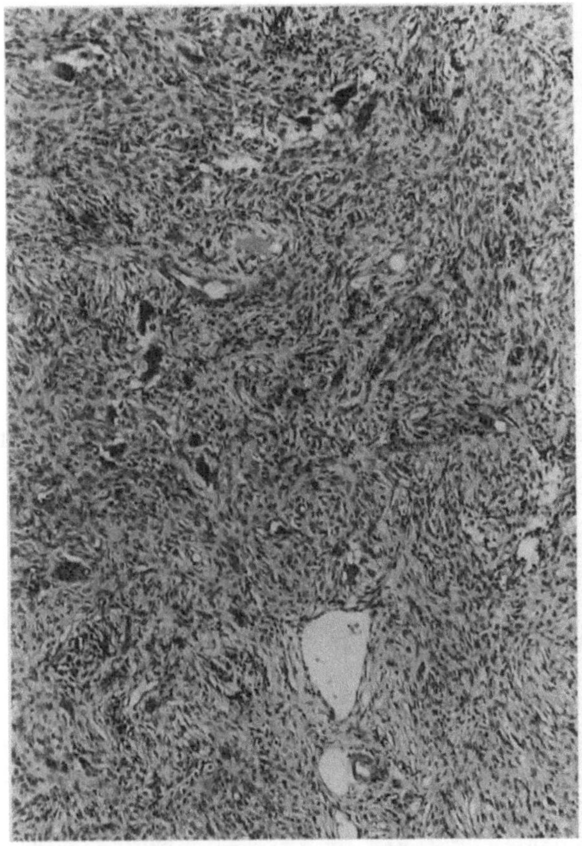

VI.5a

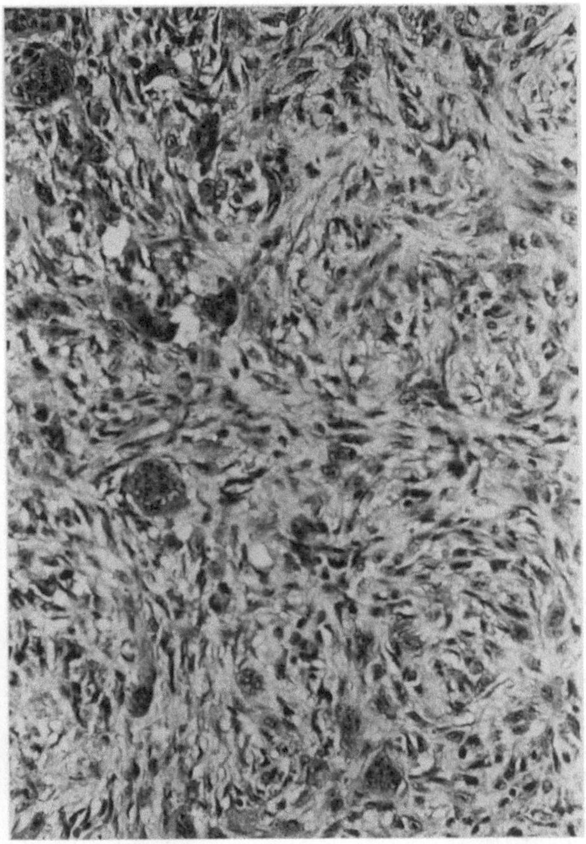

b

Fig. VI.5a,b. Photomicrographs showing at lower and higher magnification the whorled (storiform) spindle-cell stroma and a scarce number of irregularly distributed multinucleated giant cells of smaller size than in genuine giant-cell tumor. **a** ×100, **b** ×250

Fig. VI.6a–d. Photomicrographs illustrating other characteristic histologic features. Beside the spindle-celled fibrous tissue are more or less extensive areas of foam (xanthoma) cells intermingled with multinucleated giant cells. **a** ×100, **b** ×200, **c,d** ×400 ▶

Rizzoli Institute and found ten lesions with an extensive, distinct fibroblastic pattern and/or fibroxanthomatous pattern that could have been mistaken for benign fibrous histiocytoma.

The gross and histologic findings are essentially identical to those of metaphyseal fibrous defect (nonossifying fibroma) and are described in detail in Chap. IX (Figs. VI.5, VI.6). The alleged positivity of α_1-antitrypsin and α_1-antichymotrypsin (Huvos 1991), which are unstable and variable markers for histiocytic lesions, cannot be considered a definite diagnostic criterion.

Treatment. Almost universally, treatment of benign fibrous histiocytoma consists of intralesional or marginal excision. In one of our cases, located in a rib, a segmental en bloc resection was performed (Fig. VI.2). In our small series of 14 cases, as in Bertoni et al.'s (1986) seven cases from the Rizzoli Institute, there were no recurrences. However, Fechner (1984) and Clarke et al. (1985) reported local recurrences in three of eight cases.

2. Lipoma

Definition, WHO: *"A benign tumor of mature adipose tissue with no evidence of cellular atypism."*

Benign and malignant tumors of adipose tissue are among the most common soft tissue tumors. It is therefore surprising that they are among the rarest neoplasms in bone, despite the fact that adipose tissue is an important constituent of bone marrow.

There are two types of benign fatty tumors: (1) *parosteal (periosteal) lipomas*, which apparently arise from the subperiosteal tissue and

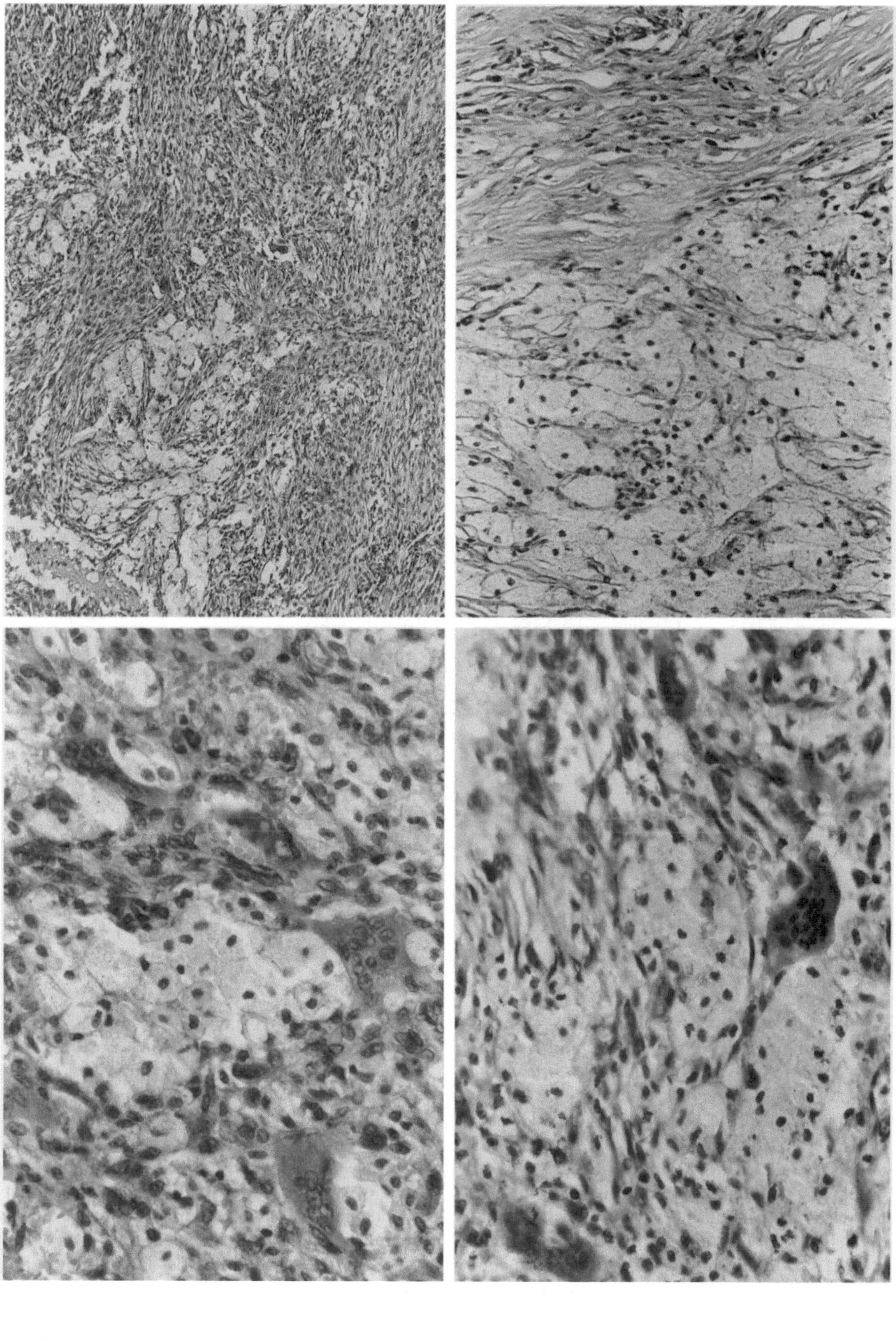

a b c d

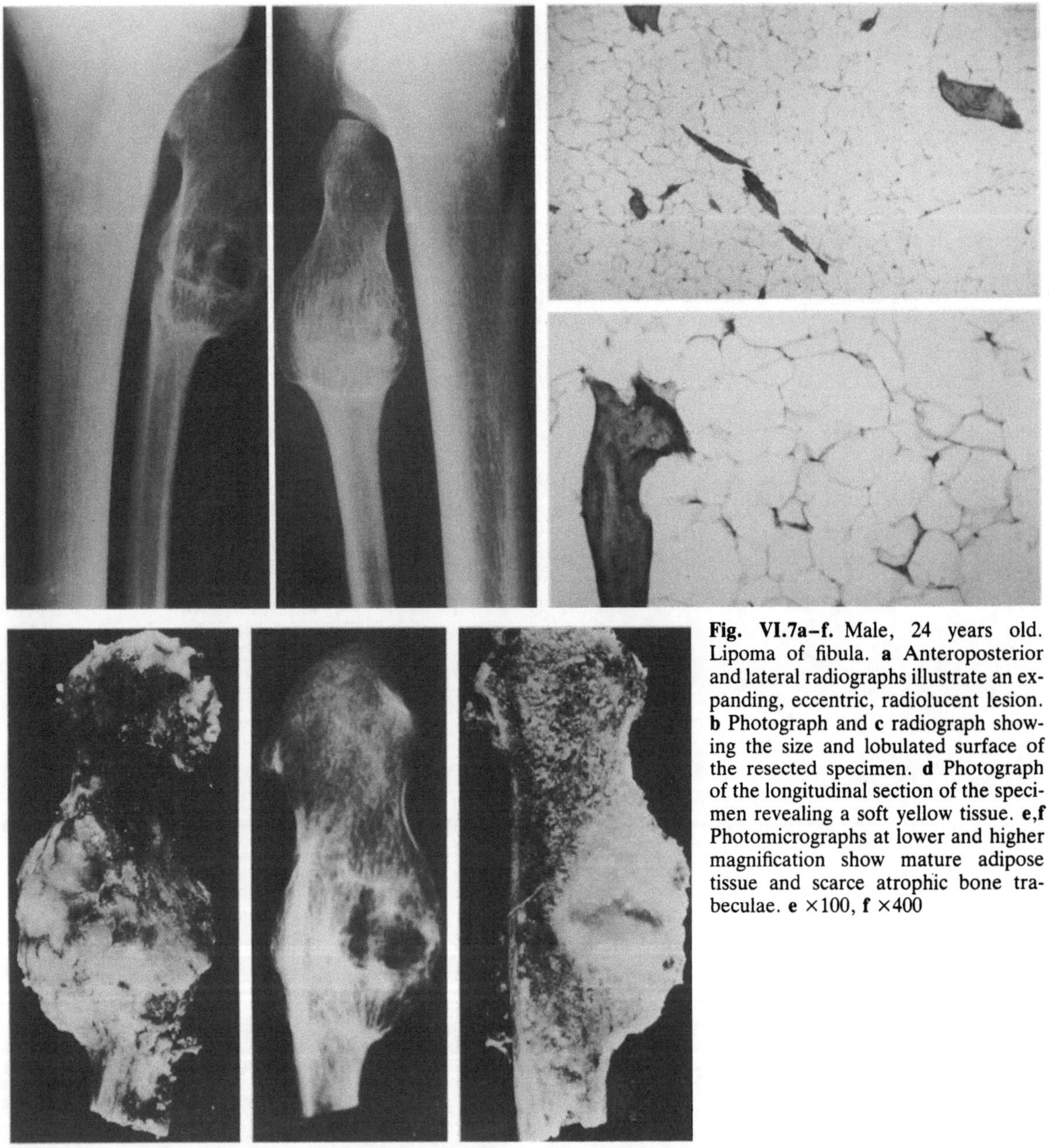

a e f b, c, d

Fig. VI.7a–f. Male, 24 years old. Lipoma of fibula. **a** Anteroposterior and lateral radiographs illustrate an expanding, eccentric, radiolucent lesion. **b** Photograph and **c** radiograph showing the size and lobulated surface of the resected specimen. **d** Photograph of the longitudinal section of the specimen revealing a soft yellow tissue. **e,f** Photomicrographs at lower and higher magnification show mature adipose tissue and scarce atrophic bone trabeculae. **e** ×100, **f** ×400

usually induce a periosteal reaction (Bartlett 1930; Fleming et al. 1962; Kurland and Kennard 1965; Schweitzer 1970), and (2) *intraosseous lipomas*, which arise from the medullary cavity and may expand the bone from within (Dickson et al. 1951; Child 1955; Azizi 1968). Most reports on this lesion have been of one or two cases (Zorn et al. 1971; Gunterberg and Kindblom 1978; DeLee 1979; Döhler and Harms 1981; Goldman et al. 1984) or of a small number of cases (Ramos et al. 1985). This entity seems to be more common than the periosteal type. "Lipomas" reported by Makrycostas (1927) with a certain frequency within vertebral bodies are probably not genuine neoplasms but circumscribed foci of fatty marrow (Schmorl and Junghanns 1971; Lichtenstein 1977).

Incidence. *Intraosseous lipomas* are among the rarest of all bone tumors. Jaffe (1958) stated that he personally had not encountered one case, and Lichtenstein (1977) mentioned only one case, located in the upper humerus. Dahlin and Unni (1986) found six cases of lipoma, an incidence of

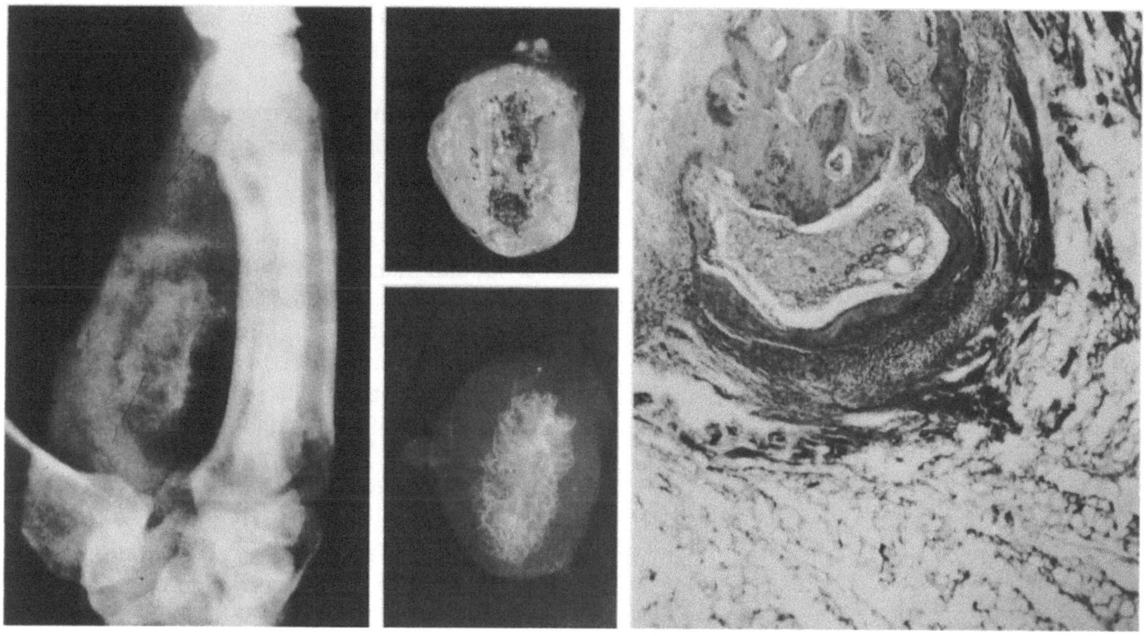

a b, c, d

Fig. VI.8a–d. Male, 55 years old. Periosteal lipoma of metacarpal bone. **a** Lateral radiograph showing an ovoid, clear, well-delimited juxtaosseous area characteristic of lipoma, with central bone density. **b** Photograph and **c** radiograph of the excised nodule, which was attached to the bone and shows centrally metaplastic bone formation. **d** Photomicrograph illustrates bone formation within fatty tissue

1 in 1000 of all bone tumors at the Mayo Clinic. A diligent search by Hart (1973) revealed 28 reported cases over a span of 100 years. A careful review made by Döhler and Harms (1981) found 14 additional cases reported after Hart's review and added four of their own to total 40 reported cases. We have seven well-documented cases of intraosseous and three of periosteal lipomas in our files.

Therefore the large series of 61 histologically verified cases reported recently by Milgram (1988) is surprising. Three additional cases not treated with surgery and two cases with multiple intraosseous sites are also recorded in this article. However, Milgram proposed that intraosseous lipomas be subdivided into three groups, depending on the degree of involution: (I) solid tumors of viable lipocytes, (II) transitional cases with partial fat necrosis and focal calcification, but also regions of viable lipocytes, and (III) late cases with variable degrees of cyst formation, calcification, and reactive new bone formation. In this author's opinion only group I and some group II cases should be classified as typical intraosseous lipomas. Most cases of group III are better defined as cases of fat necrosis or bone infarctions, and had been classified as such in the literature.

Clinical Findings. The average age of presentation was 38.5 years; there was no predilection for any age group, ages ranging from 5 to 70 years (Spjut et al. 1971). Long bones were involved in 59% of cases, the tibia, femur, and fibula being the most common sites. Three of our cases were located in the upper end of the fibula and the remainder in the femur, preferentially the upper end (Moorefield et al. 1976; Milgram 1981); the tumors usually occurred in the metaphysis. The calcaneus is also a common site.

Intraosseous lipoma is usually an incidental finding; pain and/or swelling are the most common complaints in the remaining cases.

Radiographic Features. Radiologically, a radiolucent, generally well-delimited lytic area with well-defined, sometimes sclerotic margins and endosteal scalloping was most frequently observed; in several lesions, a trabecular pattern produced a loculated appearance. In more than half the lesions, bone expansion was observed; it was a constant finding in rib and fibular lesions, as we found in our three patients with a tumor in this location (Fig. VI.7). No cortical expansion was observed in larger long bones; cortical destruction and periosteal reaction are always lacking. In the few recent cases reported, the CT values were

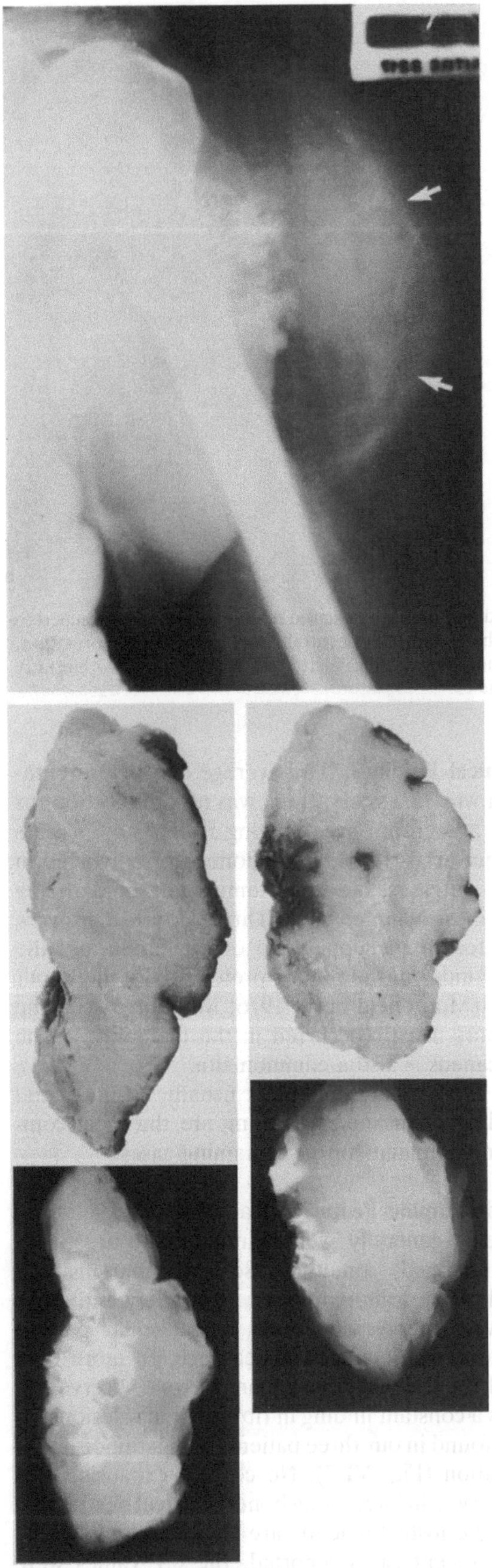

a b c

typical and characteristic of fat (Ramos et al. 1985; Leeson et al. 1983).

Pathologic Findings. *Macroscopically*, the tumors showed a lobulated, clearly demarcated soft mass, of bright yellow color, without bony consistency.

Histologically, the tumors were composed of a lobular mass of mature adipose tissue. In the majority of reported cases, atrophic bony trabeculae were found. These were an important diagnostic feature, especially when they exhibited often empty osteocytic lacunae, i.e., signs of necrosis (Hart 1973). Although we can confirm the presence of a few, thin bony trabeculae in almost all intraosseous lipomas, we did not find signs of bone necrosis (Fig. VI.7). Myxoid degeneration, fat necrosis, calcification, and ossification have been recorded in cases of intraosseous lipoma (Milgram 1988; see literature). We want to emphasize that in our opinion a diagnosis of intraosseous lipoma should be accepted only when a discrete lobulated mass is found and/or when the pathologist receives the complete resection specimen; this together with the characteristic radiologic pattern allows an unequivocal diagnosis of lipoma. Fragments of fatty tissue with atrophic bone trabeculae and areas of fat infarction and/or calcification are *not* diagnostic and may be found in localized osteoporosis or in the vicinity of other lesions.

The treatment of intraosseous lipoma consists of excision of the tumor; no recurrences have been observed.

Parosteal (periosteal) lipomas were less common in the literature and in our material. Only those cases that produced a radiologic pattern characterized by a round or ovoid well-defined soft tissue mass adjacent to the bone were included. The tumor mass was more translucent than the surrounding muscle tissue and showed depression of the cortical surface and characteristic spicular or radiating periosteal bone formation (Figs. VI.8, VI.9). Our three cases were

Fig. VI.9a–c. Female, 57 years old. Periosteal lipoma. **a** Radiograph shows the well-defined, soft tissue tumor attached with a broad base at the upper third of humerus and the conspicuous periosteal new-bone formation. **b,c** Photographs and radiographs of the longitudinal section of the specimen illustrate a dark zone at the tumor basis corresponding to the area of periosteal metaplastic bone formation

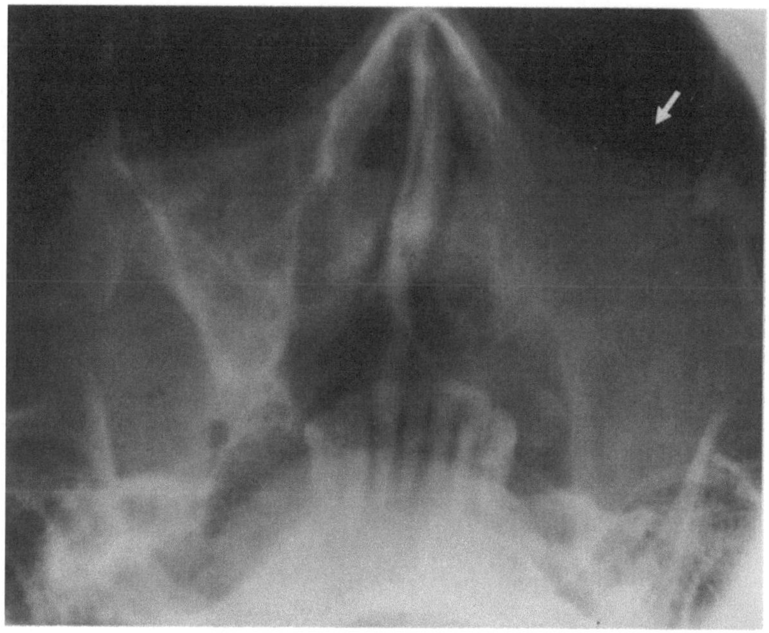

Fig. VI.10. Male, 38 years old. Desmoplastic fibroma of maxilla. Radiograph shows a large, ill-defined radiolucent lesion which partially destroyed the cortex

adults. The tumors were located in the upper part of the humerus and femur and in the metacarpal shaft. In all cases, swelling was the presenting symptom. The treatment consisted of complete excision of the tumors, which were attached to the cortex without involving it.

B. Intermediate

1. Desmoplastic Fibroma

Definition, WHO: *"A rare locally aggressive intermediate tumor characterized by the formation of abundant collagen fibers by the tumor cells. The tissue is sparsely cellular, and the nuclei are ovoid or elongated. The cellularity, pleomorphism, and mitotic activity that are features of fibrosarcoma are lacking."*

Under the term "desmoplastic fibroma" Jaffe reported in 1958 five cases of a bone lesion showing pathologic features identical to those of the desmoid tumors of soft tissues, clearly differentiating it from other "fibromas" of bone (nonossifying and chondromyxoid fibroma). This distinct entity, which is definitely uncommon, was the only benign fibrous tumor accepted by the WHO classification (1972) and the writer (1981). At present desmoplastic fibroma is included by the majority of pathologists among the group of true fibrous tumors, based exclusively on clinical and radiologic features. Only about 100 cases have been reported in the literature (Whitesides and Ackerman 1960; Dahlin and Hoover 1964; Cohen and Goldenberg 1965; Sugiura 1976; Bertoni et al. 1984; Gebhardt et al. 1985), including only a few reports with ten (Rabhan and Rosai 1968) or more cases (Nilsonne and Goethlin 1969; Campanacci 1990). We have in our files 16 cases, one of which was reported previously (Martinez Mosquera et al. 1977). Two of our cases were of periosteal origin.

Clinical Findings. Pain or swelling, sometimes of long duration before diagnosis, is the most common complaint, accompanied by functional disability. A pathologic fracture may in some cases be the presenting symptom.

Age and Sex. Although there is wide variation in age, the great majority of patients are young adults less than 30 years old. There seems to be no sex predominance. An exception is the clear male predominance in Dahlin and Unni's series of nine cases (among 8542 bone tumors) (seven males and two females).

Localization. The most common anatomic sites involved are the long bones (humerus, femur, tibia) or flat bones (ilium, scapula, mandible, and maxilla) (Hinds et al. 1969; Eisen and Butler 1984; Bertoni et al. 1986). However, desmo-

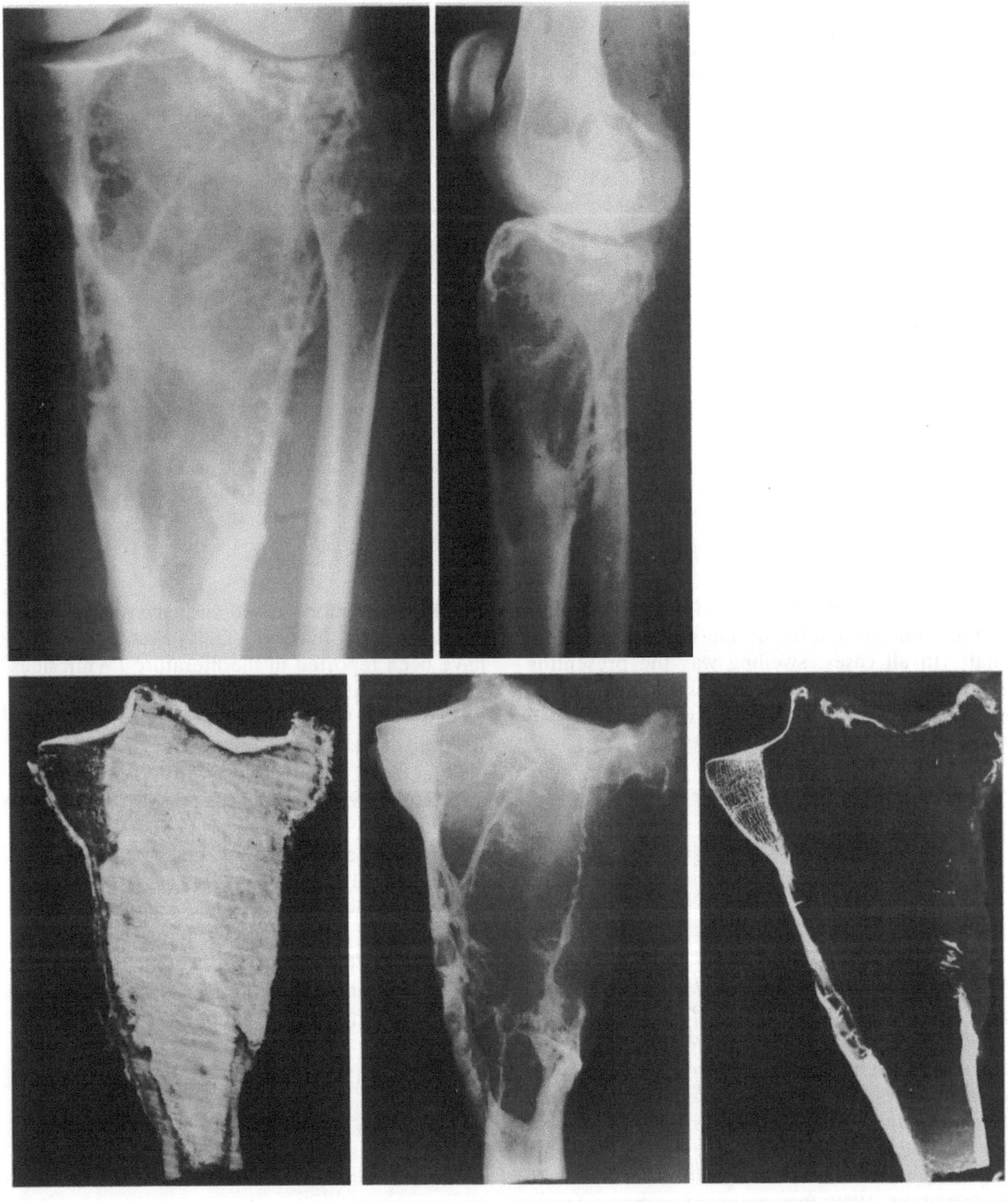

a

b, c

d

Fig. VI.11a–d. Male, 26 years old. Desmoplastic fibroma of tibia. **a** Anteroposterior and lateral radiographs illustrate a large radiolucent trabeculated lesion extending from the joint to the diaphysis, which excludes the diagnosis of giant-cell tumor. A segmental resection was performed, followed by prosthesis. **b** Photograph of the specimen showing a firm grayish-white tumor that has destroyed a great part of the lateral cortex, as is seen clearly in the radiograph of the specimen (**c**) and a thin 5-mm thick longitudinal section (**d**)

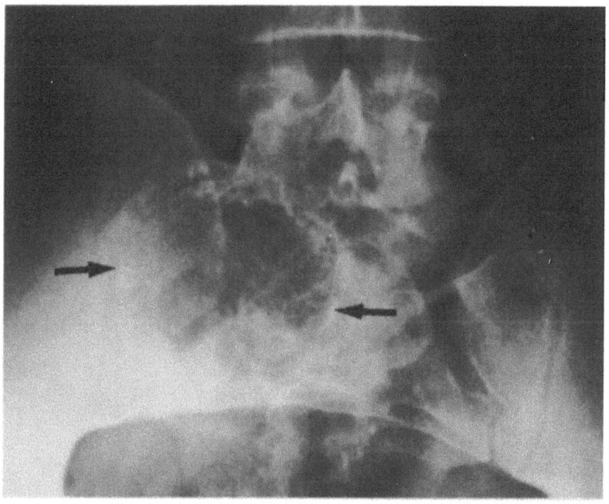

Fig. VI.12. Female, 24 years old. Desmoplastic fibroma of sacrum. Radiograph shows a roundish, well-defined radiolucent lesion. The clinical-radiologic diagnosis was osteoblastoma

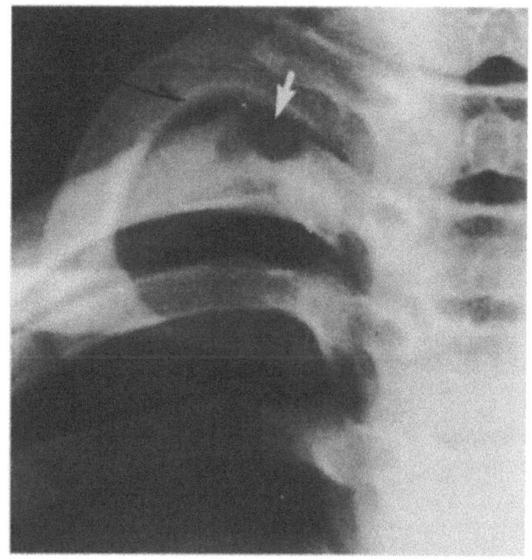

Fig. VI.13. Male, 7 years old. Desmoplastic fibroma of second rib. Radiograph reveals eccentric radiolucent lesion expanding the thinned cortex

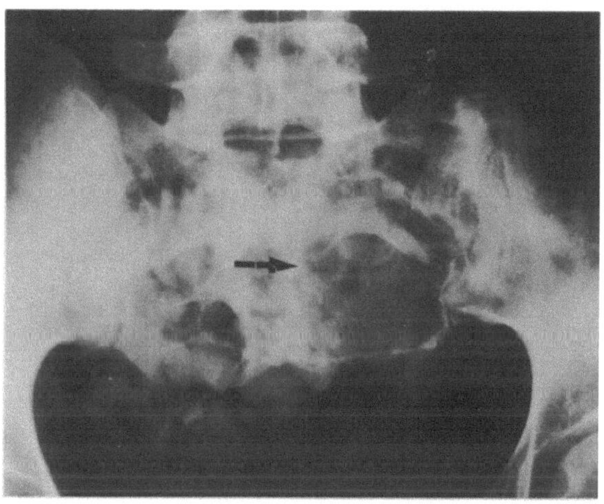

Fig. VI.14. Male, 32 years old. Desmoplastic fibroma of sacrum showing a large osteolytic lesion with ill-defined margins toward the medullary cavity

plastic fibroma may also occur in other long bones (Scheer and Kuhlman 1963); the shaft end or the metaphysis is more frequently affected. In our material, the tumor occurred in the upper tibia (three cases), femur (two cases), sacrum (three cases), humerus, rib, acetabulum, and jaw (two cases each).

Radiographic Features. The radiographs generally showed an extensive radiolucent lesion, often expanding the thinned cortex. In our material, the cortex was destroyed exceptionally (Fig. VI.10) with extension into the adjacent soft tissues, resembling a malignant tumor. In two cases, a trabeculated pattern was observed (Fig. VI.11) or the tumor was surrounded by a thin sclerotic border (Figs. VI.12–VI.14) similar to the radiographic appearance of osteoblastoma.

Pathologic Findings. *Grossly*, the tumor is grayish white, of firm elastic consistency, identical to the gross aspect of desmoid tumors of soft tissues and well-differentiated fibrosarcoma. In two of our cases the tumor was well delineated, showing a thin rim of bone in one instance (Fig. VI.11).

Histologically, the tumor is characterized by bundles of abundant collagen fibers, often forming thickened, hyalinized bands, separated by scarce spindle-shaped fibroblasts of small size, with elongated or ovoid nuclei and without evident mitotic activity. The hypocellularity and the abundant intercellular substance (Figs. VI.15, VI.16), together with the lack of multinucleated giant cells and/or lipid-bearing histiocytes (xanthoma cells), distinguish desmoplastic fibroma from metaphyseal fibrous defect (nonossifying fibroma); the absence of metaplastic bone formation distinguishes it from fibrous dysplasia. However, the most difficult problem is the histologic differentiation from well-differentiated fibrosarcoma, although the lack of mitotic activity, nuclear hyperchromatism, or atypism in desmoplastic fibroma may help in the distinction. However, some areas of this tumor may be more cellular, and, on the other hand, in some fibrosarcomas more or less extensive areas with predominant collagen tissue may occasionally be found, making differential diagnosis difficult.

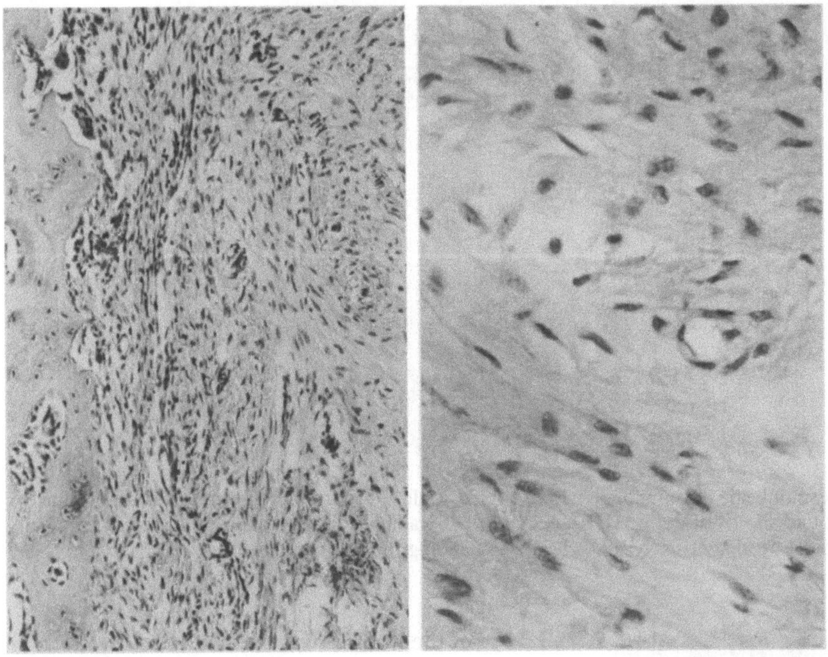

a b

Fig. VI.15a,b. Photomicrographs showing at lower and higher magnification the well-differentiated, poorly cellular fibrous tissue with abundant, partly hyalinized collagen fibers. The nuclei are ovoid or elongated, and there is no cellular pleomorphism or mitotic activity. In **a** osteoclastic resorption on the inner surface of the thin neoformed cortex is seen. **a** ×100, **b** ×300

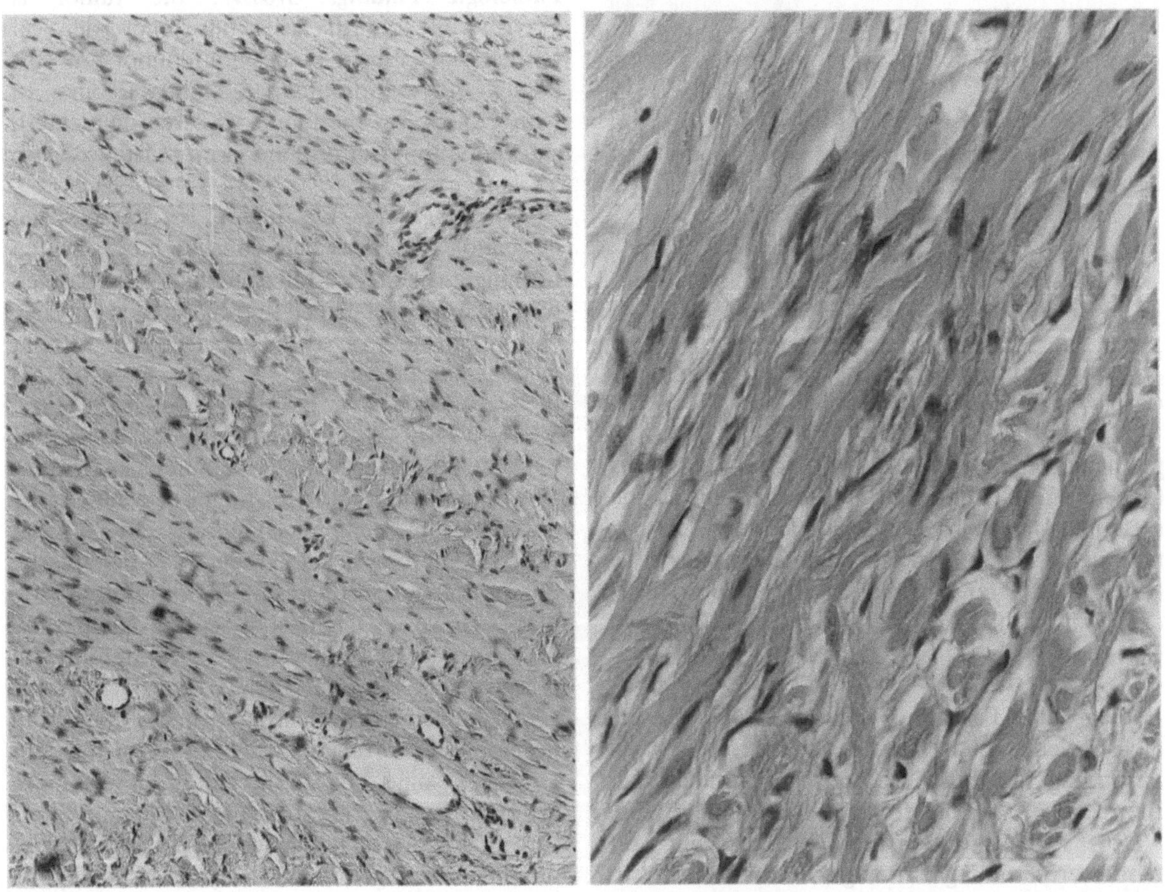

a b

Fig. VI.16a,b. Microphotographs at lower and higher magnification showing the poorly cellular fibrous tissue with abundant thick, partly hyalinized collagen fibers. **a** ×100, **b** ×400

Fig. VI.17. Photomicrograph of periosteal desmoid eroding the cortex (*top*) and showing histologic features identical to those of the centrally located desmoplastic fibroma. ×100

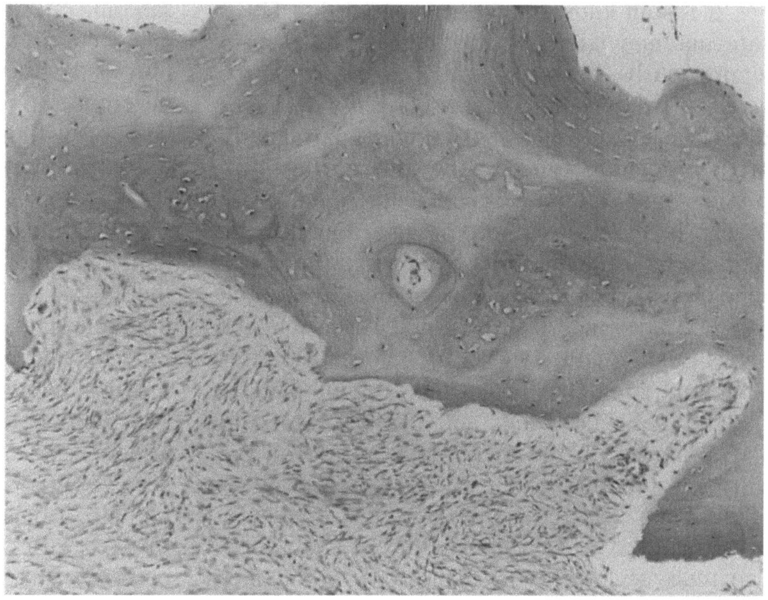

Treatment. Recurrences after curettage or incomplete excision have been reported. Therefore, the treatment indicated is complete en bloc resection or segmental resection. Amputation is generally not necessary, except for the rare extensive and destructive lesions. Metastases have not been reported to date.

The "periosteal desmoid" reported first by Kimmelstiel and Rapp (1951) has gross and microscopic features identical to those of the centrally located "desmoplastic fibroma," but is generally smaller (Marek 1955). In the writer's opinion, "periosteal desmoid" is the peripheral counterpart of desmoplastic fibroma, located beneath the periosteum and frequently producing a localized shallow defect with a sclerotic base at the underlying cortex (Fig. VI.17). The lesion possibly arises from the periosteum and differs pathologically from the common "fibrous cortical defect." The few cases reported and the two cases observed by us were in children or adolescents, and the preferred site was the lower femoral end and the tibia.

The treatment indicated is complete excision.

C. Malignant

1. Fibrosarcoma

Definition, WHO: *"A malignant tumor characterized by the formation by the spindle-shaped tumor cells of interlacing bundles of collagen fibers, and by the absence of other types of histological differentiation, such as the formation of cartilage or bone."*

In the past, some authors denied the occurrence of fibrosarcoma primary in bone, postulating that it originated in the periosteum or the adjacent parosteal soft tissues with secondary invasion of the marrow cavity (Geschickter 1932; Stout 1948) or that it is in reality a poorly differentiated osteosarcoma with only scarce osteoid or tumor bone formation, i.e., so-called fibroblastic osteosarcoma. At present, it is accepted by almost all authors, including the writer, that fibrosarcoma of bone is a distinct entity, which arises either from the supportive connective tissue of the marrow cavity (*central*, *endosteal*, *or medullary fibrosarcoma*) or much less frequently from periosteum (*periosteal fibrosarcoma*) or parosteal soft tissue (Jaffe 1958; Gilmer and MacEwen 1958; Eyre-Brook and Price 1969; Lichtenstein 1977; Pritchard et al. 1977). Although some authors (Dahlin and Unni 1986; Eyre-Brook and Price 1969) excluded the periosteal variety from their consideration, maintaining that the vast majority of cases may have arisen from extraosseous soft tissues merely abutting the bone and secondarily eroding the bone cortex, Huvos and Higinbotham (1975) found that 89 of their cases were central or medullary in location and 41 were periosteal or peripheral. These findings are in sharp contrast to those in our and all other larger series, in which "periosteal" fibrosarcoma is definitely infrequent or nonexistent (Taconis and Van Rijssel 1985).

It is well known and documented that fibrosarcoma may arise as a malignant change in a previously benign lesion (*secondary fibrosarcoma*), most commonly associated with Paget disease and giant-cell tumors of bone, particularly after irradiation, and rarely with fibrous dysplasia, bone infarct, osteomyelitis, and other benign bone lesions. Fibrosarcoma may also be induced by irradiation of a bone without preexistent disease. Secondary fibrosarcoma accounted for 23.9% of the 207 cases in the Mayo Clinic series (Dahlin and Unni 1986); 35 occurred after radiation, four developed in giant-cell tumors that had no prior radiation, and five developed in Paget disease. In the 45 fibrosarcomas from the Hospital Cochin in Paris, 80% were primary (André et al. 1983). There were preexisting bony abnormalities in 15 of the 102 cases of fibrosarcomas of long bones registered in the files of the Netherlands Committee on Bone Tumors (Taconis and Van Rijssel 1985). In our series, 13 cases occurred in preexisting Paget disease, ten in giant-cell tumors (all after prior irradiation), three in fibrous dysplasia, and two in bone infarcts.

Incidence. Fibrosarcoma was less frequent than osteosarcoma, chondrosarcoma, giant-cell tumor, and Ewing sarcoma, accounting for 6.5% (166 cases) of the malignant tumors primary in bone. The three largest reported series include: 207 cases studied at the Mayo Clinic (Dahlin and Unni 1986), that is, approximately 4% of the total number of primary malignant bone tumors (less than one-sixth as common as osteosarcoma); 130 cases treated at the Memorial Sloan-Kettering Cancer Center, during a period of more than 50 years (Huvos and Higinbotham 1975); and 118 cases filed at the Rizzoli Institute, Bologna (Campanacci 1990). From 1953 to 1976, 102 cases of fibrosarcoma were registered in the files of the Netherlands Committee, excluding fibrosarcomas of soft tissues with secondary erosion of bone. During the past two decades, since the first report of malignant fibrous histiocytoma as a primary bone tumor (Feldman and Norman 1972), the exact criteria for the microscopic diagnosis of fibrosarcoma have undergone considerable changes; it has become increasingly less frequent and many cases are at present classified as malignant fibrous histiocytoma or fibroblastic osteosarcoma. In a study made of the clinical course of 102 fibrosarcomas of long bones filed at the Netherlands Committee on Bone Tumors, 55 cases were predominantly fibroblastic osteosarcoma or pure fibrosarcomas while 47 contained extensive areas resembling so-called malignant fibrous histiocytoma. There was no significant difference in clinical behavior in fibrosarcoma with or without marked features of malignant fibrous histiocytoma.

Clinical Findings. *Age and Sex.* There is no evident sex predominance in most series, although there is a slightly higher ratio of males to females in others (Huvos and Higinbotham 1975). Eighty-four of our patients were males and 72 were females. Their age ranged from 5 to 80 years, but adults between 20 and 60 years of age were affected most frequently. These findings agreed with those of other series and were similar to the age distribution in chondrosarcoma, but contrasted with the lower age of patients with osteosarcoma (Scheme VI.1).

Some exceptional cases of congenital fibrosarcoma have been published; in a review of the literature, Wells (1940) reported five cases, all located in a tubular bone. Other single cases have been recorded by Kindblom and Angervall (1978) and Fauré et al. (1981). In our series we have two cases, localized in the radius and fibula, respectively. The prognosis of this type of tumor after amputation seems to be better than that of fibrosarcoma at other ages.

Localization. In accordance with the findings of most other observers, the most common anatomic site was long tubular bones; thus the femur (59 cases) and tibia (33 cases) accounted for 55% of cases, the tumor occurring preferentially in the metaphyseal or epiphyseal area of the lower end of the femur and the upper end of the tibia. Because most of our material comes from orthopedic departments, we have only a few cases located in the head; this contrasts with the 26% of tumors involving the skull and jaws in Dahlin's series, and the 15% in the craniofacial bones (most often the mandible) in the files of the Memorial Hospital.

Multifocal (*multicentric*) *fibrosarcoma* is exceptional. Only a few cases have been reported in the literature (Steiner 1944; Nielson and Poulsen 1962). One case that was studied ultramicroscopically (Hernandez and Fernandez 1976) has been published. We observed two such cases, one with multiple synchronous tumors in both tibiae and the other with lesions at the upper femoral end and in a lumbar vertebra, both of which were rapidly fatal. Only two cases in Dahlin and Unni's

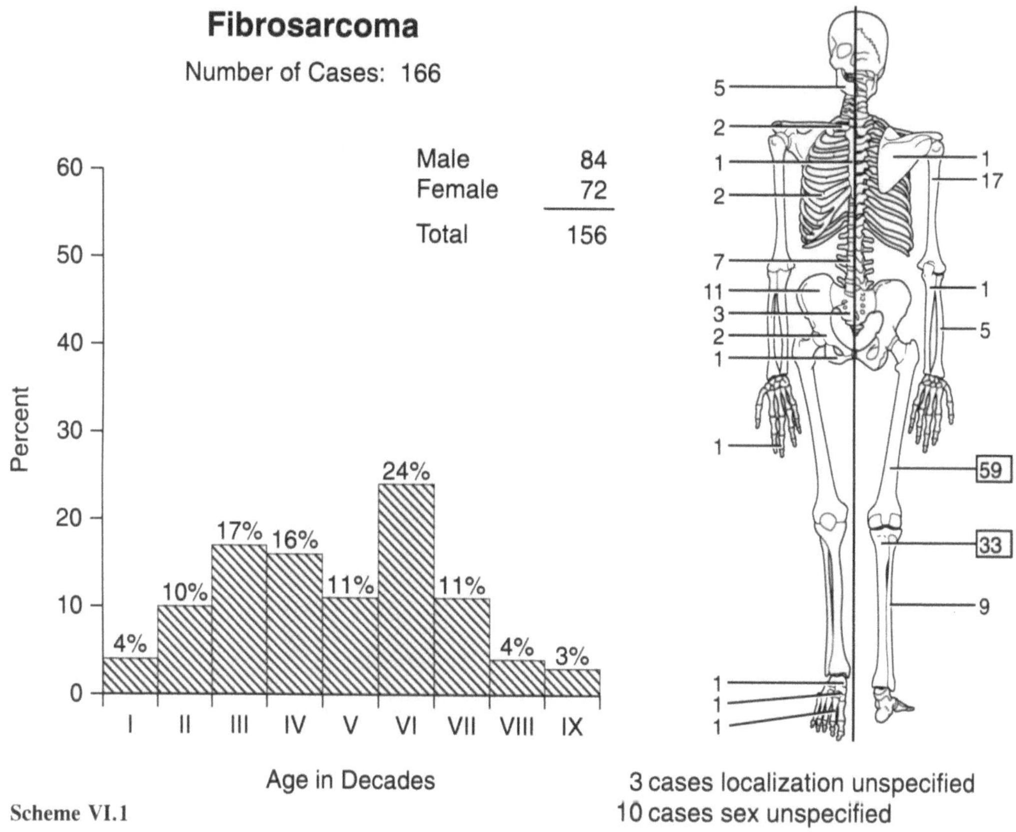

Scheme VI.1

series presented multifocal lesions. However, Dahlin (1978) stated that he has seen several other examples in material seen in consultation, in which two or more skeletal foci were present when the patient first sought medical advice.

Symptoms. Primary fibrosarcoma's symptoms are not characteristic; they are similar to those of other malignant bone tumors, the most common complaint being pain and swelling, with a palpable mass often a frequent feature in peripheral (periosteal) fibrosarcoma or in highly malignant tumors. Especially in slow-growing, low-grade tumors (Eyre-Brook and Price 1969) there is usually a long delay before diagnosis, ranging from several months to a few years. Due to the destructive character of fibrosarcoma, pathologic fracture is a frequent complication, and it constitutes the initial symptoms in some cases.

Radiographic Features. The radiographic appearance was that of a radiolucent, often permeative or mottled lesion, with ill-defined borders toward the medullary cavity, located most frequently in the metaphyseal region, extending into the epiphysis or the diaphysis. The osteolytic area was occasionally eccentric and epiphyseal, simulating the pattern of giant-cell tumor (Figs. VI.18–VI.23).

Rarely, a slightly sclerotic marginal border was observed, usually in relationship to a well-differentiated, slow-growing tumor. The bone cortex was generally thinned and disrupted over a relatively wide area, with extension into soft tissues. Expansion of the cortex or periosteal new-bone formation was rare. Like other authors, we found an evident relationship between the radiographic appearance and the rate of growth and differentiation of the tumor. The well-differentiated, generally slow-growing lesions often showed well-defined borders and, occasionally, thinning and expansion of the cortex, suggesting a diagnosis of giant-cell tumor (Figs. VI.20, VI.23), chondromyxoid fibroma (Fig. VI.24), or desmoplastic fibroma. In contrast, a poorly differentiated and rapidly invading lesion with indistinct borders and extensive cortical destruction renders very difficult the differential diagnosis with osteolytic osteosarcoma in younger patients and malignant lymphoma, malignant vascular tumors, metastatic carcinoma, and localized (solitary) myeloma in adults.

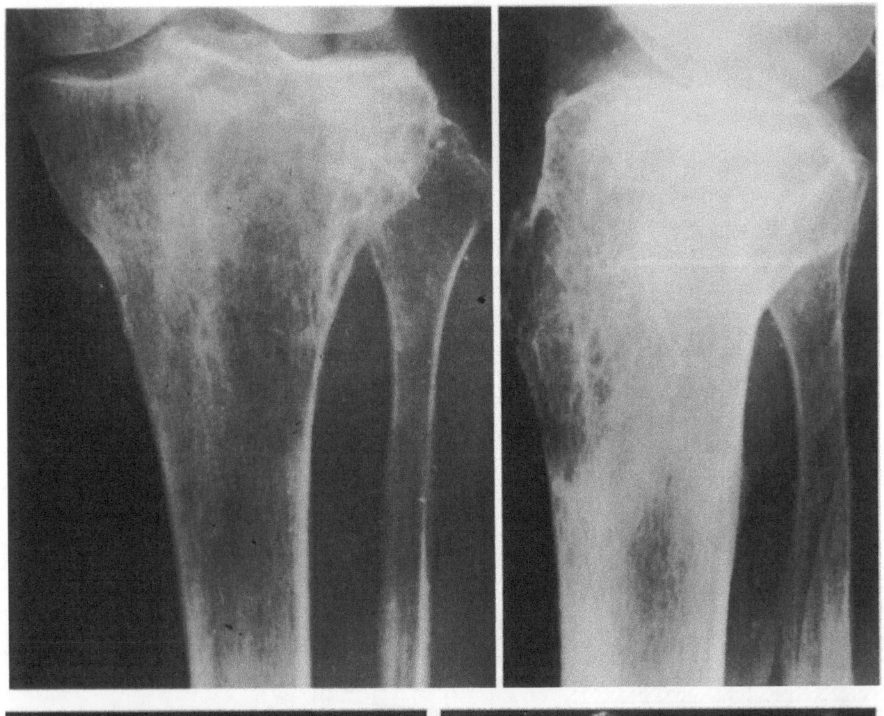

Fig. VI.18a–c. Female, 70 years old. Fibrosarcoma of tibia. **a** Anteroposterior and lateral radiographs illustrate an osteolytic lesion in the metaphyseal region, with ill-defined margins, partly destroying the cortext at its anterior aspect. **b** Photograph and **c** radiograph of the amputation specimen show the extensive invasion of soft tissues and the white color of the bulk of the tumor, with some hemorrhagic areas

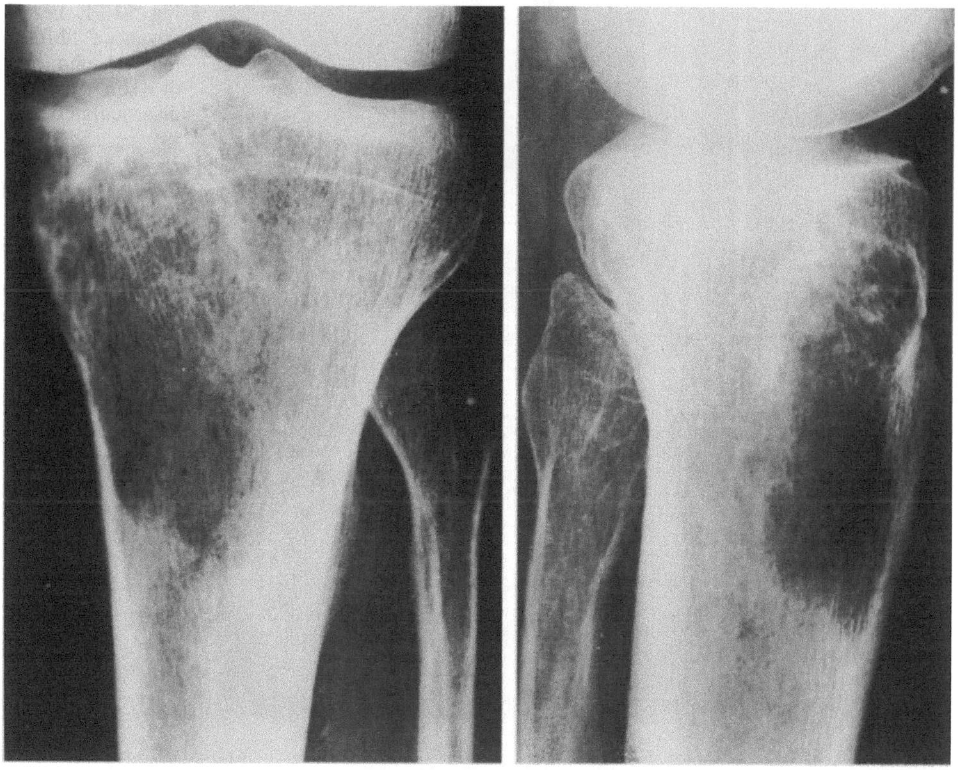

VI.19

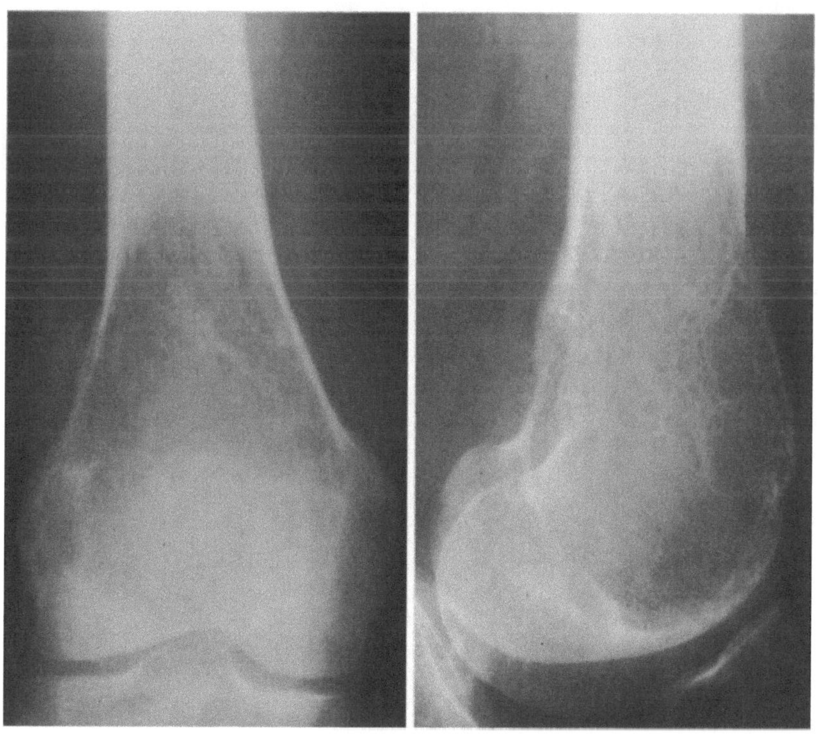

VI.20

Fig. VI.19. Female, 67 years old. Fibrosarcoma of tibia. Anteroposterior and lateral radiographs show the destructive lesion with ill-defined borders toward the medullary cavity. Note slight periosteal reaction and its lateral aspect

Fig. VI.20. Male, 26 years old. Fibrosarcoma of the lower femoral end. Anteroposterior and lateral radiographs showing a large osteolytic lesion in the meta-epiphyseal region, suggestive of giant-cell tumor

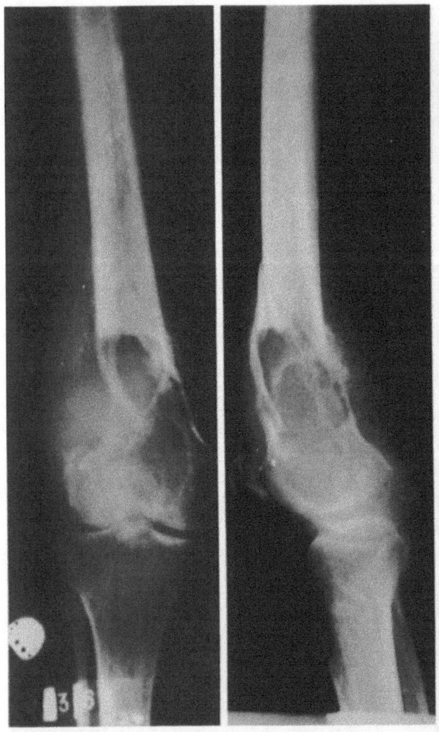

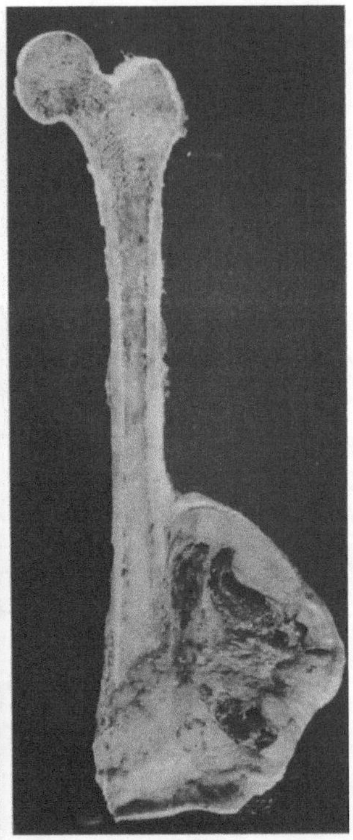

◄ **Fig. VI.21.** Female, 24 years old, with advanced fibrosarcoma of the lower femoral end and extensive invasion of soft tissue, which has been disarticulated

Fig. VI.22a–c. Male, 45 years old. ► Fibrosarcoma of the lower femoral end. Clinical radiographs and photographs of the surface and the section of the tumor show its eccentric location and the well-delimited surface of the soft tissue mass

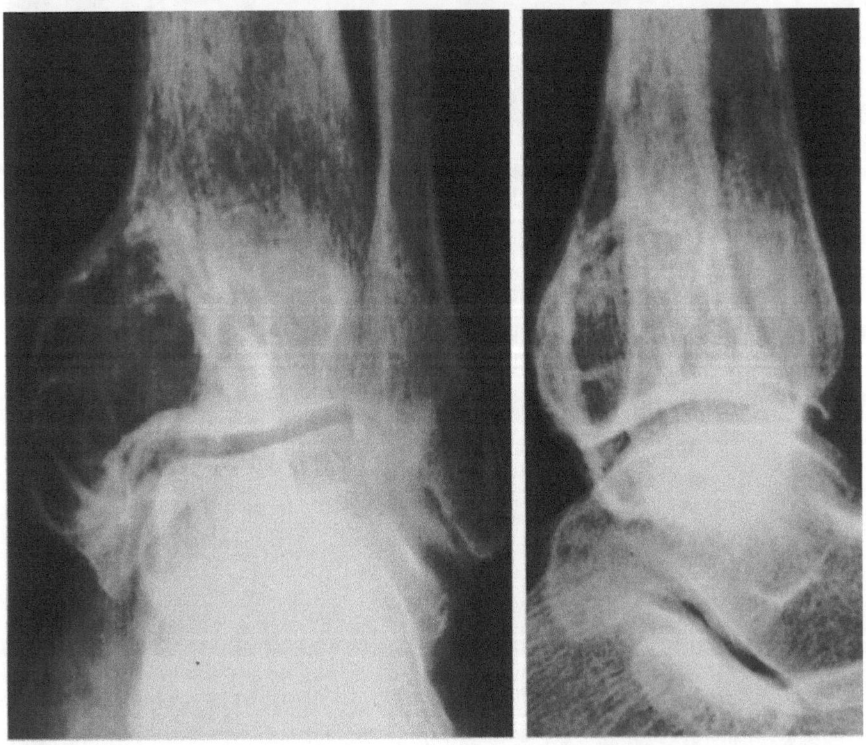

▲

Fig. VI.23. Male, 38 years old. Fibrosarcoma of distal tibia. Anteroposterior and lateral radiographs show a radiolucent, eccentric, and expanding lesion of the medial malleolus, suggesting giant-cell tumor

Fig. VI.24a–c. Male, 51 years old. Fibrosarcoma of the ► greater trochanter. **a** Anteroposterior and lateral radiographs show radiolucent lesion with well-defined, slightly sclerotic borders toward the spongiosa and partial destruction of the cortex, which is more clearly seen in the photograph and radiograph of the resection specimen (**b**,**c**)

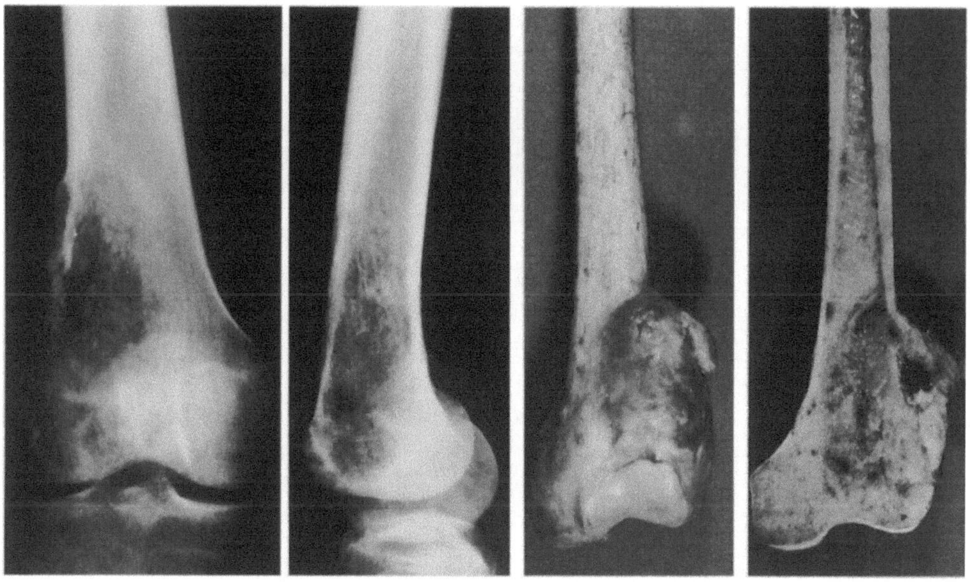

VI.22a b, c

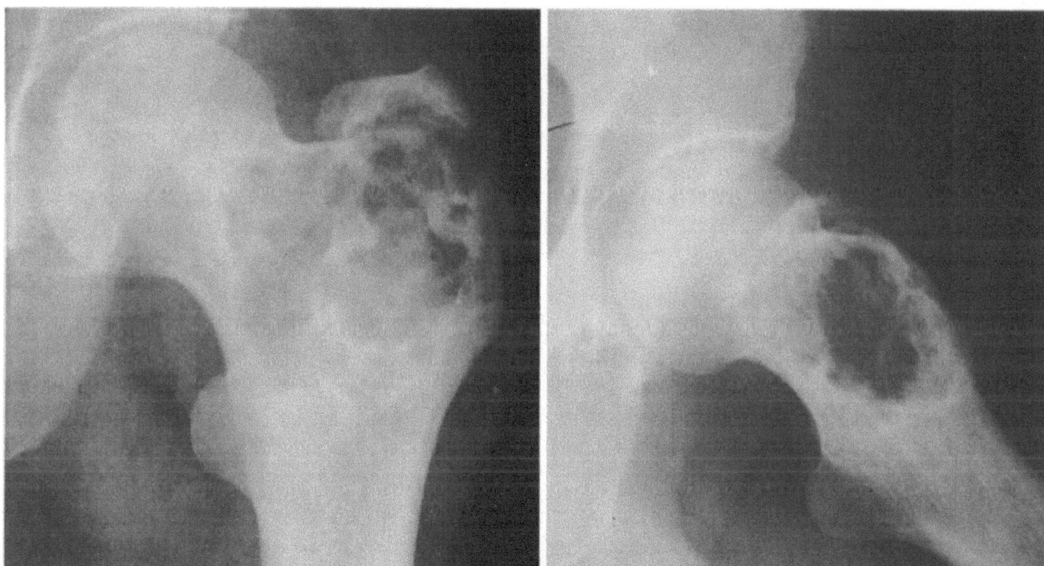

a

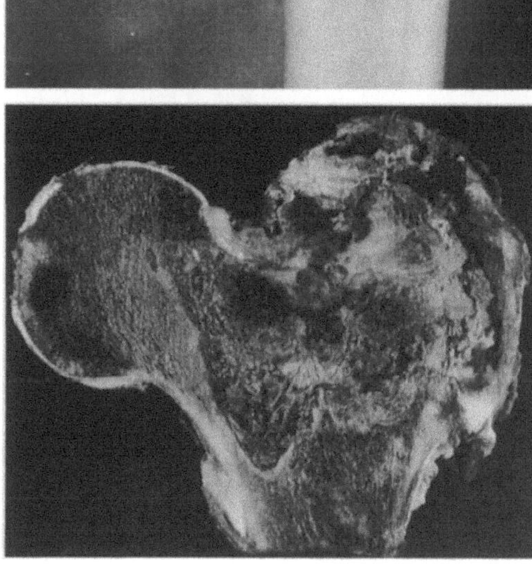

VI.24b

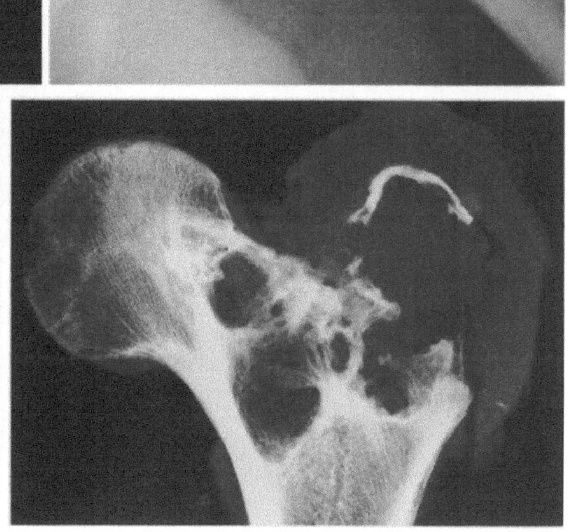

c

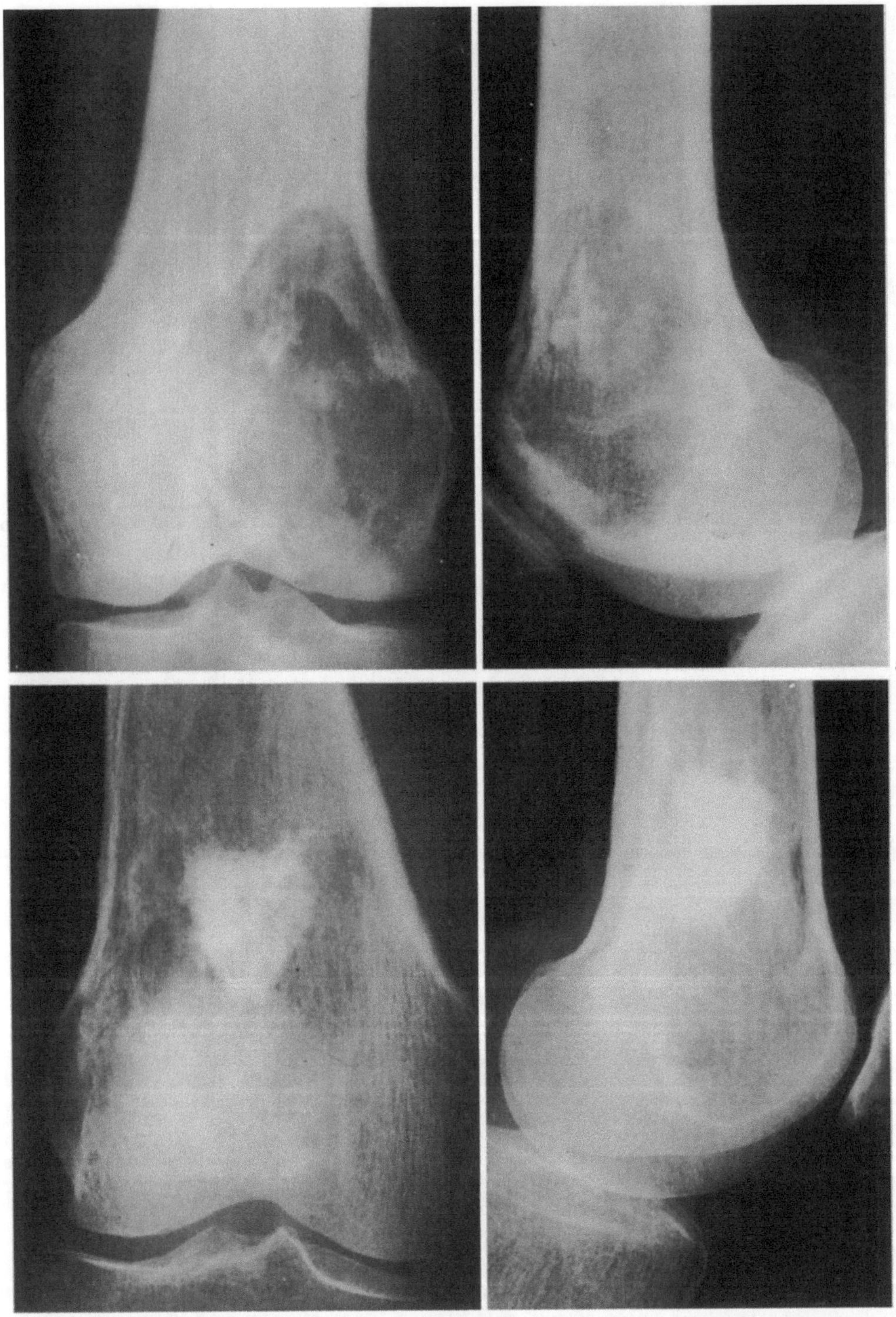

a

b

Fig. VI.25a,b. Two cases of fibrosarcoma with ischemic bone infarcts. **a** Male, 57 years old. Anteroposterior and lateral radiographs showing radiolucent eccentric lesion with rather well-defined margin. **b** Female, 69 years old. The central dense radiopacity is larger, of coarse, granular aspect

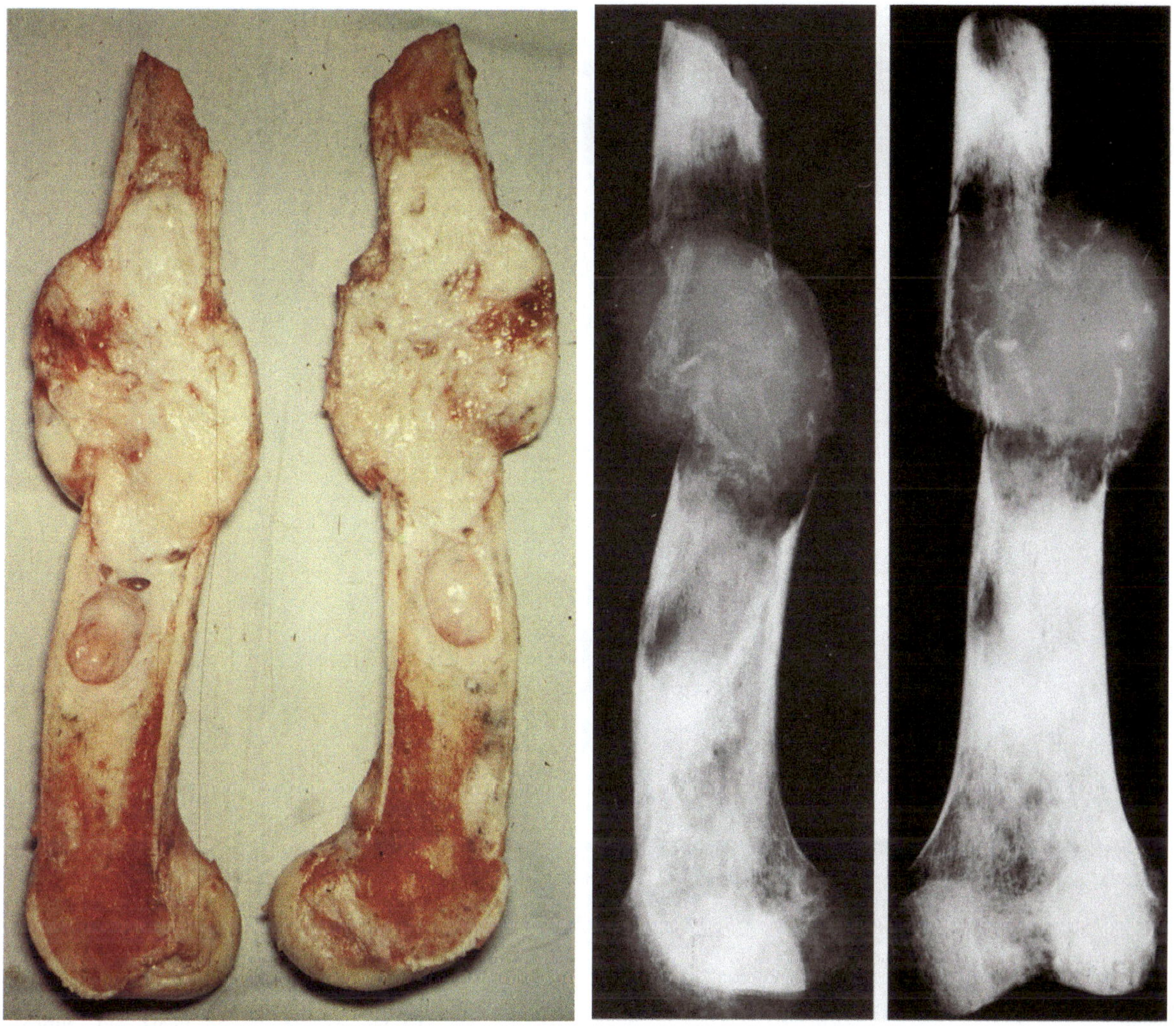

a b, c

Fig. VI.26a–c. Male, 25 years old. Fibrosarcoma developed in fibrous dysplasia of femur. **a** Photograph of the amputation specimen illustrates the extensive destruction of the cortices in the midshaft by the grayish white tumor, which blends toward the medullary cavity into the dysplastic, partly cystic tissue. **b** Lateral and **c** anteroposterior radiographs show the osteolytic destructive tumor and the ground-glass appearance of the lower part of the shaft

Figures VI.25 and VI.26 show the radiographic appearances in two cases of fibrosarcoma associated with ischemic bone infarcts, and in a patient with fibrosarcoma that developed in fibrous dysplasia of the femur.

Pathologic Findings. The *gross pattern* was variable according to the grade of tumor differentiation. The tumor is grayish-white, and the consistency varies from firm and rubbery to soft and friable, depending on the amount of collagen of the tumor stroma. Areas of hemorrhage, necrosis, or cystic degeneration or myxoid areas were occasionally observed; intratumoral bone or cartilage formation was always lacking. The tumor was of variable, generally ovoid shape, with its longest axis parallel to the bone of origin; usually it had irregular margins, with infiltration and destruction of the spongiosa and the cortex. Extension into the adjacent soft tissues was common (Figs. VI.21, VI.22, VI.27). We have seen only a few examples of peripheral fibrosarcoma of undoubtedly periosteal origin, located at the external surface of a bone; rarely there is no appreciable involvement of the cortex, but more frequently the tumor erodes the underlying bone and penetrates into the medullary cavity (Fig. VI.28). In two cases, the tumor was located in the interosseous space of the forearm and eroded extensively both the radius and the ulna;

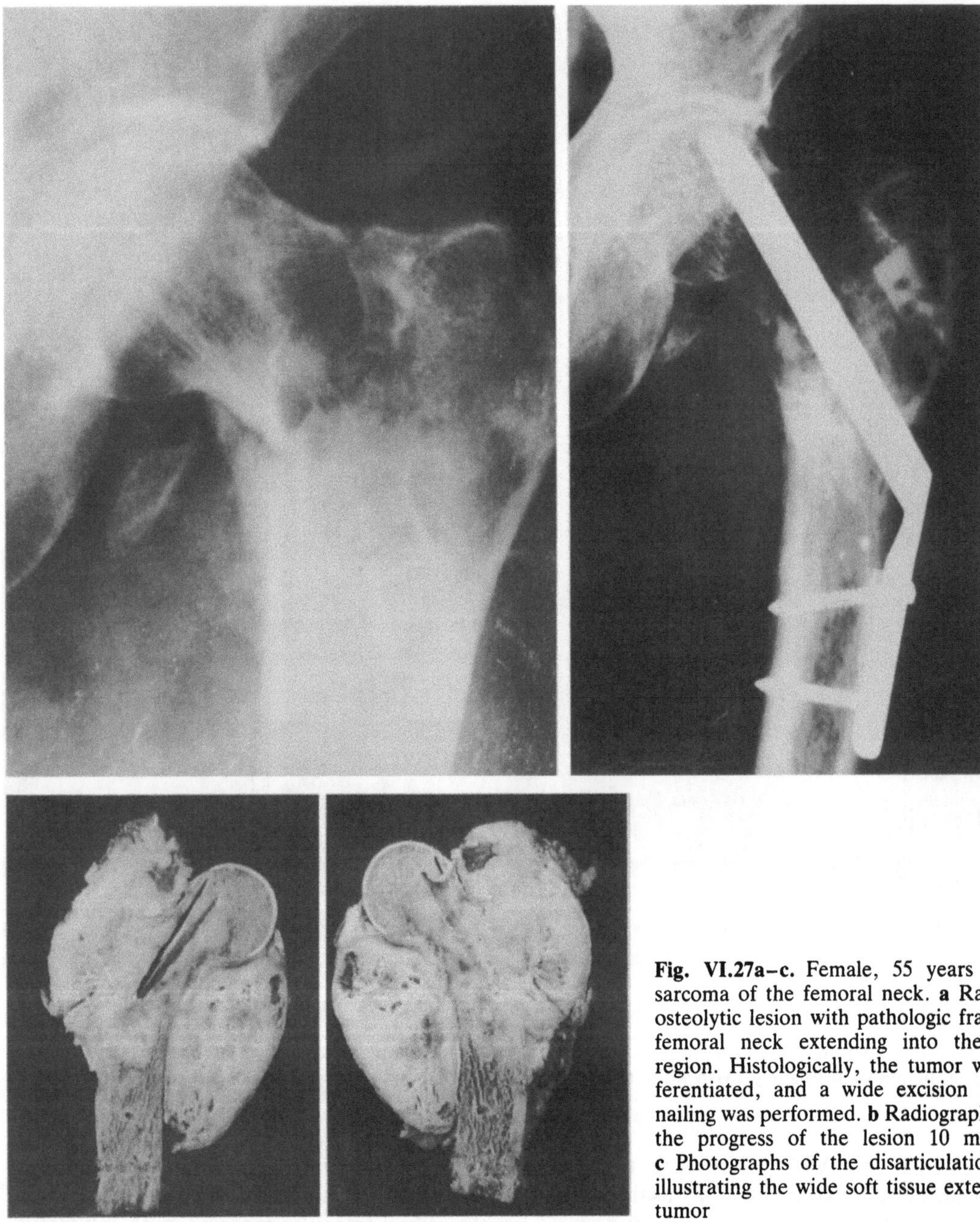

a b c

Fig. VI.27a–c. Female, 55 years old. Fibrosarcoma of the femoral neck. **a** Radiograph of osteolytic lesion with pathologic fracture in the femoral neck extending into the trochanter region. Histologically, the tumor was well differentiated, and a wide excision followed by nailing was performed. **b** Radiograph illustrating the progress of the lesion 10 months later. **c** Photographs of the disarticulation specimen illustrating the wide soft tissue extension of the tumor

in another case, it was in the intercostal space, eroding two ribs. Metastases in regional lymph nodes were rare, the common route of dissemination being hematogenous into the lung.

The *histologic structure* of fibrosarcoma of bone, like that of soft tissue, covers a wide range, which is clearly related to the aggressiveness of the tumor. Jaffe (1958) divided fibrosarcoma into two histologic types, the well-differentiated and the poorly differentiated, the latter group including some lesions that are frankly anaplastic.

Using Broder's methods, other authors (Pritchard et al. 1977; Dahlin 1978) graded fibrosarcomas into four grades on the basis of cytologic features and found most to be of the moderately well or poorly differentiated types and only a few to be well differentiated. Using the same method that we applied for chondrosarcoma, we divided our cases into three grades: *well differentiated*, *moderately differentiated*, and *poorly differentiated*. The same criteria are also applied by other authors (Taconis and Van Rijssel 1985). The his-

Fig. VI.28. Male, 13 years old. Periosteal fibrosarcoma of ulna. Radiograph shows soft tissue mass attached to and eroding the underlying bone with periosteal reactive bone formation, producing a Codman's triangle at its upper aspect ▶

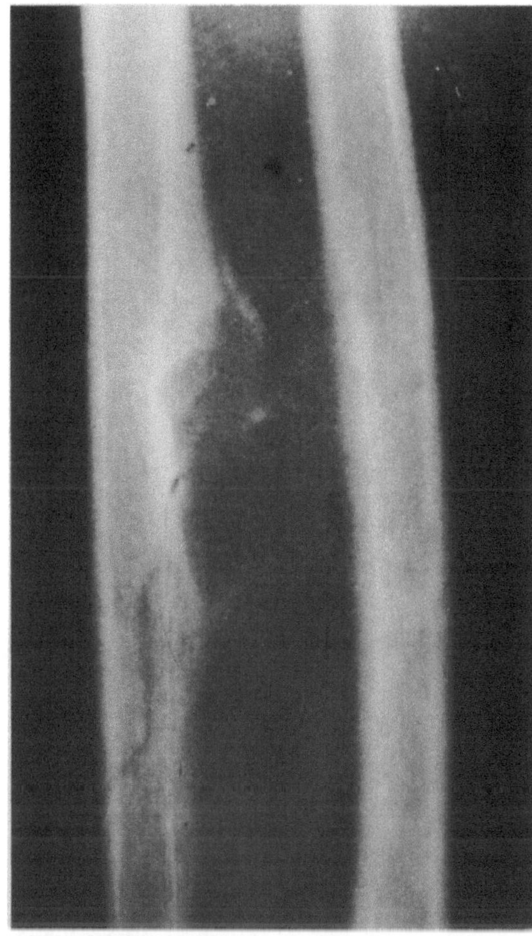

Fig. VI.29. a A topographic micrograph showing the intramedullary origin of this small fibrosarcoma, which was an incidental autopsy finding in the Pathologic Institute of Vienna, directed by Prof. J. Erdheim. **b** Same case showing the well-delimited tumor within the medullary cavity. **a** ×10, **b** ×60 ▼

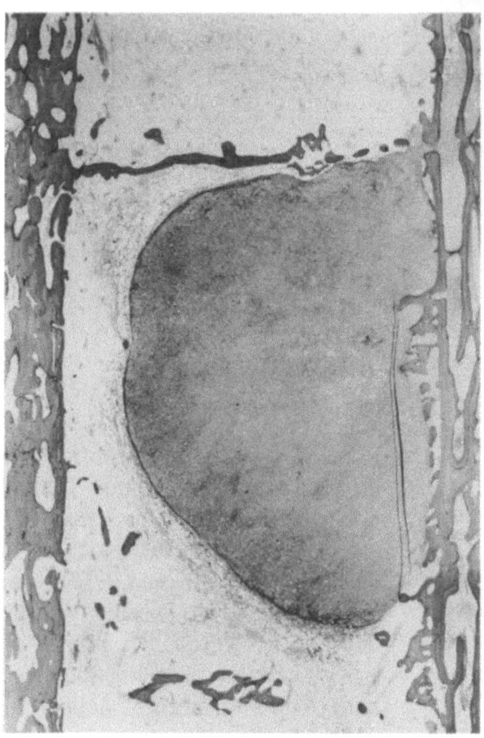

a

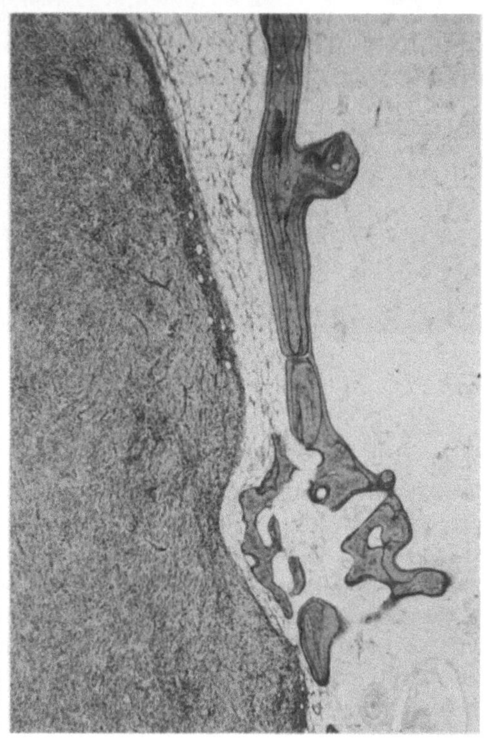

b

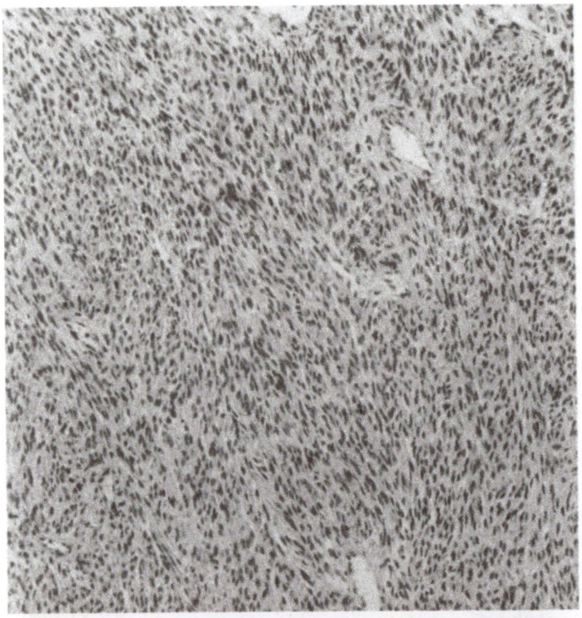

a

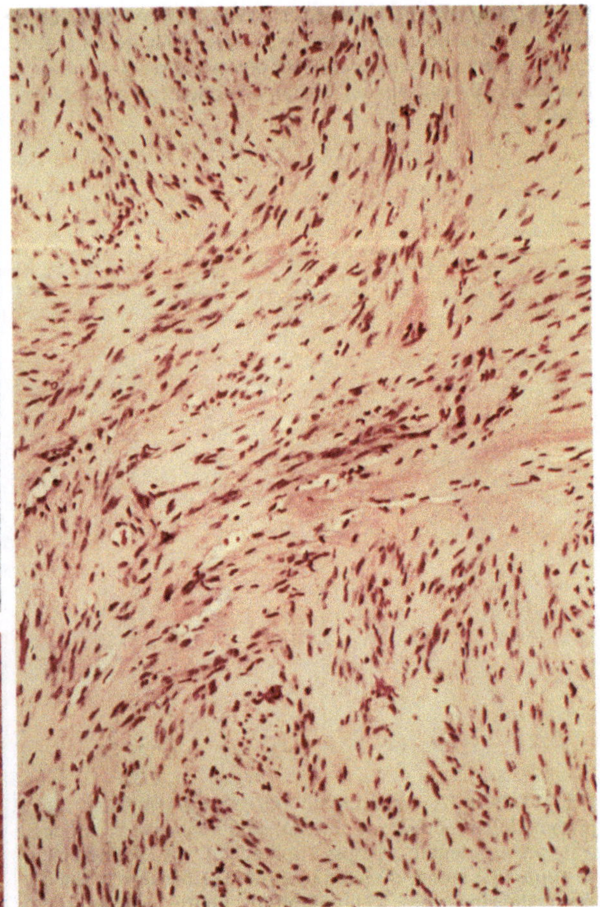

b

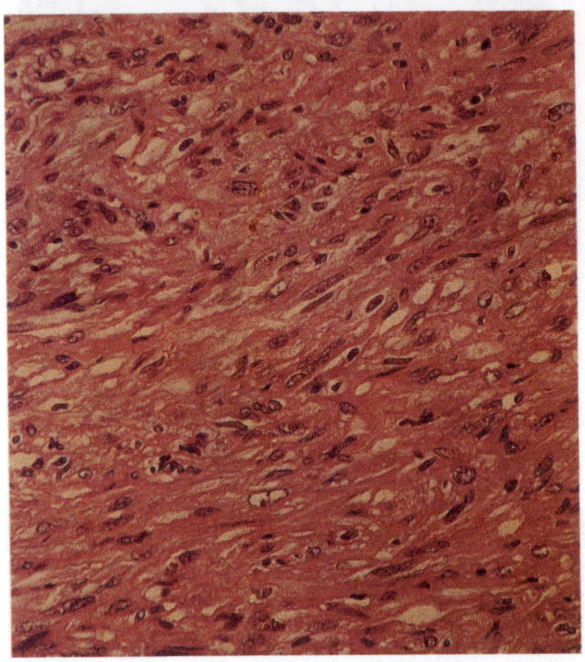

c

Fig. VI.30a–c. Photomicrographs illustrating different features of well-differentiated fibrosarcomas. The tumor cells are spindle shaped with ovoid or elongated nuclei, with only occasional larger, plump, and hyperchromatic nuclei. The intercellular collagen fibers are generally conspicuous and sometimes hyalinized (**b,c**). However, areas with this pattern may also be found in poorly differentiated fibrosarcoma. **a** ×100, **b** ×100, **c** ×300

tologic structure and grade of differentiation were usually related to biologic behavior and growth rate of the tumor. In the *well-differentiated type* (Figs. VI.29, VI.30), the fibroblastic tumor cells are spindle shaped and elongated, with ovoid or elongated nuclei; the nuclei are occasionally hyperchromatic and plump, but there is a lack of cellular atypism or mitotic activity. The number of tumor cells is scarce as compared with the relatively abundant intercellular collagen fibers, which occasionally may be dense and hyalinized. In such cases, differentiation from desmoplastic fibroma may be extremely difficult, and we could not corroborate Jaffe's finding that the nuclei of the fibroblasts are twice as large as those in desmoplastic fibroma. The well-differentiated fibrosarcoma grows slowly and is usually well delimited, whereas the *poorly differentiated type* is very cellular, with pronounced cellular atypism and evident mitotic activity, hyperchromatic nuclei, and cells with one or more bizarre nuclei. The connective stroma is generally scarce, occasionally made up only of reticulin fibers (Fig. VI.31). However, in some areas of poorly differentiated fibrosarcoma, abundant collagen fibers, often hyalinized, may be found, which explains the necessity of examining several samples from different zones before establishing the histologic grade of a tumor. This is also important in order to rule out the presence of an osteolytic osteosarcoma containing only a small amount of tumor bone, which in some fields may be completely lacking. Many tumors with an anaplastic, undifferentiated pattern, containing cells with one or more bizarre nuclei (tumor giant cells), which in the past were termed "pleomorphic fibrosarcoma," are at present classified as "malignant fibrous histiocytoma" (fibroxanthosarcoma). Poorly differentiated tumors grow more rapidly, invading and destroying the cancellous bone and the cortex, and produce frequent metastases, even after radical surgery.

Treatment and Prognosis. It is generally accepted that surgery is the most suitable method of treatment for both periosteal and medullary fibrosarcoma. The type of surgical procedure – amputation, disarticulation, or en bloc resection – depends in great part on the histologic grade of differentiation and on the local conditions and location of the tumor. In well or moderately well differentiated tumors of the extremities, without or with only limited extension into extraosseous soft tissue, segmental resection is the treatment of choice, followed by allograft or prosthetic reconstruction. In contrast, for poorly differentiated and anaplastic fibrosarcomas, the surgical treatment is the same as for osteosarcoma, i.e., amputation or disarticulation, for extensive lesions with neurovascular involvement vs wide resection and limb salvage. In tumors located at the lower femoral end – a frequent location – the functionally superior cross-bone amputation is preferred over disarticulation of the hip (Pritchard et al. 1977). In the event of recurrence after en bloc resection, amputation is indicated. In recent years limb-sparing surgery has been increasingly used, accompanied by preoperative and adjuvant chemotherapy (Huvos 1991), with beneficial results.

Radiation therapy is considered ineffective, and it is employed only in surgically unresectable, moderately or poorly differentiated tumors with or without chemotherapy.

We found, as did most other authors, a close correlation between survival rates and histologic grade of differentiation, there being a poorer prognosis in patients with poorly differentiated tumors (Jaffe 1958; Cunningham and Arlen 1968; Pritchard et al. 1977; Campanacci 1990; Huvos 1991).

The overall 5-year survival rate ranges from 28% (Eyre-Brook and Price 1969; Pritchard et al. 1977) to 34% (Huvos and Higinbotham 1975). Survival for 10 years or more was observed in 21.8% of patients in Pritchard's Mayo Clinic series and in 28% of Huvos and Higinbotham's patients treated at the Memorial Sloan-Kettering Cancer Center. In the study of the Netherlands Committee on Bone Tumors (Taconis and Van Rijssel 1985), in which treatment was similar in the group of pure fibrosarcomas and the predominantly malignant fibrous histiocytoma type, the 5-year survival was the same (34%) in both groups. Lung metastases developed in 63% of the patients with fibroblastic sarcomas and in 59% of those with malignant fibrous histiocytoma-like tumors. The histologic grade was of prognostic value in both groups; 5-year survival was 64% in 14 patients with grade I tumors, 41% in 32 with grade II tumors, and 23% in 56 with grade III tumors.

2. Malignant Fibrous Histiocytoma

In the last two decades, an increasing number of cases have been reported of a primary malignant bone tumor with histologic features essentially the same as those of a malignant fibrous histiocytoma (fibroxanthosarcoma) arising in soft tissues (Feldman and Norman 1972; Mirra et al. 1974; Newland et al. 1975; Huvos 1976; Spanier 1977; Dahlin et al. 1977; Feldman and Lattes 1977; McCarthy et al. 1979). Ghandhur-Mnaymneh et al. (1982) found 119 cases published in the literature. Larger series have been reported more recently (1986) by Dahlin and Unni (52 cases) and by Huvos et al. (1985, 130 cases). Formerly, many of these neoplasms were classed as liposarcomas, pleomorphic fibrosarcomas, osteolytic osteosarcomas, anaplastic reticulosarcomas, or malignant giant-cell tumors. In the WHO classification system (first edition), the term "*undifferentiated sarcoma*" was applied to "a malignant tumor with a pleomorphic spindle-celled structure but devoid of any specific pattern of histological differentiation." It is evident that currently a majority of this group would be classified as "malignant fibrous histiocytoma" (MFH).

Following the concepts of Stout and coworkers based on tissue culture studies of the

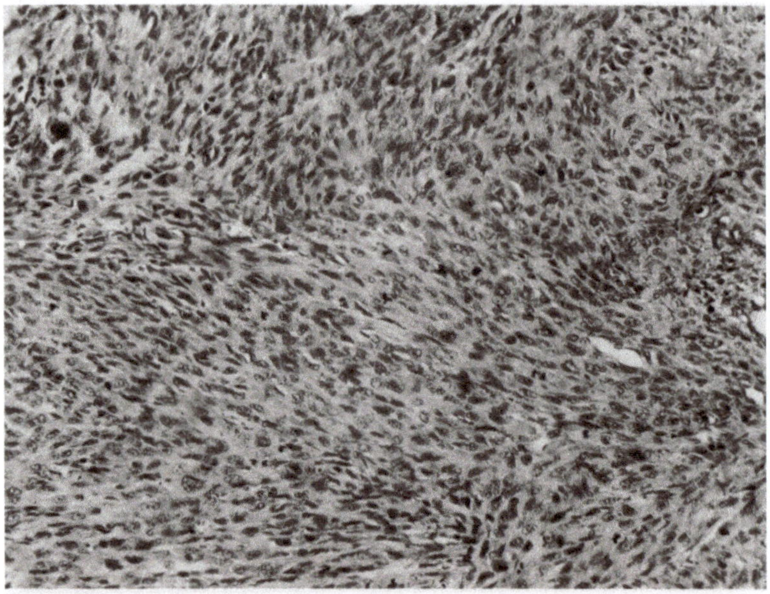

a

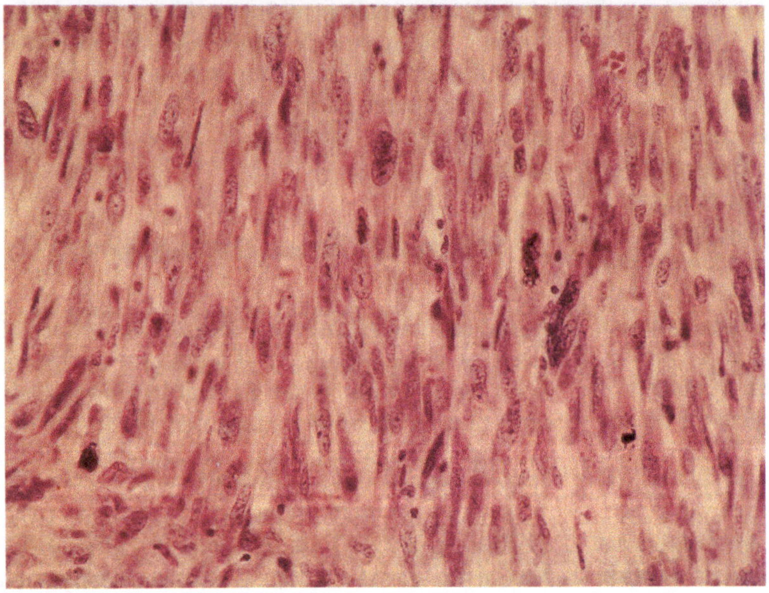

b

Fig. VI.31. **a** Photomicrograph of moderately differentiated fibrosarcoma showing the herringbone pattern of the interlacing bundles of the spindle-celled tumor cells with only scarce collagen fibers. **b** Same case, showing some typical and atypical mitoses. **c,d** Photomicrographs of poorly differentiated fibrosarcoma showing marked cellular pleomorphism with bizarre nuclei and numerous atypical mitoses. **a** ×160, **b** ×300, **c,d** ×600

"facultative fibrogenesis" of histiocytes (Ozzello et al. 1963; Stout and Lattes 1967), a wide range of lesions are thought to be derived from the tissue histiocyte or from more immature precursors with their possible potential for morphologic and functional differentiation into both histiocytic and fibroblastic lines, whereby they acquire the capacity to produce collagen – so-called facultative fibroblasts. Ultrastructural studies (Merkow et al. 1971; Fu et al. 1975) seem to support Stout's thesis.

The histologic criteria for the diagnosis of "malignant fibrous histiocytoma" (fibroxanthosarcoma) outlined by Stout and Lattes (1967) and Kempson and Kyriakos (1972) for soft tissue lesions have been applied to tumors arising in bone, and include the following:

1. Bundles of fibers and spindle-shaped fibroblastlike cells arranged in a storiform or "cartwheel" pattern and showing evident mitotic activity and features of atypism. Although the storiform pattern is characteristic, it is not pathognomonic of cells of primary histiocytic origin and may be found in other sarcomas.

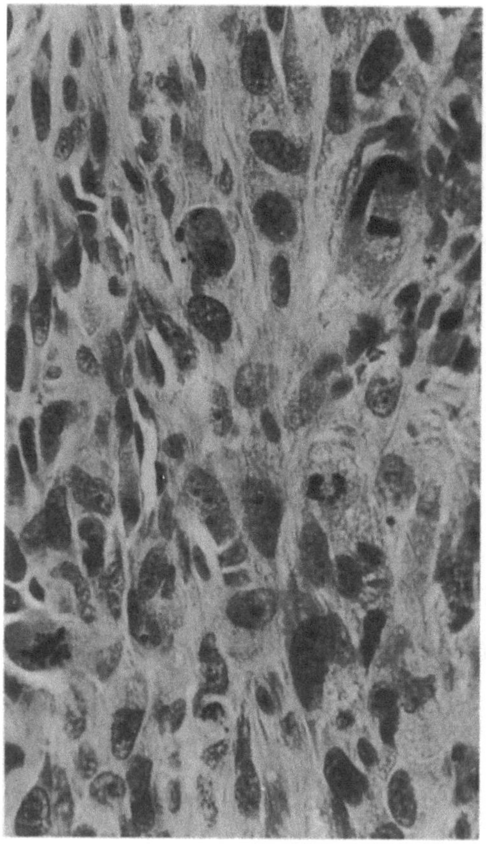

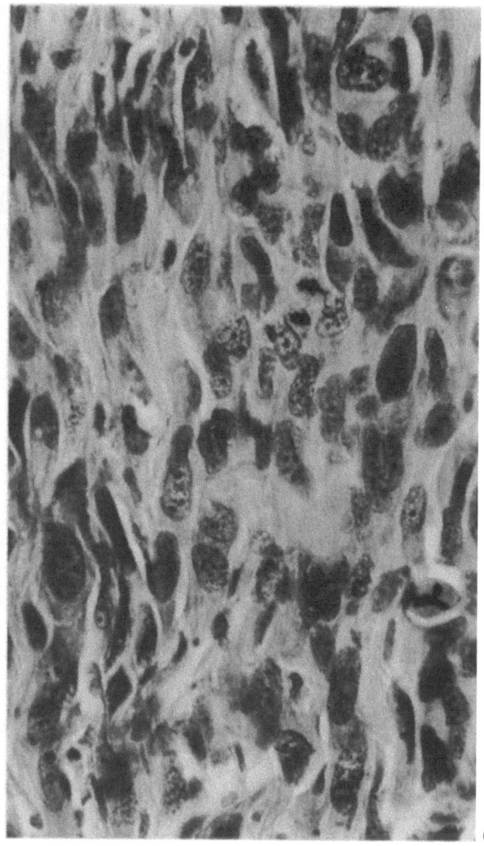

VI.31c d

2. Rounded cells exhibiting features of histiocytes with ovoid, often indented or grooved nuclei and well-defined cytoplasmic borders. These cells frequently show phagocytic activity with cytoplasmic inclusions of red blood cells, hemosiderin, and/or lipids, becoming transformed into foam (xanthoma) cells containing bizarre, pleomorphic, frequently multiple nuclei.
3. Typical multinucleated giant cells of the osteoclastic type as well as atypical ones.
4. Relatively conspicuous infiltration of inflammatory cells, predominantly lymphocytes.

Following these histologic criteria, we reviewed our older material and found among cases classified previously as undifferentiated or pleomorphic sarcoma, liposarcoma, pleomorphic fibrosarcoma of bone, or highly anaplastic osteolytic osteosarcoma, several cases that displayed the aforementioned histologic pattern and may be regarded as MFH. These cases, together with the recent cases, bring us to a total of 37 cases.

Incidence. Malignant fibrous histiocytoma is a relatively rare neoplasm. The 37 cases observed in our laboratory represent 1.6% of the malignant primary bone tumors. Spanier et al. (1975) found 11 cases in more than 400 primary tumors of bone, and Dahlin and Unni (1986) found 52 examples among 6514 primary malignant bone tumors. These cases were segregated from 207 fibrosarcomas and 1274 osteosarcomas. During a 50-year period 130 patients with primary (72%) or secondary (28%) MFH arising in bone were seen at Memorial Hospital (Huvos et al. 1985).

Clinical Findings. *Age and Sex.* There was a slight female predominance in our and Spanier's series (22:15) and a male predominance in other large series. All ages between 12 and 82 years were affected, with an average age of 50 years. No patients were under 10 years of age in our group, but Dahlin reported one 6-year-old child.

Localization. The tumor usually involved the long bones: 18 were located in the tibia and 14 in the femur, usually in the metaphyseal region, which agrees with the findings of most other

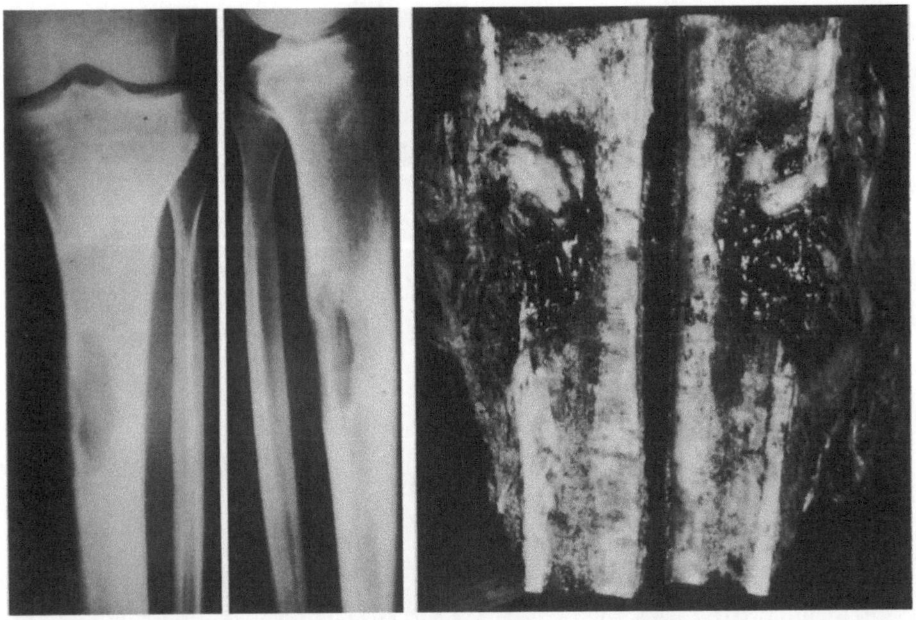

a b

Fig. VI.32a,b. Male, 26 years old. Malignant fibrous histiocytoma of tibia. **a** Anteroposterior and lateral radiographs demonstrate an eccentric osteolytic lesion with ill-defined borders. **b** Photograph of the resected specimen, modified after previous biopsy, showing destruction of the cortex and penetration into soft tissue of the predominantly hemorrhagic tumor

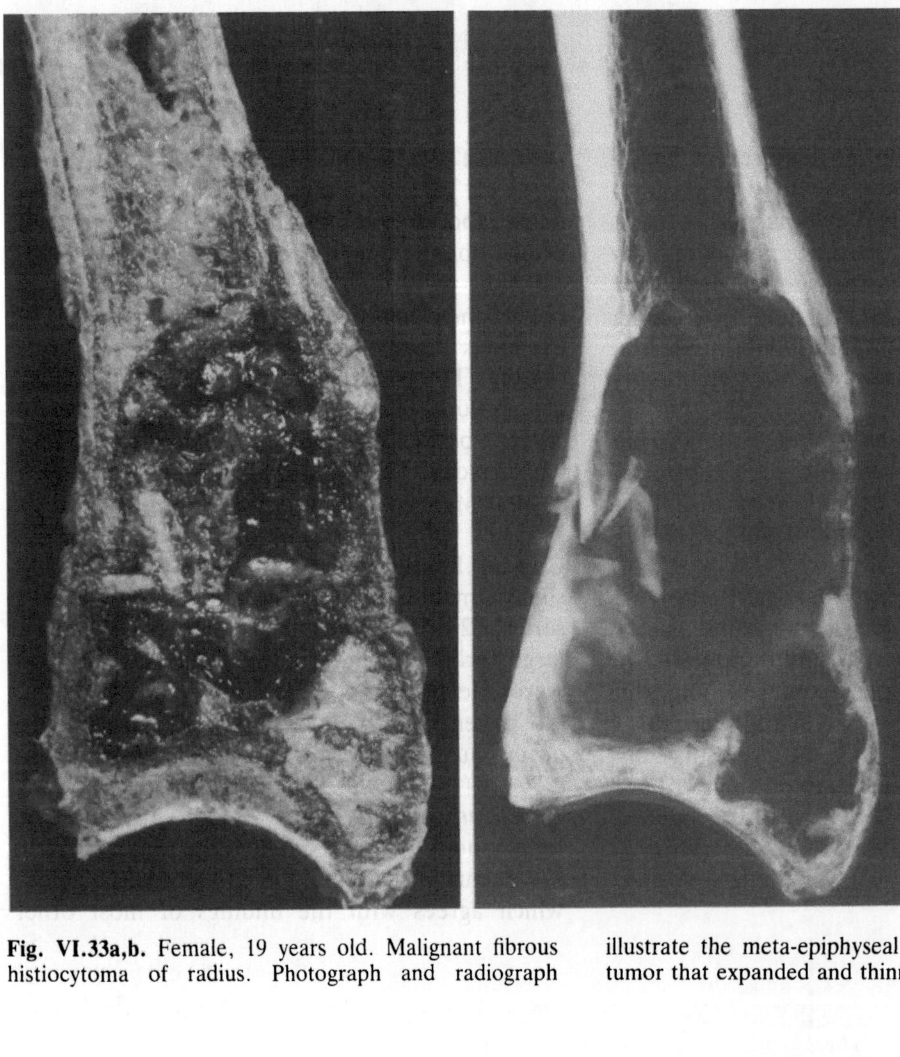

a b

Fig. VI.33a,b. Female, 19 years old. Malignant fibrous histiocytoma of radius. Photograph and radiograph illustrate the meta-epiphyseal location of this osteolytic tumor that expanded and thinned the cortex

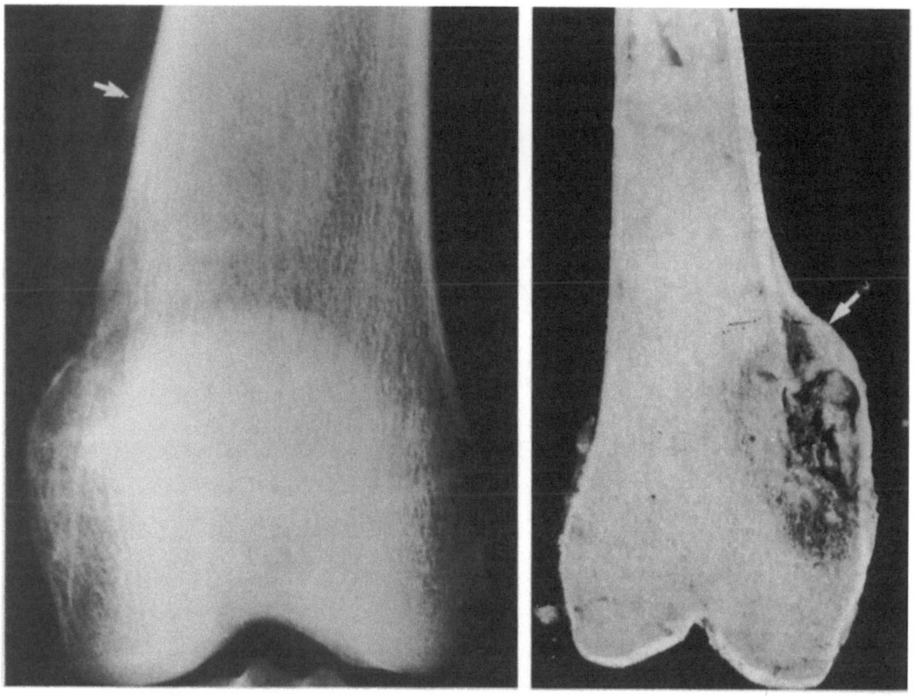

a b

Fig. VI.34a,b. Female, 23 years old. Malignant fibrous histiocytoma of femur. **a** Anteroposterior radiograph shows radiolucent lesion with ill-defined margins in the metaphysis that has partly destroyed the cortex and produced a Codman's triangle. The radiographic aspect suggested osteosarcoma. **b** Photograph shows the evident intraosseous origin of the tumor and the Codman's triangle

series. In Huvos' series, 69% affected long bones, the most common location being the femur (32%), followed by the tibia and fibula (23%), humerus (11%), shoulder girdle (12%), and craniofacial bones (11%). Involvement of the spine or ribs seems to be exceptional, and no case of this location was found in our, Dahlin's, and Spanier's series. Multifocal osseous involvement seems to be exceptional (Dahlin and Unni 1986).

Symptoms. The most common complaints were pain and swelling, with a duration ranging from a few weeks to several months. Two cases developed in bones affected by Paget disease with a long-term history of pain. Twenty cases of MFH occurred in bones affected by a previous disease, especially Paget sarcoma, following previous irradiation (Huvos 1991).

Radiographic Features. The lesion is radiolucent, with ill-defined borders. It is more frequently located in the metaphyseal region, usually destroying the cortex and penetrating extensively into soft tissues (Figs. VI.32–VI.36). A pathologic fracture is not infrequent. In advanced cases, it is sometimes difficult to establish the intra- or extraosseous origin of the tumor (Fig. VI.36). Usually, no significant periosteal reaction is found, an exception being an atypical Codman's triangle in one of our cases (Fig. VI.34). The radiographic pattern, although clearly revealing a malignant process, is not characteristic, and similar features may be found in many other primary or secondary malignant tumors. Total body scans and computed tomograms are helpful in determining the intramedullary and/or extraosseous extension of the tumor.

Pathologic Findings. The gross aspect was variable in different tumors and in different areas of the same lesion: in some cases yellowish, brownish, or hemorrhagic areas of soft consistency predominated; in others, firm white to grayish zones of fibrous aspect. Necrotic zones were frequent and sometimes extensive. Wide cortical destruction and extension into soft tissue was a frequent finding.

The above-described *histologic features*, which characterized MFH of soft tissues, were constantly found in the tumor arising in bone, but varied considerably in different zones in the same lesion. Only cases that showed a combination of

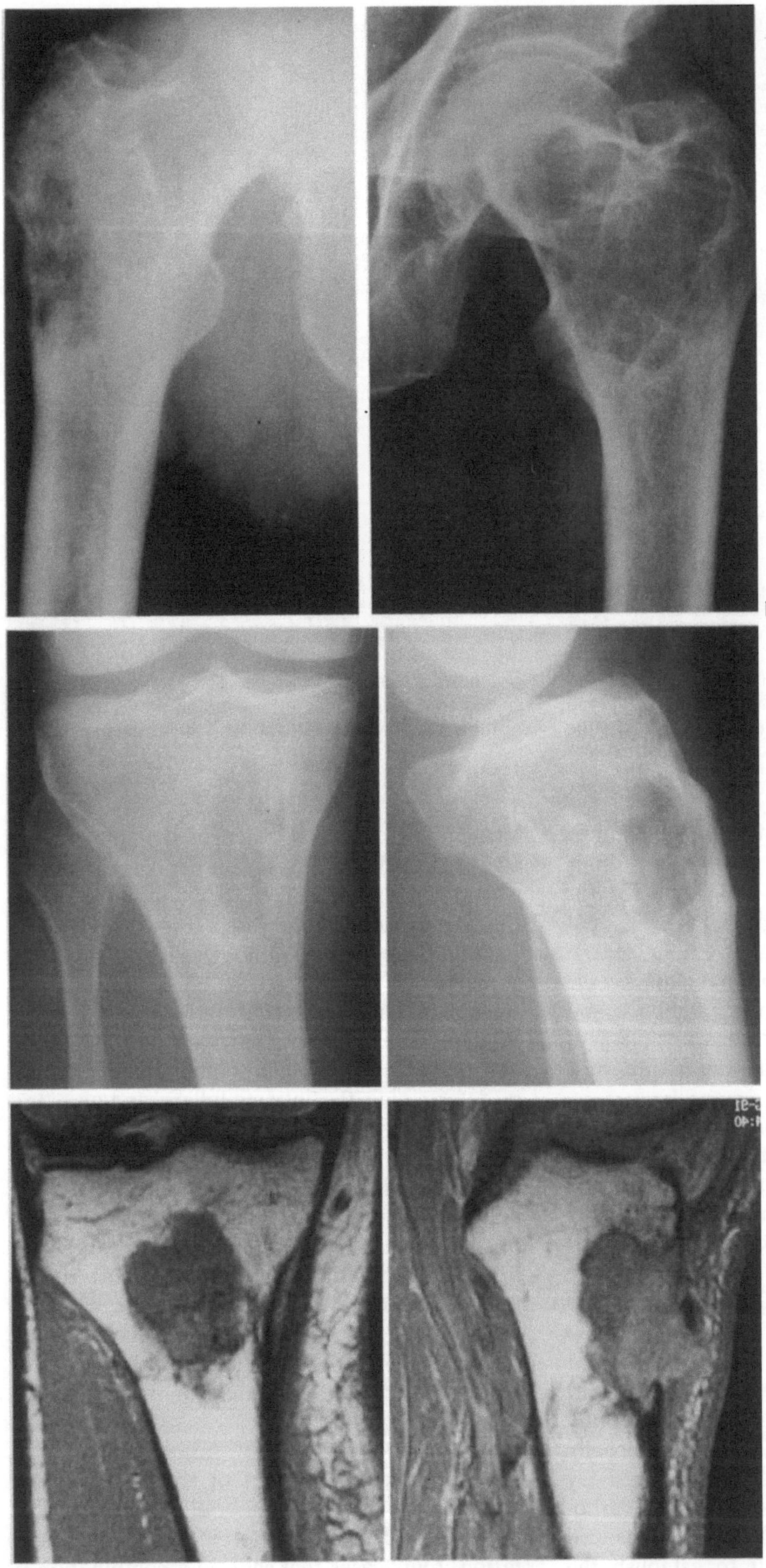

Fig. VI.35a–d. Three different cases of malignant fibrous histiocytoma. **a** Male, 54 years old. Radiograph shows an osteolytic permeative lesion in the trochanteric region. **b** Female, 22 years old with a larger radiolucent trabeculated lesion in the upper femoral metaphysis. **c,d** Male, 64 years old. **c** Anterposterior and lateral radiographs. **d** Anteroposterior and lateral T1-weighted MRI scans show the destruction of the anterior cortex and penetration into soft tissues (St. Louis University Medical Center)

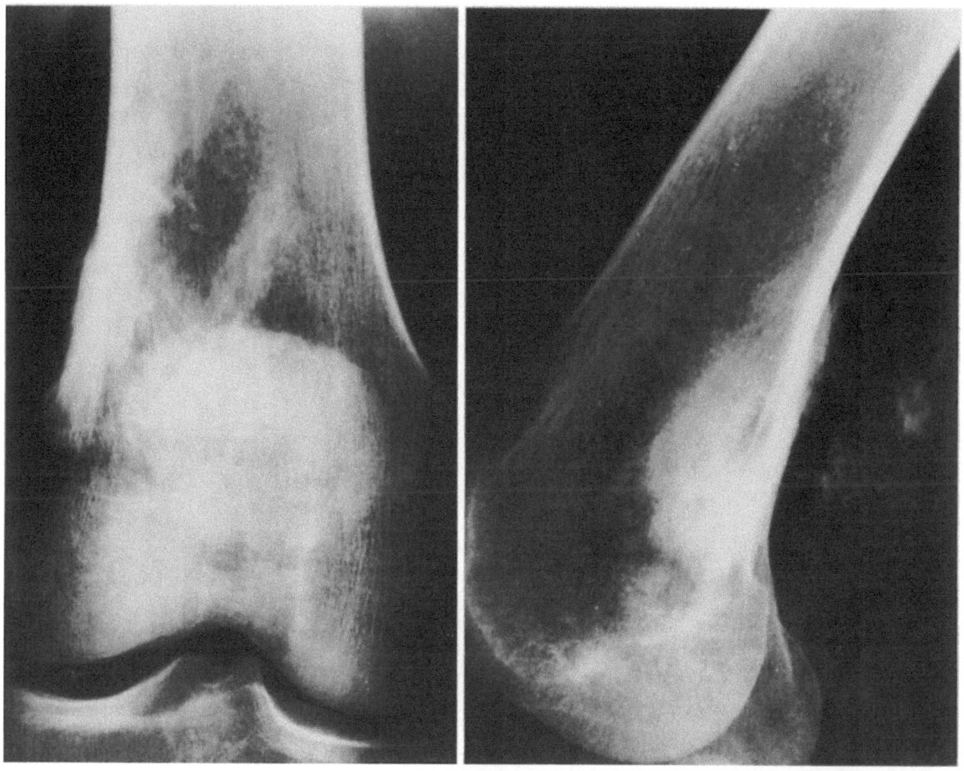

a

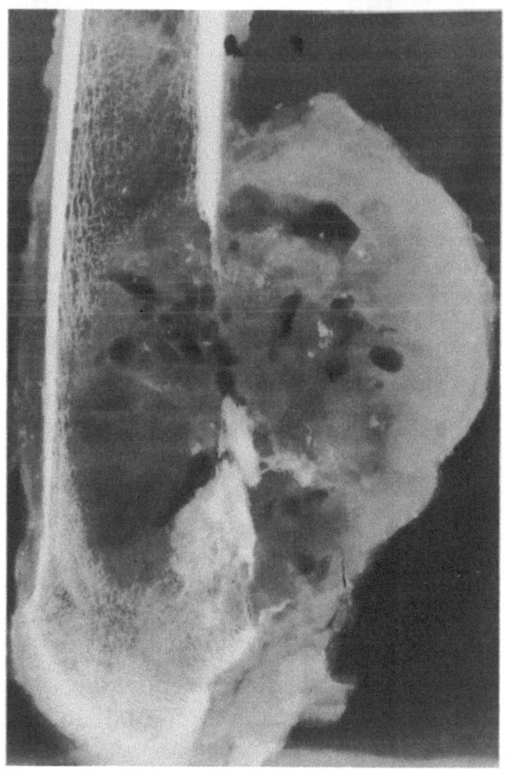

b

Fig. VI.36a,b. Female, 46 years old. Malignant fibrous histiocytoma of femur. **a** Anteroposterior and lateral radiographs demonstrate a large, osteolytic, ill-defined lesion in the lower femoral end with some ares of sclerosis invading soft tissue at its posterior aspect. **b** Radiograph of a 5-mm thick slab of the amputation specimen showing the osteolytic aspect of the tumor, which has destroyed the posterior cortex and extensively invaded soft tissues. It is difficult to determine the intra- or extraosseous origin of this tumor. The bone sclerosis was due to reactive, not tumor bone formation

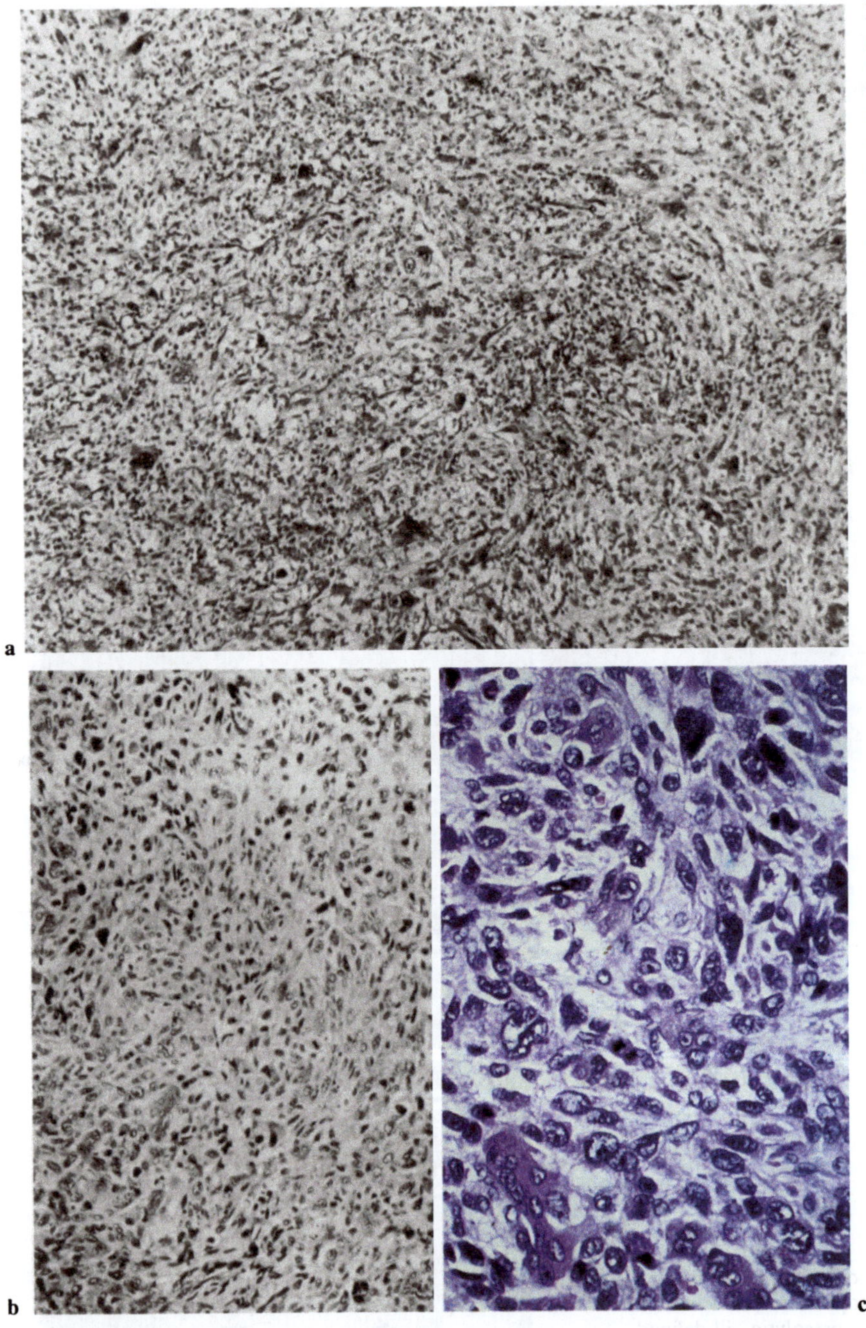

Fig. VI.37a–c. Photomicrographs of malignant fibrous histiocytoma show the pleomorphic aspect of the tumor, with a storiform pattern and evident nuclear atypism. Numerous cells with one or more hyperchromatic nuclei and small round cells are observed in **a**. In **c**, osteoclastic giant cells are seen. **a** ×100, **b** ×180, **c** ×400

a histiocytic and fibroblastic component were accepted as pertaining to this entity (Figs. VI.37, VI.38). The histiocytic elements have round to ovoid, often indented or grooved nuclei with prominent nucleoli, abundant eosinophilic cytoplasm, and well-defined borders, sometimes resembling reticulum cells. These cells frequently show evident phagocytic activity, with the cytoplasm containing red blood cells, hemosiderin, and granular debris. The cytoplasm often has a foamy appearance (xanthoma cells) and contains typical nuclei or, more commonly, one or several pleomorphic, bizarre nuclei (Fig. VI.39). Besides this atypical giant cell, multinucleated osteoclast giant cells may be found.

The fibroblastic component consists of spindle cells with varying degrees of fibrogenesis and cellularity in different lesions or areas of the same tumor, presenting a characteristic storiform pattern. The spindle cells often show evident

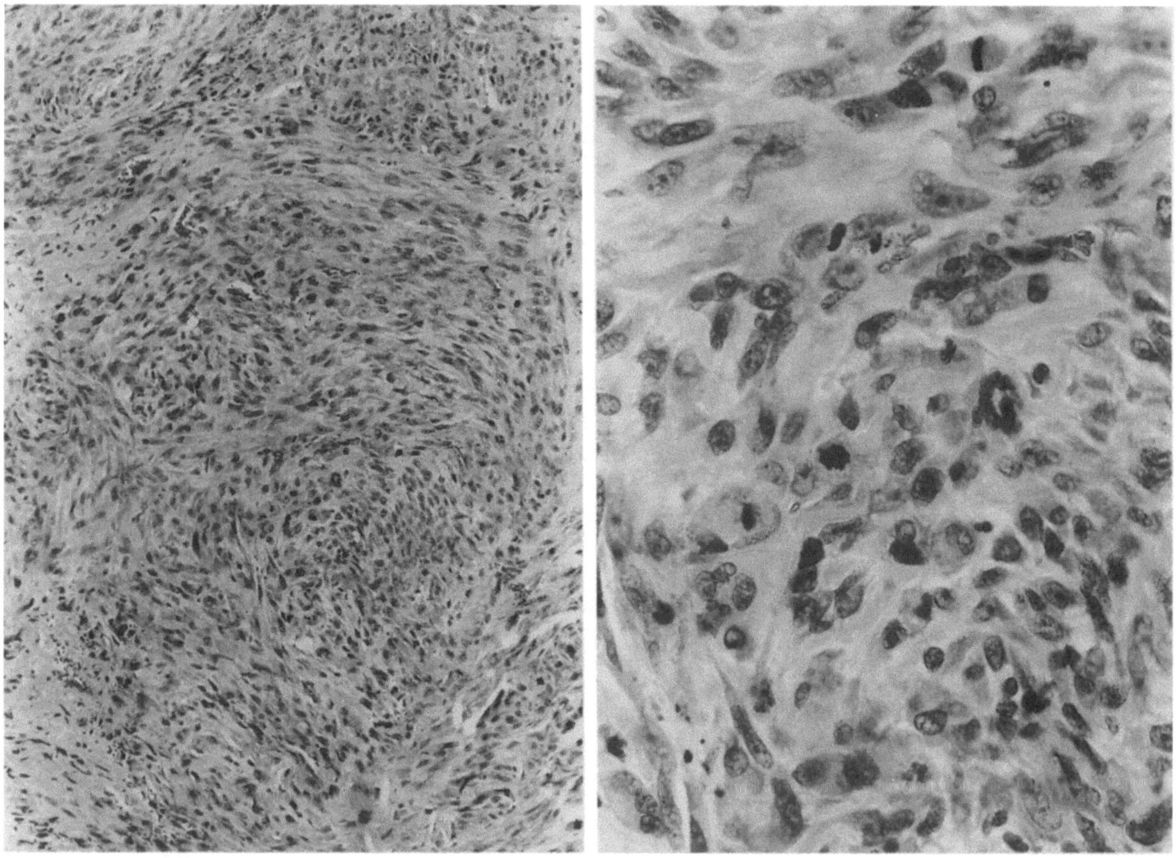

Fig. VI.38a,d. Photomicrographs showing at lower and higher magnification the storiform pattern and the pleomorphism of the fibroblastic and histiocytic cells. **a** ×150, **b** ×400

nuclear hyperchromatism and pleomorphism, sometimes with abundant, elongated eosinophilic cytoplasm containing coarse granular material, similar to the strap cells of rhabdomyosarcoma. Mitotic figures are frequent. Another frequent characteristic is focal or more diffuse infiltration of inflammatory cells, predominantly lymphocytes. In none of our cases was cartilage, tumor bone, or osteoid formation found; such cases, with even limited areas, were classified as osteosarcomas.

A characteristic finding was abundant reticulin fibers in the cellular areas of the tumor, involving individual cellular elements.

This author believes that the reports of MFH include many poorly differentiated sarcomas, so that the diagnosis of MFH is made too often. The diagnosis is frequently based on small biopsy specimens in which the characteristic but nonspecific "storiform" or "cartwheel" pattern is seen. It is possible that many cases represent some other type of pleomorphic undifferentiated neoplasm, particularly osteosarcoma and fibrosarcoma (the fibrohistiocytomatous type). In fact, in several cases diagnosed as MFH by open biopsy, study of the amputation specimen demonstrated areas of chondroid and osteoid or bone formation by the tumor cells. This finding, even in small amounts, excludes the diagnosis of MFH (Dahlin and Unni 1986). The positive identification of tumor osteoid places a sarcoma in the osteosarcoma category, even if it exhibits a storiform pattern or has other morphologic characteristics of MFH. However, McCarthy et al. (1979) classified some cases with scarce areas of tumor, osteoid, or cartilage formation as MFH. In controversial cases in which the presence of osteoid is debatable, as in 18 of the 35 cases of Dahlin et al., the demonstration of abundant tissue alkaline phosphatase is characteristic of osteosarcoma. Electron microscopic studies are also of value in these debatable cases.

Pathogenesis. In spite of numerous histologic, immunohistochemical, and ultrastructural studies, the histogenesis of MFH remains controversial.

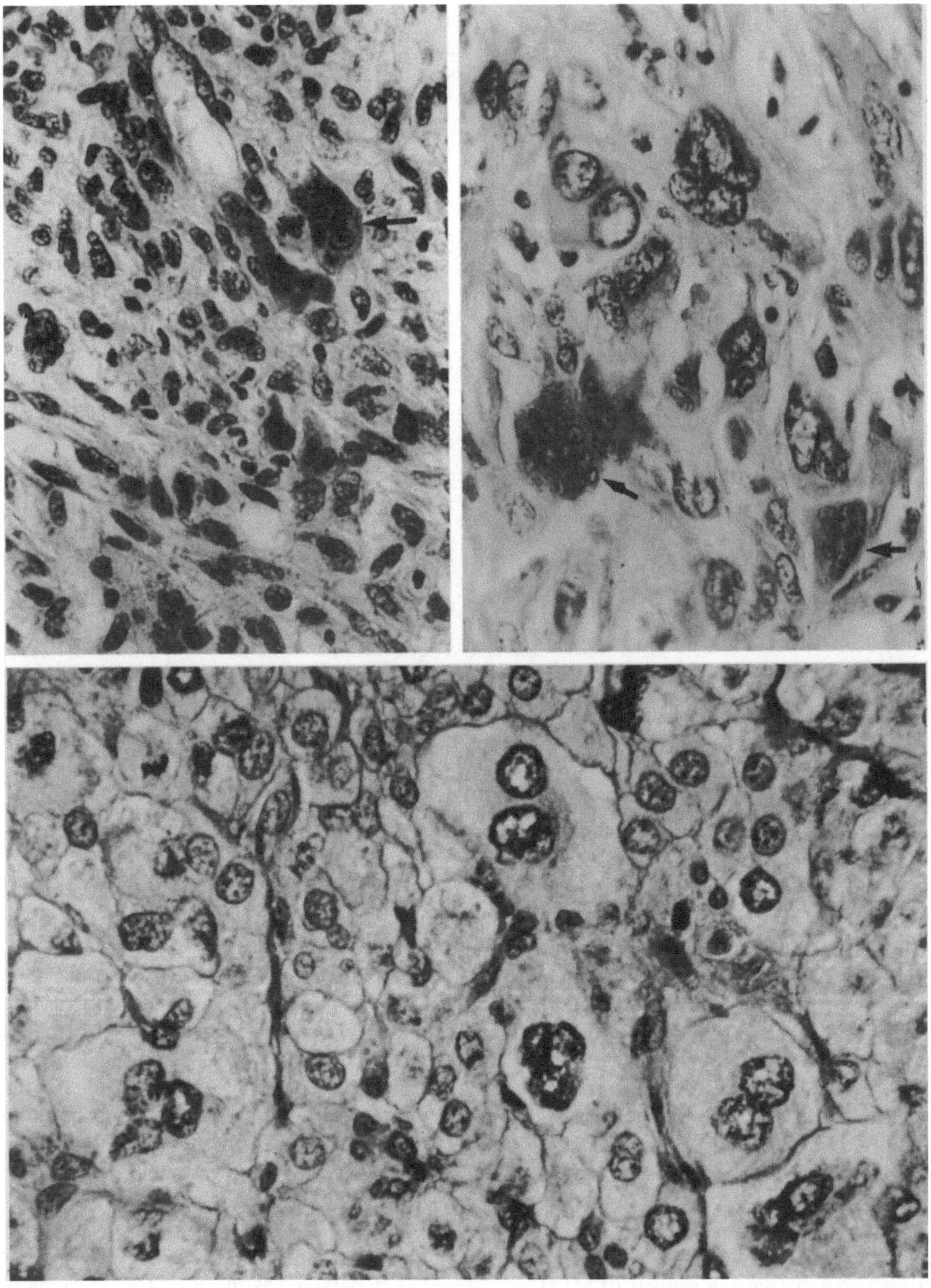

a b c

Fig. VI.39a–c. Photomicrographs showing at high magnification benign and malignant multinucleated giant cells and in **c** many large cells with abundant foamy cytoplasm and one or more bizarre nuclei. **a** ×400, **b,c** ×600

There are no clear morphologic criteria, based on light or electron microscopic studies, for the cytologic characterization of the tissue histiocyte, generally equated with the mononuclear phagocyte system.

Both MFH of the spindle-cell fibrous type with a typical storiform pattern and the histiocytic xanthomatous variant show homogeneous vimentin reactivity. The glycoproteins α_1-antitrypsin and α_1-antichymotrypsin and the bacteriolytic enzyme lysozyme have been used as classic, supposedly specific, immunohistochemical markers for cells of histiocytic origin; unfortunately, however, nonhistiocytic tissue such as adenocarcinoma of stomach and gallbladder, melanoma, or even some benign mixed tumors of salivary gland origin may also react positively with these markers. Therefore caution should be exercised in interpreting the results obtained with these markers, and the diagnosis of MFH should not be excluded because of the lack of a positive staining reaction, which is frequent in predominantly fibroblastic and myxoid variants.

The *ultrastructural* features of MFH are not diagnostically specific, and tumor cells with identical characteristics may be found in various other neoplasms (Inada et al. 1976). At least two distinct cell types may generally be observed: (1) a fibroblastic element with elongated, narrow nucleus and evident rough endoplasmic reticulum, scanty lysosomes, and lipid droplets, and (2) round cells (histiocytes) with oval or lobulated nuclei showing cytoplasmic processes, well-developed Golgi zones, and abundant cytoplasmic lysosomes and lipid droplets.

The association of MFH with other underlying bone abnormalities, e.g., Paget disease and other nonneoplastic conditions, especially ischemic bone infarct, is a relatively frequent finding (Michael and Dorfman 1976; Spanier 1977; Galli et al. 1978; McCarthy et al. 1979; Mirra et al. 1977; Campanacci 1990). Mirra proposed that MFH arises from the area of a bone infarct by transformation of a formerly benign chronic reparative process rich in mononuclear and multinuclear histiocytes and fibroblasts.

Until further investigations resolve the controversial problem concerning the histogenesis of this neoplasm, this author agrees with Weiss and Enzinger that "it is better regarded as primitive and pleomorphic sarcoma showing partial fibroblastic and histiocytic differentiation" as reflected by reticulin and/or collagen production and occasional phagocytosis.

Treatment and Prognosis. Treatment of older cases found in a retrospective review was ablative surgery in all cases located in long limb bones. In those located in bones not amenable to surgery, irradiation produced some palliation. None of the patients of this older group survived more than 2 years because of metastatic spread, pulmonary involvement being the major cause of death. In some more recent cases, treatment was a wide en bloc resection with multidrug chemotherapy; and in other cases, amputation followed by adjunctive chemotherapy. In the Memorial Hospital experience (Huvos et al. 1985), shared by Campanacci (1990), the management of spindle-cell sarcomas (high-grade fibrosarcomas) of bone, including MFH, is similar to that of osteosarcoma. Low-grade (grades I and II) MFH of bone is treated with wide surgical excision, as radical as with high-grade lesions (grades III and IV) but without the necessity of chemotherapy. Patients with a high-grade lesion are placed on preoperative (neoadjuvant) chemotherapy to reduce the size of the primary tumor and to make limb-sparing surgery possible. The best postoperative adjuvant chemotherapy regimen is the T-12 protocol of Rosen for osteosarcoma, although the choice of regimen does vary in accordance with the preoperative chemotherapy response. Amputations are employed less and less frequently and are usually reserved for patients with pathologic fractures or unusually large lesions. Campanacci (1990) and Capanna et al. (1984) obtained a good response with preoperative chemotherapy in nearly half of the cases, and when it was combined with wide or radical surgical resection and postoperative chemotherapy they noted improved survival for these patients.

The frequency of lymph node metastasis is low or zero in some series (Capanna et al. 1984; Huvos et al. 1985; Dahlin and Unni 1986) and relatively high in others (Spanier 1977; Yuen and Saw 1985). Lung metastases are common and were noted in 41 (31.5%) of the 130 patients of Huvos et al. (1985). Synchronous multifocal bone involvement is rare, but metachronous osseous metastases are not uncommon (10%).

The prognosis of MFH is difficult to judge because in many older case reports there is a lack of follow-up data or because other neoplasms with some MFH component are often included. According to the Memorial Hospital experience, patients with low-grade tumors have a better prognosis than those with high-grade lesions. On the other hand, survival also differs according to age: patients 21 years or younger had a substantially better prognosis than those who were older. This is explained by the fact that older patients are more commonly affected by secondary MFH, especially in association with Paget sarcoma or previous irradiation.

3. Liposarcoma

Definition, WHO: *"A malignant tumor characterized by lipoblastic differentiation, as shown by the presence of atypical lipoblasts in varying stages of differentiation."*

Liposarcoma, a common tumor of soft tissues, may infiltrate the underlying bone, but deep penetration is unusual. Liposarcoma arising within bone is even rarer, and only a limited number of authenticated cases have been reported. In some publications, there is no convincing evidence that the tumor originated within bone, and in others, the tumor probably will have to be reclassified as malignant fibrous histiocytoma (fibroxanthosarcoma), this being especially true of those with an evident pleomorphic histologic pattern.

Since the first report by Ewing of a primary liposarcoma originating in bone (which he later included in his revised classification of bone tumors prepared for the Bone Tumor Registry, 1939, as a distinct tumor entity arising from the fat cells of bone marrow), fewer than 20 cases have been recorded in the literature. In some of these, the osseous origin is debatable. Jaffe (1958) stated in his book that he "has not seen a neoplasm that can be accepted with certainty as primary liposarcoma of bone," although he does not entirely rule out the possibility of its existence. After studying the pathologic features of a case reported later by Retz (1961), he became convinced of the existence of this type of tumor. However, the majority of authors interested in proving the osseous origin and liposarcomatous character of the tumor have not focused their attention upon the probable existence of another cell type in addition to the lipomatous one, with different degrees of maturity and differentiation. As we shall discuss later, some published cases of liposarcoma correspond to the tumor type we described as "primary malignant mesenchymoma of bone."

The few publications report single cases of primary liposarcoma of bone, all but one arising in the extremities, with the majority in the lower extremity, the tibia being the most frequently affected bone (Pardo-Mindan et al. 1981; Larsson et al. 1975; Schneider et al. 1980; Torok et al. 1983; Campanacci 1990).

We have only two cases in our files; they were located in the lower femur and upper tibia. A few other cases (five) have been reclassified as malignant fibrohistiocytomas. The mean age of patients in the reported cases was around 30 years, with an evident male predominance.

Radiographically, liposarcomas are destructive, radiolucent, ill-defined lesions (Fig. VI.40), sometimes expanding and destroying part of the cortex.

The gross and histologic features are identical to those found in liposarcomas arising in soft tissue (Fig. VI.40b,c). The treatment indicated is similar to that for other high-grade spindle-cell sarcomas and requires wide or radical resection of the involved bone with either a limb-sparing resection or amputation. The prognosis seems to be poor in most cases, with an average survival time of 2 years.

4. Malignant Mesenchymoma

Definition, WHO: *"A malignant tumor characterized by the presence of multiple types of differentiation and structural pattern, particularly those not usually encountered in the skeleton."*

Malignant mesenchymoma arising in bone was first reported by the writer and associates in 1966 as a distinct entity not included in any existing bone tumor classification. The diagnosis of malignant mesenchymoma was based on the fact that the neoplasm showed a liposarcomatous predominance. However, there were also large areas in the central part of the tumor with all the macro- and microscopic characteristics of osteosarcoma, without clearly defined limits between the two neoplastic types.

The tumor, which involved the upper metaphysis of the tibia in a 17-year-old boy, was of unquestionable medullary origin. The roentgenographic and gross patterns showed that the tumor had broken through the cortex and formed a typical Codman spur; it invaded the soft parosteal tissues extensively, presenting an apparently well-delimited lobular surface, with an evident yellow color of most of the tumor. However, in the central part, large, radiologically sclerotic areas were found with the histologic features of osteosarcoma (Figs. VI.41–VI.43). In none

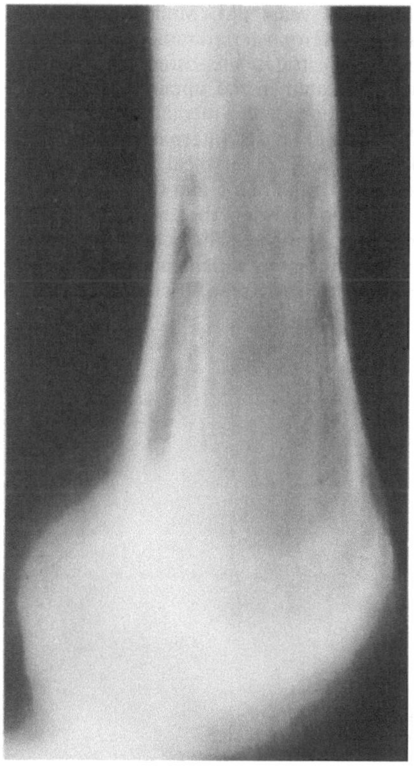

a

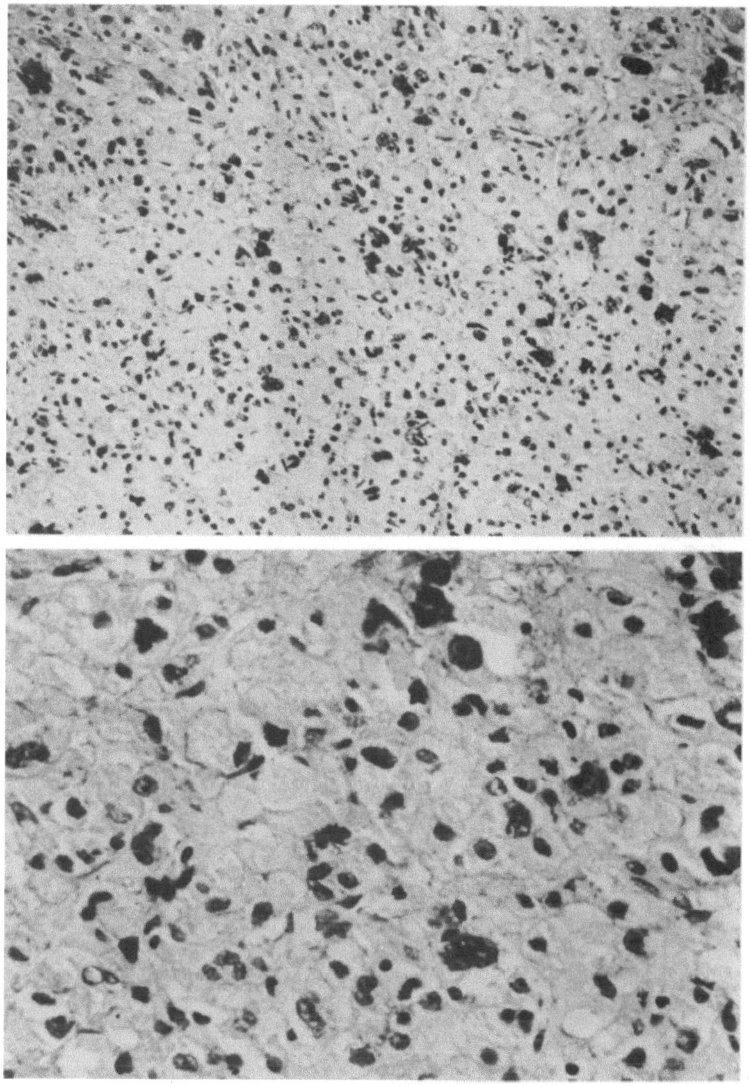

b

c

Fig. VI.40a–c. Female, 35 years old. Liposarcoma of femur. **a** Lateral tomogram shows a large osteolytic lesion in the lower femoral end; the intramedullary origin is evident. **b,c** Photomicrographs illustrating at lower and higher magnification the pattern of pleomorphic liposarcoma. **b** ×100, **c** ×400

of the examined amputation specimens for osteosarcoma were such extensive zones of liposarcoma found, nor have we found such a description in the literature, with the exception of a brief discussion in Lichtenstein's book (1965). We interpreted the case as a *mixed tumor of mesenchymal origin*, for which the designation "malignant mesenchyma" proposed by Stout (1948) appeared to be justified. Stout applied this term to those soft tissue tumors of mesenchymal origin composed of tumor cells differentiating in two or more unrelated malignant forms, retaining the multipotential capacity of the primitive mesenchyma. Because most of the tumors of mesenchymal derivation may have fibrosarcomatous areas, this tissue type is not recognized as separate in evaluating tumors.

As mentioned before in the section on liposarcoma, some of those published cases appear to show a similar combination (Mastragostino 1957; Retz 1961; Bertoni and Laus 1978). Another case with features similar to our case, involving the upper fibula, was subsequently reported by Ross and Hadfield (1968) as "osteoliposarcoma" (malignant mesenchymoma). Since our first case, we have observed three more cases of mixed mesenchymal tumors arising in bone, one of which exhibited the same combination of liposarcomatous and osteosarcomatous components (Fig. VI.44); in the other two cases, however, malignant tissues of mesenchymal origin other than osteosarcomatous tissues were present, such as extensive areas similar to Ewing sarcoma, hemangiopericytoma, or rhabdomyosarcoma. In

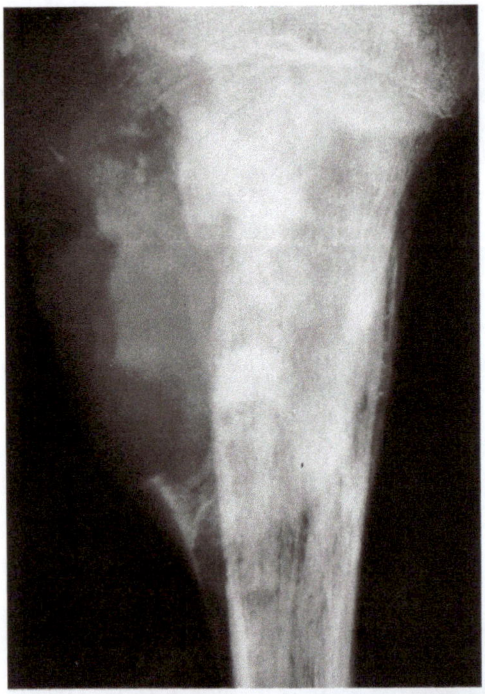

a

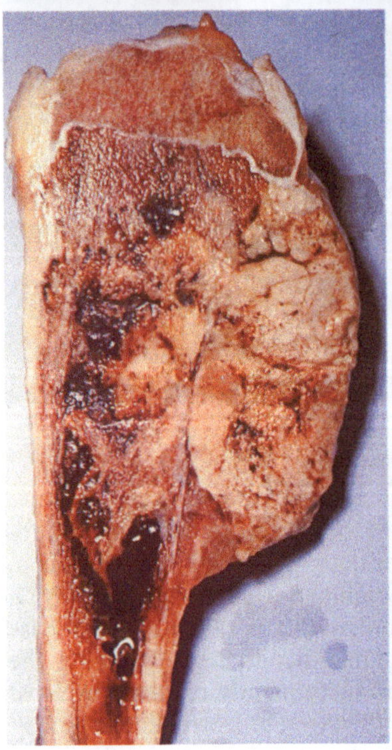

b

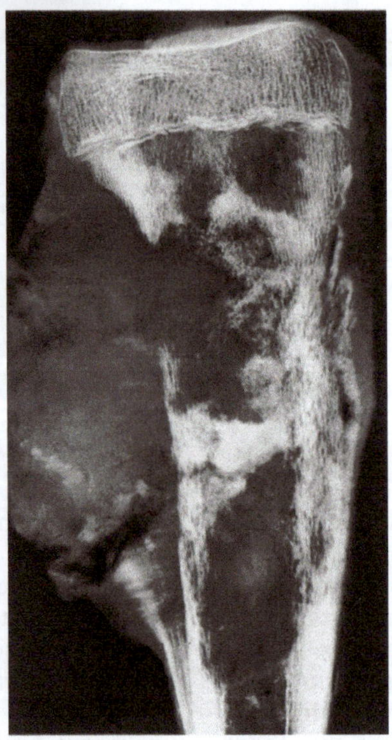

c

Fig. VI.41a–c. Male, 17 years old. Malignant mesenchymoma of tibia. **a** Anteroposterior radiograph of the amputation specimen illustrates the osteolytic-sclerotic aspect of the tumor, located in the upper metaphyseal region. There is destruction of the medial cortex and a typical Codman's triangle on its internal aspect. The radiographic aspect appears to be typical osteosarcoma. **b** Photograph and **c** radiograph of a 5-mm-thick section of the amputation specimen showing the extensive penetration of the tumor into soft tissue. The bulk of the tumor was of yellowish color, alternating with hemorrhagic areas. The Codman's triangle is clearly seen. (Schajowicz et al. 1966)

the section on mesenchymal chondrosarcoma, we mentioned that some of the cases described by McFarland et al. (1977) as "dedifferentiated chondrosarcoma" and those reported by Hutter et al. (1966) as "primitive multipotential primary sarcoma of bone" should, in our opinion, be classified as malignant mesenchymomas. Malignant mesenchymoma has been accepted by Lichtenstein as a distinct entity and was included in his classification (1977). He mentioned having observed several pertinent cases, one with the most common combination of liposarcoma and osteosarcoma. However, in another case involving the pubic bone in a 23-year-old male, in addition to fields of osteosarcoma there were large multinucleated "strap" cells (apparently

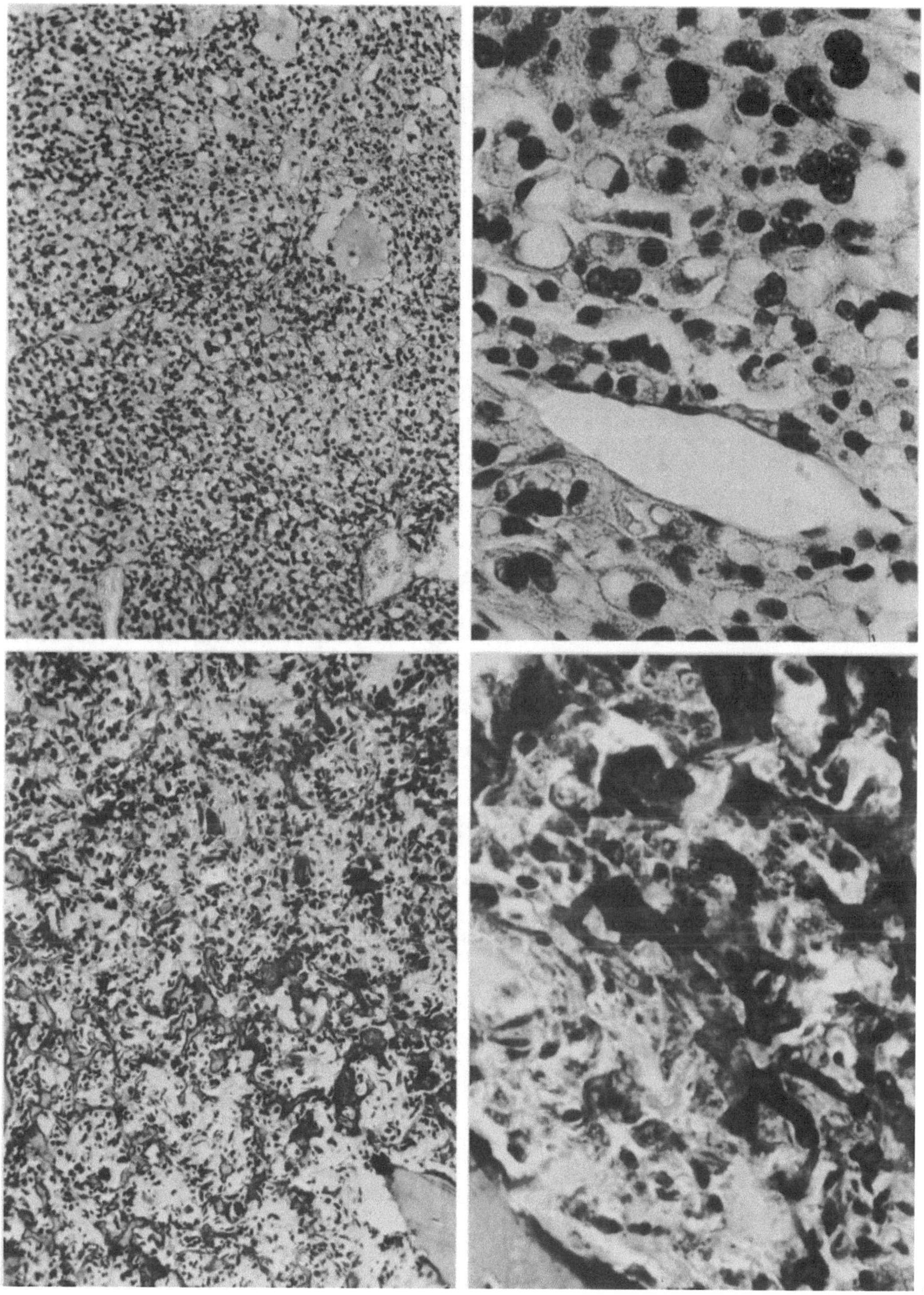

a b c d

Fig. VI.42. a,b Photomicrographs of an area of liposarcoma of the same case as in Fig. VI.41, illustrating at lower and higher magnification the characteristic signet-ring cells and lipoblasts with large hyperchromatic nuclei. **c,d** Photomicrographs of areas of osteosarcoma illustrating an irregular network of calcified tumor bone trabeculae. **a,c** ×100, **b,d** ×400

a

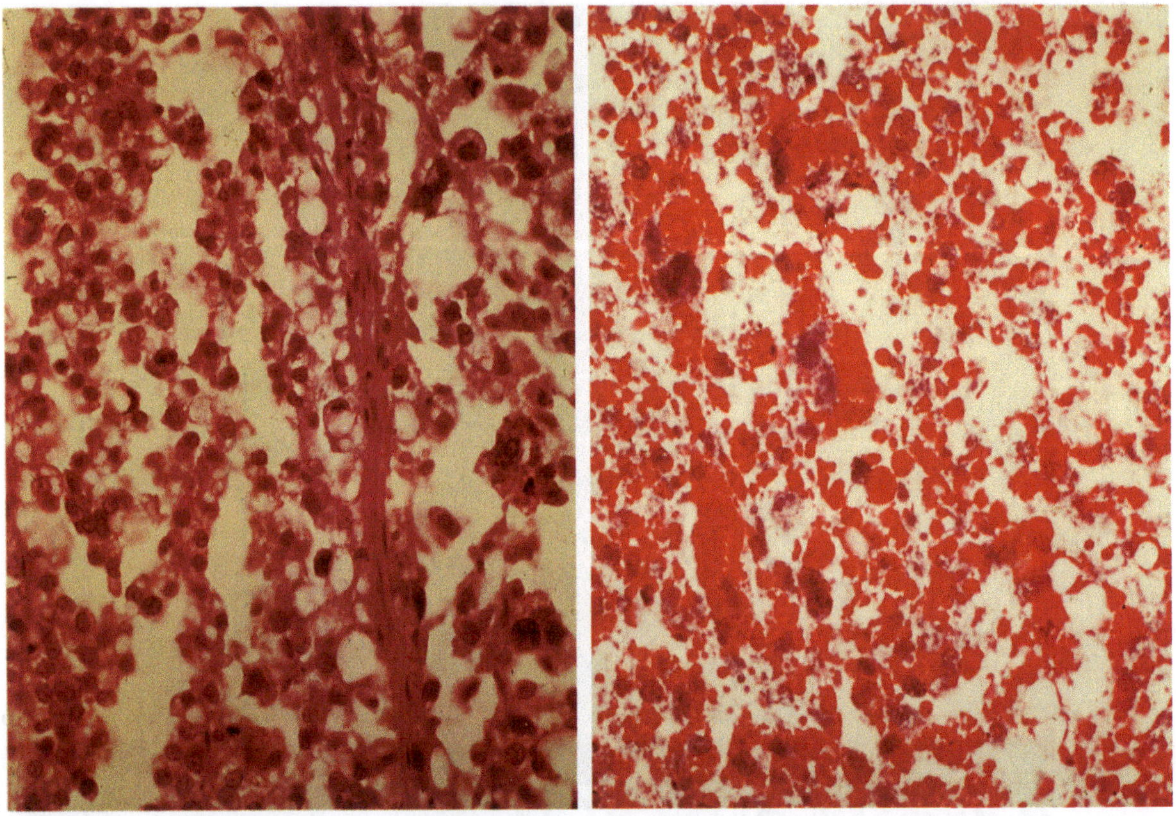

b

Fig. VI.43a,b. Photomicrograph of malignant mesenchymoma (same case as in Figs. IV.41 and VI.42), showing the liposarcomatous pattern stained with HE and special fat stain (Sudan). **a**,**b** ×320

VI.44a

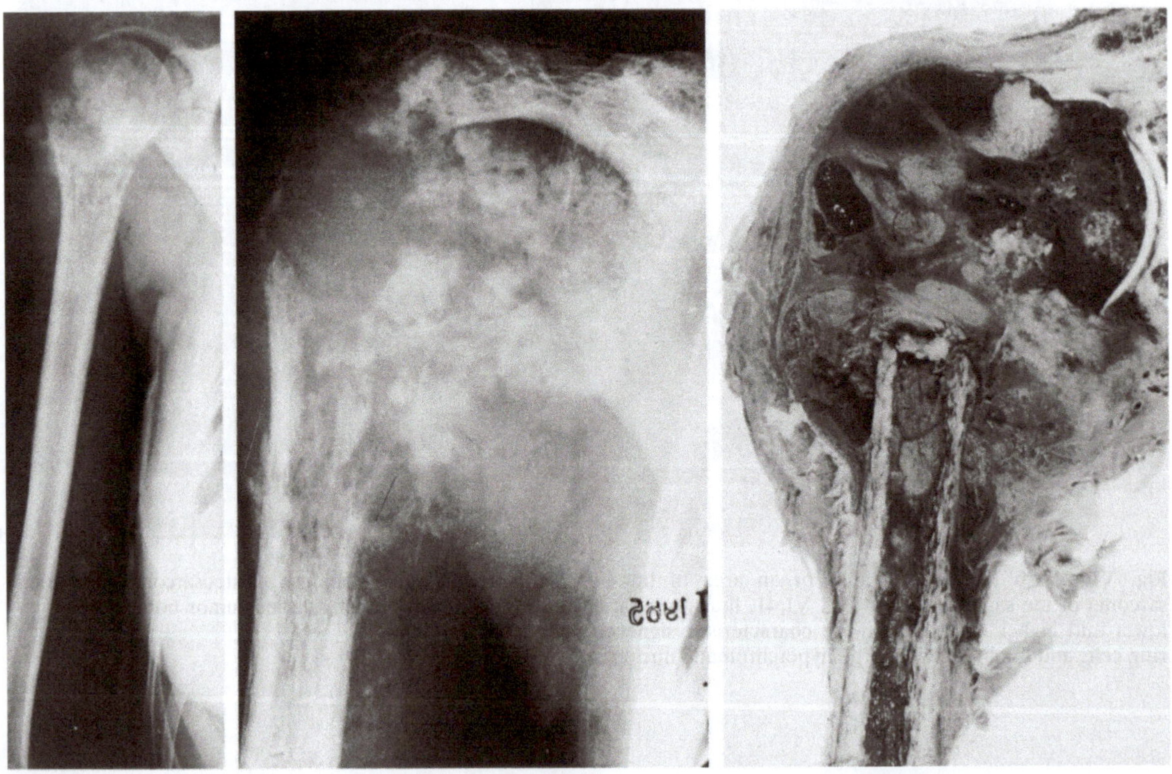

b, c

indicative of rhabdomyosarcoma) and vacuolated cells resembling lipoblasts. Two other cases, in which chondrosarcomatous, osteosarcomatous, and giant-cell tumor-like areas were observed, are not distinct from conventional osteosarcoma, in which these tissue differentiations are a common feature.

The ages of our four patients ranged from 14 to 65 years. There were three males and one female. The tumors were located in the tibia, humerus, radius, and metatarsus. The radiographic appearance was extremely variable: in our first case, the tumor exhibited malignant characteristics identical to those of osteosarcoma, while in others the tumor mimicked a metastatic carcinoma or malignant lymphoma (Fig. VI.44). The gross and microscopic features varied according to the tumor tissue component present.

The treatment was, in all cases, ablative surgery (amputation or disarticulation), the survival time being less than 2 years.

5. Primary Leiomyosarcoma of Bone

This is a rare condition and only three cases had been reported as of 1978. In 1965 Evans and Sanerkin reported an osteolytic tumor of the tibia in a 73-year-old male, who died 4 weeks after radiation therapy. An autopsy showed only metastatic nodules in the lung besides the tibial lesion. The diagnosis was particularly based on the presence of spindle cells with a cytoplasm stained with Masson's trichrome, myofibrils being demonstrated by Mallory's phosphotungstic acid-hematoxylin stain. No electron microscopic examination was made. The second case, in the femur of an 18-year-old female, was reported by Overgaard et al. (1977), and the third, in the proximal right humerus of a 75-year-old male, by Meister et al. (1978); both were studied by light and electron microscopy, which showed characteristic changes with cytoplasmic myofilaments, dense bodies, pinocytic vesicles, and basal lamina fragments.

◄

Fig. VI.44a–c. Female, 22 years old. Malignant mesenchymoma of humerus. **a** Radiograph showing radiolucent permeative lesion with irregular areas of sclerosis. **b** Radiograph 6 months after radiation therapy demonstrates the extension of the tumor with wide invasion of soft tissues. **c** Photograph of the amputation specimen illustrates the predominantly hemorrhagic appearance of this large tumor. Histologically, the lesion showed areas of liposarcoma, osteosarcoma, and angiosarcoma

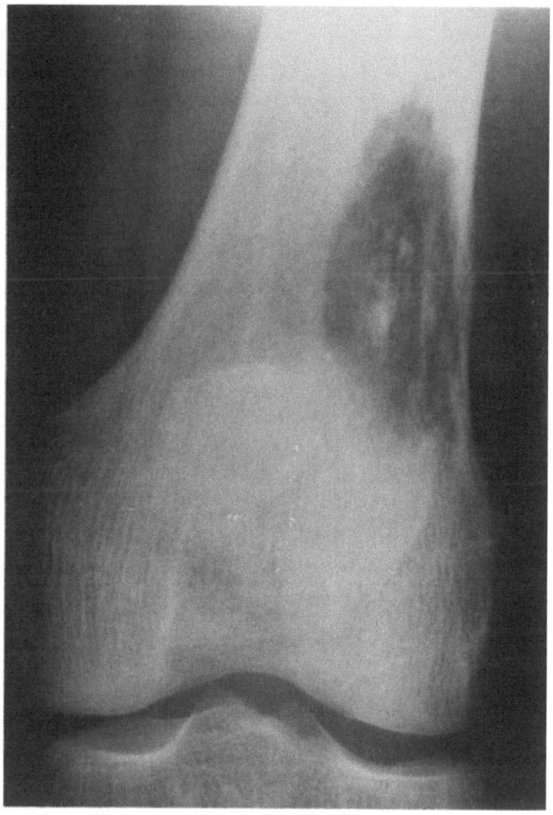

Fig. VI.45. Male, 59 years old. Leiomyosarcoma of femur. Radiograph demonstrates an eccentric, radiolucent poorly delimited lesion with scarce calcification

Two new publications appeared in 1979 (Sanerkin) and 1980 (Angervall et al.). Sanerkin reported two cases, one with a detailed cytologic and ultrastructural study, and compared them with the findings in cases of fibrosarcoma. Although he insists that there are cytologic differences, namely the undue elongation and eosinophilia of the cytoplasmic processes of leiomyosarcoma cells, he admits that certain basic similarities exist between these two tumors, manifested at the ultrastructural level by the presence of myofilaments in fibrosarcoma; "it would seem that the observed differences relate to the degree of development of the myofilamentous structures." Angervall et al. (1980) reported five cases of primary leiomyosarcoma of bone, based on the histologic and ultrastructural findings in three of their cases. They emphasized the importance of trichrome stains, such as van Gieson stain, and the finding of abundant myofilaments with elongated densities. However, it is now accepted that electron microscopy is not conclusive in differentiating leiomyosarcoma and fibrosarcoma, because myofilaments may be

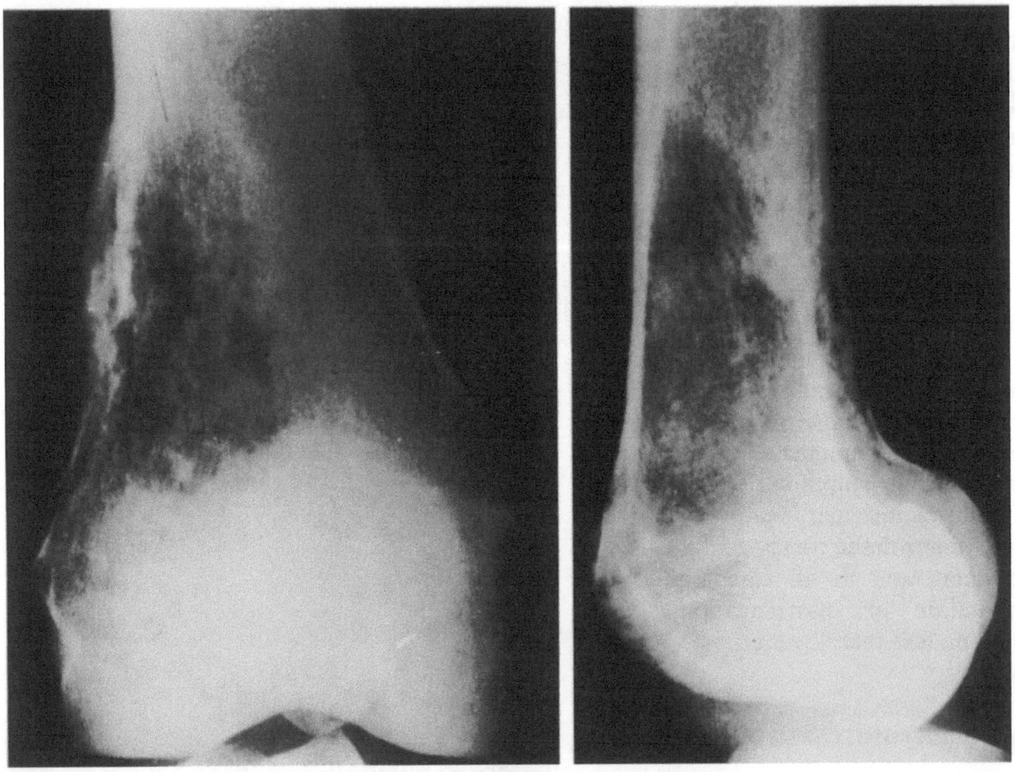

Fig. VI.46. Female, 45 years old. Leiomyosarcoma of femur. Anteroposterior and lateral radiographs illustrate a radiolucent permeative lesion with unusual periosteal new bone formation. This case was first classified as fibrosarcoma

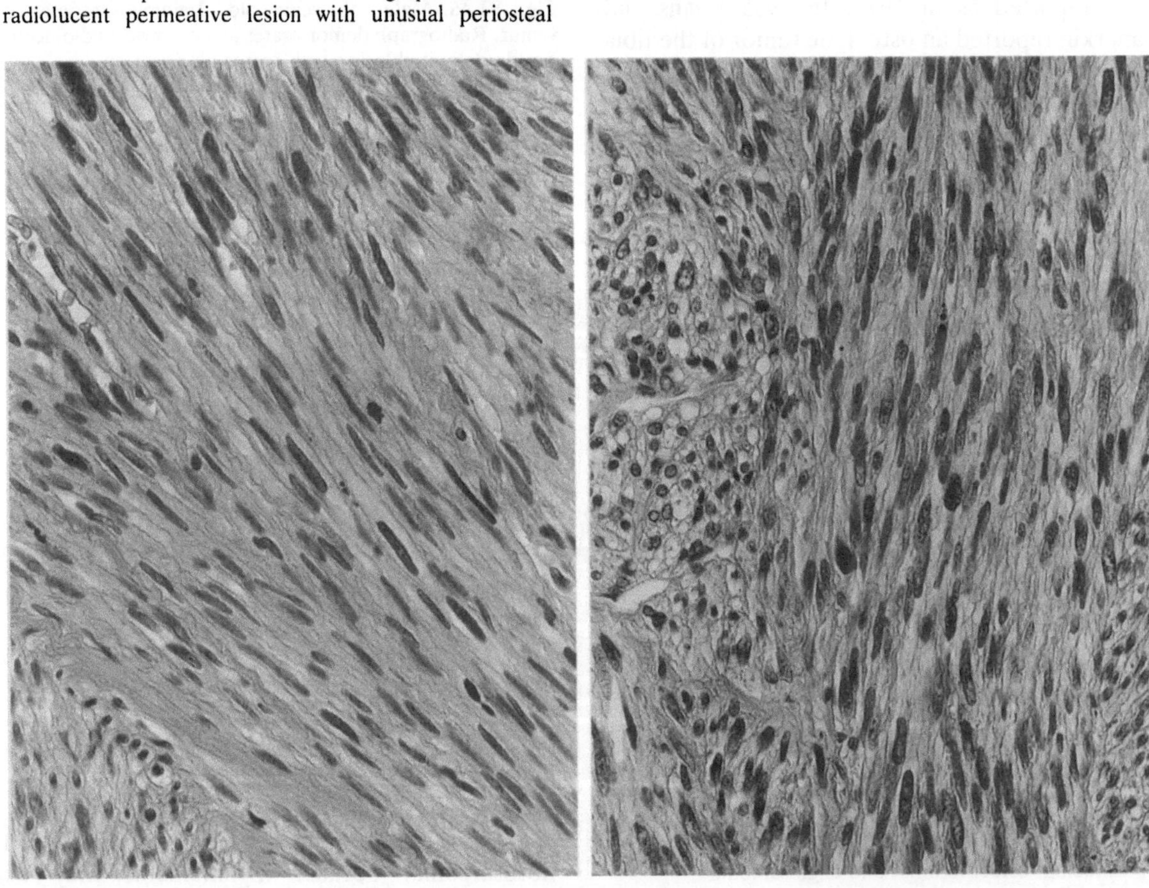

a b

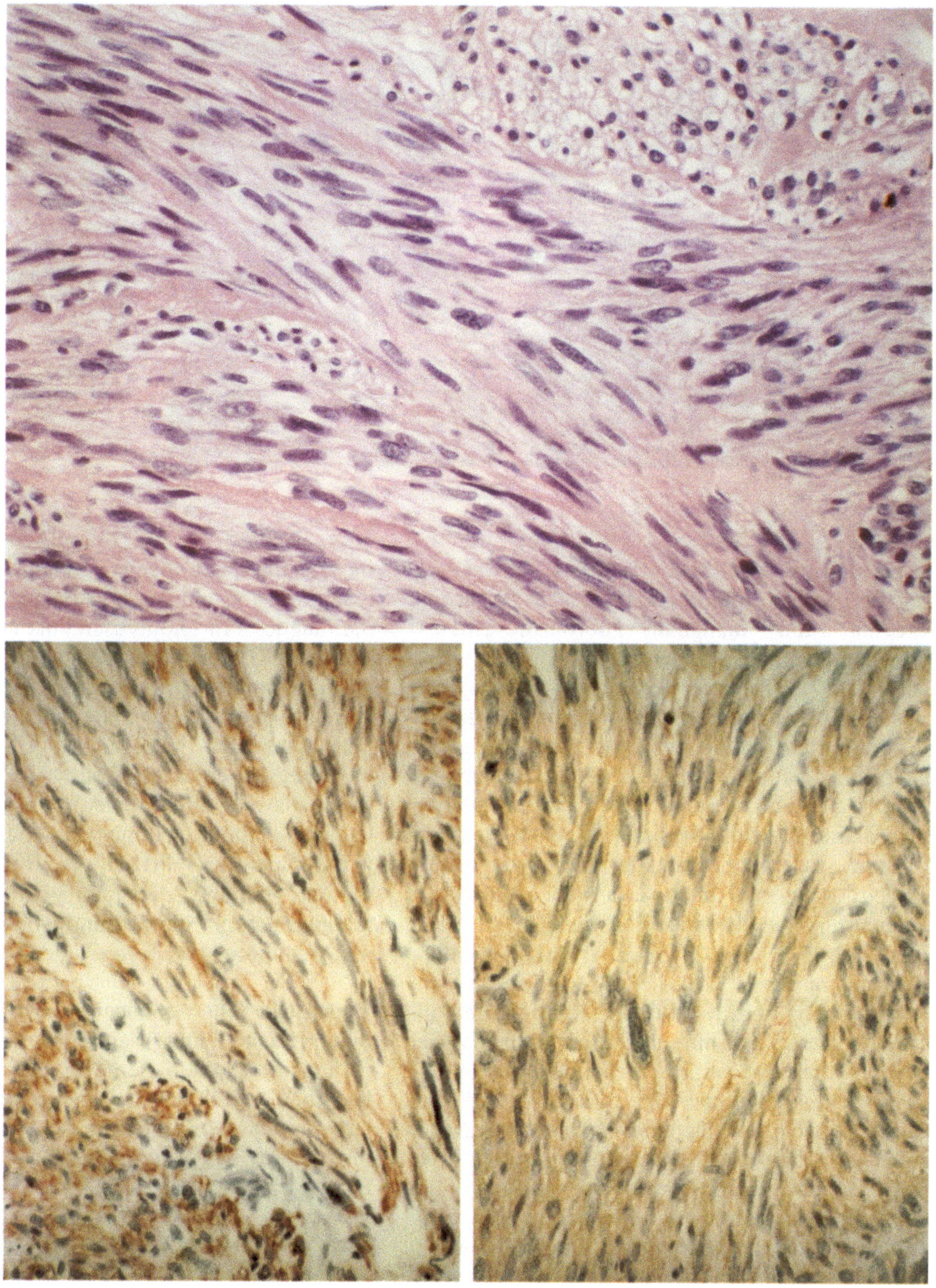

a b c

Fig. VI.47a–c. Photomicrographs show elongated spindle cells with cigar-shaped nuclei and conspicuous eosinophilic cytoplasm. There was only scarce pleomorphism and mitotic activity. **b** The immunohistochemical study revealed strong positivity for actin and **c** desmin markers. **a–c** ×200

Fig. VI.48a,b. Photomicrographs illustrate the characteristic histologic features of leiomyosarcoma, with interlacing bundles of elongated cells, cigar-shaped nuclei, and only scarce mitoses. **a,b** ×400

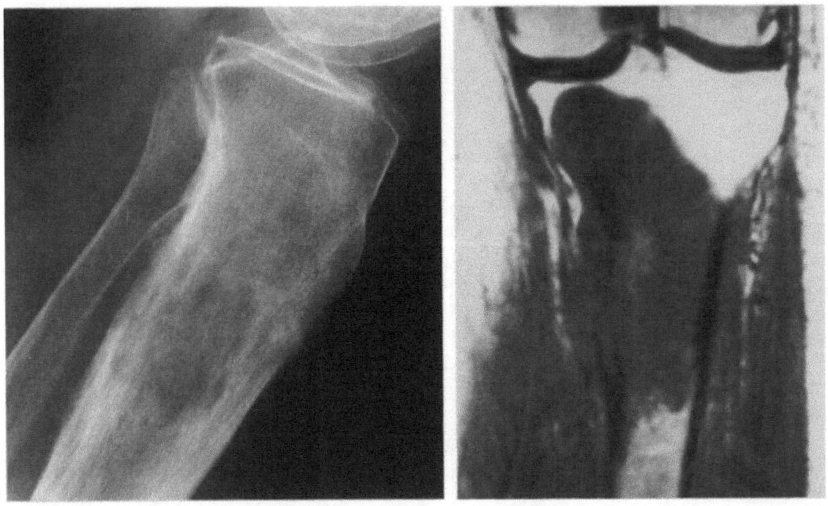

Fig. VI.49. a Lateral radiograph shows a radiolucent lesion with ill-defined margins and periosteal reaction at its posterior aspect. **b** T1-weighted MRI reveals the extension of the lesion toward the subchondral area, and destruction of the medial cortex. A wide en bloc resection followed by allograft was performed on leiomyosarcoma of the tibia. (Courtesy of K. Unni, Mayo Clinic)

found in fibroblasts ("myofibroblasts") in various reactive and neoplastic states, such as fibrosarcoma and malignant fibrohistiocytomas (Hernandez and Fernandez 1976; Churg and Kahn 1977). The latter authors concluded that these tumors contain cells showing a spectrum of differentiation from fibrocytic to myogenic. Therefore Sanerkin postulated that primary leiomyosarcoma of bone need not necessarily always arise from the media of the blood vessels: "it may also conceivably develop through advanced myogenic metaplasia of a sarcoma originating from fibroblastic tissue."

Until 1985 only 25 cases of pure leiomyosarcoma of bone had been reported in the literature; 16 of these tumors were located in the long bones and nine in the jaw bone. More recently the Swedish researchers Berlin et al. (1987) recorded the clinical and pathologic features of 16 cases of leiomyosarcoma primary in bone, including the five previously reported by Angervall et al. (1980). This figure was obtained after reviewing the Swedish series of spindle-cell sarcomas of bone filed at the Cancer Registry, and diagnosis was based on light and electron microscopic examinations. Thirteen tumors were located in a long bone of an extremity (nine around the knee joint) and three in the central skeleton. Radiographically all the tumors were osteolytic and three patients had a pathologic fracture.

In recent years immunohistochemistry has been widely used in the diagnosis of myogenic tumors. The intermediate muscle filament desmin has been studied in leiomyosarcoma of soft tissue and of the bone (Kawai et al. 1983). However, the results have been variable, since desmin immunohistochemistry is of only limited value for the diagnosis of leiomyosarcoma of bone (Berlin et al. 1987). The smooth muscle specific mononuclear antibody recognizing actin seems to be more sensitive for the identification of smooth muscle tumors.

Only three cases with the characteristic histologic and immunohistochemical features of leiomyosarcoma of bone were found in our files (Figs. VI.45–VI.48); Fig. VI.49 shows the radiographic and MRI findings in a patient with leiomyosarcoma of the tibia who was examined and treated at the Mayo Clinic.

Treatment. The clinical behavior indicates that primary leiomyosarcoma of bone is highly malignant. Eight patients of the Swedish series had died of the tumor, and of the other eight patients who were alive at follow-up, three had metastases. The remaining five patients had been free of disease for 6.5–12.3 years.

6. Undifferentiated Sarcoma

Definition, WHO: *"A malignant tumor with a pleomorphic spindle-celled structure but devoid of any specific pattern of histological differentiation."*

In a limited biopsy specimen, a poorly differentiated fibrosarcoma, an osteosarcoma with relatively little tumor bone, a lymphoma, or even an undifferentiated metastatic carcinoma, can pose practical difficulties of identification and thus be confused with cases properly belonging to this group. But even after careful study of adequate samples of tissue, including the application of newer cytomorphologic and immunohistochemical methods, and subsequent follow-up investigation, rare cases remain in which the tumor is regarded as primary in bone but where no specific pattern of differentiation can be detected. Consequently, this group is regarded as an essential part of the classification.

References

Benign Fibrous Histiocytoma

Bahls G (1936) Über cin solitares Xantom im Knochen. Zentralbl Chir 63:1041–1046
Bertoni F, Capanna R, Calderoni P, Bacchini P (1983) Case report 223. Skeletal Radiol 9:215–217
Bertoni F, Calderoni P, Bacchini P et al. (1986) Benign fibrous histiocytoma of bone. J Bone Joint Surg [Am] 68:1225–1230
Bertoni F, Unni KK, McLeod RA, Sim FH (1988) Xanthoma of bone. Am J Clin Pathol 90:377–384
Burman MS, Sinberg SE (1938) Solitary xanthoma (lipoid granulomatosis). Arch Surg 37:1017–1032
Clark TD, Stelling CB, Fechner RE (1985) Case report 328. Skeletal Radiol 14:149
Clarke BE, Xipell JM, Thomas DP (1985) Benign fibrous histiocytoma of bone. Am J Surg Pathol 9:806–815
Dahlin DC (1978) Bone tumors, 3rd edn. Charles C. Thomas, Springfield, IL
Dahlin DC, Unni KK (1986) Bone tumors: general aspects and data on 8542 cases. Charles C. Thomas, Springfield, IL
Destouet JM, Kyriakos M, Gilula LA (1980) Fibrous histiocytoma (fibroxanthoma) of a cervical vertebra: a report with a review of the literature. Skeletal Radiol 5:241–246
Dominok GW, Eisengarten W (1980) Benignes fibröses Histiozytom des Knochens. Zentralbl Allg Pathol 214:77–83
Fechner RE (1984) Benign fibrous histiocytoma in adults including three cases with recurrence. Read at the Closed Meeting of the International Skeletal Society, Sept. 9, 1984
Fechner RE, Huvos AG, Mirra JM et al. (1984) A symposium on the pathology of bone tumors. In: Sommers SC, Rosen PP (eds) Pathology annual, part I, vol 19. Appleton-Century-Crofts, Norwalk, Connecticut, pp 125–194
Hermann G, Steiner G, Sherry HH (1988) Case report 465. Diagnosis: benign fibrous histiocytoma (BFH). Skeletal Radiol 17:195–197
Huvos AG (1991) Bone tumors: diagnosis, treatment, prognosis. W.B. Saunders, Philadelphia
Roessner A, Immenkamp M, Weidner A et al. (1981) Benign fibrous histiocytoma of bone: light- and electron-microscopic observations. J Cancer Res Clin Oncol 101:191–202
Saito R, Caines MJ (1977) Atypical fibrous histiocytoma of the humerus: a light and electron microscopic study. Am J Clin Pathol 68:409–415
Spjut HJ, Fechner RE, Ackerman LV (1981) Tumors of bone and cartilage (Supplement). Atlas of tumor pathology, 2nd series, Fasc 5. Armed Forces Institute of Pathology, Washington, DC
Yagmai I (1978) Intra- and extraosseous xanthomata associated with hyperlipidemia. Radiology 128:49–54

Lipoma

Azizi D (1968) Le lipome intra-osseux. J Chir (Paris) 96:557
Bartlett EI (1930) Periosteal lipoma. Arch Surg 21:1015
Caruolo JE, Dahlin DC (1953) Lipoma involving bone and simulating malignant bone tumor. Proc Staff Meet Mayo Clin 28:361
Child PL (1955) Lipoma of the os calcis. Am J Clin Pathol 25:1050
Cowdell RH (1954) Intra-osseous lipoma of rib. Br J Surg 41:664
Dahlin DC (1978) Bone tumors, 3rd edn. Charles C. Thomas, Springfield, IL
Dahlin DC, Unni KK (1986) Bone tumors: general aspects and data on 8542 cases. Charles C. Thomas, Springfield, IL
Delee JC (1979) Intraosseous lipoma of the proximal part of the femur. J Bone Joint Surg [Am] 61:601
Demos TC, Bruno E, Armin A et al. (1984) Parosteal lipoma with enlarging osteochondroma. AJR 143:365–366
Dickson AD, Ayres WW, Mason MW, Miller WR (1951) Lipoma of bone of intra-osseous origin. J Bone Joint Surg [Am] 33:257
Döhler R, Harms D (1981) Intraosseous lipomas. Z Orthop 119:138–141
Fleming RJ, Alpert M, Garcia A (1962) Parosteal lipoma. Am J Roentgenol Radium Ther Nucl Med 87:1075
Freiberg RA, Air GW, Glueck CH et al. (1974) Multiple intraosseous lipomas with type-IV hyperlipoproteinemia. J Bone Joint Surg [Am] 56:1729–1732
Goldman AB, Marcove RC, Huvos AG et al. (1984) Case report 280. Diagnosis: intraosseous lipoma of the tibia. Skeletal Radiol 12:209–212
Gunterberg B, Kindblom LG (1978) Intraosseous lipoma. A report of two cases. Acta Orthop Scand 49:95
Hart JAL (1973) Intra-osseous lipoma. J Bone Joint Surg [Br] 55:624–632
Jaffe HL (1958) Tumors and tumorous conditions of the bones and joints. Lea & Febiger, Philadelphia
Kurland KZ, Kennard JW (1965) Parosteal lipoma arising from the proximal radius: a case report. Clin Orthop 41:140
Leeson M, Kay D, Smith B (1983) Intraosseous lipoma. Clin Orthop 181:186–190
Lichtenstein L (1977) Bone tumors, 5th edn. C.V. Mosby, St. Louis
Makrycostas K (1927) Über das Wirbelangiom-lipom und Osteom. Virchow's Arch [A] 265:259–303
Milgram JW (1981) Intraosseous lipomas with reactive ossification in the proximal femur: report of eight cases. Skeletal Radiol 7:1–13
Milgram JW (1988) Intraosseous lipomas: a clinicopathologic study of 66 cases. Clin Orthop 231:277–302
Moorefield WC Jr, Urbaniak JR, Gonzalvo AA (1976) Intramedullary lipoma of the distal femur. South Med J 69:1210–1211

Mueller MC, Robbins JL (1960) Intramedullary lipoma of bone. J Bone Joint Surg [Am] 42:517
Ramos A, Castello J, Sartoris DJ et al. (1985) Osseous lipoma: CT appearance. Radiology 157:615–619
Salzer M, Gatzmann H (1963) Parostale lipome. Bruns Beitr Klin Chir 206:501–505
Salzer M, Salzer-Kuntschik M (1965) Zur Frage der sogenannten zentralen Knochenlipome. Beitr Pathol Anat Allg Pathol 132:365
Savarese A, Donofrio G (1981) A case of parosteal lipoma of the neck of the radius. Chir Organi Mov 67:711–714
Schmorl G, Junghanns H (1971) The human spine in health and disease, 2nd edn. Grune & Stratton, New York
Schweitzer G (1970) Parosteal lipoma of the radius. S Afr Med J 44:648
Smith WE, Fienberg R (1957) Intraosseous lipoma of bone. Cancer 10:1151
Spjut HJ, Dorfman HD, Fechner RE, Ackerman LV (1971) Tumors of bone and cartilage. Atlas of tumor pathology, 2nd series, Fasc 5. Armed Forces Institute of Pathology, Washington, DC
Steiner M, Gould AR, Rasmussen J et al. (1981) Parosteal lipoma of the mandible. Oral Surg 52:61–65
Zorn DT, Cordray DP, Randels PH (1971) Intraosseous lipoma of bone involving the sacrum. J Bone Joint Surg [Am] 53:1201–1204

Desmoplastic Fibroma

Bertoni F, Calderoni P, Bacchini P, Campanacci M (1984) Desmoplastic fibroma of bone: a report of six cases. J Bone Joint Surg [Br] 66:265–268
Bertoni F, Present D, Marchetti C et al. (1986) Desmoplastic fibroma of the jaw: the experience of the Istituto Beretta. Oral Surg 61:179–184
Beskin JL, Haddad RJ Jr (1985) Desmoplastic fibroma of the first metatarsal: a case report. Clin Orthop 195:299–303
Campanacci M (1990) Bone and soft tissue tumors. Springer, Vienna New York
Cohen P, Goldenberg RR (1965) Desmoplastic fibroma of bone. J Bone Joint Surg [Am] 47:1620–1625
Dahlin DC, Hoover NW (1964) Desmoplastic fibroma of bone. JAMA 188:685–687
Dahlin DC, Unni KK (1986) Bone tumors: general aspects and data on 8542 cases. Charles C. Thomas, Springfield, IL
Eisen MZ, Butler HE (1984) Desmoplastic fibroma of the maxilla: report of a case. J Am Dent Assoc 108:608–609
Gebhardt MC, Campbell CJ, Schiller AL et al. (1985) Desmoplastic fibroma of bone: a report of eight cases and review of the literature. J Bone Joint Surg [Am] 67:732–747
Godinho FS, Chiconelli JR, Lemos C (1967) Desmoplastic fibroma of bone: report of a case. J Bone Joint Surg [Br] 49:560–561
Graudal N (1984) Desmoplastic fibroma of bone: case report and literature review. Acta Orthop Scand 55:215–219
Hinds EC, Kent JN, Fechner RE (1969) Desmoplastic fibroma of the mandible. J Oral Surg 27:271–274
Jaffe HL (1958) Tumors and tumorous conditions of the bones and joints. Lea & Febiger, Philadelphia
Kimmelstiel P, Rapp IH (1951) Cortical defect due to periosteal desmoids. Bull Hosp Joint Dis 12:286–297
Lanari A (1983) Effect of progesterone on desmoid tumors (aggressive fibromatosis). N Engl J Med 309:1523
Lichtman EA, Klein MJ (1985) Case report 302. Diagnosis: desmoplastic fibroma of the proximal end of the left femur. Skeletal Radiol 13:160–163
Makek M, Lello GE (1986) Desmoplastic fibroma of the mandible: literature review and report of three cases. J Oral Maxillofac Surg 44:385–391
Marek FM (1955) Fibrous cortical defect (periosteal desmoid). Bull Hosp Joint Dis 16:77
Martínez Mosquera V, Furneo H, Schajowicz F (1977) Fibroma desmoplástico del hueso. Bol Trab Soc Argent Ortop Traum 42:374–380
Meary R, Danan JP, Tomeno B et al. (1978) Desmoid fibroma of the limbs. Rev Chir Orthop 64:195–204
Nilsonne U, Goethlin G (1969) Desmoplastic fibroma of bone. Acta Orthop Scand 40:205–215
Rabhan WN, Rosai J (1968) Desmoplastic fibroma. J Bone Joint Surg [Am] 50:487–502
Schajowicz F (1981) Tumors and tumorlike lesions of bone and joints. Springer, New York Berlin Heidelberg
Scheer GE, Kuhlman RE (1963) Vertebral involvement by desmoplastic fibroma. JAMA 185:669–670
Sugiura I (1976) Desmoplastic fibroma: case report and review of the literature. J Bone Joint Surg [Am] 58:126–130
West R, Huvos AG, Lane JM (1983) Desmoplastic fibroma of bone arising in fibrous dysplasia. Am J Clin Pathol 79:630–633
Whitesides TE, Ackerman LV (1960) Desmoplastic fibroma. J Bone Joint Surg [Am] 42:1143–1150

Fibrosarcoma

André S, Tomeno B, Forest M et al. (1983) Fibrosarcoma of bone. Rev Chir Orthop 69:107–116
Batts M Jr (1941) Periosteal fibrosarcoma. Arch Surg 42:566–576
Bertoni F, Capanna R, Calderoni P et al. (1984) Primary central (medullary) fibrosarcoma of bone. Semin Diagn Pathol 1:185–198
Campanacci M (1990) Bone and soft tissue tumors. Springer, Vienna New York
Chung EB, Enzinger FM et al. (1976) Infantile fibrosarcoma. Cancer 38:729–739
Cronin J (1973) Fibrosarcoma of the paranasal air sinuses. J Laryngol Otol 87:667–674
Cunningham MP, Arlen M (1968) Medullary fibrosarcoma of bone. Cancer 21:31–37
Dahlin DC (1978) Bone tumors, 3rd edn. Charles C. Thomas, Springfield, IL
Dahlin DC (1982) Case report 189. Infantile fibrosarcoma (congenital fibrosarcoma-like fibromatosis). Skeletal Radiol 8:77–78
Dahlin DC, Ivins JC (1969) Fibrosarcoma of bone: a study of 114 cases. Cancer 23:35–41
Dahlin DC, Unni KK (1986) Bone tumors: general aspects and data on 8542 cases. Charles C. Thomas, Springfield, IL

Dorfman HD, Norman A, Wolff H (1966) Fibrosarcoma complicating bone infarction in a caisson worker: a case report. J Bone Joint Surg [Am] 48:528–532

Eyre-Brook AL, Price CHG (1969) Fibrosarcoma of bone: review of 50 consecutive cases from the Bristol Bone Tumor Registry. J Bone Joint Surg [Br] 51:20–37

Fauré C, Grumer M, Boccon-Gibod L (1981) Case report 149. Diagnosis: infantile congenital fibrosarcoma of humerus. Skeletal Radiol 6:208–211

Feldman F, Norman D (1972) Intra- and extraosseous malignant histiocytoma (malignant fibrous xanthoma). Radiology 104:497–508

Furey JG, Ferrer-Torelles M, Reagan JW (1960) Fibrosarcoma arising in the site of bone infarction: a report of two cases. J Bone Joint Surg [Am] 42:802–810

Galli SJ, Weintraub HP, Proppe KH (1978) Malignant fibrous histiocytoma and pleomorphic sarcoma in association with medullary bone infarcts. Cancer 41:607–619

Geschickter CI (1932) So-called fibrosarcoma of bone: bone involvement by sarcoma of neighboring soft parts. Arch Surg 24:231–291

Gilmer WS Jr, MacEwen GD (1958) Central (medullary) fibrosarcoma of bone. J Bone Joint Surg [Am] 40:121

Hall J, Tseng SC, Timpl R et al. (1985) Collagen types in fibrosarcoma: absence of type III collagen in reticulin. Hum Pathol 16:439–446

Hernandez FJ, Fernandez BB (1976) Multiple diffuse fibrosarcoma of bone. Cancer 37:939–945

Huvos AG (1991) Bone tumors: diagnosis, treatment, prognosis. W B Saunders, Philadelphia

Huvos AG, Higinbotham NL (1975) Primary fibrosarcoma of bone: a clinico-pathological study of 130 patients. Cancer 35:837–847

Jaffe HL (1958) Tumors and tumorous conditions of the bones and joints. Lea & Febiger, Philadelphia

Jeffree GM (1972) Enzymes in fibroblastic lesions. J Bone Joint Surg [Br] 54:535–546

Jeffree GM, Price CHG (1976) Metastatic spread of fibrosarcoma of bone: a report on 49 cases and a comparison with osteosarcoma. J Bone Joint Surg [Br] 58:418–425

Kindblom LG, Angervall L (1978) Congenital solitary fibromatosis of the skeleton: case report of a variant of congenital generalized fibromatosis. Cancer 41:636–640

Larsson EW, Lorentzon R, Boquist L (1976) Fibrosarcoma of bone: a demographic, clinical and histopathological study of all cases in the Swedish Cancer Registry from 1958 to 1968. J Bone Joint Surg [Br] 58:412–417

Lichtenstein L (1977) Bone tumors, 5th edn. C.V. Mosby, St. Louis

Netherlands Committee on Bone Tumours (1966) Radiological atlas of bone tumors, vol 1. Mouton, The Hague

Nielson AR, Poulsen H (1962) Multiple diffuse fibrosarcomata of the bone. Acta Pathol Microbiol Scand 55:265–273

Nilsonne U, Mazabraud A (1974) Fibrosarcoma of bone. Rev Chir Orthop 60:109–122

Pritchard DJ, Sim FH, Ivins JC, Soule EH, Dahlin DC (1977) Fibrosarcoma of bone and soft tissues of the trunk and extremities. Orthop Clin North Am 8:869–881

Schwartz DT, Albert M (1964) The malignant transformation of fibrous dysplasia. Am J Med Sci 247:1–20

Steiner E (1944) Multiple diffuse fibrosarcoma of bone. Am J Pathol 20:887–893

Stout AP (1948) Fibrosarcoma: the malignant tumor of fibroblasts. Cancer 1:30–63

Taconis WK, Mulder JD (1984) Fibrosarcoma and malignant fibrous histiocytoma of long bones: radiographic features and grading. Skeletal Radiol 11:237–245

Taconis WK, Van Rijssel TG (1985) Fibrosarcoma of long bones: a study of the significance of areas of malignant fibrous histiocytoma. J Bone Joint Surg [Br] 67:111–116

Taconis WK, Van Rijssel TG (1986) Fibrosarcoma of the jaws. Skeletal Radiol 15:10–13

Wells HG (1940) Occurrence and significance of congenital malignant neoplasm. Arch Pathol 30:535

Malignant Fibrous Histiocytoma

Abdul Karim FW, Ayala AG, Chawla SP et al. (1985) Malignant fibrous histiocytoma of the jaws: a clinicopathologic study of 11 cases. Cancer 56:1590–1596

Abrahams TG, Hull M (1986) Case report 394. Diagnosis: malignant fibrous histiocytoma (MFH) arising in an infarct of bone. Skeletal Radiol 15:578–583

Bacci G, Springfield DS, Capanna R et al. (1987) Adjuvant chemotherapy for malignant fibrous histiocytoma in the femur and tibia. J Bone Joint Surg [Am] 67:620–625

Belza MG, Urich H (1986) Chordoma and malignant fibrous histiocytoma. Cancer 58:1082–1087

Betelli G, Avella M, Capanna R et al. (1987) Neoadjuvant chemotherapy in malignant fibrous histiocytoma of the extremities: preliminary results in 10 cases treated preoperatively with methotrexate and cisplatin. Chir Organi Mov 72:111–117

Bhagavan BS, Dorfman HD (1982) The significance of bone and cartilage formation in malignant fibrous histiocytoma of soft tissue. Cancer 49:480–488

Boland PJ, Huvos AG (1986) Malignant fibrous histiocytoma of bone. Clin Orthop 204:130–134

Bonfiglio M, Platz CF (1981) Case report 141: malignant fibrous histiocytoma associated with enchondroma of bone. Skeletal Radiol 6:127–130

Brooks JP, Pascal RR (1984) Malignant giant cell tumor of bone: ultrastructural and immunohistologic evidence of histiocytic origin. Hum Pathol 15:1098–1100

Campanacci M (1990) Bone and soft tissue tumors. Springer, Vienna New York

Capanna R, Bertoni F, Bacchini P et al. (1984) Malignant fibrous histiocytoma of bone: the experience at the Rizzoli Institute. Report of 90 cases. Cancer 54:177–187

Castillo M, Tehranzadeh J, Becerra J et al. (1987) Case report 408: malignant fibrous histiocytoma of innominate bones and femur (multicentric). Skeletal Radiol 16:74–77

Dahlin DC, Unni KK (1986) Bone tumors: general aspects and data on 8542 cases. Charles C. Thomas, Springfield, IL

Dahlin DC, Unni KK, Matsuno T (1977) Malignant (fibrous) histiocytoma of bone: Fact or fancy? Cancer 39:1508–1516

Den Heeten GJ, Koops HS, Kamps WA et al. (1985) Treatment of malignant fibrous histiocytoma of bone: a plea for primary chemotherapy. Cancer 56:37–40

Dorfman HD, Norman A, Wolff H (1966) Fibrosarcoma complicating bone infarction in a caisson worker. J Bone Joint Surg [Am] 48:528–532

Dunham WK, Wilbon WH (1979) Malignant fibrous histiocytoma of bone. J Bone Joint Surg [Am] 61:939–942

Feldman F, Lattes R (1977) Primary malignant fibrous histiocytoma (fibrous xanthoma) of bone. Skeletal Radiol 1:145–160

Feldman F, Norman D (1972) Intra- and extraosseous malignant histiocytoma (malignant fibrous xanthoma). Radiology 104:497–508

Frierson HF Jr, Fechner RE, Stallings RG et al. (1987) Malignant fibrous histiocytoma in bone infarct: association with sickle cell trait and alcohol abuse. Cancer 59:496–500

Fu Y, Gabbiani G, Kaye G, Lattes R (1975) Malignant soft tissue tumors of probable histiocytic origin (malignant fibrous histiocytoma). General considerations and electron microscopic and tissue culture studies. Cancer 35:176–198

Furey JG, Ferrer-Torelles M, Reagan JW (1960) Fibrosarcoma arising at the site of bone infarcts. J Bone Joint Surg [Am] 42:802–810

Galli SJ, Wintraub HP, Proppe KH (1978) Malignant fibrous histiocytoma and pleomorphic sarcoma in association with medullary bone infarct. Cancer 41:607–619

Ghandur-Mnaymneh L, Zych G, Mnaymneh W (1982) Primary malignant fibrous histiocytoma of bone: report of six cases with ultrastructure study and analysis of the literature. Cancer 49:698–707

Hardcastle P, Nade S, Arnold W (1986) Hereditary bone dysplasia with malignant change: report of three families. J Bone Joint Surg [Am] 68:1079–1089

Harris M (1980) The ultrastructure of benign and malignant fibrous histiocytomas. Histopathology 4:29–44

Heselson HG, Price SK, Mills EED et al. (1983) Two malignant fibrous histiocytomas in bone infarcts. J Bone Joint Surg [Am] 65:1166–1171

Hoffman MA, Dickersin GR (1983) Malignant fibrous histiocytoma: an ultrastructural study of 11 cases. Hum Pathol 14:913–922

Huvos AG (1976) Primary malignant fibrous histiocytoma of bone: clinico-pathologic study of 18 patients. NY State J Med 76:552–559

Huvos AG (1991) Bone tumors: diagnosis, treatment, prognosis. W.B. Saunders, Philadelphia

Huvos AG, Heilweil M, Bretsky SS (1985) The pathology of malignant fibrous histiocytoma of bone: a study of 130 patients. Am J Surg Pathol 9:853–871

Huvos AG, Woodard HQ, Heilweil M (1986) Postradiation malignant fibrous histiocytoma of bone: a clinicopathologic study of 20 patients. Am J Surg Pathol 10:9–18

Inada O, Yumoto T, Furuse K et al. (1976) Ultrastructural features of malignant fibrous histiocytoma of bone. Acta Pathol Jpn 26:491–501

Kahn LB, Webber B, Mills E et al. (1978) Malignant fibrous histiocytoma (malignant fibrous xanthoma: xanthosarcoma) of bone. Cancer 42:640–651

Katenkamp D, Stiller D (1981) Malignant fibrous histiocytoma of bone: light microscopic and electron microscopic examination of four cases. Virchows Arch [A] 391:323–335

Kempson R, Kyriakos M (1972) Fibroxanthosarcoma of the soft tissues. Cancer 29:961–976

Kyriakos M, Kempson RL (1976) Inflammatory fibrous histiocytoma: an aggressive and lethal lesion. Cancer 37:1584–1606

Lawson CW, Fisher C, Gatter KC (1987) An inmunohistochemical study of differentiation in malignant fibrous histiocytoma. Histopathology 11:375–383

Lee YS, Pho RWH, Nather A (1984) Malignant fibrous histiocytoma at site of metal implant. Cancer 54:2286–2289

Martínez-Tello FJ, Navas Palacios J, Calvo-Asensio M et al. (1981) Malignant fibrous histiocytoma of bone: a clinicopathological and electron-microscopical study. Pathol Res Pract 173:141–158

McCarthy EF, Matsuno T, Dorfman HD (1979) Malignant fibrous histiocytoma of bone: a study of 35 cases. Hum Pathol 10:57–70

Merkow LP, Frich JC Jr, Slifkin M et al. (1971) Ultrastructure of fibroxanthosarcoma (malignant fibroxanthoma). Cancer 28:372–383

Mesiter P, Konrad E, Hohne N (1981) Incidence and histological structure of the storiform pattern in benign and malignant fibrous histiocytomas. Virchows Arch [A] 393:93–101

Michael RH, Dorfman HD (1976) Malignant fibrous histiocytoma associated with bone infarcts: report of a case. Clin Orthop 118:180–183

Mirra JM, Bullough PG, Marcove RC et al. (1974) Malignant fibrous histiocytoma and osteosarcoma in association with bone infarcts. J Bone Joint Surg [Am] 56:932–940

Mirra JM, Gold RH, Marafiote R (1977) Malignant (fibrous) histiocytoma arising in association with a bone infarct in sickle-cell disease: Coincidence or cause-and-effect? Cancer 39:186–194

Nakashima Y, Morishita S, Kotoura Y et al. (1985) Malignant fibrous histiocytoma of bone. Cancer 55:2804–2811

Newland RL, Harrison MA, Wright RG (1975) Fibroxanthosarcoma of bone. Pathology 7:203–208

Ozzello L, Stout AP, Murray M (1963) Cultural characteristics of malignant histiocytomas and fibrous xanthomas. Cancer 16:331–344

Picci P, Stilli S (1982) Malignant fibrous histiocytoma arising from an exostosis in a patient affected by multiple exostoses. Ital J Orthop Traumatol 8:205–206

Roholl PJ, Kleyne J, Pijpers HW et al. (1985) Comparative immunohistochemical investigation of markers for malignant histiocytes. Hum Pathol 16:763–771

Roholl PJM, Kleyne J, Van Basten CDH et al. (1985) A study to analyze the origin of tumor cells in malignant fibrous histiocytomas: a multiparametric characterization. Cancer 56:2809–2815

Shirasuna K, Sugiyama M, Miyazaki T (1985) Establishment and characterization of neoplastic cells from a malignant fibrous histiocytoma: a possible stem cell line. Cancer 55:2521–2532

Smith J, Botet JF, Yeh SDJ (1984) Bone sarcomas in Paget's disease: a study of 85 patients. Radiology 152:583–590

Soini Y, Miettinen M (1989) Widespread immunoreactivity for alpha-1-antichymotrypsin in different types of tumors. Am J Clin Pathol 89:131–136
Soule EH, Enriquez P (1972) Atypical fibrous histiocytoma, malignant fibrous histiocytoma, malignant histiocytoma and epithelioid sarcoma: a comparative study of 65 tumors. Cancer 30:128–143
Spanier SS (1977) Malignant fibrous histiocytoma of bone. Orthop Clin North Am 8:947–961
Spanier SS, Enneking WF, Enriquez P (1975) Primary malignant fibrous histiocytoma of bone. Cancer 36:2084–2098
Stout AP, Lattes R (1967) Tumors of the soft tissues. In: Atlas of Tumor Pathology, 2nd series, Fasc 1. Armed Forces Institute of Pathology, Washington, DC, pp 320–358, 107–115
Taconis WK, Van Rijssel TG (1985) Fibrosarcoma of long bones: a study of the significance of areas of malignant fibrous histiocytoma. J Bone Joint Surg [Br] 67:111–116
Urban C, Rosen G, Huvos AG et al. (1983) Chemotherapy of malignant fibrous histiocytoma of bone: a report of five cases. Cancer 51:795–802
Weiner M, Sedlis M, Johnston AD et al. (1983) Adjuvant chemotherapy of malignant fibrous histiocytoma of bone. Cancer 51:25–29
Weiss SW, Enzinger FM (1977) Myxoid variant of malignant fibrous histiocytoma. Cancer 39:1672–1685
Wood GS, Beckstead JH, Turner RR et al. (1986) Malignant fibrous histiocytoma tumor cells resembling fibroblasts. Am J Surg Pathol 10:323–335
Yuen WWH, Saw D (1985) Malignant fibrous histiocytoma of bone. J Bone Joint Surg [Am] 67:482–486

Liposarcoma

Addison AK, Payne SR (1982) Primary liposarcoma of bone: case report. J Bone Joint Surg [Am] 64:301–304
Barnard L (1934) Primary liposarcoma of bone. Arch Surg 29:560–565
Campanacci M (1990) Bone and soft tissue tumors. Springer, Vienna New York
Catto M, Stevens J (1963) Liposarcoma of bone. J Pathol Bacteriol 86:248–253
Dawson EK (1955) Liposarcoma of bone. J Pathol Bacteriol 70:513–520
Duffy J, Stewart FW (1938) Primary liposarcoma of bone: report of a case. Am J Pathol 14:621–626
Ewing JA (1939) A review of the classification of bone tumors. Bull Am Coll Surg 24:290–295
Goldman RL (1964) Primary liposarcoma of bone: report of a case. Am J Clin Pathol 42:503–508
Jaffe HL (1958) Tumors and tumorous conditions of the bones and joints. Lea & Febiger, Philadelphia
Larsson SE, Lorentzon R, Boquist L (1975) Primary liposarcoma of bone. Acta Orthop Scand 46:869–876
Mastragostino S (1957) Tumori lipoblastici primitivi dello scheletro. Chir Organi Mov 44:18–36
Pardo-Mindan FJ, Ayala H, Joly M et al. (1981) Primary Liposarcoma of bone: light and electron microscopic surgery. Cancer 48:274–280
Retz LD Jr (1961) Primary liposarcoma of bone: report of a case and review of the literature. J Bone Joint Surg [Am] 43:123–129
Schneider HM, Wunderlich T, Puls P (1980) The primary liposarcoma of the bone. Arch Orthop Traum Surg 96:235–239
Schwartz A, Shuster M, Becker SM (1970) Liposarcoma of bone: report of a case and review of the literature. J Bone Joint Surg [Am] 52:171–177
Stewart FW (1931) Primary liposarcoma of bone. Am J Pathol 7:87–93
Torok G, Meller Y, Maor E (1983) Primary liposarcoma of bone: case report and review of the literature. Bull Hosp Joint Dis 43:28–37

Malignant Mesenchymoma

Bertoni F, Laus M (1978) Primary malignant mesenchymoma of bone. Ital J Orthop Traumatol 4:105–108
Hutter RVP, Foote RL Jr, Francis KC, Sherman RS (1966) Primitive multipotential primary sarcoma of bone. Cancer 19:1–25
Lichtenstein L (1965) Bone tumors, 3rd edn. C.V. Mosby, St. Louis, p 314
Lichtenstein L (1977) Bone tumors, 5th edn. C.V. Mosby, St. Louis
Mastragostino S (1957) Tumori lipoblastici primitivi dello scheletro. Chir Organi Mov 44:18–36
McFarland GB Jr, McKinley GM, Reed RJ (1977) Dedifferentiation of low grade chondrosarcomas. Clin Orthop 122:157–164
Retz LD Jr (1961) Primary liposarcoma of bone: report of a case and review of the literature. J Bone Joint Surg [Am] 43:123–129
Ross CF, Hadfield G (1968) Primary osteo-liposarcoma of bone (malignant mesenchymoma): report of a case. J Bone Joint Surg [Br] 50:639–643
Schajowicz F, Cuevillas AR, Silberman FS (1966) Primary malignant mesenchymoma of bone. Cancer 19:1423–1428
Sterns EE, Haust MD, Wollin DG (1976) Malignant mesenchymoma of the mandible. Can J Surg 12:444
Stout AP (1948) Mesenchymoma, the mixed tumor of mesenchymal derivation. Am Surg 127:278–290

Primary Leiomyosarcoma of Bone

Angervall L, Berlin O, Kindblom LG, Stener B (1980) Primary leiomyosarcoma of bone: a study of cases. Cancer 46:1270–1279
Berlin O, Angervall L, Kindblom LG et al. (1987) Primary leiomyosarcoma of bone: a clinical, radiographic, pathologic-anatomic and prognostic study of 16 cases. Skeletal Radiol 16:364–376
Brooks J (1982) Immunohistochemistry of soft tissue tumors: myoglobin as a tumor marker for rhabdomyosarcoma. Cancer 50:1757–1763
Bures JC, Barnes L, Mercer D (1981) A comparative study of smooth muscle tumors utilizing light and electron microscopy, immunocytochemical staining and enzymatic assay. Cancer 48:2420–2426
Churg AM, Kahn LB (1977) Myofibroblasts in related cells in malignant fibrous and fibrohistiocytic tumors. Hum Pathol 8:205–218

Eady JL, McKinney JD, McDonald EC (1987) Primary leiomyosarcoma of bone: a case report and review of the literature. J Bone Joint Surg [Am] 69:287–289
Enneking WF, Spanier SS, Goodman MA (1980) A system for the surgical staging of musculoskeletal sarcoma. Clin Orthop 153:106–120
Enzinger FM, Weiss SW (1983) Soft tissue tumors. C.V. Mosby, St. Louis
Evans DJ, Lampert IA, Jacobs M (1983) Intermediate filaments in smooth muscle tumours. J Clin Pathol 36:57
Evans DMD, Sanerkin NG (1965) Primary leiomyosarcoma of bone. J Pathol Bacteriol 90:348–350
Fornasier VL, Paley D (1983) Leiomyosarcoma in bone: Primary or secondary? A case report and review of the literature. Skeletal Radiol 10:147–153
Hernandez FJ, Fernandez BB (1976) Multiple diffuse fibrosarcoma of bone. Cancer 37:939–945
Kawai T, Suzuki M, Mukai M et al. (1983) Primary leiomyosarcoma of bone: an immunohistochemical and ultrastructural study. Arch Pathol Lab Med 107:433–437
Loizaga JM (1976) Leiomyosarcoma primario de hueso. Informe de un caso. Patología 9:247–254
Meister P, Konrad E, Gokel JM, Romberger K (1978) Case report 59: leiomyosarcoma of the humerus. Skeletal Radiol 2:265–267
Miettinen M, Lehto VP, Ekblom P et al. (1984) Leiomyosarcoma of the mandible: diagnosis as aided by immunohistochemical demonstration of desmin and laminin. J Oral Pathol 13:373–381
Overgaard J, Frederiksen P, Helmig O, Myrejensen O (1977) Primary leiomyosarcoma of bone. Cancer 39:1664–1671
Pasquel PM, Nemelvet S, Deleon B (1976) Primary rhabdomyosarcoma of bone: a case report. J Bone Joint Surg [Am] 58:1176–1178
Sanerkin NG (1979) Primary leiomyosarcoma of bone and its comparison with fibrosarcoma: a cytological, histological and ultrastructural study. Cancer 44:1375–1387
Shamsuddin AK, Reyes F, Harvey JW et al. (1980) Primary leiomyosarcoma of bone. Hum Pathol 11:581–583
Von Hochstetter AR, Eberle H, Rüttner JR (1984) Primary leiomyosarcoma of extragnathic bones: case report and review of the literature. Cancer 53:2194–2200
Wang T, Erlandson RA, Marcove RC et al. (1980) Primary leiomyosarcoma of bone. Arch Pathol Lab Med 104:100–104
Young CL, Wold LE, McLeod RA et al. (1988) Primary leiomyosarcoma of bone. Orthopedics 11:615–618

CHAPTER VII

Other Tumors

A. Benign

1. Neurilemoma (Schwannoma, Neurinoma)

Definition, WHO: *"A benign tumor of nerve sheath origin having the same morphological features as soft tissue neurilemomas, but originating within a bone."*

In contrast to their relative frequency in soft tissues, intraosseous tumors of neurogenous origin are extremely rare. Only 36 well-documented neurilemomas originating in bone were collected by Fawcett and Dahlin in 1967, including seven personal cases, one associated with neurofibromatosis.

This neoplasm, originating in the Schwann cells of the nerve sheet, is designated indistinctly schwannoma or neurilemoma, its histogenesis having been confirmed by tissue culture techniques and electron microscopic studies (Fischer and Vuzevski 1968). Verocay, who gave the first histologic description in 1908, designated this tumor *neurinoma*. The Latin School of Del Rio Hortega (1962) and Polak (1966) prefer the term *lemmocytoma*. Despite the fact that the histologic features of this tumor have been clearly defined, there is still considerable confusion about the terminology of neurogenic tumors of the peripheral nerves. The terms neurinoma, neurilemoma, perineural fibroblastoma, and neurofibroma are often used synonymously.

The nerve supply within bone is not yet well established. The presence of nerve fibers, especially of the sensory type, in the periosteum is well recognized, but inside the bone the nerves are usually associated with blood vessels, mostly nonmyelinated and probably derived from the autonomic nervous system, and are related to the regulation of blood flow (Sherman 1963). In only a few sites, e.g., the mandible and the sacrum, do long nerve segments traverse the bones, which explains the fact that these sites are by far the most frequently involved locations of neurogenous tumors (neurilemoma and neurofibroma). In other locations, it is sometimes doubtful whether the lesion originated inside the bone or was of periosteal or subperiosteal origin with secondary erosion and penetration into the bone. The latter was the possible pathogenesis in some of our cases (located in the femur, spine, and sacrum) and in many of the reported cases (Fig. VII.1a,b).

Clinical Findings. Neurilemoma arising inside bone is rare (de Santos and Burgess 1940; Cowley and Miller 1942; Hart and Basom 1958; Samter et al. 1960; Mazingarbe and Mazabraud 1970; Lewis and Korbin 1972; Polkey 1975; Gordon 1976) and it is probable that several reported cases were actually of periosteal origin. In the recent Mayo Clinic series (Dahlin and Unni 1986), only ten cases were identified, accounting for less than 1% of benign tumors. Our material comprises 11 cases, which is less than 0.46% of benign tumors. In this number, two cases of evident periosteal or subperiosteal origin and three of possible juxtaosseous origin (one located in the sacrum and two in vertebral bodies) are included. The fact that our laboratory receives most of its material from orthopedic centers explains why we had only a limited number of mandibular tumors and no neurilemomas at this location, the most frequently involved site in other series. Approximately one-third of the reported cases involved the mandible (four of ten cases of Dahlin), followed in order of frequency by sacrum, humerus, femur, phalanges, and others. Two of our evidently intraosseous tumors were located in phalanges, one in the ilium and one in the clavicle.

As in Dahlin and Unni's series, there was a slight predominance of females (5:3). Ages ranged from 2½ to 65 years, but most reported cases fell between the second and sixth decades of life.

Symptoms. The tumor is usually of long duration before it is seen, and the most common complaint is local pain, sometimes radiating along the

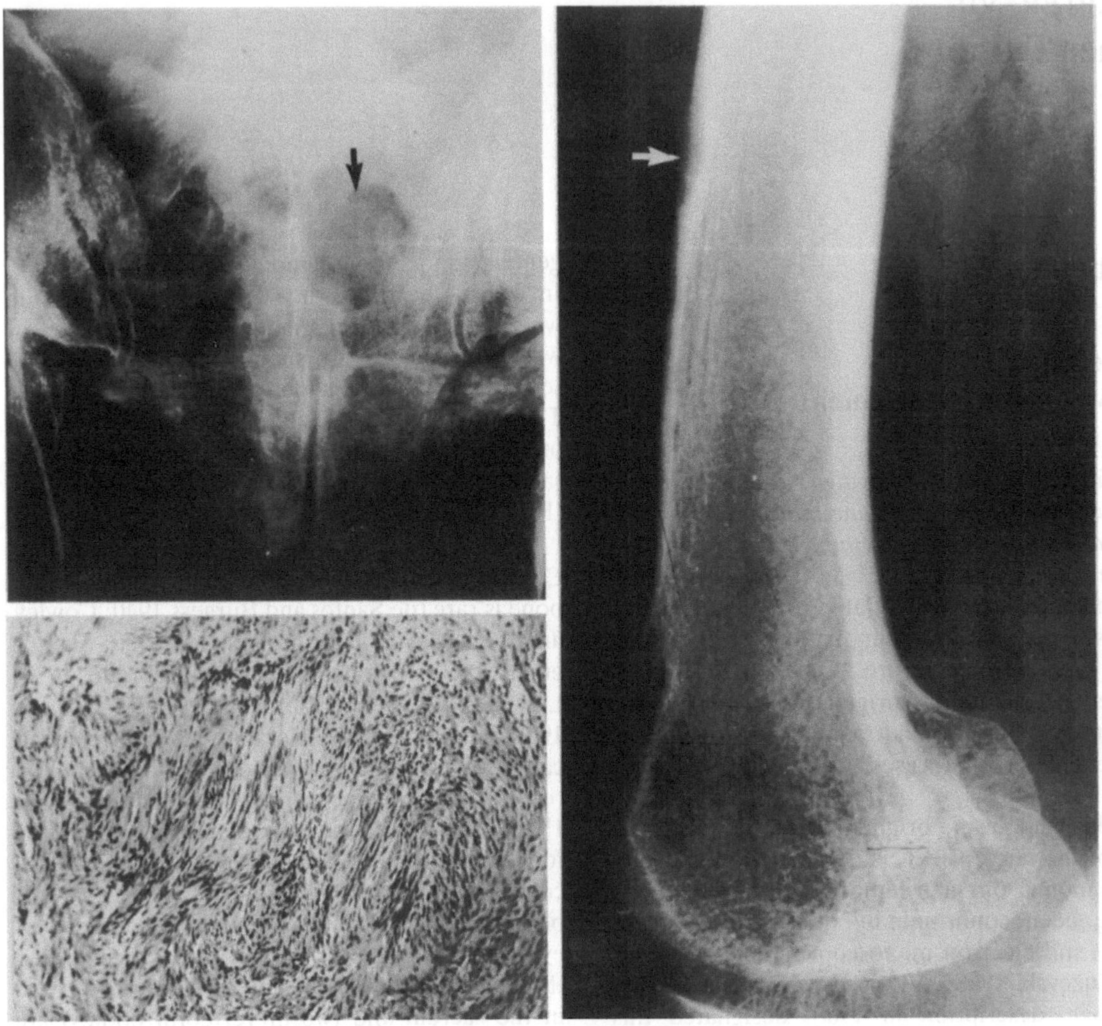

a c b

Fig. VII.1a–c. Two cases of extraosseous neurilemoma penetrating into bone. **a** Female, 51 years old, with neurilemoma of the sacrum, showing a well-defined radiolucent lesion, apparently originated by secondary penetration of an extraosseous tumor. **b** Female, 35 years old, with periosteal neurilemoma producing a small cortical defect in the femoral diaphysis. **c** Photomicrograph showing the characteristic palisaded structure of this case

affected nerve, often accompanied by local swelling and/or tenderness of the lesion, particularly in the more superficial periosteal tumors. Often the lesion is asymptomatic and may be found incidentally (Fawcett and Dahlin 1967), as in one of our cases located in the clavicle.

Radiographic Features. Radiologically, neurilemoma may appear as a central radiolucent lesion, usually in the midshaft with a discretely delineated zone of rarefaction, sometimes with a thin sclerotic border (Fig. VII.1a). The tumor is occasionally intraosseous and expands the overlying cortex (Fig. VII.2). The lesions sometimes have a multilocular appearance, which in tumors involving the jaws may closely simulate ameloblastoma. However, in the mandible the lesion is more frequently osteolytic, with a well-defined margin, and is nontrabeculated. Periosteal reaction is usually absent. Not infrequently, the lesion is located eccentrically, often at the site of a nutrient foramen, producing destruction of the cortex and slight periosteal reactive bone formation. In such cases, it is sometimes difficult to discount a possible cortical or subperiosteal origin with secondary erosion of the underlying cortex. This was evidently the pathogenesis in two of our cases (Fig. VII.1b). We have seen a large neurilemoma, apparently originating in the interosseous space of the forearm, which eroded

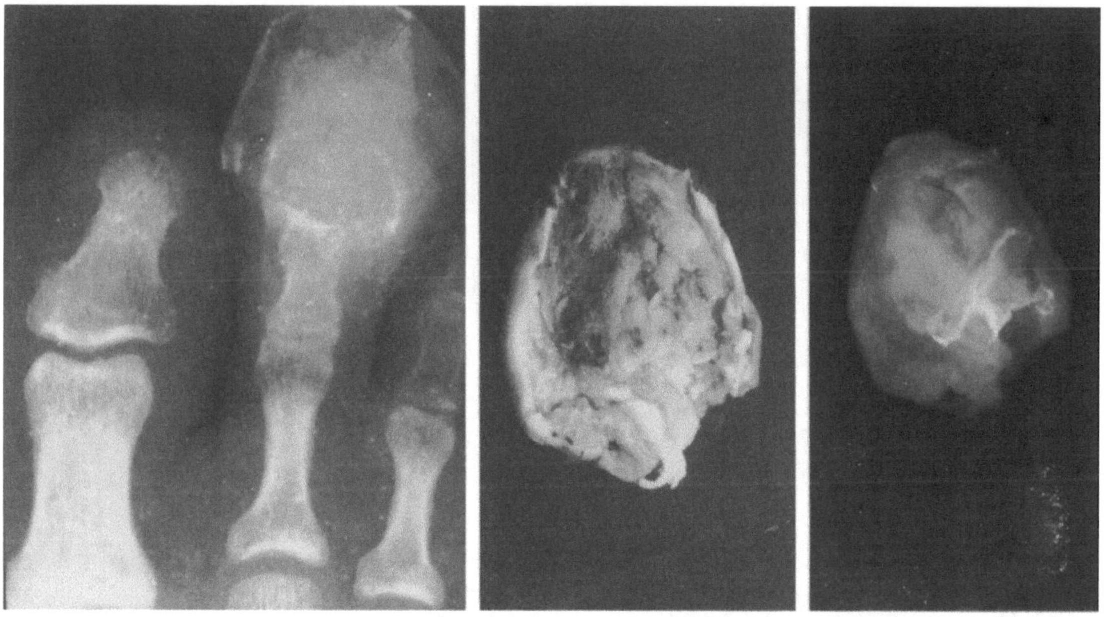

a b, c

Fig. VII.2a–c. Male, 27 years old. Neurilemoma of second terminal phalanx of foot. **a** Radiograph of osteolytic expanding intraosseous lesion with destruction of the thinned cortex. **b** Photograph and **c** radiograph showing the intraosseous origin of this solid, destructive tumor

both the radius and ulna, penetrating deeply into the spongiosa of the radius (Fig. VII.3).

Pathologic Findings. The tumor is generally encapsulated and well demarcated from the adjacent bone and may show a close association with a nerve, particularly in the mandible. The lesion is usually firm in consistency, of grayish-white color, and may contain cystic areas of different sizes.

Histologically, the tumor shows the classic combination of two patterns of tissue, the "Antoni A and B types." The first is characterized by compact bundles and whorls of Schwann cells with their nuclei aligned in rows or palisades (Figs. VII.1c, VII.3c). Occasionally the cells adopt an organoid arrangement, particularly at the periphery, similar to tactile corpuscles, called Verocay bodies. The "Antoni B" tissue consists of a loose meshwork of edematous myxomatous tissue with some microcystic areas and dispersed Schwann cells, lymphocytes, and histiocytic elements, sometimes containing hemosiderin or lipids. Blood vessels are a characteristic finding, often dilated and with thickened hyaline walls and fibrinous mural thrombi.

Most tumors show areas of both histologic types, with either the "Antoni A" or "Antoni B" pattern predominating markedly in some lesions. Cells with irregular plump hyperchromatic and sometimes bizarre nuclei may be found in some areas in the majority of these tumors and may mimic a malignant tumor. However, mitotic figures are completely lacking and apparently represent degenerative changes. Isolated cases of intraosseous malignant neurilemoma have been reported (Peers 1934; Güthert 1952; Bose et al. 1970), but none of them appear to be indisputable. No case of unequivocal intraosseous origin has been observed by the writer.

Treatment. The treatment of choice is surgical excision. Resection may be required only in larger lesions.

2. Neurofibroma

Neurofibroma is a benign tumor, characterized by the presence of peripheral nerve elements (Schwann cells and neurites) and connective tissue, which are arranged in a diffuse, haphazard manner. Del Rio Hortega (1962) and Polak (1966) designated it "lemmocito-fibroma."

The majority of neurofibromas are associated with neurofibromatosis (von Recklinghausen's disease), the incidence of solitary intraosseous neurofibroma being extremely low. By far the most frequent site is the mandible, with about 20

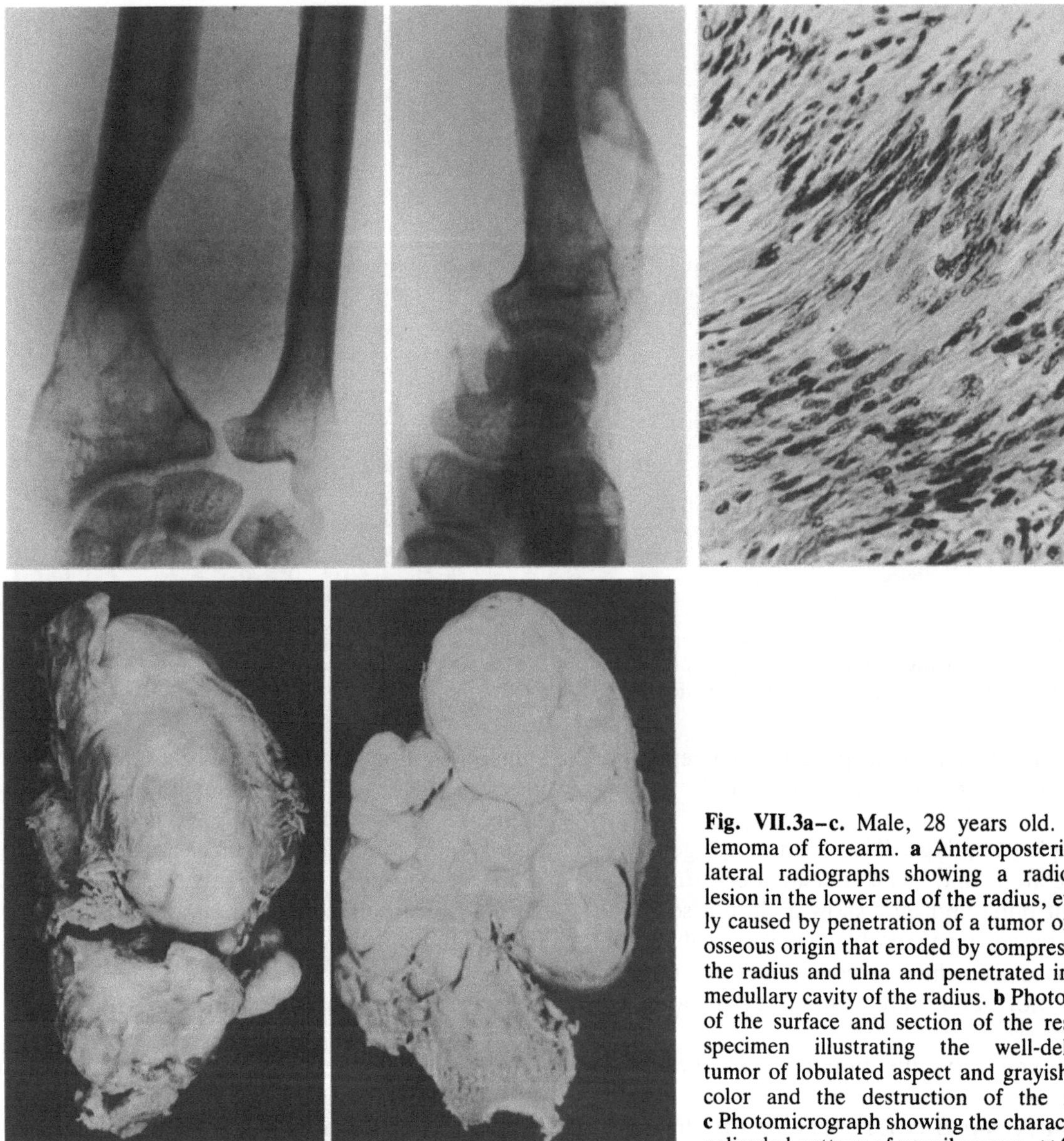

a c b

Fig. VII.3a–c. Male, 28 years old. Neurilemoma of forearm. **a** Anteroposterior and lateral radiographs showing a radiolucent lesion in the lower end of the radius, evidently caused by penetration of a tumor of interosseous origin that eroded by compression of the radius and ulna and penetrated into the medullary cavity of the radius. **b** Photographs of the surface and section of the resection specimen illustrating the well-delimited tumor of lobulated aspect and grayish-white color and the destruction of the radius. **c** Photomicrograph showing the characteristic palisaded pattern of neurilemoma. ×400

reported cases in this bone. Only two cases of intraosseous neurofibroma, both associated with neurofibromatosis, were reported in the literature (Gross et al. 1939; Baldwin and Weiner 1974); they were located in the midshaft of the humerus in a 30-year-old woman and in the ulna in a 3-year-old girl, respectively. We have eight cases in our records, all associated with neurofibromatosis. Three were located in the tibia and two in the fibula; the remainder were situated in the cranium, spine, and sacrum (Figs. VII.4, VII.5).

Macroscopically, the lesion is of firm consistency and of grayish-white color, with an irregular, poorly delimited surface, sometimes in close relationship to nerve segments. In two cases located in the tibia and fibula, the lesions were found in the area of a congenital pseudoarthrosis. The tumor sometimes can arise in the subperiosteal or periosteal tissue from nerves in this region, but a tumor in these locations produces a cortical cystic lesion without penetrating deeply into the underlying bone.

Fig. VII.4a,b. Female, 73 years old. Neurofibroma of skull in neurofibromatosis (von Recklinghausen's disease). **a,b** Radiographs in different projections showing an osteolytic expanding lesion in the skull, of evident intraosseous origin

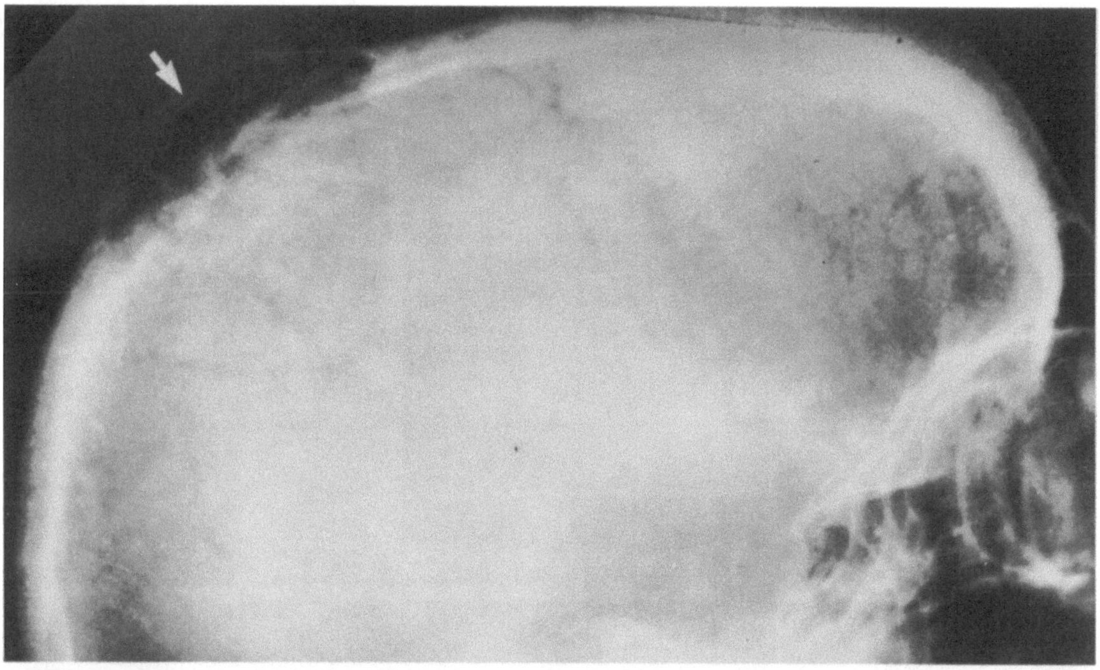

a

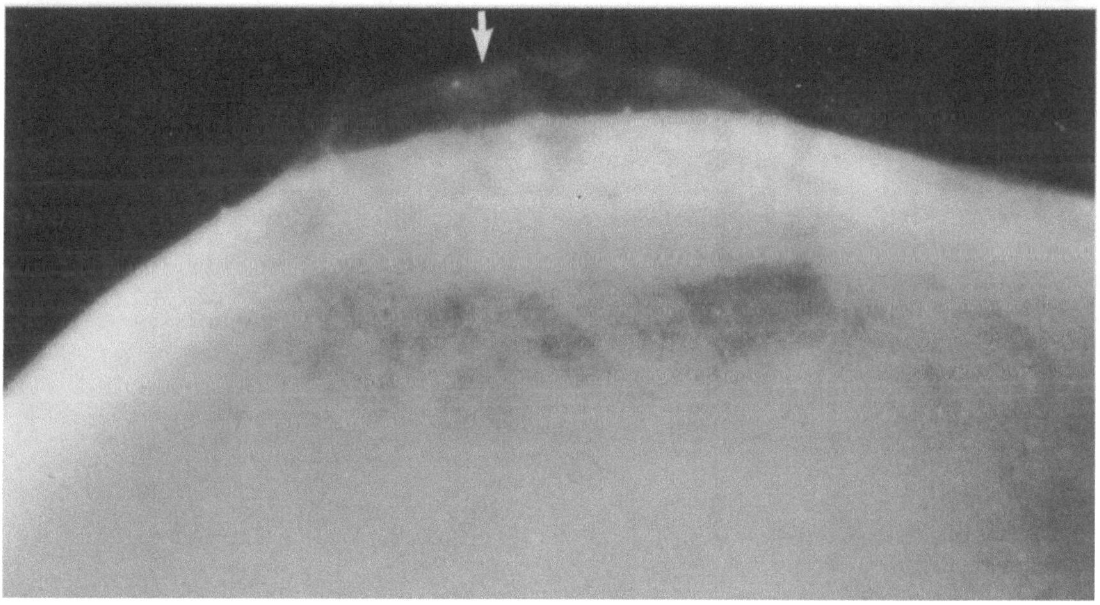

VII.4b

Although neurofibroma and neurilemoma are not clearly separated as different entities by some authors, there are sufficient criteria to distinguish the two processes histologically, a finding also confirmed by ultrastructural studies (Waggener 1966). The loose tissue structure and the shape of the tumor cells with their elongated nuclei and fibrillar cytoplasmic prolongations, the presence of an increased number of small nerve bundles with fascicles of collagen fibers, and the absence of typical palisade structures are characteristic and diagnostic findings (Figs. VII.5, VII.6). Much more common than the foregoing intraosseous solitary lesions, which are radiologically radiolucent, often with well-defined margins, and expand or perforate the cortex, are the other types of skeletal and extraskeletal changes of neurofibromatosis. These include scoliosis, growth disorders, congenital bowing and pseudoarthrosis of the lower leg, and other congenital anomalies. However, these changes are usually not associated with the presence of neurofibromatous tissues within the affected bone.

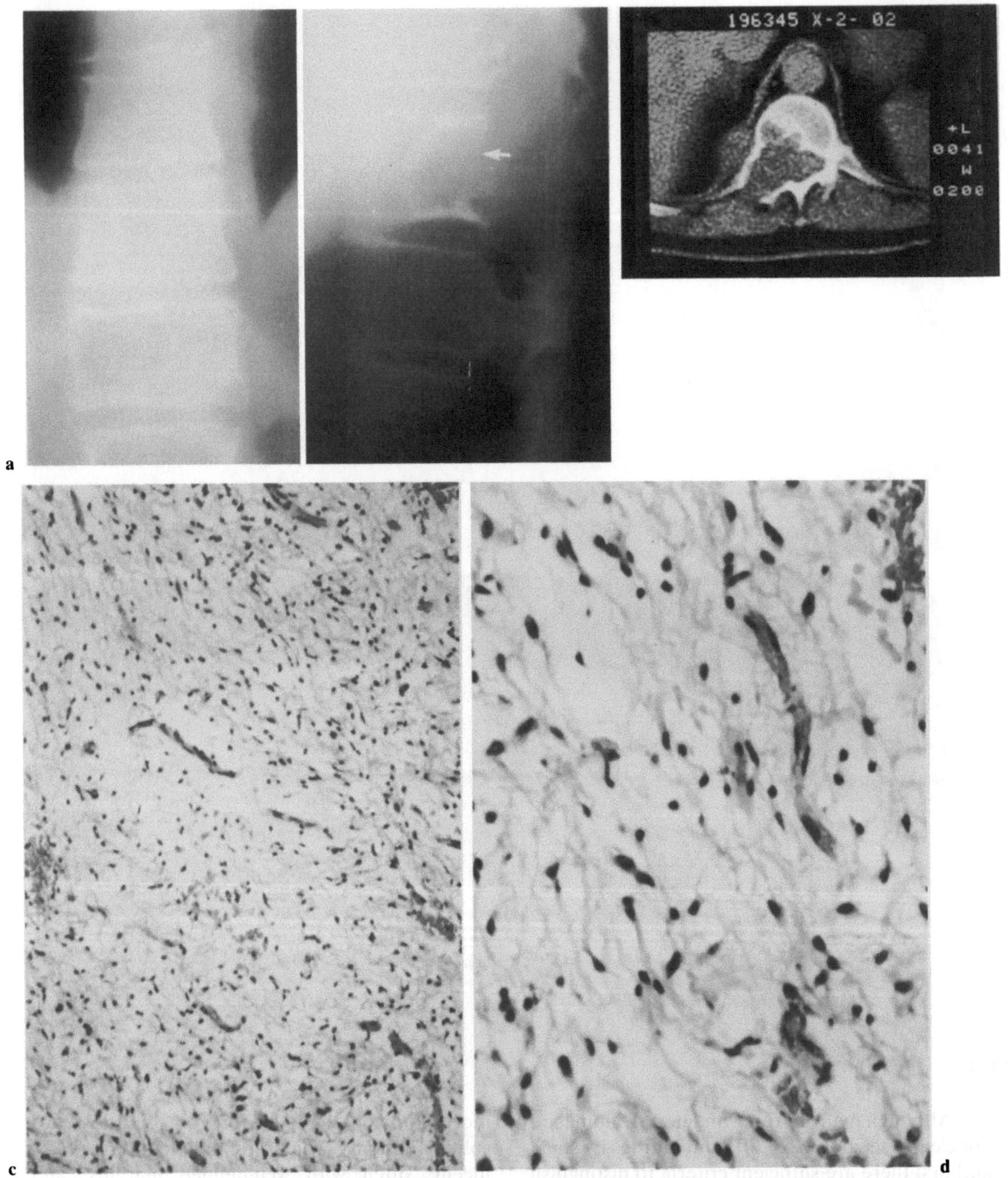

Fig. VII.5a–d. Male, 53 years old. Neurofibroma with penetration into first lumbar vertebra. **a** Anteroposterior and lateral tomograms show a radiolucent lesion with well-defined margins toward the spongiosa, which evidently has penetrated into bone at its posterior aspect. **b** The computed tomogram demonstrates clearly the extension and intraosseous penetration of the tumor, which originated in spinal nerves. **c,d** Photomicrographs showing at lower and higher magnification the histologic features. **c** ×120, **d** ×250

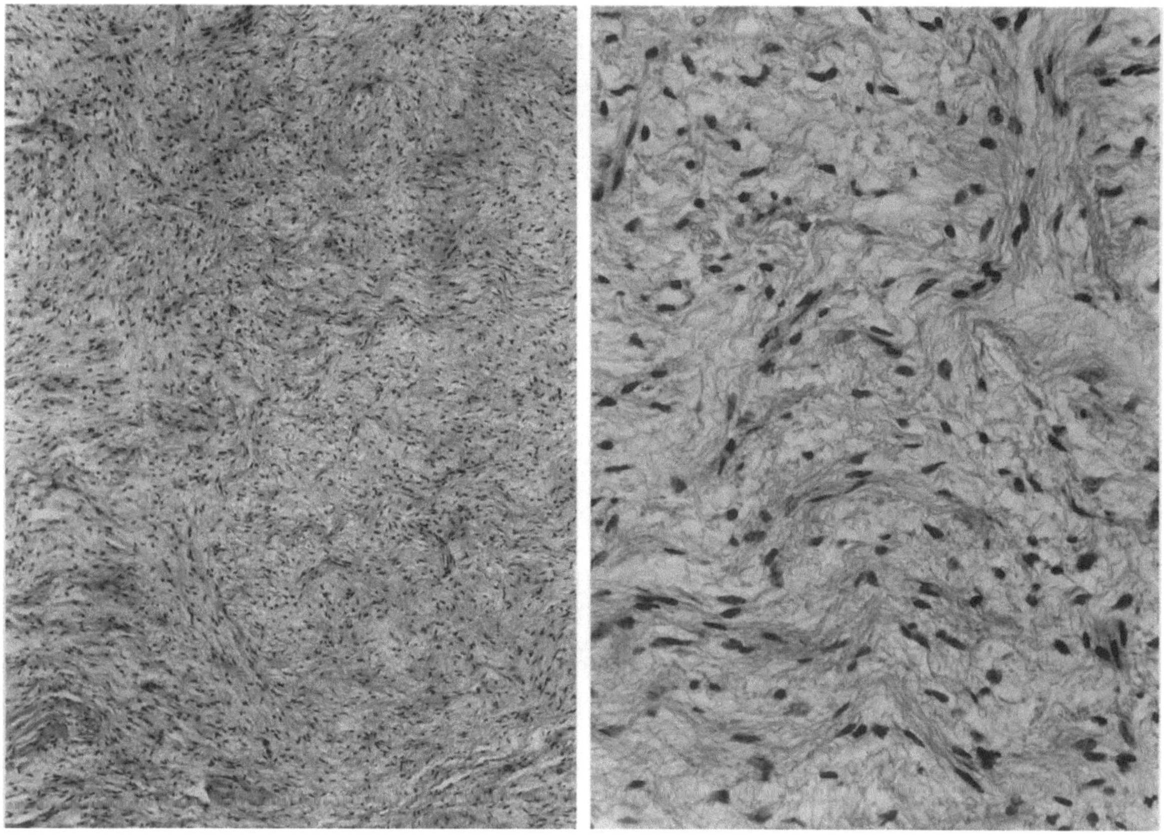

a b

Fig. VII.6a,b. Photomicrographs of neurofibroma at lower and higher magnification show the undulated aspect of the conspicuous collagen fibers and elongated nuclei. **a** ×100, **b** ×400

B. Malignant

1. Chordoma

Definition, WHO: *"A locally aggressive or malignant tumor characterized by a lobular arrangement of tissue which is usually made up of cords and sheets of highly vacuolated cells ("physaliphorous cells") and mucoid intercellular material. These tumors are restricted to the axial skeleton. This together with their histological structure suggests that they originate from notochordal tissue."*

Chordoma is a neoplasm that arises from notochordal remnants in the nucleus pulposus of the intervertebral disk, designated as normally situated chordal vestiges, and/or from abnormal ectopic remnants, because they are located where notochord should have regressed, i.e., in the spheno-occipital region (including clival ecchordosis), in the posterior part of nasopharynx, in the substance of bone in the vertebral bodies, or in the tissues surrounding them. Chordoma, therefore, occurs almost exclusively in the midline of the axial skeleton, with a distinct predilection for the distal and proximal ends of the vertebral column, i.e., the spheno-occipital and sacrococcygeal regions.

The name chordoma was originally applied by Müller in 1858 to small, proliferated excrescences that represent heterotopic notochordal tissue occurring at the base of the skull, in the region of the clivus, for which Stewart and Morin (1926) suggested the more appropriate name *ecchordosis physaliphora*. These are small gelatinous, translucent whitish nodules of no more than a few millimeters. Microscopically, these nodules show only a few cells, usually highly vacuolated and containing mucin, the same as the abundant intercellular substance. An ecchordosis does not produce clinical symptoms, and it is discovered incidentally or when a special search is made for it. Ribbert (1894) found in a series of 500 autopsies, 10 instances (2%) of clival ecchordosis, and Stewart and Morin (1926) found 4 in 350 necropsies.

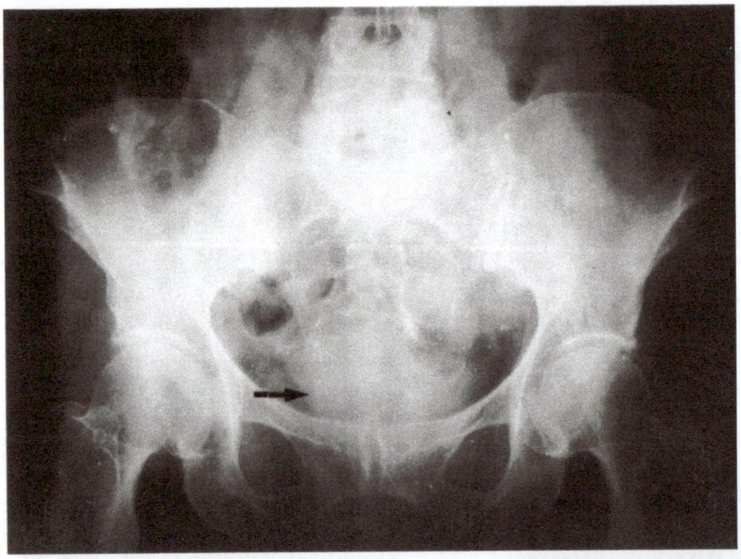

a

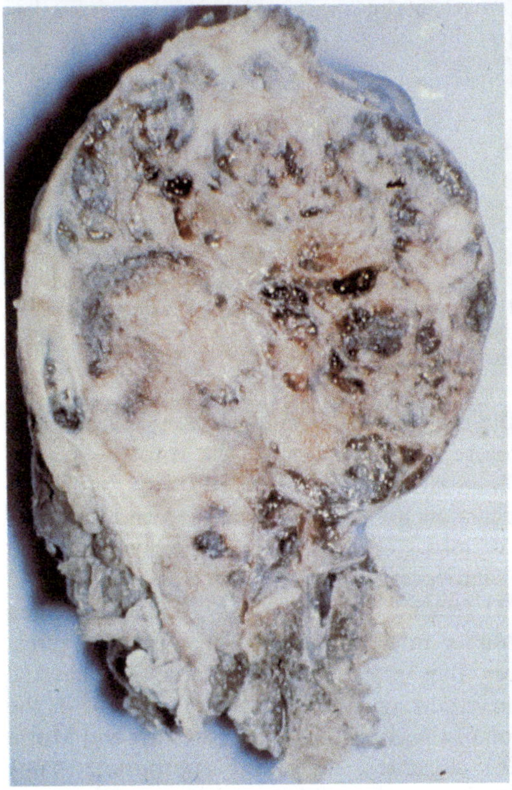

b

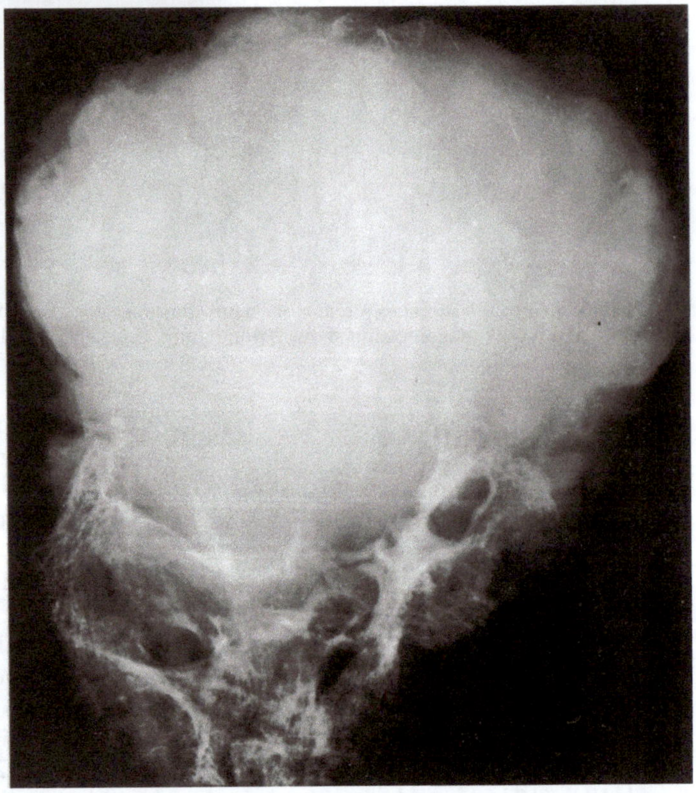

Fig. VII.7a–c. Female, 62 years old. Sacrococcygeal chordoma. **a** Radiograph shows destructive lesion with ill-defined borders involving multiple sacral segments. **b** Photograph and **c** radiograph of the specimen showing the cut surface of lobular aspect with multiple areas of cystic softening. The tumor is of grayish-blue color similar to myxoid or cartilaginous tissue. (Schajowicz et al. 1972)

In contrast to this nonneoplastic excrescence, chordomas are true neoplasms that are slow-growing but locally invasive, destroying the adjacent bone and infiltrating soft tissue structures with the formation of a large soft tissue mass containing areas of calcification or bony fragments. Although metastases are relatively rare, they may occur, usually in advanced cases or after repeated recurrences.

For details of the embryologic, clinical, and roentgenologic findings of this neoplasm, the reader is referred to the excellent and complete compilation of Firooznia and Pinto (1977).

Incidence. Chordoma is a rather infrequent tumor, and relatively few cases are reported from most institutions. In our laboratory only 31 cases have been recorded, which accounts for 1.3% of the malignant tumors in our material. Eighty patients with histologically verified chordomas were diagnosed at Memorial Hospital, New York, from 1949 through 1983. Fifty-seven of the patients (71%) were male and 23 (29%) were female. The high incidence of 262 cases in the Mayo Clinic series (more than 4% of the malignant tumors) is surprising and difficult to explain, even taking into consideration a possible selection factor (Dahlin and Unni 1986).

Clinical Findings. *Age and Sex.* Cranial chordomas occur somewhat more frequently in males than in females. The vertebral lesions do not have any significant sex predilection, but sacrococcygeal chordomas affect males (Dahlin 1978) twice as commonly as females. Chordoma is distinctly uncommon in patients less than 30 years of age.

Cranial chordomas occur predominantly in the third, fourth, and fifth decades, with a mean age of onset of 35 years, whereas sacrococcygeal chordomas are usually recognized a decade later than cranial chordomas, the mean age of onset being about 50 years in most series (Jaffe 1958; Epstein 1969; Dahlin and Unni 1986).

Localization. Chordoma is most commonly located at the proximal and distal ends of the vertebral column, i.e., the spheno-occipital and sacrococcygeal regions. These two sites account for 85%–90% of all reported tumors. Among the 80 patients studied at Memorial Hospital, in 53 cases (66%) the lesion was located in the sacrococcygeal region, in 24 (30%) the lesion involved the vertebral column at a higher level, and in 3 (4%) the tumor was situated in the spheno-occipital area (Huvos 1991). This is in contrast to the Mayo Clinic series, in which 97 cases (37%) occurred at the base of the brain. Twenty-one of our cases were located in the sacrococcygeal region. The remaining lesions occur along the rest of the spine, involving in descending order of frequency the cervical spine, particularly the C1–C2 region, the lumbar spine, and the thoracic spine.

There are a few exceptional reports of chordomas occurring in locations not adjacent to the region of the primitive notochord, such as in jaws, paranasal sinuses (Berdal and Myhre 1964), and scapula (Higinbotham et al. 1967). Most of these cases, especially those from the older literature, are questionable. These lesions, together with those situated in the deep soft tissues, reported as "chordoid tumors" by Stewart or as "parachordoma," will be discussed later.

Symptoms. The clinical symptoms vary according to the location, the onset in the majority of cases being insidious. Cranial chordomas may produce symptoms early, whereas vertebral and particularly sacrococcygeal chordomas may exist for a long period without causing significant symptoms. They are usually discovered in advanced stages of their evolution. The presenting complaints arise because the slowly expanding and infiltrating tumor mass destroys the neighboring bony structures of the base of the skull, vertebral bodies, and sacrum, and compresses the brain, spinal cord, and/or the nerves arising from them. The most common complaints in cranial chordomas are pain, headache and visual disturbances, or nasopharyngeal symptoms secondary to invasion of the nasopharynx, which may precede the onset of intracranial signs by many years and occasionally are the first manifestations of the disease.

The clinical manifestations of the vertebral and sacrococcygeal chordomas are preferentially neurologic and vary from mild to severe pain, paresthesia, and/or motor disturbances, to complete paralysis, lasting a few months to a few years prior to the discovery of the true nature of the disease.

In sacrococcygeal chordomas, the presence of a large presacral mass, palpable on rectal examination, may cause displacement and compression of rectum, bladder, and other pelvic structures, producing urinary and fecal troubles. These may also be due to neurologic problems.

Radiographic Features. Bone destruction is the most constant feature of chordoma, involving all areas and being especially relevant in sacrococcygeal tumors. A lytic lesion, with irregular scalloped margins expanding the sacrum, is the most frequent finding, associated with intratumoral calcification in 50% of cases (Utne and Pugh 1955). The osseous lesion may have an extraosseous retrosacral or pelvic mass, which displaced the bladder and rectum in 85% of Utne and Pugh's cases (Figs. VII.7, VII.8; cf. appearances in fibrosarcoma and ependymoma of the sacrum, shown in Figs. VII.9 and VII.10, respectively).

Intracranial chordomas show bone involvement in most cases, with destruction of the clivus,

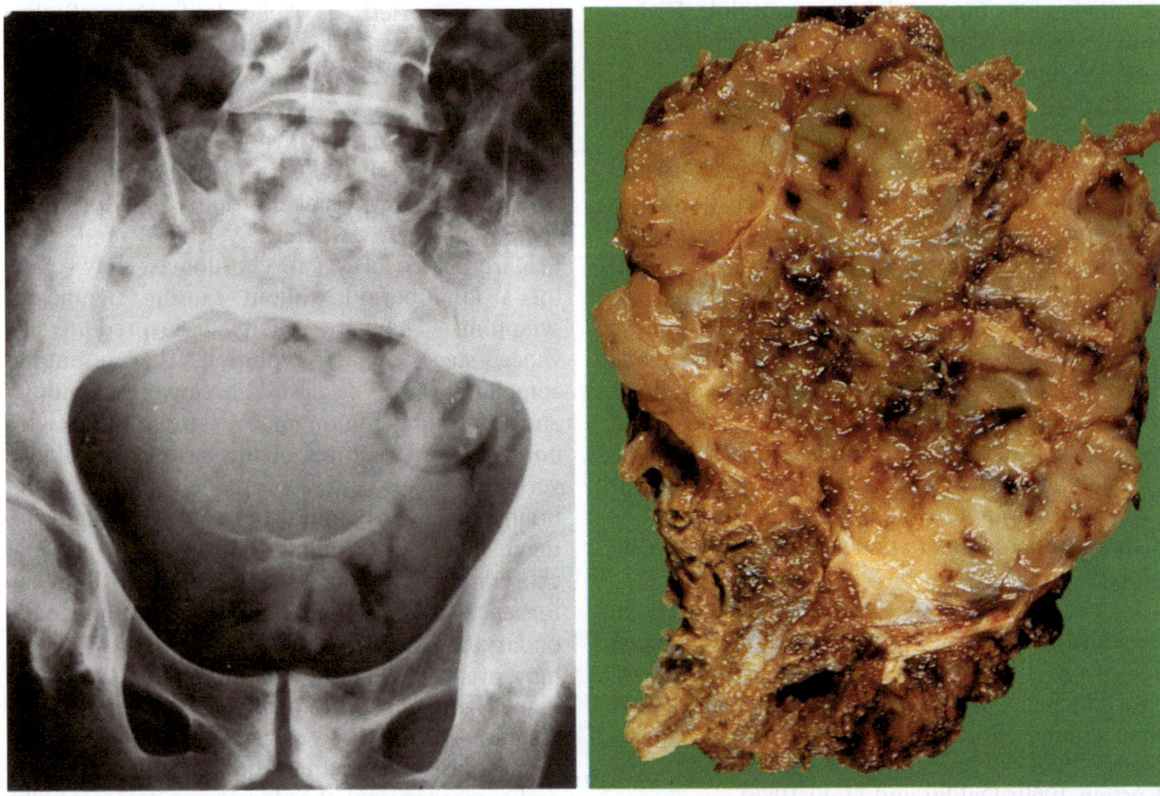

a b

▲ **Fig. VII.8a,b.** Male, 54 years old. Sacrococcygeal chordoma. **a** Radiograph shows a large radiolucent lesion partly destroying the cortex. **b** Photograph of the specimen illustrates the lobulated, partly hemorrhagic aspect of the grayish-blue fleshy tumor

Fig. VII.9a,b. Female, 29 years old. Fibrosarcoma of sacrum. Lateral and anteroposterior radiographs show a large radiolucent lesion with intrapelvic extension, suggesting chordoma
▼

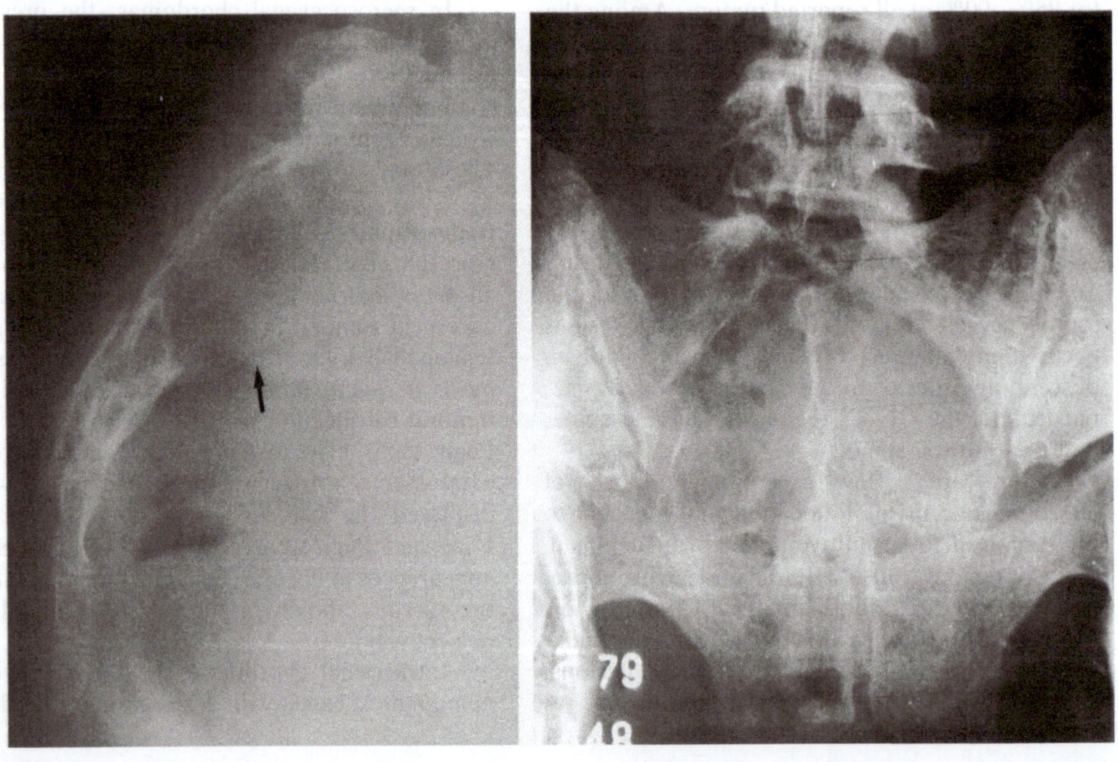

a b

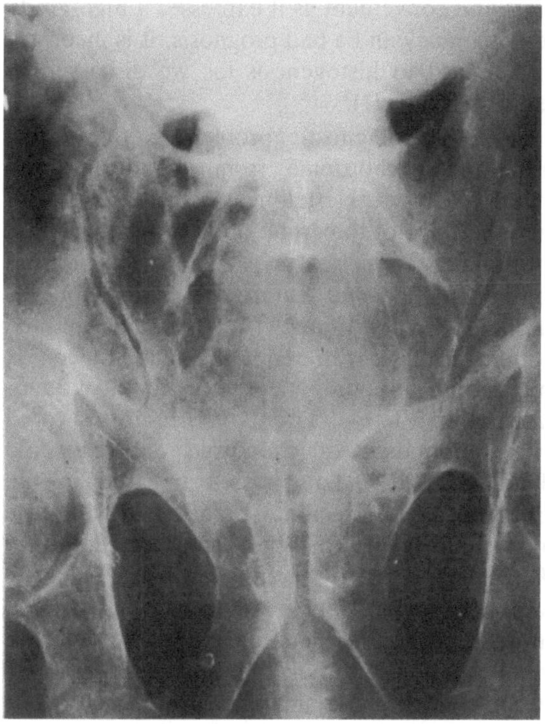

◀ **Fig. VII.10.** Male, 39 years old. Ependymoma of sacrum. Large radiolucent, apparently well-defined lesion. Patient complained of pain for 7 years

dorsum sellae, and posterior clinoids or with invasion of the sellar floor or the sphenoid sinus. Almost half of the lesions may show calcifications. Angiography, pneumoencephalography, brain scan, and more recently computed tomography and especially MRI have been of great help in detecting intracranial and vertebral chordomas. In the latter location, the involvement of two or more adjacent vertebral bodies is an important diagnostic feature reported by most radiologists (Firooznia and Pinto 1977). In half of their patients, osteosclerosis, in the absence of pathologic fracture, was observed. Abnormality of the intervertebral disk space and presence of a soft tissue mass, precervical or paravertebral, are frequent findings. Most vertebral chordomas show posterior extension into the spinal canal, which is best evaluated with a myelogram or MRI (Fig. VII.11).

a 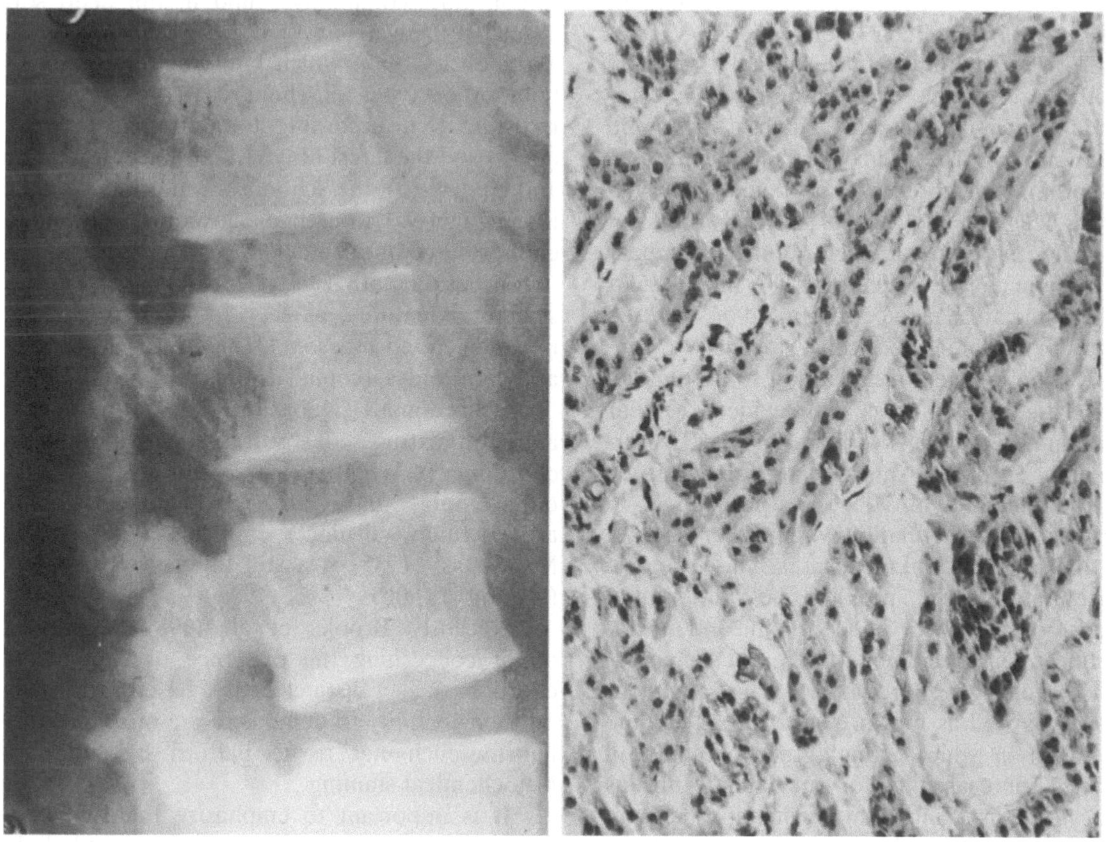 b

Fig. VII.11a,b. Female, 49 years old, with chordoma in the second lumbar vertebra. **a** Lateral radiograph shows radiolucent, ill-defined lesion in the posterior site of the vertebral body. **b** Photomicrograph demonstrates cords of cells with small dark nuclei and abundant, often vacuolated cytoplasm, separated by mucoidlike substance. ×250 (Schajowicz and Derqui 1968)

Pathologic Findings. *Grossly*, chordoma usually appears to originate within bone. After destroying the bone tissue, it extends into adjacent structures with formation of a lobulated soft tissue mass that frequently seems to be well encapsulated. The tumor infiltrates the marrow spaces without clear delimitation and may expand the cortex of the sacrum or more rarely of a vertebral body. The surface of the tumor is of a grayish or bluish-white color, with extensive gelatinous, translucent areas alternating sometimes with cystic or hemorrhagic foci. The consistency varies from firm to soft and friable. Infrequently, irregular calcified zones may be observed. Grossly, the pattern is often similar to that of chondrosarcoma or mucous carcinoma (Figs. VII.7, VII.8).

Histologically, the tumor shows a characteristic arrangement in lobules, separated by a framework of fibrous septa of different thickness, containing thin-walled blood vessels. The tumor cells vary in size and shape, being polyhedral or prismatic with eosinophilic cytoplasm and arranged in cords and sheets, resembling epithelial cells and associated with minimal to abundant amounts of intercellular mucin (Figs. VII.12, VII.13). The amount of mucin usually increases with the size of the lobules. Intracellular cytoplasmic, mucin-containing vacuoles, varying in size and number and often displacing the nucleus, are a prominent feature of chordoma ("physaliphorous cells") (Fig. VII.12c). As the process of vacuolation proceeds, the cell outlines disappear and the mucus is expelled into the intercellular spaces; some areas may be composed of scattered stellate or disintegrated cells, forming a syncytium lying in a sea of mucus. In some tumors, relatively extensive areas with evident cellular pleomorphism and cells with two or more hyperchromatic or bizarre nuclei and some mitotic activity are found, but this does not appear to have any clear correlation with either rate of growth or frequency of metastases. The histologic features may cause problems of differential diagnosis of sacrococcygeal chordoma and mucin-secreting adenocarcinoma of the rectosigmoid, but the cells of chordoma contain abundant glycogen as well as mucin (Fig. VII.12d). Some rare cases, in which a high-grade spindle cell sarcoma (fibrosarcoma or malignant fibrous histiocytoma) is found within or juxtaposed to an otherwise characteristic chordoma, have been referred to as "dedifferentiated (Miettinen et al. 1987). Although the term "dedifferentiated" is short and convenient as it expresses a high-grade of malignancy and a bad prognosis, it is incorrect with regard to histogenesis (as we discussed in detail in Chap. II).

Another diagnostic problem is the differentiation of chordoma from chondroma and chondrosarcoma. Heffelfinger et al. (1973) found that one-third of the group of 55 spheno-occipital chordomas contained a significant chondroid component that had features of either chondrosarcoma or chondroma. The stroma resembled hyaline cartilage with neoplastic cells in lacunae; the chondroid component occasionally dominated (Fig. VII.14). Twenty-two tumors showed this combination of chondroid and chordoid elements, and 19 of these originated in the spheno-occipital region. Compared with the large number of what they named "*chondroid chordomas*," true chondrosarcomas in the parasellar region were extremely rare. It is well known that chordomas are easily confused with chondromatous tumors, especially chondrosarcomas with predominant myxoid structures or with the so-called myxoid chondrosarcoma, a tumor most commonly found in the deep soft tissues (Enzinger and Shiraki 1972; Weiss 1976; Wick et al. 1988) which has a better prognosis than other types of chondrosarcoma. It is interesting that according to Heffelfinger et al. (1973) and the latest Mayo Clinic records (Dahlin and Unni 1986), the "chondroid chordoma" had a longer survival rate than chordomas without a chondroid component.

A lesion with similar histologic and ultrastructural features, as seen in the extraskeletal myxoid chondrosarcoma, has been described as "chordoid sarcoma" (Martin et al. 1973) or "parachordoma" (Dabska 1977), a tumor that arises in extraosseous soft tissues ("peripheral chordoma"). Whether "parachordoma," "chordoid sarcoma," and extraskeletal chondrosarcoma are actually distinct entities (Povysil and Matejovsky 1985) is a still unresolved problem (see Fig. II.90b).

Recently Brooks et al. (1987) expressed doubt concerning the existence of "chondroid chordoma" as a distinct entity, based principally on their inability to demonstrate a mixed epithelial–mesenchymal tissue pattern by immunohistochemical staining.

It is important to emphasize that *immunohistochemical methods* have been of great help in the differential diagnosis of chordoma. Miettinen (1984) (see also Miettinen et al. 1983; Salisbury

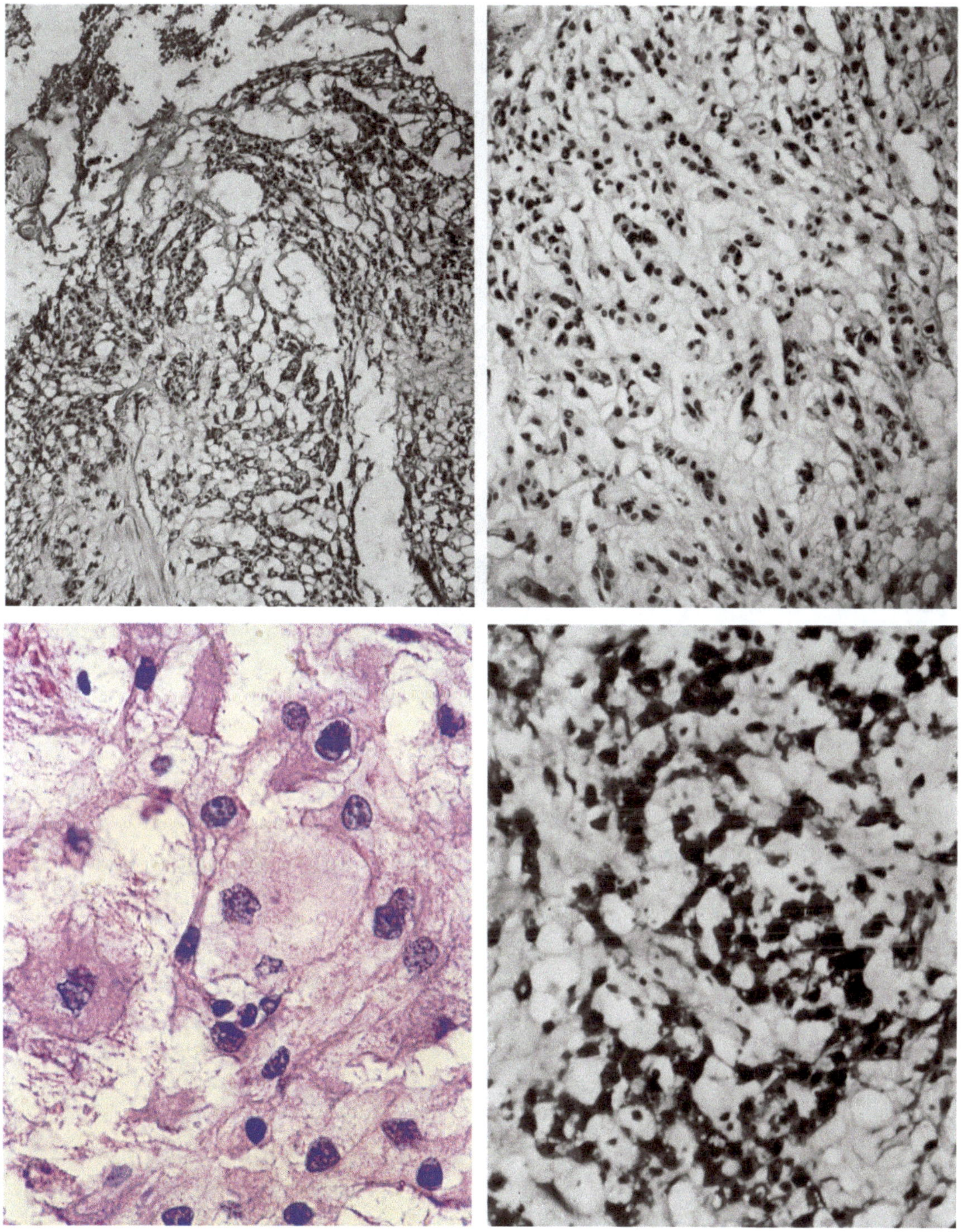

a b c d

Fig. VII.12. a,b. Photomicrographs showing cords and anastomosing strands of cells, separated by abundant mucoid substance. **c** High magnification shows the highly vacuolated cells ("physaliphorous cells") and the mucoid intercellular substance. Note the nuclear pleomorphism. **d** PAS stain reveals the presence of abundant glycogen granules (*dark-stained*) in the cytoplasm of the tumor cells. **a** ×100, **b** ×180, **c** ×600, **d** ×400

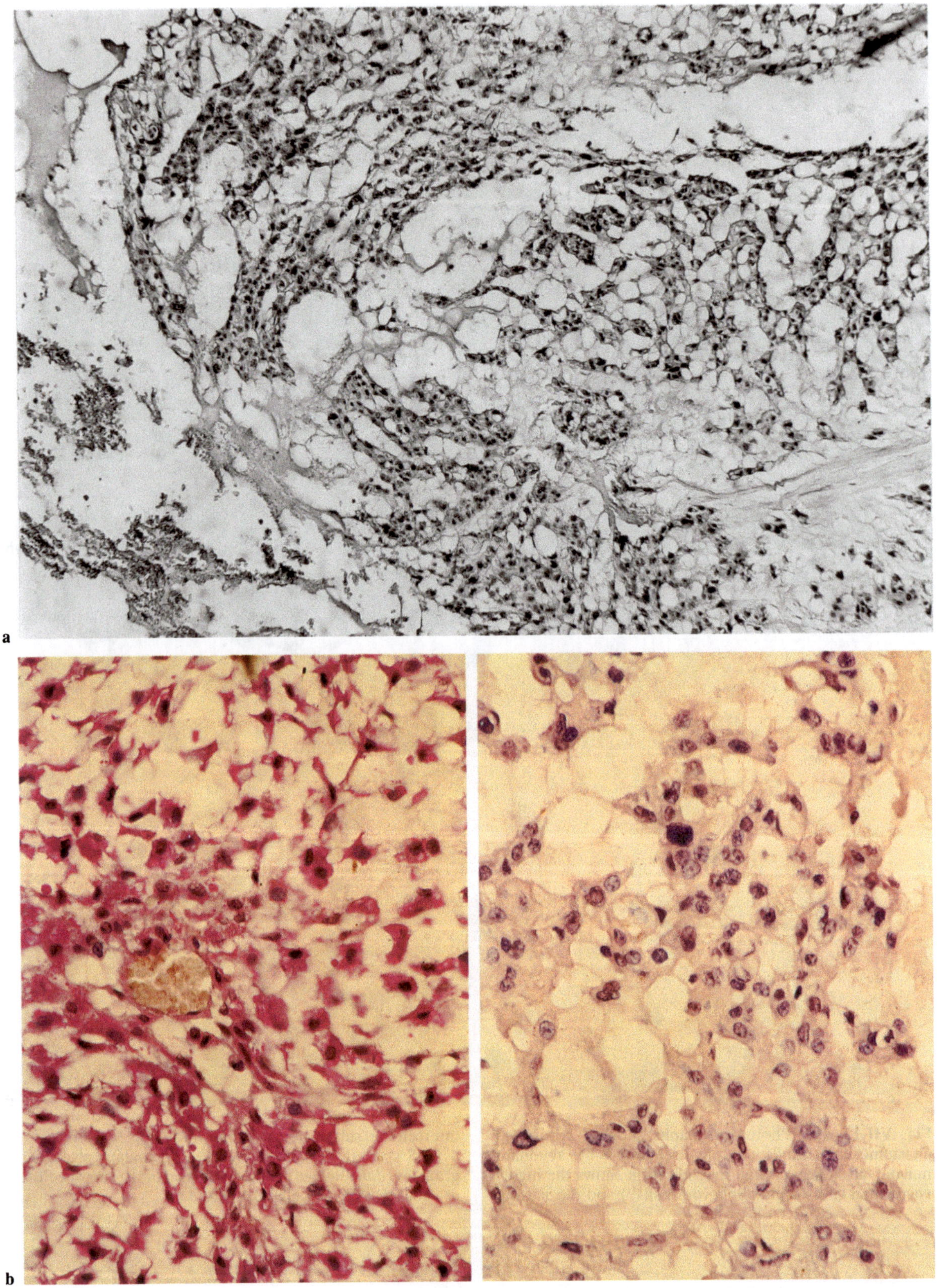

a b c

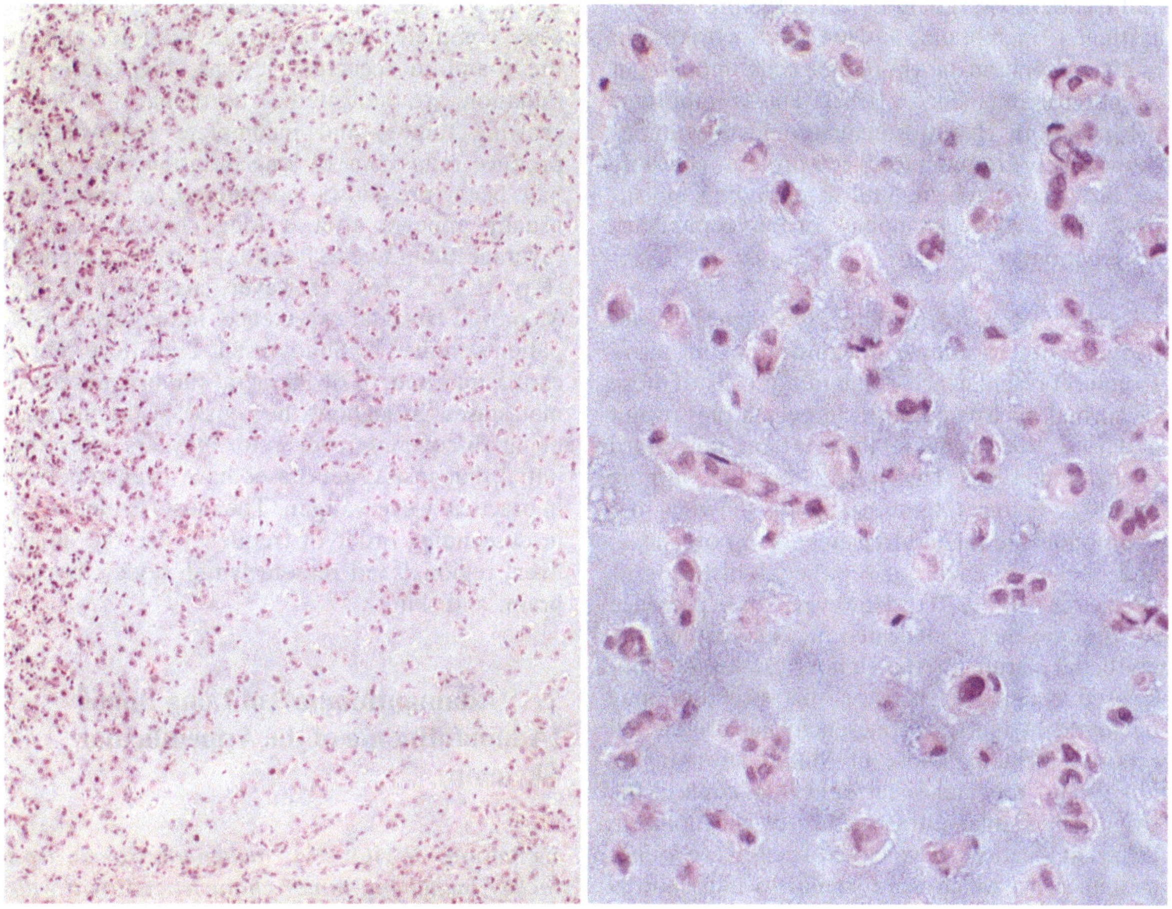

a

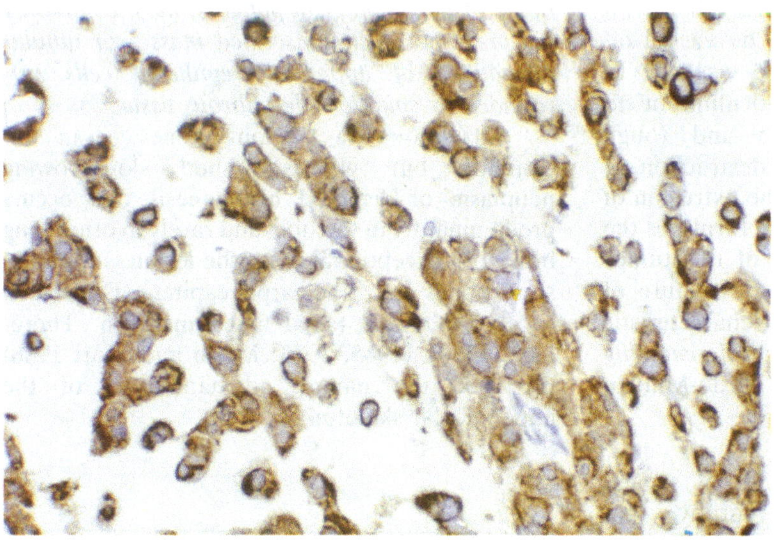

b

◄

Fig. VII.13a–c. Photomicrographs show the characteristic histologic features of chordoma at lower and higher magnification. **c** PAS stain yields strongly positive staining of the cytoplasm of tumor cells. **a** ×100, **b,c** ×400

VII.14a,b. Photomicrographs of cranial chordoma. **a** Shows abundant hyaline bluish stroma, separating single or small cords of tumor cells, similar to hyaline cartilage. It is possible that cases with these features have been referred to as chondroid chordomas. **b** However, the stain with keratin markers was conspicuously positive in this case, a finding not seen in cartilage tumors. **a** ×200, **b** ×400 and Isaacson 1985) demonstrated the presence of epithelial membrane antigen and cytokeratin in the cytoplasm of chordoma cells and not in chondrosarcoma (Fig. VII.14). This is important because both chondrosarcomas and chordomas show positive staining for S-100 protein, which is, on the other hand, helpful in excluding mucin-producing adenocarcinoma or myxopapillary ependymoma.

Electron Microscopy. The few publications dealing with chordoma demonstrated the ultrastructural resemblance of the tumor cells to those of normal nucleus pulposus in guinea pigs (Spjut and Luse 1964) and to those of rat notochord (Pena et al. 1970). This finding, together with the histologic features, tends to support the view that chordomas are related to elements of notochord, and seems to favor an epithelial histogenesis (Pena et al. 1970). However, the presence of desmosomes, advocated as supporting the epithelial nature of the tumor, cannot be considered conclusive, because this structure may be found in tumors of mesenchymal origin. All reports, including those of Murad and Murthy (1970) and Kay and Schatzki (1972), confirm the essentially similar ultrastructure of chordoma in different locations. Two types of cells were found: stellate cells, which were similar to notochordal elements, and the physaliphorous cells, with transitional types between both. The vacuolization seen by the light microscope was due to dilatation of the endoplasmic reticulum or to enzymatic lysis of mitochondria and rough endoplasmic reticulum. This self-destruction of the cell organelles contributes to the extrusion of cytoplasmic material that ultimately furnishes the abundant matrix so characteristic of this tumor (Kay and Schatzki 1972). The ultrastructure of chordoma seems to be sufficiently characteristic to aid in the diagnosis, especially in *differentiating chordoma from chondrosarcoma* (Pardo-Mindán et al. 1981; Valderrama et al. 1983).

Treatment and Prognosis. In recent years, high-dose radiation, though not curative, has been recognized as offering the possibility for significant palliation and tumor regression (Higinbotham et al. 1967; Pearlman and Friedman 1970). However, it is generally accepted that complete surgical resection offers the best chance for long-term survival. Unfortunately, this can only be accomplished in sacrococcygeal chordomas and some vertebral lesions. In many cases, due to the extension of the process, complete removal is not feasible, and in these and in recurrent lesions, high doses of radiation are indicated. Chordoma is a slow-growing tumor, and incomplete removal can produce remissions of long duration. Metastasis has been previously considered as rare and usually appears after a long clinical duration (average time 3 years) and repeated recurrences (Fox et al. 1968). However, according to the Memorial Hospital experience, in the series of 54 patients studied by Sundaresan, 11 of 18 vertebral chordomas and 10 of 36 sacral tumors presented metastases throughout the course of the disease, being discovered from 1 to 10 years after the initial diagnosis. Metastases have been reported in practically every organ. The most frequent sites in descending order of frequency are the lungs, liver, regional and remote lymph nodes, bones, brain, and skin.

2. "Adamantinoma" of Long Bones (Adamantinoma of the Appendicular Skeleton)

Definition, WHO: *"A malignant, or at least locally malignant, tumor characterized by a wide range of morphological patterns, most commonly the presence of circumscribed masses or tubular formations of apparently epithelial cells surrounded by spindle-celled fibrous tissue."*

Adamantinoma of long bones is an uncommon but well-established slow-growing neoplasm of disputed histogenesis that occurs predominantly in the tibia and rarely in other long bones. In exceptional cases the lesion is found in short bones, e.g., the carpal capitate (Diepeveen et al. 1960) and tarsal first cuneiform. Therefore, Moon (1965, 1973; Moon and Mori 1986) proposed the name "adamantinoma of the appendicular skeleton."

Fig. VII.15a–e. Fourteen-year-old boy with adamantinoma of the femur. **a** Anteroposterior and lateral radiographs show a radiolucent, ill-defined lesion in the midshaft with enlargement of the cortex at its medial aspect. **b** Photograph and **c** radiograph show the grayish-white, solid, centrally located tumor. **d,e** Photomicrographs at lower and higher magnification illustrate the characteristic histologic features of adamantinoma. **d** ×100, **e** ×300

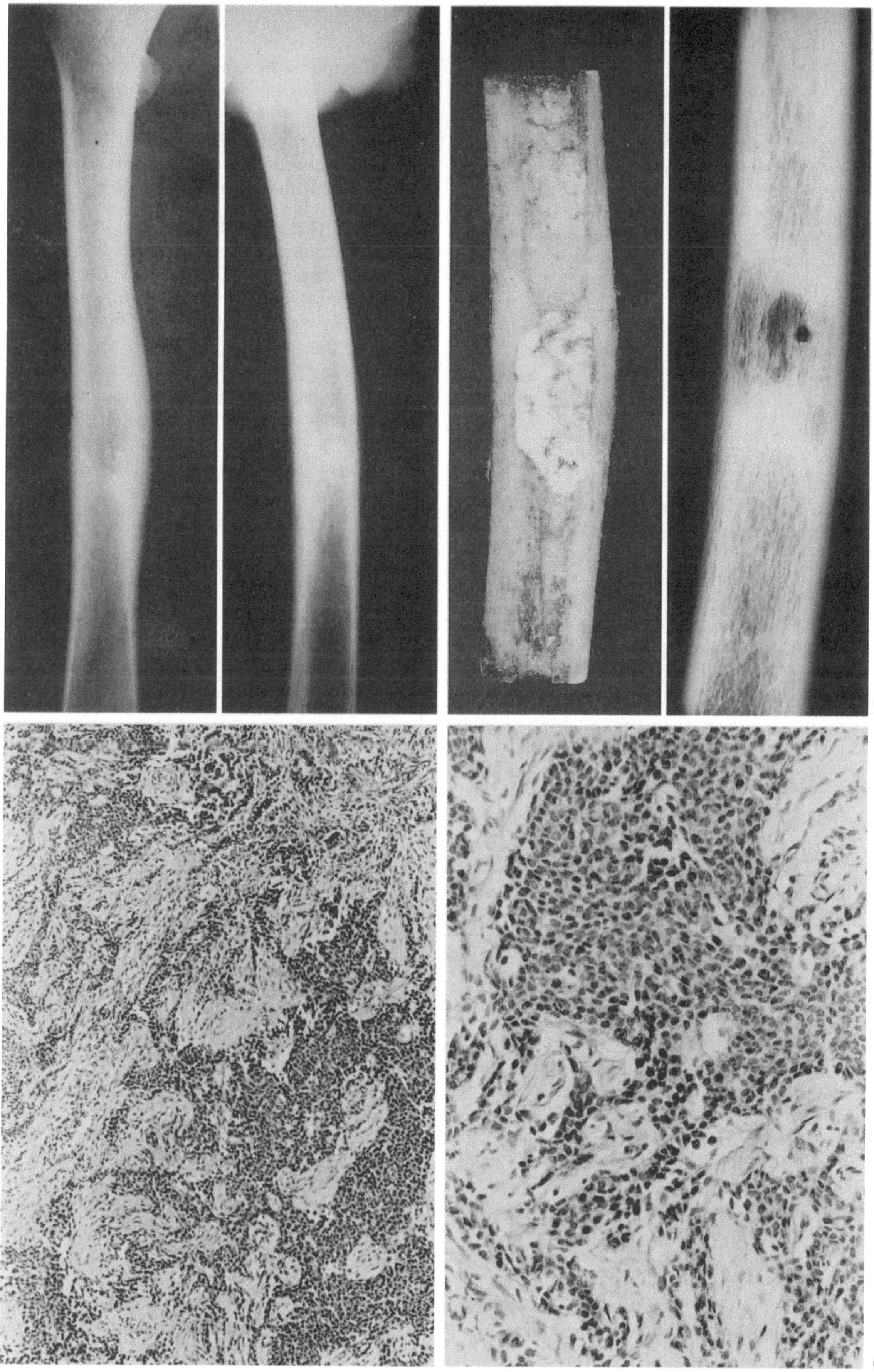

a b, c

d e

The term "primary adamantinoma of tibia" was introduced in 1913 by Fischer because of its close resemblance to the more common mandibular tumor; the similarities included the gross appearance and the histologic features, including the columnar and palisaded arrangement of the peripheral basaloid cells. Therefore, he considered a possible origin from embryonal epithelium of the enamel germ, the ectodermal elements in the legs of the embryo having the potential to develop into enamel epithelial anlage in the same manner as the gingival epithelium penetrating into the maxilla.

Because the first 17 reported cases of the lesion occurred exclusively within the tibia, until 1942 it was referred to as "adamantinoma of the tibia." After the publication of a case involving the ulna (Anderson and Saunders 1942) and of other cases located in the ulna and other long bones, the term "adamantinoma of long bones" was adopted.

Incidence. Adamantinoma of long bones is a rare tumor. Reports of one or a few cases, and only a few larger series, have been published in the last two decades by Unni et al. (1974; 29 cases), Huvos and Marcove (1975; 14 cases), Weiss and Dorfman (1977; 9 cases), and Campanacci (1990; 14 cases). The 23 cases in the last Mayo Clinic series (Dahlin and Unni 1986) represented only 0.3% of the malignant primary bone tumors. Moon and Mori (1986) carefully reviewed the literature and found 195 well-documented cases, to which they added five new cases. More recently Czerniak, Rojas-Corona, and Dorfman (1989) presented a clinicopathologic review of 25 cases, including an immunohistochemical study in seven cases. In our files 19 cases of adamantinoma of long bones were recorded, i.e., 1% of malignant bone tumors.

Clinical Findings. Age and Sex. The tumor is somewhat more frequent in males, with a total of 114 males (57%) and 86 females (43%) in Moon and Mori's review (1986) of the world literature. The ages range from 4 to 74 years, with a peak incidence in females between 10 and 30, while males seem to have a peak incidence between 31 and 50. Only six cases (3%) of Moon's review were in children under the age of 10 years. We reported recently three cases of adamantinoma of the tibia associated with and mimicking fibrous dysplasia or osteofibrous dysplasia in children aged 3, 9, and 16 years (Schajowicz and Santini-Araujo 1989), out of 14 cases. This coexistence of fibrous dysplasia-like lesions and adamantinoma of the tibia has been recognized for more than three decades (Baker et al. 1954; Cohen et al. 1962; Delarue et al. 1964; Johnson 1972; Markel 1978; Campanacci et al. 1981), but it seems to be more frequent than formerly believed.

Localization. Approximately 90% of the cases involved the tibia, most often the middle or distal end of the diaphysis. In almost 10%, the tibia and fibula were involved synchronously. A number of cases have been found in extratibial locations, including the ulna (6) (Anderson and Saunders 1942; Etchart et al. 1961), the femur (10), the fibula (13), the humerus (9), the radius (1), and the metatarsus (1) (Lipper and Kahn 1983). The short bones in which the tumor was reported include the carpal capitate (Diepeveen et al. 1960) and the tarsal first cuneiform.

The writer observed one case in a rib and one in the femur (Fig. VII.15). In two of our cases, the tumor was multifocal: In one case, there were several separated foci in the tibia and in the adjacent fibula; in the other case, there were foci in the lower and upper end of the tibia and in the lower end of the femur. The foci appeared metachronously during the long evolution of the process, finally causing this patient's death with pulmonary metastases.

Unni et al. (1974) reported a simultaneous occurrence in the tibia and the fibula in three cases. These authors also described one patient with a presenting lesion in the humerus, in whom, on autopsy, they also observed involvement of the ribs, vertebrae, and pubis. In the absence of any evidence of visceral metastases, it is probable that these are cases of multifocal origin rather than metastatic foci.

Symptoms. The most common complaint was localized swelling or enlargement of the involved bone. The tibia and other superficially located bones being most frequently involved, small tumors are often palpated, but medical attention is usually not sought until pain develops. The pain is mild at the beginning, becoming more severe when the lesion increases in size. Because of the slow growth rate of the tumor, the symptoms may be of extremely long duration, varying from months to years. Many patients presented with a history of possible or definite trauma previous to the development of the bone tumor. This is important, because trauma is supposed to play an important role in the etiology of the tumor (Ryrie 1932).

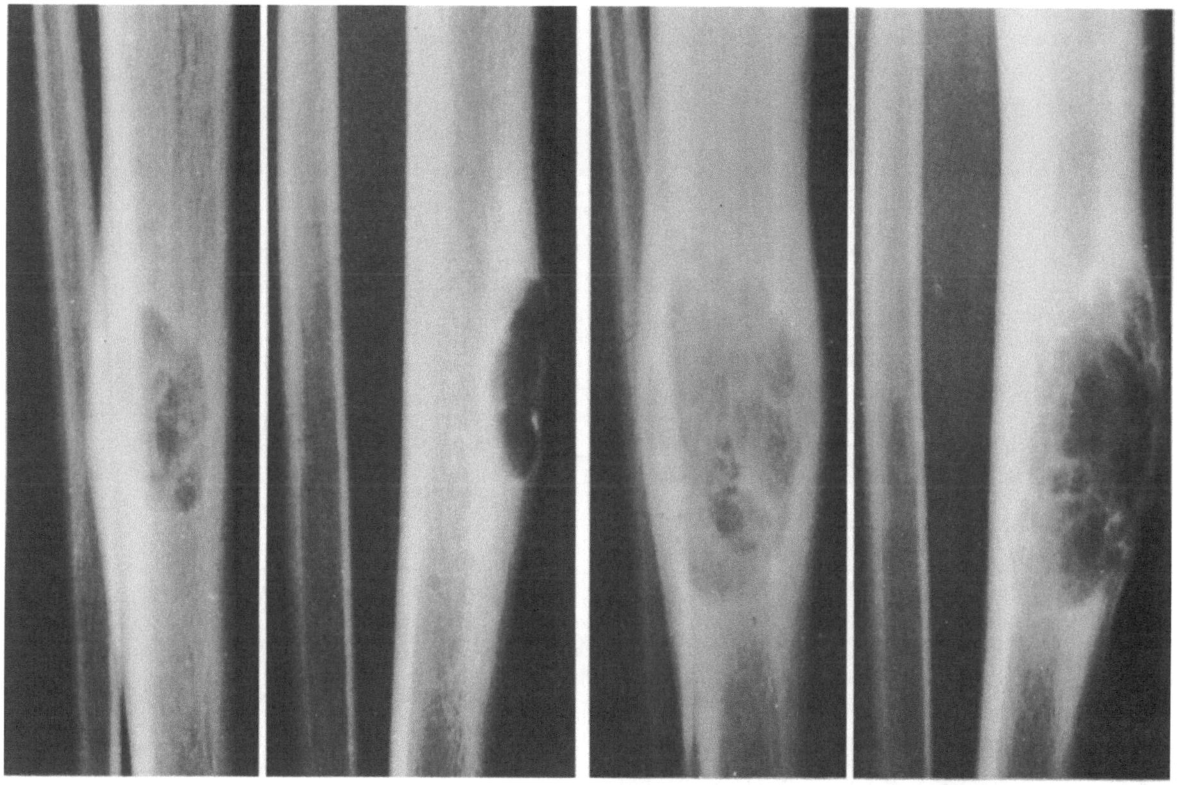

a b

Fig. VII.16a,b. Male, 12 years old. Adamantinoma of tibia. **a** Anteroposterior and lateral radiographs show an eccentric, sharply defined osteolytic lesion. The anterior cortex is thinned and slightly expanded. **b** Recurrence 1 year after curettage because of an erroneous diagnosis of bone cyst. A wide segmental resection was performed followed by cadaver bone graft. After two recurrences an amputation was performed 6 years after onset. (Schajowicz et al. 1972)

On physical examination, a firm swelling, sometimes tender, fixed to the underlying shaft of the bone, is found; occasionally the covering skin is tense or shiny, but moves easily over the tumor mass.

Radiographic Features. The radiographic appearance is that of a radiolucent, often well-delineated elongated lesion (Figs. VII.16–VII.18) (Schajowicz et al. 1972), sometimes trabeculated or multilocular, with osteolytic areas of different sizes, separated by slightly sclerotic bone. The larger lesions are sometimes eccentric and usually expand and thin the cortex, deforming

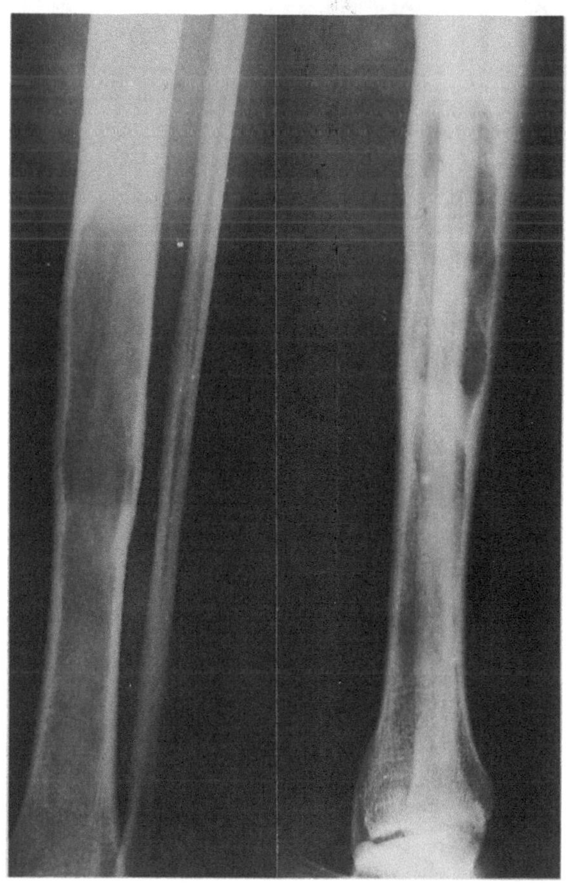

Fig. VII.17. Male, 28 years old. Adamantinoma of tibia. ▶ Anteroposterior and lateral radiographs illustrate radiolucent lesion with ill-defined margins, thinning but only slightly expanding the cortex

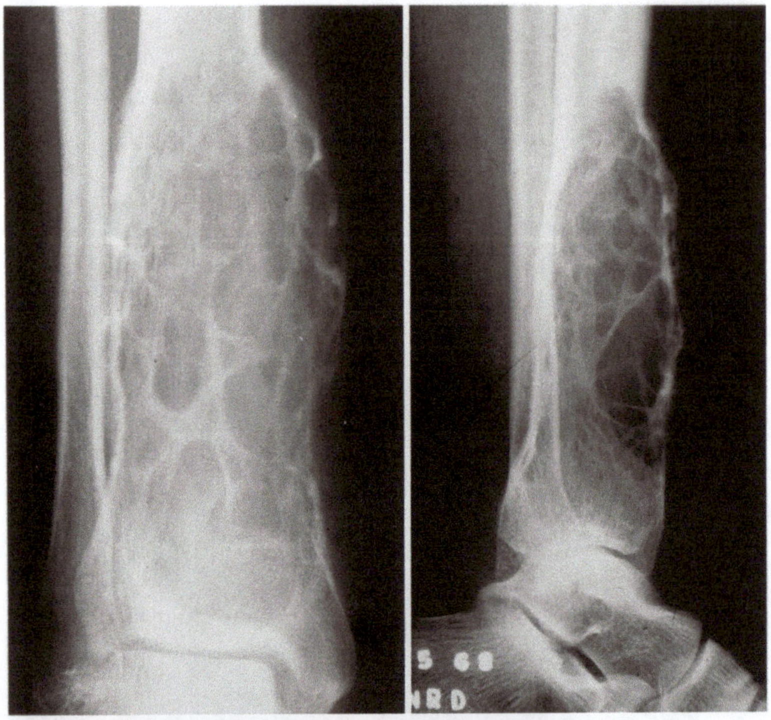

a

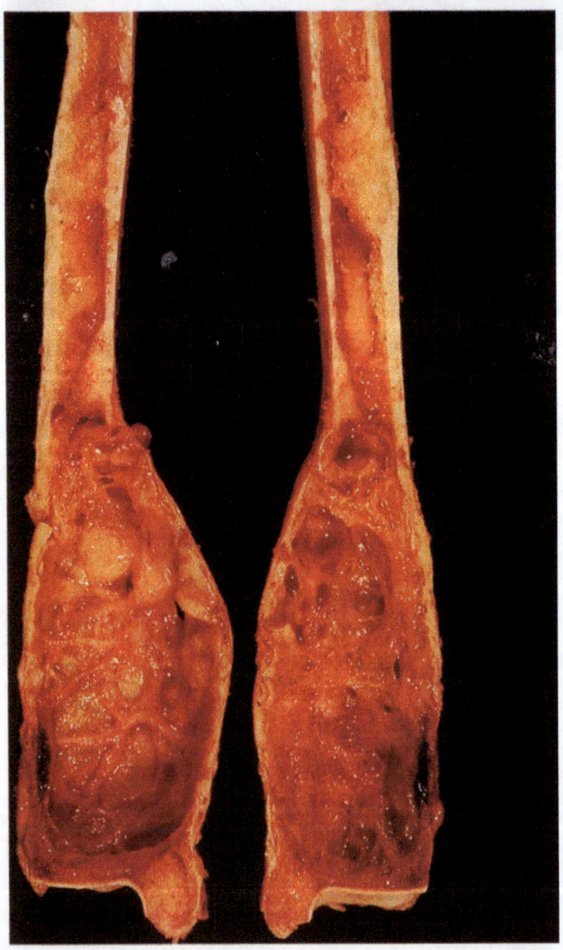

b

Fig. VII.18a,b. Adamantinoma of tibia. **a** Anteroposterior and lateral radiographs show a large, radiolucent, trabeculated lesion in the lower third, which has widely expanded the thinned cortex. **b** Photograph of the specimen shows the predominantly solid tumor with some cystic and hemorrhagic areas. A small grayish-white nodule is seen proximally, separated from the tumor, which histologically corresponds to fibrous dysplasia. (Courtesy of the late C. Lemos, Rio de Janeiro, Brazil)

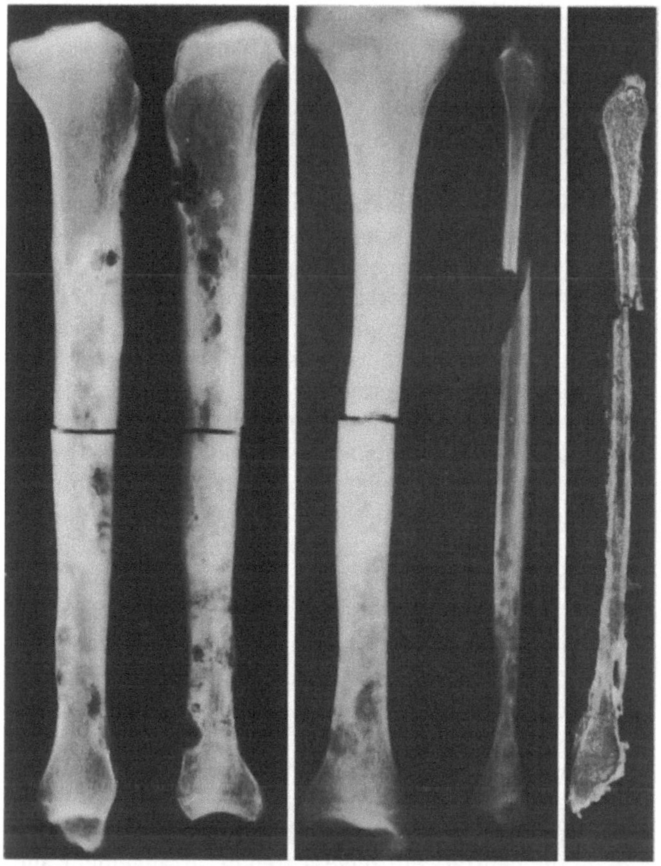

a

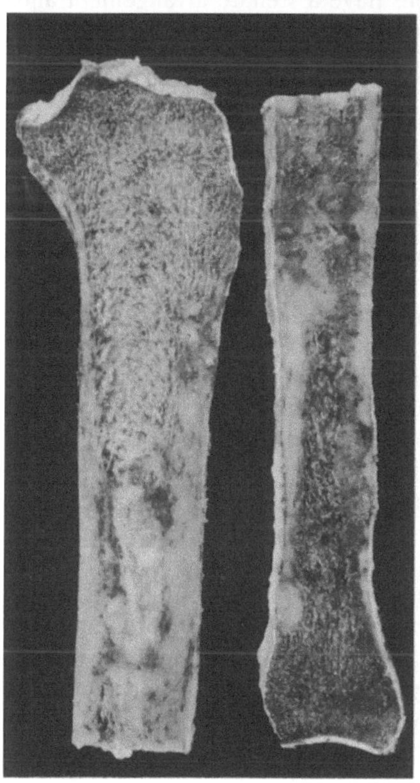

b

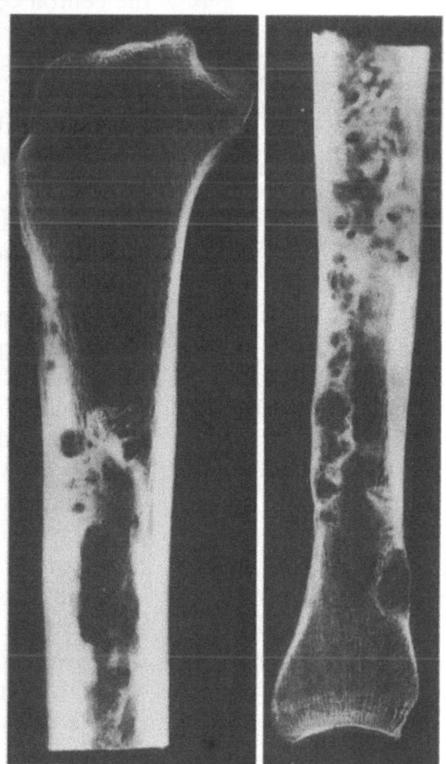

c

Fig. VII.19a–c. Female, 33 years old. Multicentric adamantinoma in tibia and fibula. **a** Anteroposterior and lateral radiographs of the amputation specimen show multiple osteolytic areas of different sizes, separated by sclerotic bone, with a "sawtooth" appearance of the cortex. **b** Photographs and **c** radiographs of a thin section of the specimen illustrate the multicentric aspect

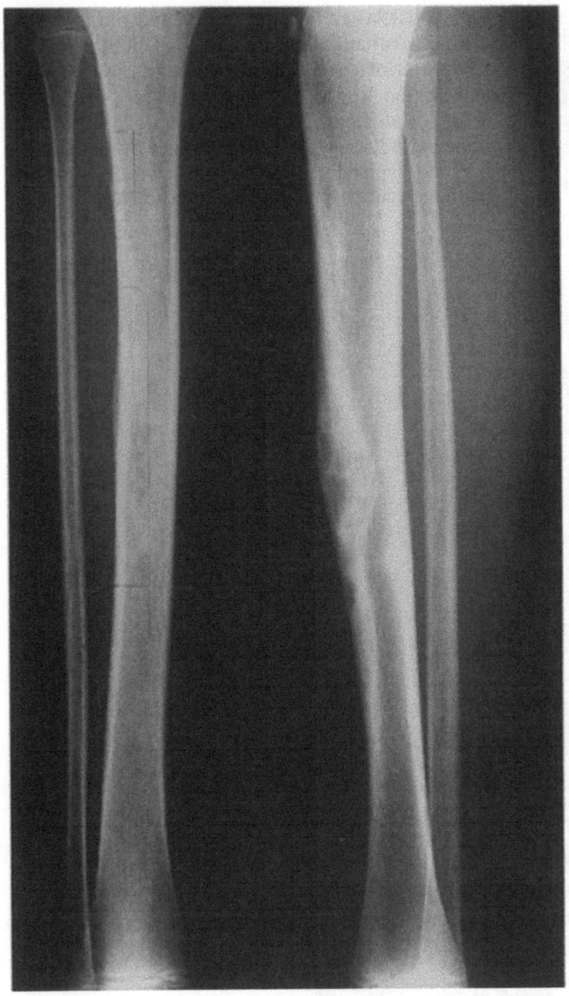

Fig. VII.20. Nine-year-old girl with adamantinoma of the tibia. Anteroposterior and lateral radiographs show a lucent, multilocular lesion with a sclerotic border on the anterior aspect of the midshaft, primarily involving the cortex. A similar, but smaller radiolucent lesion is seen on the upper one-third of the tibia

the shaft of the bone, usually in its middle or lower end. There is sometimes a "sawtooth" area of cortical destruction (Fig. VII.19).

The tumor rarely destroys the cortex extensively, but periosteal reaction or soft tissue penetration is uncommon. Larger tumors may present a "soap bubble" appearance (Fig. VII.18). In one of our cases, the tumor involved almost the entire tibial shaft, which was widened, deformed, and frankly cystic; this was demonstrated clearly in the resection specimen, in which an enormous cystic cavity was found.

Some long-standing lesions may show a more radiopaque ground-glass appearance and may be confused with fibrous dysplasia. Smaller circumscribed lytic lesions, separated from the large tumor, may correspond to areas of fibrous dysplasia (Cohen et al. 1962) or, more commonly, to separate tumoral foci (Unni et al. 1974; Schajowicz and Santini 1989) (Fig. VII.20).

Pathologic Findings. *Grossly*, the tumor is frequently circumscribed with a somewhat lobulated surface, expanding the cortex eccentrically. The cortex is thinned and only rarely destroyed. There may or may not be extension of the tumor into the soft tissues. The tumor tissue is in part solid or grayish-white or pink, and of soft and friable to firm and rubbery consistency, alternating with extensive, usually multiple cystic cavities filled with a clear and watery or brown and hemorrhagic fluid. The cystic cavity may occupy a great portion of the tumor, as in one of our cases (Fig. VII.18b).

Histologically, there is considerable variation in cellular patterns and in the relative amount of epithelial and spindle-celled fibrous tissue of different tumors or of different areas of the same tumor (Figs. VII.15d,e, VII.21). The most common appearance is that of epithelial-appearing cells, forming strands or nests, with peripheral columnar and palisaded cells, whereas the central cells have a stellate arrangement and are often separated by cystic spaces. This basaloid pattern gives the lesion some degree of resemblance to the adamantinoma (ameloblastoma) of the jaws and to other epithelial tumors of the basal cell type (basal-cell carcinoma of the skin). Infrequently, a squamous-cell appearance with keratin pearl formation (Unni et al. 1974) or a tubular pattern may resemble squamous-cell carcinoma or adenocarcinoma.

Weiss and Dorfman (1977) described four basic histologic patterns that may predominate in an individual case: basaloid, spindled, squamoid, and tubular; usually a mixture of several patterns was observed within each case.

In Weiss and Dorfman's nine cases of adamantinoma, the basaloid was the most common pattern (present in eight cases and predominant in three), and the squamous pattern was the least frequent. The spindled pattern, which was present in six cases but prominent in only two, was similar to the basaloid, except that the peripheral orientation was lacking; the spindle cells were occasionally arranged in small whorled clusters, and in three cases the spindle cells exhibited palisading of nuclei, resembling smooth muscle or neural tumors. Reticulin stain

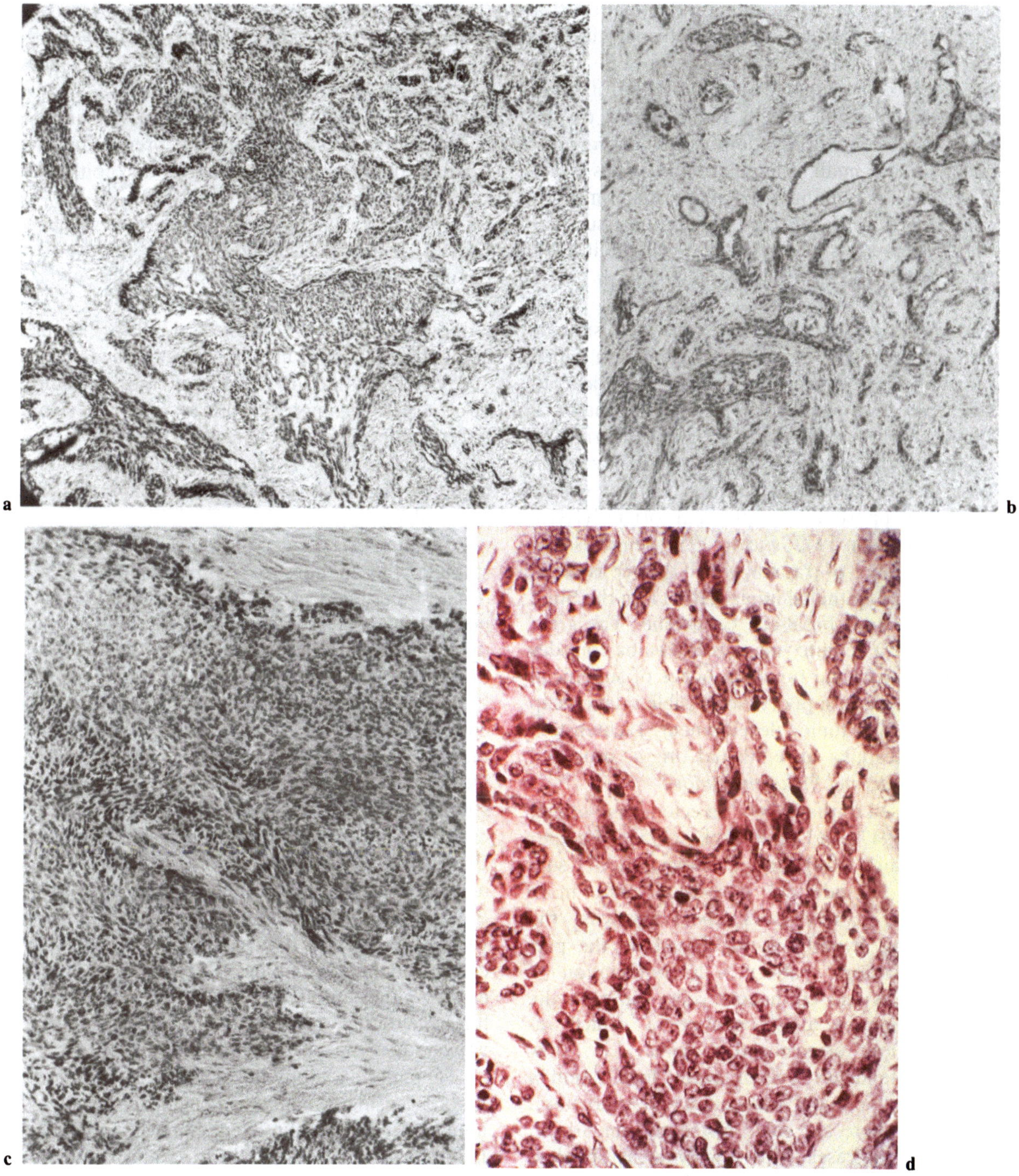

Fig. VII.21a–d. Photomicrographs showing different histologic patterns of adamantinoma of tibia. **a** At low magnification, solid zones alternating with alveolar or tubular structures separated by connective tissue are seen. **b** Cell cords or tubular structures may suggest a vascular tumor. *Solid areas* show central zones where the cells are separated by irregular spaces. **c** Large solid areas with an evident spindle-celled structure. **d** The basaloid pattern and some tubular structures at high magnification. **a** ×100, **b** ×200, **c** ×300, **d** ×400 demonstrated fibers encircling individual cells, a characteristic feature of mesenchymal tumors. The tubular pattern, which was present in six cases and prominent in four, consisted of small flattened or cuboidal cells lining spaces of different sizes, giving the impression of *vascular* channels or small glandular formations (Fig. VII.21b). The lining cells were sometimes so compressed by the surrounding fibrous tissue that they appeared as rows of single cells infiltrating the stroma.

Pathogenesis. The extreme variety of histologic patterns and the tumor's predominant tibial location are the principal reasons for the considerable controversy over the pathogenesis of this tumor. Since Fischer's original description, numerous theories of the pathogenesis have been postulated. The great majority of the earlier reports supported an epithelial origin (Ryrie 1932; Robinson 1942; Cicero 1958), emphasizing the importance of trauma, which they considered the cause of epithelial implantation into the tibia, giving rise to a basal-cell carcinoma. The great frequency of definite previous traumatic episodes and the site of the tumor in bones of superficial location seem to support the possible relationship of trauma and tumor development. Lichtenstein (1977), accepting an epithelial origin, proposed the term "*dermal inclusion tumor*."

Opposed to the idea of an ectodermal origin, Lauche (1947) and later Hicks (1954), Lederer and Sinclair (1954), and Uehlinger (1957) suggested a mesodermal derivation and, more specifically, a *synovial sarcoma* involving the tibia. Their hypothesis was based on the particular histologic pattern – a combination of spindle cells and epithelioid cells – and on the clinical features of adamantinoma, which resemble those of synovial sarcoma, i.e., slow growth, a tendency to recur locally, localization in the extremities, and insensitivity to irradiation. Although there are some histologic similarities, especially in cases with a prominent spindled aspect, we never found a typical biphasic pattern characteristic of malignant synovioma, which has a much worse prognosis than adamantinoma.

The concept of *angioblastic origin*, elaborated by Changus et al. (1957), has since found some defenders (Huvos and Marcove 1975). Based on morphologic and histochemical studies, such as the positive alkaline phosphatase reaction (similar to that occurring in the vascular endothelium) and other special histologic techniques (reticulin stain, PAS, etc.), Huvos and Marcove proposed the term "*malignant angioblastoma*."

Although it is true that in a few cases it may be extremely difficult to distinguish adamantinoma from the vascular tumors (hemangioendothelioma), especially in the predominantly tubular pattern, in most cases an epithelial structure is evident.

In contrast, *ultrastructural studies* have proved definitely that most of the tumors are of epithelial origin (Albores Saavedra et al. 1968; Rosai 1969; Schajowicz et al. 1971, 1974; Yoneyama et al. 1977; Mori et al. 1984; Pieterse et al. 1982; Knapp et al. 1982; Pérez-Atayde et al. 1985). The tissue in the three cases of Unni et al. (1974) was not well preserved for electron microscopic studies (material previously embedded in paraffin). Although they also described an epithelial structure, these findings are not fully acceptable.

In our two cases and in all other cases studied, the findings of basal membranes, of desmosomes, and especially of tonofibrils composed of fascicles of microfilaments converging upon the desmosomes, prove the epithelial origin of the tumor cells (Fig. VII.22).

Although desmosomes are also present in endothelial cells, we have not observed structures indicative of a vascular origin in our cases. However, based on the few ultramicroscopic studies of these scarce cases, such an origin cannot be entirely denied; for instance Llombart-Bosch and Ortuño-Pacheco (1978) and Povysil and Matejovsky (1981) found structures identical to Weibel-Palade bodies, characteristic for vascular elements. It is possible that the basic cells of adamantinoma have a capacity to differentiate along epithelial as well as mesenchymal lines, although the epithelial differentiation appears to be far more common.

The more recently introduced relevant tissue markers using immunohistochemical assays as applicable to formalin-fixed, paraffin-embedded tissues have helped greatly to confirm the epithelial nature of this neoplasm (Knapp et al. 1982; Mori et al. 1984; Pérez-Atayde et al. 1985). Thus immunohistochemical study showed the coexpression of cytokeratin and vimentin on the one hand, and the lack of factor VIII and

Fig. VII.22a,b. Electron micrograph of adamantinoma of ▶ tibia showing desmosomes and tonofilaments, more clearly seen in **b**

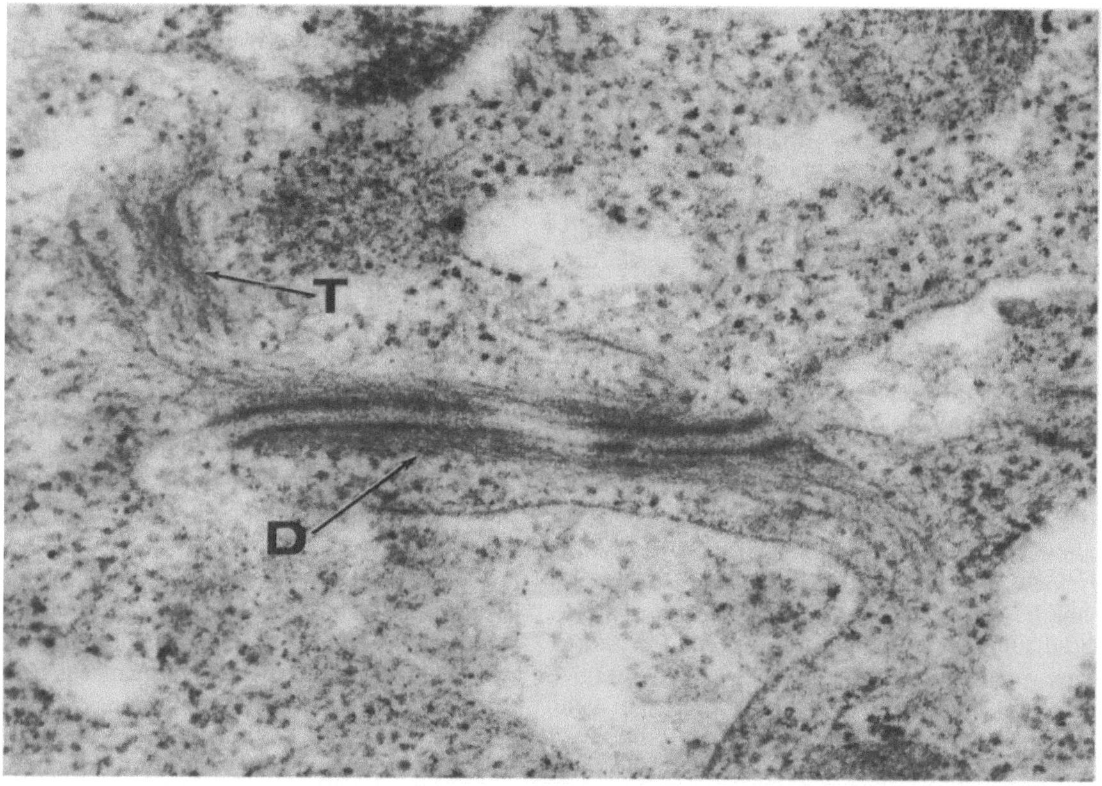

a

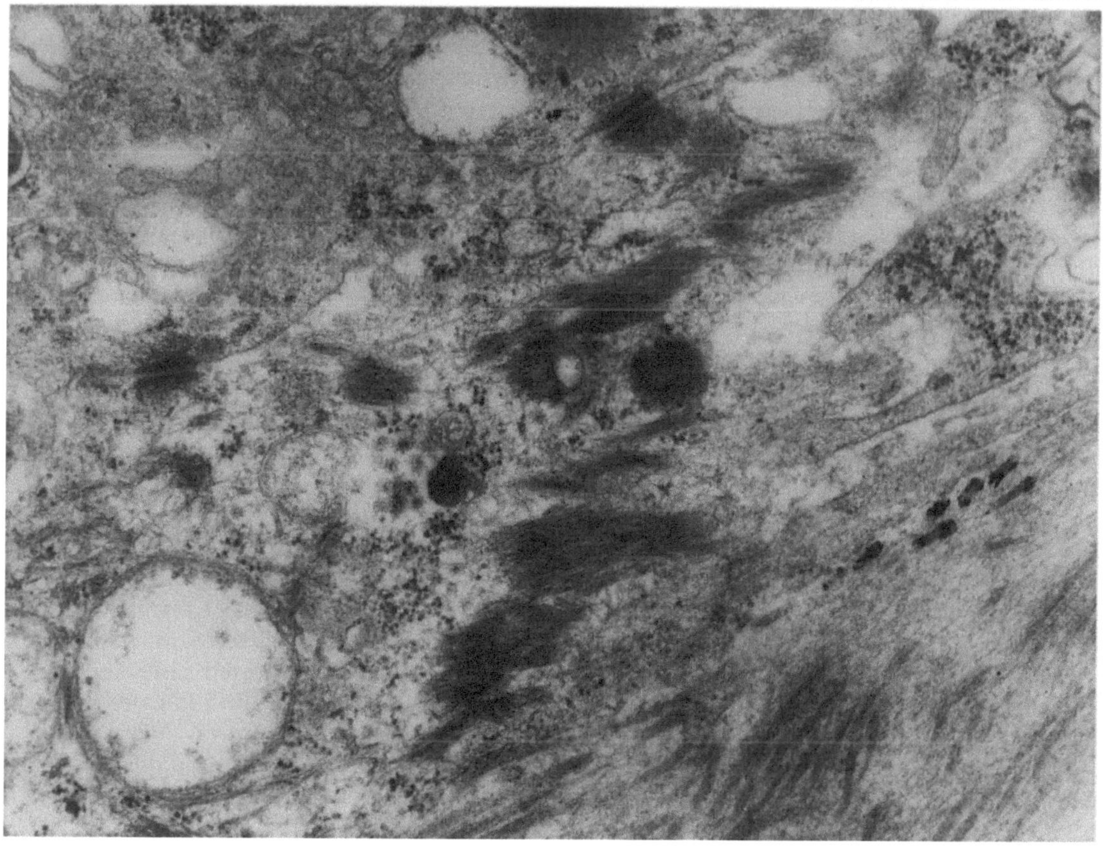

b

Ulex europaeus (markers for endothelial cells) and S-100 protein staining on the other (Knapp et al. 1982; Rosai and Pinkus 1982; Mori et al. 1984; Pérez-Atayde et al. 1985; Czerniak et al. 1989). In our laboratory we carried out a histochemical study of keratin markers in seven cases of adamantinoma (comprising 17 specimens, including the original lesions, recurrences, and metastases) and confirmed the findings of the other researchers.

Association of Adamantinoma with Fibrous (Osteofibrous) Dysplasia. In several of our cases, as in a great number of the reported cases (9 of the 25 cases of Czerniak et al. 1989), fibrous dysplasia-like areas, at present distinguished from classic fibrous dysplasia and classified as osteofibrous dysplasia (Campanacci et al. 1981) or "ossifying fibroma" (Kempson 1966), were found between the tumor strands at the periphery of the tumor or sometimes at a certain distance away, separated from the tumor by normal bone tissue. Like Johnson (1972), we prefer to call these lesions "intracortical fibrous dysplasia." We do not consider these entities two distinct diseases, but rather different histologic expressions of essentially the same process, which varies depending on location (predominantly intracortical or medullary) and age (see Chap. IX, Sect. 6, on fibrous dysplasia). In their first paper Weiss and Dorfman interpreted fibrous dysplasia-like areas (found in seven of nine cases) as part of the spectrum of dual epithelial and mesenchymal differentiation of which the tumor is capable. In some cases the fibrous dysplasia-like component predominates over the scarce epithelioid islands of tumor cells, especially in intracortical lesions and younger patients, and consequently is not recognized as adamantinoma. In three of our cases, an erroneous diagnosis of fibrous or osteofibrous dysplasia was made by the contributing pathologist (Figs. VII.23, VII.24). Also three of Dorfman's cases (Czerniak et al. 1989) had been originally diagnosed as osteofibrous dysplasia but were reclassified after further study. On the basis of distinct radiologic, histologic, and immunohistochemical patterns these authors distinguished a new type of "differentiated adamantinoma" from the classic adamantinoma (8 of 25 cases). It is characterized by the patient's age (first two decades), the intracortical location of the entire lesion, the uniform predominance of an osteofibrous dysplasia-like pattern, and the scattered positivity of epithelial elements for cytokeratin. They postulate that the predominance of an osteofibrous dysplasia-like pattern in differentiated adamantinoma is the "result of a *secondary reparative process overgrowing* matured and *regressing* tumor tissue." Therefore osteofibrous dysplasia (ossifying fibroma) may in some cases represent the spontaneous evolution of an underlying adamantinoma. Although they admit that this concept does not rule out the possibility of the existence of de novo osteofibrous dysplasia unrelated to adamantinoma, we believe their statements are premature and unproven; this is especially so with regard to their claim of a more favorable prognosis for the differentiated type of adamantinoma, being based, as it is, on such a small number of cases and insufficient follow-up data.

Treatment and Prognosis. Adamantinoma of long bones is a tumor of low-grade malignancy which is locally invasive and produces metastases relatively late. The treatment of choice is surgery. If the tumor is localized at the time of diagnosis, en bloc resection followed by bone grafts is preferred in our institute and by most authors. Amputation is indicated for a local recurrence, for lesions that have extensively invaded soft tissues, or for multifocal lesions. However, other surgeons found primary amputation more successful (Moon 1965; Huvos and Marcove 1975) because of the high incidence of local recurrence after en bloc excision. This they attributed to the fact that some of the tumors are multicentric or more extensive than is evident from the roentgenographic examination. Adamantinoma is highly radioresistant, and only exceptional cases of partial regression or apparent cure have been reported (Zand et al. 1972).

There are neither histologic nor clinicoradiologic features that aid in predicting the biologic behavior of the tumor and its potential capacity to metastasize. There is no proof that there are two different types of adamantinoma with distinct prognoses ("differentiated" and "classic"), as suggested by Czerniak et al. (1989).

Metastases occurred in approximately 15%–20% of the reported cases and more precisely in 22 (18%) of the 125 cases reviewed by Moon. The average survival time was 5.9 years. Autopsies were performed on only five patients. Metastases were found most frequently in lung, inguinal lymph nodes, and other bones.

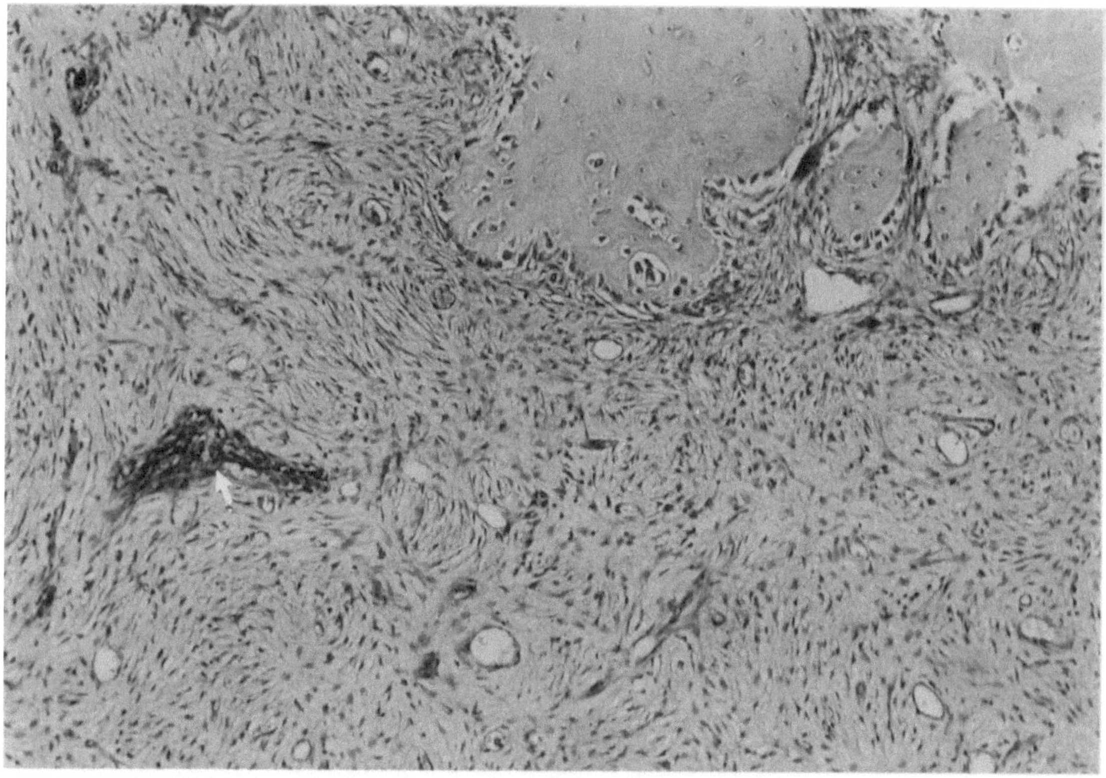

a

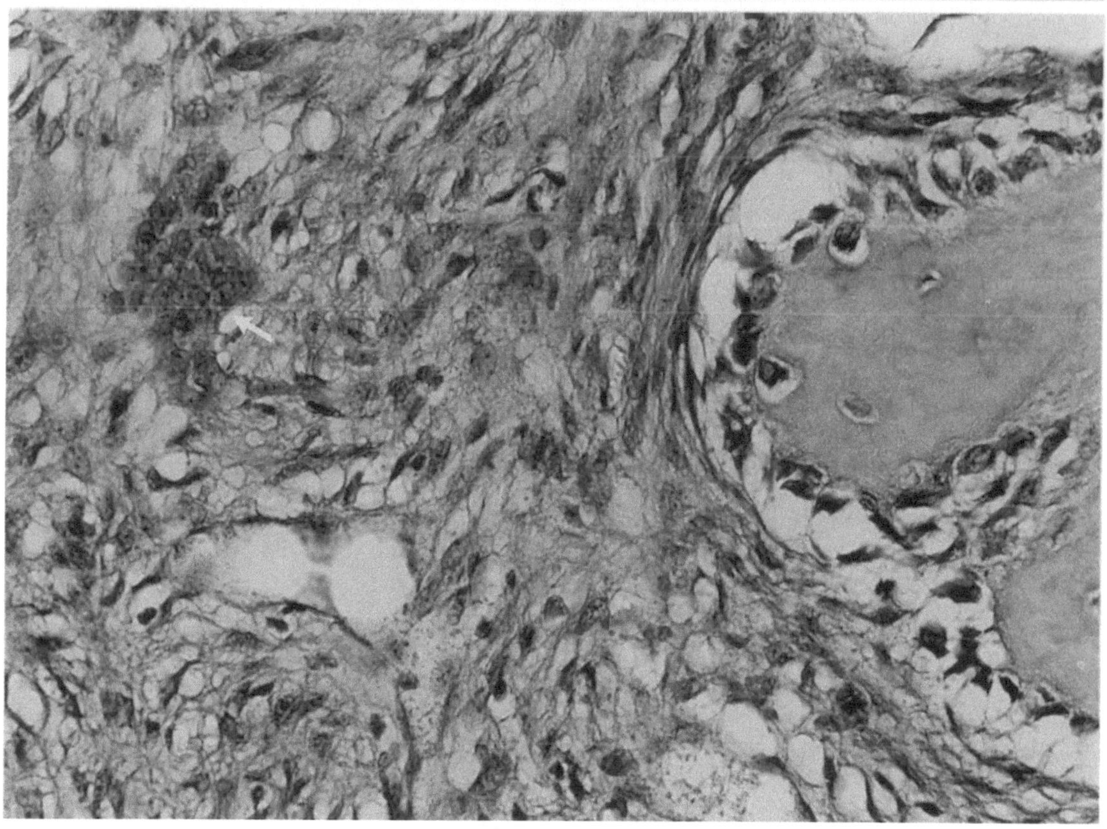

b

Fig. VII.23a,b. Photomicrographs show small isolated tumor islands (*arrow*). The lesion has a basaloid pattern within a fibrous dysplasia-like lesion; the loose fibrous stroma has a storiform pattern and newly formed bone trabeculae with rims of active osteoblasts on their surface. **a** ×100, **b** ×400

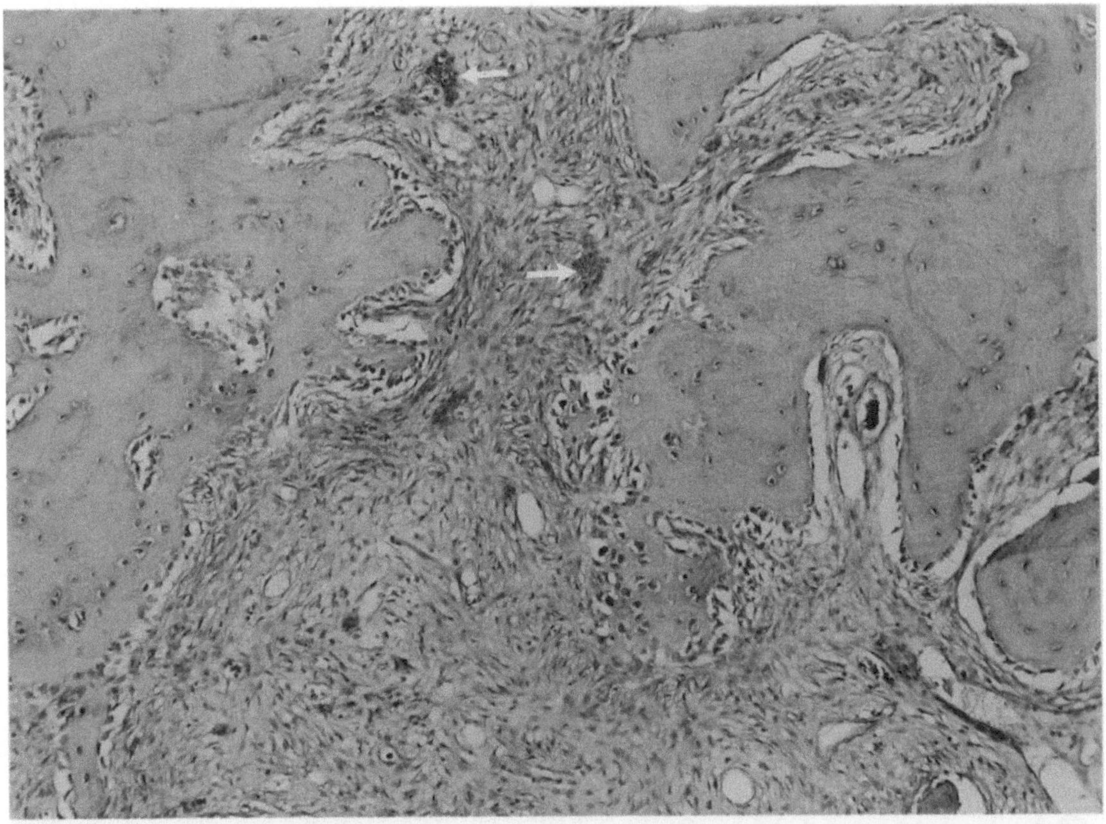

a

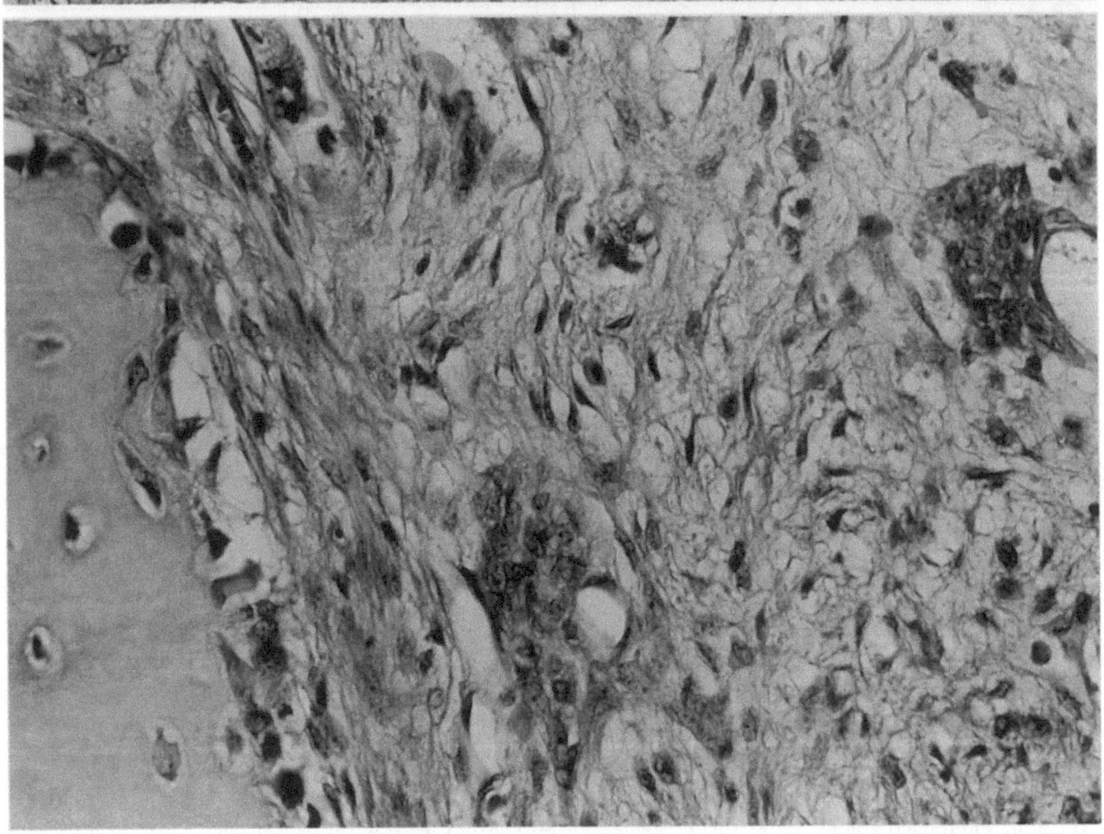

b

◀ **Fig. VII.24a,b.** Photomicrographs show similar histologic features in another case of adamantinoma associated with osteofibrous dysplasia-like pattern

References

Neurilemmoma and Neurofibroma

Aegerter EE (1950) The possible relationship neurofibromatosis, congenital pseudoarthrosis and fibrous dysplasia. J Bone Joint Surg [Am] 32:618–626

Baldwin DM, Weiner DS (1974) Congenital bowing and intraosseous neurofibroma of the ulna: a case report. J Bone Joint Surg [Am] 56:803–807

Bose KS, Thakur S, Chakbrarty S, Banerje S (1970) Intraosseous malignant schwannoma. J Indian Med Assoc 54:328–329

Brasfield RO, Das Grupta TK (1972) Von Recklinghausen's disease: a clinico-pathological study. Ann Surg 175:86–104

Cowley AH, Miller DS (1942) Neurilemmoma of bone: a case report. J Bone Joint Surg 24:684–689

Dahlin DC, Unni KK (1986) Bone tumors: general aspects and data on 8542 cases. Charles C. Thomas, Springfield, IL

Del Rio Hortega PD (1962) Tumors of the peripheral nerves. Charles C. Thomas, Springfield, IL

de Santos DA, Burgess E (1940) Primary and secondary neurilemmoma of bone. Surg Gynecol Obstet 71:454–461

Dickson JH, Waltz TA, Fechner RE (1971) Intraosseous neurilemmoma of the third lumbar vertebra. J Bone Joint Surg [Am] 53:349–355

Fawcett KJ, Dahlin DC (1967) Neurilemmoma of bone. Am J Clin Pathol 47:759–766

Fischer ER, Vuzevski VC (1968) Cytogenesis of schwannoma (neurilemmoma), neurofibroma, dermatofibroma, and dermatofibrosarcoma as revealed by electron microscopy. Am J Clin Pathol 49:141–154

Gordon E (1976) Solitary intraosseous neurilemmoma of the tibia: review of intraosseous neurilemmoma and neurofibroma. Clin Orthop 117:271–282

Gross P, Bailey FR, Jacox HW (1939) Primary intramedullary neurofibroma of the humerus. Arch Pathol 28:716–718

Güthert H (1952) Ein malignes Neurinom des Knochens. Zentralbl Allg Pathol 88:185

Hart MS, Basom WC (1958) Neurilemmoma involving bone. J Bone Joint Surg [Am] 40:465–468

Hunt JC, Pugh DG (1961) Skeletal lesions in neurofibromatosis. Radiology 76:1

Lewis HH, Korbin HT (1972) Neurilemmoma of the first metacarpal: a case report. Clin Orthop 82:67–69

Mazingarbe A, Mazabraud A (1970) A case of neurinoma of the tibia. Rev Chir Orthop 56:83–88

Peers JH (1934) Primary intramedullary neurogenic sarcoma of ulna. Am J Pathol 10:811

Polak M (1966) Blastoma del Sistema Nervioso Central y Periférico. López, Buenos Aires

Polkey CE (1975) Intraosseous neurilemmoma of the cervical spine causing paraparesis and treated by resection and grafting. J Neurol Neurosurg Psychiatry 38:776–781

Prescott GH, White RE (1970) Solitary central neurofibroma of the mandible: report of a case and review of the literature. J Oral Surg 28:305–309

Russell DS, Rubinstein LJ (1963) Tumors of the nerve roots and peripheral nerves: pathology of tumors of the nervous system, 2nd edn. Williams & Wilkins, Baltimore

Samter TG, Vellios F, Shafer WG (1960) Neurilemmoma of bone: report of three cases with a review of the literature. Radiology 75:215–222

Sane S, Yonis R (1971) Subperiosteal or cortical cyst and intramedullary neurofibromatosis: uncommon manifestations of neurofibromatosis. J Bone Joint Surg [Am] 53:1194–1201

Sherman MS (1963) The nerves of bone. J Bone Joint Surg [Am] 45:522–528

Waggener JD (1966) Ultrastructure of benign peripheral nerve sheath tumors. Cancer 19:699–709

Wilber MC, Woodcock JA (1957) Ganglioneuromata in bone: report of a case. J Bone Joint Surg [Am] 39:1385

Chordoma

Abenoza P, Sibley RK (1987) Chordoma: an immunohistochemical study. Hum Pathol 17:744–747

Baker HW, Coley BL (1953) Chordoma of lumbar vertebra. J Bone Joint Surg [Am] 35:403–408

Berdal P, Myhre E (1964) Cranial chordomas involving the paranasal sinuses. J Laryngol Otol 78:906–919

Brooks JJ, LiVolsi VA, Trojanowski JQ (1987) Does chondroid chordoma exist? Acta Neuropathol (Berl) 72:229–235

Cogdon CC (1952) Benign and malignant chordomas: a clinicoanatomic study of 22 cases. Am J Pathol 28:793–821

Crawford T (1958) The staining reactions of chordoma. J Clin Pathol 11:110–113

Dabska M (1977) Parachordoma: a new clinicopathologic entity. Cancer 40:1586–1592

Dahlin DC (1978) Bone tumors, 3rd edn. Charles C. Thomas, Springfield, IL

Dahlin DC, Unni KK (1986) Bone tumors: general aspects and data on 8542 cases. Charles C. Thomas, Springfield, IL

Enzinger F, Shiraki M (1972) Extraskeletal chondrosarcoma: an analysis of 34 cases. Hum Pathol 3:421–435

Epstein B (1969) The spine: a radiological text and atlas, 3rd edn. Lea & Febiger, Philadelphia

Firooznia H, Pinto RS (1977) Chordoma. In: von Diethelm L (ed) Encyclopedia of medical radiology, vol 5, part 6. Springer, Berlin Heidelberg New York, pp 354–416 (bibliography)

Fox JE, Batsakis JG, Owano LR (1968) Unusual manifestations of chordoma: a report of two cases. J Bone Joint Surg [Am] 50:1618–1628

Friedmann I, Harrison DFN, Bird ES (1962) The fine structure of chordoma with particular reference to the physaliphorous cell. J Clin Pathol 15:116–125

Graf L (1944) Sacrococcygeal chordoma with metastases. Arch Pathol Lab Med 37:136–139
Healy JH, Lane JM (1989) Chordoma: a critical review of diagnosis and treatment. Orthop Clin North Am 20:417–426
Heffelfinger MJ, Dahlin DC, McCarty CS, Beabout JW (1973) Chordomas and cartilaginous tumors at the skull base. Cancer 32:410–420
Herndon JH, Cohen J (1970) Chondroma of a lumbar vertebral body resembling a chordoma. J Bone Joint Surg [Am] 52:1241–1247
Higinbotham NL, Philips RF, Farr HW, Hustu HO (1967) Chondroma: thirty-five-year study at Memorial Hospital. Cancer 20:1841–1850
Horowitz T (1941) Chordal ectopia and its possible relation to chordoma. Arch Pathol Lab Med 31:354–362
Husain F (1960) Chordoma of the thoracic spine. J Bone Joint Surg [Br] 42:560
Huvos AG (1991) Bone tumors: diagnosis, treatment, prognosis. W.B. Saunders, Philadelphia
Jaffe HL (1958) Tumors and tumorous conditions of the bones and joints. Lea & Febiger, Philadelphia
Kamrin RP, Potanos JN, Pool JL (1964) An evaluation of the diagnosis and treatment of chordoma. J Neurol Neurosurg Psychiatry 27:157–165
Kay S, Schatzki PF (1972) Ultrastructural observations of a chordoma arising in the clivus. Clinico-pathology reports. Hum Pathol 3:403–413
Luschka H (1837) Über gallertartige Auswüchse am Clivus Blumenbachii. Virchows Arch [A] 11:8
Martin RF, Melnick PJ, Warner NE et al. (1973) Chordoid sarcoma. Am J Clin Pathol 59:623–635
Meis JM, Raymond AK, Evans HL et al. (1987) "Dedifferentiated" chordoma: a clinicopathologic and immunohistochemical study of three cases. Am J Surg Pathol 11:516–525
Miettinen M (1984) Chordoma: antibodies to epithelial membrane antigen and carcinoembryonic antigen in differential diagnosis. Arch Pathol Lab Med 108:891–892
Miettinen M, Lehto VP, Dahl D et al. (1983) Differential diagnosis of chordoma, chondroid, and ependymal tumors as aided by anti-intermediate filament antibodies. Am J Pathol 112:160–169
Miettinen M, Karaharju E, Jarvinen H (1987) Chordoma with a massive spindle-cell sarcomatous transformation. A light- and elecron-microscopic and immunohistological study. Am J Surg Pathol 11:563–570
Müller H (1858) Über das Vorkommen von Resten der Chorda dorsalis beim Menschem nach der Geburt und Über ihr Verhältnis zu den Gallertgeschwülsten am Clivus. Z Rationelle Med 2:202–229
Murad TM, Murthy MSN (1970) Ultrastructure of chordoma. Cancer 25:1204–1215
Pardo-Mindán FJ, Guillen FJ, Villas C et al. (1981) A comparative ultrastructural study of chondrosarcoma, chordoid sarcoma, and chordoma. Cancer 47:2611–2619
Pearlman AW, Friedman M (1970) Radical radiation therapy of chordoma. Am J Roentgenol Radium Ther Nucl Med 108:333–341
Pena CE, Horvat BL, Fischer ER (1970) The ultrastructure of chordoma. Am J Clin Pathol 53:544–551
Povysil C, Matejovsky Z (1985) A comparative ultrastructural study of chondrosarcoma, chordoid sarcoma, chordoma and chordoma periphericum. Pathol Res Pract 179:546–559
Ribbert H (1984) Über die Ecchondrosis physalifora spheno-occipitalis. Zentralbl Allg Pathol 5:457–461
Rich TA, Schiller A, Suit H et al. (1985) Clinical and pathologic review of 48 cases of chordoma. Cancer 56:182–187
Salisbury JR, Isaacson PG (1985) Demonstration of cytokeratins and an epithelial membrane antigen in chordomas and human fetal notochord. Am J Surg Pathol 9:791–797
Schajowicz F, Derqui JC (1968) Puncture biopsy in lesions of the locomotor system: review of results in 4050 cases, including 941 vertebral punctures. Cancer 21:531–548
Schajowicz F, Ackerman LV, Sissons HA (1972) Histological typing of bone tumors. International histological classification of tumors, No. 6. World Health Organization, Geneva
Schmorl G (1928) Über Chordareste in den Wirbelkorpern. Zentralbl Chir 55:2305
Spjut H, Luse SA (1964) Chordoma: an electron microscopic study. Cancer 17:643–646
Stewart MJ, Le F, Burrow J (1923) Ecchondrosis physaliphora spheno-occipitalis. J Neurol Psychopathol 4:218–220
Stewart MJ, Morin JE (1926) Chordoma: a review with report of a new sacroccygeal case. J Pathol Bacteriol 29:41–60
Sundaresan N (1986) Spinal chordomas. Clin Orthop 204:135–142
Utne JR, Pugh DG (1955) The roentgenologic aspects of chordoma. Am J Roentgenol Radium Ther Nucl Med 74:593–608
Valderrama E, Kahn LB, Lipper S et al. (1983) Chondroid chordoma: electron-microscopic study of two cases. Am J Surg Pathol 7:625–632
Wang CC, James AE (1968) Chordoma with a brief review of the literature and report of a case and widespread metastases. Cancer 22:162–167
Weiss SW (1976) Ultrastructure of the so-called "chordoid sarcoma." Evidence supporting cartilaginous differentiation. Cancer 37:300–306
Wick MR, Burgess JH, Manivel JC (1988) A reassessment of "chordoid sarcoma." Ultrastructural and immunohistochemical comparison with chordoma and skeletal myxoid chondrosarcoma. Modern Pathol 1:433–443

Adamantinoma of Long Bones

Adler CP (1990) Case report 587. Adamantinoma of the tibia mimicking osteofibrous dysplasia. Skeletal Radiol 19:55–58
Albores Saavedra J, Diaz Gutierrez D, Altamirano Dimas M (1968) Adamantinoma de la tibia. Observaciones ultrastructurales. Rev Med Hosp Gen Mexico City 31:241–252
Alguacil-Garcia A, Alonso A, Pettigrew NM (1984) Osteofibrous dysplasia (ossifying fibroma) of the tibia and fibula and adamantinoma. A case report. Am J Clin Pathol 82:470–474
Anderson CE, Saunders JB (1942) Primary adamantinoma of the ulna. Surg Gynecol Obstet 75:351–356

Baker PL, Dockerty MB, Coventry MB (1954) Adamantinoma (so-called) of the long bones: review of the literature and a report of three new cases. J Bone Joint Surg [Am] 36:704–720

Baud P, Tomeno B, Courpied JP et al. (1987) A peculiar tumor: adamantinoma of the long bone. Apropos of 7 consecutive cases followed up after resection. Rev Chir Orthop 73:3–13

Bullough PG, Goldenberg VM (1971) Multicentric origin of adamantinoma of the tibia: a case report. Rev Hosp Spec Surg 1:71–74

Campanacci M (1990) Bone and soft tissue tumors. Springer, Vienna New York

Campanacci M, Giunti A, Bertoni F et al. (1981) Adamantinoma of the long bones. The experience at the Istituto Ortopedico Rizzoli. Am J Surg Pathol 5:533–542

Campanacci M, Giunti A, Leonessa C (1970) Adamantinoma delle ossa lunghe. Chir Organi Mov 58:385–394

Changus GW, Speed JS, Stewart FW (1957) Malignant angioblastoma of bone: a reappraisal of adamantinoma of long bone. Cancer 20:540–559

Cicero AH (1958) El llamado adamantinoma de los huesos largos. Arch Cuban Cancer 17:190–200

Cohen DM, Dahlin DC, Pugh DG (1962) Fibrous dysplasia associated with adamantinoma of the long bones. Cancer 15:515–521

Czerniak B, Rojas-Corona RR, Dorfman HD (1989) Morphologic diversity of long bone adamantinoma: the concept of differentiated (regressing) adamantinoma and its relationship to osteofibrous dysplasia. Cancer 64:2319–2334

Dahlin DC (1978) Bone tumors, 3rd edn. Charles C. Thomas, Springfield, IL

Dahlin DC, Unni KK (1986) Bone tumors: general aspects and data on 8542 cases. Charles C. Thomas, Springfield, IL

Delarve J, Chomette G, Brocheriou C (1964) Adamantinome du tibia et "dysplasie fibreuse." Ann Anat Pathol 9:373–378

Diepeveen WP, Hjort GH, Pock-Steen OC (1960) Adamantinoma of the capitate bone. Acta Radiol 53:377–384

Elliot GB (1962) Malignant angioblastoma of long bone, so-called "tibial" adamantinoma. J Bone Joint Surg [Br] 44:25–33

Etchart M, Viviani G, Behn K (1961) Adamantinom der Ulna. Fortschr Roentgenstr 95:415–418

Evans RW, Thomas GE, Walker NM (1960) A congenital malignant synovial tumour of bone. J Bone Joint Surg (Br) 42:742–748

Fischer B (1913) Über ein primares Adamantinom der Tibia. Frank Z Pathol 12:422–441

Hicks JD (1954) Synovial sarcoma of the tibia. Pathol Bacteriol 67:151–161

Huvos AG, Marcove RC (1975) Adamantinoma of long bones: a clinico-pathological study of fourteen cases with vascular origin suggested. J Bone Joint Surg [Am] 54:148–154

Johnson LC (1972) Congenital pseudoarthrosis, adamantinoma of long bone and intracortical fibrous dysplasia of the tibia. J Bone Joint Surg [Am] 54:1355

Keeney GL, Unni KK, Beabout JW, Pritchard DJ (1989) Adamantinoma of long bones: a clinicopathologic study of 85 cases. Cancer 64:730–737

Kempson R (1966) Ossifying fibroma of the long bones. A light and electron microscopic study. Arch Pathol 82:218

Knapp RH, Wick MR, Scheithauer BW et al. (1982) Adamantinoma of bone: an electron microscopic and immunohistochemical study. Virchows Arch [A] 398:75–86

Lasda NA, Hughes EC Jr (1979) Adamantinoma of the ischium. Case report. J Bone Joint Surg [Am] 61:599–600

Lauche H (1947) Zur Kenntnis von Pathologie und Klinik der Geschwülste mit synovialmembranartigem Bau (Synovialome, oder synoviale Endothelio-Fibrome und Sarkome). Frankf Z Pathol 59:2–29

Lederer H, Sinclair AJ (1954) Malignant synovioma simulating "adamantinoma of the tibia." J Pathol Bacteriol 67:163–168

Lichtenstein L (1977) Bone tumors, 5th edn. Mosby, St. Louis, Missouri

Lipper S, Kahn LB (1983) Case report 235. Diagnosis: Ewing-like adamantinoma of the left radial head and neck. Skeletal Radiol 10:61–66

Llombart-Bosch A, Ortuño-Pacheco G (1978) Ultrastructural findings supporting the angioblastic nature of the so-called adamantinoma of the tibia. Histopathology 2:189–200

Maier C (1900) Ein primares myelogenes Platten-Epithelcarcinoma der Ulna. Bruns Beitr Chir 26:552–566

Markel SF (1978) Ossifying fibroma of long bone: its distinction from fibrous dysplasia and its association with adamantinoma of long bone. Am J Clin Pathol 69:91–97

Mills SE, Rosai J (1985) Adamantinoma of the pretibial soft tissue. Clinicopathologic features, differential diagnosis, and possible relationship to intraosseous disease. Am J Clin Pathol 83:108–114

Mirra JM, Kameda N (1985) Myxoid angioblastomatosis of bones: a case report of a rare, multifocal entity with light, ultramicroscopic, and immunopathologic correlation. Am J Surg Pathol 9:450–458

Moon NF (1965) Adamantinoma of the appendicular skeleton: a statistical review of reported cases and inclusion of 10 new cases. Clin Orthop 43:189–213

Moon NF (1973) Adamantinoma of the appendicular skeleton. Sound/Slide Program for the American Academy of Orthopedic Surgeons

Moon NF, Mori H (1986) Adamantinoma of the appendicular skeleton updated. Clin Orthop 204:214–237

Mori H, Yamamoto S, Hiramatsu K et al. (1984) Adamantinoma of the tibia: ultrastructural and immunohistochemic study with reference to histogenesis. Clin Orthop 190:299–310

Naji AF, Murphy JA, Stasney RJ, Neville WE, Chrenca P (1964) So-called adamantinoma of long bones: report of a case with massive pulmonary metastasis. J Bone Joint Surg [Am] 46:151–158

Pérez-Atayde AR, Kozakewich PW, Vawter GF (1985) Adamantinoma of the tibia: an ultrastructural and immunohistochemical study. Cancer 55:1015–1023

Pieterse AS, Smith PS, McClure J (1982) Adamantinoma of long bones: clinical, pathological and ultrastructural features. J Clin Pathol 35:780–786

Plump D, Haponik EF, Katz RS et al. (1986) Primary adamantinoma of rib: thoracic manifestations of a rare bone tumor. South Med J 79:352–355

Povysil C, Matejovsky Z (1981) Ultrastructure of adamantinoma of long bones. Virchows Arch [A] 393:233–244

Robinson HGB (1942) Adamantinoma of the tibia. JAMA 119:1524

Rosai J (1969) Adamantinoma of the tibia. Electron microscopic evidence of its epithelial origin. Am J Clin Pathol 51:786–792

Rosai J, Pinkus GS (1982) Immunohistochemical demonstration of epithelial differentiation in adamantinoma of the tibia. Am J Surg Pathol 6:427–434

Ryrie BJ (1932) Adamantinoma of the tibia. Aetiology and pathogenesis. Br Med J 2:1000–1003

Schajowicz F, Gallardo H (1967) Adamantinoma de tibia. Rev Ortop Traumatol Lat Am 12:105–118

Schajowicz F, Cabrini RL, Simes RJ (1971) Microscopia electrónica de "adamantinoma" de los huesos largos. Rev Ortop Traumatol Lat Am 16:185–194

Schajowicz F, Ackerman LV, Sissons HA (1972) Histological typing of bone tumors. International histological classification of tumors, No. 6. World Health Organization, Geneva

Schajowicz F, Itoiz ME, Santini Araujo E, et al. (1974) Immunohistochemical investigation of keratins as a marker for an epithelial differentiation of "adamantinoma" of long bones. Latin American Registry of Bone Pathology and Department of Radiobiology, National Atomic Energy Commission, Buenos Aires, Argentina

Schajowicz F, Santini Araujo E (1989) Adamantinoma of the tibia masked by fibrous dysplasia. Report of three cases. Clin Orthop Rel Res 238:294–301

Sowa DT, Dorfman HD (1986) Unusual localization of adamantinoma of long bones: report of a case of isolated fibular involvement. J Bone Joint Surg [Am] 68:293–296

Spjut HJ, Dorfman HD, Fechner RE, Ackerman LV (1971) Tumors of bone and cartilage. Atlas of tumor pathology, 2nd series, Fasc 5. Armed Forces Institute of Pathology, Washington, DC

Uehlinger EA (1957) Das Skelettsynoviom (Adamantinom). In: Roentgendiagnostik Ergebnisse, 1952–1956. Thieme, Stuttgart, pp 96–103

Unni KK, Dahlin DC, Beabout JW, Ivins JC (1974) Adamantinoma of long bones. Cancer 34:1796–1805

Weiss SW, Dorfman HD (1977) Adamantinoma of long bones: an analysis of nine new cases with emphasis on metastasizing lesions and fibrous dysplasia-like changes. Hum Pathol 8:141–153

Yoneyama T, Winter WG, Milsow L (1977) Tibial adamantinoma: its histogenesis from ultrastructural studies. Cancer 40:1138–1142

Zand A, Chamber GH, Street DM (1972) So-called "adamantinoma of long bone." Clin Orthop 86:178–182

CHAPTER VIII
Tumors Arising at Site of Preexisting Bone Lesions

1. Sarcoma Developing in Paget Disease of Bone

The development of sarcoma is the most serious complication of Paget disease. In fact, Paget's original case (1877) developed a fibrosarcoma in the radius after 22 years, and five of his 23 patients died of sarcoma. Although well recognized as a possible complication of Paget disease, the exact incidence of malignancy is difficult to establish because there is no reliable statistical information on the frequency of uncomplicated disease; in the world literature the reported incidence of malignancy ranges from 0.15% to 20%.

Incidence. The incidence of Paget disease is high in some countries (United Kingdom and Australia), average in some (North America, Germany, France, and Italy), and low in others (Sweden, Africa, and Asia). In Argentina and Brazil the incidence is similar to that in the United States.

The only reliable data on frequency come from the necropsy studies of Schmorl in Germany (1932). He found 138 cases of Paget disease out of 4614 necropsies on randomly selected people over 40 years of age, an incidence of 3%. Similar figures were reported by Collins (1956): 3.7% of 650 necropsies in patients aged over 40 revealed Paget disease.

Until the incidence of the disease itself is known, the frequency of malignant change cannot be established with certainty. The published data vary widely. In those series which consider only patients with advanced and clinically obvious disease the percentage with sarcoma is high – between 5% and 20% (Schajowicz 1942; Jaffe 1958; Goldenberg 1961; Lichtenstein 1977); when the large number of asymptomatic patients with mild Paget disease is considered, the complication rate is obviously much less, ranging from 0.15% (Price 1962; Sissons 1965; Price and Goldie 1969) to 0.9% and even 2% (Porretta et al. 1957; McKenna et al. 1964; Barry 1969). In a paper from the Mayo Clinic (Wick et al. 1981), out of 3964 patients with Paget disease seen between 1927 and 1977, 38 had primary malignant bone tumors; this represents an incidence of sarcomatous change of 0.95%. In more recent publications from the same institution (Greditzer et al. 1983), the figure was even lower. Our files contain 987 cases of Paget disease registered between April 1940 and the end of July 1981; 62 of these patients had developed sarcomas (6.28%) and two had giant-cell tumors without histologic signs of malignancy (Schajowicz et al. 1983).

Clinical Findings. *Sex and Age.* Most series report that Paget sarcoma is more common in men. In their review of the literature McKenna et al. (1964) reported 117 men and 52 women. Barry (1969), in his review of teaching hospitals in Australia, found that sarcoma occurred in 78 men and 38 women, though histologic proof was sometimes lacking. The largest series, collected from registries in Bristol, London, and Leeds, was reported by Ross, Middlemiss, and Fitton (1973); there were 145 cases of histologically proven sarcoma arising in Paget disease, with a sex ratio of 1.9 males to 1 female. In our 62 cases, however, there was only a slight male predominance (1.6:1). This was also true for Huvos et al. (1983), who diagnosed 65 cases of Paget osteosarcoma (36 men and 29 women) at Memorial Hospital, New York, during a 60-year span from 1921 through 1981. The Mayo Clinic (Dahlin and Unni 1986), in a series of 50 cases, had 32 males and 18 females.

Only one of our cases was observed before the age of 50, the tumor occurring most often between the ages of 50 and 70, the average age being 66 years. This agrees with the figures reported by Ross et al. (1973) (average age, 67.4 years) and Wick et al. (1981) (average age, 64 years).

Localization. The site of involvement and the type of sarcoma are shown in Table VIII.1. The most frequent sites, in descending order, were the

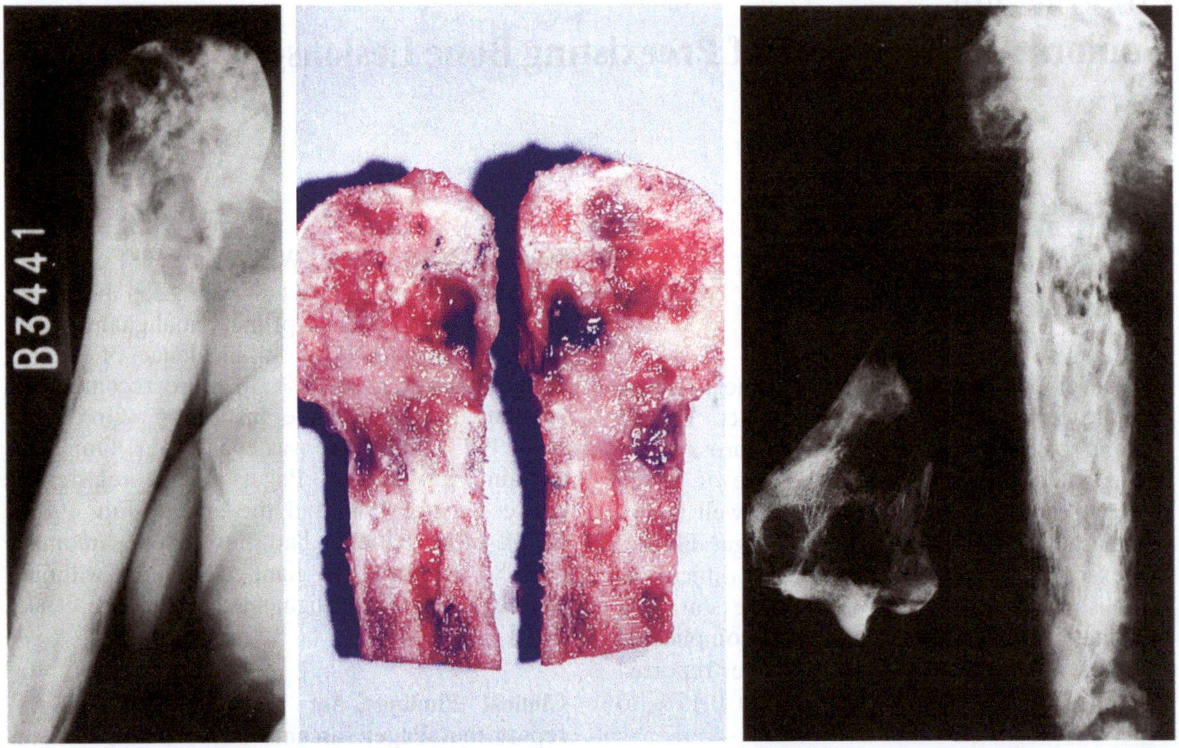

a, b c

Fig. VIII.1a–c. Male, 50 years old. Polyostotic Paget disease with multicentric osteosarcoma. **a** Radiograph showing Paget disease of the humerus with an osteolytic, ill-defined lesion at its upper end that destroyed the inner aspect of the cortex. **b** Photograph of a sagittal section of the amputation specimen showing the fleshy and hemorrhagic aspect of the tumor, the cortical destruction, and the evident hyperemia of the pagetic bone. **c** Radiograph of a thin section of the whole humerus reveals other osteolytic foci of sarcoma in the lower humeral end (at *left*, separated due to a pathologic fracture)

Table VIII.1. The varieties of sarcoma and their anatomic distribution (Schajowicz et al. 1983)

Site	Osteosarcoma	Fibrosarcoma	Chondrosarcoma	Malignant fibrohistiocytoma	Malignant lymphoma	Total
Femur	14	6	2	1	–	23
Humerus	4	5	–	–	–	9
Innominate bone	8	1	–	1	–	10
Tibia	5	2	2	–	–	9
Vertebra	2	1	1	–	1	5
Jaw	2	–	–	–	–	2
Cranium	2	–	–	–	–	2
Clavicle	1	–	–	–	–	1
Scapula	1	–	–	–	–	1
Total	39	15	5	2	1	62

femur (37%), the pelvis (16%), the humerus (14.5%), and the tibia (14.5%). Unlike other series (Barry 1961; McKenna et al. 1964; Huvos et al. 1983), in which the skull and facial bones were frequently involved, we had only four such cases; this is evidently due to the fact that we receive most of our material purely from orthopedic departments. That the humerus (Fig. VIII.1) is commonly affected has been pointed out by most authors (Lake 1951; Porretta et al. 1957; Barry 1969; Wick et al. 1981). Ross et al. (1973), in their series of 145 cases, found that sarcoma arose most frequently in the femur (39%), followed by the humerus (14.5%); our own findings were similar. On the other hand, Wick et al. (1981) and Huvos et al. (1983) found that the bone most commonly affected was the pelvis, followed by the humerus and the femur.

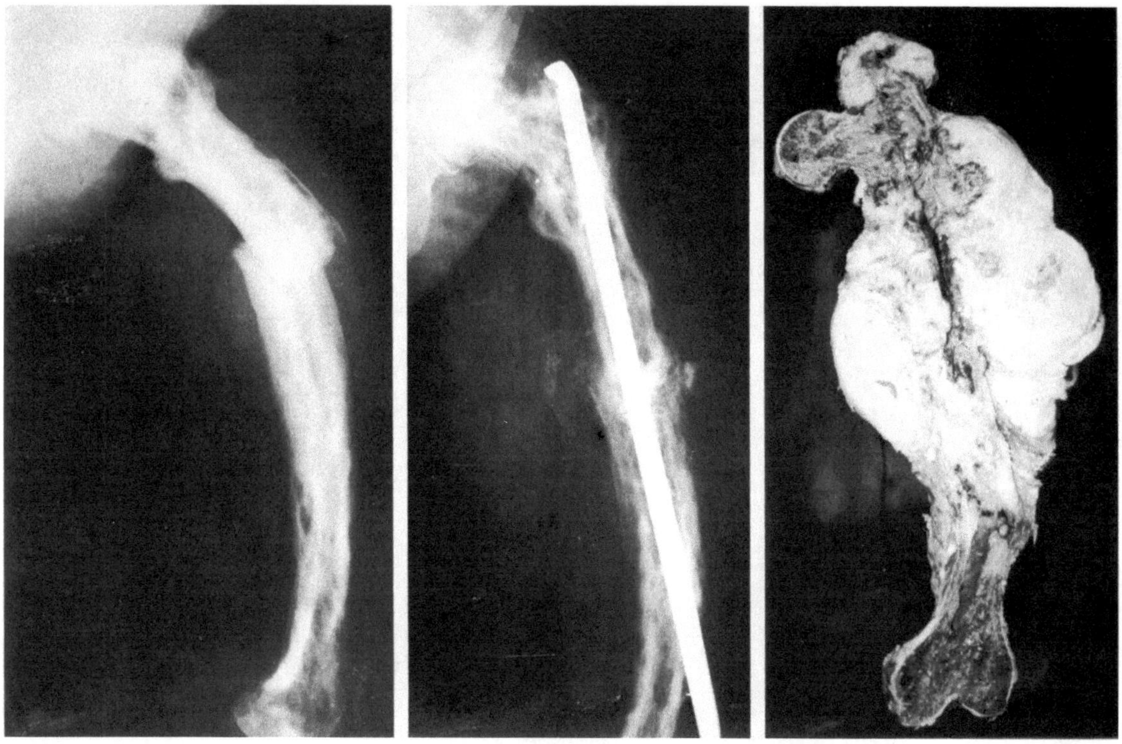

a, b c

Fig. VIII.2a–c. Female, 70 years old, who had polyostotic Paget disease for 21 years. Osteosarcoma arising in previous pathologic fracture of the femoral shaft. **a** Radiograph illustrates transverse fracture in femur shaft showing the characteristic alteration of bone structure. **b** Radiographic aspect 6 months after nailing. **c** Photograph of the amputation specimen illustrating the large tumor mass that developed 10 months later at the site of the previous fracture

The low incidence of vertebral sarcoma is evident in our series (only five cases) and in other large series – four of the 116 sarcomas in the Australian series (Barry 1969), three of the 145 reported by Ross et al. (1973), only one of Huvos' 65 cases (1983), and 1% in Wilner's (1982) review of 192 cases. The high proportion of sarcoma of the humerus, found in all series, is interesting and is in sharp contrast with uncomplicated Paget disease, which, according to Schmorl's necropsy studies, occurred most commonly in the sacrum (56%) and the spine (50%), followed by the right femur (31%) and the cranium (25%). We had no examples of sarcoma involving the distal parts of the upper and lower extremities.

Most cases of sarcoma developed in patients with polyostotic disease (Fig. VIII.2); it was rare in monostotic Paget disease. An interesting feature is the occurrence of multiple sarcomatous foci, which often developed simultaneously (or within short intervals) in different bones, or in different areas of the same bone. The incidence in our series, as in others (Ross et al. 1973), was between 16% and 30%, and the tumors occurred most frequently in the femur and skull. We wish to emphasize that whenever single or multifocal sarcoma developed in our series, it always occurred in a bone showing the characteristic changes of Paget disease. This agrees with the findings of Coley and Sharp (1931) and Huvos et al. (1983), and seems to favor a multicentric origin of the sarcomatous lesions rather than a metastatic spread, at least in the majority of cases.

Symptoms. The most constant symptoms are swelling, which is generally visible early, especially in the skull, and an increase in the existing pain which is so characteristic of Paget disease.

The effect of local injury, especially of fracture, on the development of sarcoma is not convincing; it occurred in only one of our cases, in which a neoplasm arose at the site of a healed fracture (Fig. VIII.2). Pathologic fracture through the sarcomatous area (Figs. VIII.3, VIII.4), on the other hand, was a frequent finding (20%, Schajowicz 1981).

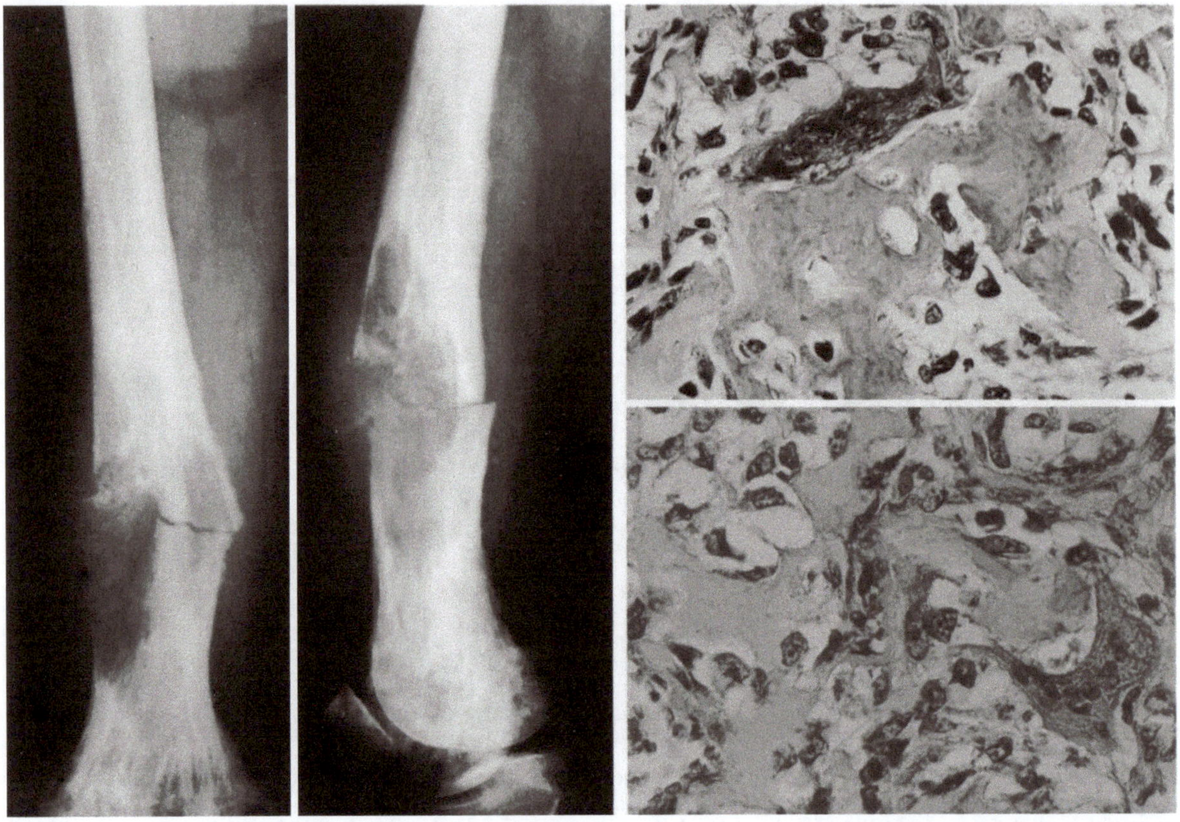

a

b

▲ **Fig. VIII.3a,b.** Male, 70 years old. Osteosarcoma arising in Paget disease of the femur at the site of a pathologic transverse fracture. **a** Anteroposterior and lateral radiographs showing the typical structural alterations with a pathologic fracture and a large ill-defined osteolytic lesion that destroyed part of the thinned cortex at its anterior aspect. **b** Photomicrographs illustrate tumor osteoid trabeculae surrounded by atypical osteoblasts, alternated with osteoclasts. ×400

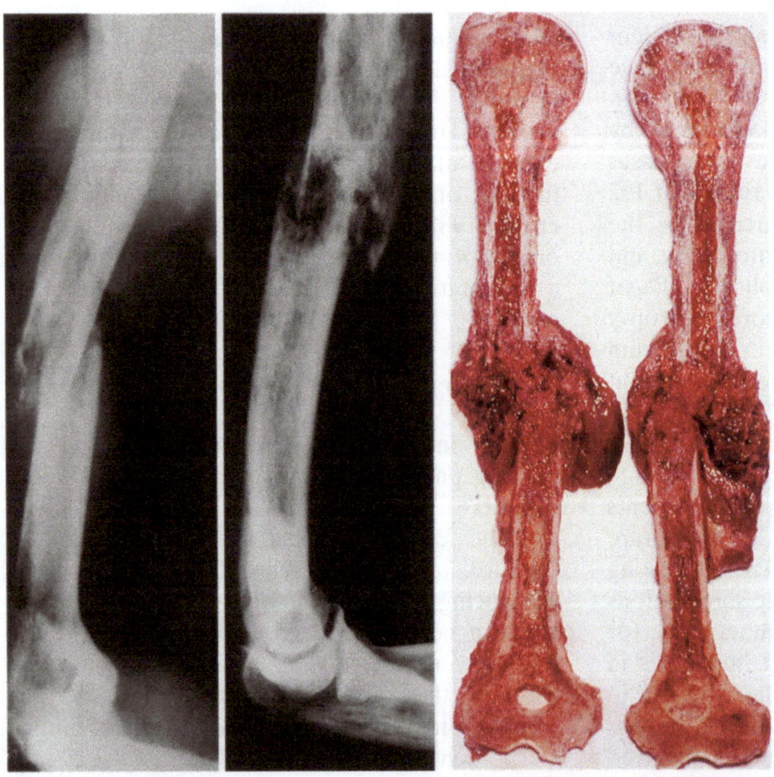

a, b

Fig. VIII.4a,b. Osteosarcoma in Paget disease of humerus in a male, 71 years old. **a** Anteroposterior and lateral radiographs show an osteolytic lesion in the midshaft with pathologic fracture. **b** Photograph of specimen illustrates typical Paget lesion in the upper end and the tumor mass of hemorrhagic aspect with soft tissue invasion

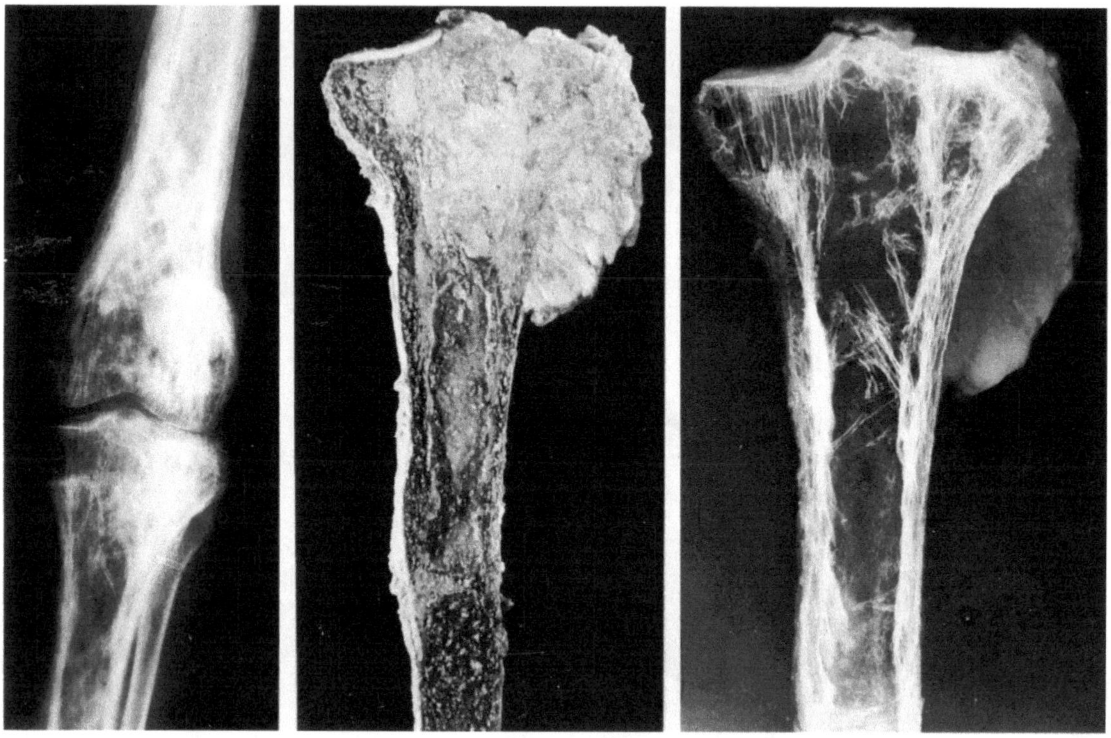

a b, c

Fig. VIII.5a–c. Female, 60 years old. Polyostotic Paget disease and secondary chondrosarcoma in the upper end of tibia. **a** Radiograph showing the characteristic changes of Paget disease of femur and tibia. The tumor, which has produced soft tissue swelling, is not clearly distinguishable in the radiograph. **b** Photograph of the amputation specimen reveals the extension of the tumor, involving the upper end of tibia and extending into soft tissues. Note the hyperemic aspect of the pagetic bone. **c** Radiograph of a 5-mm-thick section reveals that the tumor invaded the medullary cavity without conspicuous destruction of the cancellous bone

The alkaline phosphatase level usually rises abruptly above the already high values in uncomplicated Paget disease. But, because of the marked variation in alkaline phosphatase levels, this finding has no definite diagnostic value. The same considerations hold for the levels of urinary hydroxyproline excretion.

Radiographic Features. The radiographic appearances depend largely on the histologic type of the tumor, which, in 63% of our series and in 60% of Ross' series, was an osteosarcoma. In most instances the radiographs showed an ill-defined osteolytic lesion of the medulla with varying degrees of destruction of the cortex and penetration into the surrounding soft tissues (Figs. VIII.2, VIII.5). In Ross' series, soft tissue tumors occurred in 78 cases (57%) and destruction, either cortical or medullary, in nearly 90%. Only rarely was the tumor predominantly osteoblastic with intraosseous and extraosseous sclerosis. More often it was osteolytic with occasional irregular areas of reactive bone formation. With fibrosarcomas and with the other uncommon varieties of malignancy, the lesion was usually purely osteolytic (Fig. VIII.6), though two of the chondrosarcomas showed spots of calcification. The predominantly destructive nature of the lesions explains the frequency of pathologic fractures, which occurred in 20% of our cases and in 36% of Ross' series.

Pathologic Findings. The most common histologic type of tumor was osteosarcoma: this tumor type was found in 39 cases (63%) in our series, in 60% of cases in Ross' series (1973), and in 32 of the 38 sarcomas in the Mayo Clinic series (Wick et al. 1981). The next most common tumor type was a fibrosarcoma, with 15 cases (24%) in our series and 19% in that of Ross. The distribution of the other rarer tumor types (chondrosarcoma, five cases; malignant fibrohistiocytoma, two cases; and malignant lymphoma, one case), together with their location, is shown in Table VIII.1. We would emphasize that among these rare tumor types the diagnosis was definite in only two cases of chondrosarcoma, in which the complete amputation specimens were available;

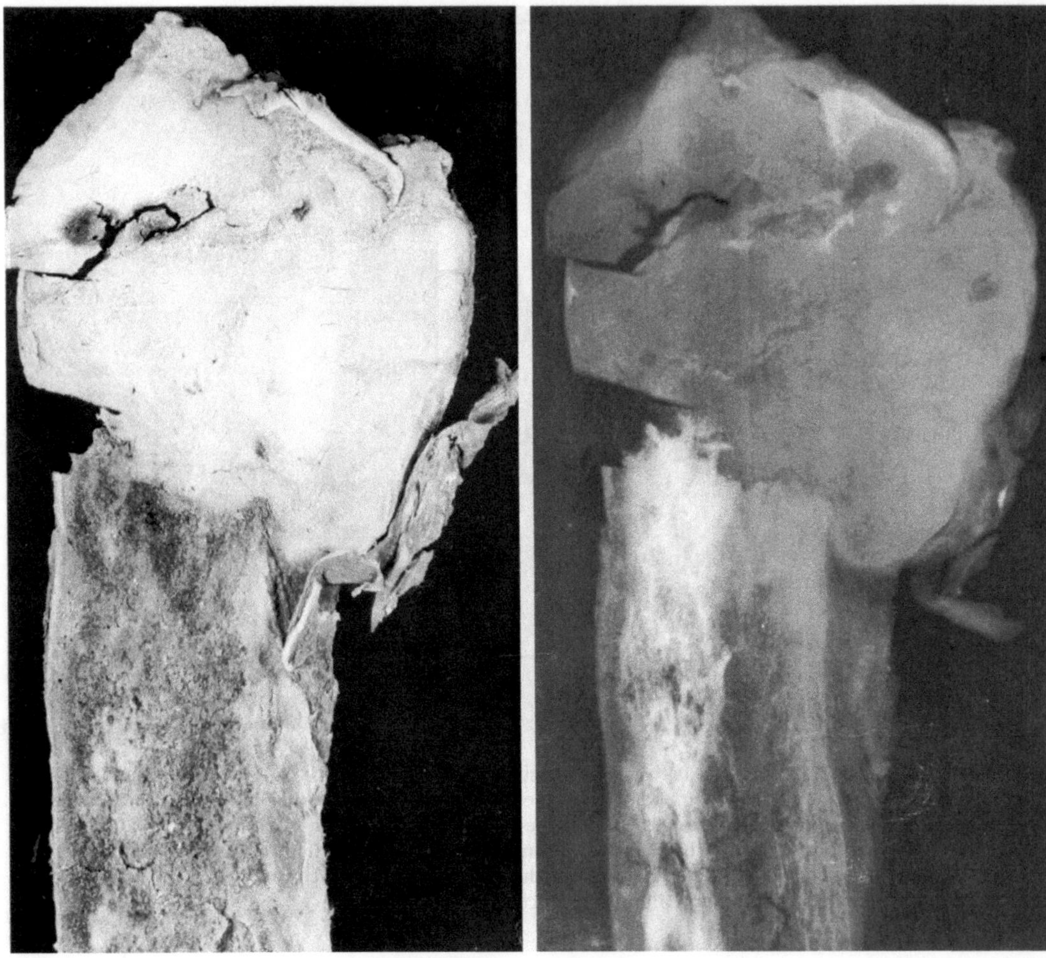

a b

Fig. VIII.6a,b. Male, 62 years old. Fibrosarcoma arising in monostotic Paget disease of tibia. **a** Photograph and **b** radiograph of the amputation specimen illustrate a large grayish-white osteolytic tumor of the upper end of the tibia

in the other cases only open or aspiration biopsies were performed, so that the presence of bone-forming tissue in other areas of the tumor (that is, an osteosarcoma) could not be definitely excluded. Only four instances of histologically verified malignant fibrohistiocytoma at the site of Paget disease have been previously reported, one by Spanier, Enneking, and Enriquez (1975) and three by Dahlin (1978). The number of malignant fibrohistiocytomas developing in Paget disease observed by us and by others is evidently low because by present standards of diagnosis, several pleomorphic fibrosarcomas would now be classified as malignant fibrohistiocytoma.

The histologic features are similar to those of the same type of sarcoma arising in normal bone, but frequently there is more anaplasia (Figs. VIII.7, VIII.8). However, in a large number of osteosarcomas complicating Paget disease, a particular histologic pattern was observed; it was characterized by a great number of osteoclast giant cells, alternating with numerous, often atypical, osteoblasts on the surface of the newly formed bone trabeculae (Figs. VIII.3b, VIII.7c). Thus the process of anarchic remodeling with alternation of osteoclastic bone resorption and osteoblastic bone apposition (the characteristic features of Paget disease; Fig. VIII.9) is reproduced or even exaggerated. The fact that a fairly large number of giant cells of osteoclastic type can often be seen in sarcomas arising in Paget disease (Schajowicz and Oleaga Alarcon 1945; Schajowicz 1981) means that great care is needed when making the differential diagnosis from an ordinary giant-cell tumor. Although extremely rare, *giant-cell tumors with no histologic signs of malignancy* may be associated with Paget disease. However, in contrast to osteosarcomas rich in

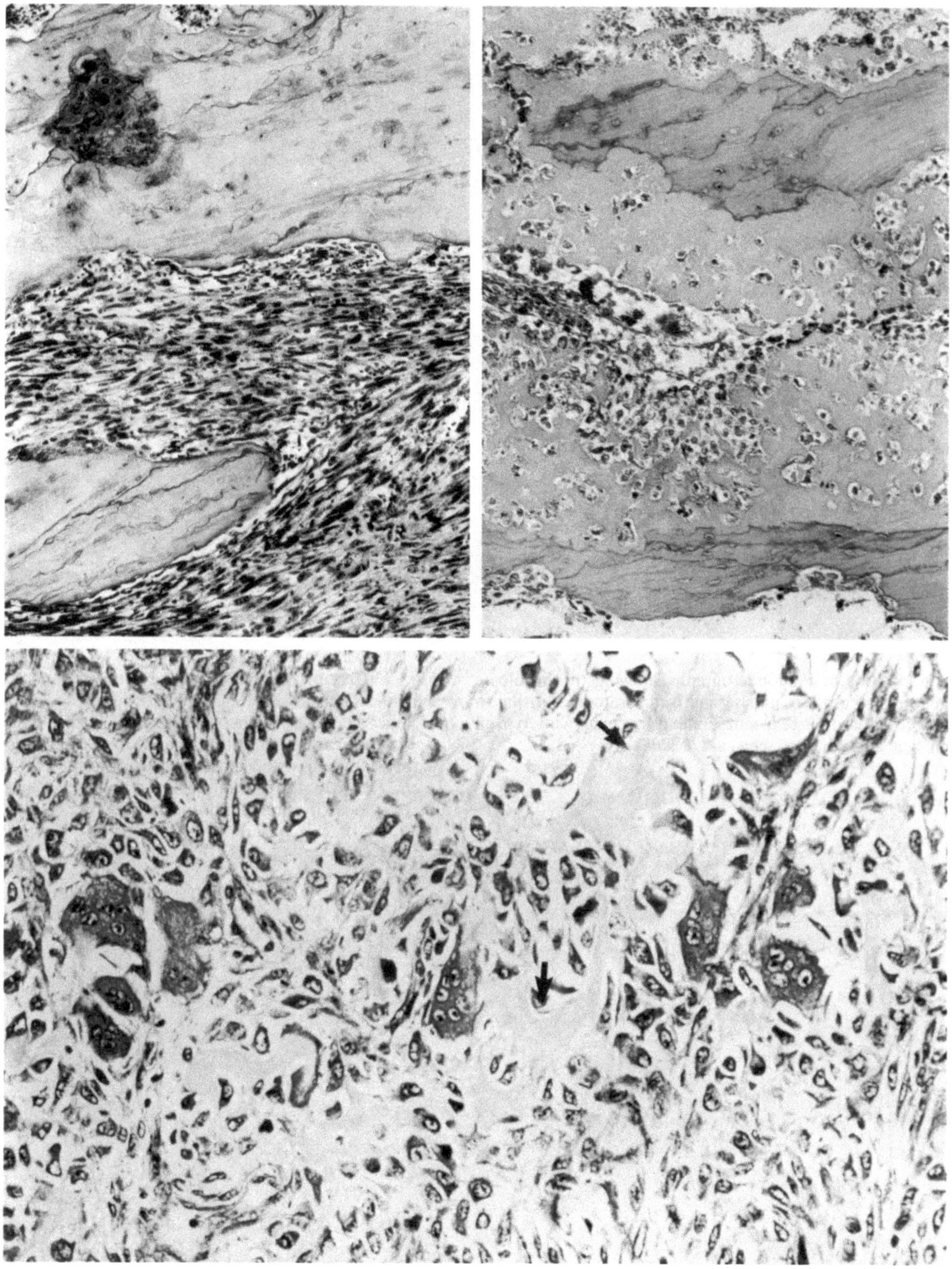

Fig. VIII.7a–c. Photomicrographs illustrating **a** highly cellular fibrosarcoma arising in Paget disease, **b** osteosarcoma with tumor bone and osteoid formation surrounding bone trabeculae with typical mosaic structure, and **c** osteosarcoma showing osteoid trabeculae surrounded by rows of osteoblasts, alternating with numerous osteoclasts, similar to the pattern of Paget disease. **a**,**b** ×120; **c** ×400

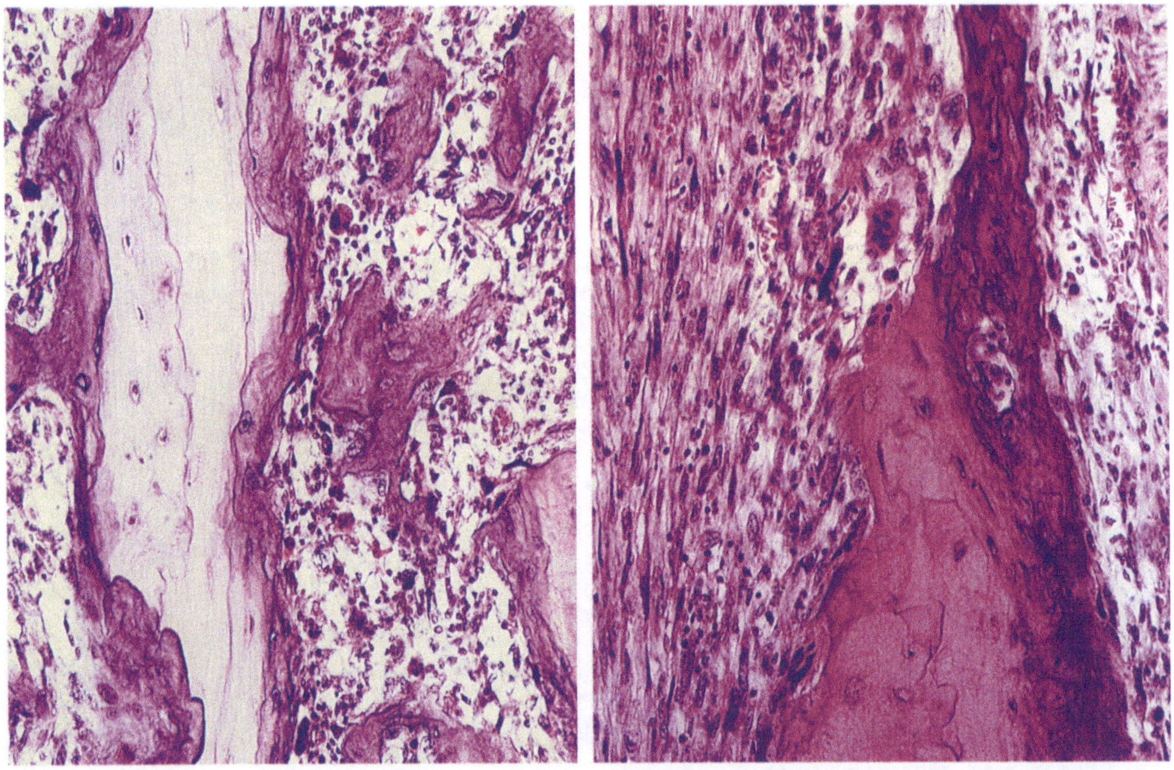

a b

▲ **Fig. VIII.8a,b.** Photomicrographs showing the histologic features of **a** osteosarcoma and **b** fibrosarcoma arising in Paget disease. Preexistent bone trabeculae with typical mosaic structure are seen. **a**,**b** ×200

Fig. VIII.9a,b. Photomicrographs at low and higher magnification showing the characteristic histologic features of Paget's disease of bone. The typical "mosaic" structure, due to the anarchic alteration of bone formation by rows of osteoblasts and osteoclastic bone resorption, is clearly seen. Between the thickened lamellar bone trabeculae, there is loose hyperemic fibrous marrow. **a** ×100, **b** ×300 ▼

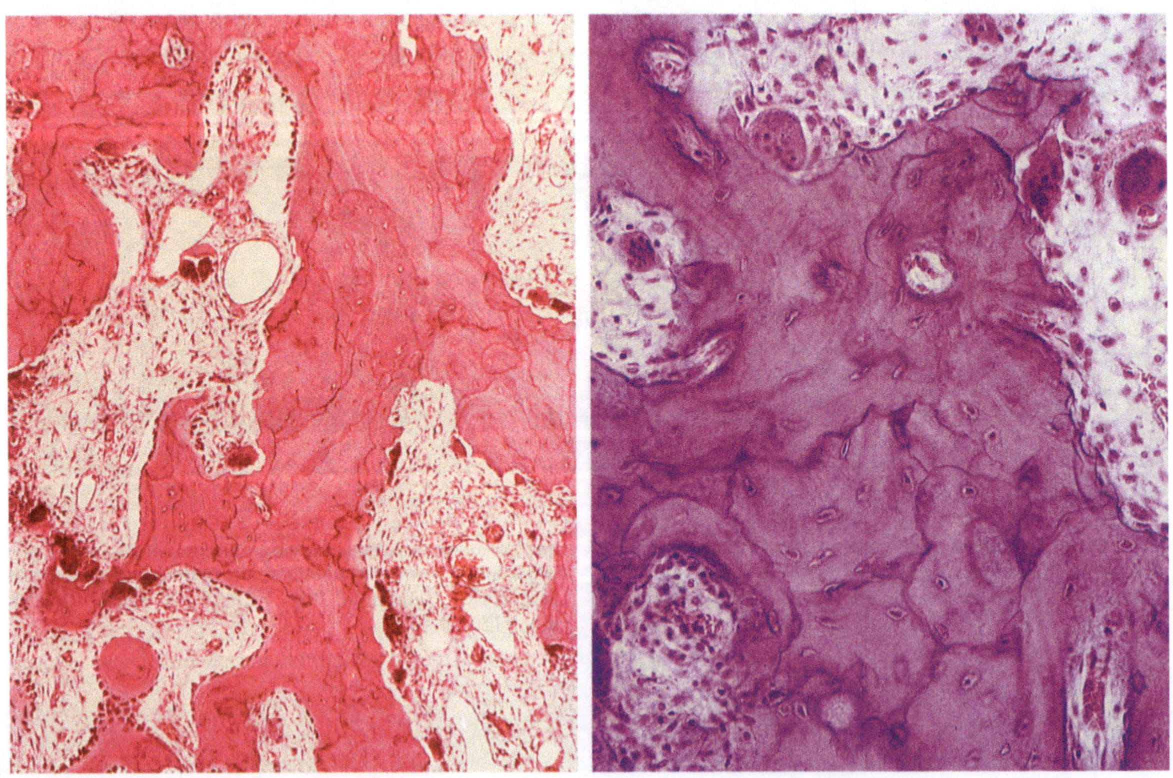

a b

giant cells, they have a relatively good prognosis; they are in fact less aggressive than giant-cell tumors originating in normal bones. To the small number of such cases found in the English literature by McKenna et al. (1964), we added another situated in the diaphysis of the tibia (a monostotic lesion) of a 45-year-old patient who was followed up for more than 4 years (Schajowicz and Slullitel 1966) (see Fig. III.46), and a second case affecting the clavicle, a rare site for Paget sarcoma; this tumor was resected and had not recurred after 3 years (Schajowicz et al. 1983).

The majority of such giant-cell tumors occur in the craniofacial bones (Jaffe 1958; Brooke 1970) and only a few cases have been found in the ilium (Campanacci 1990), humerus, or tibia. It is interesting that those arising in long bones do not involve the epiphyseal end of the bone.

In the last two decades viral-like intranuclear inclusions have been reported in the osteoclasts of Paget disease (Rebel et al. 1974; Mills and Singer 1976; Gherardi et al. 1980; Schajowicz et al. 1985). If we accept a viral etiology for Paget disease, and this has been supported by Mills et al. (1981), the same mechanism might cause the sarcomas which supervene. Mills and Singer (1976) have, in fact, reported identical inclusions in a sarcoma with giant cells arising in a case of Paget disease of the maxilla, and Mirra and coworkers (1981) described similar inclusions in a giant-cell tumor associated with Paget disease. Similar findings have previously been reported in isolated cases of giant-cell tumor (osteoclastoma) without Paget disease (Welsh and Meyer 1970; Le Charpentier et al. 1977; Vacher-Lavenu et al. 1981; Schajowicz et al. 1985; Fornasier et al. 1985). However, in the only case of osteosarcoma arising in Paget disease studied ultrastructurally by Reddick et al. (1980), no such inclusions were found in the giant-cell osteoclasts. Future studies investigating the presence of similar inclusions in osteoclast giant cells in Paget sarcoma are needed; if they are found, this would support a viral etiology.

The few cases reported as malignant giant-cell tumors are in our opinion examples of osteosarcomas rich in giant cells or malignant fibrous histiocytomas; a positive histochemical finding of alkaline phosphatase could help to establish the diagnosis of osteosarcoma in those cases in which tumor osteoid tissue is rare or apparently nonexistent (Schajowicz and Cabrini 1954; Sanerkin and Jeffree 1980). Another conspicuous finding was the increased number of osteoclasts in the areas of pagetic bone adjacent to the tumor. All these histologic findings in osteosarcoma associated with Paget disease are responsible for the most common osteolytic pattern and seem to support a close histogenetic relationship between the two.

Pathogenesis. It seems clear that a close histopathogenetic relationship exists between Paget disease and the associated sarcoma. This supposition is based on three separate observations.

Firstly, osteosarcoma complicating Paget disease occurs at an age when osteosarcoma is otherwise rare. Coley and Sharp (1931) first emphasized that 28% of osteosarcomas occurring in patients of more than 50 years of age had Paget disease. Sissons (1965) found that 26% of all primary malignant bone tumors occurring in patients over 40 years of age were associated with Paget disease and that this percentage rose progressively with increasing age. In our series Paget sarcoma was most common after 55 years of age.

Secondly, in our series, whenever sarcoma (whether single or multiple) developed, this always occurred in bones which were already affected by Paget disease: this agrees with the findings of Coley and Sharp (1931). When sarcomas were multiple, they were frequently more or less synchronous, and they affected different areas of one single, already pagetic, bone or several already pagetic bones (Huvos et al. 1983). This also suggests that, in most instances at least, there is a multicentric origin of the sarcomatous change rather than a metastatic spread.

The third feature was that, in the pagetic bone or the sarcoma, there was a conspicuous increase in the cellular activity involved in the remodeling process, especially in the number of osteoclast giant cells. Frequently the osteosarcoma developing in pagetic bone showed a great number of giant cells of osteoclastic type, accompanied by active and atypical osteoblasts, thus imitating in an exaggerated manner the process of anarchic remodeling characteristic of Paget disease. In our opinion these observations constitute important findings favoring a close pathogenetic relationship between Paget disease and its sarcomatous transformation.

In a few cases, we found an increase in the number and activity of the fibroblasts in the fibrous marrow in the vicinity of the sarcoma (especially with fibrosarcomas); this finding has been reported previously by von Albertini (1928). We also agree with him that the cellular features

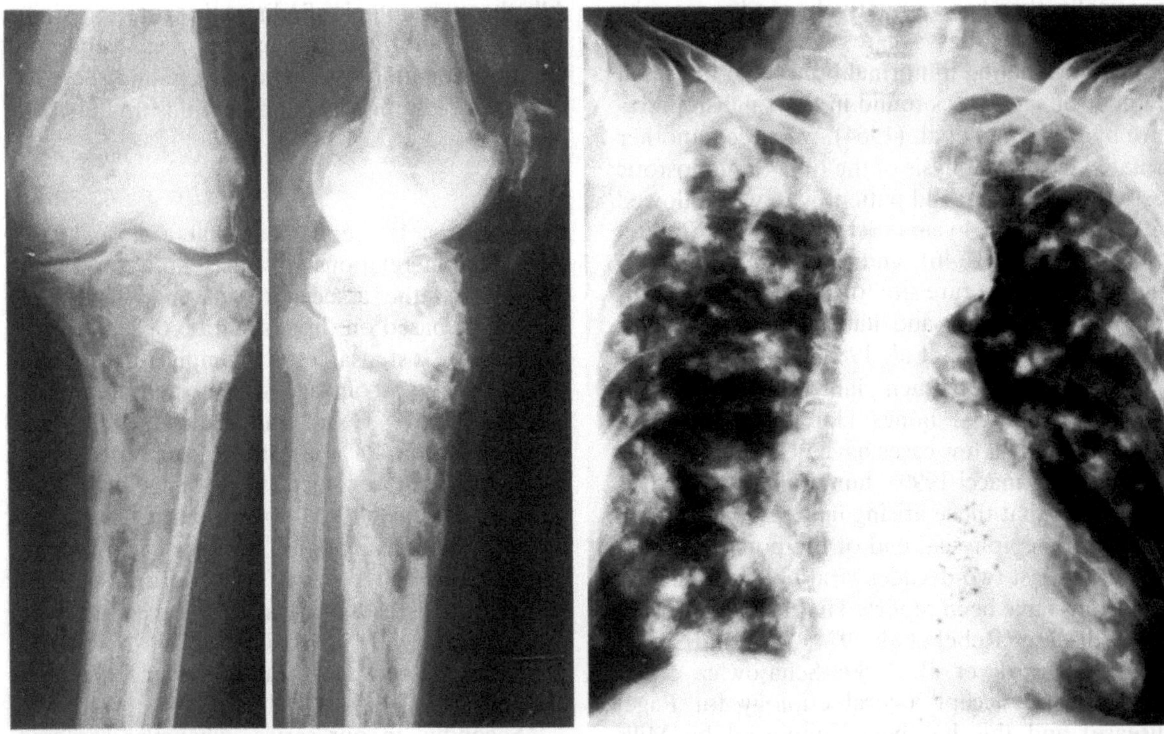
a b

Fig. VIII.10a,b. Female, 60 years old. Osteosarcoma arising in the tibia after internal therapeutic use of radium. **a** Anteroposterior and lateral radiographs illustrate the extensive osteolytic and permeative lesions with areas of sclerosis in the upper tibia. **b** Numerous pulmonary metastatic nodules. (Courtesy of Dr. J. Petasnick, Chicago)

suggest that Paget disease may possibly be considered a presarcomatous lesion.

Finally, it should be pointed out that although sarcomas arising in Paget disease are relatively rare, the absolute number of patients with this complication is significant, because Paget disease is so common.

Treatment and Prognosis. The prognosis of Paget sarcoma is poor. It is particularly bad in patients with (a) tumors not amenable to operation, (b) pathologic fractures, (c) multicentric lesions, or (d) histologically anaplastic and pleomorphic tumors. In the Australian series of 116 patients (Barry 1969), none survived more than 5 years; most cases were rapidly fatal, death occurring within 12 months of the onset of the sarcoma.

Only a few cases have been reported with a survival of more than 5 years. All were treated by amputation or disarticulation, with or without radiotherapy: one by Russell (1949), two by Platt (1947), followed up and reported by Stevens and Lennox (1958), one by Cowie et al. (1958), two by Schatzki and Dudley (1961), two by Price and Goldie (1969), three by Dahlin (1978), and three by Huvos et al. (1983). Russell reported a malignant osteoclastoma arising in Paget disease. This patient, a woman of 59, had a tumor of the tibia treated by midthigh amputation and was alive and well after more than 10 years; this tumor was probably a giant-cell-rich osteosarcoma. In our series we had only one patient who survived more than 5 years; the tumor was a fibrosarcoma in the upper tibia (which was the only bone affected by Paget disease) and was treated by midthigh amputation (Fig. VIII.6).

2. Postradiation Sarcoma of Bone

Ionizing radiation in the form of radionuclides or external radiation may cause serious damage to the musculoskeletal system, such as growth disturbances, necrosis of the osseous tissue, radiation osteitis, and, on rare occasions, bone sarcomas.

Sarcoma related to internal radiation was first reported as an industrial hazard by Martland (1929, 1931), who noted the appearance of osteosarcomas several years after the ingestion of radioactive particles of radium 226 by watch painters who had the habit of pointing their brushes in their mouths. Another cause of skeletal sarcomas after radiation was the ingestion of radium salts and/or mesothorium, administered for therapeutic purposes in the United States in the 1920s to numerous patients affected with various medical disorders, including rheumatic diseases (Fig. VIII.10) (Looney 1955, 1966) and bone tuberculosis (Spiess and Mays 1970; Hasterlik and Finkel 1965). Intravenous injection of Thorotrast has produced malignant tumors, such as the Thorotrast-induced osteosarcoma (Altner et al. 1972) and the chondrosarcoma of the axilla in a 38-year-old male reported by Schajowicz et al. (1967). The potential danger of bone-seeking radionuclides in the induction of bone tumors has been established in experimental animals by a number of workers and has been studied in humans, especially after the use of long-range β-emitters such as strontium 90.

The first cases of sarcoma as a result of overexposure to *external* radiation were reported several years after x-ray therapy given for osteoarticular tuberculosis (Beck 1925; Kuttner 1931). In 1945, Hatcher published a report of the development of sarcoma in normal bone in the field of irradiation.

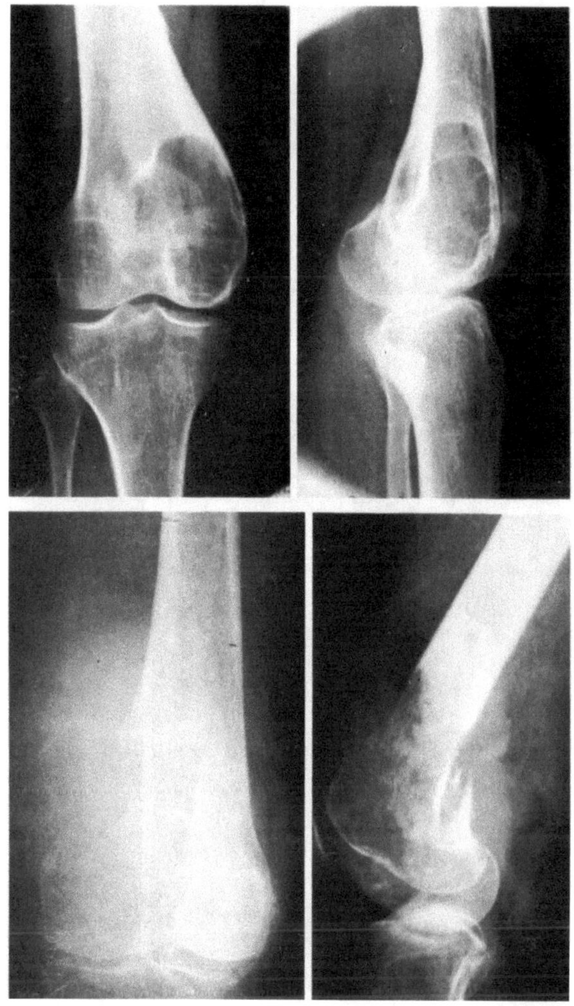

a

b

Fig. VIII.11a,b. Female, 41 years old. Fibrosarcoma arising in giant-cell tumor of lower femoral end 8 years after curettage and conventional radiation therapy. **a** Anteroposterior and lateral radiographs illustrate typical giant-cell tumor of medial femur condyle. **b** Anteroposterior and lateral radiographs show the large destructive ill-defined lesion with pathologic fracture. The patient died a few months later with pulmonary metastases

The most common types of radiation-induced sarcoma are osteosarcoma, fibrosarcoma, and malignant fibrous histiocytoma. Steiner (1965) reported 92 cases, half of which were osteosarcomas and half, fibrosarcomas. The Mayo Clinic's series (Dahlin and Unni 1986) of 103 postradiation sarcomas included 52 osteosarcomas, 35 fibrosarcomas, eight malignant fibrous histiocytomas, four chondrosarcomas, one Ewing sarcoma, one malignant lymphoma, and one metastasizing chondroblastoma. The tumors are related to the dosage, type, and site of irradiation, the age of the patient, and other factors. The interval between time of irradiation and development of sarcoma is variable, ranging from 2.75 to 55 years, with an average of 15.9 years in the Mayo Clinic series and 11 years in other series. Ninety-four cases of postradiation sarcomas of bone and soft tissues were seen in the Memorial Hospital, New York (Huvos et al. 1985, 1986; Huvos 1991), including 66 osteosarcomas, 20 malignant fibrous histiocytomas, four fibrosarcomas, and four chondrosarcomas. The time interval between radiation and sarcoma varied from 3.5 to 33 years for osteosarcomas and from 4 to 47 years for malignant fibrous histiocytomas. The radiation dosage and the incidence of sarcoma seem to be related. In general, larger doses seem to result in a higher number of malignant tumors, the lowest dose in adults having been recorded by Cahan et al. (1948) – 30 Gy. The risk of damage is higher in young children, and in addition to malignant bone tumors, growth disturbances or benign bone lesions, such as osteochondromas, are often produced.

The following criteria for diagnosing postradiation sarcoma were established by Cahan et al. (1948): (1) the initial bone or soft tissue in which the radiation-induced sarcoma develops is nonmalignant; (2) the sarcoma must have arisen within the irradiated region; (3) there is a rela-

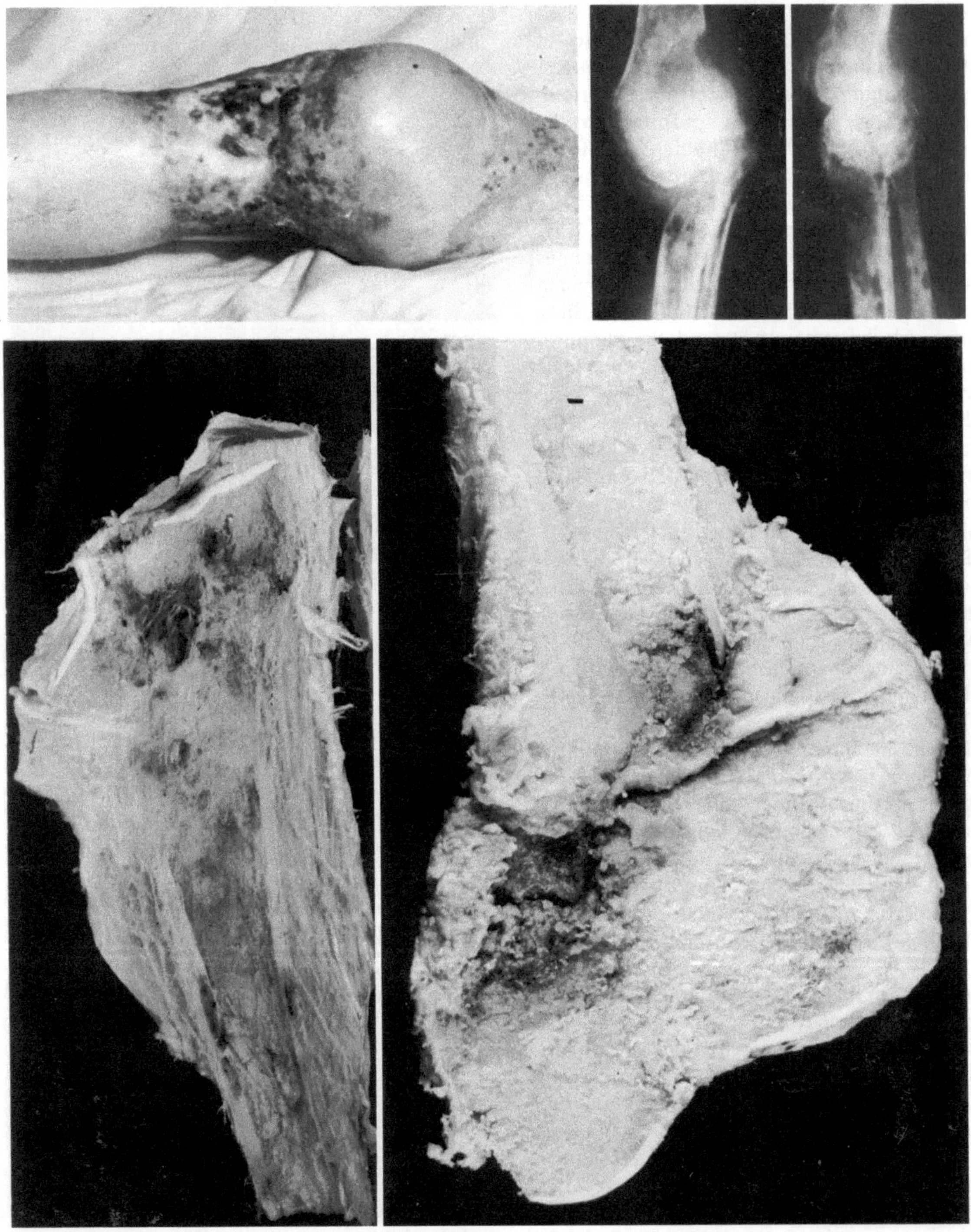

a b c

Fig. VIII.12a–f. Female, 18 years old, who developed fibrosarcoma 5 years after conventional radiotherapy for giant-cell tumor of tibia. **a** Photograph of the amputation specimen shows the extensive skin alteration and a large swelling at the knee region. **b** Anteroposterior and lateral radiographs illustrate the extensive destructive lesions in the upper tibia and lower end of the femur, with sclerotic margins. **c** Photographs of a section of the amputation specimen show the large grayish-white tumor mass in the lower femur and upper tibia and the deformation of this bone.

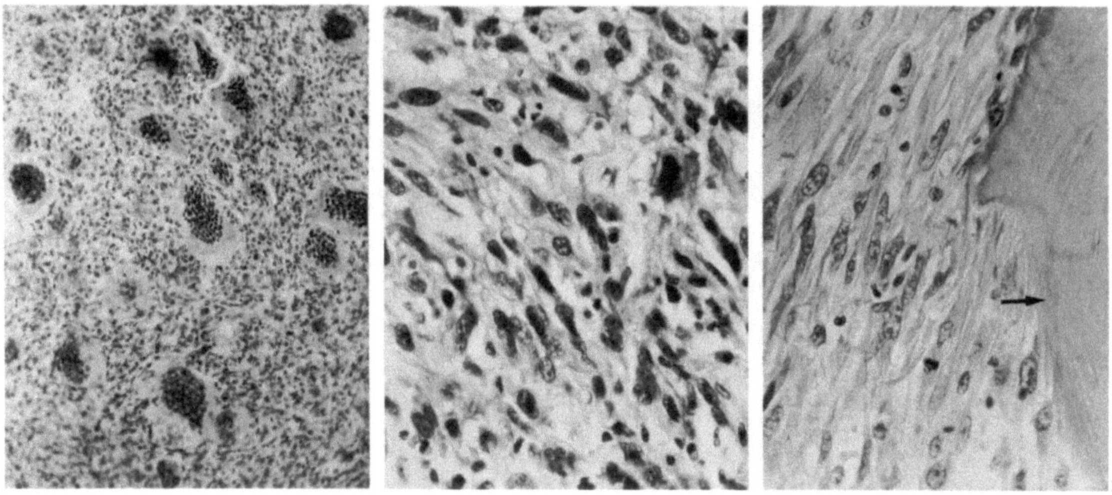

d, e f

Fig. VIII.12 (continued). **d** Photomicrograph showing the characteristic histologic pattern of the giant-cell tumor before treatment. **e,f** Pleomorphic high-grade fibrosarcoma after curettage and irradiation. In **f**, necrotic bone trabecula at *left*. **d** ×100, **e,f** ×400

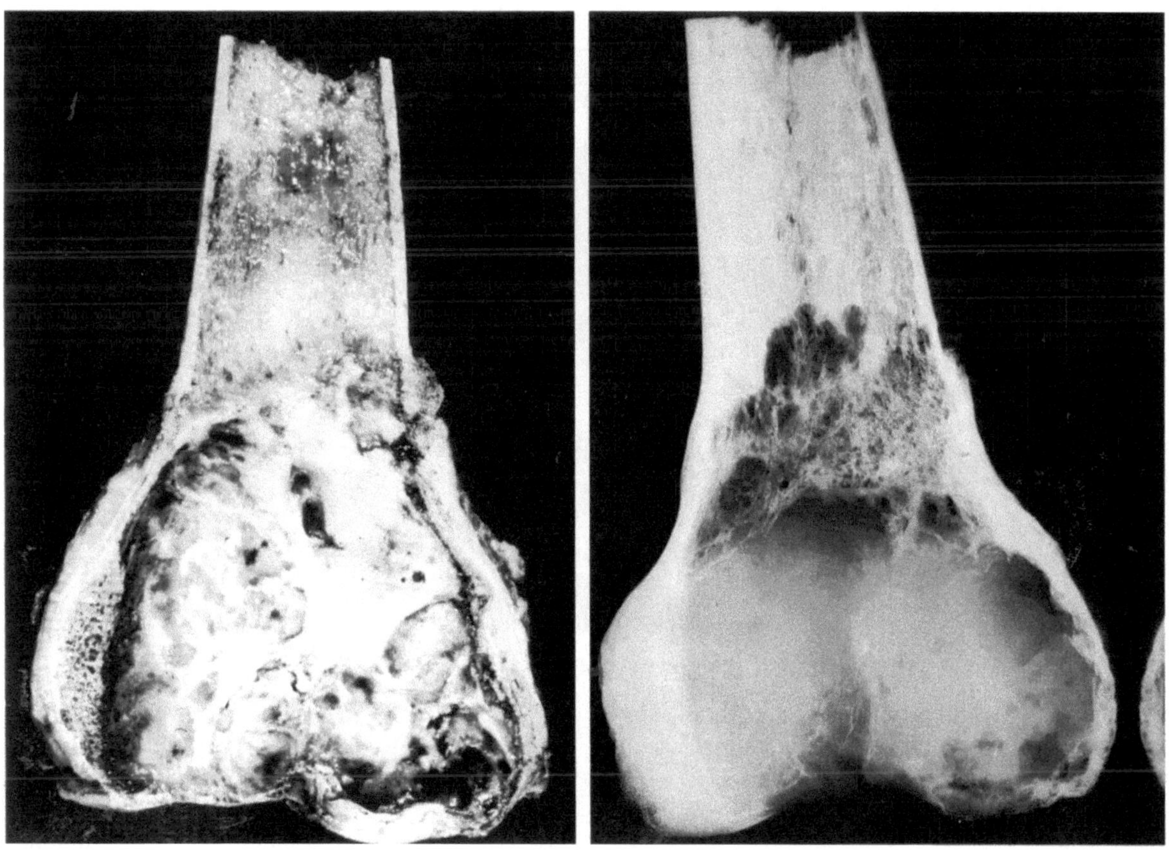

a b

Fig. VIII.13a,b. Male, 35 years old. Fibrosarcoma developing in giant-cell tumor of femur. **a** Photograph and **b** radiograph of amputation specimen illustrate a large tumor of grayish-white color involving the lower end of femur, with partial destruction of the joint borders and ill-defined margins toward the medullary cavity

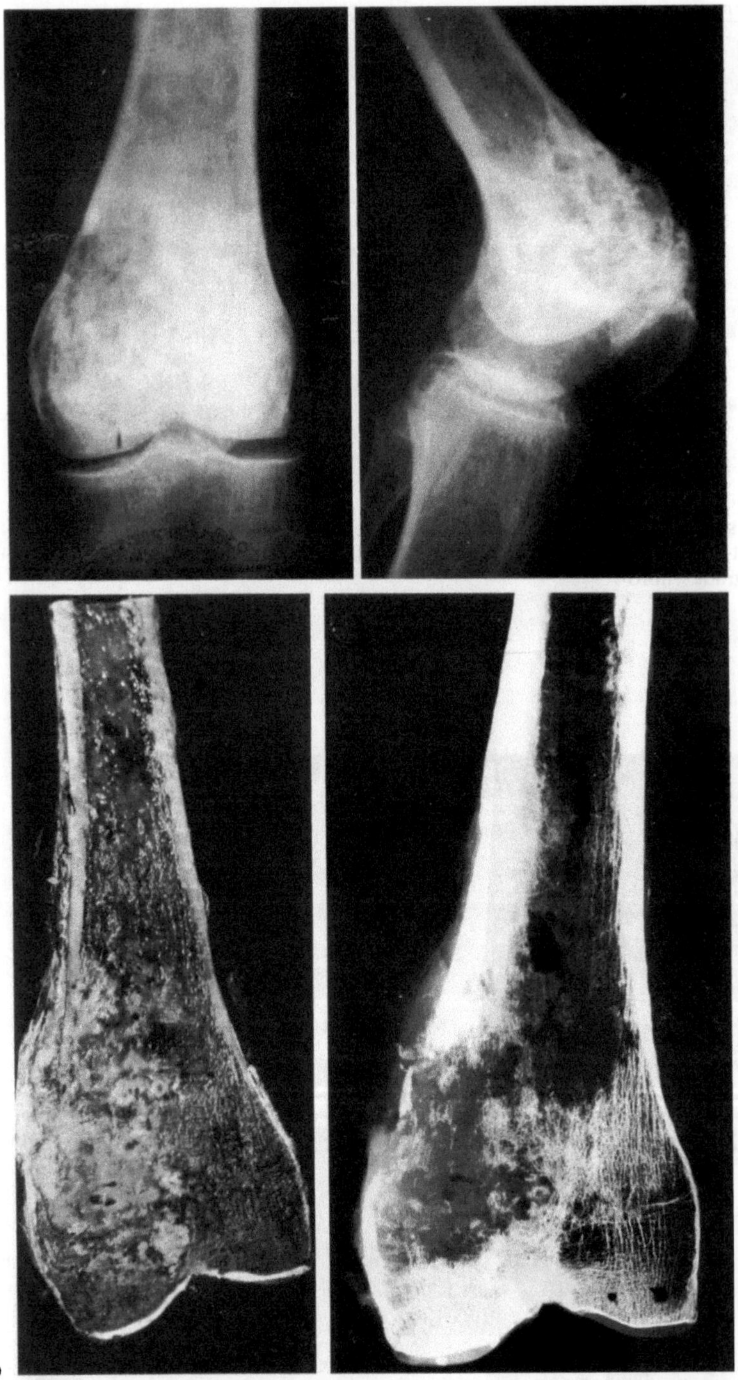

a b c

Fig. VIII.14a–c. Male, 27 years old. Osteosarcoma arising in irradiated giant-cell tumor of femur. **a** Anteroposterior and lateral radiographs 12 years after curettage and irradiation of giant-cell tumor showing eccentric osteolytic lesion in the femur condyle, alternating with irregular areas of sclerosis. **b** Photograph and **c** radiograph of the amputation specimen demonstrating the ill-defined borders of the predominantly osteolytic tumor. The patient developed inguinal lymph gland and pulmonary metastases 10 months later

tively long asymptomatic latent period; (4) the sarcomatous nature of the postradiation lesion must be established histologically.

The development of increasing pain, swelling, edema, and tenderness, in addition to radiographic, mostly osteolytic changes, leads the clinician to suspect the development of malignant change.

In our files there are 16 cases of postradiation sarcoma, ten of which occurred after irradiation of giant-cell tumors as the sole treatment or combined with curettage; the interval between irradiation and development of the sarcoma ranged from 5 to 18 years (Figs. VIII.11–VIII.15). Most cases were fibrosarcomas. It is possible that, following present criteria, several

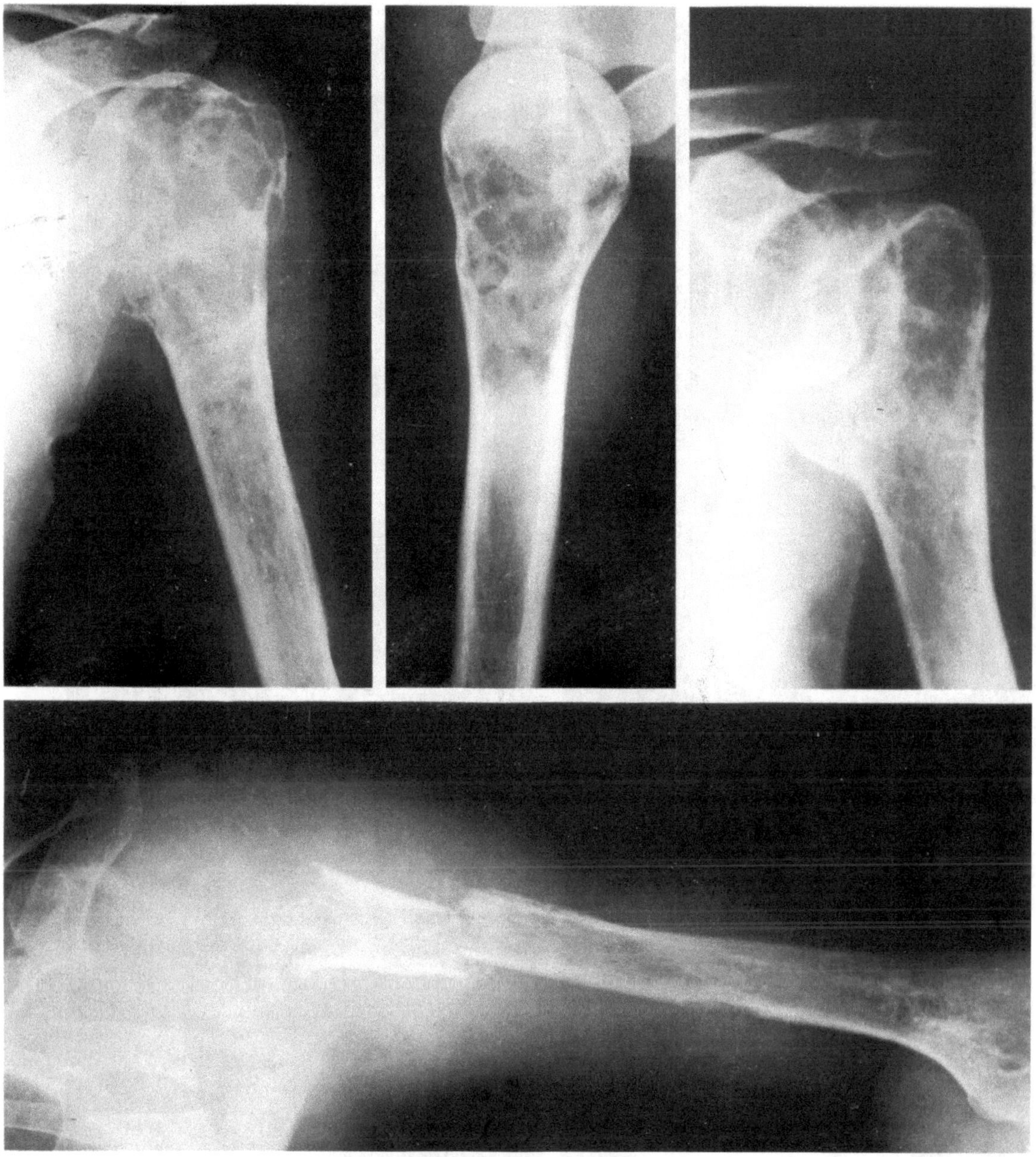

a b, c d

Fig. VIII.15a–d. Male, 44 years old. Osteosarcoma of humerus arising in giant-cell tumor 11 years after irradiation. **a** Radiograph of the giant-cell tumor before treatment. **b,c** Radiographs 8 months and 5 years after irradiation, showing the apparent complete regression of the lesion. **d** Radiograph 11 years after irradiation. A huge tumor developed which destroyed the upper end of the humerus and extensively invaded the shaft, producing a pathologic fracture

of the pleomorphic fibrosarcomas would be classified as malignant fibrous histiocytoma. In a case of metaphyseal fibrous defect, a fibrosarcoma developed 15 years after repeated curettages and radiotherapy (see Fig. IX.52). In another case, a multicentric osteosarcoma developed 10 years after radiation of the humerus because of suspicious metastases of a breast cancer with sarcomatous foci in the humerus and radius (Fig. VIII.16).

Once the sarcoma has developed, the prognosis is poor; the tumor usually metastasizes and causes death in a short period. The *treatment* indicated is surgical ablation (amputation or disarticulation) for lesions in the extremities. Sim et al. (1972) had only two long-term survivors

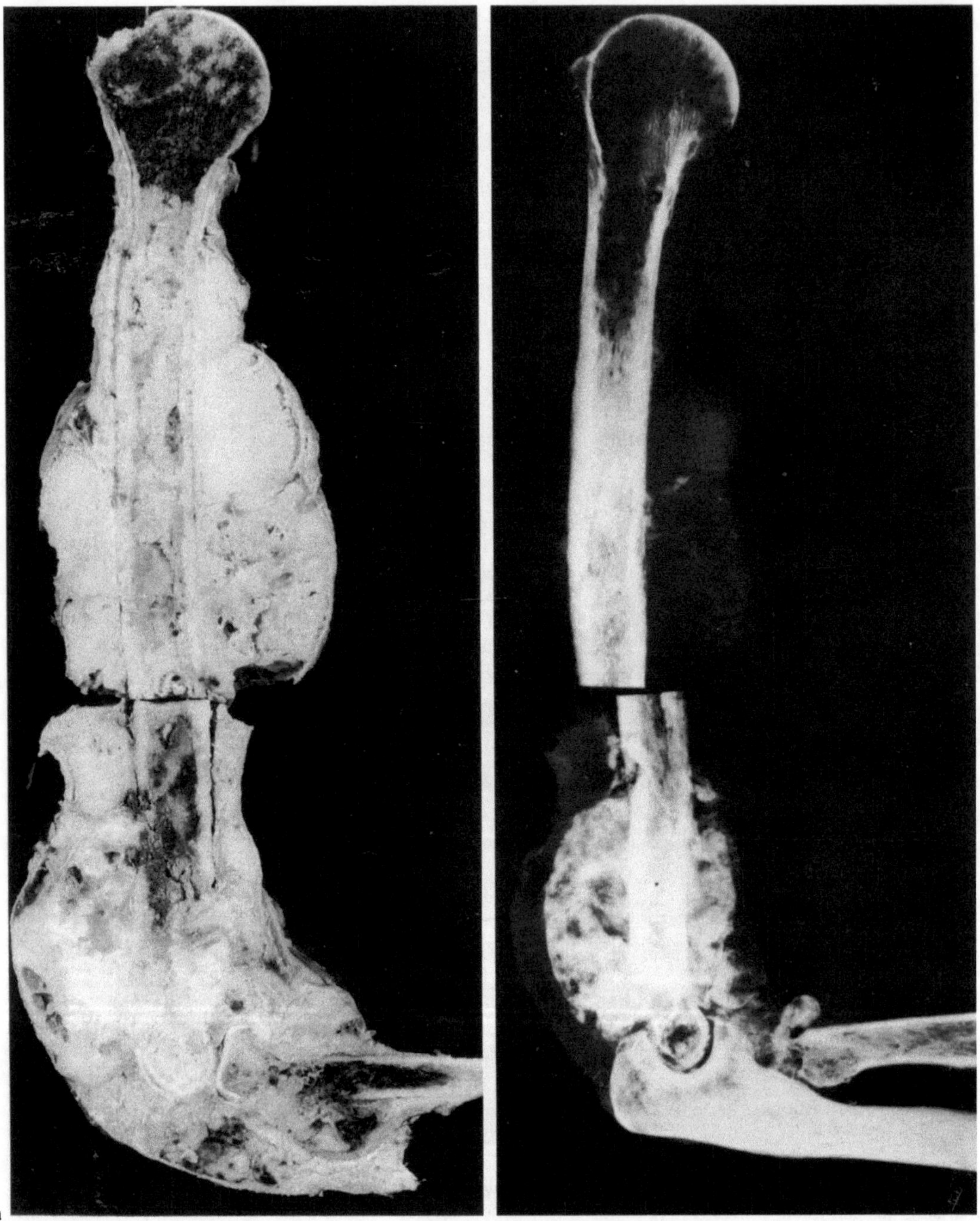

a b

Fig. VIII.16a,b. Female, 69 years old. Multicentric postradiation osteosarcoma in humerus and upper end of radius. The patient was irradiated because of suspicion of metastases from breast cancer in the humeral shaft without histologic proof. Ten years after radiation she developed osteosarcoma involving the major part of the humerus and the upper end of the radius, that is, in the field of irradiation as seen in the photograph and radiograph of the amputation specimen (**a**,**b**) among 50 patients with postradiation sarcomas, the average survival being a little over 1 year. Arlen et al. (1971), from the Memorial Hospital and Cancer Center (New York), had more favorable results, reporting nine 5-year survivors among 28 patients, following early aggressive surgical treatment for accessible lesions. In lesions located in surgically inaccessible regions, such as the trunk and pelvis, the prognosis was extremely poor in all series. The role of preoperative chemotherapy followed by surgery and adjuvant chemotherapy, which seems to only slightly improve the 5-year survival of the patient, has not yet been established.

References

Sarcoma Developing in Paget Disease of Bone

Agha FP, Norman A, Hirschl S et al. (1976) Paget's disease: coexistence with metastatic carcinoma. NY State J Med 76:734–735

Anderson JT, Dehner LP (1976) Osteolytic form of Paget's disease: differential diagnosis and pathogenesis. J Bone Joint Surg [Am] 58:994–1000

Barry HC (1961) Sarcoma in Paget's disease of bone in Australia. J Bone Joint Surg [Am] 43:1122–1134

Barry HC (1969) Paget's disease of bone. Williams & Wilkins, Baltimore

Brooke RI (1970) Giant cell tumor in patients with Paget's disease. Oral Surg 30:230–241

Campanacci M (1990) Bone and soft tissue tumors. Springer, Vienna New York

Choquette D, Haraoui B, Altman RD et al. (1983) Simultaneous multifocal sarcomatous degeneration in Paget's disease of bone: a hypothesis. Clin Orthop 179:308–311

Coley BL (1960) Neoplasms of bone and related conditions, 2nd edn. Paul Hoeber, New York

Coley BL, Sharp GS (1931) Paget's disease. A predisposing factor to osteogenic sarcoma. Arch Surg 23:918–936

Coley BL, Sharp GS, Ellis EB (1931) Diagnosis of bone tumors by aspiration. Am J Surg 13:215–224

Collins DH (1956) Paget's disease of bone: incidence and subclinical forms. Lancet II:51–57

Cowie RS, Barr JS, Dudley HR Jr (1958) Bone sarcoma in Paget's disease: report of a case with long survival. J Bone Joint Surg [Br] 40:730–734

Dahlin DC (1978) Bone tumors, 3rd edn. Charles C. Thomas, Springfield, IL

Dahlin DC, Unni KK (1986) Bone tumors: general aspects and data on 8542 cases. Charles C. Thomas, Springfield, IL

Fornasier VL, Flores L, Hastings D et al. (1985) Virus-like filamentous intranuclear inclusions in a giant-cell tumor, not associated with Paget's disease of bone. J Bone Joint Surg [Am] 67:333–336

Gherardi G, Lo Cascio V, Bonucci E (1980) Fine structure of nuclei and cytoplasm of osteoclasts in Paget's disease of bone. Histopathology 4:63–74

Goldenberg RR (1961) Neoplasia in Paget's disease of bone. Bull Hosp Joint Dis 22:1–38

Grader J, Moynihan JW (1961) Multiple myeloma and osteogenic sarcoma in a patient with Paget's disease. JAMA 176:685–687

Greditzer HG III, McLeod RA, Unni KK et al. (1983) Bone sarcomas in Paget disease. Radiology 146:327–333

Hutter RVP, Foote FW, Frazell EL, Francis KC (1963) Giant cell tumors complicating Paget's disease of bone. Cancer 16:1044–1056

Huvos AG (1986) Osteogenic sarcoma of bones and soft tissues in older persons: a clinicopathologic analysis of 117 patients older than 60 years. Cancer 57:1442–1449

Huvos AG, Butler A, Bretsky SS (1983) Osteogenic sarcoma associated with Paget's disease of bone: a clinicopathologic study of 65 patients. Cancer 52:1489–1495

Jacobs TP, Michelsen J, Polay JS et al. (1979) Giant cell tumor in Paget's disease of bone. Cancer 44:742–747

Jaffe HL (1958) Tumors and tumorous conditions of the bones and joints. Lea & Febiger, Philadelphia

Lake M (1951) Studies of Paget's disease (osteitis deformans). J Bone Joint Surg [Br] 33:323–335

Le Charpentier Y, Le Charpentier M, Forest M et al. (1977) Inclusions intranucléaires dans une tumeur osseuse à cellules géantes. Nouv Presses Med 6:259–262

Lichtenstein L (1977) Bone tumors, 5th edn. C.V. Mosby, St. Louis

McKenna RJ, Schwinn CP, Soong KY, Higinbotham NL (1964) Osteogenic sarcoma arising in Paget's disease. Cancer 17:42–45

Mills BG, Singer FR (1976) Nuclear inclusions in Paget's disease of bone. Science 194:201–202

Mills BG, Singer FR, Weiner LP, Holst PA (1981) Immunohistological demonstration of respiratory syncytial virus antigens in Paget's disease of bone. Proc Natl Acad Sci USA 78:1209–1213

Mirra JM, Bauer FC, Grant TT (1981) Giant cell tumor with viral-like intranuclear inclusions associated with Paget's disease. Clin Orthop 158:243–251

Paget J (1877) On a form of chronic inflammation of bones (osteitis deformans). Trans R Med Chir Soc London 60:37–63

Platt H (1947) Sarcoma in abnormal bones. Br J Surg 34:232–239

Porretta CA, Dahlin DC, Janes JM (1957) Sarcoma in Paget's disease of bone. J Bone Joint Surg [Am] 39:1314–1329

Powell N (1983) Metastatic carcinoma in association with Paget's disease of bone. Br J Radiol 56:582–585

Price CHG (1962) The incidence of osteogenic sarcoma in south-west England and its relationship to Paget's disease of bone. J Bone Joint Surg [Br] 44:366–376

Price CHG, Goldie W (1969) Paget's sarcoma: a study of 80 cases from the Bristol and the Leeds bone tumour registries. J Bone Joint Surg [Br] 51:205–224

Putschar WGJ (1972) Circulation in Paget's disease of bone. N Engl J Med 287:717–718

Rebel A, Malkani K, Basle M (1974) Anomalies nucléaires des ostéoclastes de la maladie osseuse de Paget. Nouv Presse Med 3:1299–1301

Reddick RL, Michelitch HJ, Levine AM, Triche TJ (1980) Osteogenic sarcoma: a study of the ultrastructure. Cancer 45:64–71

Reich C, Brodsky AE (1948) Coexisting multiple myeloma and Paget's disease of bone treated with stilbamidine. J Bone Joint Surg [Am] 30:642–646

Ross FGM, Middlemiss JH, Fitton JM (1973) Paget's sarcoma in bone: a radiological study. In: Price CHG, Ross FGM (eds) Bone: certain aspects of neoplasia. Colston Papers, vol 24. Butterworth, London, pp 41–62

Russell DS (1949) Malignant osteoclastoma and the association of malignant osteoclastoma with Paget's osteitis deformans. J Bone Joint Surg [Br] 31:281–290

Schajowicz F (1942) La degeneración sarcomatosa de la osteítis deformante de Paget. Rev Ortop Traumatol 12:131–148

Schajowicz F (1981) Tumors and tumorlike lesions of bone and joints. Springer, New York Berlin Heidelberg

Schajowicz F, Cabrini RL (1954) Histochemical studies of bone in normal and pathological conditions: with special reference to alkaline phosphatase, glycogen and mucopolysaccharides. J Bone Joint Surg [Br] 36:474–489

Schajowicz F, Oleaga Alarcon F (1945) La transformación sarcomatosa de la osteitis deformante de Paget. Bol Trab Soc Argent Cirug Ortop 10:116–130

Schajowicz F, Slullitel I (1966) Giant-cell tumor associated with Paget's disease of bone: a case report. J Bone Joint Surg [Am] 48:1340–1349

Schajowicz F, Slullitel JA (1978) Sarcoma complicating Paget's disease of the clavicle. Report of a case. Rev Chir Orthop 64:691–693

Schajowicz F, Santini Araujo E, Berenstein M (1983) Sarcoma complicating Paget's disease of bone: a clinicopathological study of 62 cases. J Bone Joint Surg [Br] 64:299–307

Schajowicz F, Ubios AM, Santini Araujo E et al. (1985) Virus-like intranuclear inclusions in giant cell tumor of bone. Clin Orthop 201:247–250

Schatzki SC, Dudley HR (1961) Bone sarcoma complicating Paget's disease: a report of 3 cases with long survival. Cancer 14:517–523

Schmorl G (1932) Über Osteitis deformans Paget. Virchow's Arch [A] 283:694

Sissons HA (1965) Epidemiology of Paget's disease. Clin Orthop 45:73

Smith J, Botet JF, Yeh SDJ (1984) Bone sarcomas in Paget disease: a study of 85 patients. Radiology 153:583–590

Spanier SS, Enneking WF, Enriquez P (1975) Primary malignant fibrous histiocytoma of bone. Cancer 36:2084–2098

Stevens J, Lennox B (1958) Long survival after amputation for Paget's sarcoma of bone. J Bone Joint Surg [Br] 40:735–739

Upchurch KS, Simon LS, Schiller AL et al. (1983) Giant cell reparative granuloma of Paget's disease of bone: a unique clinical entity. Ann Intern Med 98:35–40

Vacher-Lavenu MC, Louvel A, Daudet-Monsac M et al. (1981) Inclusions tubulofilamenteuses intranucleaired dans les cellules multinuclees des tumeurs a cellules geantes des os. Etude ultrastructurale d'une serie de 31 tumeurs. CR Acad Sci Paris 293:639–644

von Albertini A (1928) Über Sarkombildung auf dem Boden der Ostitis deformans Paget. Virchow's Arch [A] 268:259

Welsh RA, Meyer AT (1970) Nuclear fragmentations and associated fibrils in giant cell tumor of bone. Lab Invest 22:63–72

Wick MR, Siegal GP, McLeod RA et al. (1981) Sarcomas of bone complicating osteitis deformans (Paget's disease): fifty years' experience. Am J Surg Pathol 5:47–59

Wilner D (1982) Radiology of bone tumors and allied disorders. W.B. Saunders, Philadelphia, pp 3048–3079

Postradiation Sarcoma of Bone

Altner PP, Simmons DJ, Lucas HJ, Cummins H (1972) Osteogenic sarcoma in a patient injected with Thorotrast. J Bone Joint Surg [Am] 54:670–675

Arlen M, Higinbotham NL, Huvos AG, Marcove RC, Miller T, Shah IC (1971) Radiation-induced sarcoma of bone. Cancer 28:1087–1099

Beck A (1925) Zur Frage des Röntgensarkoms, zugleich ein Beitrag zur Pathogenese des Sarkoms. Muench Med Wochenschr 69:623–625

Bleaney B, Vaughan J (1971) Distribution of ^{239}Pu in the bone marrow and on the endosteal surface of the femur of adult rabbits following injection of $^{239}Pu(NO_3)_4$. Br J Radiol 44:67–73

Cahan WG, Woodard HQ, Higinbotham NL, Stewart FW, Coley BL (1948) Sarcoma arising in irradiated bone: report of eleven cases. Cancer 1:3–29

Casarett GW, Tuttle LW, Baxter RC (1962) Pathology of imbibed ^{90}Sr in rats and monkeys. In: Dougherty FF, Jee WSS, Mays CW et al. (eds) Some aspects of internal irradiation. Pergamon, New York, pp 329–336

Cobb LM (1970) Radiation-induced osteosarcoma in the rat as a model for osteosarcoma in man. Br J Cancer 24:294–299

Cruz MN, Coley BL, Stewart FW (1957) Post irradiation bone sarcoma: report of eleven cases. Cancer 10:72–88

Dahlin DC, Unni KK (1986) Bone tumors: general aspects and data on 8542 cases. Charles C. Thomas, Springfield, IL

Delgado E, Rodriguez JI, Serrada A et al. (1985) Radiation-induced osteochondroma-like lesion in young rat radius. Clin Orthop 201:251–258

Dougherty TF (1962) Incidence of bone cancer in internally irradiated dogs. In: Dougherty TF, Jee WSS, Mays CW et al. (eds) Some aspects of internal irradiation. Pergamon, New York, p 47

Evans RD (1974) Radium in man. Health Phys 27:497–510

Finkel MP, Reilly CA Jr, Biskis BO (1976) Pathogenesis of radiation and virus-induced bone tumors. In: Grundmann E (ed) Malignant bone tumors. Springer, New York Berlin Heidelberg, pp 92–103

Hasterlik RJ, Finkel AJ (1965) Diseases of bones and joints associated with intoxication by radioactive substances, principally radium. Med Clin North Am 49:285–296

Hatcher CH (1945) The development of sarcoma in bone subjected to roentgen or radium irradiation. J Bone Joint Surg 27:179–195

Huvos AG (1986) Osteogenic sarcoma of bones and soft tissues in older persons: a clinicopathologic analysis of 117 patients older than 60 years. Cancer 57:1442–1449

Huvos AG (1991) Bone tumors: diagnosis, treatment and prognosis, 2nd edn. W.B. Saunders, Philadelphia

Huvos AG, Higinbotham NL, Miller TR (1972) Bone sarcomas arising in fibrous dysplasia. J Bone Joint Surg [Am] 54:1047–1056

Huvos AG, Woodard HQ, Cahan WG et al. (1985) Postradiation osteogenic sarcoma of bone and soft tissue: a clinicopathologic study of 66 patients. Cancer 55:1244–1255

Huvos AG, Woodard GQ, Heilweil M (1986) Postradiation malignant fibrous histiocytoma of bone: a clinicopathologic study of 20 patients. Am J Surg Pathol 10:9–18

Jaffe N, Ried HL, Cohen M et al. (1983) Radiation induced osteochondroma in long-term survivors of childhood cancer. Int J Radiat Oncol Biol Phys 9:665–670

Jee WSS (1971) Bone-seeking radionuclides and bones. In: Berdjis CC (ed) Pathology of irradiation. Williams & Wilkins, Baltimore, pp 186–212

Kim HJ, Chu FCH, Woodard HQ et al. (1983) Radiation induced sarcomas of bone following therapeutic radiation. Int J Radiat Oncol Biol Phys 9:107–110

Kuttner H (1931) Zur Frage der Geschwülstentstehung nach Roentgenbestrahlung von Gelenk- und Knochentuberkulosen. Arch Klin Chir 164:5–38

Looney WB (1955) Late effects (25–40 years) of the early medical and industrial use of radioactive materials: their relation to the more accurate establishment of maximum permissible amounts of radioactive elements in the body (part I). J Bone Joint Surg [Am] 37:1169–1187

Looney WB (1956) Late effects (25–40 years) of the early medical and industrial use of radioactive materials: their relation to the more accurate establishment of maximum permissible amounts of radioactive elements in the body (parts II and III). J Bone Joint Surg [Am] 38:175–218, 392–406

Loutit JF (1976) Vasoformative non-osteogenic (angio) sarcomas of bone-marrow stroma due to strontium-90. Int J Radiat Biol 30:359–383

Martland HS (1929) Occupational poisoning in manufacture of luminous watch dials. JAMA 92:466–473

Martland HS (1931) The occurrence of malignancy in radioactive persons. Am J Cancer 15:2435–2515

Martland HS, Humphries RE (1929) Osteogenic sarcoma in dial painters using luminous paint. Arch Pathol 7:406–417

Mays CW (1973) Cancer induction in man from internal radioactivity. Health Phys 25:585–592

Mays CW, Spiess H, Gerspach A (1978) Skeletal effects following ^{224}Ra injections into humans. Health Phys 35:83–90

Milgram JW (1983) The origins of osteochondromas and enchondromas: a histopathologic study. Clin Orthop 174:264–284

Mindell ER, Shah NK, Webster JH (1977) Post-radiation sarcoma of bone and soft tissues. Orthop Clin North Am 8:821–834

Rowland RE, Stehney AF, Lucas HF (1983) Dose-response relationships for radium-induced bone sarcomas. Health Phys 44[Suppl 1]:15–31

Sabanas AO, Dahlin DC, Childs DS Jr, Ivins JC (1956) Postradiation sarcoma of bone. Cancer 9:528–542

Sanerkin NG, Jeffree GM (1980) Cytology of bone tumours: a colour atlas with text. Wright, Bristol

Schajowicz F, Defillippi Novoa CA, Firpo CA (1967) Thorotrast induced chondrosarcoma in the axilla. Am J Roentgenol Radium Ther Nucl Med 100:931–937

Sim FH, Cupps RE, Dahlin DC, Ivins JC (1972) Post-radiation sarcoma of bone. J Bone Joint Surg [Am] 54:1479–1489

Spiess H, Mays CW (1970) Some cancers induced by ^{224}Ra in children and adults. Health Phys 19:713–729

Steiner GC (1965) Postradiation sarcoma of bone. Cancer 18:603–612

Vaughan JM (1973a) The effects of irradiation on the skeleton. Oxford University Press (Clarendon), London

Vaughan JM (1973b) Skeletal tumors induced by internal radiation. Proc Symp Colston Res Soc 24:377–384

Wick RR, Gössner W (1983) Follow-up study of late effects in ^{224}Ra treated ankylosing spondylitis patients. Health Phys 44[Suppl 1]:187–195

CHAPTER IX
Tumorlike Lesions

1. Solitary Bone Cyst (Simple or Unicameral Bone Cyst)

Definition, WHO: *"A unicameral cavity filled with clear or sanguineous fluid and lined by a membrane of variable thickness, which consists of loose vascular connective tissue showing scattered osteoclast giant cells and sometimes areas of recent or old hemorrhage or cholesterol clefts."*

Solitary bone cyst is a common nonneoplastic process of uncertain pathogenesis. Although generally easily recognized radiologically, a pathologist who does not know its clinical and radiologic features can occasionally confuse this process with giant-cell tumor because of the presence of a certain number of osteoclast giant cells. In the older literature, this entity was classified in the general group "osteitis fibrosa," "osteitis fibrosa cystica localizata," or "localized fibrous osteodystrophy" (Freund and Moffert 1936), from which at present fibrous dysplasia and other fibrous lesions have been separated.

Incidence. Over a period of nearly 45 years, we recorded 289 cases of unicameral bone cysts in our laboratory, i.e., fewer than the number of metaphyseal fibrous defects (357 cases).

Clinical Findings. *Age and Sex.* There was a great preponderance of young children, with the highest frequency in the first two decades of life (91%); overall, the age range was from 1 year to 53 years. The infrequent lesions observed in adults are apparently processes initiated in childhood that have remained latent for several years

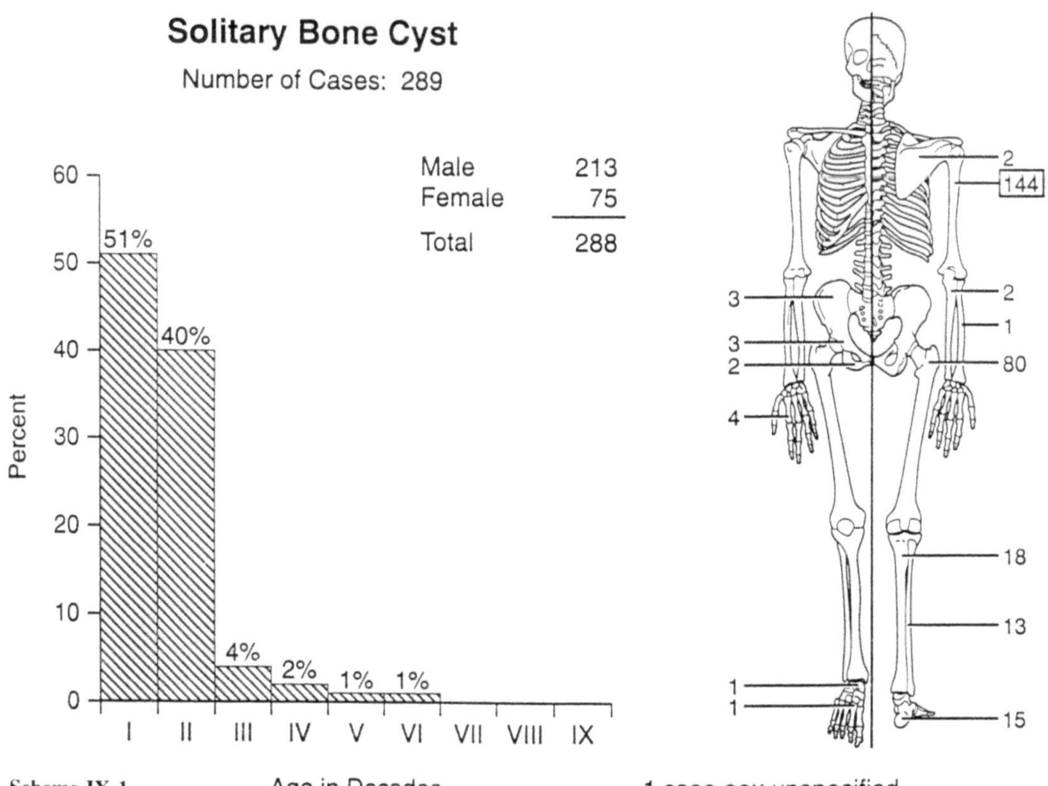

Scheme IX.1

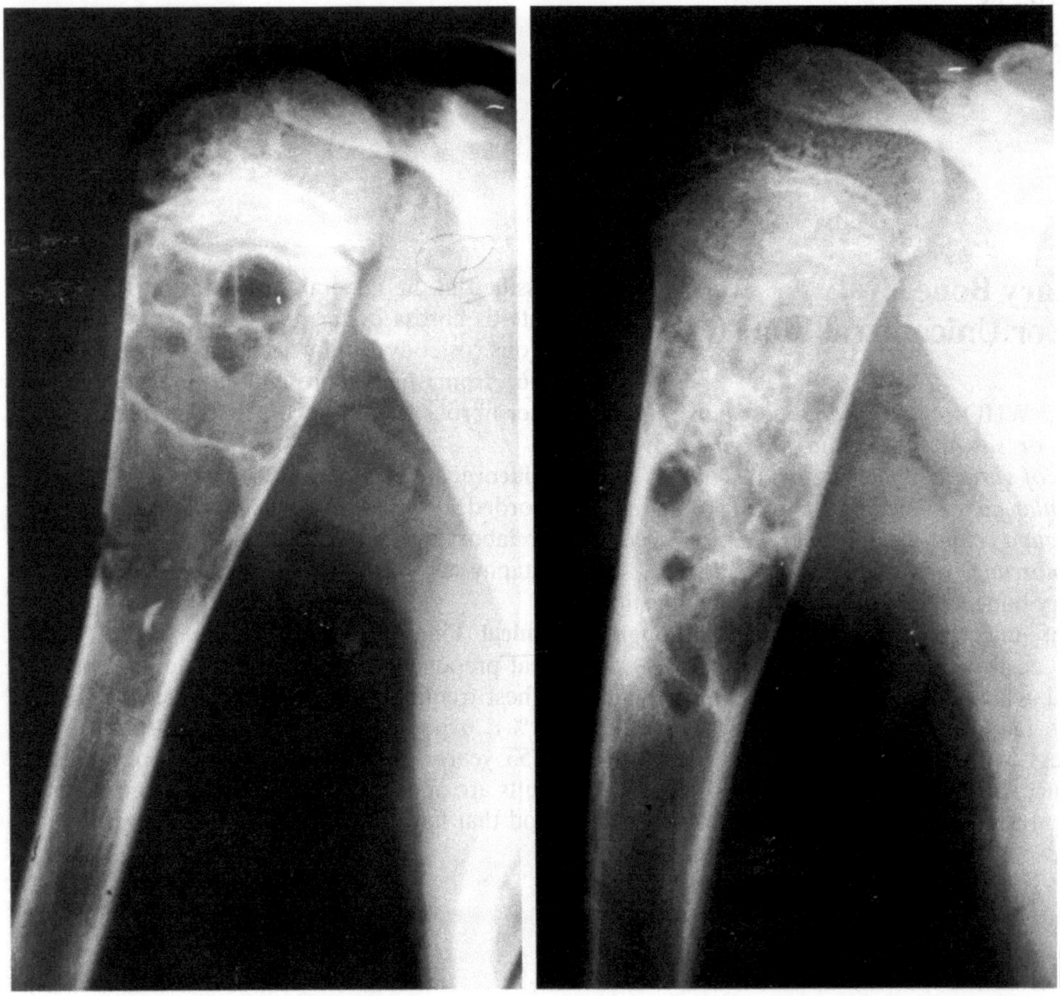

a b

Fig. IX.1a,b. Male, 11 years old. Solitary bone cyst in the upper metaphysis of humerus. **a** Radiograph shows the lytic area with a slightly trabeculated appearance and thinning of the cortex. Note a fissure at its distal end. **b** Two years after curettage, cyst had moved away from the growth plate, but showed some cystic spaces and was curetted again

or are lesions of unusual sites. Thus, most of the cysts located in the calcaneus were found in adults and seem to have a different pathogenesis (Scheme IX.1).

As in other series, such as in Campanacci's (1990) with 563 cases, there was a marked male predominance (2.7:1).

Localization. The majority of large series, including ours, indicate a predilection for the humerus, particularly the upper metaphysis, close to the growth cartilage. Fifty percent of our cases were located in the humerus, the great majority at its upper end and the remainder in the shaft. The next most common site was the upper end of the femur (75 cases, i.e., 26%), only a few cases (five) being located at the lower metaphysis.

We found only one reported case with two simultaneous localizations in humerus and tibia, in a 10-year-old patient (Sadler and Rosenheim 1964). Another patient with two single cysts was reported by Boseker et al. (1968); the second appeared in the upper humerus end after the initial treatment of a cyst in the proximal femoral end. One of our cases had cysts in both calcanei.

Symptoms. Unicameral bone cysts are generally discovered because of a fracture due to an insignificant trauma or incidentally after a roentgenographic examination for other reasons. However, some patients may experience mild pain or limitations of motion at variable times prior to the diagnosis.

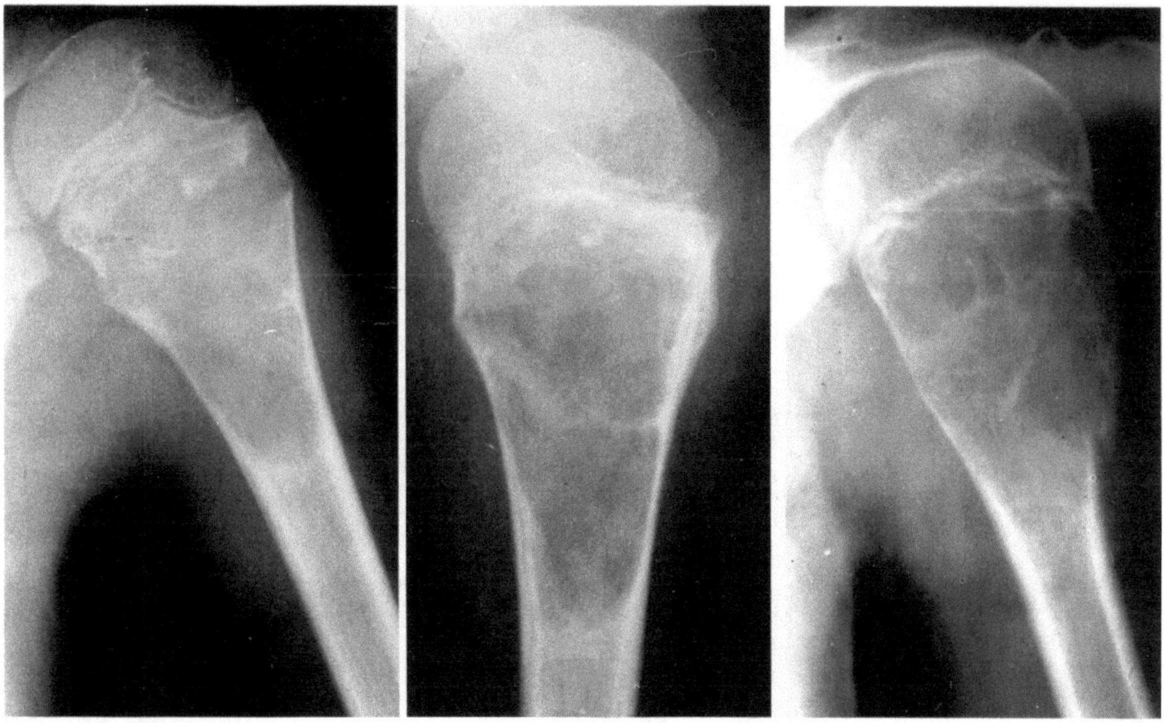

a b

Fig. IX.2a,b. Radiographs of two different cases of solitary bone cyst in the upper humeral metaphysis abutting the growth cartilage (so-called active bone cyst). **a** Male, 10 years old; **b** female, 9 years old

Fig. IX.3a,b. Two different cases of solitary bone cysts in the upper end of the femur. **a** Female, 9 years old; **b** male, 10 years old
▼

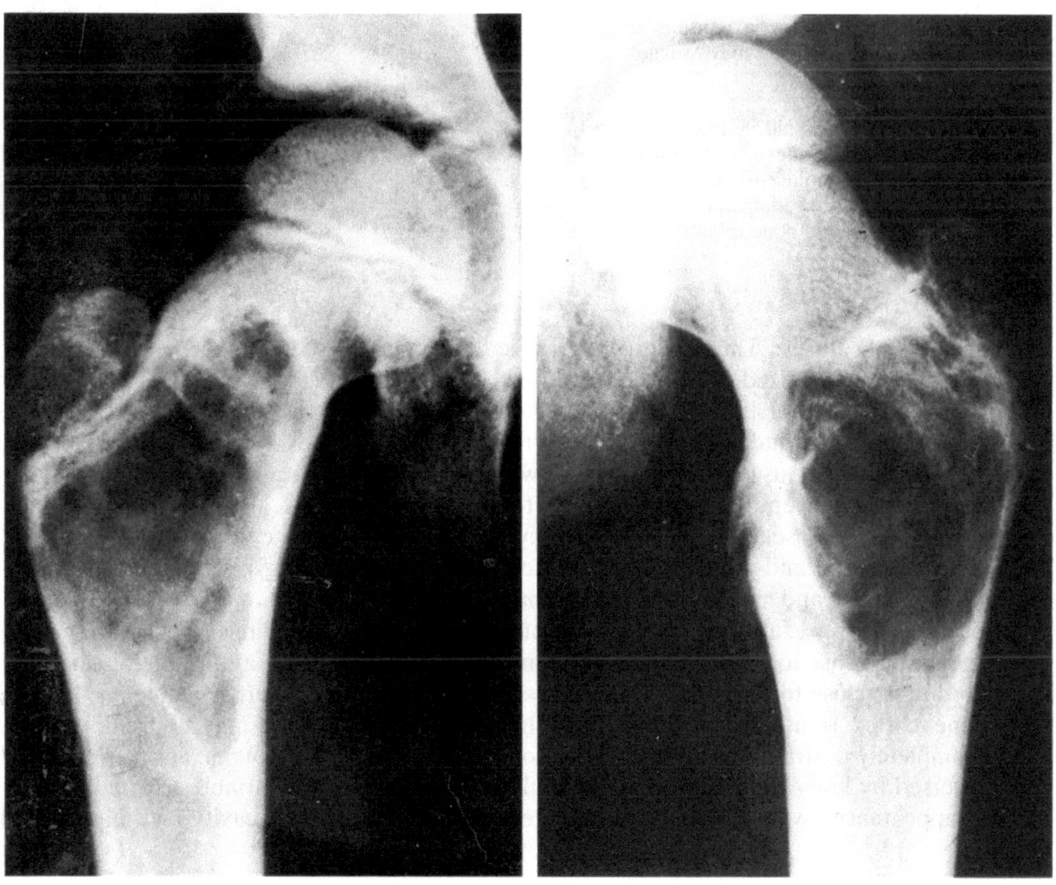

a b

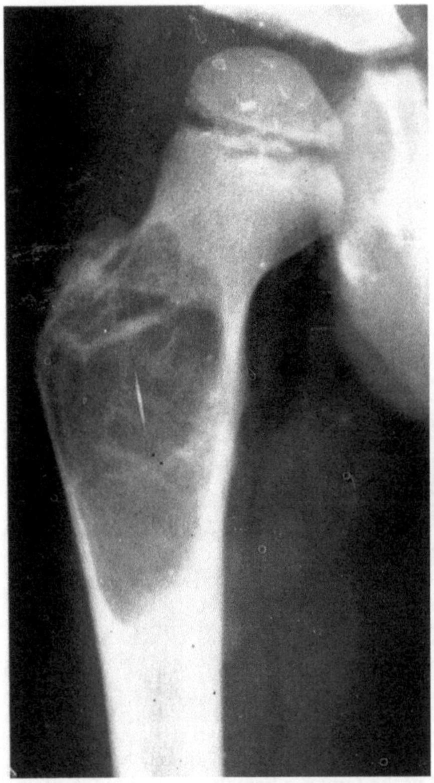

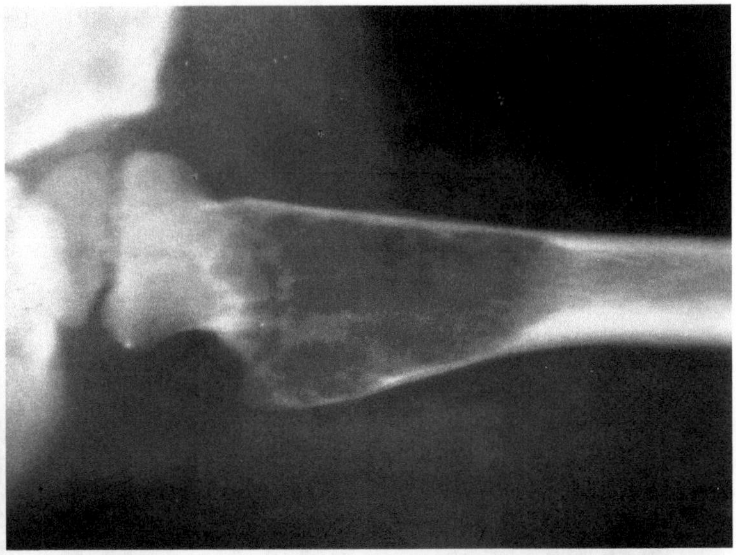

Fig. IX.4. Male, 8 years old. Anteroposterior and lateral radiographs of solitary bone cyst in the upper end of the femur. The lateral view shows a conspicuous expansion of the thinned cortex, which may suggest aneurysmal bone cyst

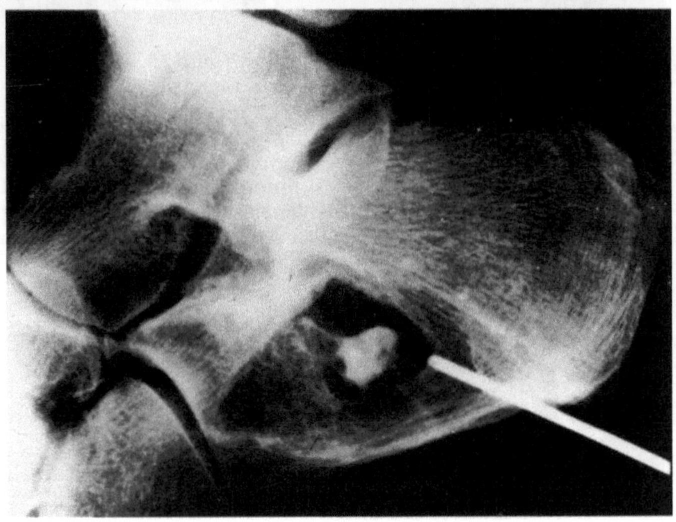

Fig. IX.5. Male, 40 years old. Solitary bone ▶ cyst of calcaneus with bone infarct. Radiograph illustrates radiolucent triangular-shaped lesion with dense radiopaque area in the central part (ischemic bone infarct)

Radiographic Features. The roentgenographic features are characterized by a well-outlined, radiolucent metaphyseal lesion, usually located centrally, expanding and thinning the cortex (Figs. IX.1–IX.4). It usually abuts the growth cartilage, but only exceptionally transgresses the plate (Hutter 1950; Boseker et al. 1968). The cyst has its broader base and greatest diameter near the epiphyseal plate and may be found in the shaft at variable distances. Jaffe called these lesions, which generally cease to increase in size, "latent" cysts, and those close to the plate, "active" cysts. The bone cortex is usually extremely thin but never completely destroyed. The cyst is occasionally traversed by bony trabeculae giving a multilocular appearance, which is due to prominent bony ridges of the cortical wall and not to true bony septa (Fig. IX.1). The most important complication is a pathologic fracture whereby the thinned cortex is crushed, giving origin to the so-called fallen fragment sign described by Reynolds (1969) (Fig. IX.1). Periosteal reaction is generally absent in bone cysts, except at sites of infarction (Figs. IX.2, IX.5).

Pathologic Findings. The *gross appearance* is characterized by a unicameral cavity filled with a clear serous or serosanguineous fluid, which after a recent fracture may be frankly sanguineous or contain blood clots or fibrin. The wall may show bony ridges of variable size and thickness that do not traverse the cavity (see Fig. IX.7a) and that

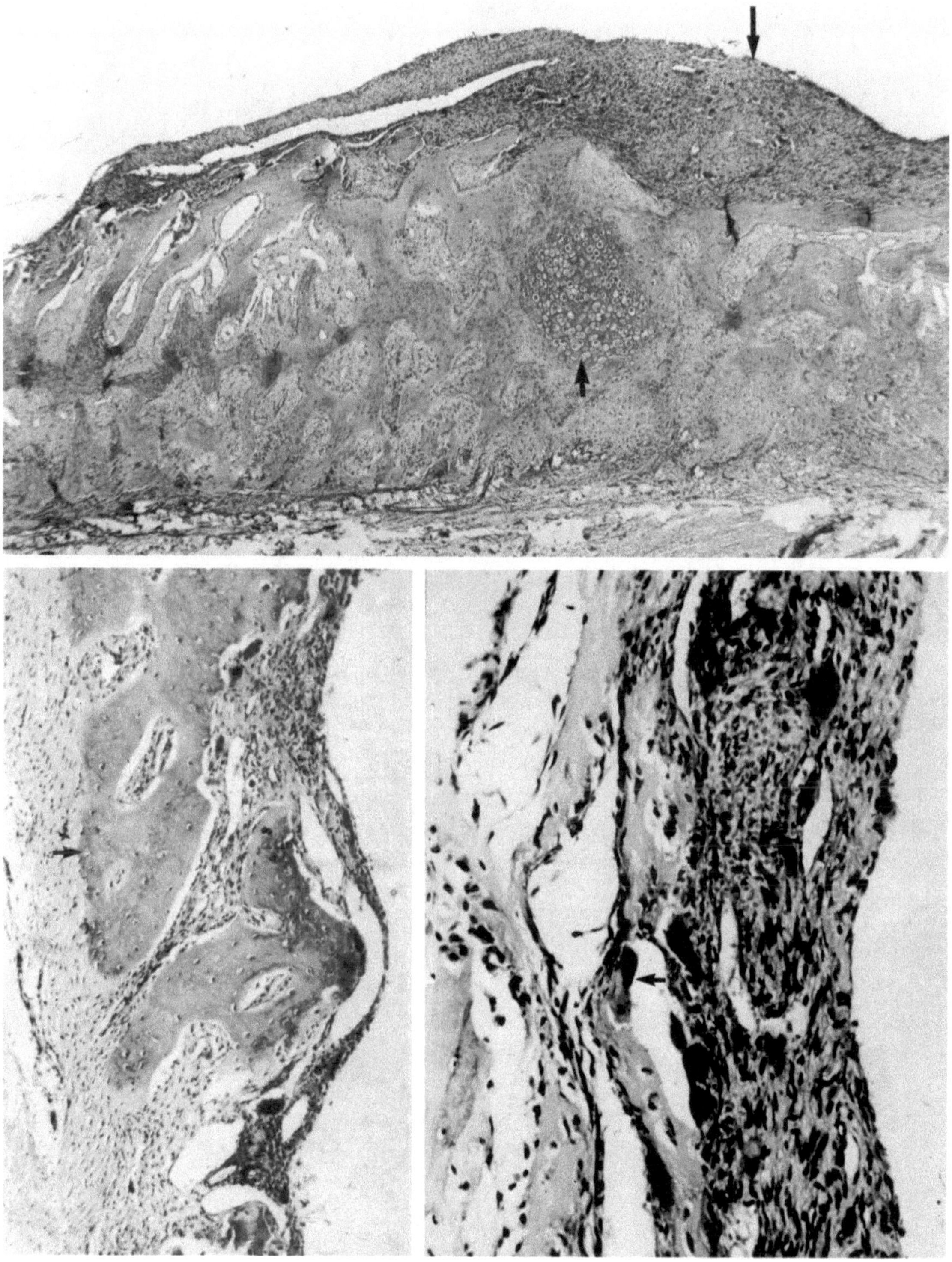

a b c

Fig. IX.6. **a** Topographic photomicrograph shows at *top* the cyst wall covering the endosteal surface of the newly formed thin cortex with cartilage callus formation. **b** Newly formed, thin cortex, composed of immature bone trabeculae covered at the outer aspect by periosteum and at the inner surface by a thin fibrous membrane. **c** At higher magnification, the newly formed cortex, lined on its inner surface by a thin fibrous membrane, rich in capillary vessels, and containing some multinucleated giant cells of osteoclast type, some located at the inner surface of the newly formed immature bone trabeculae. **a** ×40, **b** ×180, **c** ×400

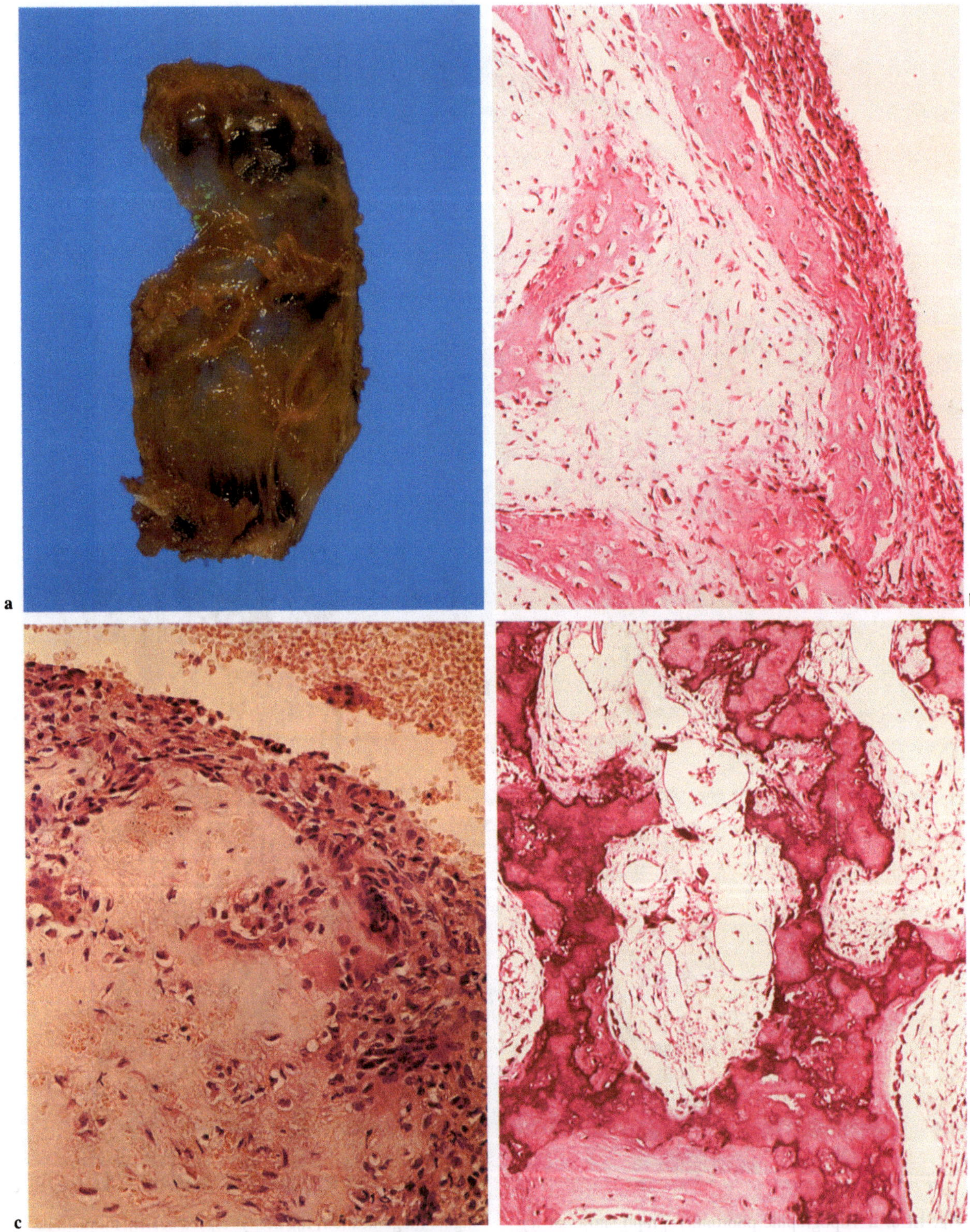

Fig. IX.7. a Photograph of the thin cortical wall of a solitary bone cyst showing prominent bony ridges, giving a radiologic aspect of trabeculation. **b–d** Photomicrographs illustrating the characteristic histologic features of the thin cyst wall, which contains scarce multinucleated giant cells, newly formed osteoid, woven bone trabeculae, and fibrinoid material. Calcified fibrinoid is stained in dark blue and surrounded by osteoid and rows of osteoblasts. The loose fibrous tissue is rich in dilated capillaries. **b** ×100, **c,d** ×250

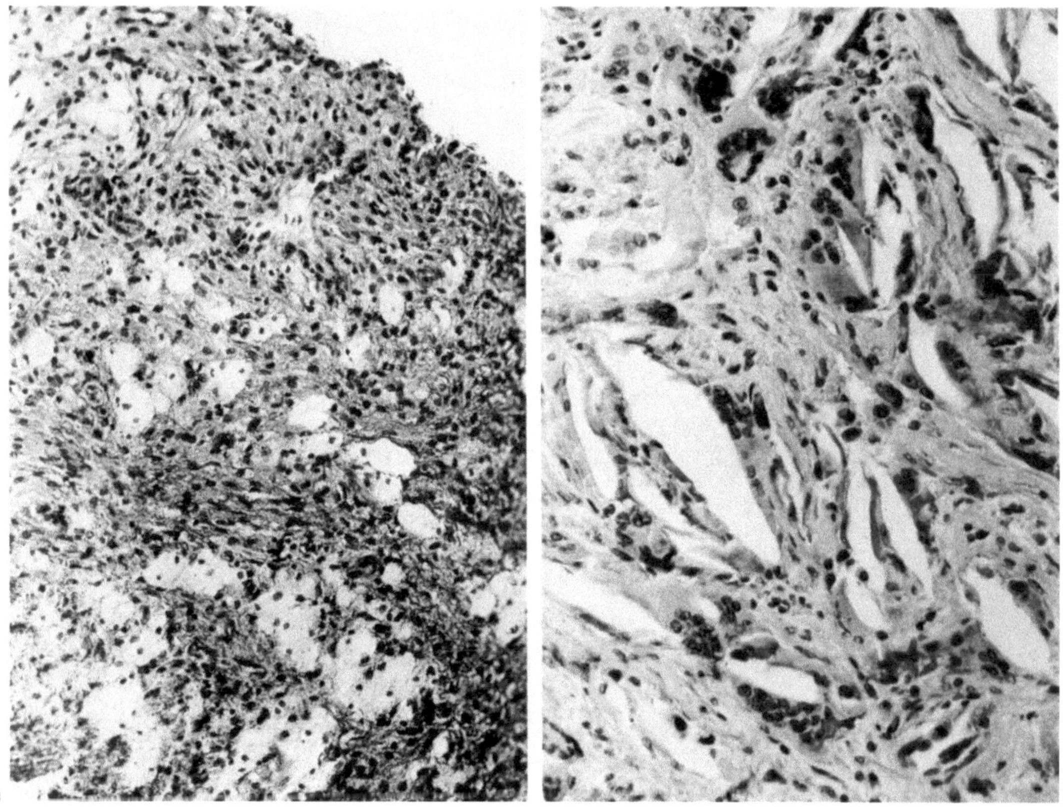

Fig. IX.8a,b. Photomicrographs showing numerous foam cells (xanthoma cells) in the cyst wall (**a**) and cholesterol crystals surrounded by foreign body giant cells (**b**). This pattern is frequently observed in older cysts and in lesions of the calcaneus

radiographically may exhibit the trabeculated or multiloculated aspect described previously. The inner surface of the cyst is lined by a usually smooth membrane that is of variable thickness and grayish white, reddish brown, or occasionally yellow in color. The cortex is often reduced to a thin translucent membrane resembling an eggshell that can be cut relatively easily with the knife.

Histologically, the cyst wall is composed of trabeculae of immature bone formed by the periosteum to the degree that the old cortex has been resorbed on its endosteal surface by osteoclasts. In areas of fracture, periosteal osteocartilaginous callus formation is a common finding (Fig. IX.6a). The cyst membrane consists of loose vascular connective tissue, showing scattered osteoclast giant cells and newly formed immature bone or osteoid trabeculae, usually oriented parallel to the surface of the cyst wall (Figs. IX.6, IX.7). Areas of recent or old hemorrhages, cholesterol clefts, and groups of xanthoma cells, particularly in older "latent" lesions or in those located in calcaneus, are observed (Fig. IX.8). In general, we have not found significant histologic differences between "latent" and "active" bone cysts (Ottolenghi et al. 1969).

A frequent and, in our opinion, characteristic feature was the presence of irregular bands or masses of fibrinlike material, often calcified and resembling odontogenic cement; they are frequently surrounded by osteoid tissue or immature bone with a rim of osteoblasts (Figs. IX.7, IX.9). Areas of mucoid degeneration and small cystic cavities resembling those observed in intraosseous ganglia were occasionally seen. In two cases, the cyst wall presented foci with an aspect similar to that of fibrous dysplasia. The newly formed cortex is rich in dilated and hyperemic capillaries and venous vessels; an identical process of venous stasis is also observed in the fibrous marrow, between the spongious trabeculae near the cyst.

Pathogenesis. The etiology of the simple bone cyst is still unresolved. In 1876 Virchow supported the concept that simple bone cysts are formed

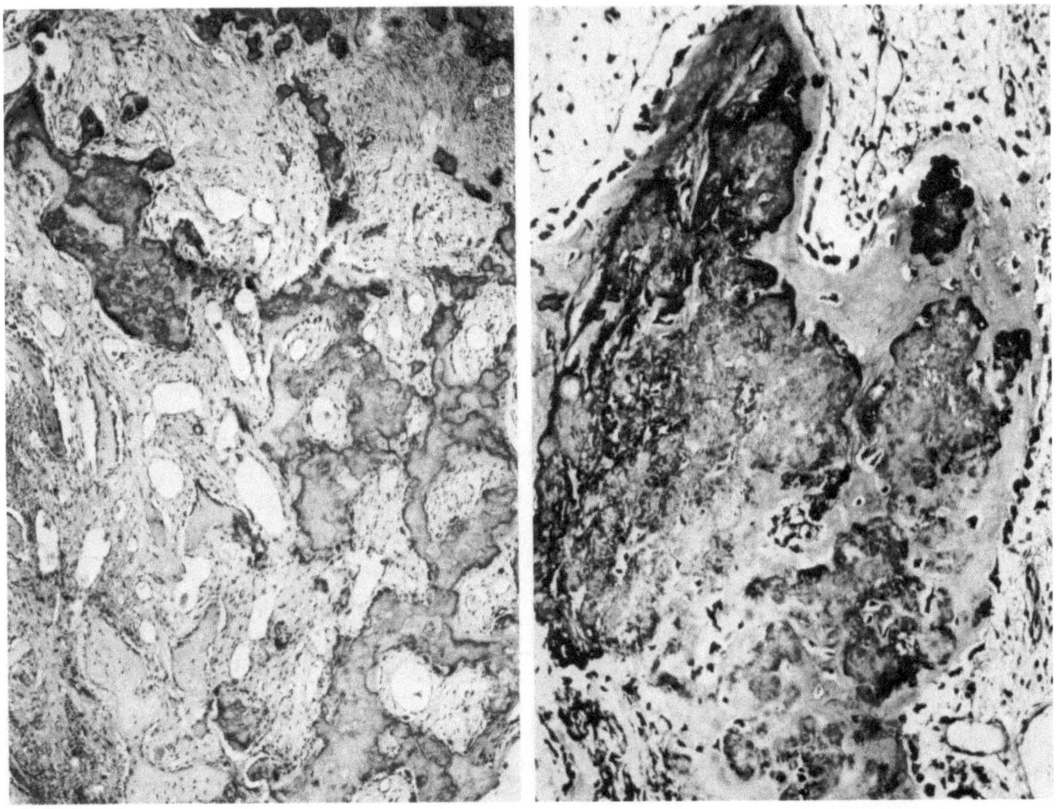

a b

Fig. IX.9a,b. Photomicrographs showing strands and irregular masses of calcified fibrinoid surrounded in part by osteoid and rows of osteoblasts. Calcified or uncalcified fibrinoid is a common and characteristic finding in solitary bone cyst. **a** ×180, **b** ×300

by a process of central cystic softening of an enchondroma, and Mönckeberg (1904) and Geschickter and Copeland (1949) advocated a similar mechanism in giant-cell tumors. Johnson and Kindred (1958), supporting Virchow's interpretation, advocated the neoplastic nature of the bone cyst, which begins as a solid lesion of the myxochondroid, fibromatous, or lipomatous type, based on the common finding of these structures in the cyst wall. Another hypothesis is the partial or total cystic softening of an "osteitis fibrosa" or "fibrous osteodystrophy" (von Recklinghausen 1891; Konjetzny 1922). One of the most widely accepted hypotheses is that of Pommer (1919) and his pupils Lang (1922), Haselhofer (1937), and others, who postulated a post-traumatic intramedullary hematoma that provokes venous stasis ("phlegmasiae") in its periphery, thus favoring the osteoclastic resorption of the cancellous tissue and cortex. The cystic cavity is formed posteriorly through liquefaction of the hematoma, which is surrounded by a fibrous membrane. To this concept, other authors (Jaffe and Lichtenstein 1942) added further factors, i.e., a local disturbance in bone growth and development (osteodystrophy), a thesis formerly postulated by Mikulicz in 1905. This would explain the predilection for sites of most active growth.

Based on the similarity between the bone cyst fluid and serum and extracellular fluid, Cohen (1960, 1970) proposed as the cause, "a transient circulatory compromise attributed to a developmental anomaly in the veins of the affected bone" (Cohen 1977). Campanacci (1990) found a high intracystic pressure in the active cysts (more than 30 cm H_2O with a pulsating column), while the intracystic pressure in inactive cysts is equal to venous pressure (6–10 cm H_2O).

Treatment and Prognosis. The standard treatment of simple bone cyst has been curettage and autogenous or homogeneous bone grafts of different types (Fig. IX.10). However, the rate of failure to cure due to recurrences in approximately 30%–45% of cases has stimulated the development of more radical therapy. It is difficult to judge the results of treatment because of the

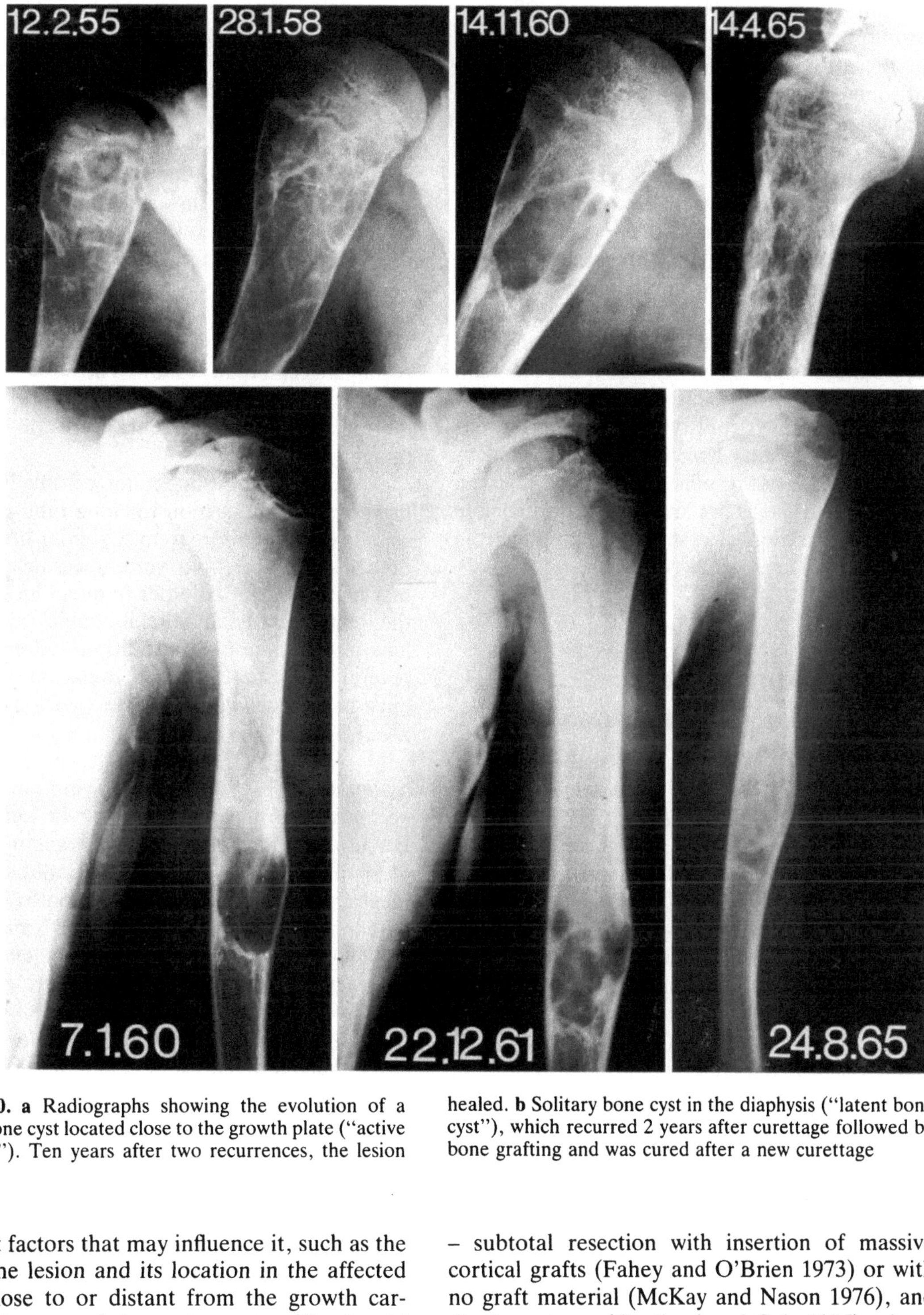

Fig. IX.10. a Radiographs showing the evolution of a solitary bone cyst located close to the growth plate ("active bone cyst"). Ten years after two recurrences, the lesion healed. **b** Solitary bone cyst in the diaphysis ("latent bone cyst"), which recurred 2 years after curettage followed by bone grafting and was cured after a new curettage

different factors that may influence it, such as the site of the lesion and its location in the affected bone (close to or distant from the growth cartilage), the age of the patient, etc. (Ottolenghi et al. 1969).

Cohen (1977) published an excellent review with a critical synthesis of the different types of treatment, based on his own experience and that gleaned from some of the largest published series (Neer et al. 1973; Spence et al. 1976; Campanacci et al. 1976). The more radical forms of treatment – subtotal resection with insertion of massive cortical grafts (Fahey and O'Brien 1973) or with no graft material (McKay and Nason 1976), and diaphysectomy (Gartland and Cole 1975) – have practically disappeared since the introduction of injections of methylprednisolone (Depo-Medrol), advocated by Scaglietti (1974; Scaglietti et al. 1976, 1979, 1982) and Campanacci et al. (1977) in the treatment of unicameral bone cysts and other benign bone lesions (e.g., eosinophilic granuloma).

Campanacci et al. (1986) compared 178 cases of solitary bone cysts treated with curettage and bone grafting with 141 cases treated with cortisone injections. The end results were comparable in the two groups. Local risk factors in the surgical group were active cysts and previous operations. In the other group they were multiloculation of the cyst, active cyst, and size of the cyst. The treatment consists in penetrating the cavity with two needles used for skeletal biopsy, extracting the fluid, using physiologic solutions to cleanse with pressure, and finally removing one needle and injecting with the other a quantity of Depo-Medrol approximately equal to the fluid extracted. This treatment is repeated every 2 months. Generally from two to five infiltrations are required. Solitary bone cysts of the calcaneus and in adults do not respond to local steroids. The action of cortisone is not known, but even simple repeated extraction of cystic fluid may have the same effect (Chigira et al. 1983).

2. Aneurysmal Bone Cyst (Multilocular Hematic Bone Cyst)

Definition, WHO: *"An expanding osteolytic lesion consisting of blood-filled spaces of variable size separated by connective tissue septa containing trabeculae of bone or osteoid tissue and osteoclast giant cells."*

The name aneurysmal bone cyst was introduced by Jaffe and Lichtenstein in 1942 in their paper on solitary bone cysts. They described in detail two cases with the conspicuous "blown-out" distension of the contour of the affected bone, so characteristic in the radiographic picture. In 1950, Jaffe and Lichtenstein, in separate articles, gave further details of this benign lesion, which became well established as a distinct clinicopathologic entity. Prior to these publications, examples of aneurysmal bone cyst were classified as variants of giant-cell tumor, atypical or subperiosteal giant-cell tumor, subperiosteal ossifying hematoma, hemangioma, hemangiomatous or hemorrhagic bone cyst, or telangiectatic osteosarcoma. Despite the large number of publications on the subject, the etiology remains unknown.

Incidence. It is difficult to establish the real incidence of aneurysmal bone cyst because, in addition to the several hundred cases reported, many others are still unpublished. Only a few authors have reported series of more than 50 cases (Tillman et al. 1968; Biesecker et al. 1970; Levy et al. 1975; Lichtenstein 1957). In the last series of the Mayo Clinic (Dahlin and Unni 1986), 208 cases were reported, i.e., half the number of giant-cell tumors. Campanacci (1990) recorded 332 cases. In our laboratory, 217 cases of aneurysmal bone cysts are registered, compared with 460 genuine giant-cell tumors.

Clinical Findings. The lesion was slightly more common in females, which agrees with other series (Campanacci et al. 1986). The great majority occurred in the first three decades (81%), and more than 50% of patients were 10–20 years of age.

Almost every bone may be involved, but there was a predilection for long tubular bones, usually of the lower extremity (femur in 33 cases, tibia in 32 cases), and vertebrae, including the sacrum (29 cases). Another frequent location was the pelvis, especially the iliopubic ramus. We have seen no case with multiple lesions, but in several cases in the spine, adjacent vertebrae have been involved by direct extension (Scheme IX.2).

Symptoms. The presenting symptoms varied according to the involved bone. In long bones, the most common complaint was swelling, usually accompanied by tenderness and mild to severe local pain of several weeks' or months' duration and sometimes radiating to the proximal joints. When vertebrae are affected, pain and muscle contracture of the involved segment, associated later with neurologic symptoms due to compression of nerve roots or of the cord, are frequent complaints; if the affected vertebrae collapse, the complaints are accentuated and paraplegia may develop.

Radiographic Features. The characteristic radiographic appearance is that of a radiolucent expanding "blown-out" or "ballooned out" eccentric or, less commonly, central lesion which usually arises in the metaphysis or diaphysis of a long bone (Figs. IX.11–IX.14); cf. Figs. IX.15–IX.17 for appearances of aneurysmal bone cysts of the calcaneus, talus, and iliopubic ramus, respectively.

Campanacci et al. (1986) reported on 198 cases of aneurysmal bone cyst treated at the Rizzoli Institute up until 1982. They divided

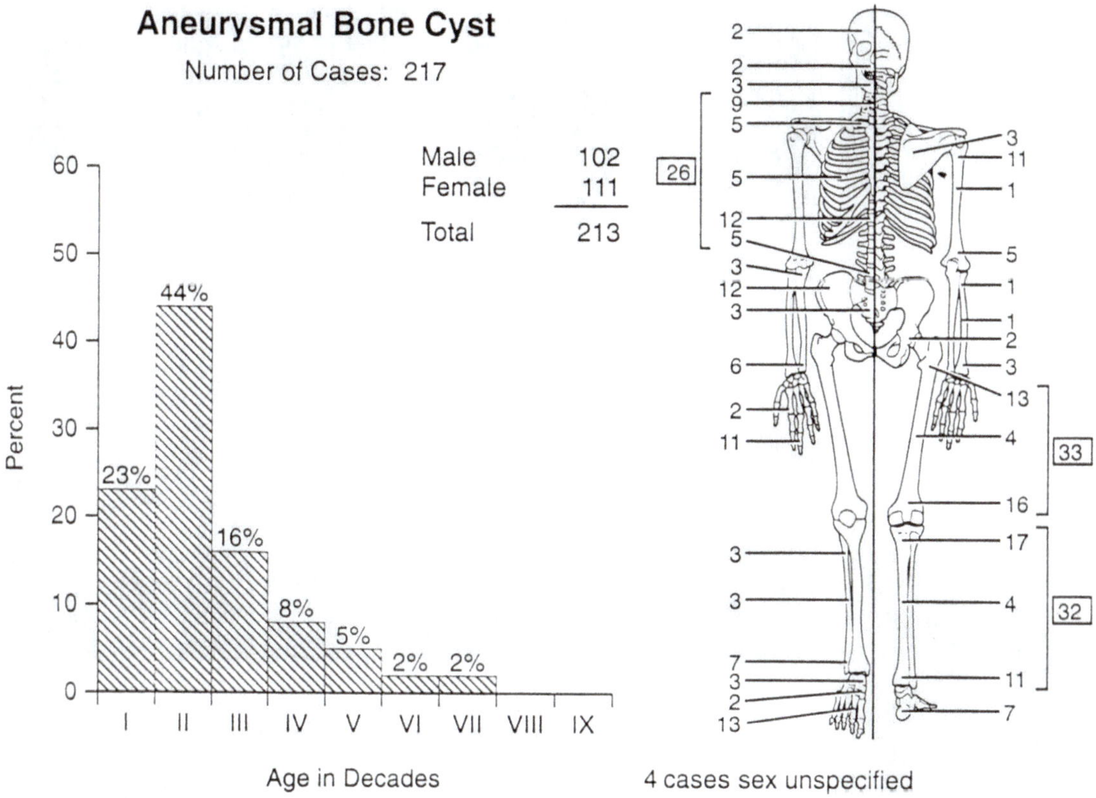

Scheme IX.2

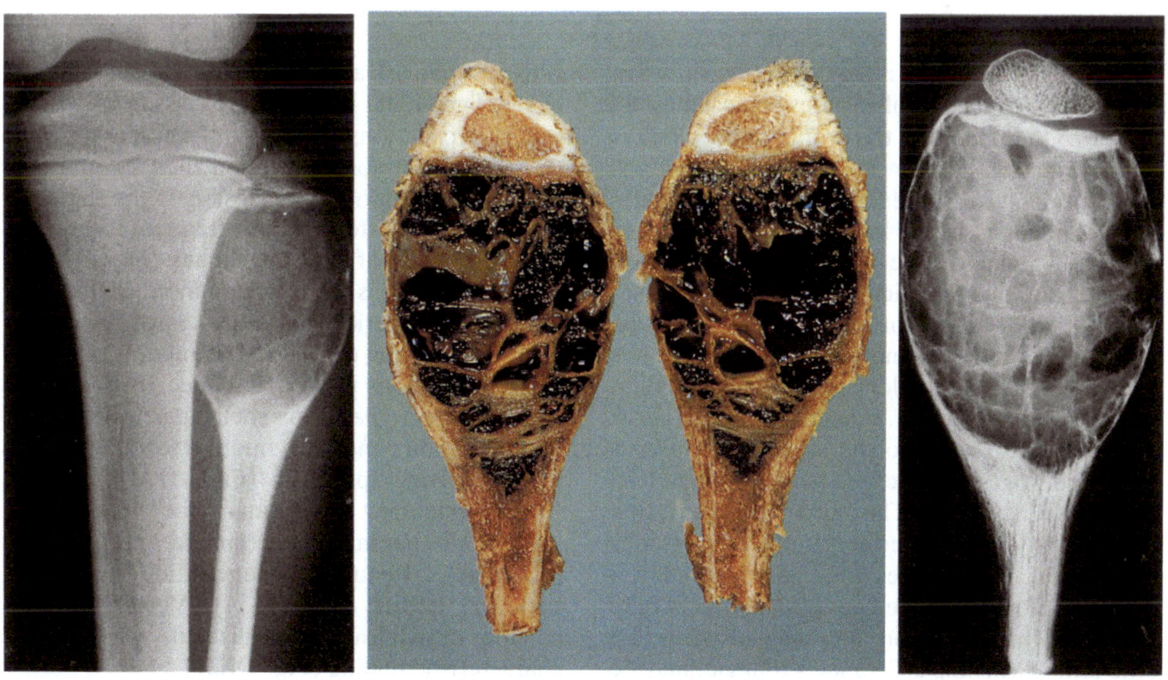

Fig. IX.11a–c. Male, 11 years old. Aneurysmal bone cyst of fibula. **a** Radiograph showing radiolucent lesion in the upper metaphysis with expansion of the thinned cortex. **b** Photograph and **c** radiograph reveal the multiloculated blood-filled cavities separated by thin-walled septa

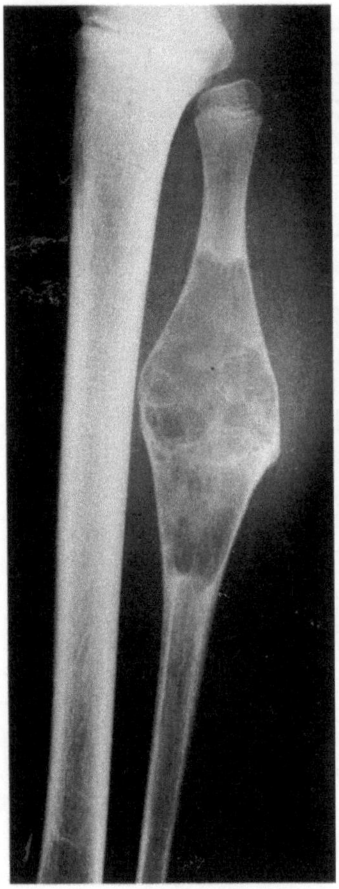

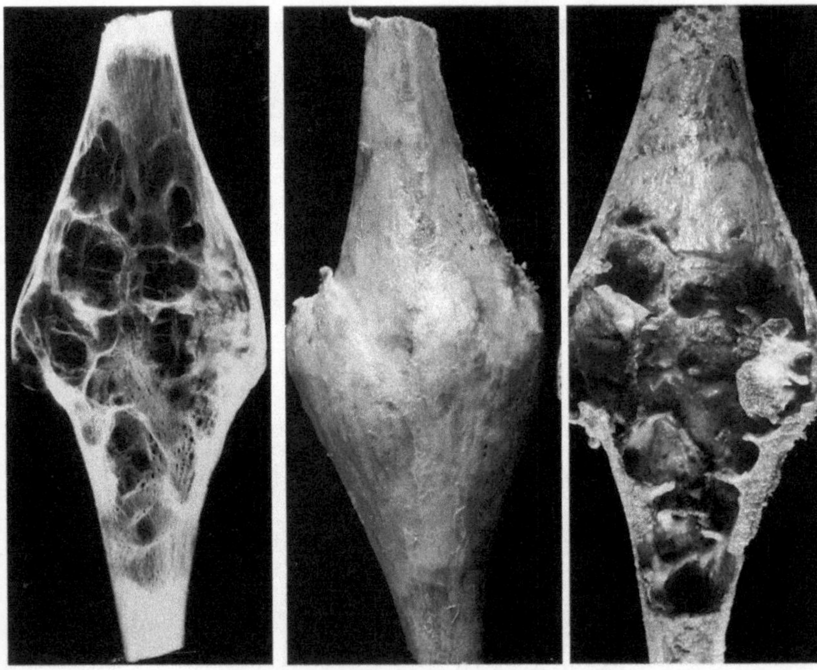

c

a, b

Fig. IX.12a–c. Male, 14 years old with aneurysmal bone cyst of fibula. **a** Clinical radiograph and **b** radiograph of the resected specimen show the expanding and trabeculated radiolucent lesion. **c** Photographs of the surface and longitudinal section illustrate the multilocular, hemorrhagic well-limited lesion

aneurysmal bone cysts radiographically into five types: In *type I* the radiolucent lesion occupies the center of the bone and the profile of the bone is either intact or slightly expanded. The cortex is more or less attenuated. Normally it is found in the metaphysis of long bones and closely resembles a simple bone cyst. In *type II* the lesion substitutes the entire width of the involved bone, which is "blown out" or "ballooned out." Type II is seen more commonly in the metaphysis and diaphysis of thin long bones (fibula, ulna, metacarpal, metatarsal), though it may also occur in flat bones. The osteolytic area often contains septa and ridges, producing a honeycomb pattern (Figs. IX.11, IX.12). The borders of the lesion are generally well defined at its inner intraosseous margin and at its surface, where it is covered by a thin shell of newly formed periosteal bone. At the border of this expansion, a laminated periosteal reaction, resembling a Codman's triangle, may be seen (Fig. IX.14). The epiphysis is only affected after closure of the growth plate and/or in large lesions (Fig. IX.18) (Dabska and Buraczewski 1969; Dahlin et al. 1955; Sherman and Soong 1957). Type I and II lesions are classified by us as central-type lesions. In *type III* the cyst appears as an *eccentric* intraosseous lesion showing minimal or wide ("blown-out") expansion of the thinned, newly formed cortex; its most frequent location is the metaphysis of the long bones (Figs. IX.14, IX.19). *Type IV* is the least common; in this type the cyst is subperiosteal, with superficial erosion of the underlying cortex and formation of a thin shell of reactive periosteal bone. In more advanced stages (*type V*) this shell is partly destroyed and the lesion penetrates into the soft tissues and the underlying spongiosa (Figs. IX.18, IX.20). In the vertebrae, aneurysmal bone cysts usually arise in the neural arches (lamina and/or spinal processes), frequently penetrating into the vertebral bodies (Fig. IX.21). Vertebral body collapse or extension into adjacent vertebrae is a characteristic finding (Fig. IX.21).

Arteriographic studies have shown delayed emptying of contrast medium, thus indicating probable stasis of blood in the cyst (Lindbom et

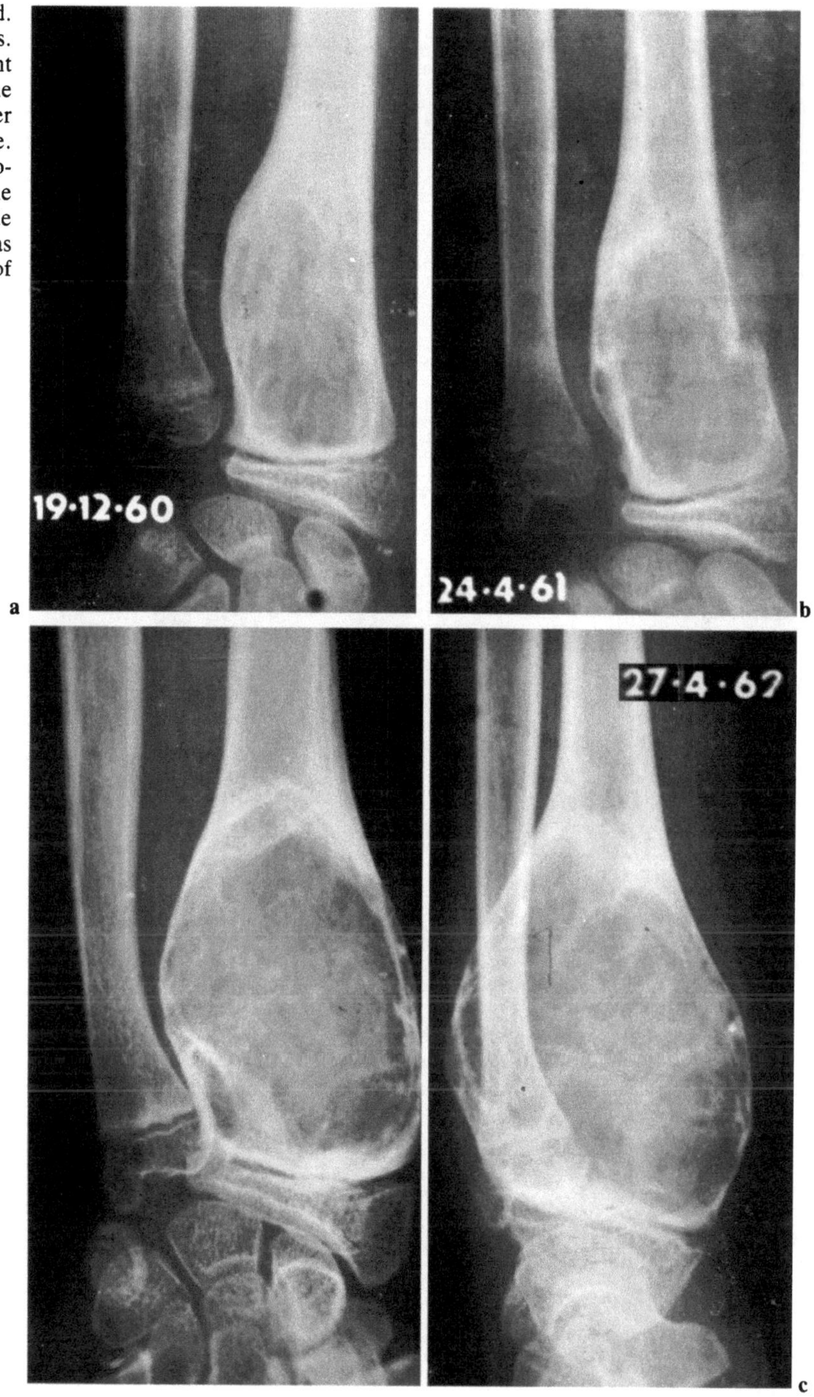

Fig. IX.13a–c. Male, 12 years old. Aneurysmal bone cyst of radius. **a** Radiograph showing radiolucent central lesion with expansion of the lateral cortex. **b** Recurrence after curettage showing pathologic fracture. **c** Anteroposterior and lateral radiographs illustrate the progress of the lesion after a second curettage. A wide excision followed by bone grafting was performed. The patient was free of disease 6 years later

al. 1961; Schobinger and Stoll 1957). However, arteriography does not seem to be helpful in the diagnosis and particularly does not permit differentiation of giant-cell tumor and aneurysmal bone cyst.

Pathologic Findings. *Grossly*, in addition to the fragmented material obtained by curettage, we studied many entirely resected or excised specimens (Figs. IX.11, IX.12, IX.18, IX.22–IX.26). The affected expanded bone is surrounded by a thin bony shell interrupted in some areas and covered by the raised periosteum. The cut surface showed the characteristic hemorrhagic multilocular appearance, consisting of spaces filled with unclotted blood of variable size, separated

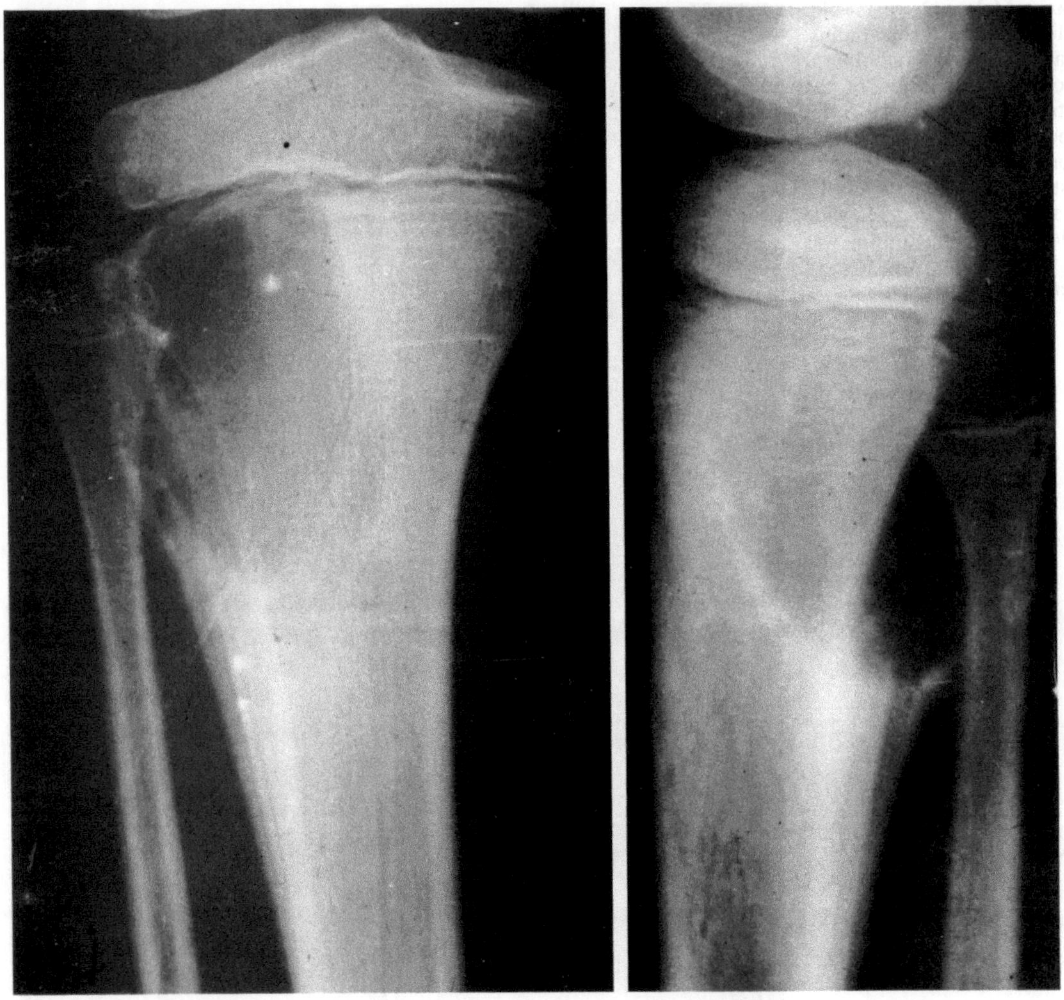

Fig. IX.14. Male, 8 years old. Aneurysmal bone cyst of the tibia. Anteroposterior and lateral radiographs show an eccentric radiolucent lesion with slightly sclerotic inner border and blown-out distension at its lateral aspect. Note the periosteal laminated bone reaction, resembling a Codman's triangle

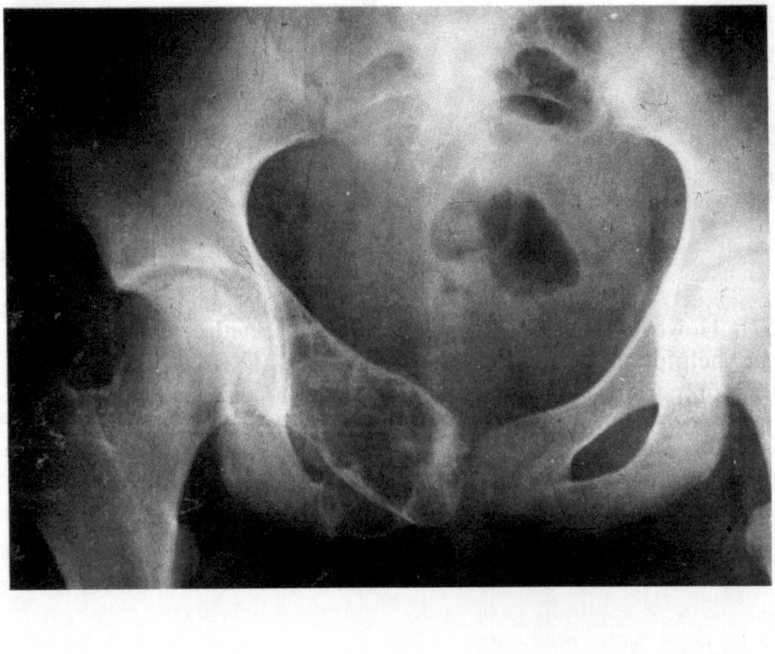

Fig. IX.15. Female, 18 years old with aneurysmal bone cyst of the iliopubic ramus. Radiograph shows expanding radiolucent lesion. Similar radiologic features can be seen in giant-cell tumors at this location

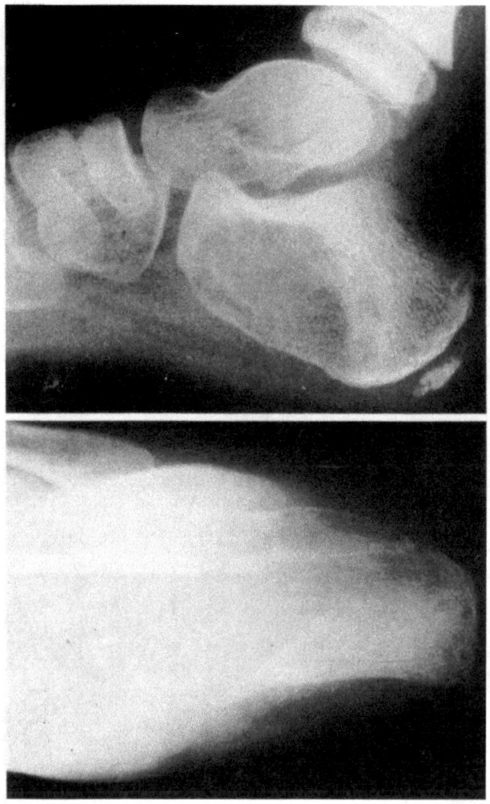
a

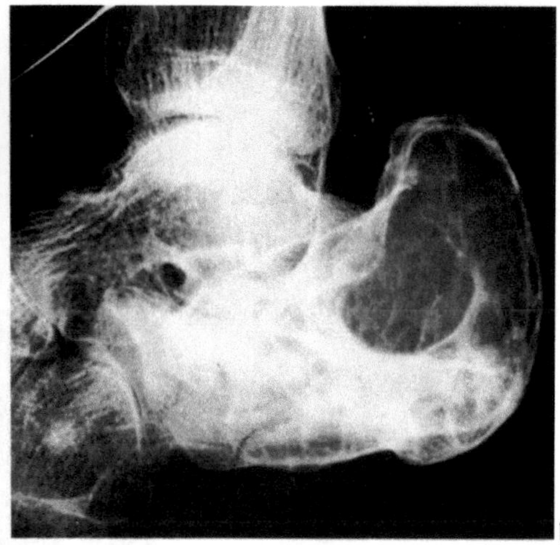
b

Fig. IX.16a,b. Two cases of aneurysmal bone cyst in the calcaneus showing radiologic patterns in different stages of evolution. **a** Female, 6 years old; **b** male, 18 years old

Fig. IX.17. Male, 9 years old. Aneurysmal bone cyst of talus

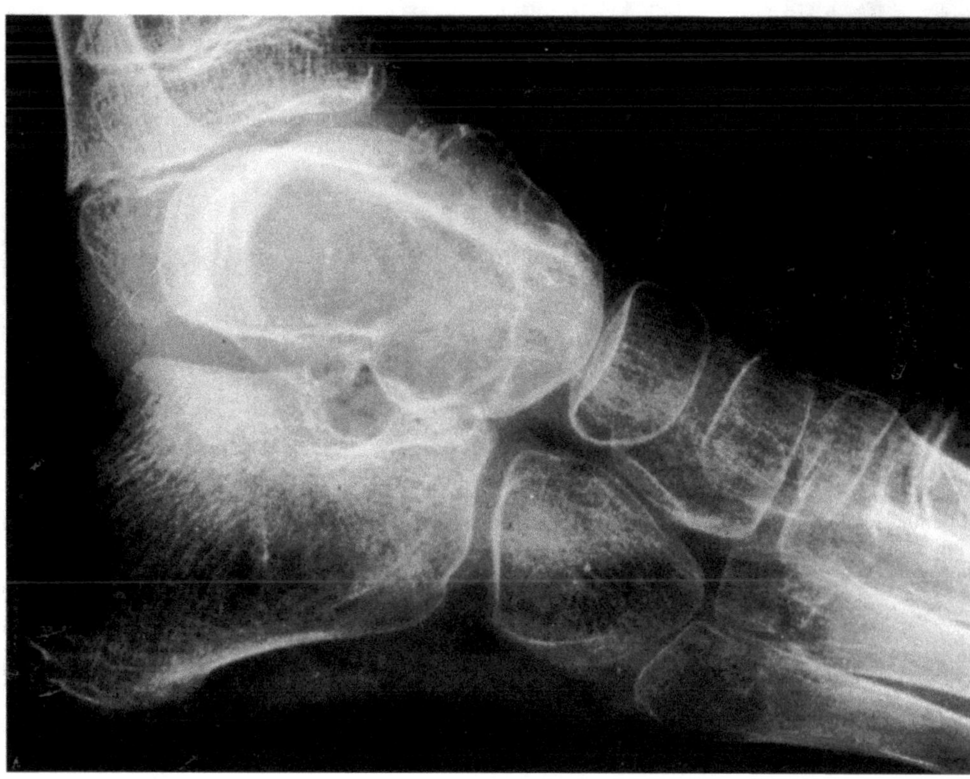

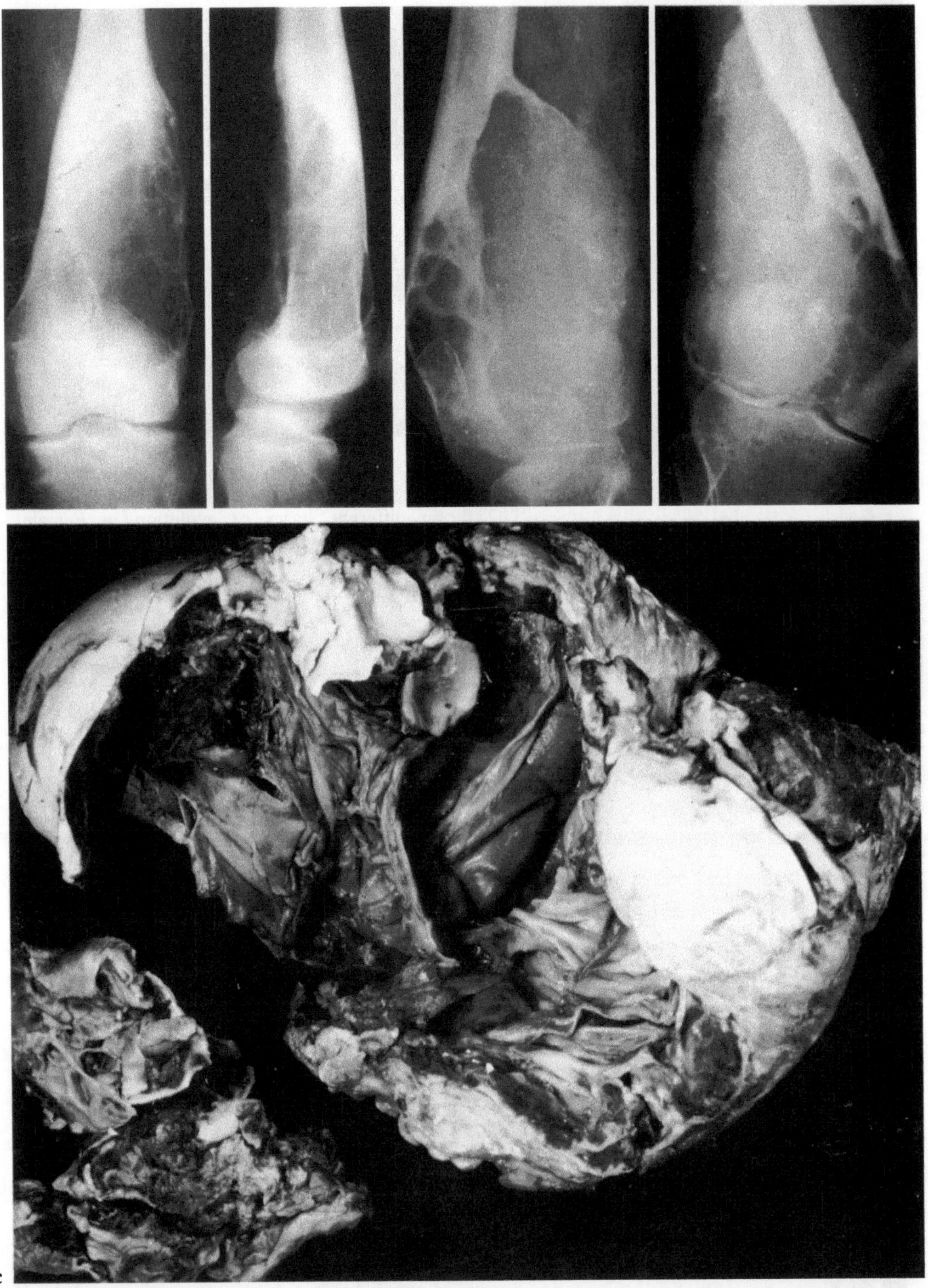

a b

c

Fig. IX.18a–c. Male, 26 years old. Aneurysmal bone cyst of femur. **a** Anteroposterior and lateral radiographs reveal a large radiolucent eccentric lesion expanding and thinning the cortex. **b** Recurrence 18 months after curettage showing the progress and blown-out distension of the lesion. **c** A wide segmental resection was performed, including both condyles

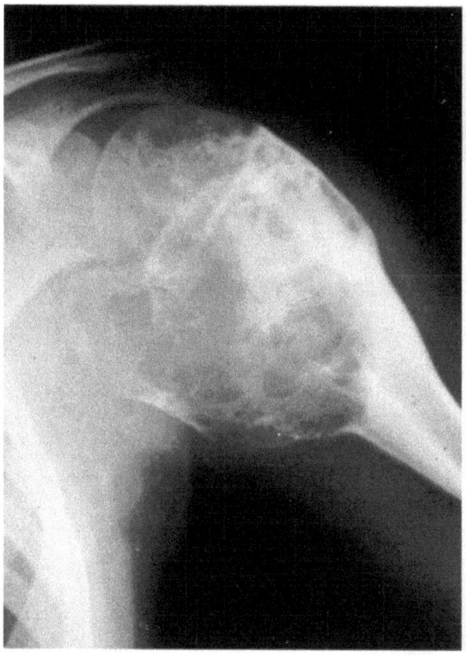

a

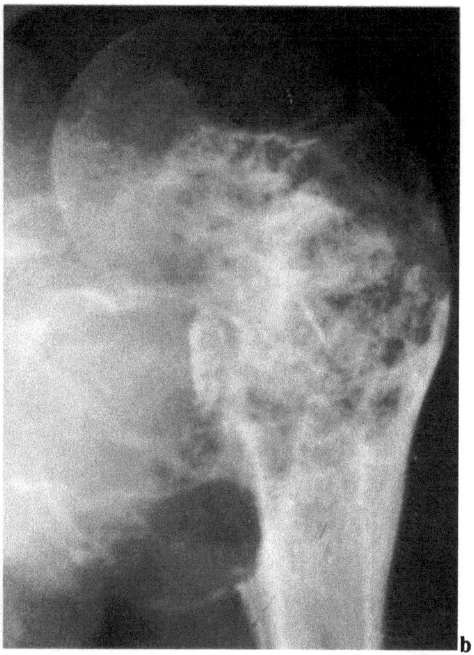

b

▲ **Fig. IX.19a,b.** Female, 11 years old. Aneurysmal bone cyst of humerus. **a** Radiograph shows an eccentric radiolucent lesion with ballooned-out distension of the thinned cortex. **b** Recurrence 6 months after an incomplete curettage. The lesion has increased in size and the thinned blown-out cortex has partially disappeared

Fig. IX.20. Male, 30 years old. Aneurysmal bone cyst of femur. Anteroposterior and lateral radiographs show large eccentric lesion of the femoral shaft with blown-out distension and vaguely trabecular appearance. Periosteal reaction is observed at its lower border ▼

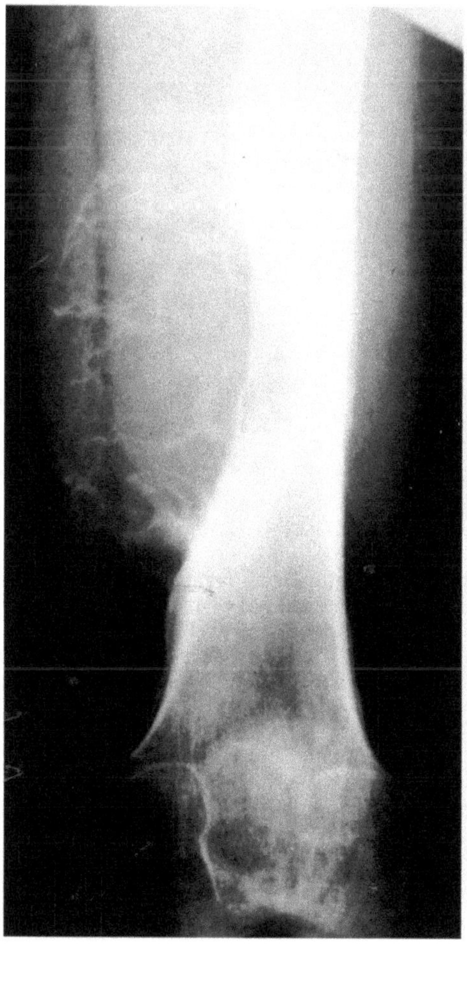

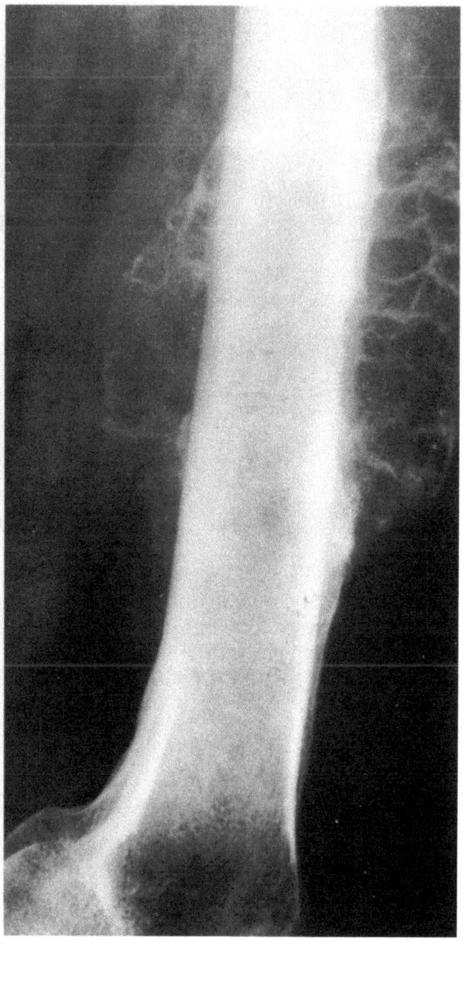

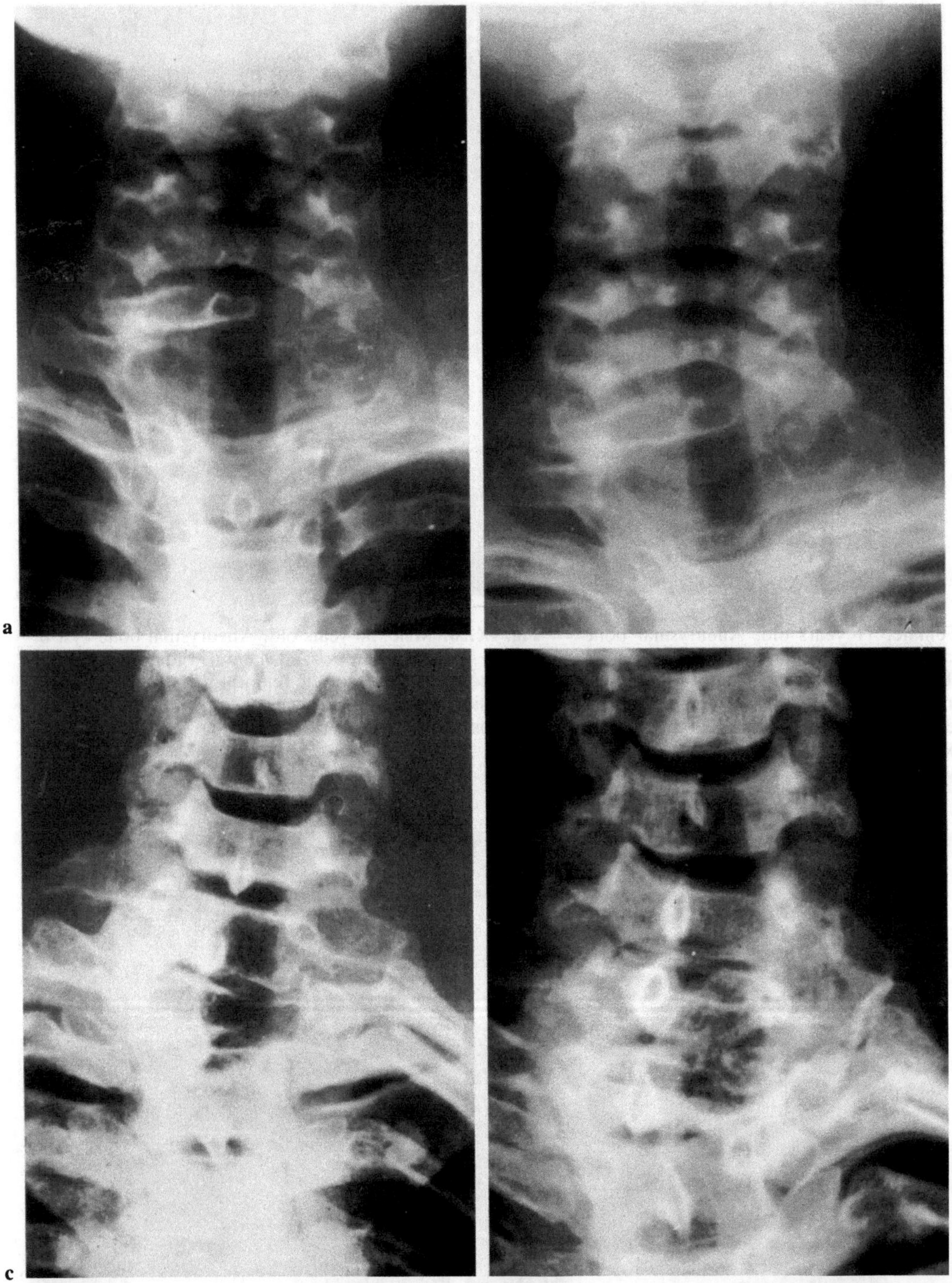

a b c d

Fig. IX.21a,b. Female, 9 years old. Aneurysmal bone cyst of the seventh cervical vertebra. **a** Radiograph illustrates a large rediolucent, ballooning lesion of the seventh cervical vertebra involving the vertebral body and neural arches, extending into the sixth vertebra. **b** Same lesion 3 months after radiotherapy; the limits are now better visible. **c,d** Female, 18 years old. Aneurysmal bone cyst involving the seventh cervical and first thoracic vertebrae. **c** Original lesion, **d** Appearance 6 years after radiotherapy, showing healing of the lesion. The patient was free of symptoms

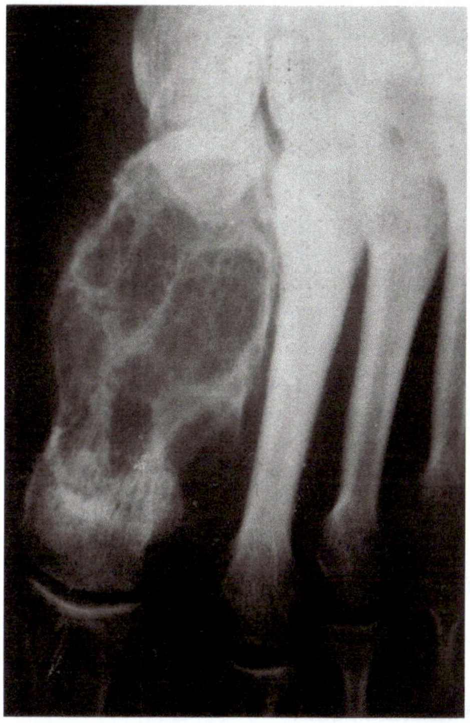
a

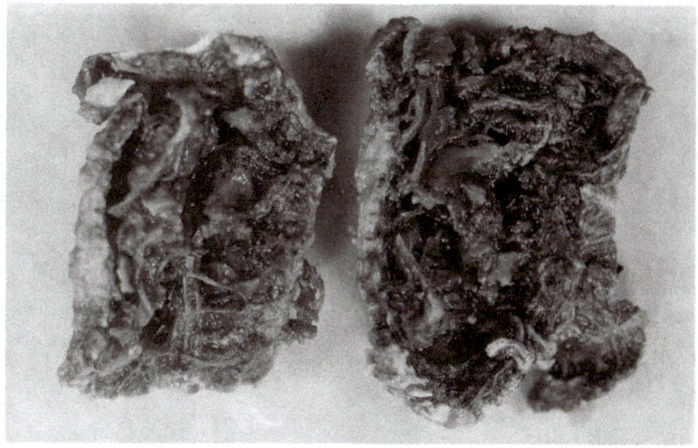
b

Fig. IX.22a,b. Male, 9 years old. Aneurysmal bone cyst of the scapula. **a** Radiograph shows a large radiolucent lesion with ballooned-out distension of the thinned cortex, involving almost the entire scapula. **b** Photograph of the resected scapula illustrates multiloculated blood-filled cavities separated by thin-walled septa

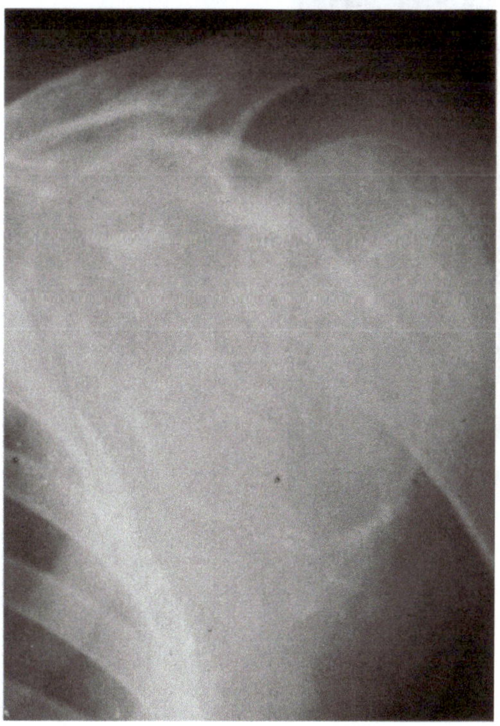
a

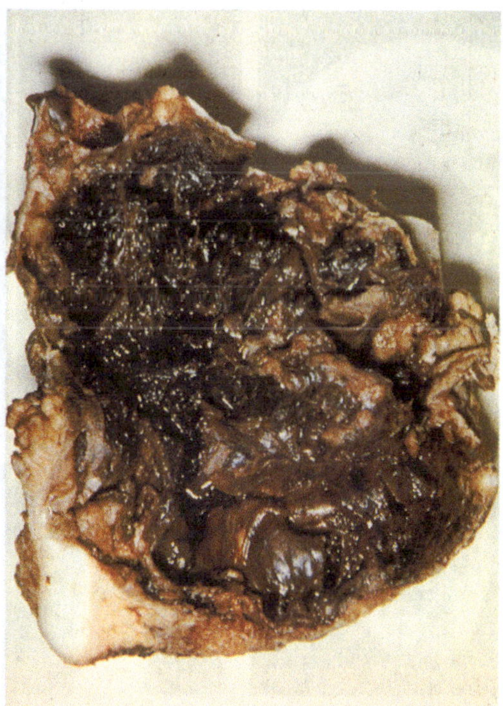
b

Fig. IX.23a,b. Male, 9 years old. Aneurysmal bone cyst of the scapula. **a** Radiograph shows a large radiolucent lesion with ballooned-out distension of the thinned cortex, involving almost the entire scapula. **b** Photograph of the resected scapula illustrates multiloculated blood-filled cavities separated by thin-walled septa

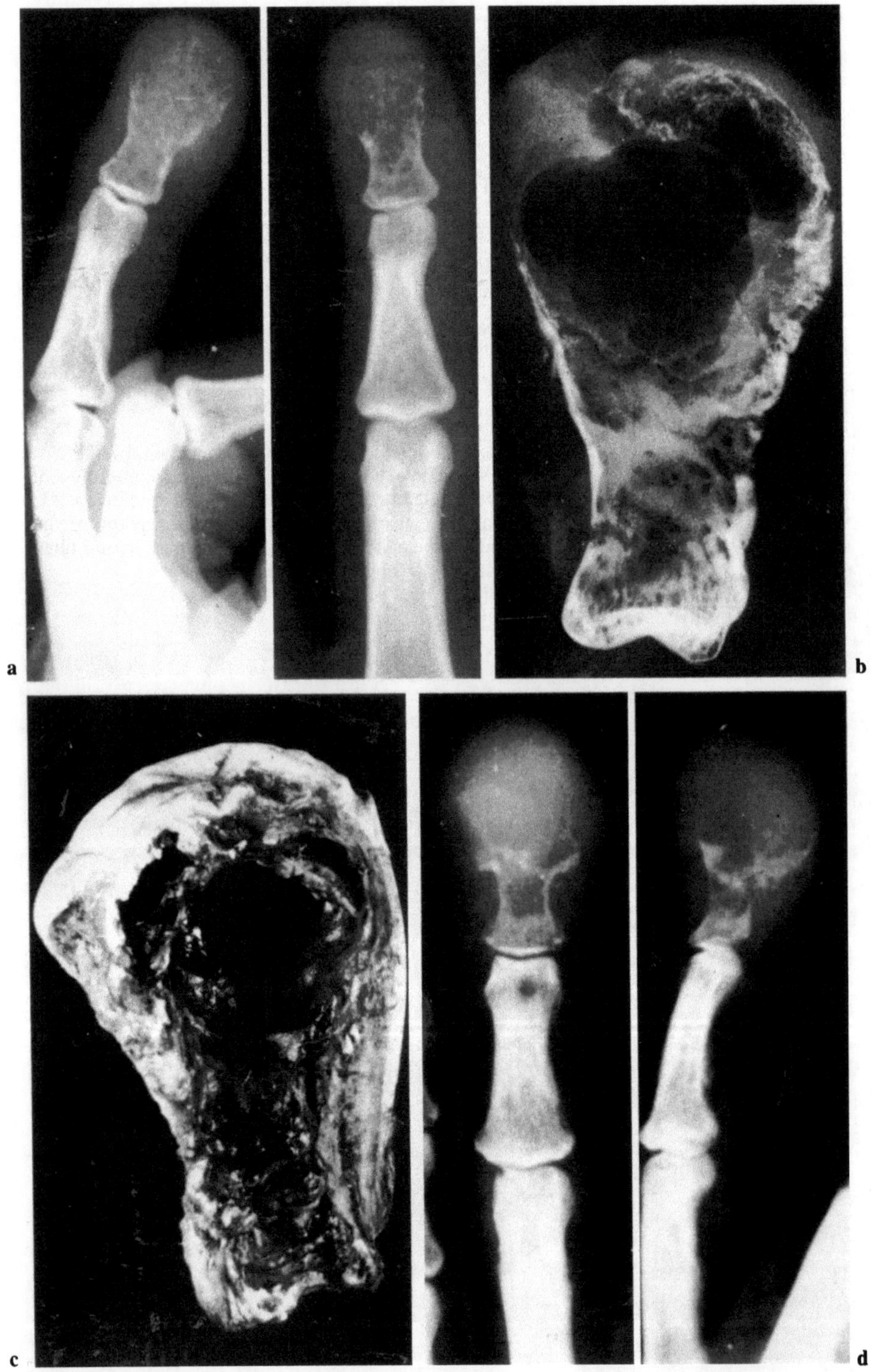

Fig. IX.24a,b. Two cases of aneurysmal bone cyst of terminal phalanges expanding and destroying the cortex, simulating a malignant tumor. **a** Female, 19 years old. **b** Radiograph and **c** photograph of the disarticulation specimen showing a multiloculated hematic cavity. **d** Female, 40 years old, showing a similar lesion. (Schajowicz et al. 1970)

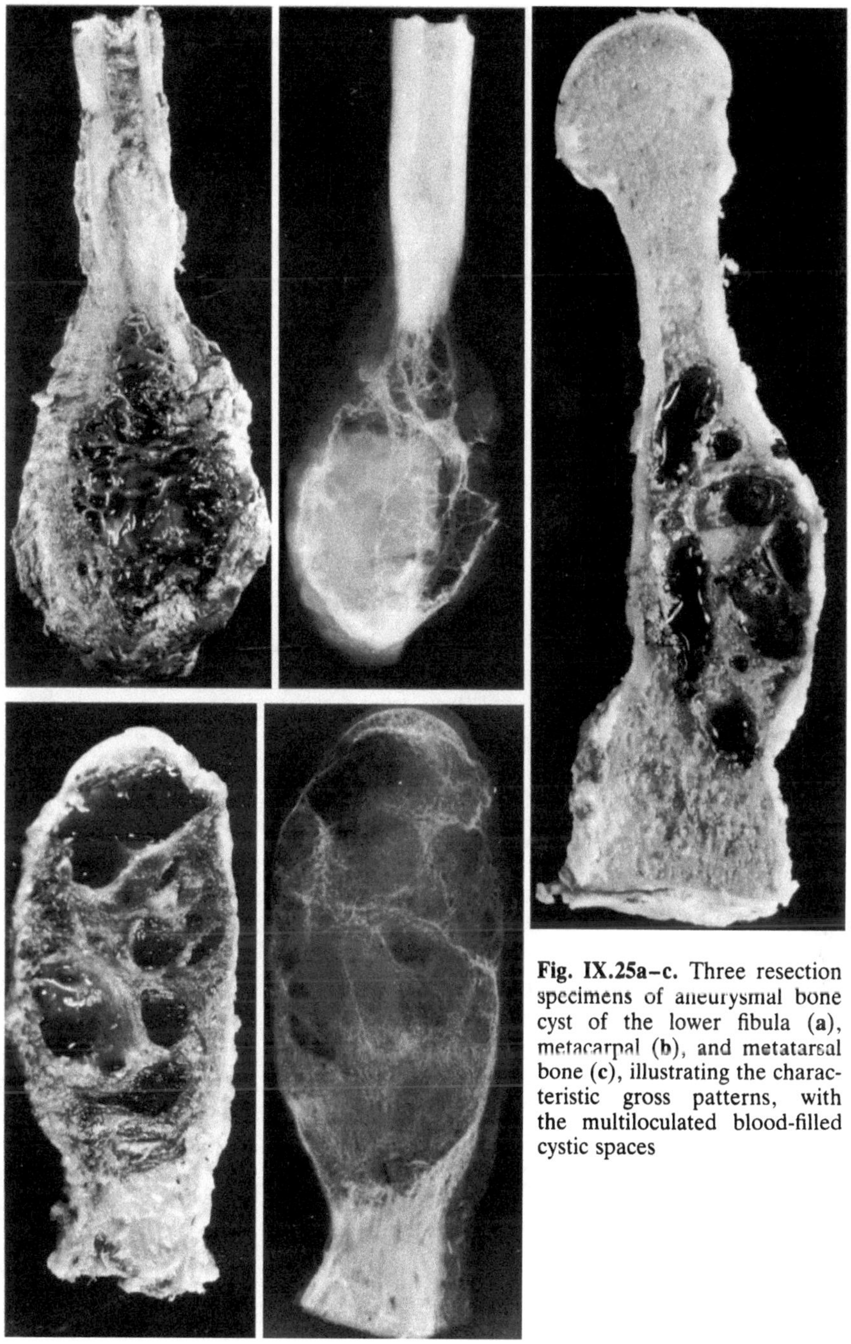

a

b

c

Fig. IX.25a–c. Three resection specimens of aneurysmal bone cyst of the lower fibula (**a**), metacarpal (**b**), and metatarsal bone (**c**), illustrating the characteristic gross patterns, with the multiloculated blood-filled cystic spaces

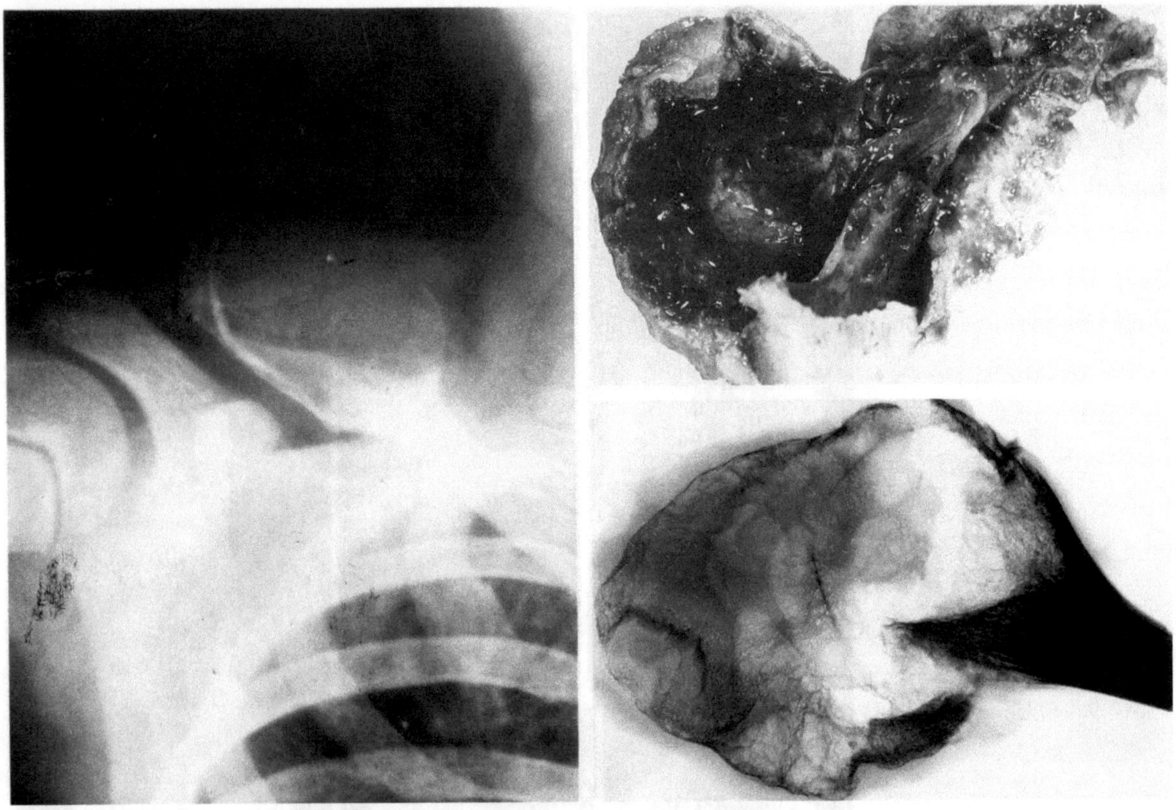

Fig. IX.26a–c. Four-year-old girl with a large aneurysmal bone cyst in the external end of the clavicle. The characteristic blown-out hemorrhagic aspect is evident in **b** and **c**

by fibrous septa of different thickness. Extensive areas of the lesion may be solid, grayish-white or reddish, and of fleshy or fibrous appearance. When the eggshell-like cortex is opened at surgery, there may be profuse venous blood; the blood contained in the cystic cavities indicates continuous drainage (Fig. IX.18). This author proposed the term "multilocular hematic bone cyst," which seems more descriptive than "aneurysmal bone cyst."

Histologically, the blood spaces are not lined by endothelium but by flattened fibroblasts, and the fibrous septa do not contain elastic fibers or a smooth muscle layer. The septa are composed of loose or more dense collagen fibers and contain osteoid or immature bone trabeculae of different sizes and a variable number of osteoclast giant cells. The stroma may show hemosiderin, extravasated blood, and histiocytic elements. The solid portions may be predominantly fibrous and present a lacework of osteoid or newly formed bone trabeculae, or may be more cellular with conspicuous numbers of osteoclast giant cells, resembling an osteoblastoma or a giant-cell tumor, respectively. It is of fundamental importance that the pathologist be familiar with the radiographic aspect and the clinical information when the diagnosis must be based on small fragments, because some areas may be indistinguishable from the tissue lining a simple bone cyst or from a true giant-cell tumor (Figs. IX.27–IX.29).

Pathogenesis. The origin and pathogenesis of aneurysmal bone cyst is still disputed. It is accepted that it may occur as a primary lesion in a previously normal bone or as a secondary feature engrafted upon a preexisting bone lesion that is replaced to a greater or lesser degree. Jaffe wrote in 1958 that in none of the cases studied did examination reveal anything in the tissue sections that would favor the latter hypothesis, nor did aneurysmal bone cyst result even from modification of the usual solitary bone cyst. However, he later changed his mind, saying at a symposium held at the University of Texas in 1962: "I am increasingly of the opinion that the aneurysmal

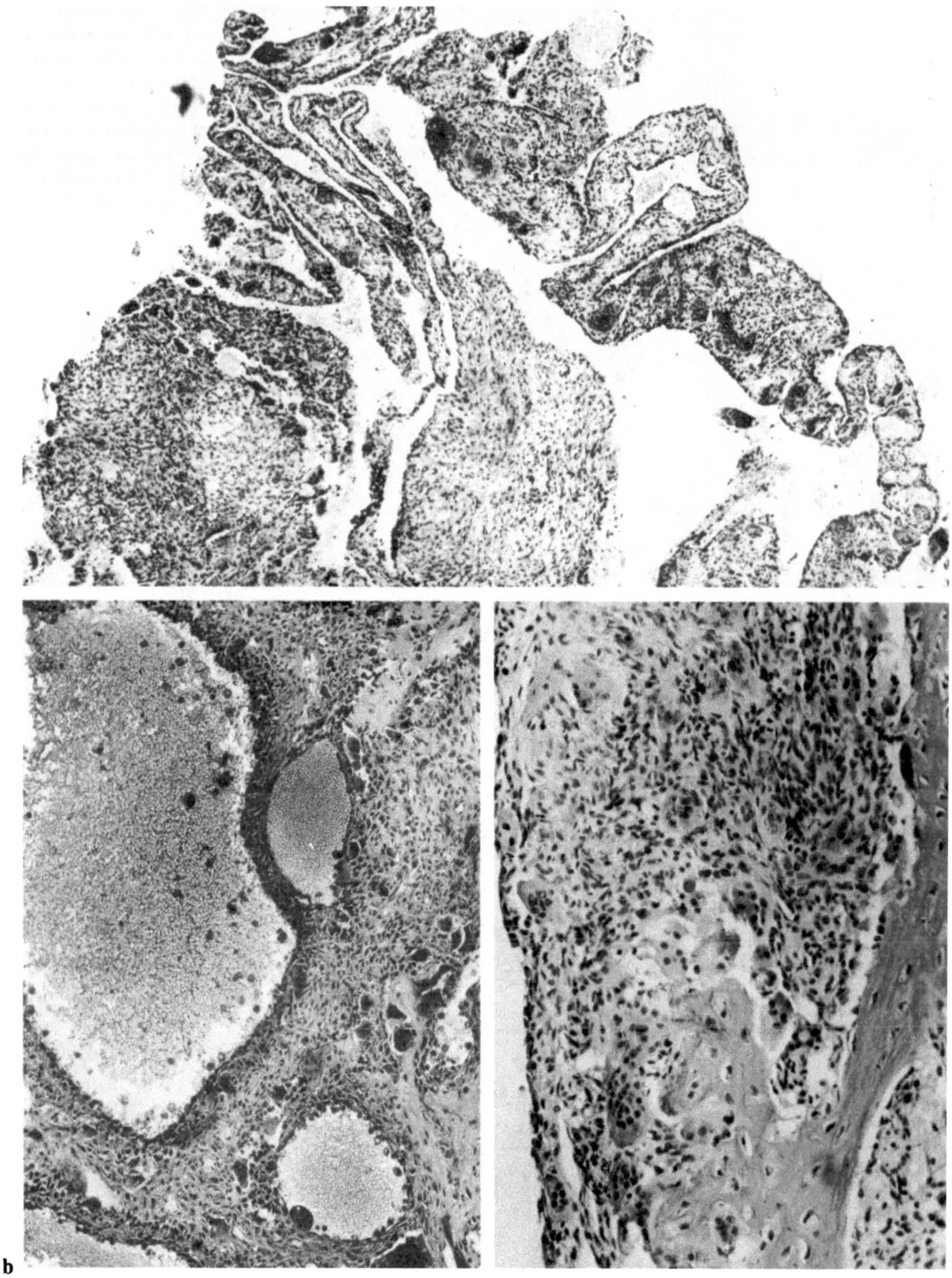

Fig. IX.27a–c. Photomicrographs illustrating the microscopic features of aneurysmal bone cyst. **a** Irregular vascular spaces, separated by connective septa of different widths containing osteoclast giant cells. **b** Vascular spaces and connective septa containing osteoid or immature bone trabecula and osteoclast giant cells. **c** Cyst wall seen at higher magnification, showing more clearly osteoclast giant cells and newly formed osteoid and immature bone trabeculae. **a** ×110, **b** ×100, **c** ×200

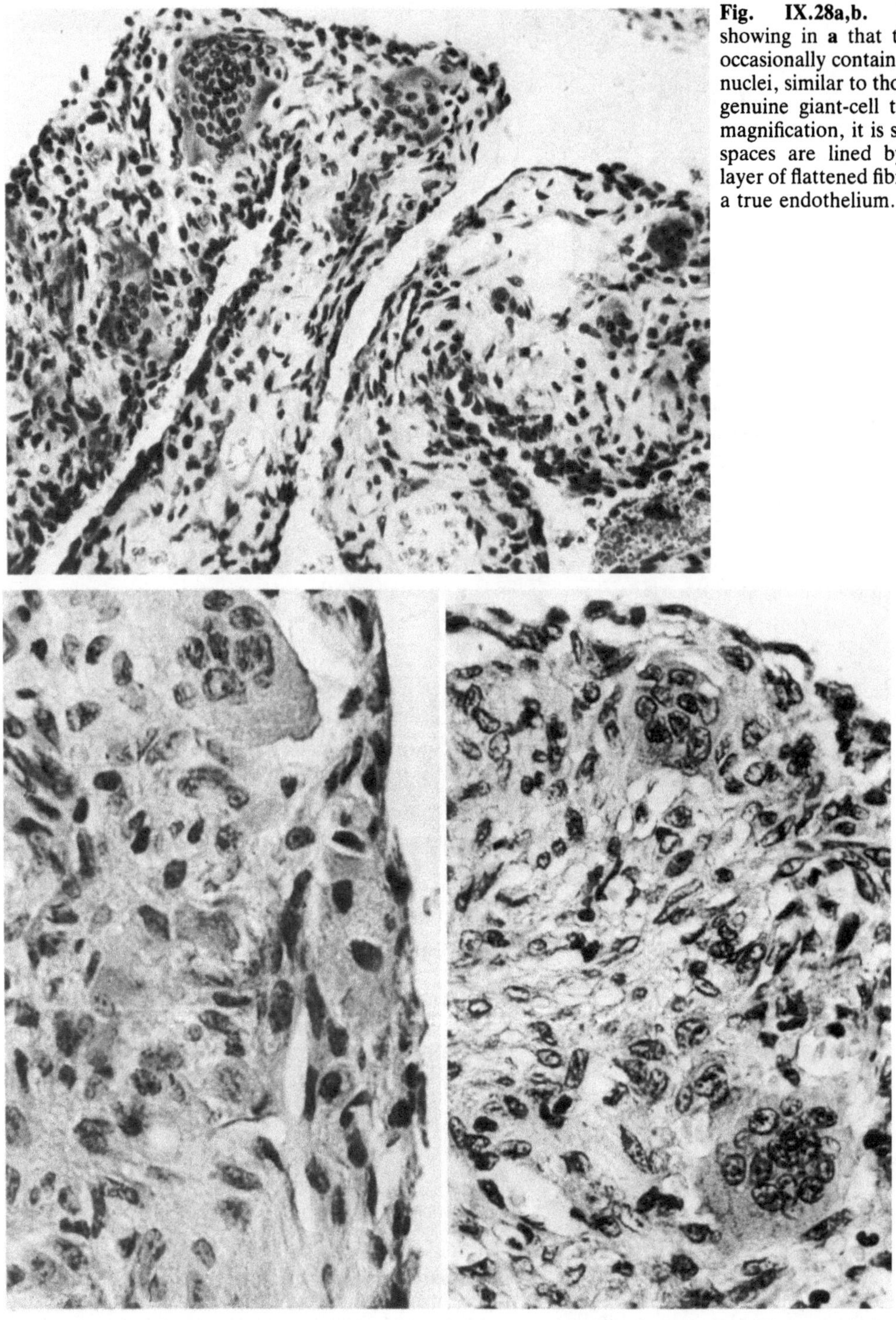

Fig. IX.28a,b. Photomicrographs showing in **a** that the giant cell may occasionally contain a great number of nuclei, similar to those observed in the genuine giant-cell tumors. **b** At high magnification, it is seen that the cystic spaces are lined by a discontinuous layer of flattened fibroblasts and not by a true endothelium. **a** ×200, **b** ×400

bone cyst constitutes a clinical-radiological complex resulting from a secondary change occurring in a preexisting lesion which is often obliterated."

The nature of the preexisting lesion varies, and in several publications an increasing number (32%–35%) of aneurysmal bone cysts have been associated with a preexisting benign or malignant bone lesion (Biesecker et al. 1970; Bonakdarpour et al. 1978). Aegerter and Kirkpatrick (1975) frequently found it superimposed on osteosarcoma, solitary bone cysts, and giant-cell tumors. Levy et al. (1975) reported from Aegerter's laboratory 57 secondary aneurysmal bone cysts in 54 patients: 18 cases were associated with solitary bone cysts,

Fig. IX.29a,b. Photomicrographs showing at lower and higher magnification the septa of different size, containing multinucleated giant cells and newly formed bone trabeculae. **a** ×100, **b** ×400

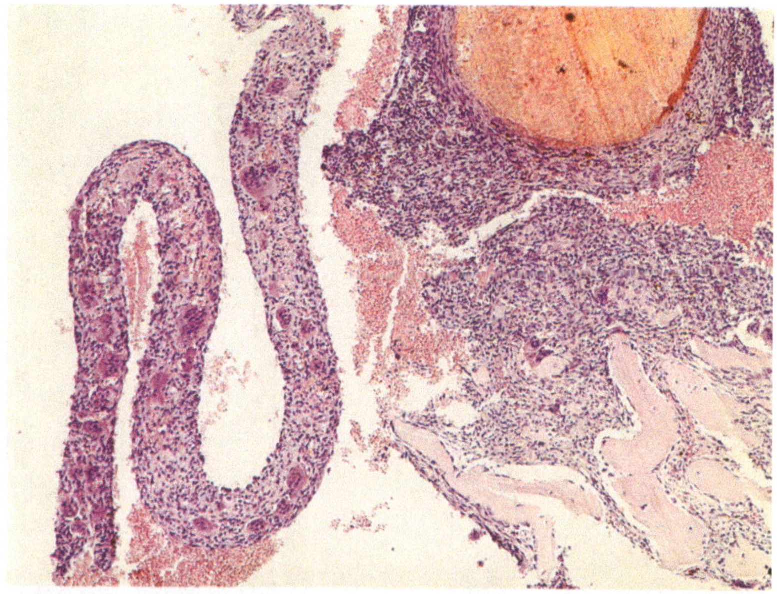

a

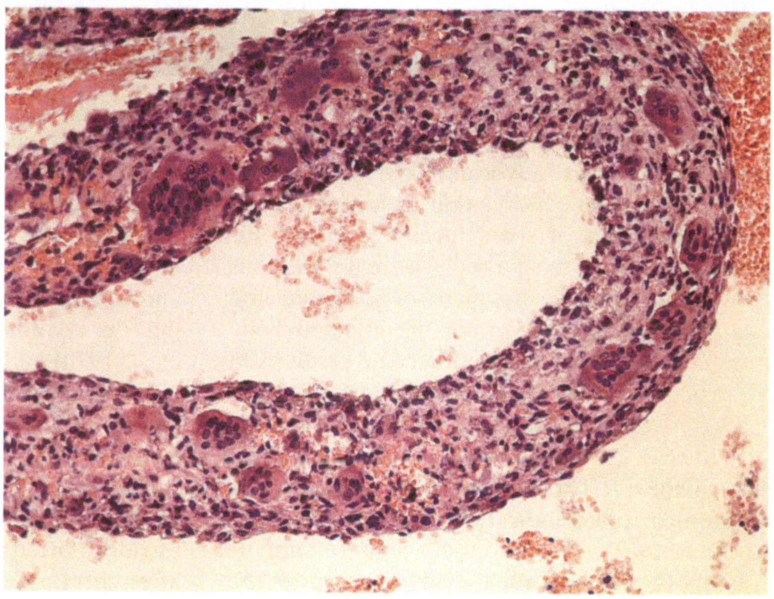

b

14 with giant-cell tumor, and 12 with osteosarcoma. Other associated lesions were nonossifying fibroma, osteoblastoma, hemangioma, and hemangioendothelioma. It is true that areas showing structures similar to those of aneurysmal bone cyst may be found in many bone lesions, neoplastic or not; they are probably the result of hemorrhage and usually occupy only a minor portion of the process. We have observed this pattern in different lesions, e.g., in about 20% of our chondroblastomas (which we designated "cystic chondroblastoma"), in fibrous dysplasia (Fig. IX.30), osteoblastoma, giant-cell tumors, and osteosarcoma. The combined study of the clinicoradiologic features permitted the correct diagnosis in the great majority of cases, which were treated according to the basic process. However, in about 80%, there was no preexisting process.

The term "solid" variant of aneurysmal bone cyst, introduced by Sanerkin et al. (1983) and used in some recent reports, is in this author's view a misnomer and a contradiction, and should be eliminated from the nomenclature. The term was in most cases applied to secondary aneurysmal bone cysts, e.g., aneurysmal bone cyst-like lesions associated with predominantly solid areas of unclassified benign giant-cell lesions.

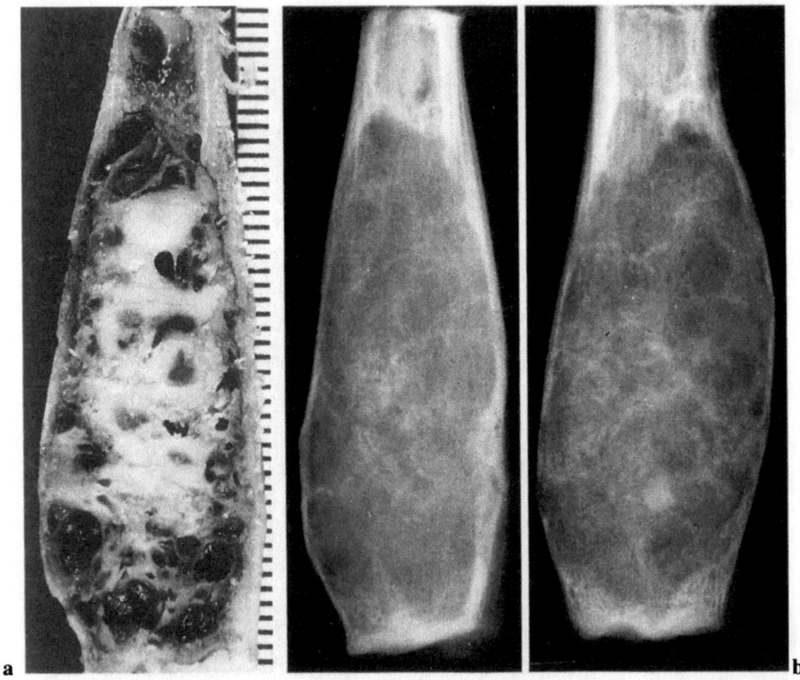

Fig. IX.30a,b. Three-year-old girl with aneurysmal bone cyst-like areas in fibrous dysplasia (secondaiy aneurysmal bone cyst). **a** Photograph and **b** radiographs of the resected specimen show solid grayish-white areas besides multiloculated, cystic, blood-filled cavities. Similar cases are sometimes referred to as "solid aneurysmal bone cyst"

The most widely accepted pathogenetic hypothesis is that advocated by Lichtenstein (1950, 1977), who believes that aneurysmal bone cyst is the result of some local circulatory disturbance, leading to markedly increased venous pressure and the development of a dilated and enlarged vascular bed within the affected bone area. The anomalous circulation could result from intraosseous arteriovenous shunts.

Arteriographic studies (Lindbom et al. 1961; Dos Santos 1950; Schobinger and Stoll 1957) showed the presence of unclotted blood in the cyst, which would indicate free circulation. The rapid extension of some cysts seems to support this hypothesis. Additional evidence includes the manometric measurement of the blood pressure within the cysts showing elevation to arteriolar levels consistent with an arteriovenous shunt (Biesecker et al. 1970) and the fact that the local change in hemodynamics is situated in a highly vascular area of the growing skeleton, i.e., metaphyses.

However, contrary to the hypothesis of arteriovenous shunts is the fact that neither histologic nor ultrastructural studies have demonstrated lining of the cyst walls by endothelial cells (Steiner and Kantor 1978). Furthermore, Ruiter et al. (1975) found increased fibrinolytic activity in the cyst fluid, which would explain the fact that fibrinolysis is an important factor in the dissolution of the clot and expansion of the lesion.

Treatment and Prognosis. The site and size of the lesion and the imminent risk of pathologic fracture or spinal cord involvement are factors that should be considered in selecting the method of treatment. The preferred treatment is surgical and consists of curettage, phenol, and bone grafting or cryotherapy after curettage (Biesecker et al. 1970) and bone grafting. Resection or wide excision is indicated in cysts located in bones where this treatment does not interfere with function, i.e., in ribs, fibula, ulna, patella, and metacarpal or metatarsal bones. The recurrence rate after resection was zero in our cases and in those reported by Clough and Price (1973), but after curettage it was 16.6% in their series.

At times, complete curettage can be difficult or impossible because of problems in exposure (some vertebral cysts) or profuse bleeding (large pelvic cysts). In the latter case, a temporary clamp of the common iliac artery is used, or embolization is performed, followed or not by surgery (Chuang et al. 1981; Murphy et al. 1982).

Although roentgenotherapy has been used successfully in the management of aneurysmal bone cyst by Nobler et al. (1968) and others, with a tumor dose of 20–30 Gy given within 2–3 weeks, curettage is preferred by most authors to avoid the potential risk of interference with the growth plate and the hazard of postirradiation sarcoma.

A few cases of malignant change after radiotherapy have been reported (Lichtenstein 1953; Dabska and Buraczewski 1969). Dahlin (1978) mentioned three cases and we observed one case located in the lumbar spine. Therefore, radiation therapy should be used preferentially in cysts that are surgically inaccessible, or in lesions of large size or so situated that a complete curettage would be difficult (spine, sacrum, ilium). Recurrences are unusual after 2 years and exceptional after 4 years (Clough and Price 1973). In cysts that continue to grow after curettage and/or after repeated recurrences, irradiation may be considered. Spinal cord complications necessitate additional decompression, which may be followed by fusion. No authentic case of malignant change of aneurysmal bone cyst has been reported in the absence of previous irradiation. Some published cases were possibly telangiectatic osteosarcomas, misdiagnosed as aneurysmal bone cysts.

3. Juxta-articular Bone Cyst (Intraosseous Ganglion)

Definition, WHO: *"A benign cystic and often multiloculated lesion made up of fibrous tissue with extensive mucoid change, situated in the subchondral bone adjacent to a joint."*

Cystic defects of bone not related to joint lesions, especially osteoarthritis (Harrison et al. 1953; Landells 1953; Rhaney and Lamb 1955; Lloyd-Roberts 1955; Ondruch 1963), have been reported under different denominations, according to the interpretation of their pathogenesis. Thus we find "bone cavity caused by a ganglion" (Fisk 1949), "necrobiotic pseudocyst or cysts caused by capsular herniation of the carpal bones" (Bugnion 1951), "synovial cysts in bone" (Hicks 1956; Crane and Scarano 1967), "subchondral bone cysts" (Woods 1961), "intraosseous ganglia" (Crabbé 1966; Seymour 1968; Mainzer and Minagi 1970; Feldman and Johnston 1973; Menges et al. 1977), "capsulo-synovial intraosseous inclusions" (Nezelof and Laurent 1966), "ganglia affecting bone" (Salzer and Salzer-Kuntschik 1968), "ganglion cysts of bone" (Sim and Dahlin 1971; Willems et al. 1973), "intraosseous mucous cysts" (Campanacci and Cervellati 1971), "ganglionic cystic defects of bone" (Kambolis et al. 1973), "*geodi isolati sottocondrali*" (Scaglietti and Stringa 1960), and "*geodi subcondrali nonatrosici*" (Catalano 1969).

Such a large number of different terms for a lesion with the same gross and microscopic characteristics, although of still disputed pathogenesis and possibly of varying etiology, is confusing. This is especially true when some authors, like Spjut et al. (1977), separate into distinct entities a "subchondral bone cyst" (p. 353) and a "synovial cyst of bone" (p. 355).

Incidence. Although these lesions are not common, there is no doubt that they are more frequent than reported in earlier publications. This is clearly shown by the large number of reports devoted to the subject in the last few years; however, with few exceptions, these reports have comprised a small number of cases. Nevertheless, in 1951 Bugnion (of Rutishauser's school) reported a significant number of cystic lesions based on specific anatomic research of carpal bones. This suggests that these lesions are much more frequent than is evident from the literature, due to the existence of minimal and totally asymptomatic lesions that are often discovered only accidentally during a radiologic examination. Only in the last few years have some reports dealt with more than ten cases (Kambolis et al. 1973, with 15 cases; Feldman and Johnston 1973, with 38 cases; and Menges et al. 1977, with 19 cases). Over a period of 17 years, we studied 88 well-documented cases in our laboratory (Schajowicz et al. 1979). This number had increased to 136 cases by the end of 1985 (Table IX.1).

Table IX.1. Site and pathogenesis of juxta-articular bone cysts in 88 well-documented cases observed over a period of 17 years (Schajowicz et al. 1979)

Site	Idiopathic	Penetrating	Total
Acetabulum	11	1	Hip 21
Upper end of femur	7	2	
Upper end of tibia	10	3	Knee 16
Upper end of fibula	3	–	
Medial malleolus	12	1	Ankle 16
Lateral malleolus	1	2	
Carpal bones	14	2	16
Scapula	1	–	Shoulder 6
Acromioclavicular joint	2	–	
Humeral head	3	–	
Olecranon	3	2	5
Tarsal bones	3	1	4
Distal end of ulna	2	–	2
Talus	2	–	2
Total	74	14	88

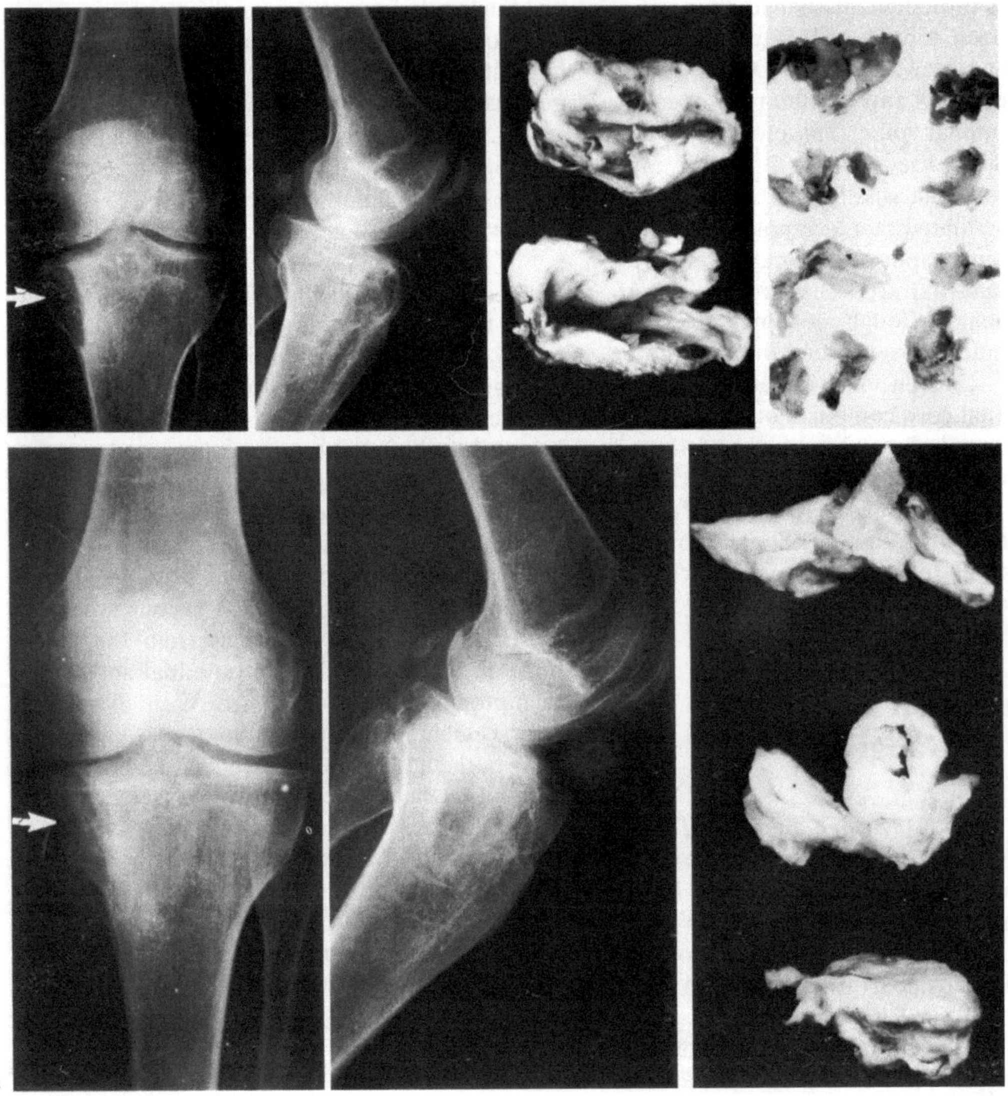

a b, c d e

Fig. IX.31a–e. Male, 34 years old, with bilateral juxta-articular bone cysts of tibia. **a** Anteroposterior and lateral radiographs of the *right* knee showing a well-defined radiolucent lesion of the medial site of the upper tibial epiphysis with a slightly sclerotic inner border. **b** Photograph of the soft tissue ganglion adjacent to the radiolucent lesion. **c** Fragments of the intraosseous multiloculated mucoid cystic lesion obtained by curettage. **d** Anteroposterior and lateral radiographs of the *left* knee of the same patient, showing radiographic and macroscopic findings. **e** At the *top*, the juxtaosseous ganglion and at the *bottom*, the intraosseous cyst. (Schajowicz et al. 1979)

Clinical Findings. *Age and Sex.* The lesions occur more frequently in adults between 20 and 59 years of age (79%) and are rare in younger subjects. The youngest patient in our series was 12 years of age and the oldest, 73, with an average age of 41 years. Lesions located in the tibial and fibular malleolus, hip joint, and carpal and tarsal bones occur more commonly below 40 years of age.

Although some authors (Nezelof and Laurent 1966) have reported a higher incidence in females, most have cited a male predominance (Hicks 1956; Woods 1961; Campanacci and Cervellati 1971; Feldman and Johnston 1973). This is in accordance with our series: we observed 77 cases in males and 54 in females.

Localization. A characteristic feature is the juxta-articular, subchondral location, commonly in long tubular bones. Multiple, especially bilateral and symmetric lesions have been reported (Hicks 1956; Crabbé 1966; Dominok and Crasselt 1967; Feldman and Johnston 1973; Campanacci and Gulino 1974; Menges et al. 1977) and were

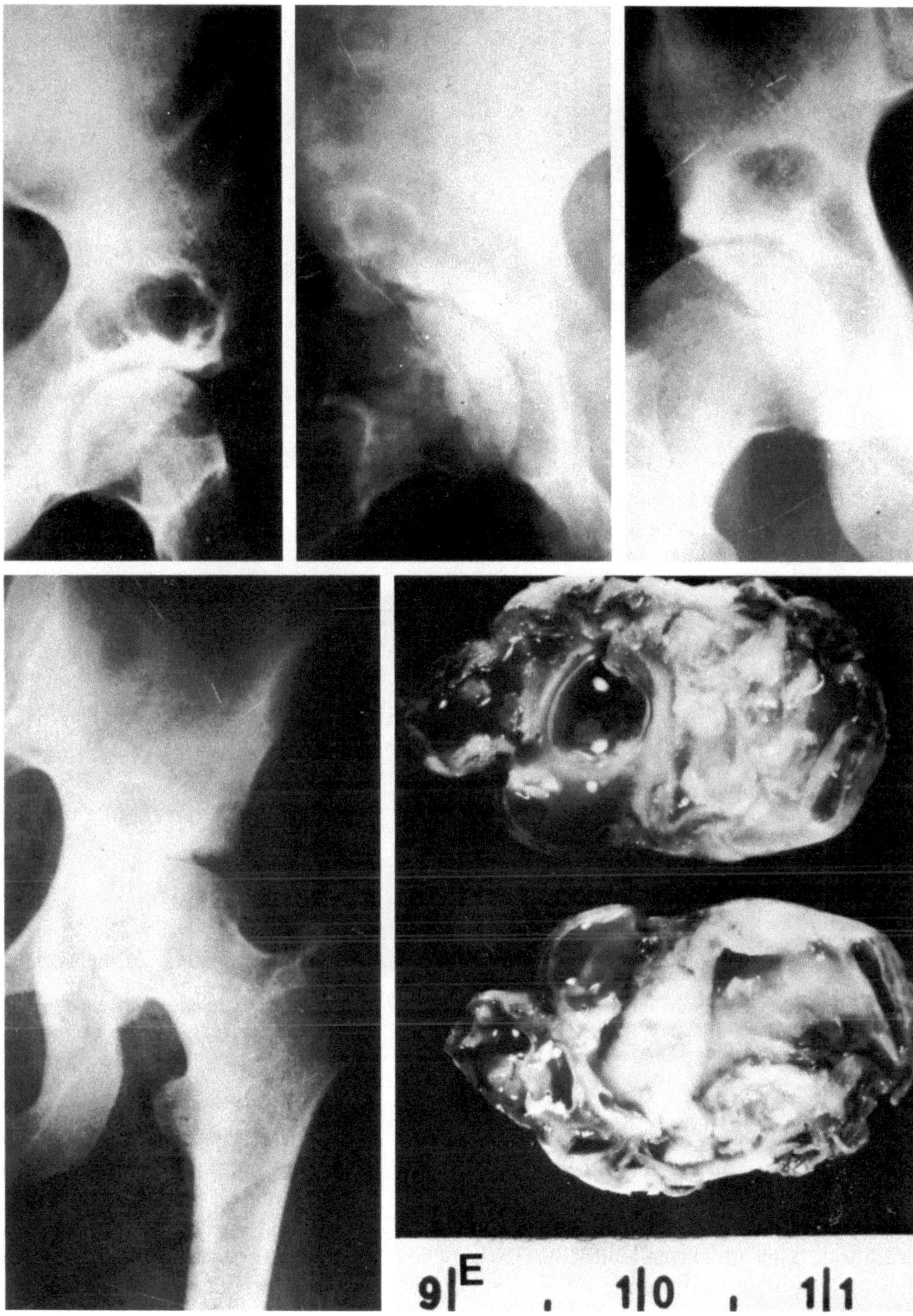

a b, c d e

Fig. IX.32a–e. Four different acetabular cysts, all in young patients with no evidence of joint disease. **a** Female, 17 years old; **b** female, 15 years old; **c** male, 27 years old; **d** female, 29 years old; **e** the specimen removed from the patient shown in **d**. (Schajowicz et al. 1979)

a
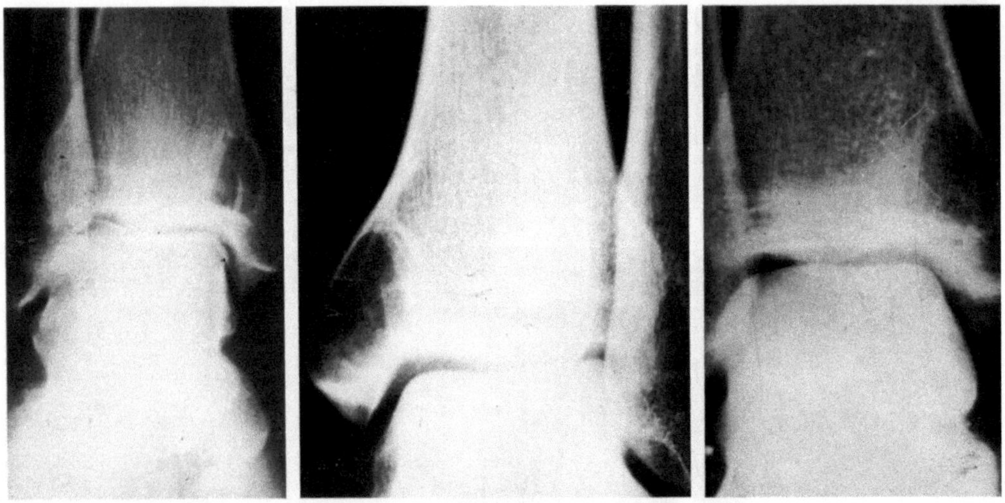
b, c

Fig. IX.33a–c. Three different cystic lesions in one of the most frequent locations, the medial malleolus, all showing thinned cortex and a slightly sclerotic inner border

a, b
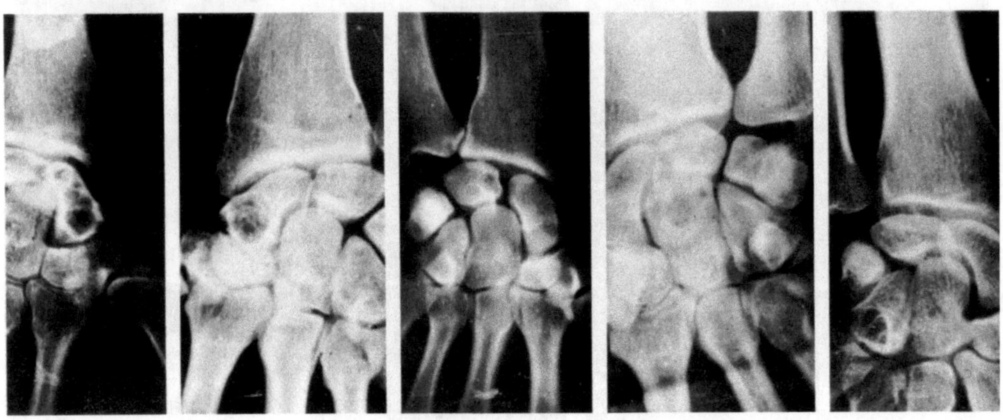
c, d, e

Fig. IX.34a–e. Radiographs of five cases with cystic lesions in different carpal bones. **a** Male, 37 years old (scaphoid); **b** female, 44 years old (scaphoid); **c** male, 35 years old (lunate); **d** male, 38 years old (capitate); **e** female, 26 years old (triquetrum). (Schajowicz et al. 1979)

also observed by us. They occurred in four of our patients: a 34-year-old man with lesions in both internal tibial condyles (Fig. IX.31); a 43-year-old woman with cystic lesions in the radius, olecranon, and tibial malleolus; a 35-year-old man with cysts in both lunate bones; and a 35-year-old man with lesions in both carpal scaphoid bones. The most common sites were the bones adjacent to the hip joint (Fig. IX.32), knee joint (Fig. IX.31), and ankle joint (Fig. IX.33), and carpal bones (Fig. IX.34). Nineteen cases were located in the tibial malleolus, 21 in the acetabulum, and 17 in the tibial plateau.

Symptoms. In many cases the bone lesion is a silent condition and is accidentally discovered by a radiograph taken for other reasons. However, even in the absence of an extraosseous ganglion, the most common symptom is pain (present in approximately 60% of our cases) in close relationship to a joint, sometimes increasing with effort and/or exercise. The symptoms may range over a widely variable period (months to several years).

Radiographic Features. Radiographs show a well-defined oval or round osteolytic area usually located eccentrically in the epiphysis of a long tubular bone, close to the thinned and sometimes expanded cortex (Figs. IX.31, IX.33). The cystic defect is generally in close relationship to a subchondral layer of the affected bone and is outlined by a thin rim of sclerotic bone. The cyst may be unicameral or multilocular; the latter presentation is not infrequent and is more commonly

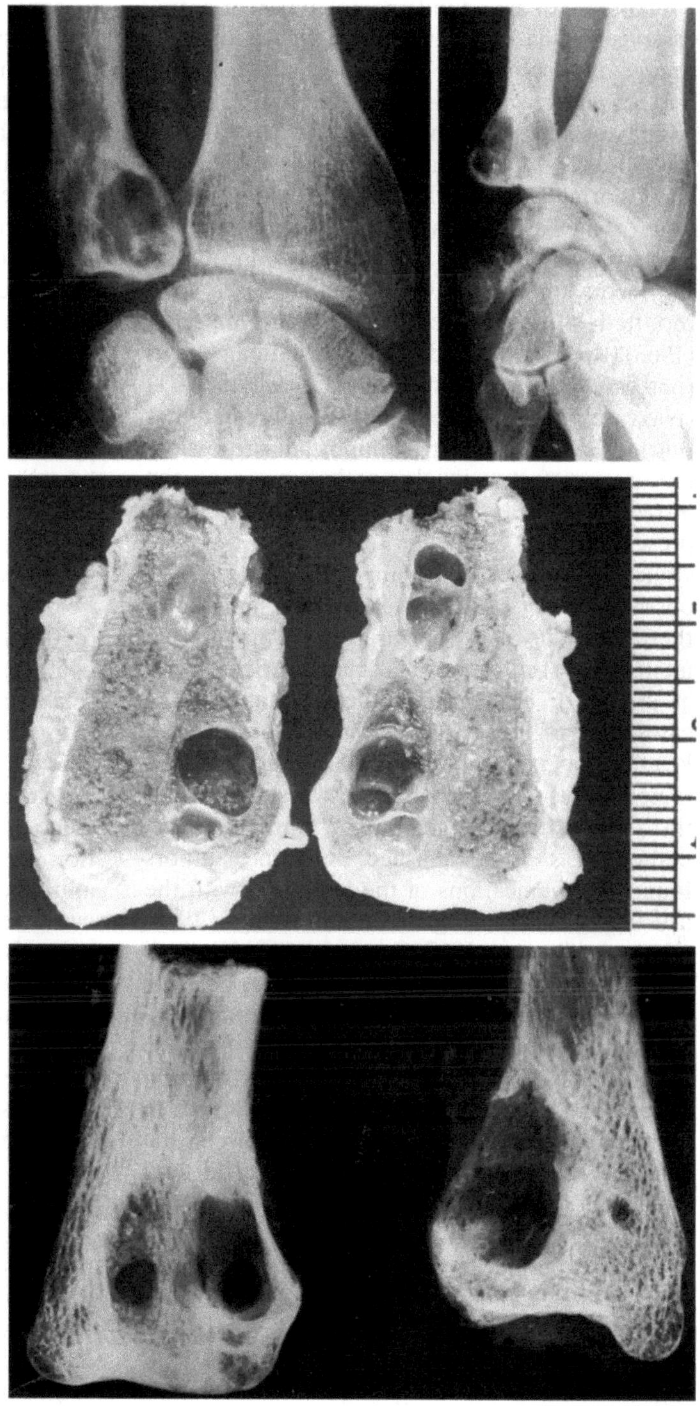

Fig. IX.35a–c. Male, 54 years old. Juxta-articular bone cyst of ulna. **a** Oblique and anteroposterior radiographs showing the osteolytic, apparently septated lesion, in the subchondral zone of the distal ulnar end, with slightly distended and thinned cortex. **b** Photograph of the resection specimen showing, besides the larger multilocular subchondral cyst, filled with mucoid substance, another apparently separated, smaller cyst; in other sections, they communicated with each other. **c** Radiographs of the specimen

encountered in the case of larger cysts. Sometimes (usually in later stages), radiographs show a communication between the bone cyst and the adjacent joint, which is better seen in tomograms (Menges et al. 1977) as a lucent line. The lesions are generally of small to moderate size (1–2 cm) but may attain a diameter of up to 5 cm. The radiographic appearance and size of the bone defect are not related to the clinical findings.

Pathogenesis. Although well recognized as a clinical entity, the pathogenesis of intraosseous ganglia is still obscure. It is generally accepted that the gross and histologic features of intraosseous ganglia are identical or at least similar to those of juxta-articular soft tissues. It is probable that they also share a common pathogenesis, that is, the mucoid degeneration of connective tissue.

There are two fundamental types of intraosseous ganglia, *one of which originates by penetration or intrusion of an extraosseous ganglion into the underlying bone* (Figs. IX.31, IX.32) due to pressure erosion. The most striking examples are those reported by Fairbanks and Lloyd (1934) and Ghormley and Dockerty (1943) with penetration of meniscus cysts into the tibial plateau, and especially the case of Fisk (1949), located at the medial malleolus. Other similar cases were reported later by Salzer and Salzer-Kuntschik (1968) (two cases), Goldman and Friedman (1969) (one case), and Campanacci and Cervellati (1971) (two cases). Kambolis et al. (1973) suggested that this mechanism is the most important or possibly the unique factor in the pathogenesis of the intraosseous cyst, although the mechanism was present in only 7 of their 14 cases. In our previously published series, this pathogenesis was possible in only 14 of 88 cases (16%), and one of these cases involved penetration of an internal meniscus cyst into the tibial plateau (Schajowicz et al. 1979). However, in the vast majority of cases, the ganglion cyst was *primarily intraosseous*, located in the juxta-articular (subchondral) region (Figs. IX.33–IX.35). We suggest that this type be termed "idiopathic" until the exact pathogenesis is established. Several authors found communications of the bone cyst with the articular cavity (Scaglietti and Stringa 1960; Crane and Scarano 1967; Catalano 1969; Nigrisoli and Beltrami 1971) and suggested a possible traumatic origin, owing to the preferential location of the cyst in sites particularly subject to trauma (malleolus region). Nigrisoli and Beltrami observed in two of their four cases a small crack in the articular cartilage that extended between the cyst and the adjacent joint. Thus, synovial fluid would be driven by the pumping action of the joint movement into the subchondral spongiosa, similar to the mechanism suggested by Harrison et al. (1953), Landells (1953), and others for the origin of the osteoarthritic cyst.

Menges et al. (1977) described a communicating channel that was recognizable in tomographic cuts as a lucent line between the cyst and a joint in 57% of their cases, but they admitted that injection of contrast substance into the ganglion failed to penetrate into the joint. However, the majority of authors (Woods 1961; Nezelof and Laurent 1966; Sim and Dahlin 1971; Goldman and Friedman 1969; Campanacci and Cervellati 1971; Kambolis et al. 1973; Feldman and Johnston 1973) did not find such communication. For these reasons the direct extrusion of synovial fluid and/or synovium through the articular cartilage defect into the subchondral bone, a mechanism postulated by Crane and Scarano (1967), has no evident anatomic basis. On the other hand, the cyst lining, described as "synovial in type," lacks a characteristic synovial cell surface. Thus, the term "synovial cyst" in bone (Hicks 1956; Crane and Scarano 1967; Spjut et al. 1971) is a misnomer and should be discarded, whether these communications exist or not.

It is generally accepted that the histogenesis of the "idiopathic" juxta-articular cyst is a mucoid transformation of connective tissue, possibly preceded by intramedullary metaplasia and proliferation of fibroblastic elements ("fibroplasia"), followed by a degenerative stage with mucoid secretion and accumulation that enlarges the ganglionic cyst (Goldman and Friedman 1969; Feldman and Johnston 1973). However, the cause of this intramedullary "fibroplasia" and myxoid degeneration is still disputed. In view of the close relationship of many bone cysts to periarticular capsuloligamentous insertions, Bugnion (1951), who studied cystic lesions in carpal bones radiographically and histologically, maintained that some of these cysts develop as a result of herniation of capsuloligamentous structures into bone, and that others originate as a consequence of cystic degeneration of a focal area of aseptic bone necrosis. Like Bugnion (1951) and Woods (1961), we favor a localized vascular disturbance as the primary cause of the cyst formation, with or without the presence of joint communications (Schajowicz et al. 1979). However, there exists the possibility of the obliteration of a connection between the cyst and the joint cavity, which may explain the relative rarity of such connections in our experience and that of other authors. Although we have not found signs of aseptic bone necrosis in our cases, we believe that this is due to the fact that generally only fully developed cysts with few or no surrounding spongiosa are excised. Small foci of bone necrosis, present at an earlier stage, have subsequently been eliminated through a process of bone resorption and remodeling. Mechanical factors and repeated minor trauma at the superficial bone areas may contribute to these intramedullary vascular disturbances.

Intraosseous ganglia display great clinical and pathologic similarities to the subchondral cysts of osteoarthritis. It is sometimes difficult to establish whether a juxta-articular cyst is secondary to a degenerative joint process or whether the articular lesions are the consequence of the cyst. In a number of cases reported as ganglion cysts, advanced osteoarthritic lesions were present, especially in the hip, such as in eight cases of Feldman and Johnston (1973). Also in rare cases of rheumatoid arthritis, the bone cysts are probably secondary to the joint lesion. However, in other cases the bone cysts, usually located in the knee and hip region and generally large, were evidently precursors of the degenerative joint disease, possibly as a consequence of partial collapse or intra-articular communication through small breaks in the articular cartilage, as Eggers et al. (1963) suggested. All of our few cases that were accepted and included as true primary juxta-articular cysts, despite evidence of articular changes, occurred in a younger age group (less than 30 years), and moderate joint lesions were confined to the site of the cyst. There was no progress of the joint lesions after excision of the cyst. We agree that the pathologic (gross and microscopic) differences are often insignificant or impossible to establish with certainty. The presence of several small cysts or pseudocysts in the "pressure" zone, in addition to one cyst of great size, numerous joint communications due to loss of or extensive defects in the articular cartilage, and the microscopic finding in their interior of necrotic bone and cartilage debris or foci of cartilaginous metaplasia are features absent in "idiopathic" juxta-articular cysts and common findings in osteoarthritis.

Differential Diagnosis. Intraosseous ganglion must always be included in the differential diagnosis of cystic epiphyseal bone lesions located in the vicinity of a joint. Only a few tumoral and tumorlike lesions, such as chondroma, aneurysmal bone cyst, and especially chondroblastoma, may occur in this area, and they generally show more conspicuous thinning and expansion of the cortex and/or stippled calcification. Other osteolytic lesions, such as solitary (unicameral) bone cysts, nonossifying fibroma, and chondromyxoid fibromas, are typically located in the metaphysis. However, it is important to distinguish cystic lesions in inflammatory (rheumatoid arthritis) or degenerative joint disease (osteoarthritis), including those secondary to aseptic necrosis. On the other hand, in a relatively high percentage of cases of "pigmented villonodular synovitis," intraosseous penetration may occur (Schajowicz and Blumenfeld 1968), the hip, ankle, and knee joint being most commonly affected. For the differential diagnosis, it is important to emphasize that in contrast to ganglion cysts, the bone lesions in pigmented villonodular synovitis are frequently located in both bony ends of the affected joint (see Chap. X).

Pathologic Findings. *Macroscopically*, there are no major differences between the intraosseous cysts and the classic ganglia commonly observed in juxta-articular connective tissue. The size of the cysts (intra- and juxtaosseous) ranged from less than 1 cm in carpal bones (Fig. IX.34) to a maximum of 4 cm (Fig. IX.31). They were uni- or more frequently multilocular and surrounded by a fibrous membrane of variable thickness, always easily separable from the adjacent spongiosa. They were filled with a viscous whitish or yellowish mucoid jellylike material. In 14 cases (16%), we found cysts of different sizes but with identical gross features in the connective tissue adjacent to the involved bone and in close relationship with the underlying intraosseous cyst, penetrating through the thinned and/or interrupted cortex. In the remaining cases, we found no juxtaosseous ganglia and only exceptionally communications with the articular cavity.

Histologically, the structure is identical to that of soft tissue ganglia. The major cystic or "mature" cavity is surrounded by a connective tissue membrane, formed by parallel fascicles of collagen fibers with a relatively small number of fibroblasts (Fig. IX.36). These cells cover the inner surface of the cavity discontinuously and are often flattened, acquiring an aspect similar to that of synovium, although an evident and continuous synovial layer was lacking in our cases. Besides the larger "mature" cysts, there are always numerous and extensive foci of myxoid transformation of the connective tissue, with stellate cells, separated by abundant mucoid ground substance. These foci evidently represent new cysts in formation (Fig. IX.37). A number of cells in these areas are round with abundant vacuolar cytoplasm, filled with PAS-positive material and apparently secreting mucoid material. Similar elements are found floating freely in the smaller or larger cystic cavities. Sometimes, adjacent to the newly formed cysts, an increased number of fibroblasts is observed, which seems to suggest that the proliferation of fibroblasts ("fibroplasia") may precede or accompany the mucoid degeneration. The cancellous bone that surrounds the cyst cavity shows, besides areas of osteoclastic bone resorption apparently corresponding to still-growing cysts, predominant new bone formation, giving origin to a rim of slight bone sclerosis.

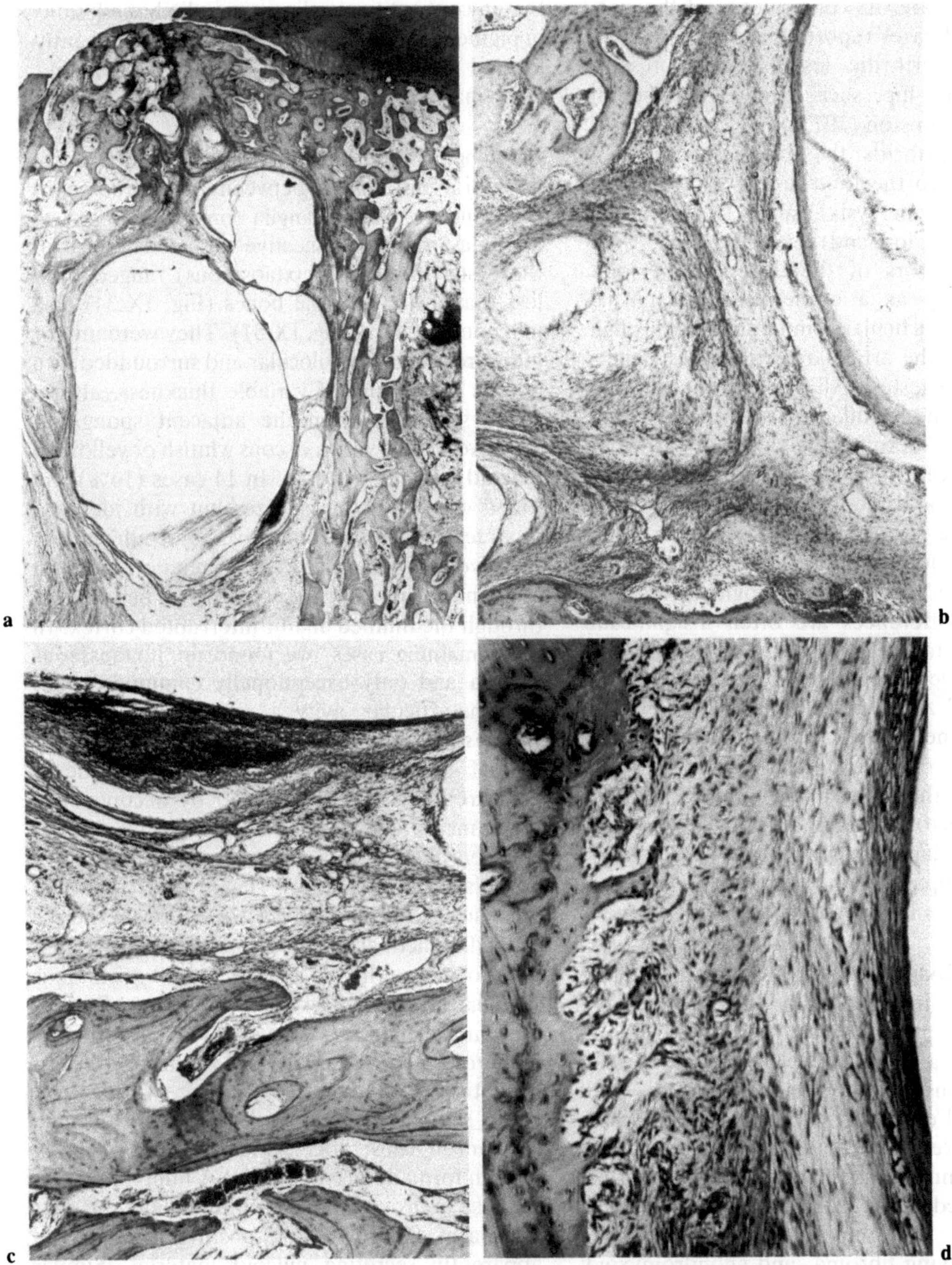

Fig. IX.36a–d. Photomicrographs of case shown in Fig. IX.35 illustrate the multiloculated nature of the cyst, in part "mature," that is, lined by membrane of fibrous tissue of different thickness, and in part showing focal areas of myxoid degeneration with formation of smaller cysts (**b**), surrounded by slightly sclerotic bone. **c**,**d** Cyst wall in two different cases consisting of fibrous tissue with some hemorrhages (**c**), surrounded by newly formed bone. (**a**, **b**, and **d**, from Schajowicz et al. 1979) **a** ×10, **b**,**c** ×100, **d** ×200

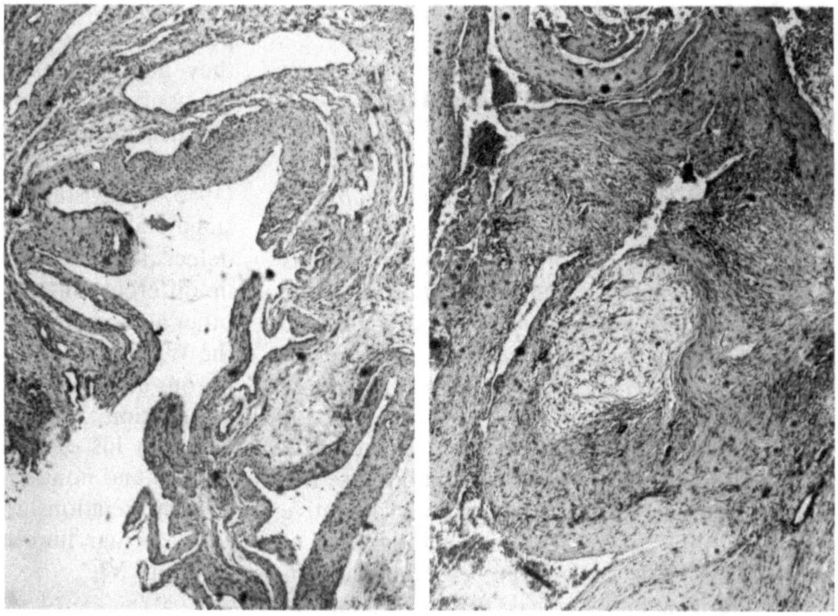

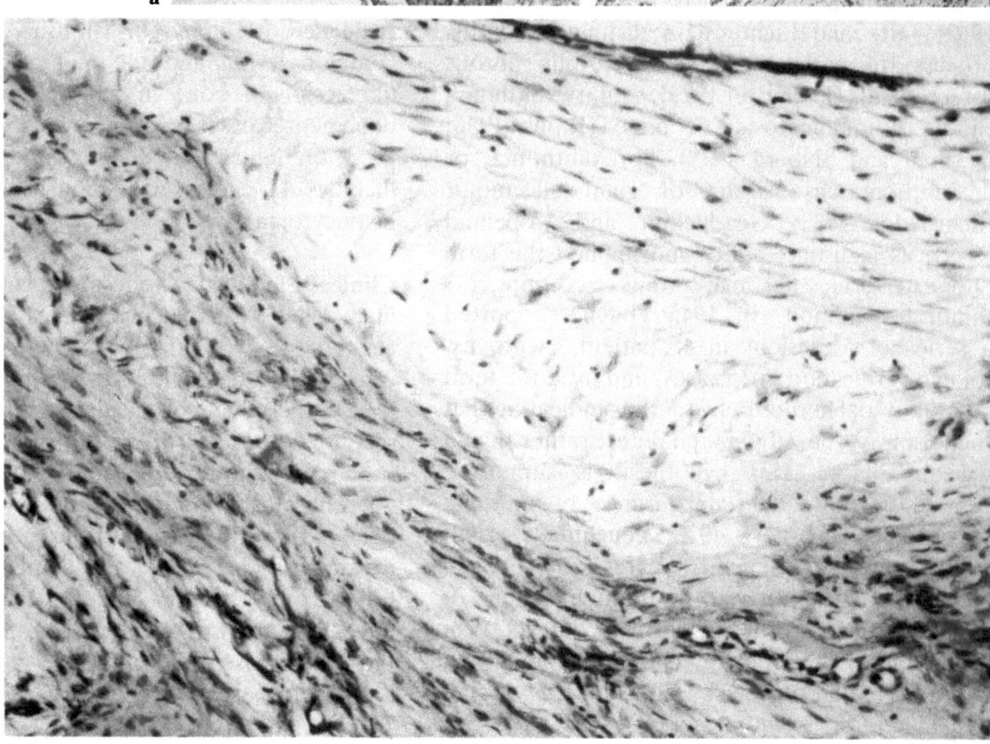

Fig. IX.37a–c. Photomicrographs showing the multiloculated aspect of the cyst, formed by folded membranes of fibrous tissue showing areas of myxoid degeneration in **a** and **b**. **c** At higher magnification, besides areas of dense connective tissue, other looser myxoid zones are observed. Unlike in synovial membrave, there is no continuous cell lining at the surface of the cyst. **a**,**b** ×60, **c** ×180

Treatment and Prognosis. Excision of the extraosseous ganglion, accompanied by curettage or excision of the bone cyst, followed by bone grafting of the cavity whenever the cyst had attained a considerable size, was the treatment in most cases. In large lesions located in a non-weight-bearing bone end, a segmental resection was performed.

The lesions generally heal without any sequelae or complications. However, some cases of one or more recurrences have been reported in the literature (Crabbé 1966; Feldman and Johnston 1973); the case of Sim and Dahlin (1971) with six recurrences and our case with five recurrences remain unique. In addition to this last case, we observed only one other recurrence.

4. Metaphyseal Fibrous Defect (Nonossifying Fibroma, Histiocytic Xanthogranuloma)

Definition, WHO: *"A well defined non-neoplastic bone lesion, characterized by essentially the same histological features of benign fibrous histiocytoma, that is, spindle-celled fibrous tissue with a storiform pattern and containing a variable number of multinucleated giant cells, hemosiderin pigment, and lipid-bearing histiocytes (xanthoma cells)."*

"Metaphyseal fibrous defect" is the term preferred by the WHO Classification because it is only descriptive and does not imply a definitive position on the still controversial pathogenesis of the process. This controversy explains the different designations applied to the lesion. In 1942, Jaffe and Lichtenstein distinguished this process [formerly classified as chronic fibrous osteomyelitis (Phemister 1929), solitary xanthoma (lipoid granulomatosis) of bone (Bahls 1936; Burman and Sinberg 1938), fibroxanthoma, or a xanthomatous variant of giant-cell tumor (Schroeder 1932; Geschickter and Copeland 1949)] as a distinct entity and applied the term "nonosteogenic fibroma," thus accepting its tumoral condition. In 1945 Hatcher reported a series of 51 lesions in 45 patients, with histologic verification in 15 cases, and used the term "metaphyseal fibrous defect," thus indicating that the lesion is a developmental defect rather than a true neoplasm. This hypothesis is supported by the not-infrequent appearance of multiple foci (Evans and Park 1978; Peuchmaur et al. 1985), their spontaneous regression (Ponseti and Friedman 1949), and the frequent finding of similar lesions ("fibrous cortical defects") in roentgenograms of healthy children: Sontag and Pyle (1941) observed such lesions in 22% of girls and 53% of boys, and in Caffey's study (1955) of 154 children they were present in 23% of girls and 42% of boys; however, in Selby's (1961) report on 151 children, no evident sex predominance was found. It is interesting that in these reports no fibrous cortical defects were found under 21 months of age, and only exceptionally after 10 years.

Jaffe (1958) later changed the term "nonosteogenic fibroma" and applied the name "nonossifying fibroma," thus insisting on its neoplastic nature. However, he used the term "cortical fibrous defect" for the smaller subperiosteal or cortical lesions, and he admits that they may increase in size and develop into a nonossifying fibroma, both entities having identical histologic features. Spjut et al. (1971) used both terms interchangeably, and Caffey (1955, 1972) stated that probably in their earlier stage, all nonossifying fibromas are cortical defects and that these lesions are the same entity in different phases. This opinion is shared by other authors and by the writer, who prefers, with the WHO, the noncommitted term "metaphyseal fibrous defect." The writer proposed the alternate designation "histiocytic xanthogranuloma," which in his opinion best reveals the histologic pattern and nonneoplastic nature of this lesion.

The relationship to and proposed distinction from "benign fibrous histiocytoma" are discussed in Chap. VI.

Incidence. Metaphyseal fibrous defect is a common lesion and the most frequent tumorlike lesion of bone in our files, i.e., 357 well-documented cases recorded over 45 years (Scheme IX.3; the figure of 368 cases cited in the scheme includes 11 cases reclassified as benign fibrous histiocytoma – see below).

Clinical Findings. The lesion was more common in males (61%) than in females (39%). In four cases the sex was unknown. The age ranged from 7 months to 69 years, but the highest incidence was in the first two decades, with a peak in the second decade (64%). Only 6% of cases were found after the third decade.

The most common anatomic location was in the femur (157 cases), preferentially the lower metaphysis (112 cases) and diaphysis (25 cases), followed by the tibia with 144 cases, most frequently in the upper (66 cases) and lower metaphyses (50 cases). Therefore, 84% of cases were located in these two bones.

The fibula (28 cases) was also frequently involved. In contrast to the common involvement of the long bones of the lower extremities, long bones of the upper extremities and short or flat bones were rarely involved, the most common site among them being the humerus (14 cases). Because of their unusual sites and clinical features, the six cases located in the pelvis, together with the two rib and three cranial lesions, have actually been reclassified as benign fibrous histiocytoma, following the more recent criteria of interpretation. Ten patients had multiple lesions: seven

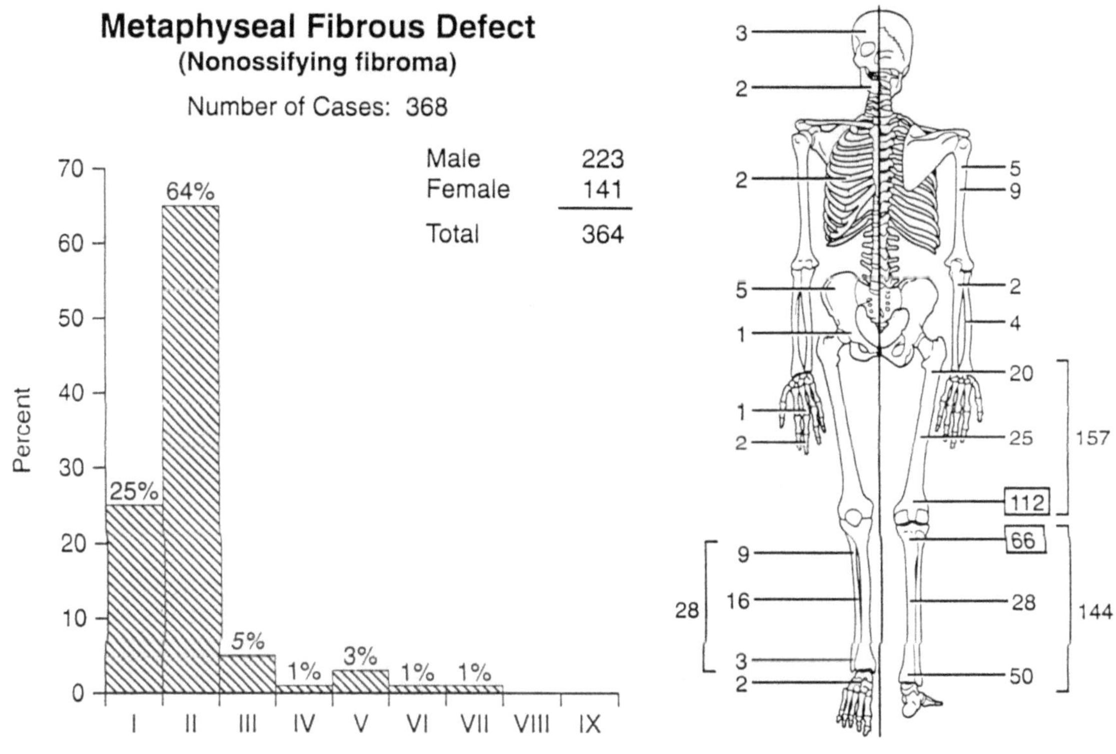

7 cases multiple
4 cases sex unspecified
11 cases located in the skull, ribs and pelvic bones were reclassified as benign fibrous-histiocytoma

Scheme IX.3

with two foci, two with three, and one with four foci, all located in the lower femoral and/or upper tibial metaphysis (Figs. IX.38, IX.39). Multiple lesions may on rare occasions be associated with extraskeletal anomalies and are referred to as Jaffe-Campanacci's syndrome (Campanacci et al. 1983; Mirra et al. 1982).

Symptoms. Pain was the principal complaint in approximately 40% of patients, and a pathologic fracture was the initiating symptom in 18%. In about 36%, the lesion was an incidental radiographic finding.

Radiographic Features. The radiographic appearance is distinctive and usually diagnostic (Cunningham and Ackerman 1956; Compere and Coleman 1957). The lesion is radiolucent and located eccentrically, usually in the metaphysis of a long bone (Figs. IX.40–IX.43); however, as growth proceeds it becomes more separated from the epiphyseal plate, moving toward the diaphysis. The inner border was usually well defined and slightly sclerotic; infrequently the lesion was traversed by some trabeculae, which gave it a multilocular appearance (Figs. IX.41, IX.43). The cortex was sometimes thinned and slightly expanded, but there was no periosteal reaction, except in cases with pathologic fracture. Particularly in small bones (fibula, ulna, radius), but also in the humerus, the process occasionally occupied the medullary cavity and the whole diameter of the long bone (Figs. IX.44–IX.46). In these cases one has to consider in the radiologic differential diagnosis fibrous dysplasia, solitary bone cyst, and eosinophilic granuloma. There are intermediate stages between small cortical or subperiosteal lesions a few centimeters in size with slight excavation of the cortex (generally classified as fibrous cortical defect) (Fig. IX.42) and the larger lesions, and it is generally recognized that they are basically different manifestations of the same disorder. We employ for both types, which present identical histologic fea-

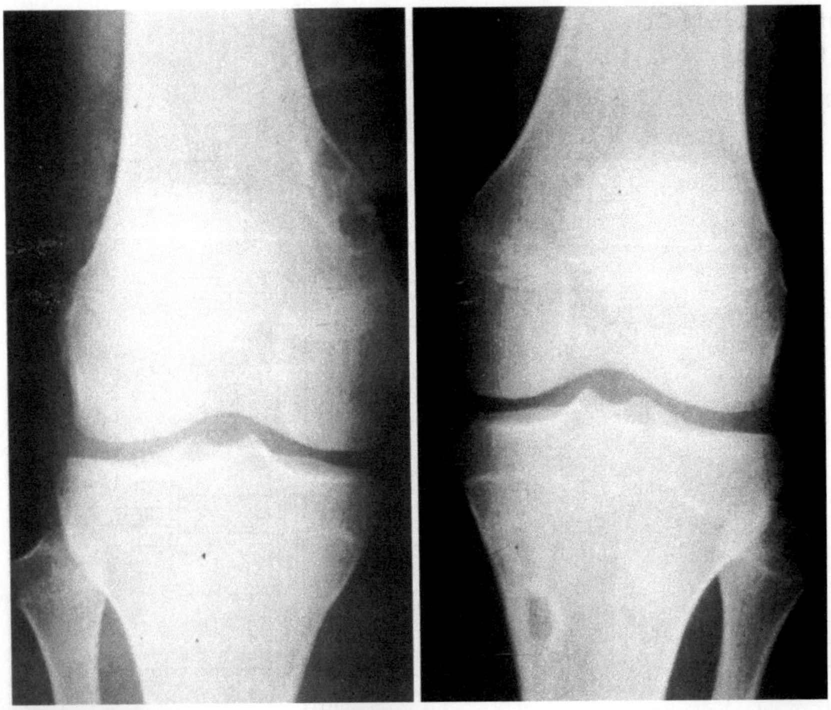

a

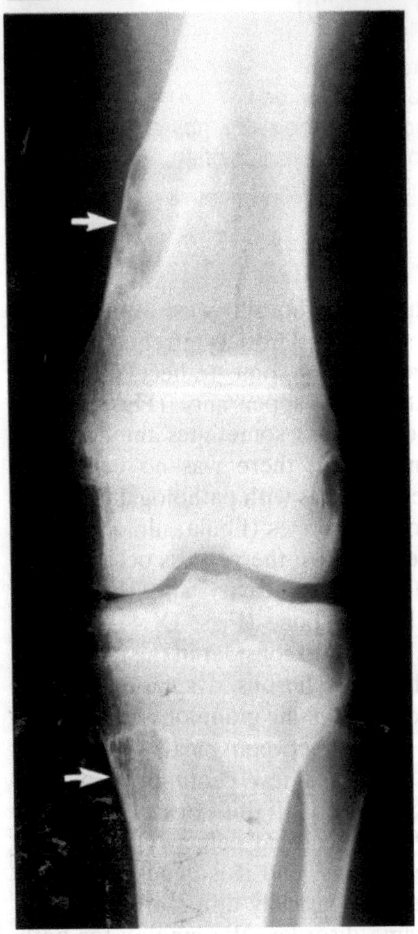

b

◀ **Fig. IX.38a,b.** Two cases with *multiple* metaphyseal fibrous defects. **a** Female, 12 years old, with small lesion in lower metaphysis of the left femur and upper metaphysis of the right tibia. **b** Female, 14 years old, with lesions in the lower femur and upper tibia of the same side (*arrows*)

Fig. IX.39. Male, 33 years old. Multiple radiolucent, well-defined lesions with a radiologic aspect similar to that of metaphyseal fibrous defect, located in both upper femoral ends and in the left ilium. There were no lesions in the ▼ skull or in other bones

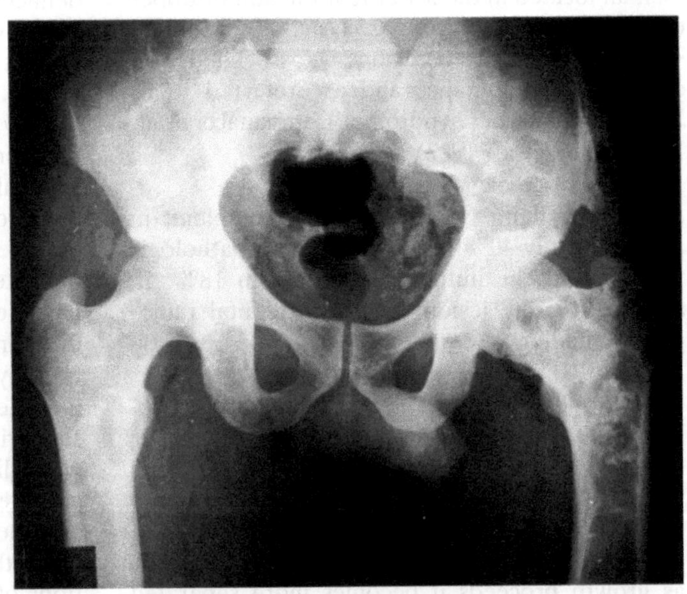

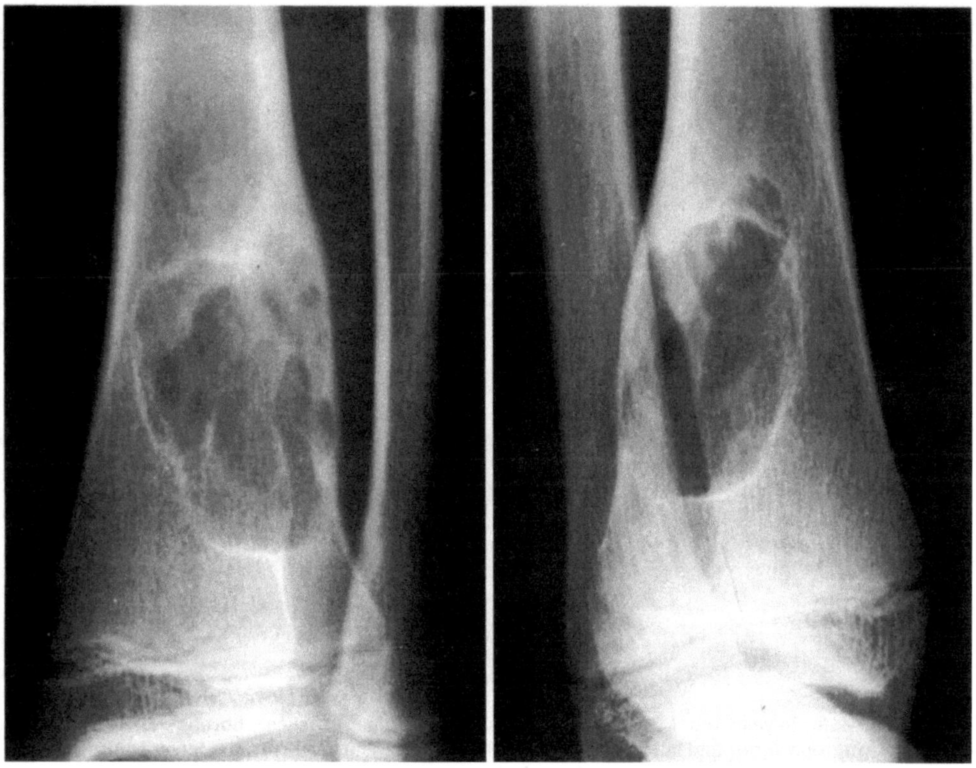

▲
Fig. IX.40. Male, 8 years old. Metaphyseal fibrous defect in lower metaphysis of tibia. Anteroposterior and lateral radiographs show a radiolucent eccentric lesion with well-defined, slightly sclerotic inner border

▶
Fig. IX.41. Female, 13 years old. Metaphyseal fibrous defect of tibia. Anteroposterior and lateral radiograms illustrate an unusually large lesion that occupies the whole width of the bone, with a pathologic fracture

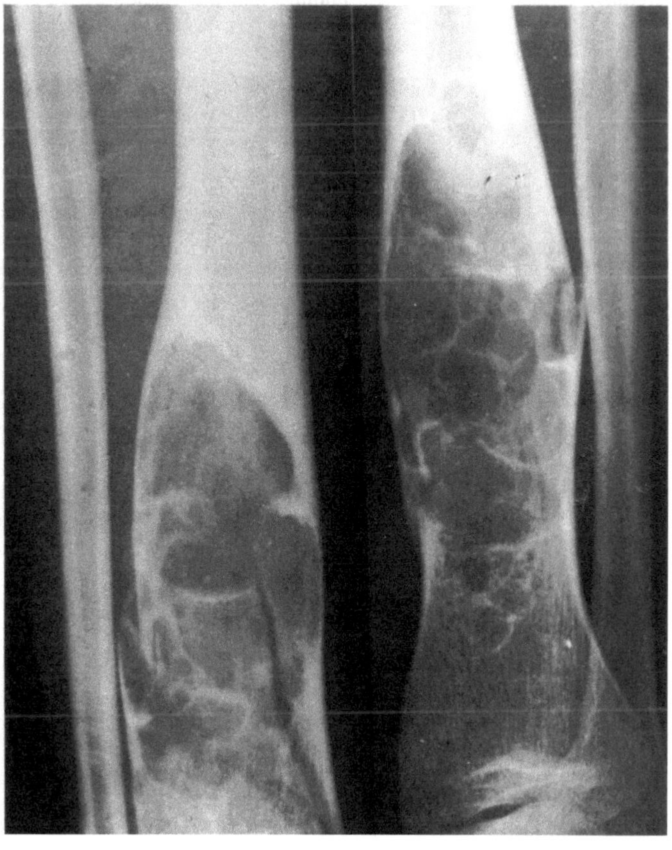

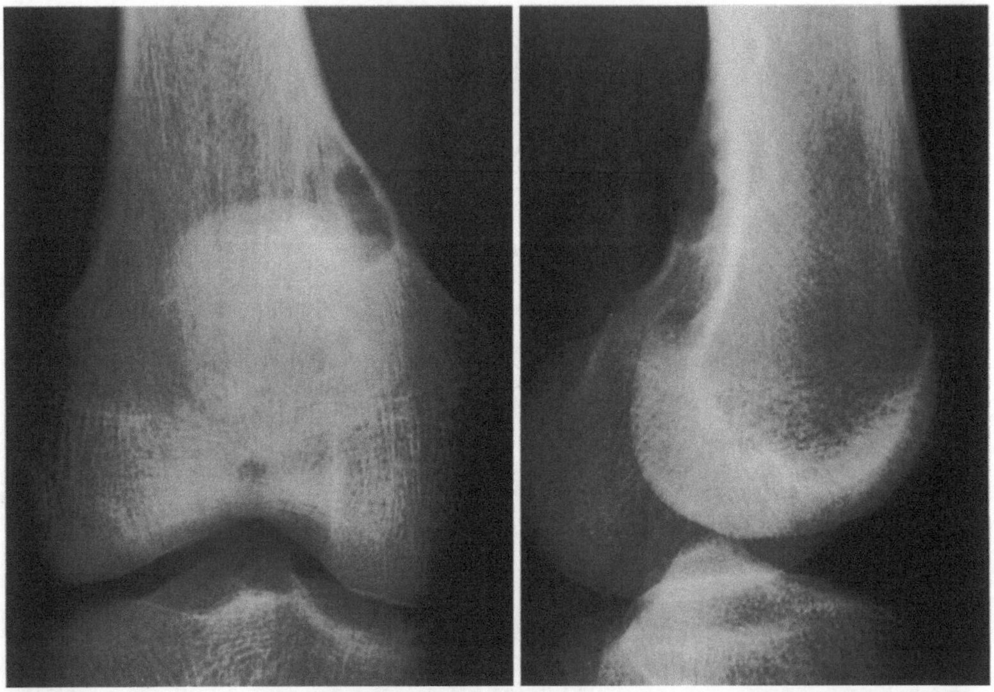

Fig. IX.42. Male, 16 years old. Metaphyseal fibrous defect of femur. Anteroposterior and lateral radiographs showing a small subcortical well-defined lesion. Such lesions are frequently incidental radiologic findings and are classed as "cortical fibrous defect." Transitional stages from "cortical fibrous defect" into metaphyseal fibrous defect (histiocytic xanthogranuloma or "nonossifying" fibroma) or spontaneous healing may occur

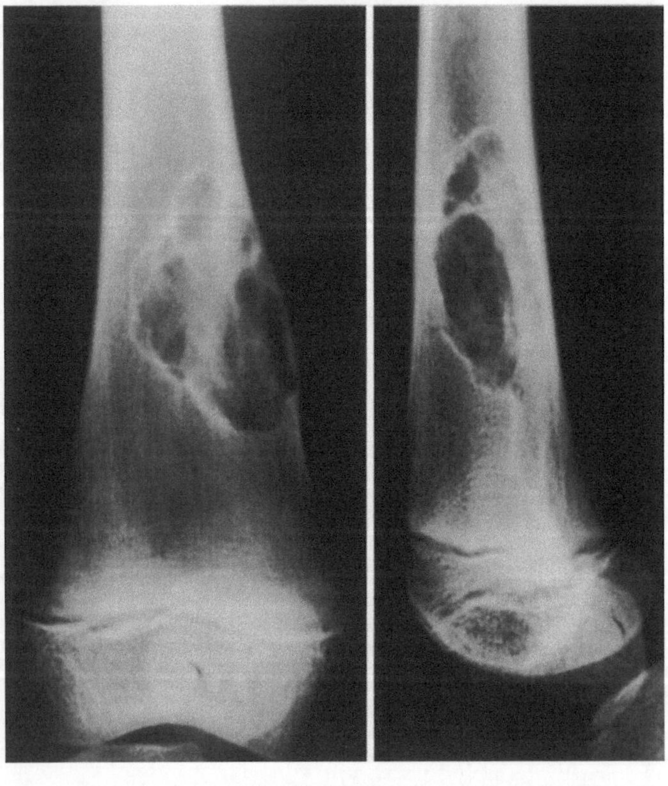

Fig. IX.43. Male, 11 years old. Metaphyseal fibrous defect of femur. Anteroposterior and lateral radiographs showing a larger lesion with the characteristic pattern, moved up toward the diaphysis

Fig. IX.44. Female, 11 years old. Metaphyseal fibrous ▶ defect in the upper third of humerus. The lesion involves the whole width of the bone. Note the conspicuous sclerotic borders

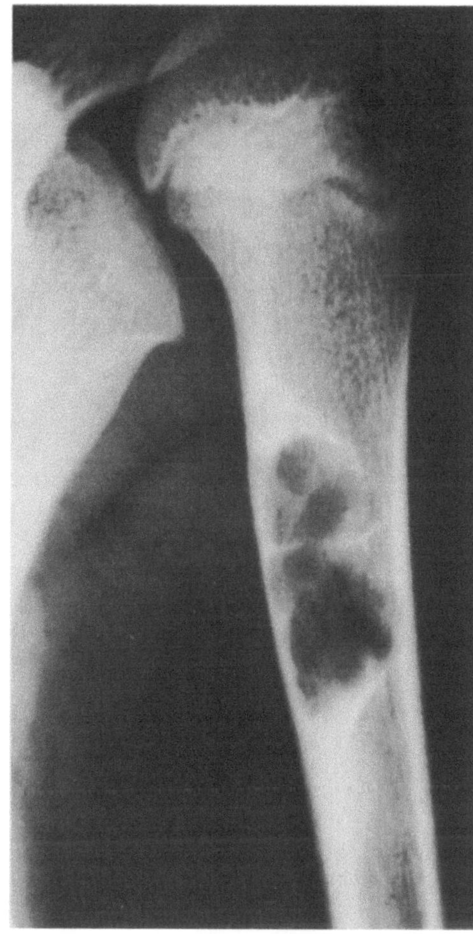

Fig. IX.45a–c. Two different cases of metaphyseal fibrous defect. **a** Female, 12 years old, with a small fibrous defect in the lower part of the radius with evident sclerotic inner border. **b** Male, 15 years old, with a large radiolucent lesion involving the entire width of the ulna, expanding and thinning the cortex. A diagnosis of fibrous dysplasia was suggested. **c** Photograph of the resected segment showing dark brownish areas alternating with white and yellowish zones ▼

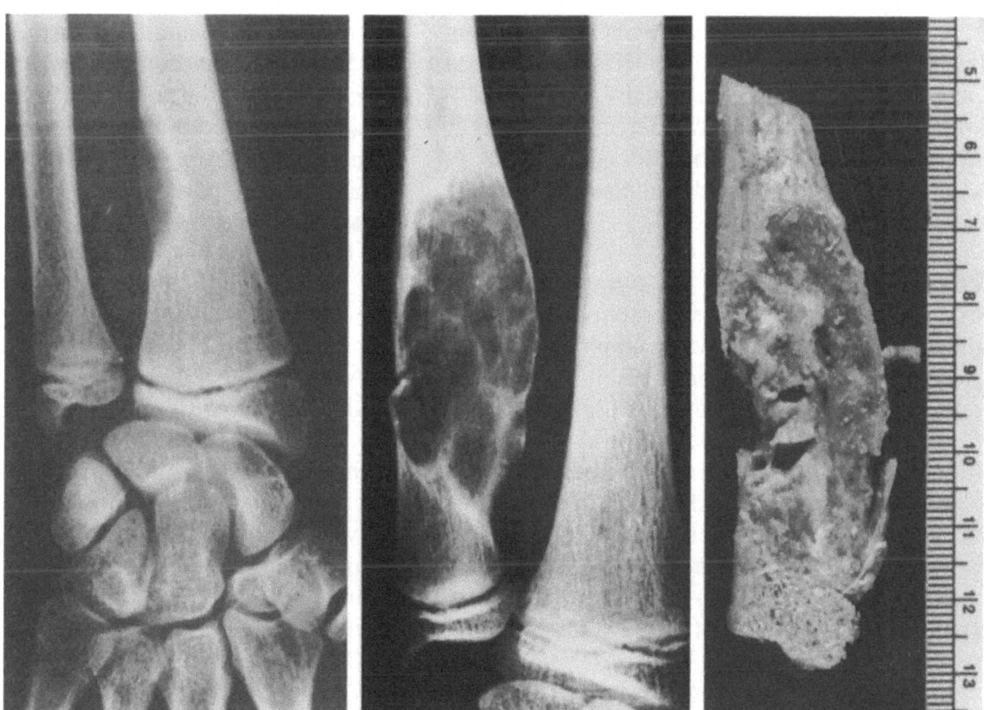

a, b **c**

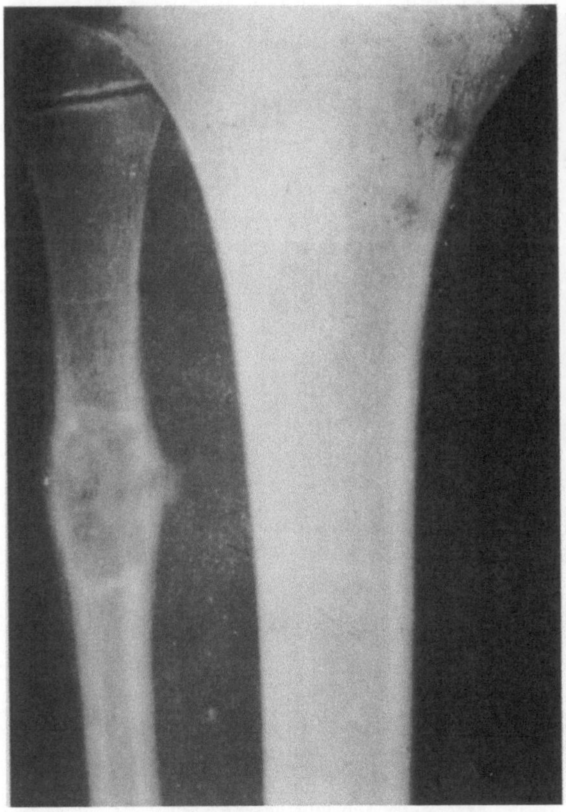
a

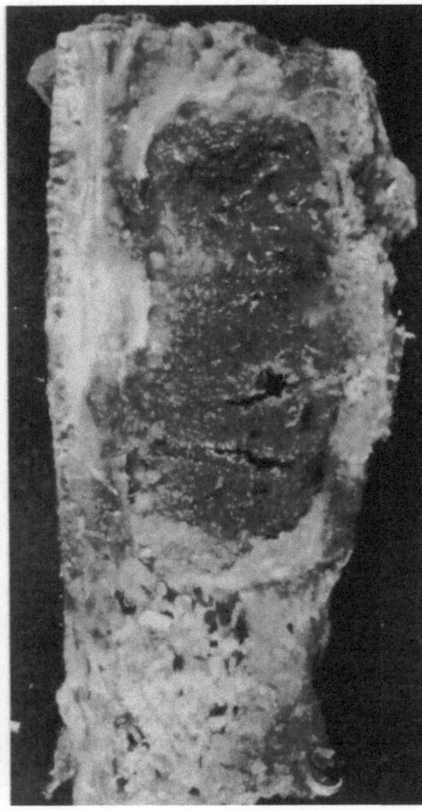
b

Fig. IX.46a,b. Male, 11 years old. **a** Metaphyseal fibrous defect of the fibula that occupies the entire width of the bone with pathologic fracture. **b** Photograph of the specimen reveals the brownish color of the lesion

tures, the term "metaphyseal fibrous defect" or "histiocytic xanthogranuloma." The process classified by Kimmelstiel and Rapp (1951) as "periosteal desmoid," although radiologically similar to the small cortical defects, presents a different histologic pattern and is included by us in the rare group of desmoplastic fibromas, periosteal type (see Chap. VI).

Pathologic Findings. Our material comprises, besides small fragments, several specimens obtained by complete excision or en bloc resection. The *gross aspect* varied considerably in different areas of the same and in different lesions, zones of grayish-white color and of firm consistency alternating with others of yellow or reddish-brown color and generally soft and fragile. In a few cases the yellow (xanthomatous) areas predominated. In some cases the lesion occupied the entire medullary cavity and was limited by a slightly expanded, thinned cortex (Figs. IX.45–IX.47).

Histologically, the process is characterized by a spindle-celled fibrous tissue with a whorled (storiform or cartwheel) pattern, a varying amount of collagen fibers and fibroblasts alternating with lipid-bearing (xanthoma cells) and hemosiderin pigment-loaded histiocytes. A variable number of multinucleated giant cells of osteoclastic type with scarce intermingled inflammatory elements (lympho- and plasmacytes) is another characteristic finding (Figs. IX.48–IX.50; see Fig. IX.51 for the general histologic pattern of a lesion in the fibula). The spindle cells in the lesion are interpreted as histiocytes adopting the pose of facultative fibroblasts. Occasionally, especially in older lesions, the collagenous fibrous tissue predominates, with only scarce areas containing histiocytic elements showing phagocytosis of hemosiderin or lipids and with few or no osteoclast giant cells. In some cases unusually heavily lipidized fibroxanthomatous areas are predominant; such cases were referred to as "fibroxanthoma" or "xanthoma" in the older literature, but also more recently (Bertoni et al. 1988). The predominance of fibrous areas and the lack of new bone formation except in the margins of the lesion were the reasons for its designation

Fig. IX.47a–c. Male, 11 years old. Metaphyseal fibrous defect of femur. **a** Radiograph showing a well-defined, radiolucent lesion that has slightly expanded the cortex and is abutting the growth plate. **b** Photograph and **c** radiograph of the resected specimen illustrate the dark brownish color of a large part of the lesion, its well-defined borders, and the thinned cortex

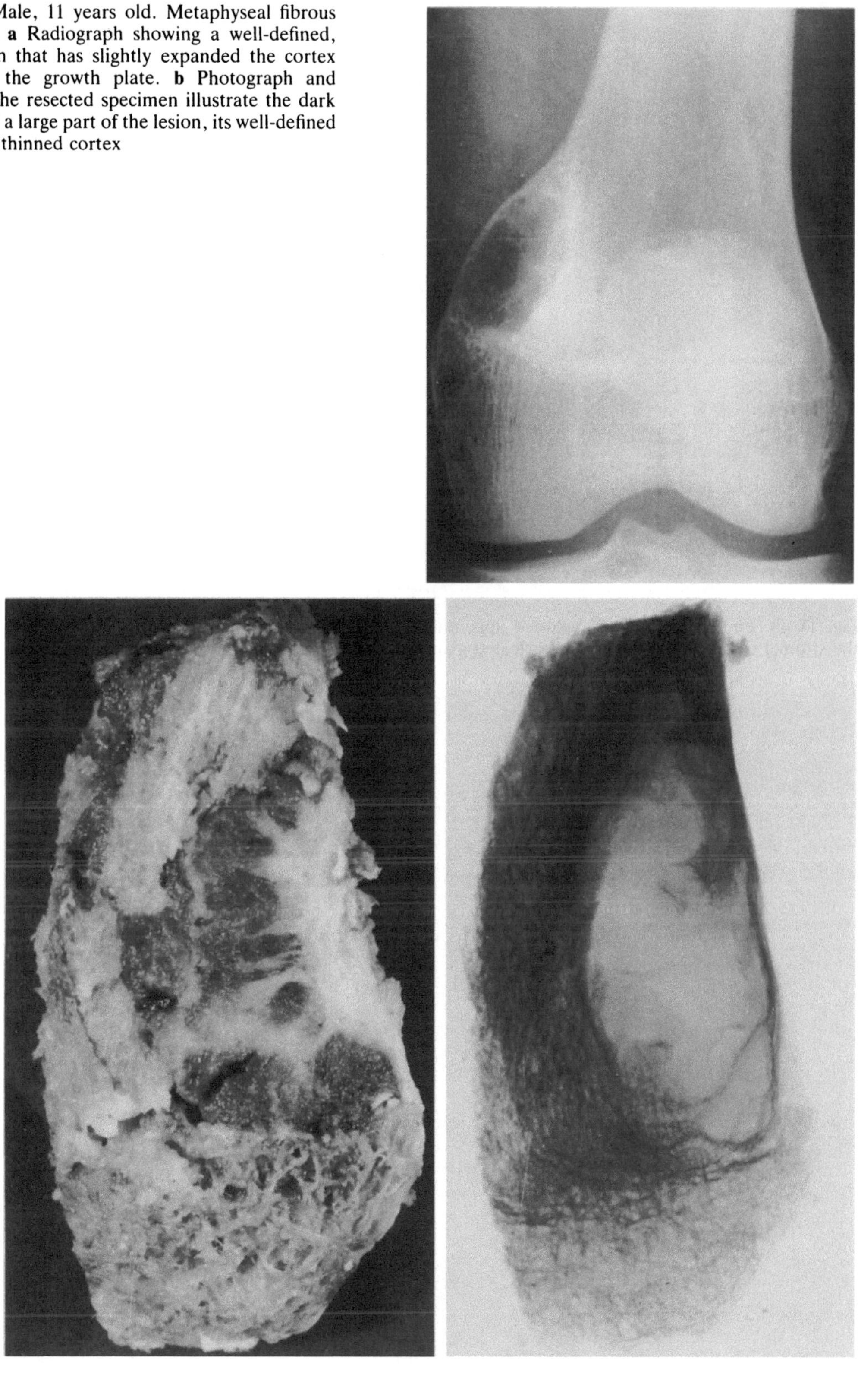
a b c

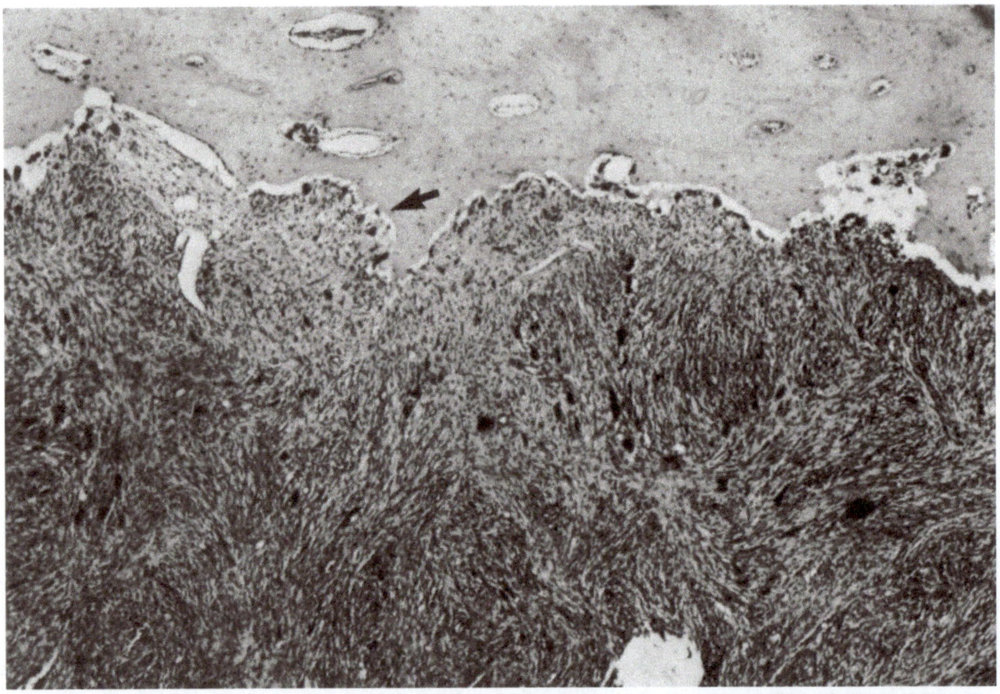

Fig. IX.48. Photomicrograph of whorled appearance of the stromal cells with scattered multinucleated giant cells within the lesion (*dark spots*) and numerous osteoclasts at the inner border of the cortex above. ×60

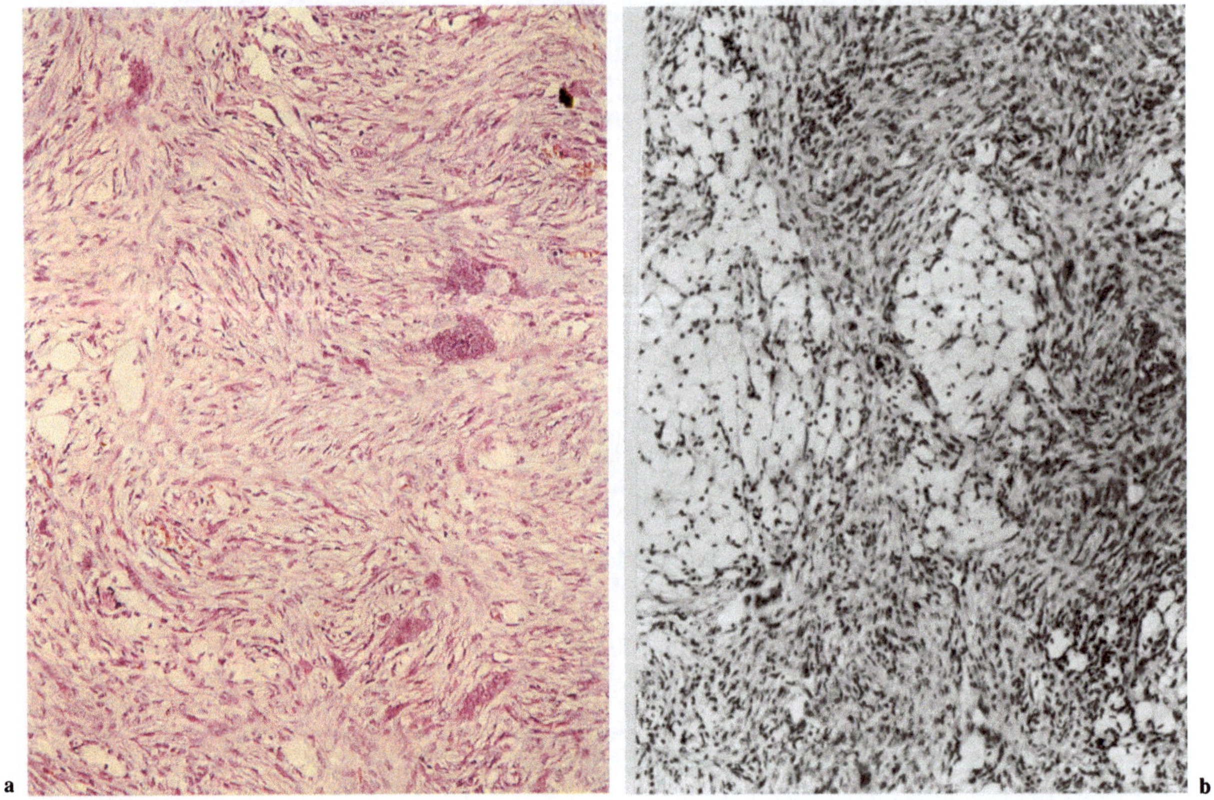

Fig. IX.49a,b. Photomicrographs showing the whorled ("storiform") spindle-celled stroma, the small number of small multinucleated giant cells, and some groups of foam cells. In **b**, there is a greater number of lipid-bearing foam cells, separated by spindle-shaped cells of fibroblastic type and only isolated giant cells. **a** ×100, **b** ×160

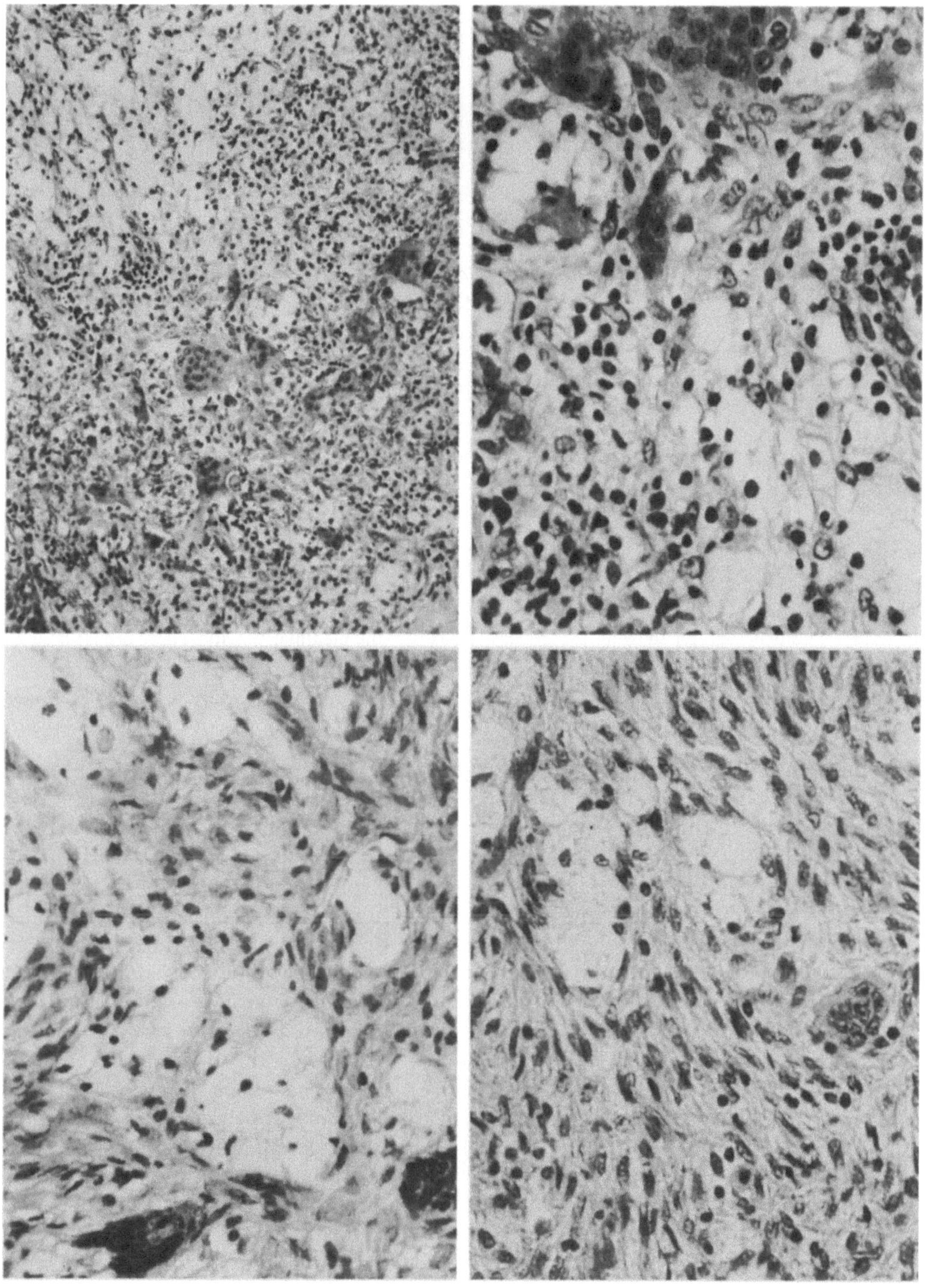

a b c d

Fig. IX.50a–d. Photomicrographs illustrating the characteristic histologic features. Besides the fibroblast-like spindle cells, foam cells, multinucleated giant cells, and small round cells, predominantly lymphocytes, are observed (**a**,**b**). **a** ×100, **b–d** ×400

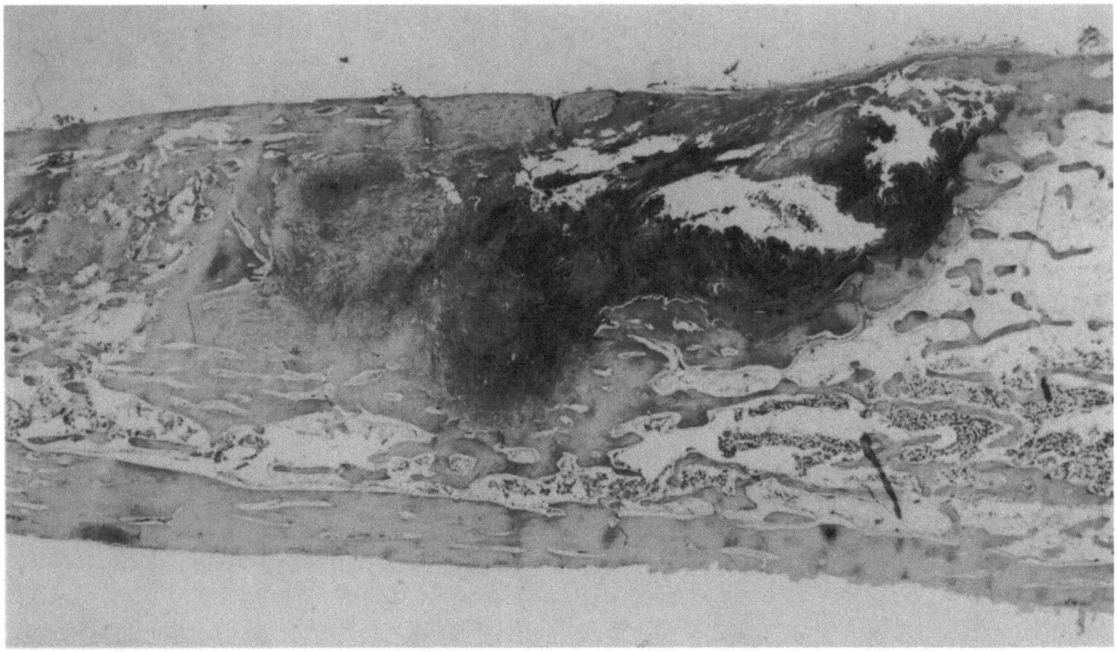

Fig. IX.51. Photomicrograph showing the general histologic pattern of a lesion in the fibula, illustrating the eccentric location and the halo of bone sclerosis toward the medullary cavity. There are no bone trabeculae within the lesion. ×10

as "nonosteogenic or nonossifying fibroma" by Jaffe and Lichtenstein (1942). This lack of metaplastic bone formation distinguishes the lesion from fibrous dysplasia. Steiner (1974), studying the ultrastructure of a fibrous cortical defect and two nonossifying fibromas of bone, confirmed the similar histologic and ultrastructural features of these lesions and their nonneoplastic nature. They were composed of fibroblasts in different stages of proliferation, of elaboration of extracellular material, and of accumulation of lipids and hemosiderin. The xanthoma cells derived from fibroblasts.

Pathogenesis. The clinical and pathologic features, particularly the presence of multiple foci, location in the metaphysis, migration away from the growth plate, and above all the possibility of spontaneous regression or self-limitation, favor the nonneoplastic, hyperplastic nature of the process. Its probable histiocytic origin would justify the designation fibroxanthoma or histiocytic xanthogranuloma, which we prefer. The intimate cause of this hyperplastic process is still unknown, but the most probable causes are a developmental defect associated with a vascular disturbance, as advocated by Hatcher, or an intraosseous hemorrhage in resorption and organization.

Treatment and Prognosis. Metaphyseal fibrous defects are benign lesions that may regress spontaneously. Treatment, which is indicated only in large lesions, with or without clinical symptoms, or when the risk of a pathologic fracture exists, consists of curettage or excision followed by bone grafting when necessary. Some metaphyseal fibrous defects may disappear or become sclerotic (ossified), and a very few recur in the same site. Malignant transformation is extremely rare. Only one case (Bhagwandeem 1966) has been reported: an aggressive fibrosarcoma appeared at the curetted site in a 21-year-old male 18 months after curettage. The published microphotographs give the impression of a malignant fibrous histiocytoma, not a fibrosarcoma, in the recurrent lesion as well as the primary. Another case of osteosarcoma arising in a nonosteogenic fibroma has been reported by Hastrup and Jensen (1965). In other cases the presence of a metaphyseal fibrous defect and an osteosarcoma in the same bone was merely coincidental (Kyriakos and Murphy 1981). In one case we observed fibrosarcomatous transformation of a lesion located in the lower end of the fibula after 15 years, which recurred twice and was treated by curettage and radiotherapy (Fig. IX.52). Only three other cases recurred, and in none of these did malignant change occur.

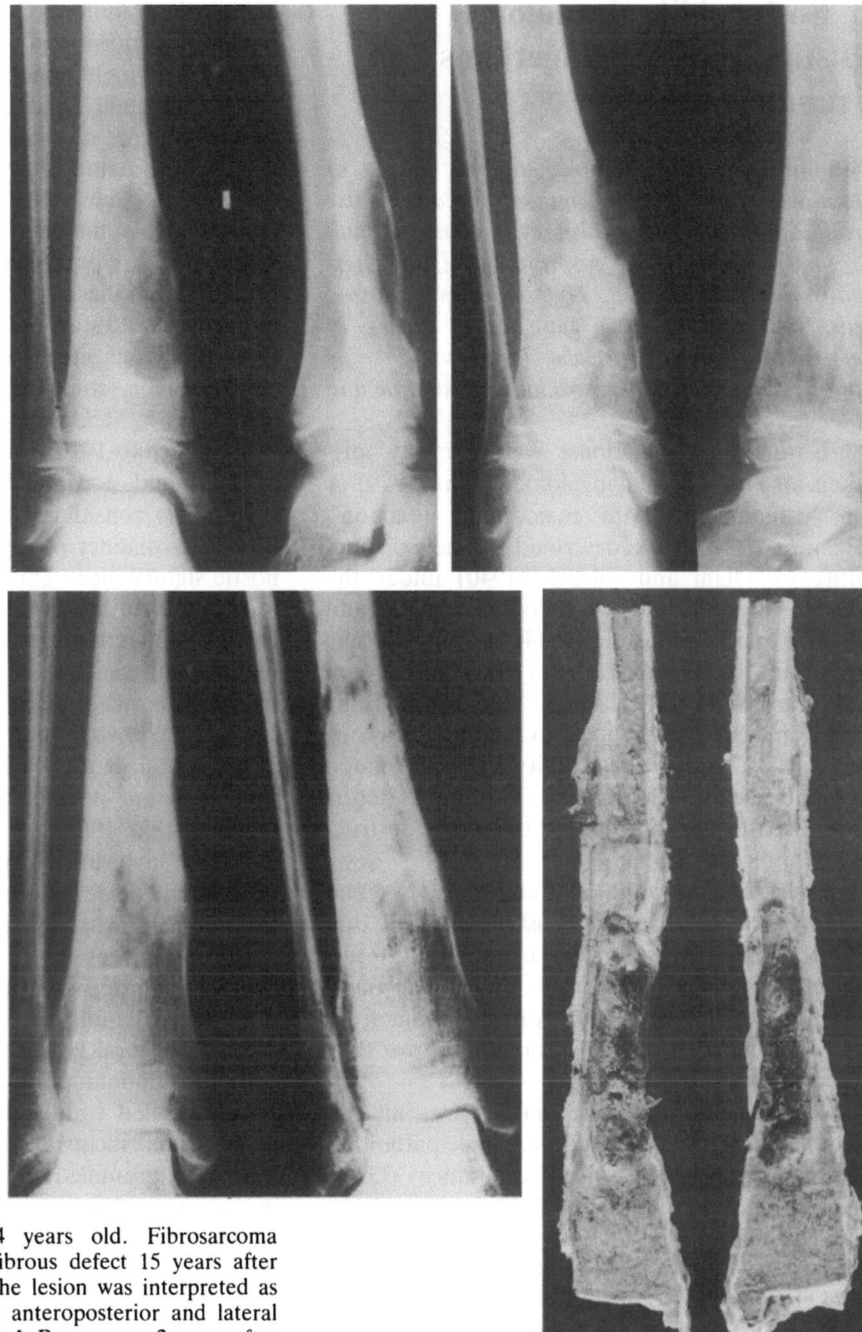

a b c d

Fig. IX.52a–d. Female, 24 years old. Fibrosarcoma developed in metaphyseal fibrous defect 15 years after curettage and irradiation. The lesion was interpreted as giant-cell tumor. **a** Original anteroposterior and lateral radiograph at 9 years of age. **b** Recurrence 2 years after curettage, showing extension of the lesion and areas of sclerosis. **c** Radiologic aspect after two further recurrences and radiotherapy showing irregular osteolytic areas alternating with conspicuous sclerosis, with the features of radiation osteitis. **d** Photograph of the amputation specimen reveals grayish-white tumor mass with extensive necrotic and hemorrhagic areas; the histologic diagnosis was fibrosarcoma and radiation osteitis

5. Eosinophilic Granuloma (Histiocytosis X, Langerhans Cell Granulomatosis)

Definition, WHO: *"A non-neoplastic lesion of unknown etiology, characterized by an intense proliferation of reticulo-histiocytic elements with varying numbers of eosinophilic leukocytes, neutrophilic leukocytes, lymphocytes, plasma cells, and multinucleate giant cells. Zones of necrosis are frequent, as also is the presence of lipid-bearing foam cells, especially in multiple and older lesions."*

Eosinophilic granuloma was formerly mistaken for "eosinophilic myeloma" (Finzi 1929) or for "osteomyelitis with eosinophilic reaction" (Schairer 1938). It was described as a new distinct entity by Otani and Ehrlich (1940) under the denomination "solitary granuloma of bone" and by Jaffe and Lichtenstein (1944) as "eosinophilic granuloma of bone." Farber (1941) and Green and Farber (1942) showed that eosinophilic granuloma could also appear in multiple locations and did not represent an entity but was related to Hand-Schüller-Christian disease and Letterer-Siwe disease. They introduced the term "destructive granuloma of bone."

Galeotti-Flori and Parenti (1937) and Wallgren (1940) had previously suggested that Hand-Schüller-Christian disease and Letterer-Siwe disease were the chronic and acute manifestations of the same basic process, namely, a systemic reticuloendothelial granulomatosis; they described transitional cases.

The concept that these entities are only different clinical manifestations of a single pathologic disorder has gained wide acceptance (Gross and Jacox 1942; Jaffe and Lichtenstein 1944; Engelbreth-Holm et al. 1944; Schajowicz and Polak 1947; Schajowicz and Slullitel 1973; Mickelson and Bonfiglio 1977; Ponseti 1948; Nezelof and Guibert 1963; Enriquez et al. 1967; Cheyne 1971). Schajowicz and Polak proposed the general term "*histiocytic granuloma*" for this group of disorders, which may appear without or with only isolated eosinophils (*pure histiocytic granuloma*) or, more commonly, with numerous eosinophilic leukocytes (*eosinophilic histiocytic granuloma*), and may involve a single or several bones. On the other hand, some of the histiocytes may be transformed into lipid-bearing xanthoma cells (*histiocytic xanthogranuloma*). These authors pointed out the different modes of presentation of histiocytic granuloma and emphasized that intermediate or transitional stages of different clinical importance might occur.

Lichtenstein, one of the most enthusiastic supporters of the unified concept, proposed in 1953 the name "*histiocytosis X*" as a broad designation under which the different types of clinical involvement could be grouped and differentiated for purposes of treatment and prognosis. He emphasized that an increasing number of lesions could start outside bone or be restricted to extraosseous sites (Lichtenstein 1964).

However, some dissenting opinions persist (Otani 1957; McGavran and Spady 1960; Fowles and Bobechko 1970). From a retrospective study of fatal and nonfatal cases, Lieberman et al. (1969) also considered the unifocal and multiple lesions as distinct processes with different prognostic significance. This divergence of opinion is in part due to the fact that the etiology of these entities still remains unknown, although several features suggest that they represent some kind of immunoallergic process (Schajowicz and Polak 1947; Schajowicz and Slullitel 1973; Rewald 1960; Avioli et al. 1963) or other type of reaction to some peculiar infection, possibly viral (Lichtenstein 1964). Certain histologic features and the favorable response to corticosteroids (Bass et al. 1953; Avioli et al. 1963) and antibiotic treatment (Aronson 1951; Fisher 1953; Dargeon 1967) in some cases seem to confirm these hypotheses, which are also supported by earlier electron microscopic studies reporting cellular inclusions of possible viral type (Basset et al. 1966). However, subsequent ultramicroscopic investigations have revealed rodlike or tennis racquet-shaped cytoplasmic inclusions in the histiocytic cells (Birbeck granules) identical to those found in the normal Langerhans cells of the dermis, which are now considered histiocytic elements (Cancilla et al. 1967; Friedman and Hanaoka 1969; Morales et al. 1969; Newton and Hamoudi 1973). Therefore the denomination "Langerhans cell granulomatosis" is actually preferred by some authors.

This term and "histiocytosis," "eosinophilic granuloma," "histiocytic granuloma," and "reticuloendotheliosis" are now the ones most frequently applied to the general disease, including all variants. It has been emphasized that the subdivisions are not sharply defined, with transitional forms existing between the different entities, especially in those multiple lesions for which arbitrary criteria often have to be adopted to classify them as pertaining to a determinate syndrome.

The term *Hand-Schüller-Christian syndrome*, which originally referred to the classic triad of skull defects, exophthalmos, and diabetes insipidus, is now more broadly used to include instances of more chronic evolution occurring generally in children older than 3 years, with multiple cranial lesions and sometimes involvement of other systems or with one of the other classic symptoms (exophthalmos or diabetes insipidus). The complete triad was only rarely found in the reported cases [six cases in the series of 129 reviewed by Cheyne (1971)] and was lacking in all but one of our cases.

The following criteria, suggested by Doede and Rappaport (1967) in a study of long-term survival, have been adopted for the diagnosis of *Letterer-Siwe syndrome*: age of onset less than 3 years; clinical findings of fever, otitis media, and recurrent bacterial infection; anemia, hemorrhages, hepatosplenomegaly, and diffuse nontender lymphadenopathy; osteolytic bone lesions; and most characteristically, cutaneous manifestations often suggestive of seborrheic eczema. According to all authors, the course is acute or subacute and the evolution commonly fatal, long survival being an exception (five instances among 96 adequately documented cases reviewed by Doede and Rappaport).

We want to emphasize that we do not consider these entities as diseases but rather as *syndromes*, that is, as different, often not well-delimited, clinical manifestations of the same basic disorder, characterized fundamentally by the proliferation of differentiated reticulohistiocytic elements of the granulomatous type and usually accompanied by numerous eosinophilic granulocytes and other inflammatory cells. The histiocytes may show secondary changes such as transformation into lipid-bearing foam cells (xanthoma cells) or phagocytosis of blood pigment and cellular debris.

Incidence. To facilitate the study, we divided our material into different categories according to the classification shown in Table IX.2. In some cases precise classification was difficult or even impossible. For these cases, the denomination "intermediate or transitional" type was adopted. According to this classification, the distribution of our 242 cases was as follows: solitary eosinophilic granuloma, 196 cases (81%); multiple eosinophilic granuloma, 16 cases (6.6%); Hand-Schüller-Christian syndrome, 23 cases (9.5%); Letterer-Siwe syndrome, 3 cases (1.2%); intermediate or transitional, 4 cases (1.7%).

Table IX.2. Classification of histiocytic granuloma (Langerhans cell granulomatosis)

Solitary	Multiple or disseminated
Eosinophilic granuloma	Chronic – With Hand-Schüller-Christian syndrome – Without Hand-Schüller-Christian syndrome Acute and subacute (Letterer-Siwe syndrome) Intermediate or transitional

The large number of solitary bone lesions is due to the fact that our laboratory receives material principally from orthopedic departments rather than from pediatric clinics, where the multiple or widely disseminated lesions generally predominate (Batson et al. 1955; Avery et al. 1957; Oberman 1961; Fowles and Bobechko 1970).

Clinical Findings. *Age and Sex.* Scheme IX.4 shows the age incidence of solitary lesions. The age of predilection for the solitary lesions was between 1 and 20 years (75%), with a peak between 5 and 10 years. The overall range was from 1 to 53 years. Only 25% of patients were over 20 years of age. Lesions in older patients (over 20 years) are more commonly found in ribs, mandible, clavicle, and scapula. In the cases of multiple locations, including those of the Hand-Schüller-Christian syndrome and Letterer-Siwe syndrome, there was a clear predominance of occurrence under 15 years of age (30 of 42 cases) with a predilection for the first 5 years (25 of 42 cases).

In several patients, the process started as a solitary lesion, but multiple foci, with or without the features of Hand-Schüller-Christian or Letterer-Siwe syndrome, developed after a few months, usually before 6 months. In none of our cases did a new focus appear in a solitary lesion after 1 year, which allows us to predict a favorable prognosis if no other lesion occurs during this period.

There was an evident male predominance in the occurrence of solitary lesions, with 136 cases in males out of a total of 196 (a ratio of 2.2:1).

Localization. The anatomic sites affected by the solitary lesions are shown in Scheme IX.4. There was a clear predominance in ribs and mandible

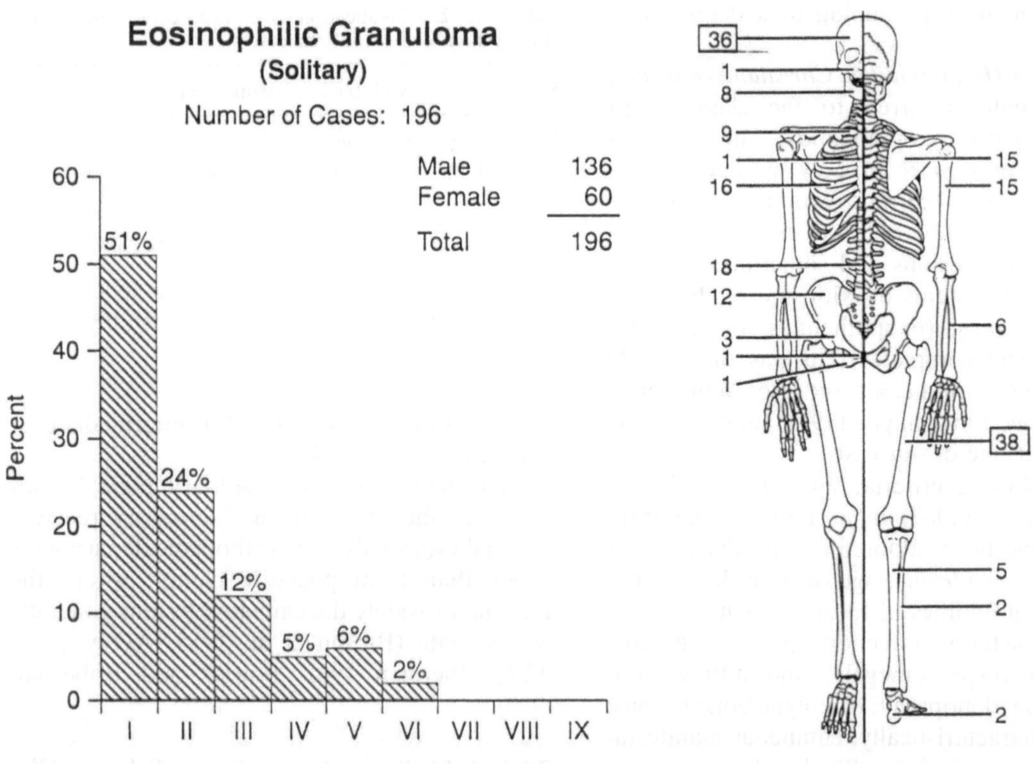

Scheme IX.4

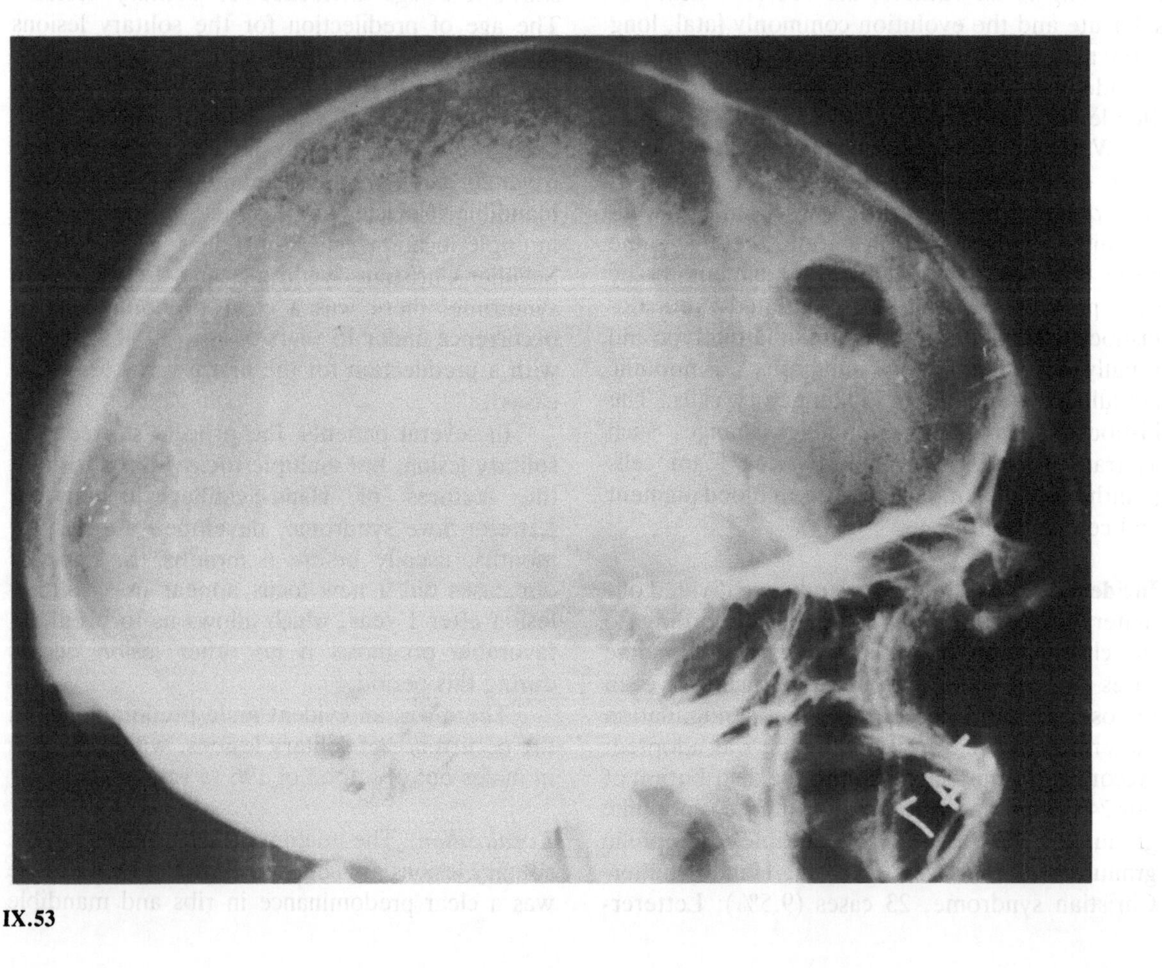

IX.53

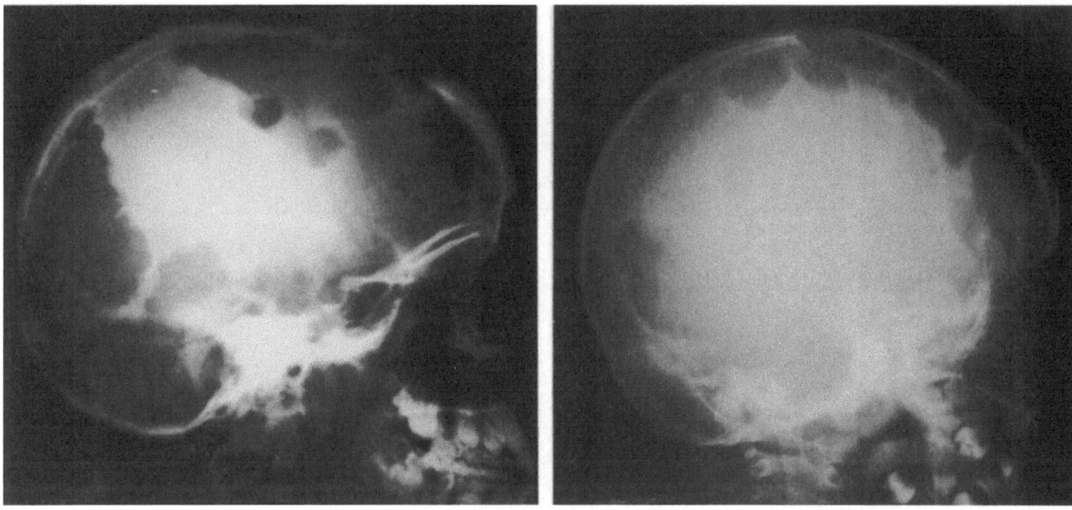

a b

▲ **Fig. IX.54a,b.** Two cases of Hand-Schüller-Christian syndrome showing the typical "geographic map" aspect of the skull. Both patients had several lesions in other bones and exophthalmos, but not diabetes insipidus. **a** Male, 12 years old; **b** male, 3 years old

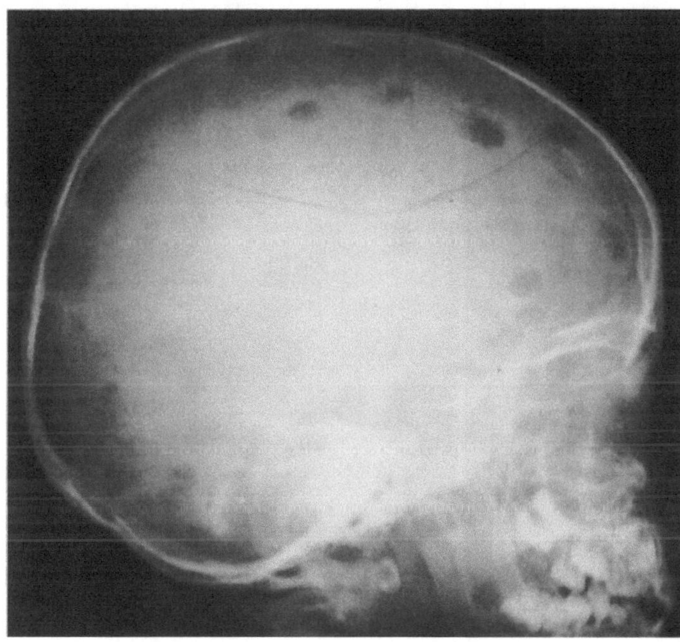

Fig. IX.55. Male, 10 months old, with Letterer-Siwe syndrome, showing multiple radiolucent lesions in the skull ▶

◀

Fig. IX.53. Male, 20 years old. Solitary eosinophilic granuloma of skull. Lateral radiograph reveals osteolytic, sharply defined lesions

over the age of 20 years, and a predominance in the skull under 20 years (70%). All the long limb bones were liable to be involved in patients under 20 years of age; lesions also occurred in the vertebrae and ilium.

In multiple lesions, with and without the features of Hand-Schüller-Christian or Letterer-Siwe syndrome, the bones most frequently affected were the skull and femur. For this reason, it seems to us that in every case of eosinophilic granuloma of the skull, a radiograph of at least both femurs is indicated, and, vice versa, that a radiograph of the skull should be taken in all cases of eosinophilic granuloma of the femur.

Symptoms. The clinical symptoms were not characteristic for solitary or multiple lesions without an accompanying syndrome. Pain, with increased local tenderness, was the most common initial complaint, followed by swelling or a tumor nodule, especially in the skull. Rarely, limping accompanied a lesion of a long limb bone or the pelvis.

In two cases located in ribs, a pathologic fracture occurred. The laboratory findings were usually negative, though there was leukocytosis in eight cases, with slight eosinophilia (over 4%) in four of them, as well as in two other cases without leukocytosis.

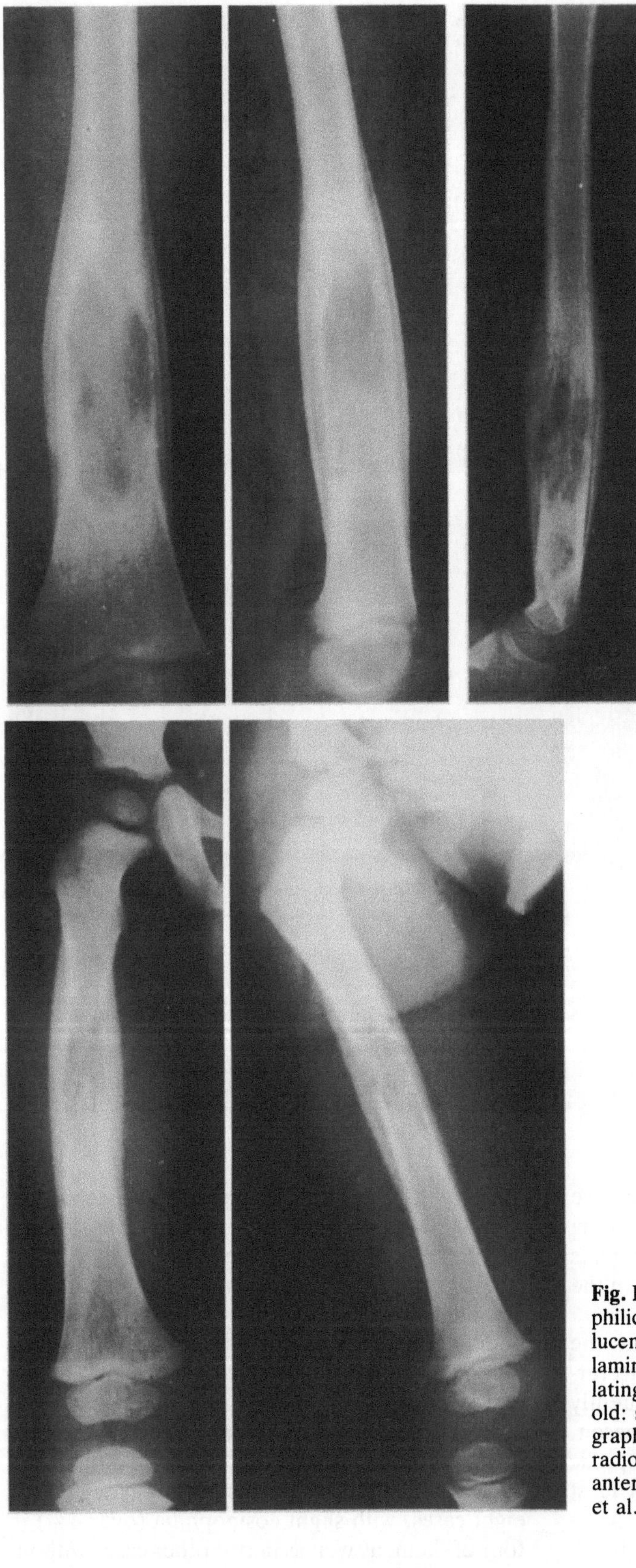

a b c

Fig. IX.56a–c. Three different cases of solitary eosinophilic granuloma of long limb bones, showing translucent, ill-defined lesions of the shaft with conspicuous laminated periosteal reactive bone formation, simulating osteomyelitis or Ewing sarcoma. **a** Male, 6 years old: shaft of femur, anteroposterior and lateral radiographs. **b** Male, 7 years old: shaft of humerus, lateral radiograph. **c** Female, 6 years old: shaft of femur; anteroposterior and lateral radiographs. (**a**, Schajowicz et al. 1972)

In 40 cases (two of them multiple), the sedimentation rate was moderately elevated, usually with a Katz index around 25. In one of the few cases in which a sternal marrow puncture was performed, 15% eosinophilic leukocytes were found.

Radiographic Features. Radiographically, the lesions usually appeared as ovoid or rounded, well-defined, translucent defects generally within the medullary cavity and surrounded by slightly denser, often scalloped edges (Figs. IX.53–IX.55). In long limb bones, the lesion was usually located in the diaphysis and less commonly in the metaphysis; in only one case was it situated in an upper femoral epiphysis. The cortex was often eroded, but generally only slightly distended. An evident periosteal reaction with new bone formation of the onion-skin type was a frequent finding, simulating osteomyelitis or Ewing sarcoma (Fig. IX.56) (Schajowicz et al. 1972).

In the spine the vertebral body was usually partly or completely collapsed (Figs. IX.57, IX.58), so that finally a flat disk of bone similar to "vertebra plana" was produced. This was described by Calvé (1925) as an osteochondrosis analogous to Perthes disease and was first identified with eosinophilic granuloma by Compere et al. (1954).

The skull lesions had a characteristic punched-out appearance; they were of variable size, were frequently multiple, and in Hand-Schüller-Christian syndrome were often confluent (Fig. IX.54). In Letterer Siwe syndrome, the osteolytic defects of the skull, like those of other bones, were generally smaller and not as conspicuous, the extraskeletal manifestations predominating (Fig. IX.55).

Figures IX.59 and IX.60 illustrate the radiographic appearances in cases of eosinophilic granuloma of the pubis and multiple eosinophilic granuloma, respectively.

Pathologic Findings. *Grossly*, in most cases the material was obtained by curettage and consisted of numerous small, irregular fragments of grayish-pink or sometimes brownish color, alternating with hemorrhagic or yellowish zones. The latter were normally scanty but occasionally they predominated, such as in the extensive osteolytic lesions of the skull, especially in the multiple lesions of Hand-Schüller-Christian syndrome, that is, in processes of apparently long evolution. In these cases, wide areas of frankly fibrous appearance have also been observed.

In addition to this fragmented material, we studied a number of complete resection specimens, especially of ribs (eight) and clavicles (five), which permitted us to observe more clearly the gross aspects. In these cases, the process was usually located centrally, the cavity being occupied by a hemorrhagic, friable, granulation-like tissue, often showing necrotic, puriform zones and frequently well delimited toward the neighboring spongiosa by a scalloped sclerotic border (though sometimes a clear border was absent). The cortex was thinned or broken in some cases, with infiltration of the soft tissue by a friable, partly puriform material, occasionally simulating a suppurative process. In three cases, reactive periosteal bone formation was observed.

The *histologic sections* showed a mixture of pale-stained reticulohistiocytic elements (histiocytes), often forming more or less compact areas or cords, and a variable number of eosinophilic leukocytes and lymphocytes, plasma cells, neutrophil granulocytes, and fibroblasts. The reticulohistiocytic cells had large ovoid, indented, or reniform pale nuclei, with inconspicuous nucleoli, and usually well-defined cytoplasmic borders (Fig. IX.61). Mitotic figures were rare. The structure, however, was not uniform, varying in different cases, as also in different fields in the same case. In many cases, eosinophils were so abundant that the diagnosis could be made without difficulty, but in others they were scarce or completely lacking in many fields. The intense histiocytic proliferation predominated, thus producing problems of differential diagnosis with malignant lymphoma (reticulosarcoma) (Fig. IX.61a). This mistake was made in the case of a lesion in a rib after examination of a specimen obtained by aspiration biopsy (Fig. IX.62). Later examination of the resected rib revealed the correct diagnosis. Most of the histiocytes were mononucleated, but transitions to multinucleated giant cells with few or several nuclei, sometimes disposed peripherally, were observed (Figs. IX.61, IX.63). With special fat stains, abundant droplets of sudanophilic fat in the middle or periphery of the cytoplasm could be demonstrated in some giant cells ("Touton cells") (Fig. IX.63c).

Patchy zones of hemorrhage and necrosis were usually present, with phagocytosis of blood pigment (hemosiderin) or lipids by the histiocytes,

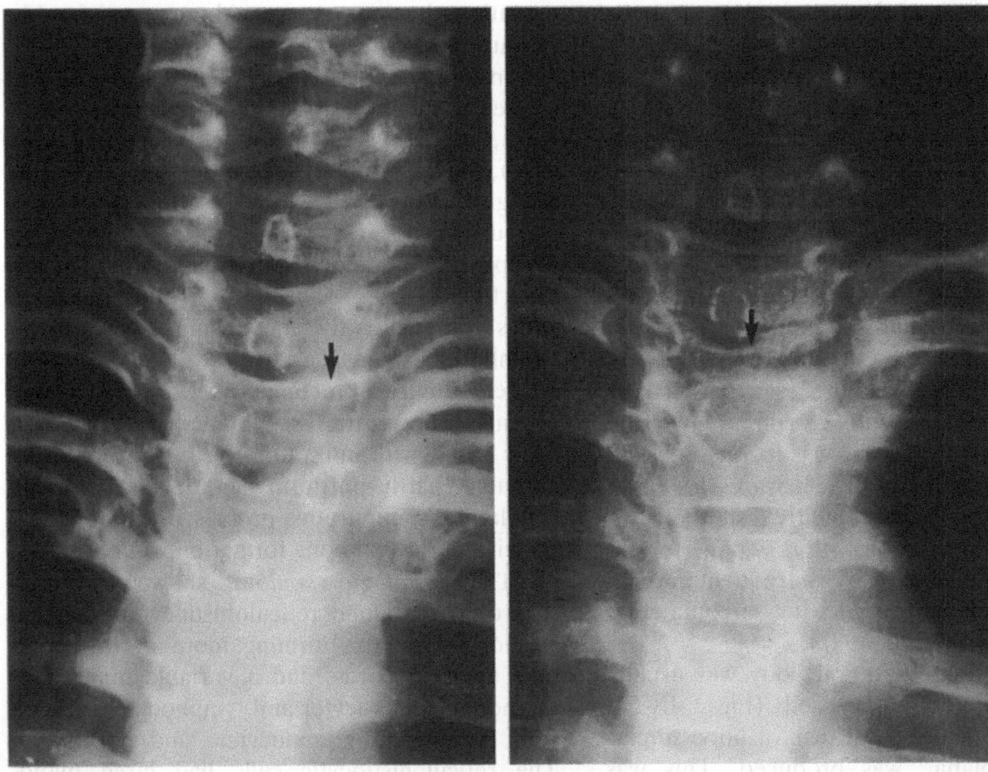

a b

Fig. IX.57a,b. Male, 12 years old. Solitary eosinophilic granuloma of second thoracic vertebra. **a** Radiograph shows a radiolucent lesion involving part of the vertebral body. **b** Radiograph 3 months later shows the collapse of the vertebral body, which is now entirely involved

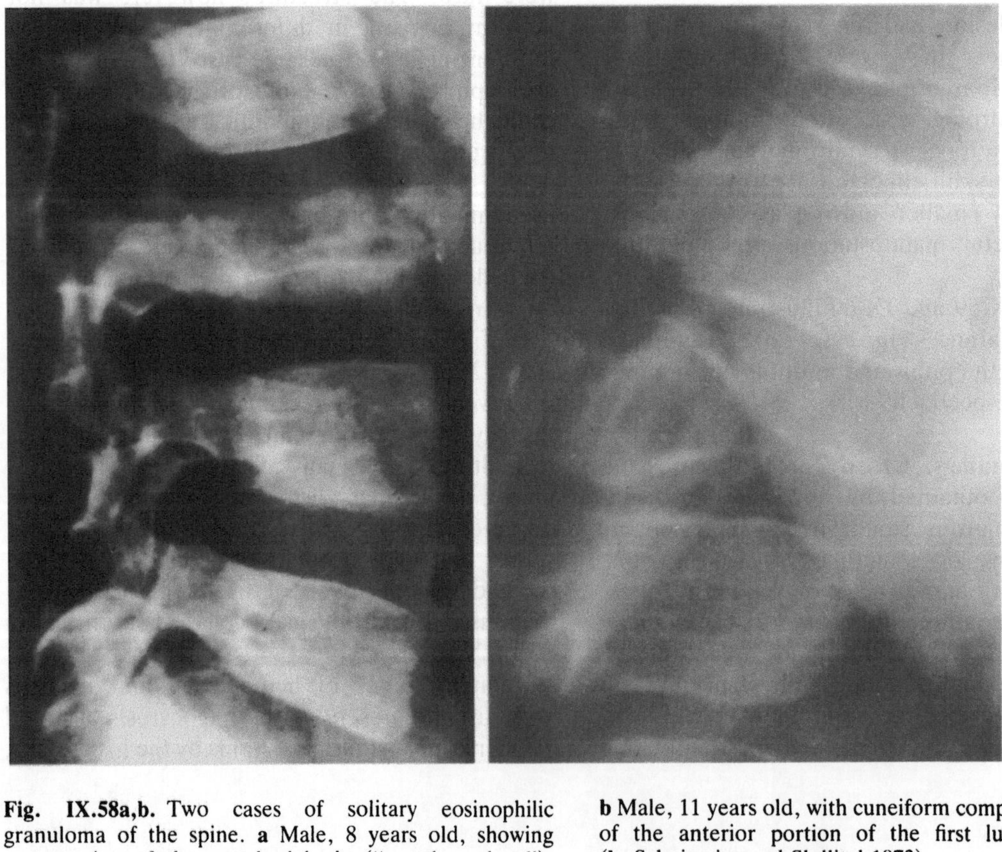

a b

Fig. IX.58a,b. Two cases of solitary eosinophilic granuloma of the spine. **a** Male, 8 years old, showing compression of the vertebral body ("vertebra plana"). **b** Male, 11 years old, with cuneiform compression fracture of the anterior portion of the first lumbar vertebra. (**b**, Schajowicz and Slullitel 1973)

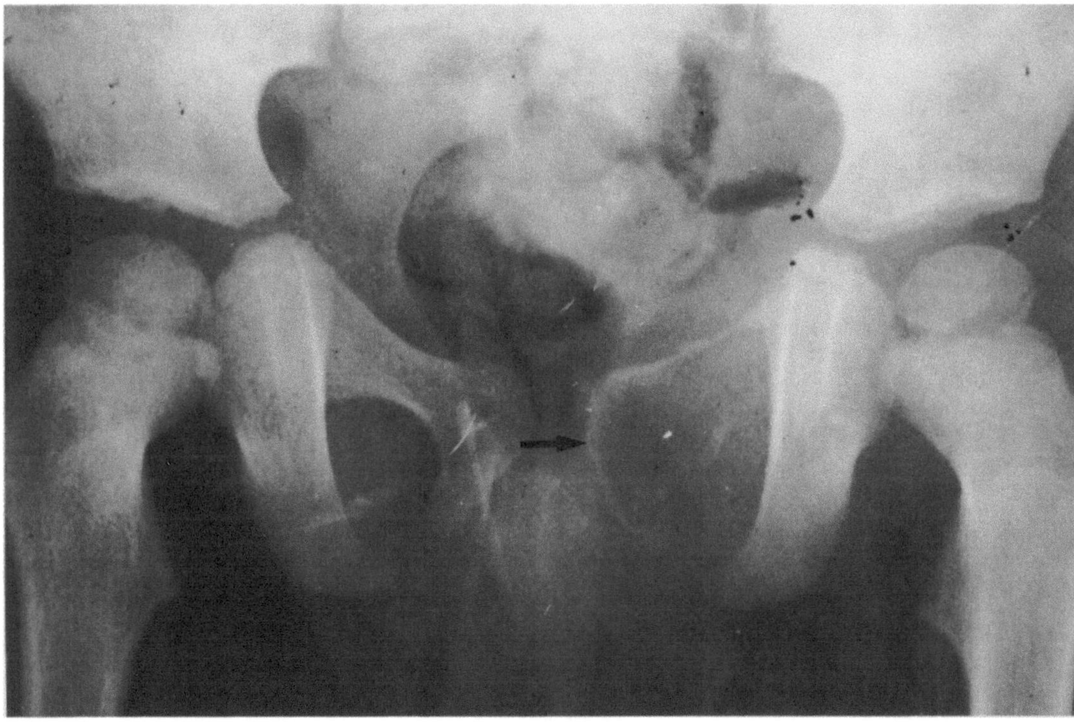

▲
Fig. IX.59. Male, 2 years old, with eosinophilic granuloma of the pubis. A large destructive lesion is seen. Five months later other lesions appeared in the skull and femur

Fig. IX.60. Male, 2 years old, with multiple eosinophilic granuloma, showing lesions in the scapula and upper and lower ends of the femur, with periosteal reactive bone formation in the femoral lesions
▼

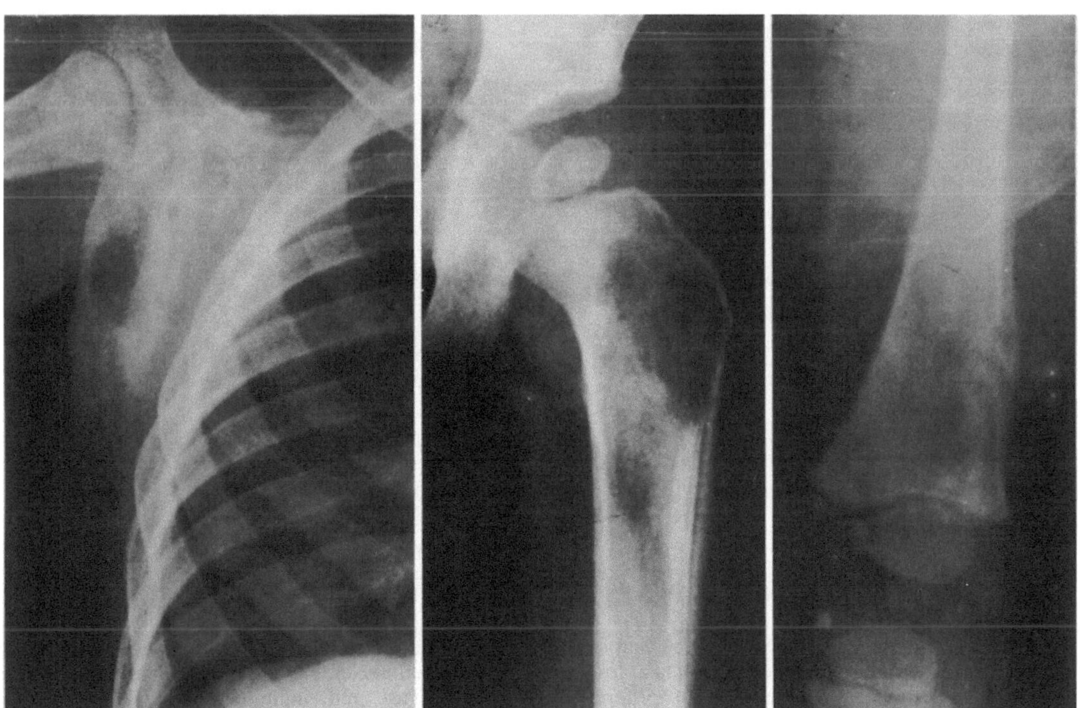

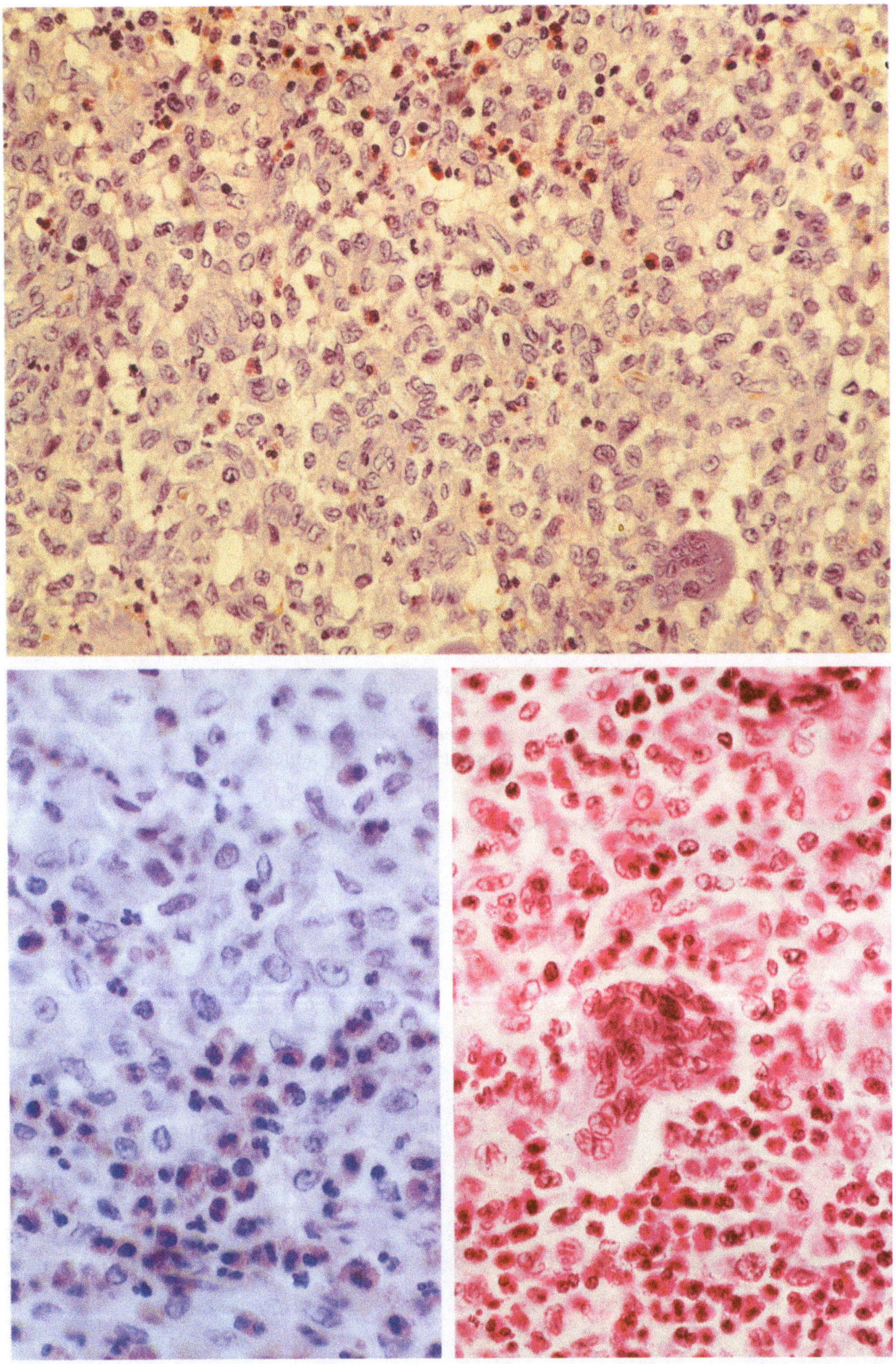

a b c

Fig. IX.61a–c. Photomicrographs show the characteristic histologic features of eosinophilic granuloma at lower and higher magnification. **a** Proliferation of differentiated histiocytes with only scarce eosinophils and isolated multinucleated giant cells. **b** Histiocytes with pale ovoid or indented nuclei, **c** alternating with numerous eosinophilic leukocytes and multinucleated giant cells. **a** ×200, **b**,**c** ×400

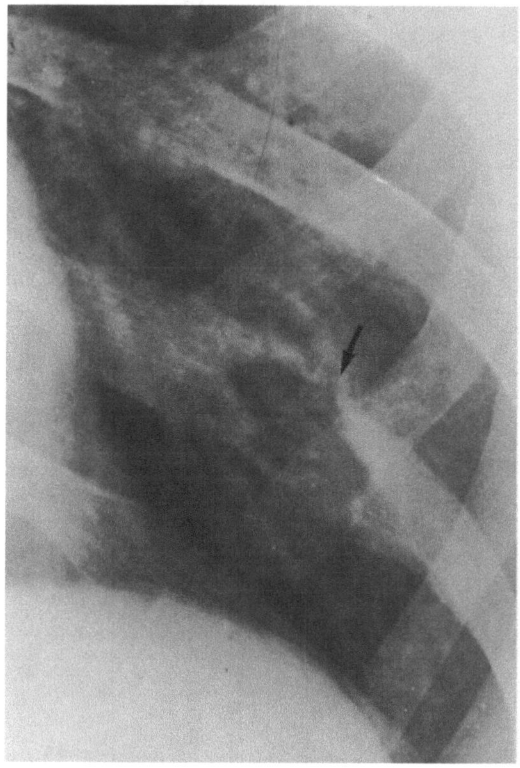
a

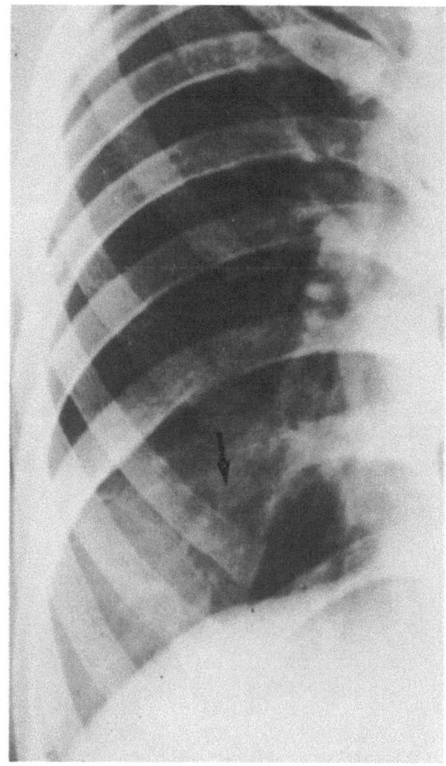
b

Fig. IX.62a,b. Two different cases of solitary eosinophilic granuloma of rib, simulating malignant tumor. **a** Male, 37 years old, with destructive, ill-defined lesion. **b** Male, 12 years old, with large lesion that completely destroyed an extensive area of the rib. Radiologically and histologically a diagnosis of reticulosarcoma was made, followed by radiotherapy. There was an evident regression of the lesion, and after 6 months a segmental resection was performed, revealing the histologic pattern of a typical eosinophilic granuloma. The patient was well and without other lesions 5 years later

which became transformed into typical lipid-bearing foam cells (xanthomatous cells). Foam cells were more abundant in the vicinity of necrotic areas, which were more extensive in the older and more widespread lesions, possibly because of deficient circulation due to hyperplasia of the arterial endothelium with evident narrowing of the vascular lumen.

However, foam cells were found not only in the vicinity of necrotic zones but also independently of them and in solitary lesions. Nevertheless, it was evident that they were more abundant in cases of Hand-Schüller-Christian syndrome, especially in the extensive skull lesions. Thus, in several cases we observed a predominance of xanthomatous areas in the skull and only scarce foam cells in other more recent foci, where the histiocytes and eosinophils predominated. The histiocytes are later replaced by fibroblastic elements with formation of connective tissue that may be intermingled with foam cells; these fibroblastic elements replace the granulomatous tissue, as we were able to observe in some cases in which repeated biopsies were performed (Fig. IX.64).

However, in Letterer-Siwe syndrome, which is almost always of acute evolution, histiocytic proliferation, accompanied by a variable number of eosinophils and other inflammatory elements, predominates. Foam cells are either lacking or are extremely scarce, apparently due to the rapid evolution of this process.

Using Rio Hortega's silver stain, a dense net of reticular fibers surrounding individual or small groups of histiocytes was often observed; sometimes, however, there were only large nests of histiocytes, giving rise to a folliclelike pattern (Fig. IX.65a). The Del Rio Hortega technique, specific for reticuloendothelial elements, confirmed the histiocytic nature of the basic cell, showing its characteristic ramified or ameboid aspect (Fig. IX.65b).

Reactive bone formation was frequently found in the periphery of the lesion as well as on the surface of the destroyed cortex of long limb bones, which often showed an onion skin pattern.

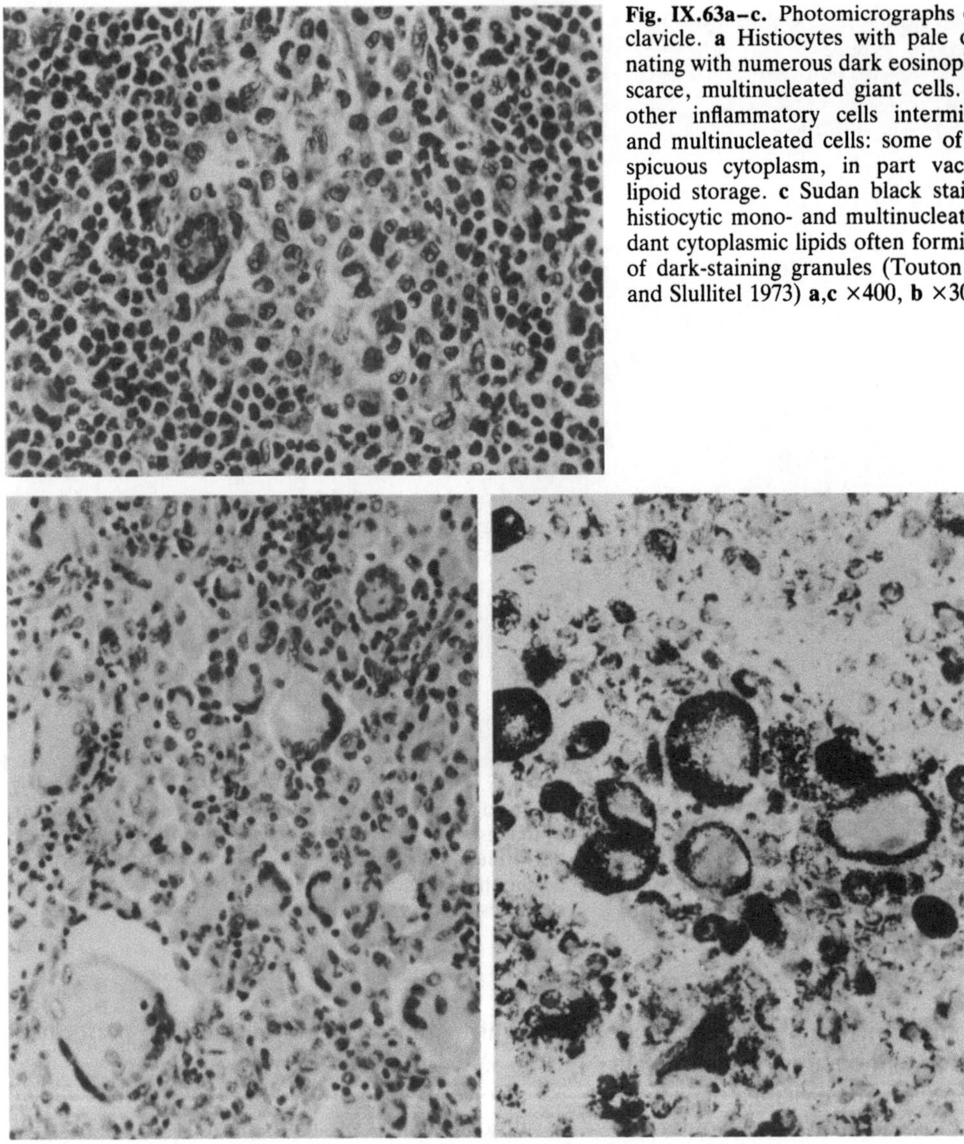

a b c

Fig. IX.63a–c. Photomicrographs of solitary lesion in clavicle. **a** Histiocytes with pale ovoid nuclei, alternating with numerous dark eosinophilic leukocytes and scarce, multinucleated giant cells. **b** Eosinophils and other inflammatory cells intermingled with mono- and multinucleated cells: some of them present conspicuous cytoplasm, in part vacuolated, indicating lipoid storage. **c** Sudan black stain shows numerous histiocytic mono- and multinucleated cells with abundant cytoplasmic lipids often forming a peripheral rim of dark-staining granules (Touton cells). (Schajowicz and Slullitel 1973) **a,c** ×400, **b** ×300

Our findings confirmed that the histologic aspect does not permit one to establish the anatomoclinical type of any particular lesion – and so predict its future evolution – without knowing the complete clinical and radiologic picture. This is in contrast to the findings of Newton and Hamoudi (1973), who supported a close relationship between histopathology and clinical course.

The comparative clinical and pathologic study of our cases strongly supports the view that eosinophilic granuloma, Hand-Schüller-Christian syndrome, and Letterer-Siwe syndrome represent only different clinical and anatomic manifestations of a single pathologic disorder, frequently occurring in transitional or intermediate types. Although it was generally impossible to predict the evolution of a particular case from the histologic picture, the dissemination of an initially solitary lesion usually occurred during the first 6 months and was more common in children under 5 years of age. Therefore, if a bone lesion remains solitary for 12 months, it may be expected with confidence that no other focus will appear in the future and cure can be said to be permanent with conservative treatment (curettage or radiotherapy in low doses). According to Enriquez and colleagues (1967) and Cheyne (1971), apart from the age of onset, the main difference between the patients who died and those who recovered was in the pattern with which the disease involved the soft tissue. A clear correlation exists between age and the bone involved, with an evident predilection for certain bones, especially the ribs and mandible, after the age of 20 years. Another important finding was the frequent presence of a variable number of lipid-bearing histiocytes (xanthoma cells) in cases of solitary and multiple eosinophilic granuloma without Hand-Schüller-Christian disease; these xanthoma cells were often found in relation to necrotic zones, but also independently of them. Thus, the presence of xanthoma cells is not diagnostic of Hand-Schüller-Christian disease. Such cells are also found occasionally in Letter-Siwe syndrome; however, they are scarce or completely lacking in this process, probably due to the short duration of this more acute disease (Wallgren 1940).

Another feature in support of the unified concept was the presence of different histologic patterns in biopsy specimens taken from different sites of multifocal lesions. In one patient we observed a predominance of xanthoma cells and fibrous areas in some cranial lesions, while material obtained from other, apparently more recent, bone lesions contained abundant eosinophils with only isolated xanthoma cells. One case started with a femoral lesion but became rapidly generalized (in less than 6 months), the patient finally developing a complete Hand-Schüller-Christian triad (Fig. IX.64). In the first biopsy, an intense histiocytic proliferation with only a few eosinophils was found, but in a second biopsy taken 2 years later from the same femoral lesion, a typical fibroxanthomatous lesion, almost completely lacking eosinophils, was observed (Fig. IX.64f). Mercer and Duthie (1956) reported similar pathologic evidence, from biopsies carried out consecutively in a patient, of the transformation from a histiocytic granulomatous stage with predominant eosinophils to a lipid granulomatous stage with predominant foam cells.

These findings, as well as the occurrence of intermediate types (especially cases in children around 3 years of age that could not be precisely classified as Hand-Schüller-Christian syndrome with conspicuous extraskeletal lesions or as a milder, less acute form of Letterer-Siwe disease), seem to confirm the unified concept and induced Rewald to call both entities "Letterer-Christian's disease." There are many features that suggest that the entities represent some type of immunoallergic (hypersensitive) reaction to a still unknown peculiar infection, possibly viral. This may explain the histologic picture (folliclelike structures and intense eosinophilia) and the favorable therapeutic effects of corticosteroids or antibiotics on some of the multiple lesions. This hypothesis would explain the well-known fact that the earlier the age of onset of the disease (under 3 years), the more acute is its evolution and the less favorable its prognosis (Enriquez et al. 1967; Cheyne 1971). We disagree with those authors who try to divide the cases into fatal and nonfatal entities (Lieberman et al. 1969), which can be done only retrospectively after knowing the complete evolution of the disease. On the other hand, we could not confirm the relationship between different histologic types and clinical behavior, as supported by Newton and Hamoudi (1973). These authors proposed dividing the group of histiocytosis into type I and type II, of benign or malignant course, on the basis of histopathologic criteria rather than on clinical grounds. Type I lesions involve the reticulo-endothelial system diffusely and show infiltrates consisting of mature histiocytes, *without* necrosis, fibrosis, eosinophilia, or giant cells. Type II lesions are either localized or generalized but are pathologically always focal and characterized by the constant presence of eosinophils, giant cells, and frequent areas of necrosis and fibrosis. However, their ultrastructural studies were not conclusive. The Birbeck granules in the cytoplasm of the histiocytes (Langerhans cells), which were reported as a characteristic finding in the different variants of histiocytosis, were present in material from patients of types I and II. The function and significance of the Birbeck granules in the Langerhans cells, which are rod-shaped structures with central filaments and periodic cross-striations, are not known (Fig. IX.66). However, these granules are not found in all histiocytes, and the histochemical demonstration of S-100 protein (although not specific for Langerhans cells) and peanut agglutination binding seem to be the most useful markers for the identification of Langerhans cells (Hajdu et al. 1986; Ree and Kadin 1987).

Treatment and Prognosis. The type of treatment varies according to the different clinical manifestations of the disease. In easily accessible unifocal lesions, the treatment of choice is curettage, especially in long bones, followed by grafting in osteolytic lesions of larger size. Except in deeply located lesions (vertebrae, ilium), radiation alone or combined with curettage is not indicated, and the dose should not be

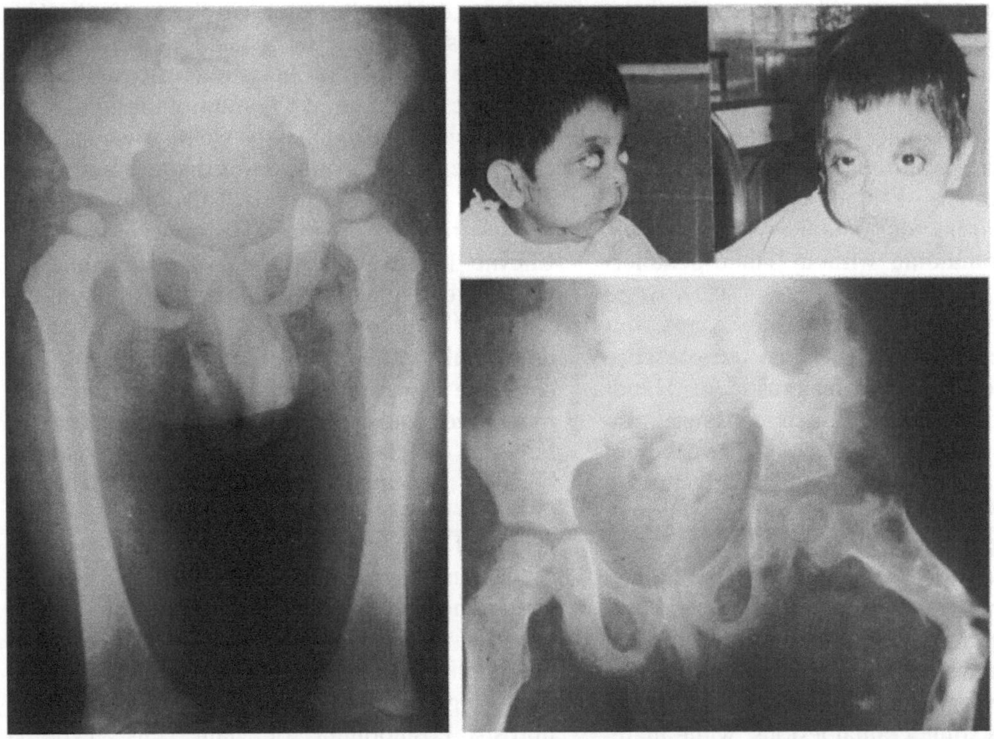

a b c

Fig. IX.64a–f. Male, 22 months old, with complete Hand-Schüller-Christian triad. **a** Radiograph taken in October, 1964, showing translucent lesion of upper third of femur. **b** Photograph and **c** radiograph of the same patient in December 1969, showing bilateral exophthalmos and bowing of the femur with radiolucent and sclerotic areas. Another osteolytic lesion is observed in the iliac bone of the same side. **d,e** Photomicrographs at lower and higher magnification showing intense histiocytic proliferation with only scarce eosinophilic and inflammatory elements. **f** Same case, biopsy taken 2 years later from the same lesion, showing numerous lipoid-bearing foam cells with single or multiple nuclei (Touton cells). (Schajowicz and Slullitel 1973) **d** ×120, **e,f** ×600

higher than 10 Gy. In larger lesions of the rib or clavicle, segmental resection may be performed. Cases with spontaneous regression have been reported and have also been observed by us. Some authors referred to the cure of cases of solitary eosinophilic granuloma by intralesional injection of corticoids (Scaglietti et al. 1976; Cohen et al. 1980). Eosinophilic granuloma of bone involving multiple sites and/or soft tissues, with or without Hand-Schüller-Christian or Letterer-Siwe syndrome, requires a more aggressive treatment. In the earliest cases, radiotherapy (3–6 Gy) was used. Occasionally it was accompanied by curettage or resection of one focus (in a rib) or by administration of hypophyseal extracts or chlorpropamide (Diabinese) in cases of diabetes insipidus, with a moderate improvement of the urine density and diminution of excretion. In subsequent cases of multiple and disseminated disease, corticosteroids in variable doses were used alone (Avioli et al. 1963) or combined with methotrexate (amethopterin) (Jones 1974). Other authors (Vogel and Vogel 1972) obtained good results with a combination of nitrogen mustard and cyclophosphamide (Cytoxan). Excellent results have been recorded by Dr. Derqui of the Children's Hospital in Buenos Aires with the antimitotic agent vinblastine sulfate (Velbe or Velban) in low doses, after the failure of surgery and radiotherapy or as primary treatment, with complete disappearance or diminution in size of the osteolytic lesions. Over a period of years, several other authors reported (Beier et al. 1963; Siegel and Coltman 1966; Kondi et al. 1972; West 1973) similar good results with vinblastine sulfate in the treatment of multiple and disseminated eosinophilic granuloma. Vinblastine and methotrexate, as well as other chemotherapeutic agents in the form of multidrug treatment, have been reported to produce occasional success in the treatment of acute disseminated histiocytosis (Beier et al. 1963; Jones 1974).

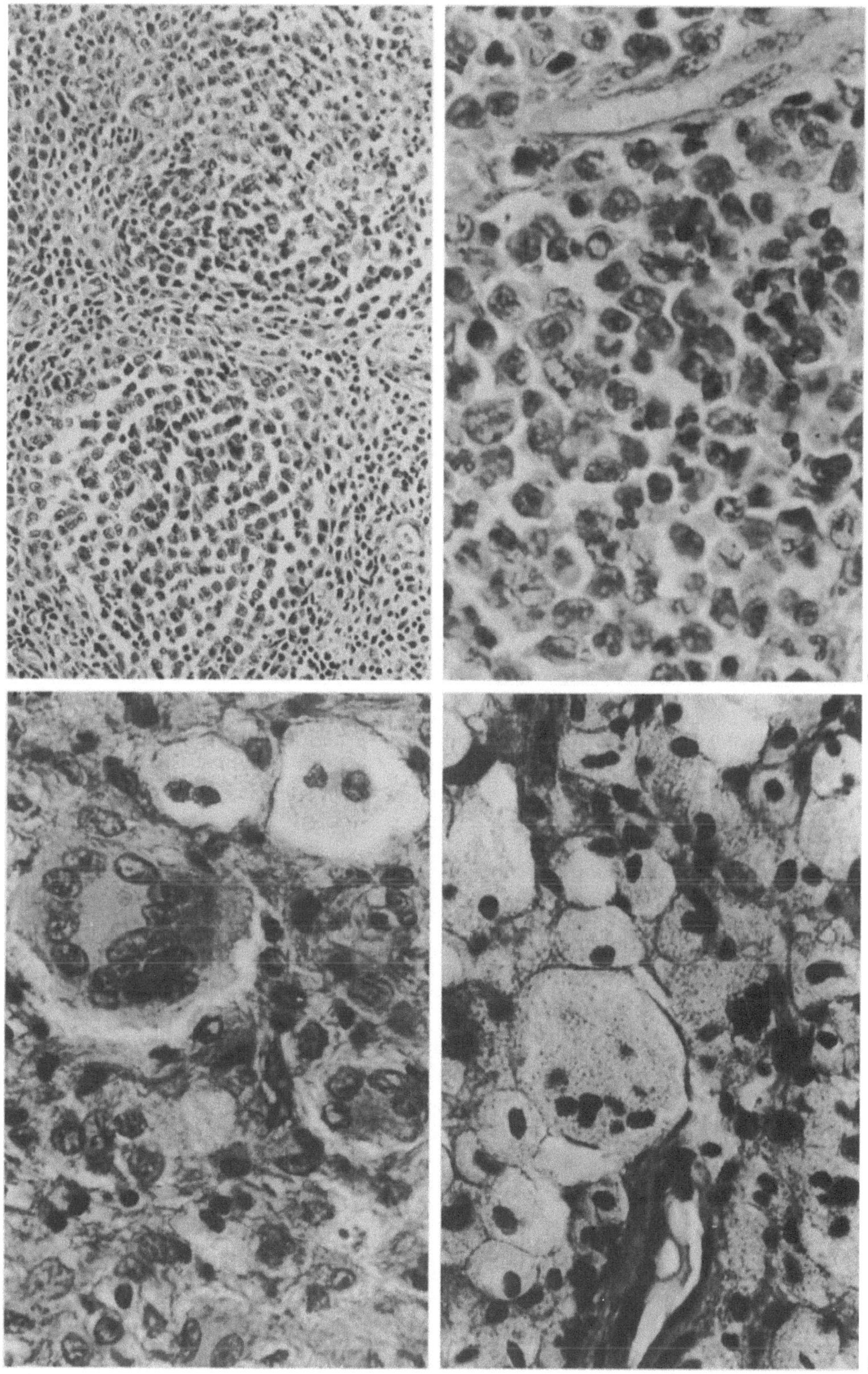

d e

f

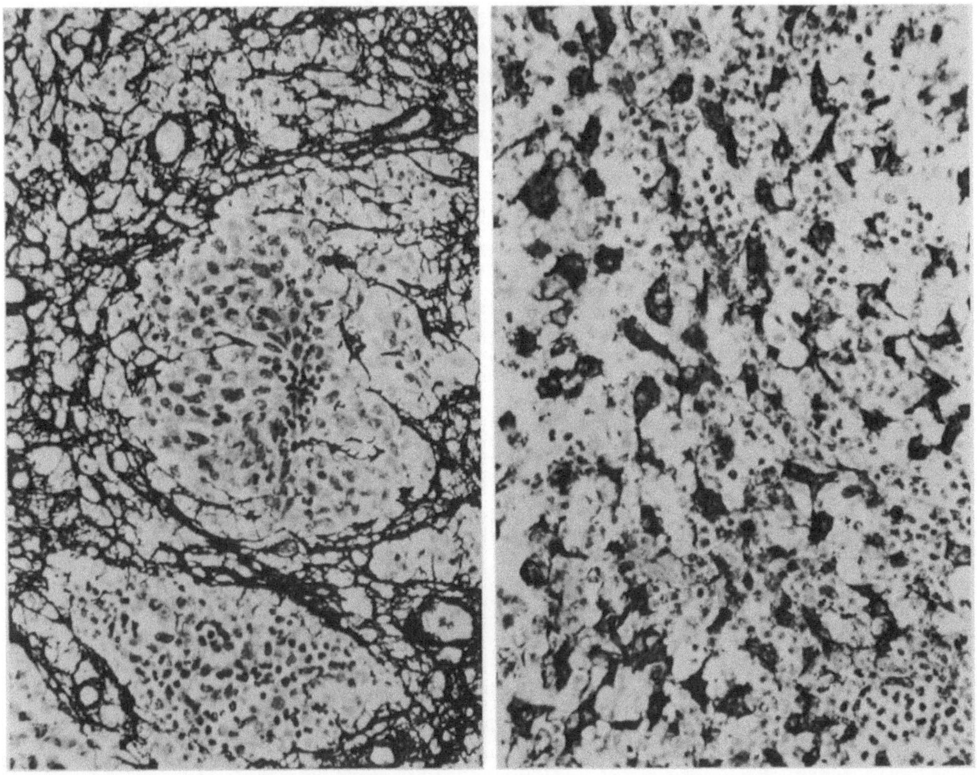

a b

Fig. IX.65. **a** Photomicrographs showing the richness of reticulin fibers and the presence of folliclelike structures, lacking reticulin fibers (Del Rio Hortega's silver stain). **b** The reticulohistiocytic nature of the cells, which are ramified or ameboid in form, is evident (Del Rio Hortega's stain for reticuloendothelial elements). (Schajowicz and Slullitel 1973) **a**,**b** ×200

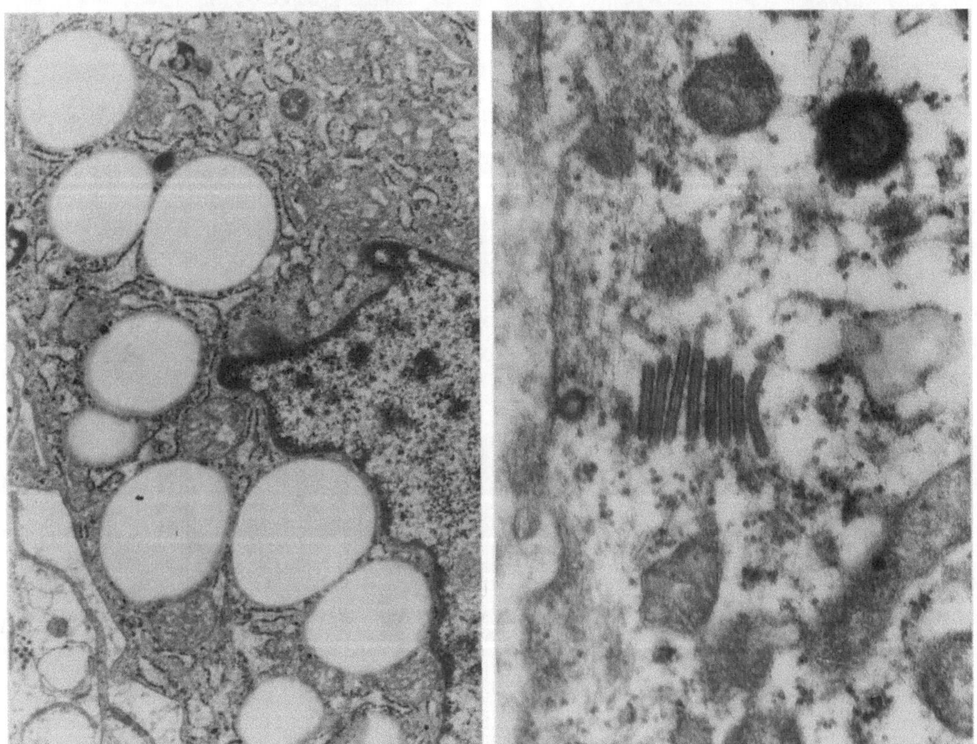

a b

Fig. IX.66a,b. Electron micrographs showing **a** histiocyte with large cytoplasmic vacuoles, lipid-bearing foam cell (xanthoma cell), and **b** typical Birbeck granules in the cytoplasm of histiocytes (Langerhans cell). **a** ×15000, **b** ×22000

6. Fibrous Dysplasia and Osteofibrous Dysplasia

A. Fibrous Dysplasia. Definition, WHO: *"A benign lesion, presumably developmental in nature, characterized by the presence of fibrous connective tissue with a characteristic whorled pattern and containing trabeculae of immature non-lamellar bone."*

In 1938, Lichtenstein described fibrous dysplasia as a distinct entity of unknown etiology involving several bones (polyostotic fibrous dysplasia). Later, Lichtenstein and Jaffe (1942) reported the existence of different clinical manifestations, i.e., solitary (monostotic) and multiple (polyostotic) forms, sometimes associated with extraskeletal symptoms; in particular, cutaneous pigmentation was more common in the polyostotic forms. Some of the more severe forms of polyostotic disease may be accompanied not only by areas of cutaneous pigmentation, but also by endocrine dysfunction with precocious puberty in females, a syndrome described by Albright et al. in 1937. Fibrous dysplasia appears to be a developmental anomaly of the bone-forming mesenchyme (Lichtenstein 1938) without consistent hereditary or familial factors. Because of the combined presence of fibrous and osseous tissue in varying proportions, Jaffe suggested in 1958 the term "fibro-osseous dysplasia" as a synonym for this entity, which in the older literature was termed "osteitis fibrosa localizata or disseminata" or "osteodystrophia fibrosa" (Freund 1934).

Clinical Findings. *Monostotic fibrous dysplasia* affects a single bone, usually with one focus and rarely with more foci of different sizes and degree of extensiveness. Occasionally, a separate focus later appears in another bone of the same extremity (monomelic type) or in other bones. Monostotic lesions were far more frequent in our laboratory, which receives cases preferentially from orthopedic departments; 296 cases were recorded compared with only 36 polyostotic lesions.

Although fibrous dysplasia usually begins in childhood, the disease is often asymptomatic and is only recognized in adult life, generally during

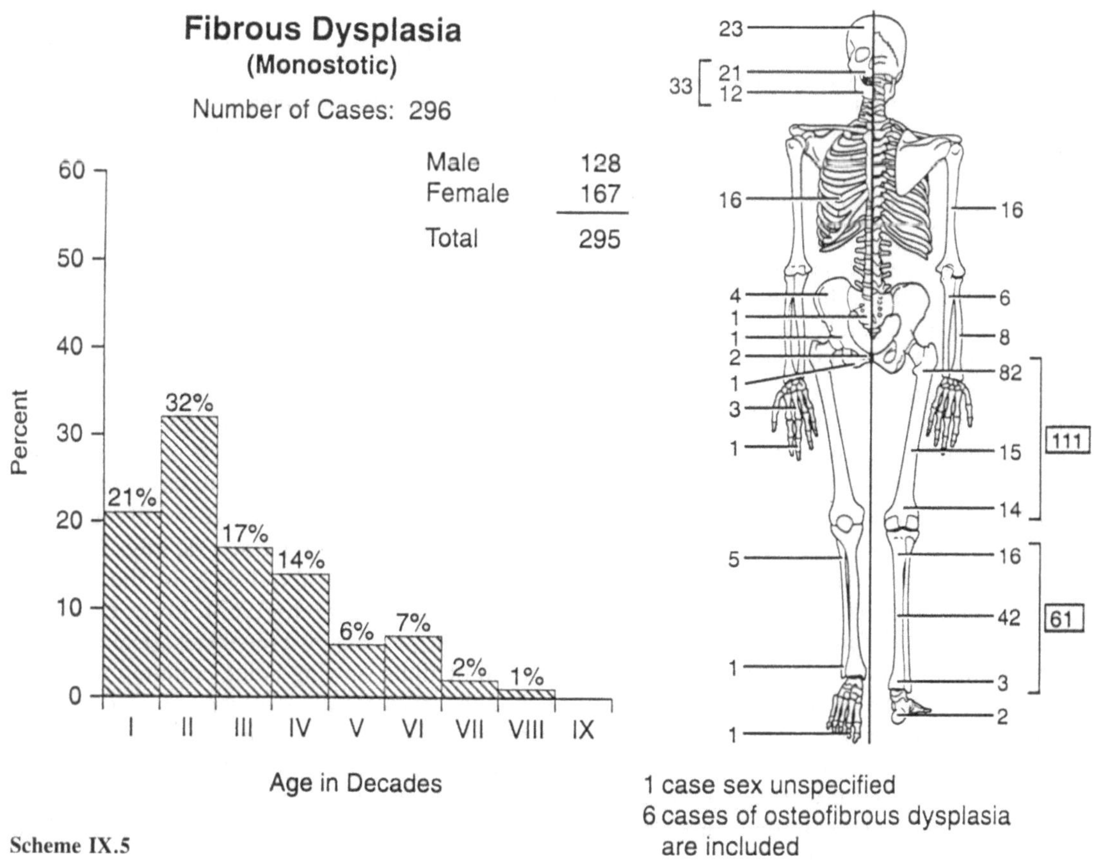

Scheme IX.5

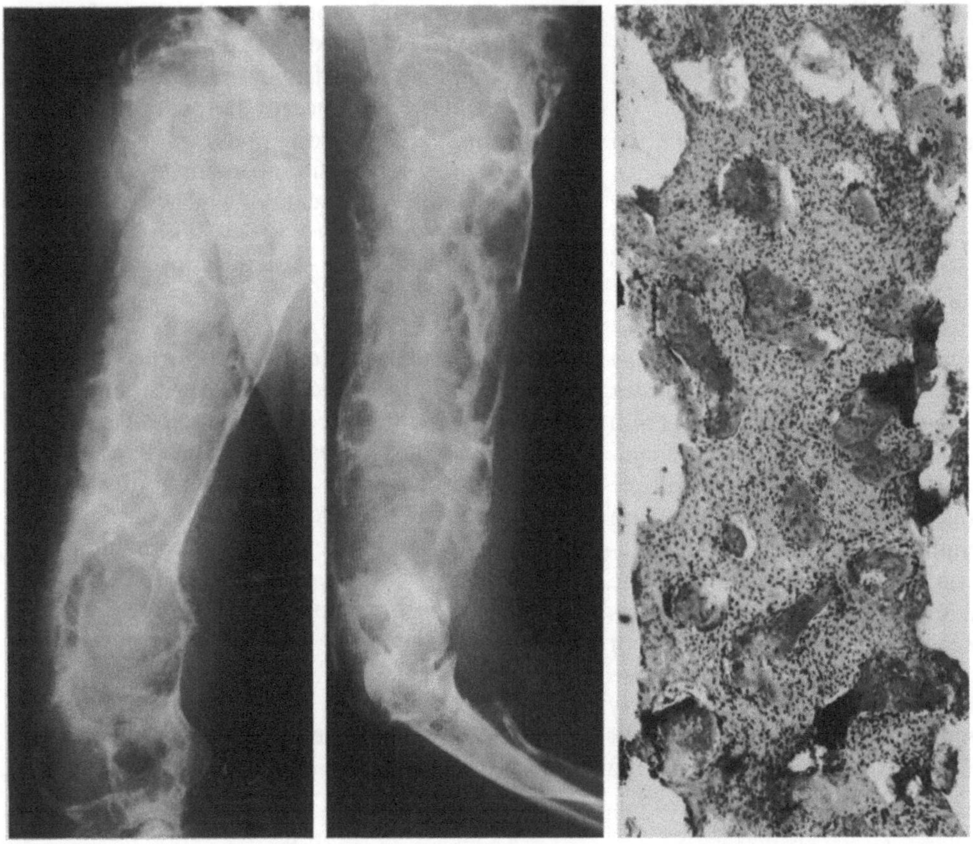

Fig. IX.67a,b. Female, 24 years old, with polyostotic fibrous dysplasia. **a** Anteroposterior radiographs demonstrate a multiloculated expanding lesion of the entire humerus; the upper end of the radius shows a similar lesion, suggesting hydatidosis. **b** Photomicrograph of the cylinder obtained by puncture biopsy illustrates the fibrous marrow with metaplastic formation of immature bone. (Schajowicz and Derqui 1968) **b** ×40

an incidental radiographic examination (Henry 1969) (Scheme IX.5).

Most patients in our series were in the first three decades of life (70%), the range being from 10 months to 76 years. There was a slight female predominance for the solitary lesion, which became more evident for polyostotic disease (2:1). Any bone of the skeleton may be involved, but the most common sites were the femur (111 cases), preferentially the upper third, tibia (61 cases), maxillary bones (33 cases), skull (23 cases), and ribs (16 cases).

Monostotic lesions may be entirely asymptomatic. The most common clinical complaints are swelling or deformity, particularly in craniofacial lesions or in those located in the femur, tibia, or ribs; occasionally there is accompanying mild or more severe pain. Pathologic fracture is often the initial symptom, particularly in bones of the extremities. Cranial lesions may progress slowly until adulthood and affect the optic nerve or the middle ear structures. Abnormal cutaneous pigmentation, found in about 50% of polyostotic cases, is rarely observed in solitary lesions. The site of the pigmentation often, but not always, corresponds to that of severe bone involvement.

The distribution and extension of *polyostotic lesions* varies widely, from involvement of a few bones of a single extremity (Fig. IX.67) to severe lesions that affect more than 50% of the skeleton. In these severe cases, symptoms begin early in life, generally before 10 years of age, and the disease usually progresses rapidly. Multiple fractures occurred in about 85% of the patients reported by Harris et al. (1962), lower extremity deformities and leg discrepancies secondary to femoral or tibial bowing being common features. Although craniofacial involvement is common, vertebral lesions are rare and exceptionally associated with neurologic symptoms. According to Grabias and Campbell (1977), puberty seems to have a quieting effect on disease activity, which is in contrast to the opinion of Harris et al. (1962)

in a report on material from the same institution (Massachusetts General Hospital).

In a small number of patients, polyostotic fibrous dysplasia with or without abnormal cutaneous pigmentation may be associated with precocious puberty in females (*Albright syndrome*) (Fig. IX.68) or with other endocrine dysfunctions, such as acromegaly, hyperthyroidism, hyperparathyroidism (Ehrig and Wilson 1972), and Cushing syndrome (Benjamin and McRoberts 1973; Danon et al. 1975). The bone lesions tend toward a preferred unilateral distribution. Albright made a distinction between the pigmented macules in fibrous dysplasia and the similar ones in neurofibromatosis. According to him, the macules of fibrous dysplasia with their irregular and dented borders look like a map of the coast of Maine, whereas the irregular but smooth borders of the pigmented nevi in neurofibromatosis resemble the coast of California.

A complete and extensive autopsy study of the first case of Albright syndrome was reported by MacMahna (1971), who discussed in detail the few other autopsied cases. Despite several reports, the pathogenesis remains unsolved, hypersecretion of hypothalamic releasing hormones having been suggested as the most probable explanation of the endocrine manifestations of this syndrome (Hall and Warrick 1972).

Albright syndrome is observed most commonly in females. It begins in infancy with vaginal bleeding, sometimes starting as early as 3 years of age, as in one of our and in other reported cases. Precocious sexual development and early bone maturation with premature closure of the growth cartilage and consequent short stature are characteristic features.

Radiographic Features. The radiographic appearance in solitary and multiple lesions is essentially the same. It varies widely from area to area and depends greatly on the proportion of bone and fibrous components of the diseased tissue, which occupies extensive areas of the interior of the affected bone. In lesions where the bony compound predominates, the radiologic aspect has a ground-glass pattern (Fig. IX.69) or may be radiopaque, a pattern common in facial and cranial bones, especially the maxilla and base of the skull (Fig. IX.70). On the other hand, when the connective tissue predominates, a radiolucent cystic appearance may be produced (Figs. IX.71, IX.72). In long bones, the dysplastic tissue erodes and expands the newly formed cortex, often resulting in a diffuse enlargement of the bone contour. Infrequently, the radiographic picture may be frankly osteolytic, corresponding to areas of cystic degeneration, or show spotty calcification when cartilage is interspersed with the fibrosseous tissue, which is rare in solitary lesions but not uncommon in polyostotic disease. Enchondroma or enchondromatosis may present diagnostic problems in these cases.

Pathologic Findings. *Grossly*, the bone tissue is replaced by solid masses of fibrous tissue of grayish-white color, firm, and more or less gritty (Figs. IX.68, IX.71). In some areas, the lesion is definitely hard, and in others, smaller or larger cystic cavities filled with serous fluid may be observed. Scarce but sometimes more extensive cartilage foci may be found occasionally in polyostotic and rarely in solitary lesions. Hemorrhage or hemosiderin pigment is usually found after a fracture (Fig. IX.71b).

Histologically, the lesion is composed of spindle cells and connective fibers, with a characteristic whorled or storiform pattern containing newly formed trabeculae of immature bone and/or osteoid of different sizes and distribution, often with an alphabetic letter-like pattern (Figs. IX.73, IX.74). In some areas, the trabeculae are sparse (Fig. IX.75) while in others they are large and more abundant, dominating the histologic picture, as is common in lesions of the craniofacial bones (Fig. IX.70). In these locations, cementlike rounded formations are frequently seen, a process classified by some authors as "fibro-osteoma" or "ossifying fibroma" (Schlumberger 1946a). Several times we found lesions with this aspect associated with typical lesions of "fibrous dysplasia" in long bones (Fig. IX.76b). The connective tissue may be loose with scarce collagen fibers and plump or stellate cells, resembling myxoid or undifferentiated mesenchymal tissue. This pattern appears to correspond to newer lesions, whereas in older ones the fibrous tissue is usually denser and sometimes hyalinized. The osteoblasts on the surface of the bone are usually flat and atrophic (Figs. IX.74, IX.76c)

Cartilage may be present, rarely in solitary and more frequently in multiple lesions; sometimes the amounts are considerable, complicating the differentiation from enchondroma or multiple enchondromatosis. Such lesions are referred to as fibrocartilaginous dysplasia. The presence of more or less abundant cartilage in polyostotic fibrous dysplasia raises the possibility of an

Fig. IX.68a–f. Female, 8 years old, with Albright syndrome. **a–e** Radiographs show polyostotic involvement with characteristic sclerosis of the cranial bone and groundglass appearance in the long-limb bones. **f** Photograph and radiograph of a resected segment of the fibula show the expansion of the bone, which is replaced by a grayishwhite fibro-osseous tissue of gritty consistency. The girl had vaginal bleedings when 5 years old and multiple cutaneous pigmented macules

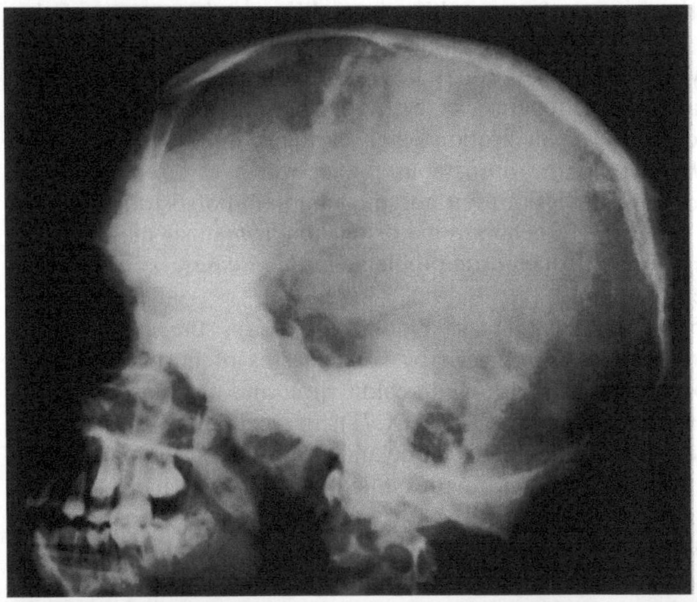

a

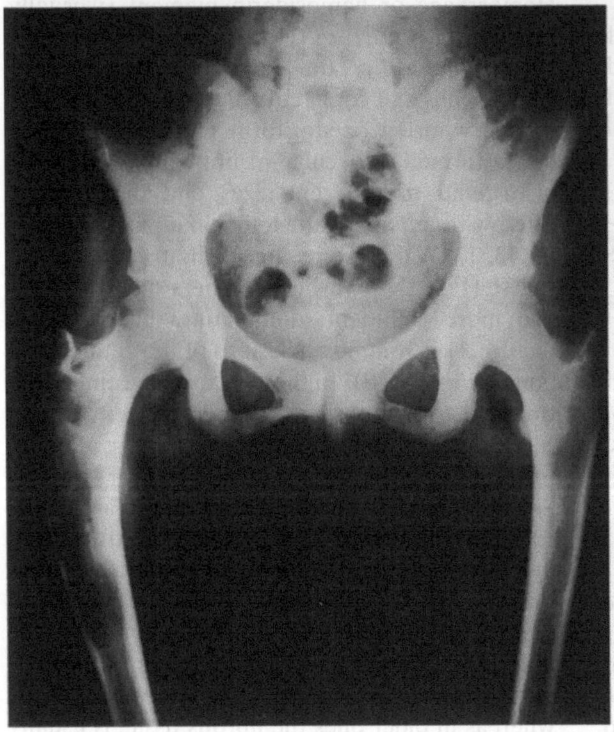

b

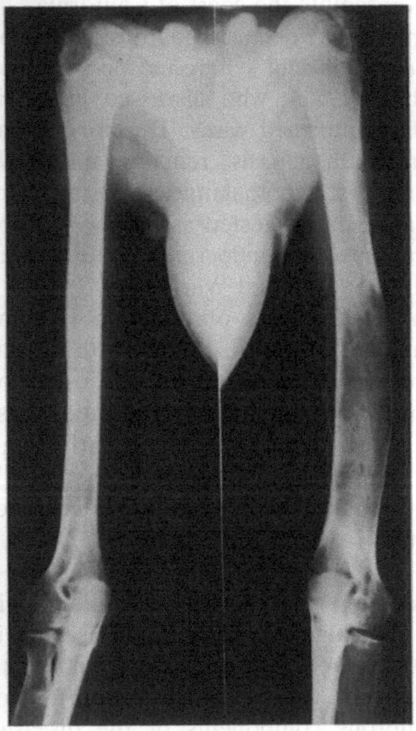

c

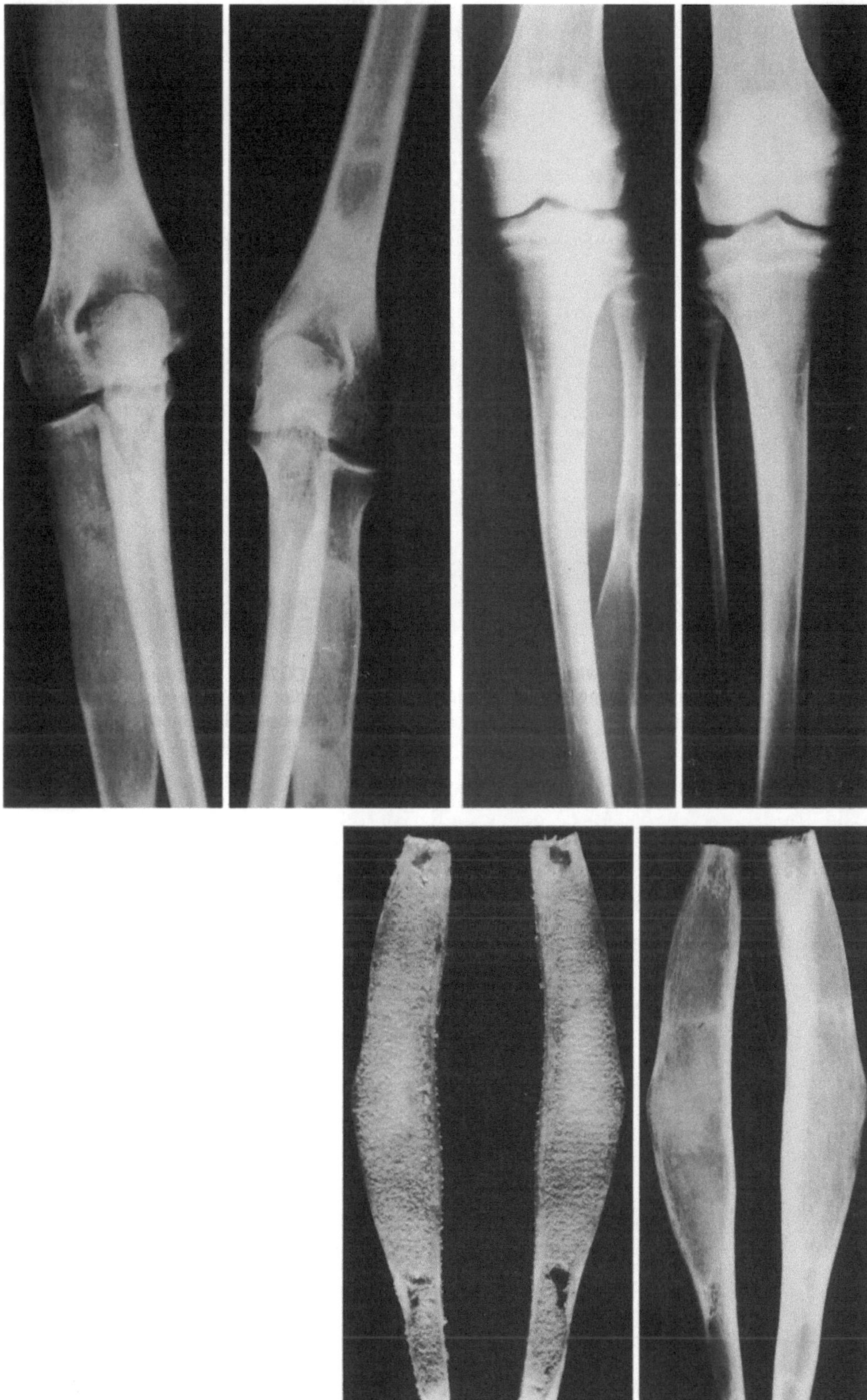

d

e

f

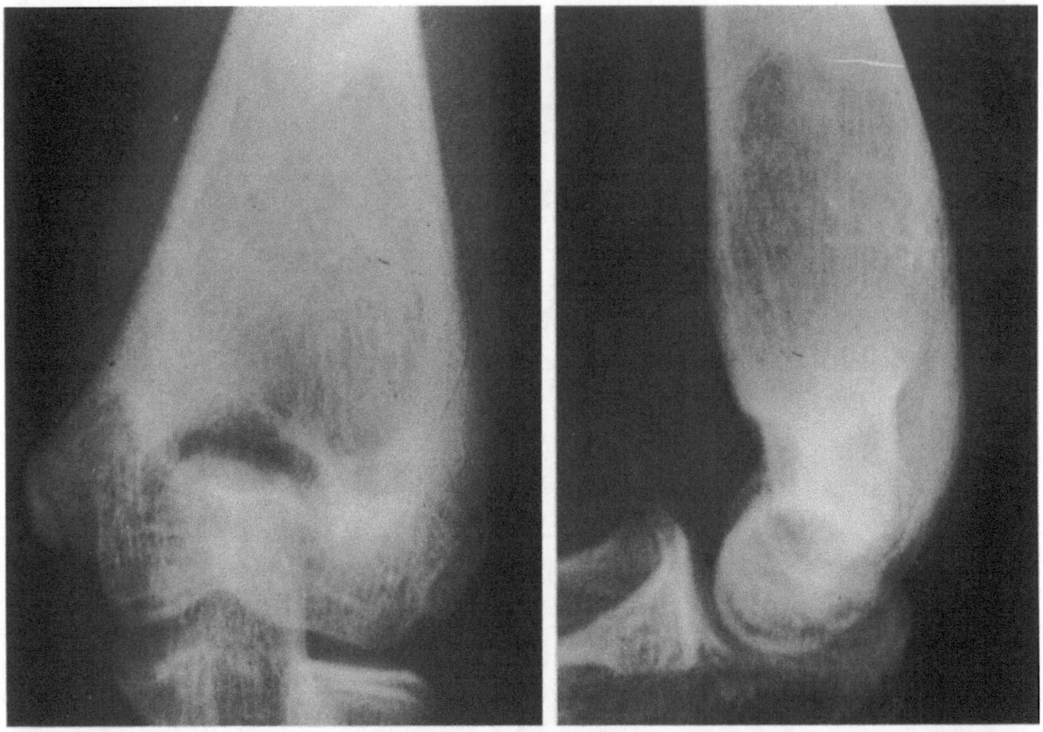

▲ **Fig. IX.69.** Male, 14 years old, with monostotic fibrous dysplasia of the humerus showing typical ground-glass appearance

▼ **Fig. IX.70a,b.** Photograph and radiograph of autopsy specimen with a section of the skull showing marked asymmetric enlargement of the frontal and parietal bone. There is intense bone sclerosis with some small osteolytic areas

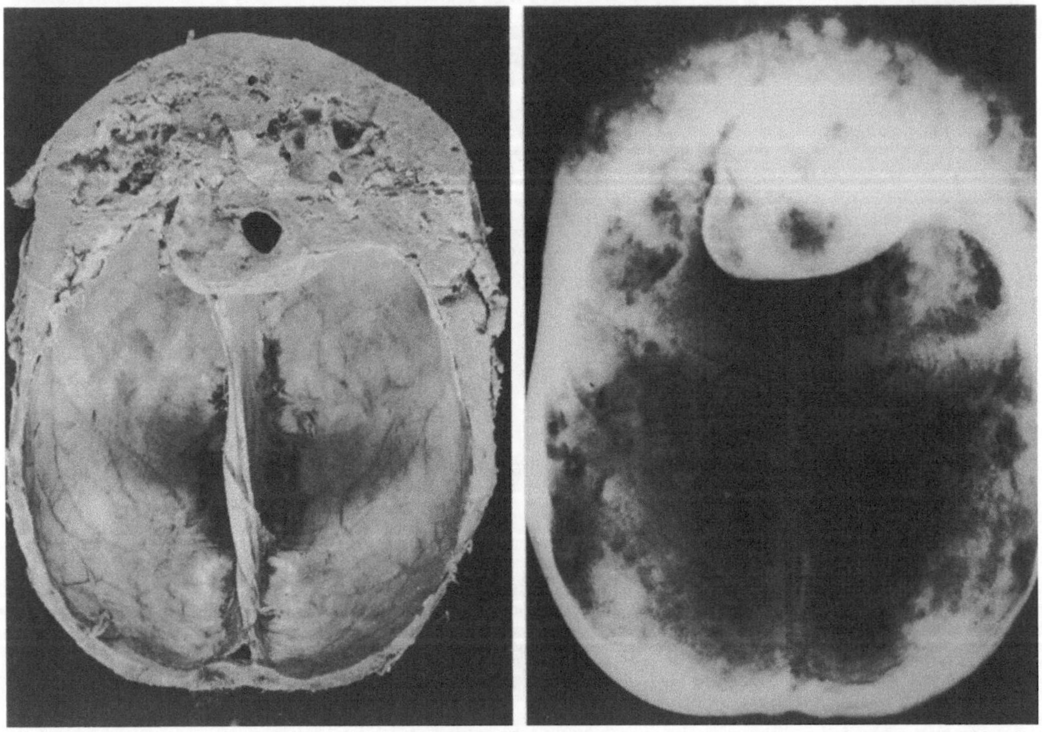

a **b**

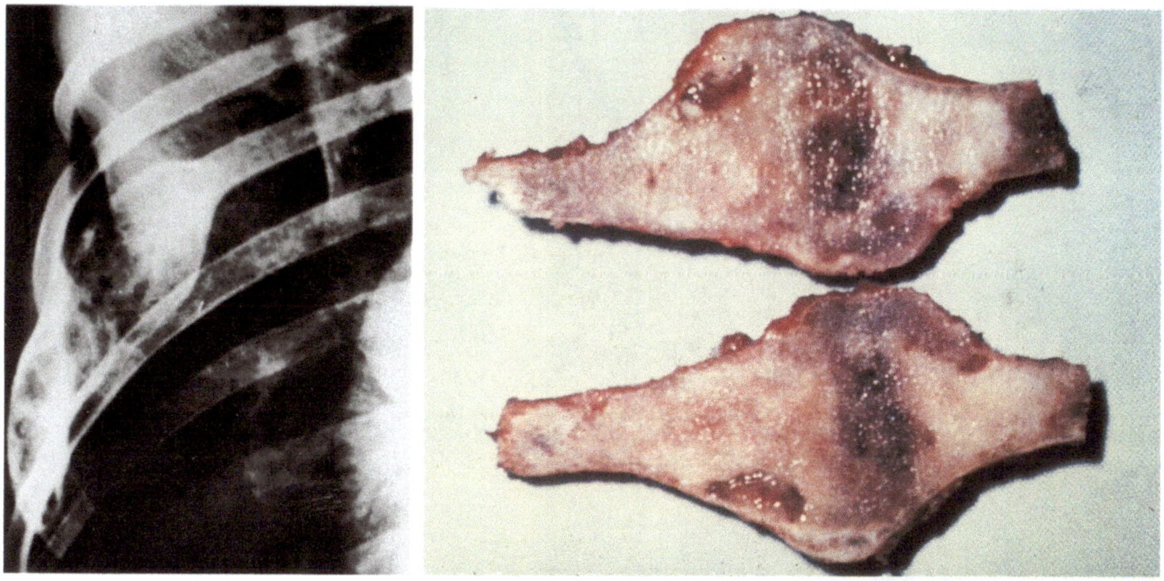

a b

Fig. IX.71. a Female, 25 years old. Monostotic fibrous dysplasia of rib, with a large expanding radiolucent lesion. **b** Photograph of the specimen shows the grayish-white color with a hemorrhagic area due to a previous fracture. **c–e** Male, 58 years old. Monostotic fibrous dysplasia of rib. Radiographs and photograph of the resected specimen show an expanding trabeculated radiolucent lesion that extends into the unexpanded portion of the rib; this is shown more clearly in the longitudinal section (**d**,**e**), where the grayish-white color of the major part of the lesion is seen

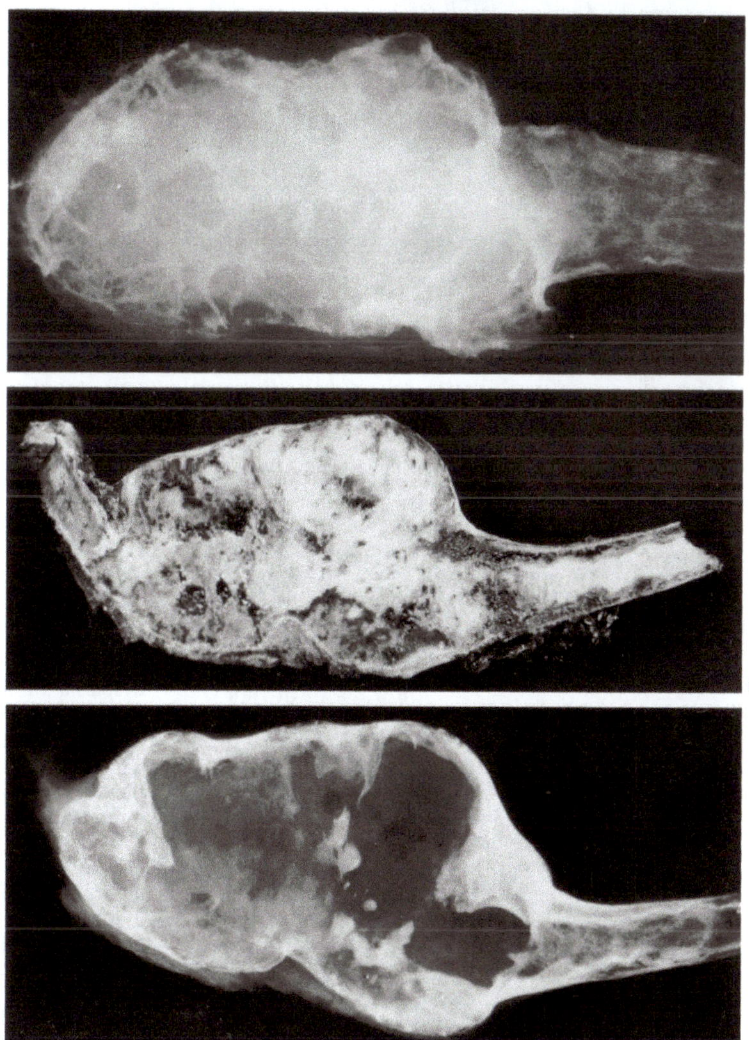

c d e

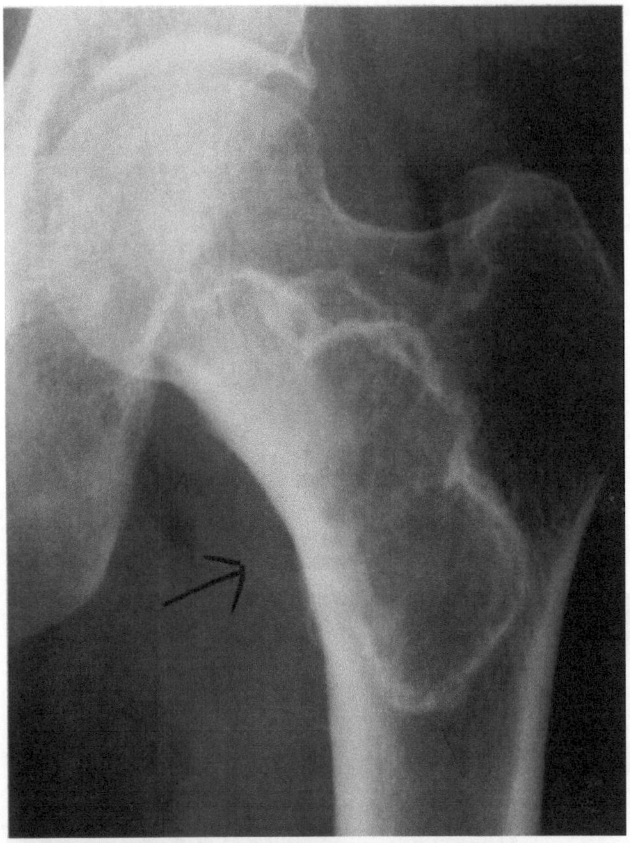

a

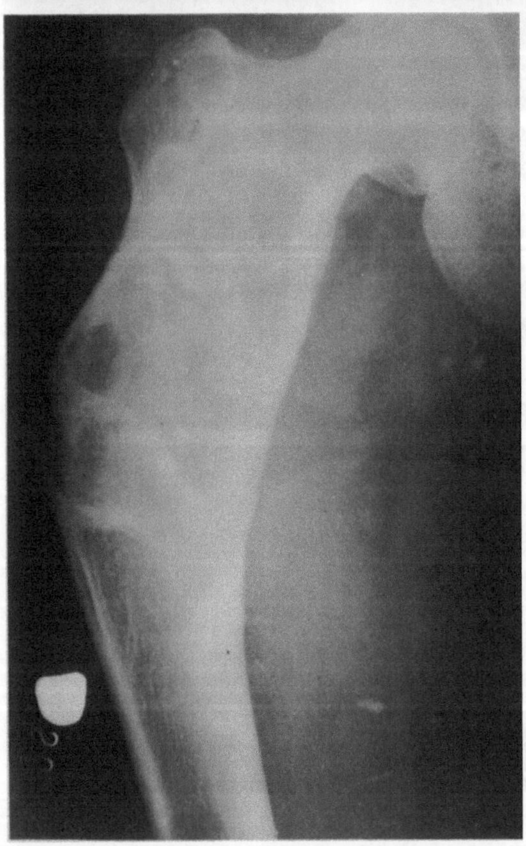

b

◀ **Fig. IX.72a, b.** Two different cases of monostotic fibrous dysplasia of the upper third of the femur. **a** Female, 30 years old. Radiograph illustrates a radiolucent lesion of ground-glass appearance with sclerotic borders. **b** Female, 22 years old. Radiograph shows bowing of the femur after a pathologic fracture and additional radiopaque areas

Fig. IX.73a–d. Photomicrographs showing at lower and ▶ higher magnification the histologic pattern of fibrous dysplasia. **a,b** Metaplastic formation of immature bone trabeculae in spindle-cell connective tissue. In **a** the bone formation is more conspicuous than in **b**, which is common in craniofacial lesions. **c,d** At higher magnification, one sees the whorled pattern of the connective tissue containing immature (woven) bone trabeculae, surrounded by flattened, apparently inactive osteoblasts. In **d** the bone trabeculae are more mature. **a,b** ×60, **c,d** ×200

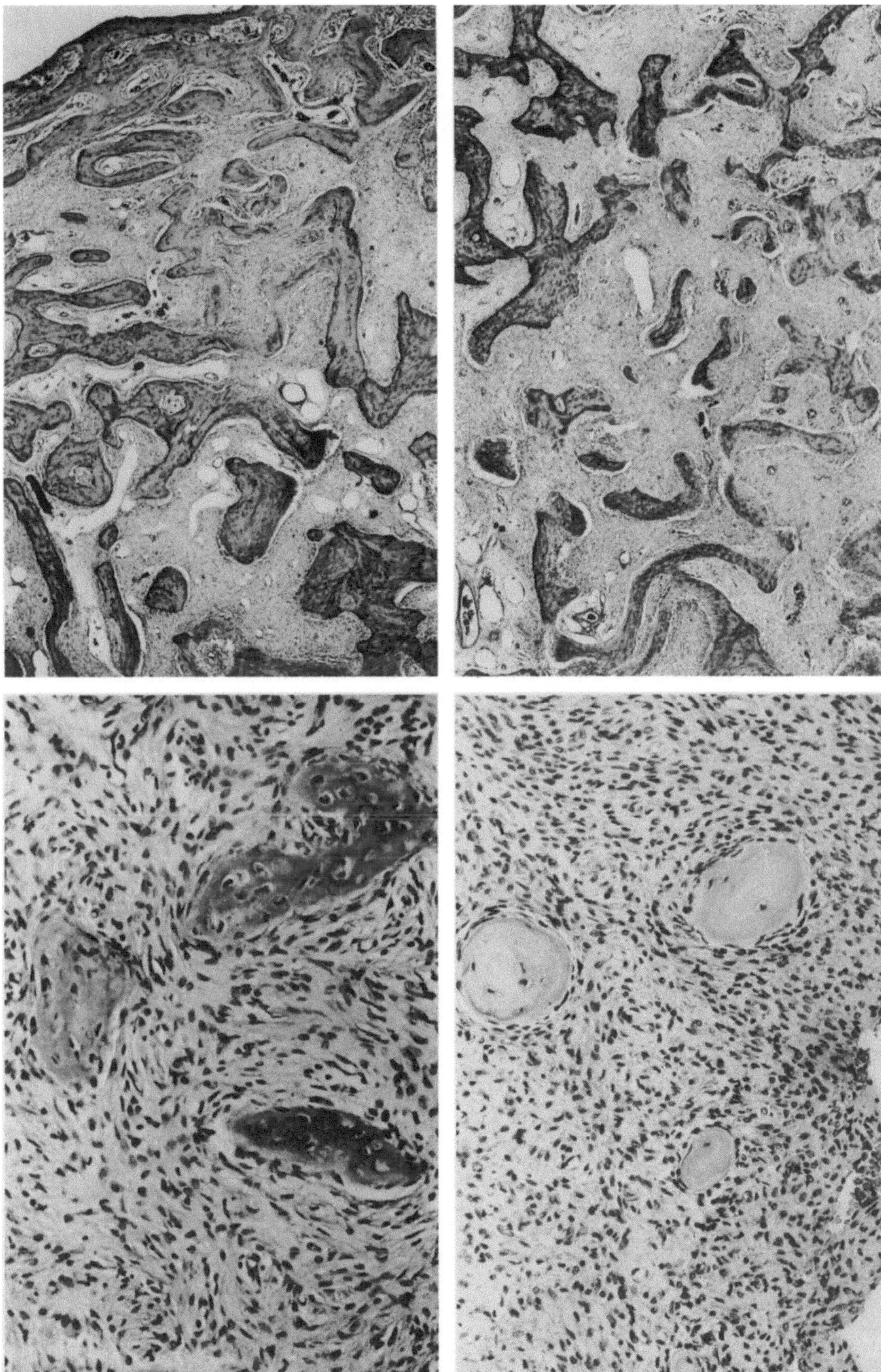

a b c d

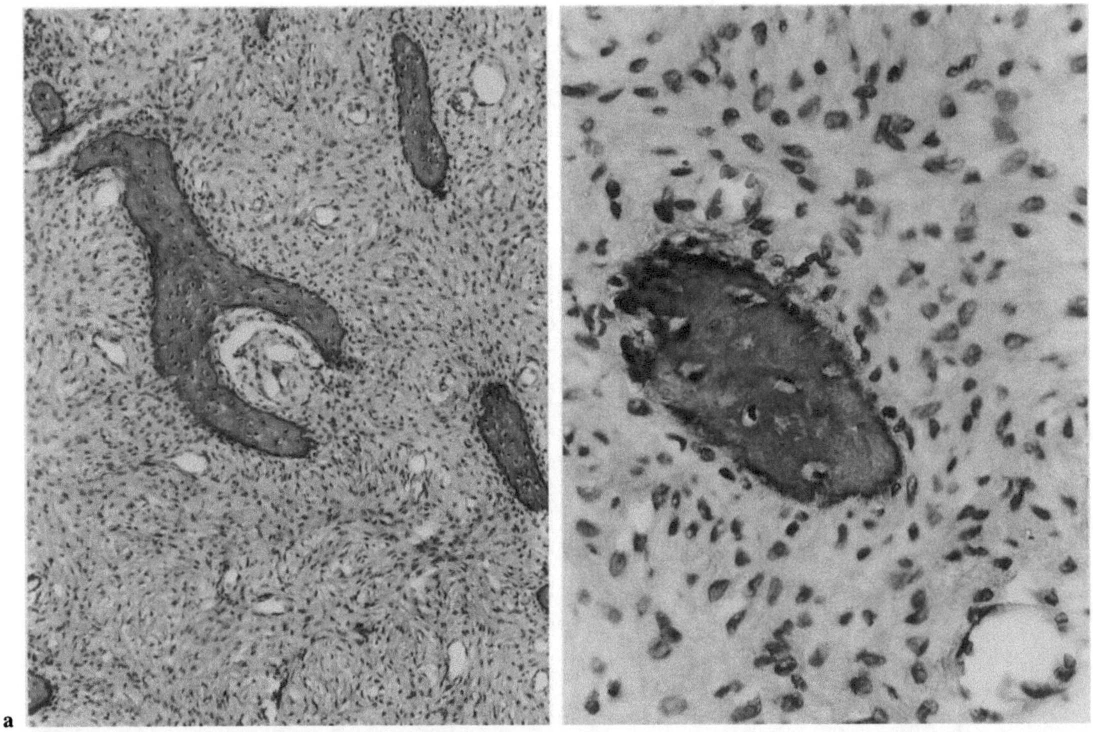

Fig. IX.74a,b. Photomicrographs showing woven bone trabeculae, in part U-shaped and surrounded by flattened osteoblasts in a fibrous storiform stroma. **a** ×100, **b** ×400

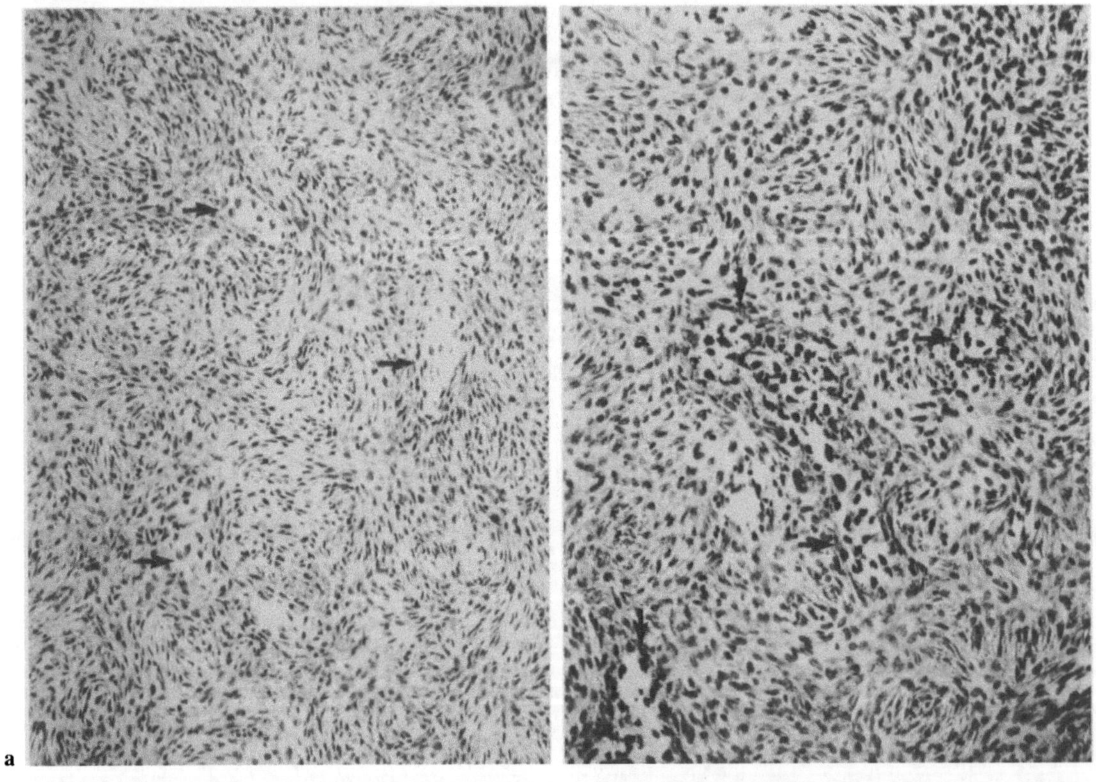

Fig. IX.75a,b. Photomicrographs showing areas with a predominant connective tissue component, with the whorled arrangement of the spindle cells and beginning formation of bone trabeculae within the dysplastic tissue. (Del Rio Hortega's nuclear-plasmatic stain). **a,b** ×180

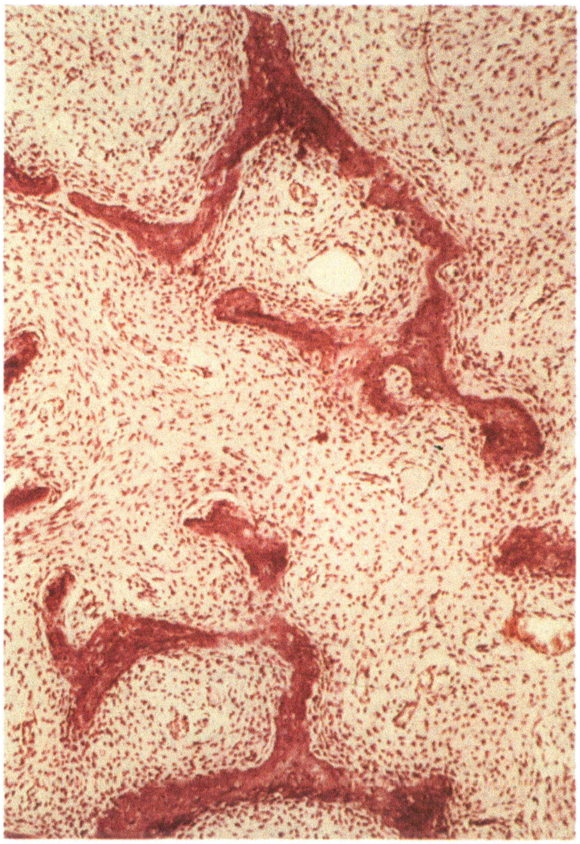

a

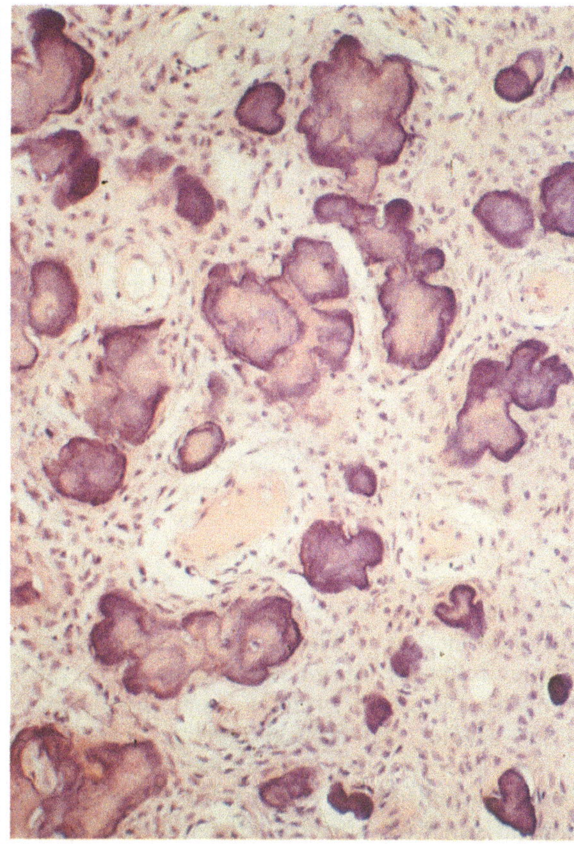

b

Fig. IX.76a–c. Photomicrographs show **a** characteristic alphabetic-letter-shaped bone trabeculae of woven bone pattern, rimmed by **c** flattened atrophic osteoblasts. **b** Several rounded and irregular cementlike formations within the fibrous stroma of fibrous dysplasia of tibia. Such cementicles are common in maxillary bone but not exceptionally rare in long bones. **a**,**b** ×100, **c** ×300

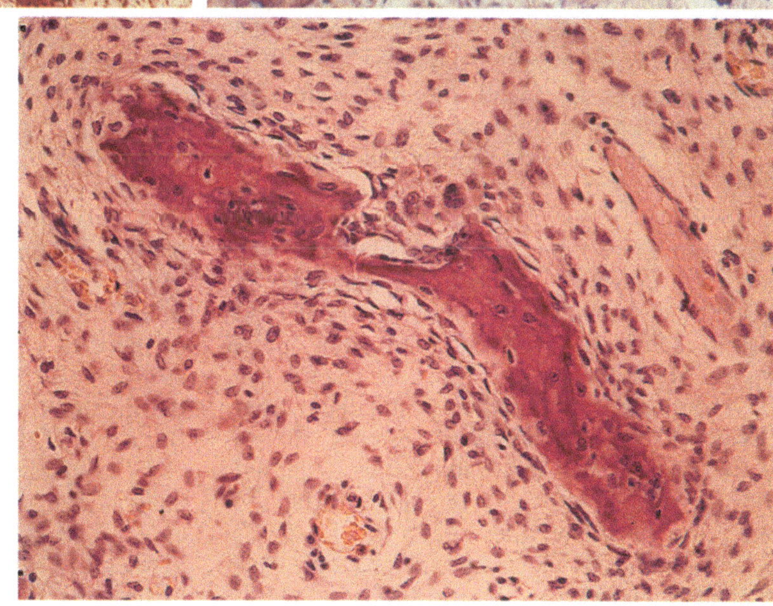

c

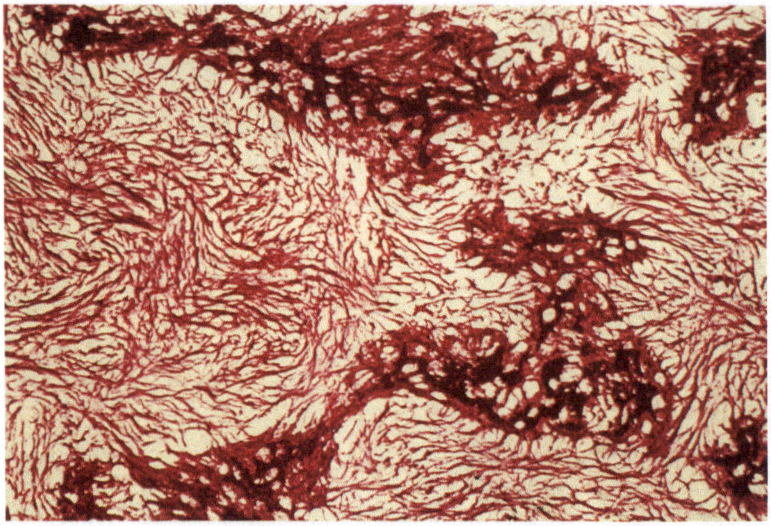

Fig. IX.77. Del Rio Hortega's stain for reticulin fibers shows the continuity between fibrils of the stroma (dysplastic tissue) and those that form the matrix of the immature (woven) bone trabeculae, which present coarse, granular calcification. ×400

interrelationship between this process and enchondromatosis (Ollier's dyschondroplasia), another dysplastic lesion. Foci of cystic degeneration with formation of small, sometimes confluent, cavities are frequent findings, justifying in part the old term "osteitis fibrosa cystica." Hemorrhages with the presence of hemosiderin pigment, especially after pathologic fractures, are not uncommon, and are sometimes associated with giant cells of the osteoclast type. However, in some cases we found these elements independent of hemorrhages or cysts.

Rarely, small groups of foam cells were seen, generally situated around blood vessels or small hemorrhages. Their numbers were always insignificant in relation to the remainder of the tissue of dysplastic aspect. The presence of metaplastic formation of immature bone and osteoid allows the differentiation from metaphyseal fibrous defect.

Thannhauser (1944) postulated that "localized and disseminated osteitis fibrosa cystica" (the former names for fibrous dysplasia) and neurofibromatosis (von Recklinghausen 1882) are related entities, because of various clinical (cutaneous pigmentation) and histologic similarities. However, our investigations (Valls et al. 1950), in which we used special silver impregnation techniques of Ramón and Cajal and Bielschowsky (quoted by Rio Hortega 1934) for nerve elements, did not show in dysplastic tissue the existence of nerve fibrils or of schwannian elements (lemmocytes) among the connective tissue cells or in the whorl formations. In any event, the presence of nerve fibers would not justify the diagnosis of neurofibromatosis, because such fibers, either normal or degenerated, can be observed in any tissue, be it tumorous or normal. Using silver stains for reticulin fibers, it could be seen that the newly formed osteoid and woven bone trabeculae corresponded to a compressed network of enlarged preexisting and newly formed reticulin fibrils, which were later impregnated with calcium granules and were continuous with those of the stroma encircling them (Fig. IX.77).

Malignant Transformation of Fibrous Dysplasia. This complication does not seem to be as rare as was previously supposed. Lichtenstein and Jaffe (1942) did not report any cases in their classic publication, but in 1958 Jaffe illustrated two cases of osteosarcomatous and chondrosarcomatous transformation. In recent years, the number of reported cases has been increasing (Milgram 1975), but it is difficult to give exact figures on the incidence of this complication (Dabska and Buraczewski 1956), which seems to occur in about 0.5% (Schwartz and Alpert 1964), more frequently after irradiation (Slow et al. 1971). Nineteen of 48 patients received roentgenotherapy to the area prior to the onset of the sarcoma (Schwartz and Alpert 1964). The interval between the diagnosis and the occurrence of the sarcoma varied from 2 to 30 years. In our files we have three cases of fibrosarcoma that developed in monostotic lesions which had not been irradiated; these lesions were located in the diaphyses of the femur (see discussion of fibrosarcoma in Chap. VI, and Fig. VI.26) and humerus and the lower end of the fibula. Besides fibrosarcoma, which

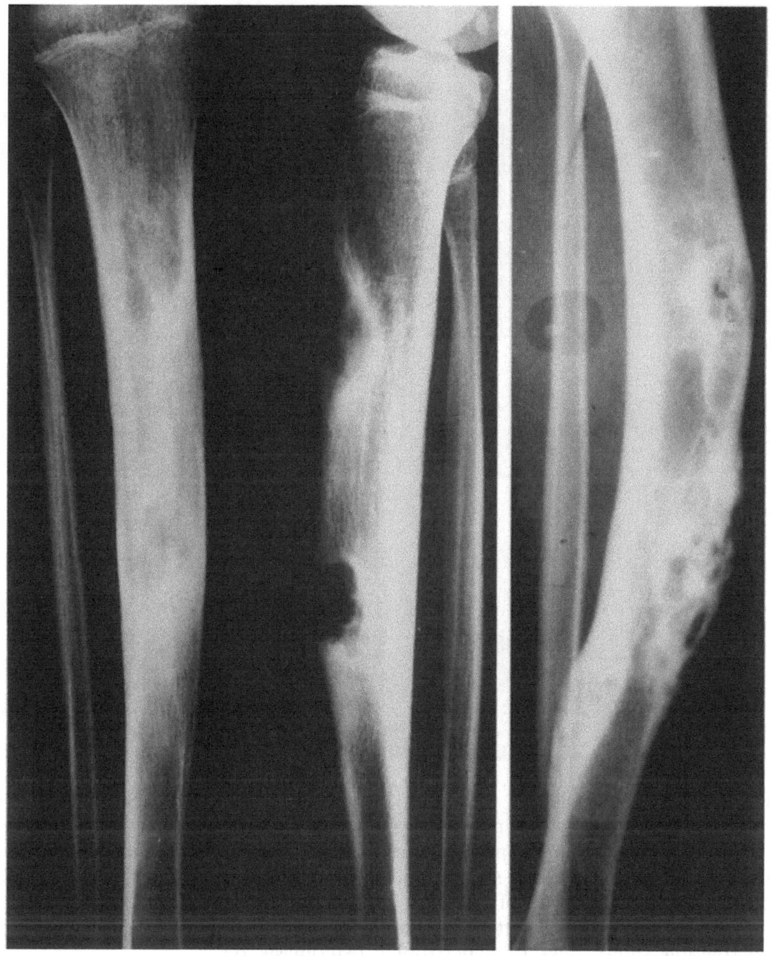

a b

Fig. IX.78a,b. Two different cases of so-called osteofibrous dysplasia. **a** Eight-year-old girl. Anteroposterior and lateral radiographs show an osteolytic, intracortical lesion with a sclerotic endosteal border at the tibial diaphysis and a similar separated lesion at the proximal end. **b** Twelve-year-old boy. Lateral radiograph demonstrates multiple osteolytic areas of different size separated by sclerotic bone, with a "sawtooth" appearance of the involved cortex, which shows conspicuous bowing. A similar radiographic pattern may be seen in cases of "adamantinoma" (see Chap. VII)

seems to be the most common type of malignant tumor (Huvos et al. 1972), osteosarcomas and, more rarely, chondrosarcomas or malignant giant-cell tumors have been reported.

There is no specific age or sex predilection, and the facial bones and the femur seem to be the areas most frequently involved. Huvos et al. (1972) reported a 52% 5-year survival rate after radical surgery, demonstrating the relatively good prognosis as compared with malignant tumor of the same type arising in normal bones.

Treatment and Prognosis. No medical or radiation therapy is effective in fibrous dysplasia. In fact, radiation therapy may increase the risk of malignant change. The surgical treatment consists primarily in the correction of deformity (especially coxa vara or shepherd's crook deformity of the upper femoral end) through different orthopedic procedures such as osteotomy, curettage followed by bone grafting (auto- or allografts), and/or nail-plate fixation (Enneking and Gearen 1986).

Pathologic fractures are treated with skeletal traction and then allowed mobilization in a functional orthosis; additional curettage and bone grafting and/or the use of a fixation device may be necessary in some cases and locations (e.g., the femoral neck). Monostotic lesions that are not painful or of small size do not always require treatment, because some cases may heal spontaneously (Grabias and Campbell 1977). On the other hand, the risk of local recurrence or pathologic fracture exists after curettage. In lesions of the ribs, fibula, ulna, or tubular bones, and in some larger lesions of the mandible, segmental resection was the preferred treatment in our institution.

B. Osteofibrous Dysplasia (Ossifying Fibroma). Definition, WHO: "*A rare benign lesion, almost exclusively localized in the tibia and fibula of young children. As in fibrous dysplasia, it is characterized by the presence of fibrous connective tissue and trabeculae of immature non-lamellar*

a, b
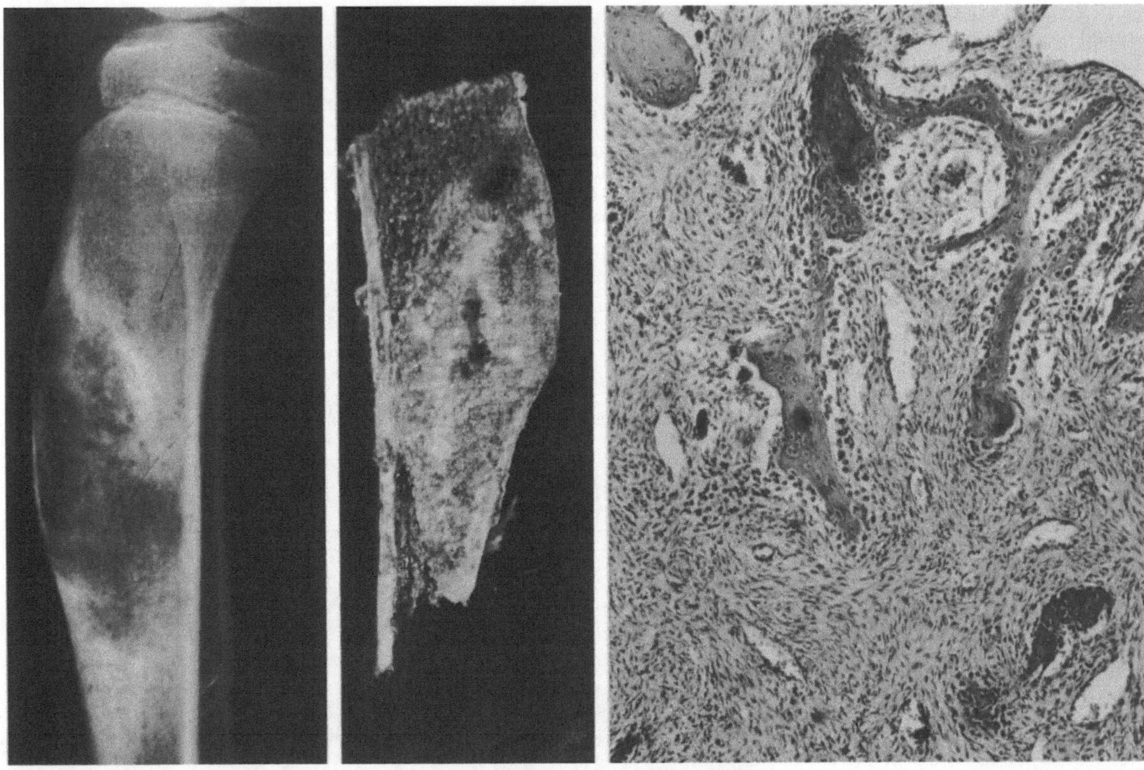
c

Fig. IX.79a–c. Female, 11 years old. Fibrous dysplasia of tibia, active stage. **a** Lateral radiograph shows a radiolucent ill-defined lesion expanding the anterior cortex. Because of the active bone formation a resection was performed. **b** Photograph of resection specimen showing the gross fibrous gritty pattern of the lesion. **c** Photomicrograph shows rows of hypertrophic osteoblasts on the surface of many bone trabeculae, separated by the whorled connective tissue seen in conventional fibrous dysplasia. Such lesions in the tibia of young children have been classified as "ossifying fibroma" by Kempson, in analogy with the process in the maxillary bone, and as "osteofibrous dysplasia" by Campanacci. **c** ×100

bone. In contrast to fibrous dysplasia, the surfaces of the woven bone trabeculae are usually covered by rows of active osteoblasts."

Kempson (1966) classified cases in the tibia of young children in which histologically the woven bone trabeculae were surrounded by rows of active osteoblasts as "ossifying fibroma," in analogy to the process of the maxillary bones that presents similar histologic features, but in contrast to fibrous dysplasia, an encapsulated growth (Pindborg et al. 1971). Kempson emphasized the more aggressive behavior of the so-called ossifying fibroma of the tibia, with the possibility of local recurrence after limited excision. Campanacci (1976) delineated the essential features of a similar lesion localized nearly exclusively in the tibia and at times in the fibula, often associated with anterior tibial bowing, and proposed the designation "osteofibrous dysplasia" of the long bones. In Campanacci and Laus' (1981) series of 44 cases there was a male predominance, and nearly all cases were observed prior to 10 years of age, most commonly within the first 5 years.

In the tibia the most common localization is the midshaft of the diaphysis, followed by the distal and proximal thirds. In rare cases the lesions are multiple in the same tibia. In the fibula the distal third of the diaphysis is usually involved.

Osteofibrous dysplasia is generally painless and revealed by palpation of the bulged, bowed anterior tibial bone profile. Radiologically, osteofibrous dysplasia shows a characteristic intracortical multiloculated bubbly appearance, with a rim of sclerosis around the lytic lesion, which sometimes extends to a great part of the diaphysis (Fig. IX.78). More infrequently the osteolysis is single and may expand the thinned cortex and/or extend towards the medullary canal (Fig. IX.79).

Histologically a certain "zonal architecture" besides the rimming of the woven bone trabeculae

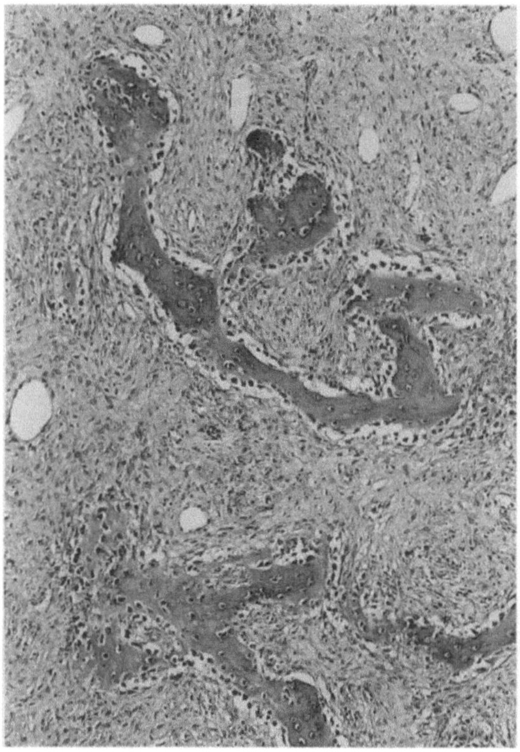

a

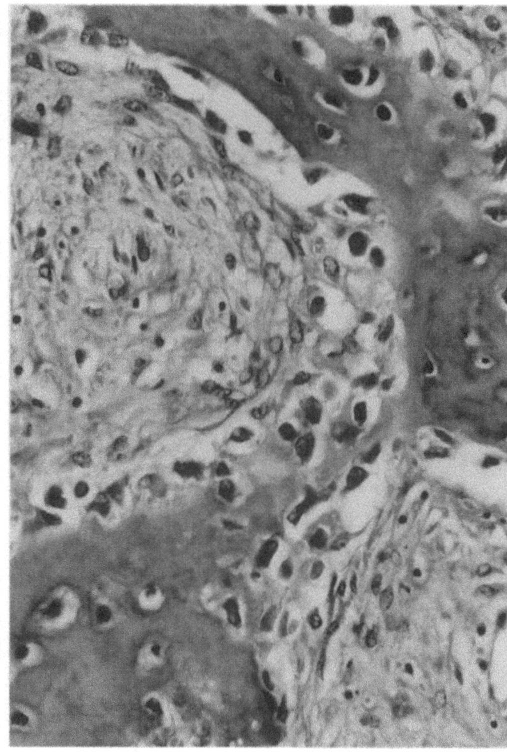

b

Fig. IX.80a,b. Photomicrographs at lower and higher magnification show the characteristic features of so-called osteofibrous dysplasia. The rims of hypertrophic osteoblasts surrounding the woven bone trabeculae are clearly seen. **a** ×100, **b** ×400

by hypertrophic, active osteoblasts has been described as characteristic (Campanacci 1976, 1990) (Figs. IX.79, IX.80); that is, sparse newly formed woven bone trabeculae are present at the center, becoming more numerous, thicker, and mature (lamellar) towards the periphery.

In a number of cases (not only those located in the tibia) we found hypertrophic osteoblasts rimming the bone trabeculae; most such cases were in younger children. We share the experience of Grabias and Campbell (1977) that this pattern indicates activity or aggressiveness of an otherwise typical fibrous dysplasia, and do not feel that the introduction of new terms is justified. We would prefer to designate these lesions as "intracortical fibrous dysplasia," as proposed by L. Johnson (1972).

Treatment. According to Campanacci, during the first 5 years of life no surgery is indicated, as the lesion tends to regress spontaneously and because there is little probability of recurrence. As we emphasized in Chap. VII, it seems possible that some cases of osteofibrous dysplasia mimicked lesions of adamantinoma of the tibia, which seems not to be as rare in young children (Schajowicz and Santini-Araujo 1989).

Surgical treatment consisting of marginal excision is indicated in extended lesions with conspicuous bowing and danger of spontaneous fractures, and in cases of pseudoarthrosis.

7. "Myositis Ossificans" (Heterotopic Ossification)

Definition, WHO: *"A non-neoplastic lesion, sometimes associated with trauma, characterized by proliferation of fibrous tissue and by formation of large amounts of new bone. Cartilage may also be present. The lesion may occur on the external surface of a bone or in soft tissues at a distance from the periosteal surface."*

The designation "myositis ossificans," although widely used, is misleading because muscle is not always involved and the lesion is not inflammatory in nature. In the writer's opinion, a better term would be "*heterotopic bone formation*" or "extraosseous localized non-

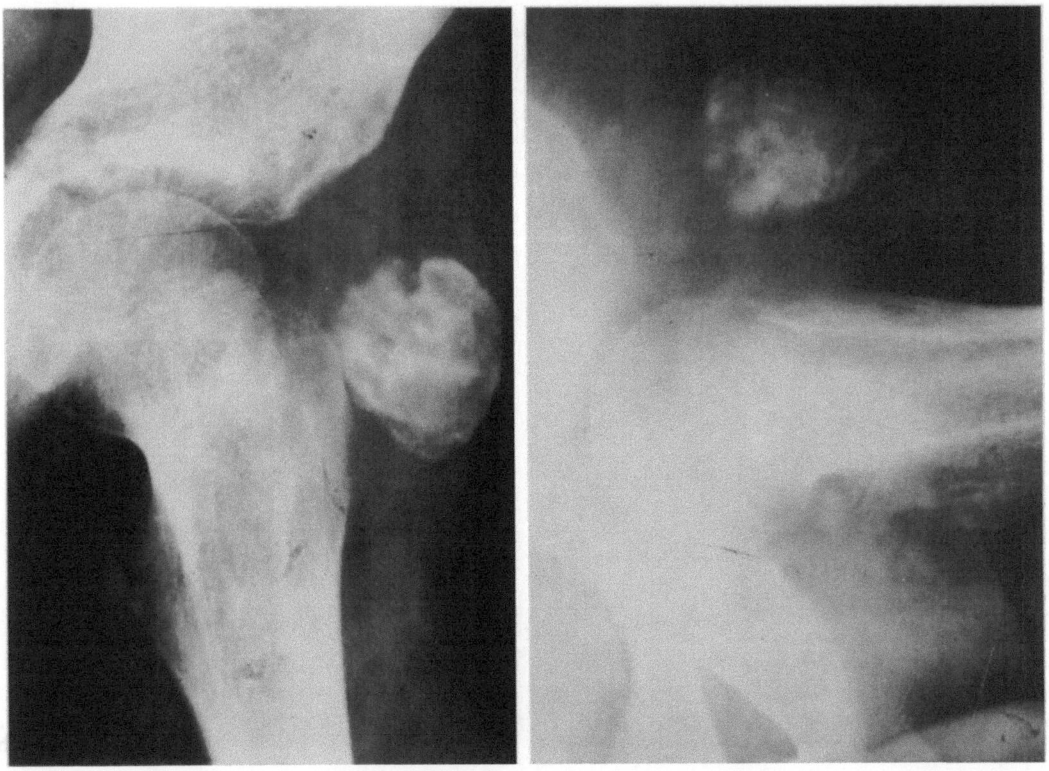

Fig. IX.81. Female, 18 years old. Pseudomalignant osseous tumor of soft tissue in hip region, without previous trauma. Anteroposterior and lateral radiographs show a round, well-delimited dense nodule in soft tissues at a certain distance from bone

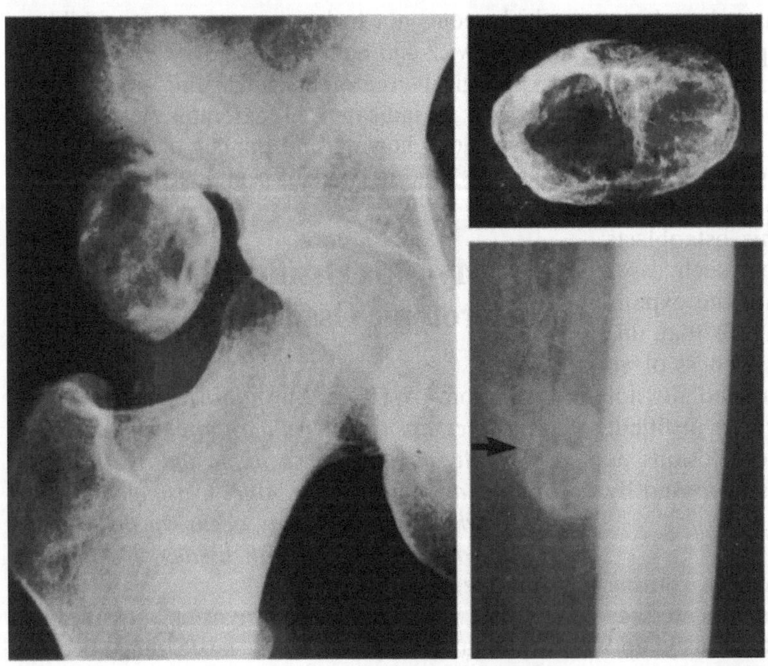

a b c

Fig. IX.82a–c. Two cases of pseudomalignant osseous tumor of soft tissue. **a** Female, 24 years old, with circumscribed calcified nodule of bony aspect with a central radiolucent core, apparently in contact with the ilium. **b** Male, 38 years old, with roundish nodule abutting at the posterior aspect of the femur, only slightly radiodense. **c** The nodule was excised 3 months later and showed radiographically a dense peripheral ossified area

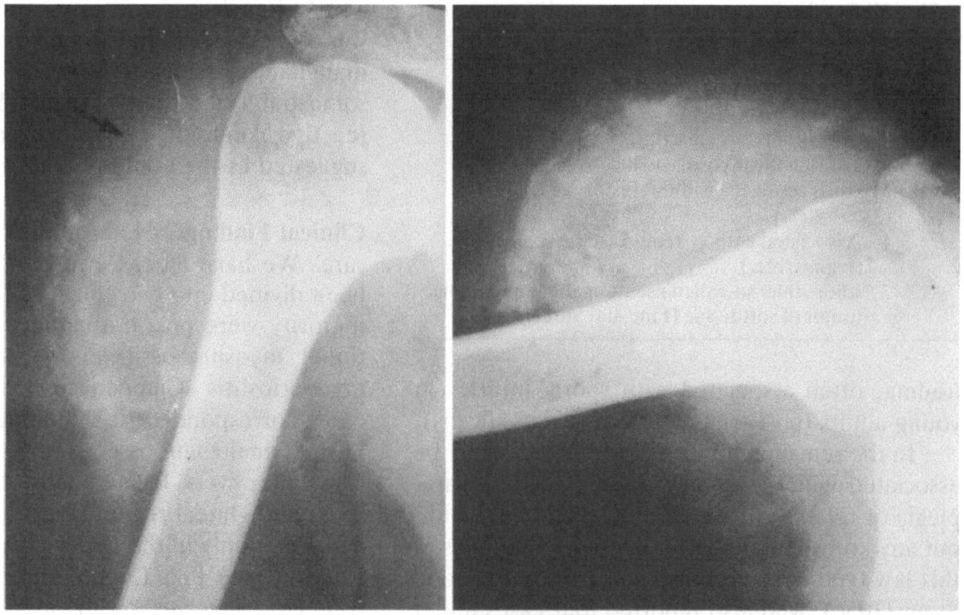

a

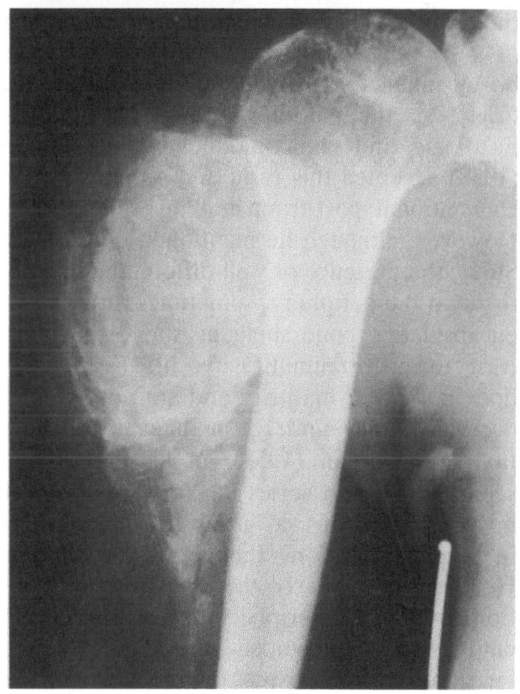

b

Fig. IX.83a,b. Female, 65 years old. Pseudomalignant osseous tumor of the arm, simulating juxtacortical osteosarcoma. **a**,**b** Anteroposterior and lateral radiographs illustrating a large, slightly calcified soft tissue shadow, with ill-defined contours, attached to the upper end of the humerus, suggesting malignant tumor. A biopsy was performed, and after 2 months the lesion showed increased density and better defined contours, slightly separated from the humerus. A complete excision was performed, confirming the diagnosis of pseudomalignant osseous tumor of soft tissue. The patient was without recurrence 3 years later

neoplastic bone and cartilage formation," as suggested by Ackerman (1958). The shorter and sufficiently precise term "heterotopic bone formation," also applied by Dahlin in his monograph (1978), seems to us preferable because of its wider application to traumatic and nontraumatic lesions. However, the term "myositis ossificans" was retained in the WHO classification because it is widely used by clinicians and pathologists.

Myositis ossificans is a disorder of obscure etiology classically divided into two different clinical entities: "myositis ossificans progressiva," which is a congenital hereditary fatal disease, and "myositis ossificans circumscripta or localizata" (Table IX.3). The localized form has been subdivided into different types according to the existence or absence of preceding trauma. In about 60% (Dorfman and Norman 1970) to 75% (Paterson 1970) of cases, there is a history of prior

Table IX.3. Classification of heterotopic ossification ("myositis ossificans")

I. Myositis ossificans progressiva (fibrositis ossificans progressiva)
II. Myositis ossificans circumscripta
  A. Post-traumatic myositis ossificans (60%–75%)
  B. Myositis ossificans without history of trauma (25%–40%)
    1. Associated with systemic disease (paraplegia, tetanus, etc.)
    2. Idiopathic: so-called pseudomalignant osseous tumor of soft tissue (Fine and Stout)

trauma, often associated with sports injuries in young adults (post-traumatic myositis ossificans).

In the remaining patients, the process may be associated with a systemic disease such as paraplegia or tetanus, or develop independently without any known etiology (idiopathic). Examples of this last type were first distinguished by Fine and Stout (1956), who also reported four cases under the term *"pseudomalignant osseous tumor of soft tissues,"* thus emphasizing that these lesions may be mistaken for an osteosarcoma of soft tissue origin by the pathologist unfamiliar with the histologic and clinicoradiologic features. Jaffe (1958) accepted this term and separated it from conventional post-traumatic myositis ossificans. However, although he mentioned, like Fine and Stout, the presence of well-differentiated osseous tissue at the periphery, sometimes forming a thin encapsulating bone shell, he stated that in contrast to post-traumatic myositis ossificans, "it does not reach maturity and stop growing, and eventually may undergo malignant transformation." Ackerman (1958), in his classic paper, separated from a series of 26 cases of so-called myositis ossificans a group of "large lesions in atypical locations thought to be sarcoma." He described clearly the direction of maturation toward the periphery or the *zoning effect*, emphasizing its diagnostic importance in the differentiation from osteosarcoma arising in soft tissues.

Other similar cases of "pseudomalignant osseous tumor of soft tissues" have been reported by Jeffreys and Styles (1966), Angervall et al. (1969), and Chaplin and Harrison (1972), who in a review of the literature found 19 published cases. However, the real number is evidently much higher, because in many publications this type of lesion is included in the general category of localized myositis ossificans (Spjut et al. 1971; Dorfman and Norman 1970) or reported as "myositis ossificans circumscripta without history of injury" (Paterson 1970).

Although in some cases a history of trauma was mentioned, in the great majority of "pseudomalignant osseous tumors" it was lacking. In some published cases (Angervall et al. 1969), a reactive condition initiated by an infection was suggested as the etiologic source.

Clinical Findings. Heterotopic ossification is not rare. We have 85 cases in our files, which have been divided into two clinical varieties. The great majority were post-traumatic lesions of conventional myositis ossificans, also referred to as myoperiostitis (Campanacci 1990), and only 22 cases corresponded to the clinicoradiologic type "pseudomalignant osseous tumors of soft tissue." The latter were located most frequently in the thigh and gluteal region (Figs. IX.81, IX.82) and less commonly in the upper arm (Fig. IX.83) and forearm (see Fig. IX.85). In conventional post-traumatic myositis or myoperiostitis, the large muscle groups of the thigh, buttocks, and upper arms, particularly the elbow region, were most frequently involved. In both types of heterotopic ossification, males predominated (2:1), and the preferred age groups were the second and third decades. Forty-five cases (54%) occurred in individuals under 30 years of age.

Symptoms. The most common complaint was localized painful swelling, frequently associated with limitation of motion of the adjacent joints.

Radiographic Features. A few weeks after the onset of pain, a firm tender mass in the soft tissues may be palpated, and the roentgenogram may still be negative or show a soft tissue mass with calcific densities (second to fourth week) and a periosteal reaction may appear in the underlying bone. Bone formation that shows the characteristic elongated "dotted veil" pattern may begin as early as 5–6 weeks after the injury and fully develop to maturity after a few months. The bony mass then becomes stationary or partially regresses or becomes attached to the underlying bone ("post-traumatic periosteoma," or periostitis ossificans). Occasionally, however, it may become separated from the underlying cortex or periosteal region by a radiolucent zone of soft tissue (Fig. IX.84).

In contrast to the dotted veil aspect or the presence of an irregular elongated bony mass, seen in post-traumatic myositis or myoperiostitis ossificans, our cases of "pseudomalignant osseous tumor" were always of ovoid or rounded shape. Although it showed similar stages of maturation,

Fig. IX.84a–c. Male, 5 years old. Post-traumatic myositis ossificans at thigh. **a** Anteroposterior and lateral radiographs showing an elongated, irregular soft tissue radiopacity abutting the femur; it is separated by a translucent line from the underlying cortex, which shows slight periosteal reactive bone formation. **b** Topographic photomicrograph of the same case illustrating intramuscular heterotopic bone formation without a clear zoning phenomenon. **c** Mature and immature bone trabeculae surrounded by layers of active osteoblasts within skeletal muscular tissue. **b** ×8, **c** ×100

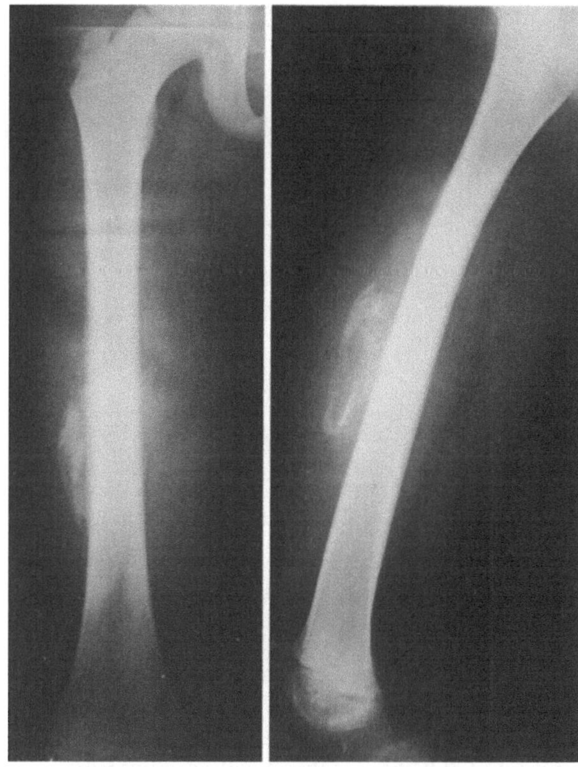

a

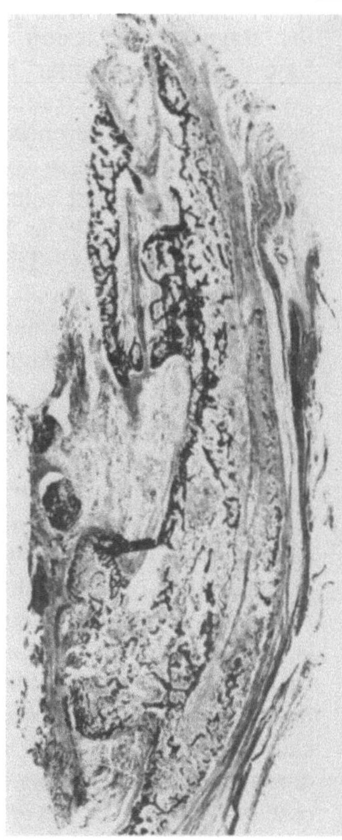

b

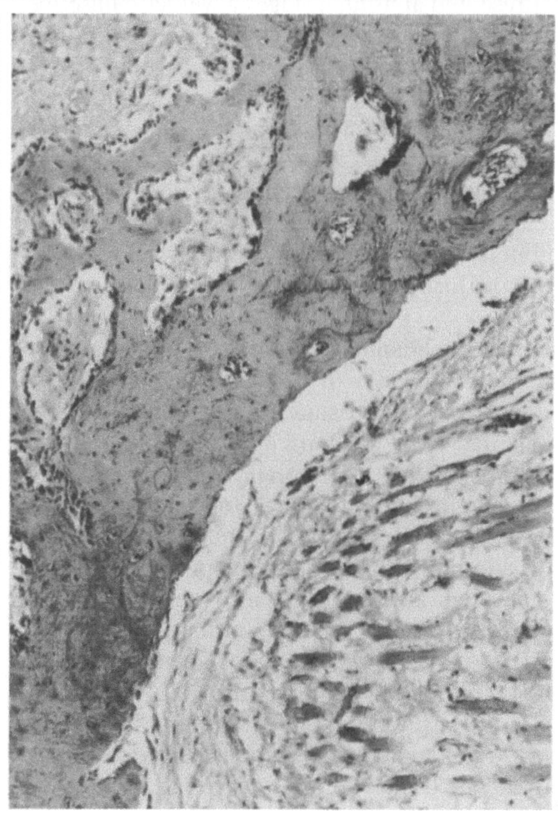

c

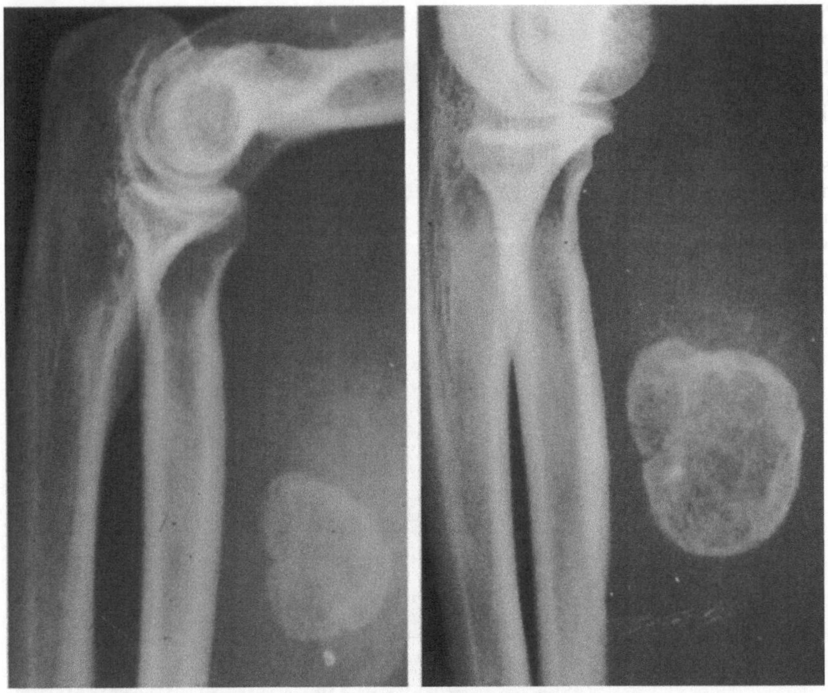

a b

Fig. IX.85a,b. Female, 36 years old. Pseudomalignant osseous tumor of soft tissue of forearm. **a** Radiograph illustrates a roundish, well-circumscribed soft tissue shadow, more radiopaque at its periphery. The patient was aware of a soft tissue swelling for 3 months without previous trauma. **b** Radiograph 1 month later shows that the nodule is now more radiopaque, with a well-delimited peripheral zone of bony density

it presented at its final stages a well-circumscribed rounded mass with a central radiolucent core surrounded by a densely calcified zone of bony aspect (Figs. IX.81–IX.83). In most of our cases, the lesion was located at some distance from the underlying bone (Fig. IX.85), as reported by other authors. However, in three cases it abutted at the bone cortex, and two of these cases exhibited laminated periosteal reaction (Fig. IX.84) (myoperiostitis).

Pathologic Findings. The *gross* appearance was similar in all cases of "pseudomalignant osseous tumors of soft tissues" and showed a well-demarcated ovoid hard mass, 3–10 cm in size, within skeletal muscle or in soft tissue. The cut surface presented two distinguishable zones, one peripheral and hard, with a relatively large area of cancellous bone or a thin, partly interrupted bone shell, and another central zone, soft with a grayish-white or yellowish-reddish appearance. Hemorrhagic areas or zones of cystic softening were found in the central part of some of our cases (Figs. IX.82, IX.86). In the cases of post-traumatic myositis ossificans we observed irregular, usually elongated areas of calcification and bony spicules, occasionally surrounding softer zones of grayish-white or reddish color, but the ovoid, well-circumscribed formations were not seen.

The *histologic* picture varies according to the stage of the lesion. In earlier stages, the biopsy shows vascular connective tissue with proliferating undifferentiated mesenchymal cells in fibroblastic differentiation, presenting some nuclear pleomorphism and occasional mitoses. Multinucleated giant cells may be found, sometimes in relationship to hemorrhages or sometimes independently. The amount of collagen fibers varies, and some less cellular areas are partly myxoid with evidence of cystic degeneration. Some remaining damaged muscle fibers were often seen at this stage. An evident osteoblastic differentiation of the mesenchymal cells with formation of osteoid or woven bone trabeculae may appear after a few days or weeks (Figs. IX.87, IX.88). In this early proliferative phase, confusion with a soft tissue sarcoma, particularly osteosarcoma, is possible if the pathologist receives only small fragments of tissue and/or is not aware of the clinicoradiologic features. In both forms of heterotopic ossification, the histologic features in the initial stages are similar, except that muscle fibers with or without signs of damage are often lacking in the pseudomalignant osseous tumor. However, the zoning phenomenon, although sometimes also present in post-traumatic heterotopic ossification, is not as striking and as regularly organized. Toward the periphery, osteoid and woven bone trabeculae

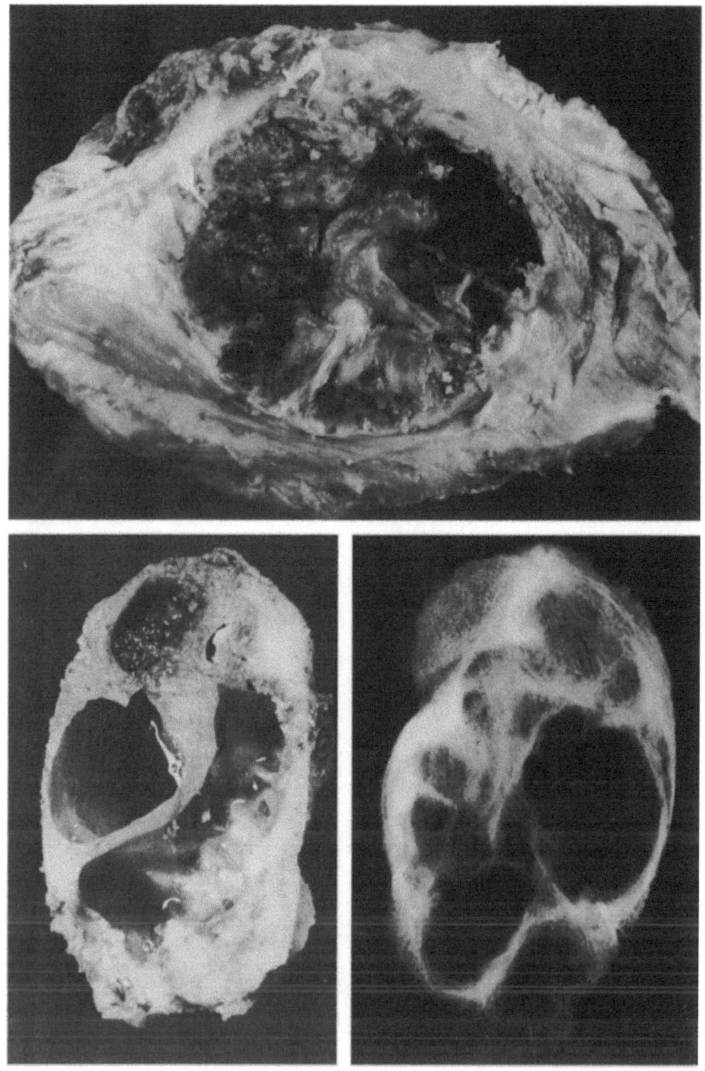

Fig. IX.86a–c. Two different cases of pseudomalignant osseous tumors of soft tissues, localized in the buttock (**a**) and groin (**b**), demonstrating the gross and radiologic features of the specimen. **a** Photograph shows a central hemorrhagic area of soft consistency surrounded by a shell of bone and skeletal muscle. **b** Photograph and **c** radiograph show central cystic cavities with scarce whitish areas surrounded by a dense rim of bone tissue

increase in size and number. The marginal zone consists of more organized woven or lamellar bone surrounded by layers of active osteoblasts, with loose connective tissue between the trabeculae (Figs. IX.87, IX.89). Zones of cartilage in different stages of differentiation and endochondral ossification are occasionally present. This characteristic peripheral maturation is of fundamental importance in the differential diagnosis with soft tissue osteosarcomas, where the periphery is the most actively proliferating and immature zone, infiltrating the surrounding tissues.

Treatment and Prognosis. The treatment of myositis ossificans depends on the stage of evolution. Excision of the fully developed, mature lesion is curative. When a lesion is recognized clinically and radiologically, it is preferable to await maturation because a certain percentage may regress spontaneously. Only in cases presenting clinical symptoms, e.g., pain or restriction of motion because of the size or location of the mass, is surgery indicated. Rarely, there may be a recurrence in a case treated surgically in an early florid stage, but malignant transformation seems to be extremely uncommon and has not been observed in our series.

Periostitis Ossificans

Periostitis ossificans comprises reparative and injury-related lesions of the periosteum. It is the periosteal equivalent of myositis ossificans, with clinicopathologic features similar to those of

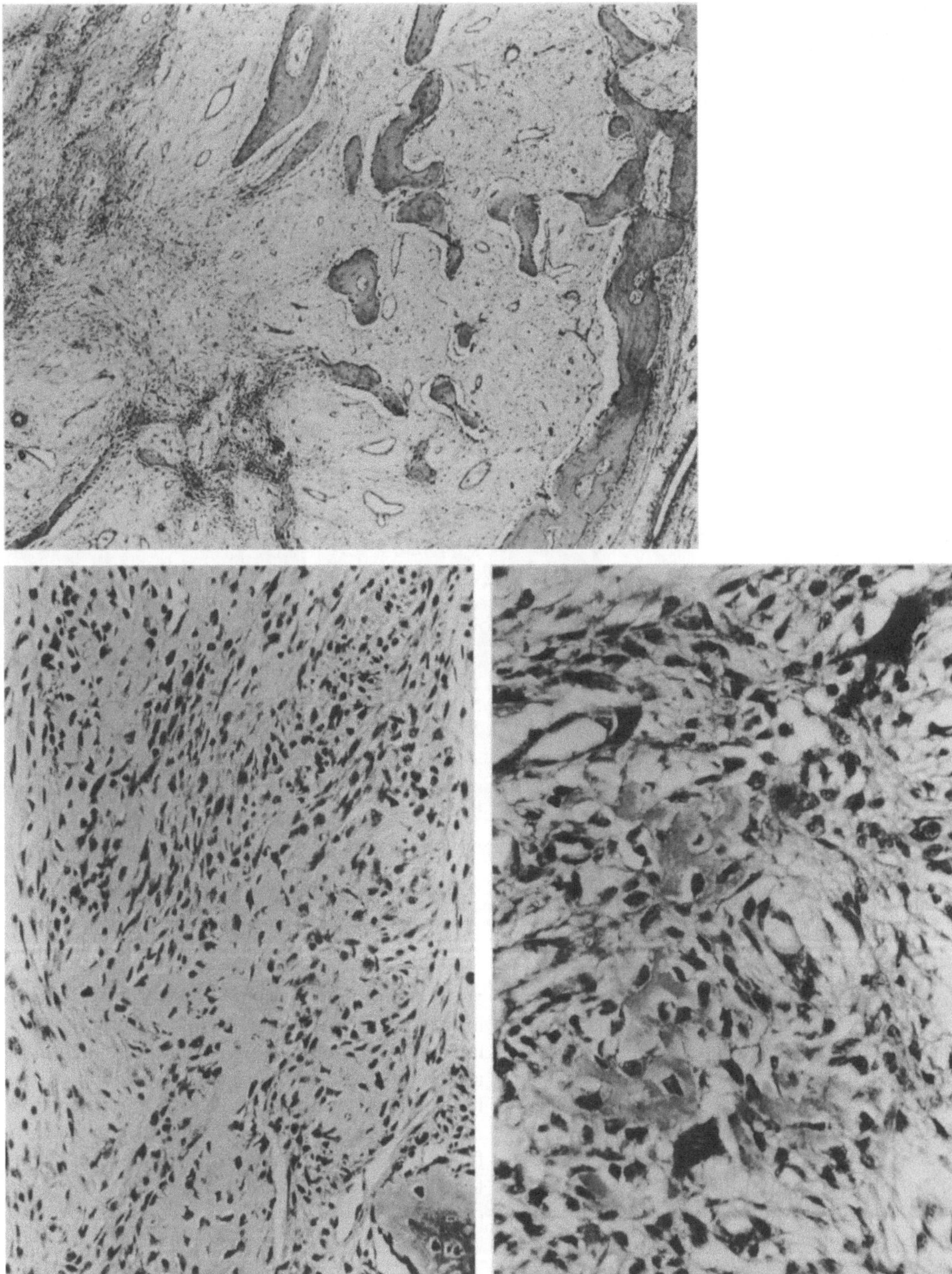

a b c

Fig. IX.87a–c. Photomicrographs showing the histologic pattern of pseudomalignant osseous tumor of soft tissues. **a** Appearance at low magnification, showing a capsule of fibrous tissue and well-formed osseous tissue, with a thin bony shell at the surface and bone trabeculae separated by loose connective tissue; the inner zone shows cellular tissue with osteoid trabeculae. **b** Osteoid formation within a stroma rich in spindle-shaped cells. **c** Another area of the central zone showing some multinucleated giant cells and osteoid trabeculae within a loose connective tissue. **a** ×100, **b** ×250, **c** ×330

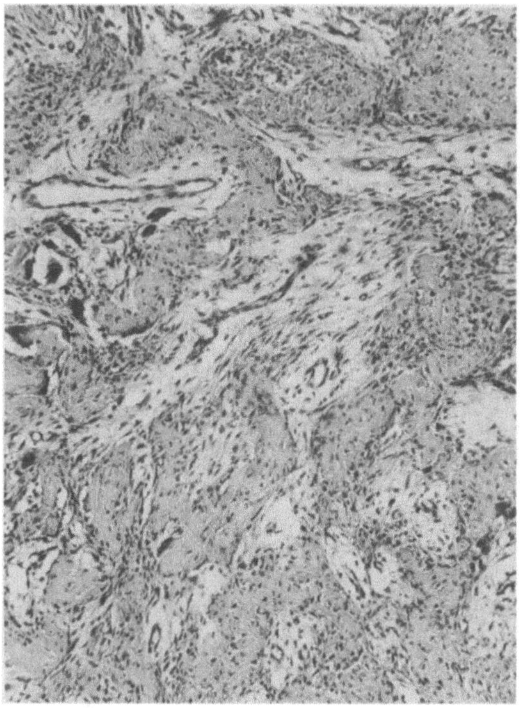

a

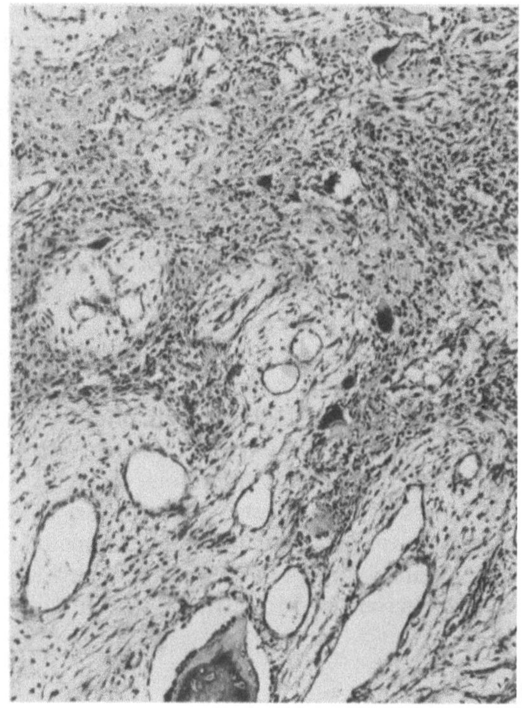

b

Fig. IX.88a,b. Photomicrographs of the inner zone at higher magnification demonstrating the active new formation of numerous osteoid trabeculae within a vascular fibrous tissue, which is edematous around the abundant capillary vessels; note also several osteoclast giant cells. Such areas have been misinterpreted as malignant, but cellular pleomorphism and atypical mitosis are lacking. × 150

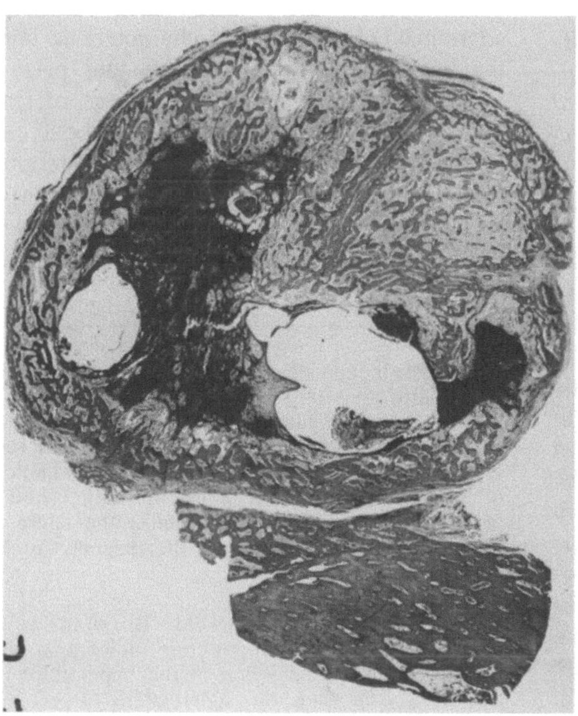

a

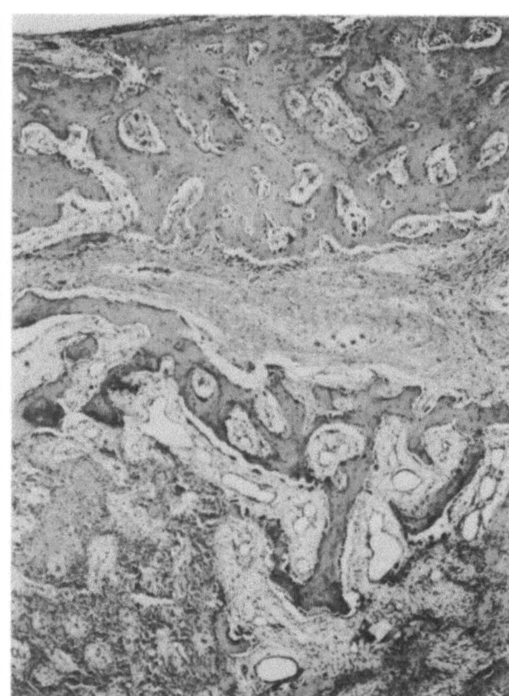

b

Fig. IX.89. a Photomicrograph showing at low magnification the peripheral zone forming a shell of bone trabeculae surrounding a central, *partly* hemorrhagic area with cystic spaces. The nodule is separated from the underlying bone (*left*), which reveals periosteal reactive bone formation (×8). **b** This photomicrograph shows the characteristic zoning phenomenon, with a marginal zone (*right*) of more organized woven and lamellar bone, surrounded by layers of active osteoblasts, and a deeper zone (*left*) showing active osteoid formation in a richly cellular stroma. **a** ×8, **b** ×100 myositis ossificans and fracture callus. As with myositis ossificans, the suffix "itis" is misleading since it is not an inflammatory disorder. This process is more common in long and flat bones, and a distal femoral variant is referred to as "cortical irregularity syndrome." A similar lesion located in hands and feet has been reported by Spjut and Dorfman (1981) under the term "florid reactive periostitis" and by Dupree and Enzinger (1986) as "fibro-osseous pseudotumor of the digits."

Thirty-five cases of another lesion of hands and feet, resembling periostitis ossificans, osteochondroma, or parosteal osteosarcoma, were reported by Nora et al. (1983) as "bizarre parosteal osteochondromatous proliferations of hands and feet." However, the exact pathogenesis of this process must still be defined, and some of the cases possibly correspond to secondary peripheral chondrosarcoma (see Fig. II.97).

8. "Brown Tumor" of Hyperparathyroidism

Definition, WHO: *"A circumscribed non-neoplastic lesion characterized by the presence of large numbers of osteoclast giant cells, usually arranged in groups and separated by richly vascularized fibrous tissue with areas of new bone and osteoid formation. The surrounding bone frequently shows evidence of increased osteoclastic resorption. Areas of recent and old hemorrhage are common."*

It is not our purpose to describe here the clinical and physiopathologic features of primary hyperparathyroidism. Instead we will focus on the radiologic and pathologic aspects of the skeletal changes (parathyroid osteosis), particularly the localized cystlike areas most commonly found in tubular and maxillary bones, the so-called brown tumor. Radiologically and histologically the brown tumor can simulate a primary or secondary neoplasm of bone. Because of the histologic similarities, diagnostic problems may arise, particularly with true giant-cell tumors in long bones and the "reparative giant-cell granuloma" of the jaws, especially when the pathologist does not possess the necessary clinical and biochemical information.

Primary hyperparathyroidism is caused by excessive production of parathyroid hormone due to a single (80%–85%) or more parathyroid adenomas, primary and diffuse hyperplasia of the parathyroid glands, or secreting parathyroid carcinoma (less than 1%). The skeletal changes due to the excess of parathyroid hormone are mainly the product of the increased diffuse osteoclastic bone resorption associated with hypercalcemia. The excess bone loss is partly compensated by new bone or osteoid formation, resulting in an increase in alkaline phosphatase. We have recorded 32 cases with the radiologic and histologic features of "brown tumors" in patients ranging from 22 to 62 years of age, most in the third and the fourth decades. There was an evident predominance of females (Black 1953; Hellström 1957; Campanacci 1990).

Radiographic Features. Radiologically, brown tumors are characterized by an osteolytic lesion with generally indistinct margins, which frequently expands the cortex and is surrounded by a thin shell of newly formed periosteal bone. The cystlike cavity may be trabeculated, giving a multiloculated appearance. Brown tumors involve more frequently the shaft and, less commonly, the ends of long limb bones or tubular bones of hands and feet (Figs. IX.90, IX.91; see Figs. IX.92 and IX.93 for the radiographic appearance at various sites in a patient with two parathyroid adenomas). Frequent and characteristic findings that accompany brown tumors and permit an accurate diagnosis are: the presence of smaller multiple cystic areas and other bone manifestations such as generalized osteoporosis (osteopenia), subperiosteal bone resorption, especially of distal phalanges and the distal end of the clavicle, disappearance of the lamina dura,

Fig. IX.90a,b. Female, 35 years old, with "brown tumor" in the fifth and third metatarsal bones. **a** Radiograph illustrates a radiolucent trabeculated lesion, slightly expanding the thinned cortex. A similar, smaller lesion is seen in the diaphysis of the third metatarsus. **b** Photograph of the excised metatarsus shows the dark brown color of the lesion, which involves almost the entire bone. Biochemical studies confirmed the diagnosis of hyperparathyroidism

Fig. IX.91. a Female, 45 years old. "Brown tumor" of the tibia. Lateral and anteroposterior radiographs show a radiolucent ill-defined lesion in the upper third of the diaphysis, expanding the anterolateral aspect of the cortex. There is evident osteopenia of the tibia and fibula. **b** Female, 52 years old. "Brown tumor" of femur. Radiograph shows a large, osteolytic, trabeculated and expanding lesion of the femoral midshaft and pathologic fracture

IX.90a
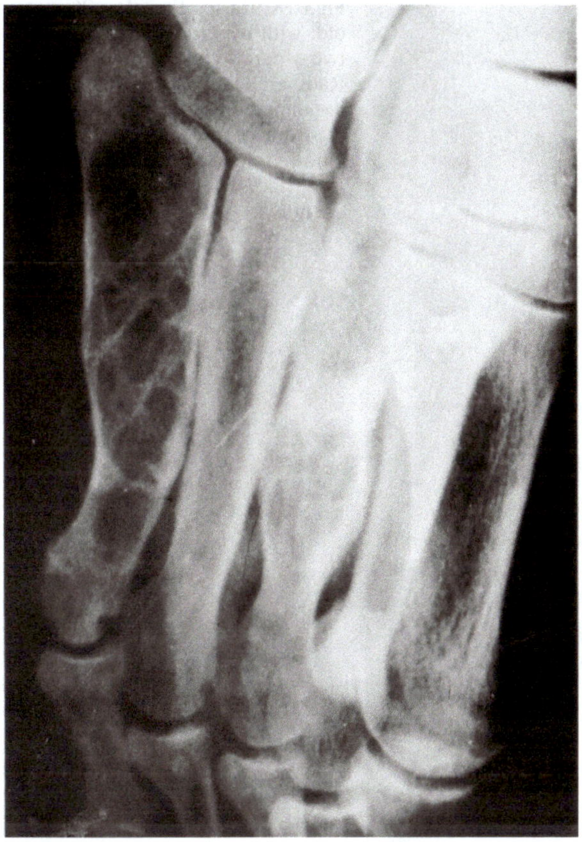

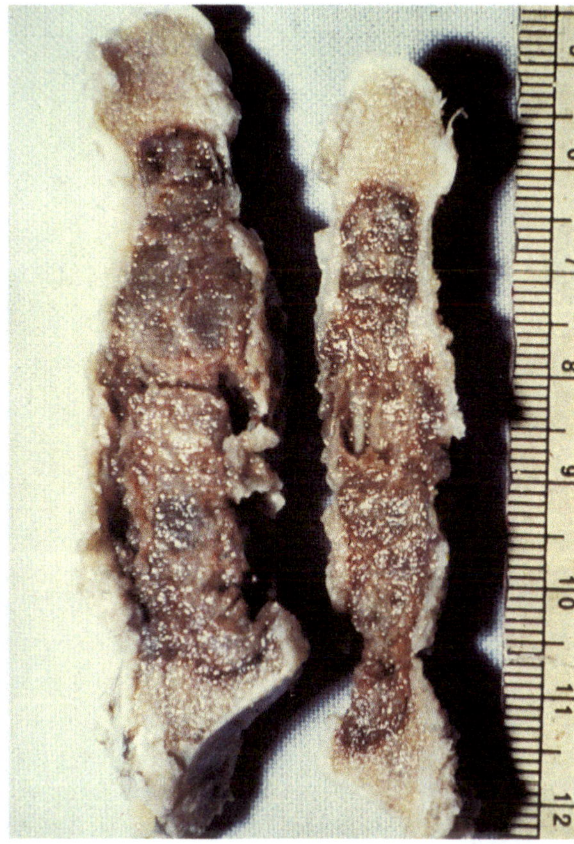

b

IX.91a
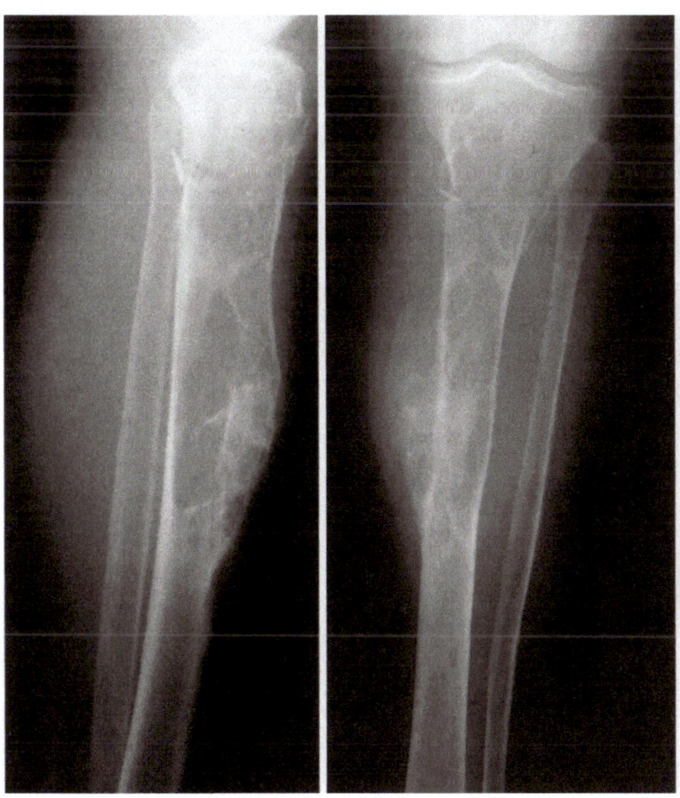

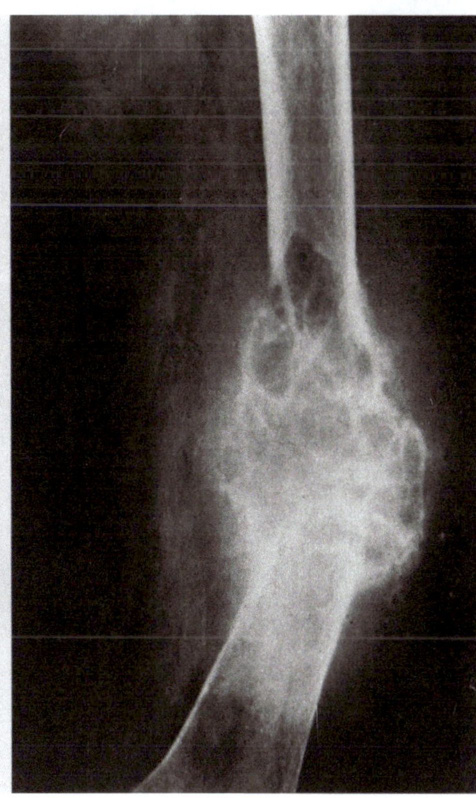
b

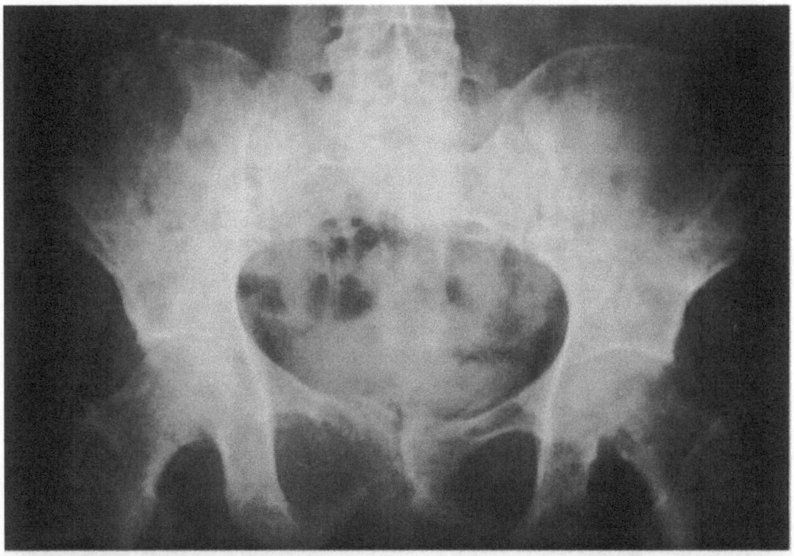

a

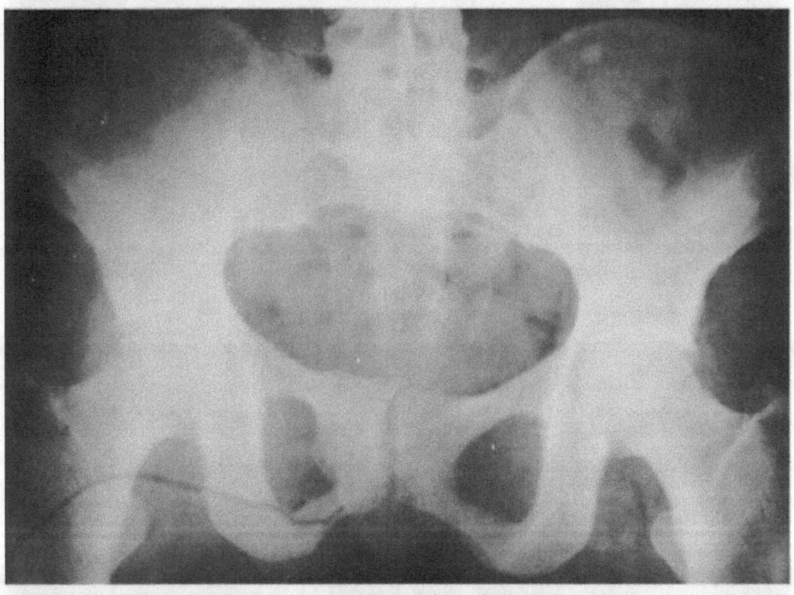

b

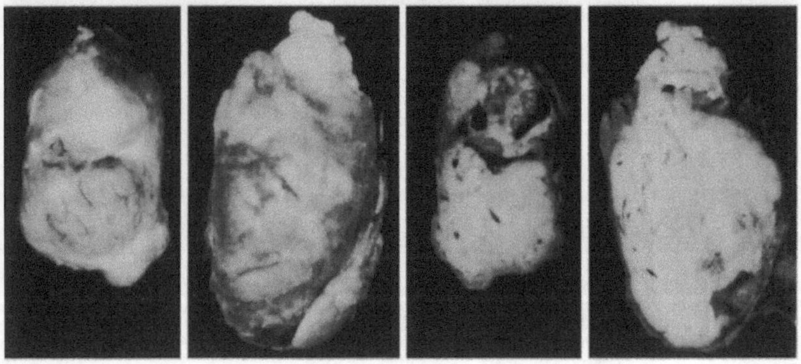

c

Fig. IX.92a–c. Female, 26 years old, with hyperparathyroidism with two parathyroid adenomas. **a** Radiograph shows a radiolucent, ill-defined lesion of the pubis. **b** Radiograph 3 months after parathyroidectomy. **c** Photographs of surface and section of the two adenomas

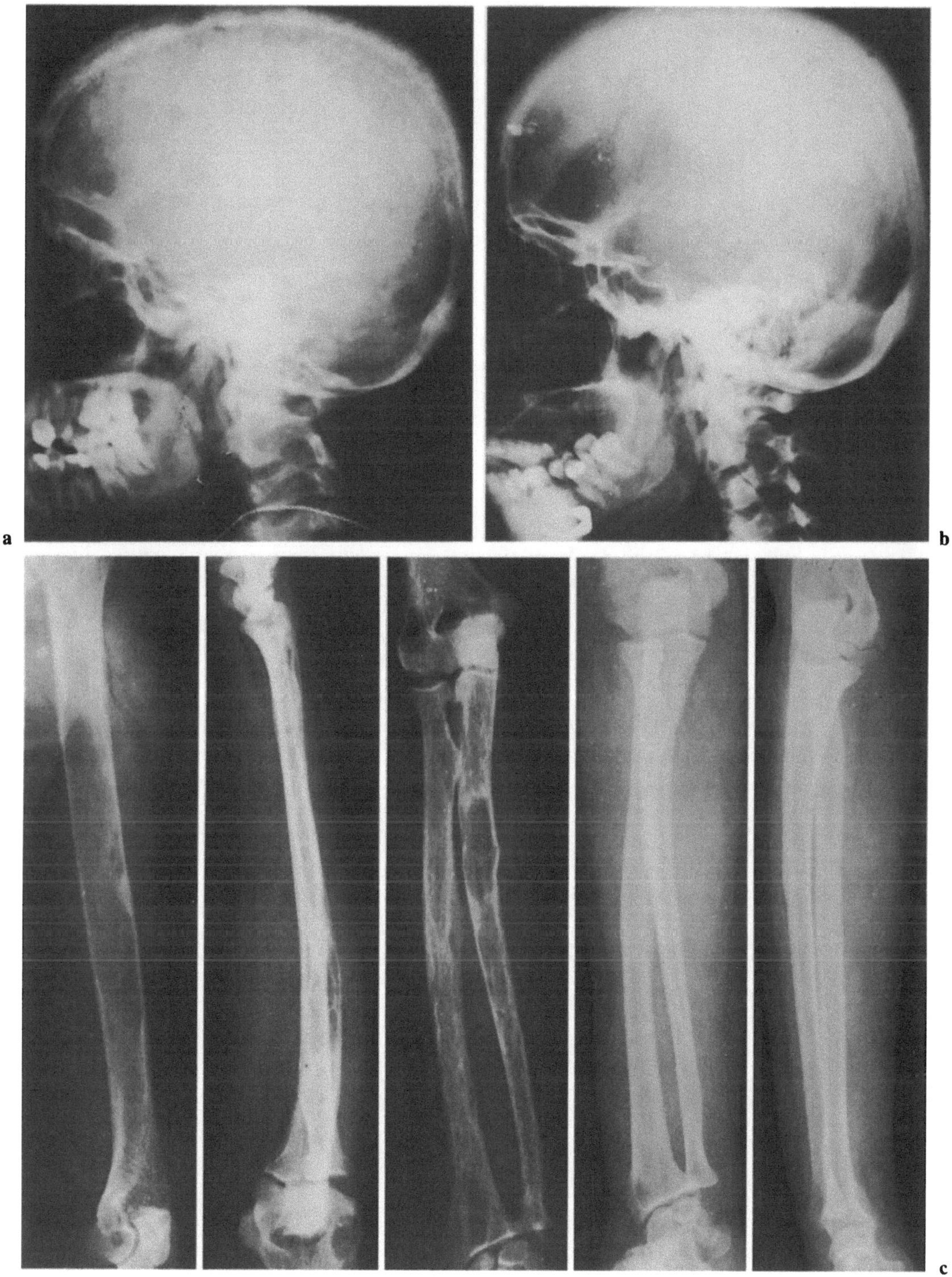

Fig. IX.93a–c. Same patient as in Fig. IX.92. Radiographs of the cranium, humerus, radius, and ulna before and after treatment, showing disappearance of the radiolucent cystlike lesions

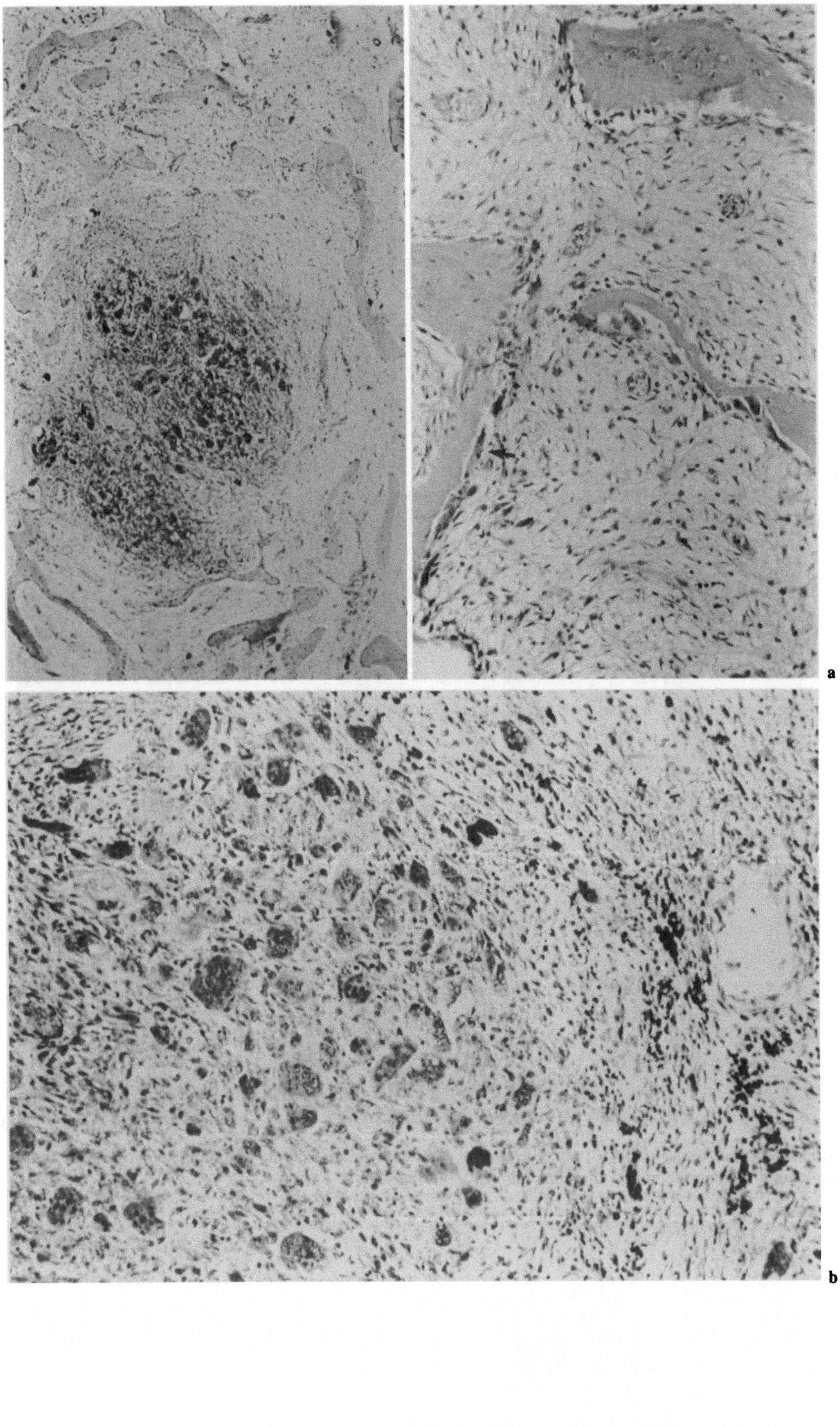
a
b

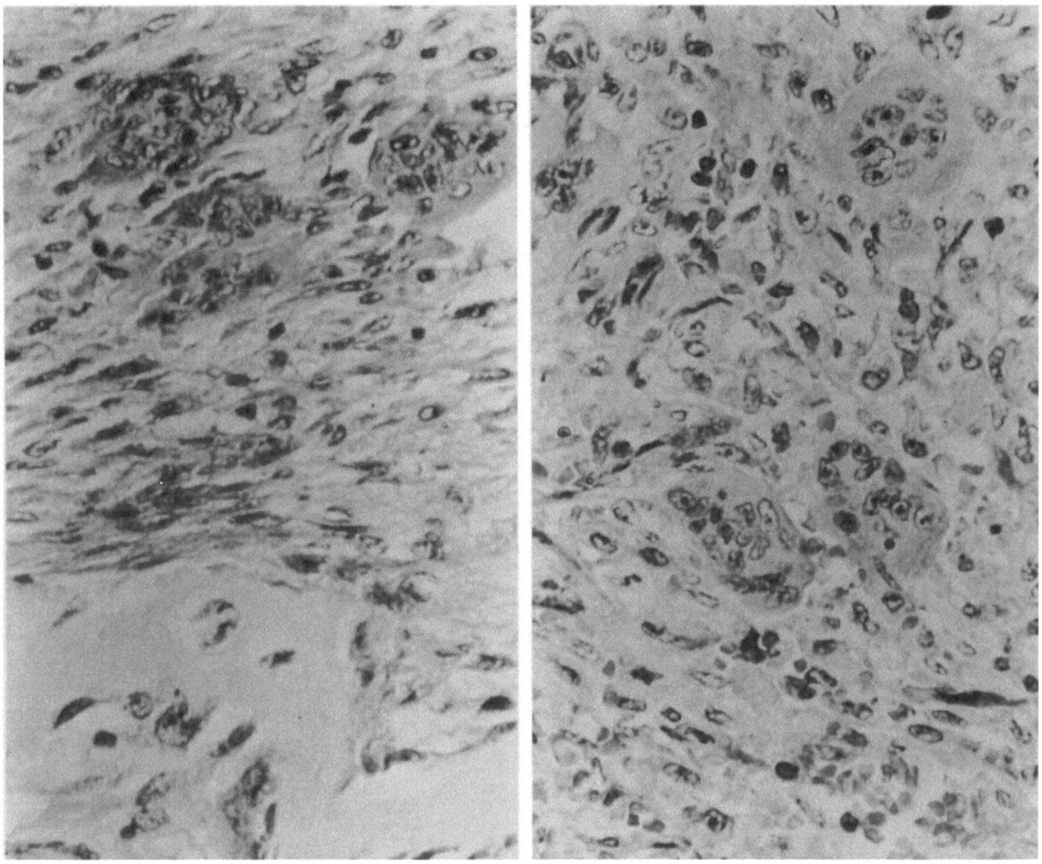

c d

Fig. IX.94a–d. Photomicrographs showing the histologic pattern of hyperparathyroidism. **a** Conglomerate of giant cells of osteoclast type within a loose vascular fibrous tissue, surrounded by bone trabeculae, which at higher magnification (**b**) show numerous osteoclasts at their surface. **c** Aggregates of numerous multinucleated giant cells, generally smaller than in giant-cell tumors, within a fibrous stroma, with mature fibroblastic elements. Dark spots at *left* correspond to hemosiderin pigment. **d** At higher magnification, the pattern of the multinucleated giant cells and the fibrous stroma with the differentiated fibroblastic spindle cells is shown. At the *bottom* and *left* are osteoid trabeculae. **a** ×50, **b** ×120, **c** ×100, **d** ×400

and diffuse granular radiolucent areas of the skull (Pugh 1958). The biochemical findings of increased serum levels of calcium and alkaline phosphatase and of low phosphate establish the definite diagnosis.

Pathologic Findings. *Grossly*, brown tumors are characterized by a circumscribed mass of reddish-brown tissue of soft consistency, presenting hemorrhagic and cystic areas of different size. The cancellous bone of the area is destroyed, and the limiting cortex is generally thinned and often distended (Fig. IX.91).

Histologically, the marrow is replaced by richly vascular loose connective tissue, showing increased osteoclastic activity on the surface of the remaining cancellous bone trabeculae (Fig. IX.94). In contrast, the weakening of the bone structure may lead to multiple fractures with abundant blood pigment in great part phagocytized by histiocytic elements. The osteoclast giant cells are generally small and irregularly distributed in smaller or larger aggregates, often but not always around hemorrhages. The mononuclear cells of the fibrous stroma, rich in collagen fibers, are more differentiated and less conspicuous than the proliferating cells of giant-cell tumors (Fig. IX.94). The spongiosa surrounding the lesion is composed in part of newly formed osteoid and immature bone trabeculae with rows of active osteoblasts (which explains the increase in serum alkaline phosphatase). This area alternates with preexistent lamellar bone trabeculae, which present an increased number of osteoclasts at their surface. Although infrequently and in contrast to the statements of other observers, we occasionally found osteoclasts also at the surface of osteoid tissue.

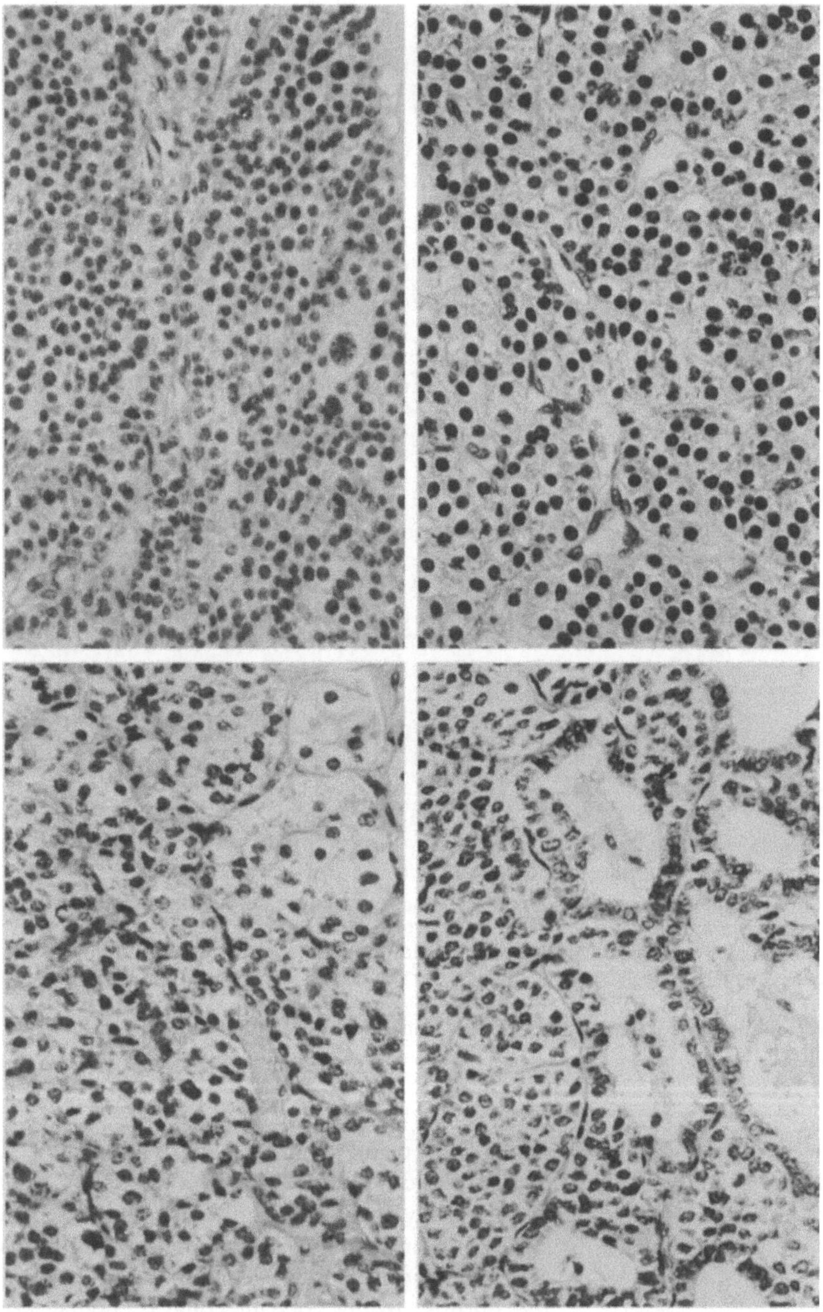

a b c d

Fig. IX.95a–d. Photomicrographs showing different histologic patterns of the parathyroid adenoma of the case illustrated in Figs. IX.92 and IX.93. The adenoma is composed principally of chief cells (**a**,**b**), with some areas of clear cells and acinous formations. ×200

The bone trabeculae may show the characteristic pattern of "dissecting fibro-osteoclasia" (Uehlinger 1940), that is, osteoclastic resorption and fibrosis inside the trabeculae, producing irregular intratrabecular spaces.

In all our cases, a single or, exceptionally, two parathyroid "adenomas" were found, ranging from 1.5 to 4 cm in diameter (Fig. IX.95). Most adenomas were composed predominantly of chief cells, as in other series. Clear cells, oxyphil cells, transitional types, or combinations of all these were sometimes found in association with chief cells (Castleman and Mallory 1935; Castleman 1952) (Fig. IX.95). No case of oxyphilic adenoma was found in our or in Castleman's series.

Differential diagnosis with true giant-cell tumors may be extremely difficult without knowledge of the clinical features in brown tumors located at the ends of long bones or in maxillary bones. In jaw bones a brown tumor may be histologically indistinguishable from giant-cell reparative granuloma. In these cases, investigation of the calcium metabolism is mandatory. Two of our patients had functioning parathyroid carcinomas; one patient who presented with vascular and thyroid invasion without showing cellular pleomorphism or atypical mitosis had a single metastatic pulmonary nodule of similar histologic aspect and died 1 year later due to spread of the tumor. An autopsy could not be performed.

9. Intraosseous Epidermoid Cyst

Definition, WHO: *"A relatively infrequent nonneoplastic lesion, characterized histologically by a membrane consisting of squamous epithelium, covered by laminated mass of keratin that may occupy part of the cavity."*

Intraosseous epidermoid cysts, also called keratin, sebaceous, or squamous epithelial cysts, do not seem to be as rare as the small number of published cases would indicate, in view of the relatively large number of cases filed in our laboratory. This may be due to diagnostic errors or to the fact that many isolated observations are actually not reported. If we exclude the epithelium-lined cysts in the jaws, epidermoid cysts are found exclusively in the distal phalanges (Byers et al. 1966; Lerner and Southwick 1968) and in the skull (Roth 1964). Dahlin (1978) found numerous epidermoid cysts in the skull and only three in distal phalanges. In contrast, in our laboratory, which receives material mostly from orthopedic departments, lesions involving the phalanges predominate. In a paper published by the writer and colleagues (1970), 11 cases among a group of 38 cystic and pseudocystic lesions of the terminal phalanx of hands and feet were diagnosed as intraosseous epidermoid cysts, including 13 cases of chondroma (12 enchondromas and one periosteal chondroma), six cases of osteoid osteoma, two aneurysmal bone cysts, and two glomus tumors, one with secondary bone penetration. Only one epidermoid cyst was located in the distal phalanx of the hallux, the third case reported in the literature (Goldsmith 1966; Roth 1964). In two cases, the cyst arose at the stump of the second phalanx remaining after traumatic amputation, and in a third case, it arose in the third phalanx after amputation of its distal end. These cases, together with a preceding trauma in the majority of cases, constitute strong evidence in favor of the traumatic etiology of intraphalangeal cyst. The number of our observations has increased to 31, compared with only eight cases located in the skull. Although there are no pathologic diagnostic problems in the phalanges, the roentgenograms show a roundish osteolytic area with no trabecular pattern (Fig. IX.96) that is not distinctive.

When the lesion reaches a certain size, the cortex becomes expanded and thinned, and fissures or fractures may be observed. In the latter cases, the healing of the fracture may modify the characteristic aspects of the cyst. In several of our cases of enchondromas, which did not show the characteristic spotty calcification, the correct radiologic diagnosis was impossible. Only pathologic study permitted a definite diagnosis; sufficient material may be obtained by a simple aspiration biopsy.

Clinically, the great majority of cases occurred in males, and the age of onset was between 19 and 54 years. Most of the patients were manual workers. The most common location was the end phalanx of the hand (Fig. IX.96); one case was in the hallux (Fig. IX.97). The symptoms included an increase in finger size, intermittent pain, which later became continuous, and curving of the nail.

Macroscopically, the cystic unilocular cavity reached a diameter of 10–20 mm. The limiting membrane was 1–5 mm thick, and it could easily be separated from the surrounding bone. On some occasions, the cavity was almost empty, or it was filled in great part by a whitish-yellow caseumlike substance. When a peripheral granulomatous reaction occurred, this area acquired a fleshy appearance (Fig. IX.97).

Histologically (Fig. IX.98), the cyst presents a peripheral zone consisting of squamous malpighian epithelium with a well-defined granulose layer covered by laminated masses of keratin that may occupy part of the cavity. The epithelium is generally thin, formed by a few cellular layers only, possibly due to the pressure of its contents. It is separated from the surrounding cortex by connective tissue, which may show a moderate inflammatory reaction. The cortex is thinned by osteoclastic resorption and rarely destroyed, the cyst coming into direct contact with the superficial dermis or epidermis. Sometimes the cyst wall is interrupted and the keratin masses come into contact with the pericystic connective tissue, followed by formation of small

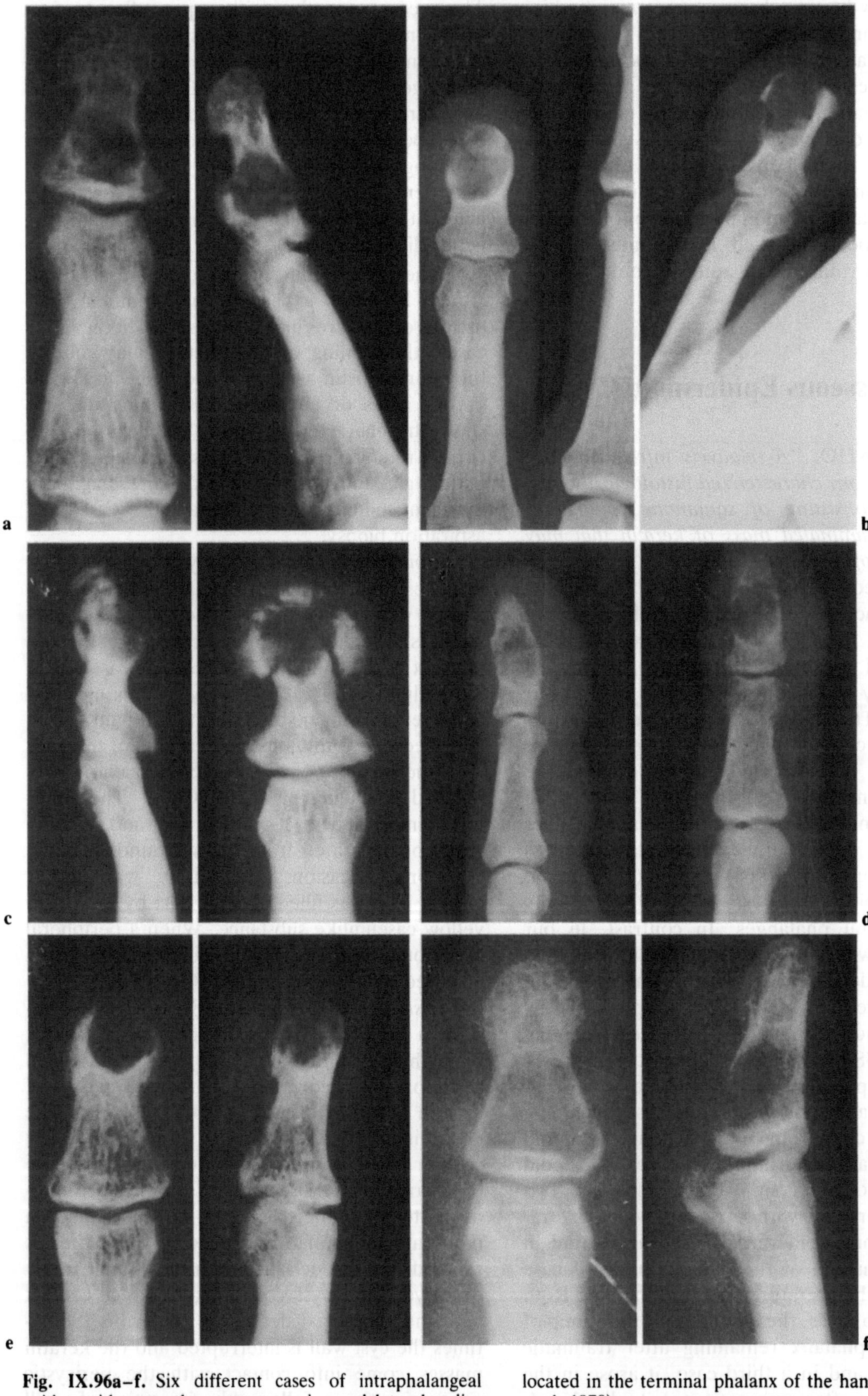

Fig. IX.96a–f. Six different cases of intraphalangeal epidermoid cysts, the anteroposterior and lateral radiographs showing the characteristic osteolytic lesions, all located in the terminal phalanx of the hand. (Schajowicz et al. 1970)

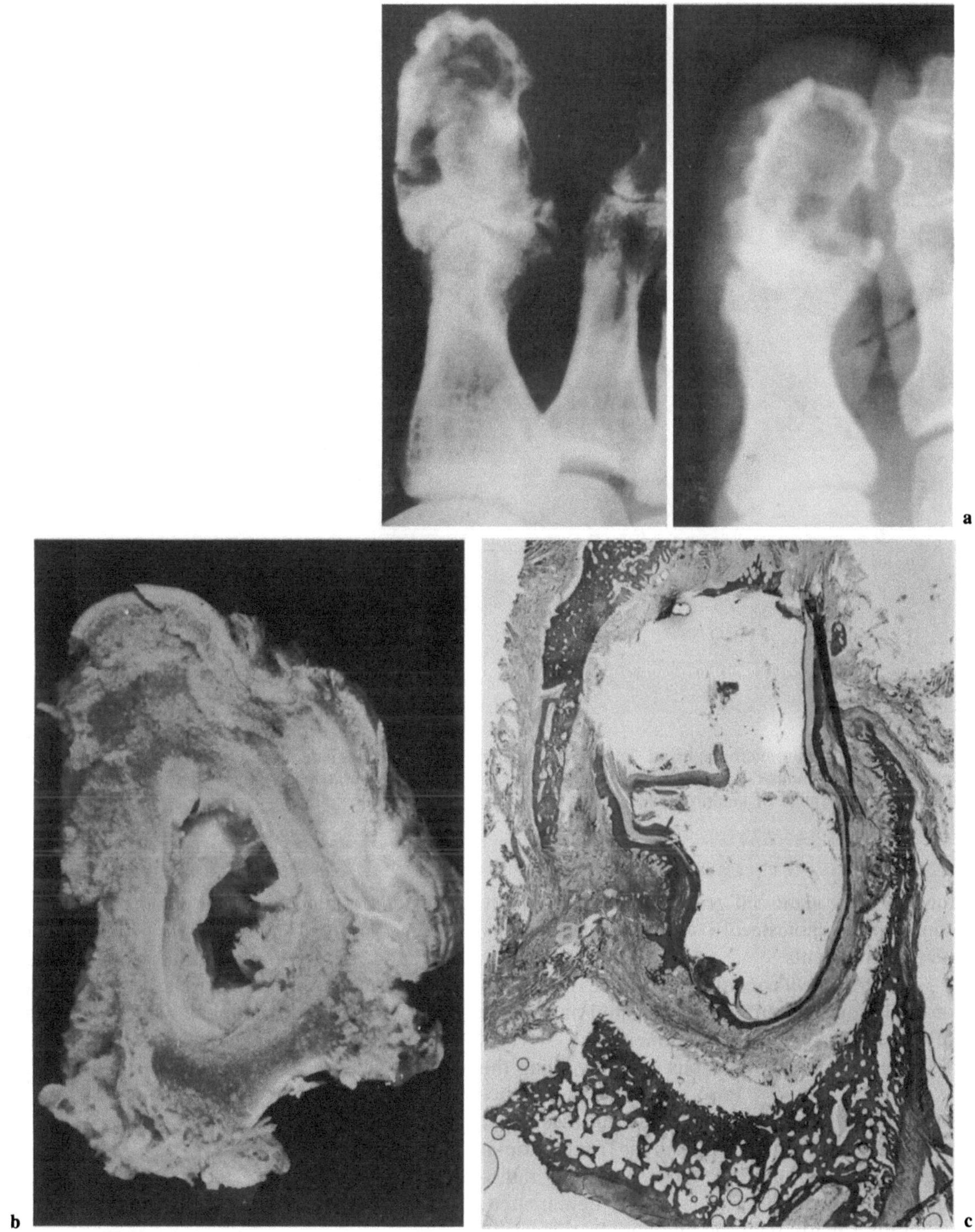

Fig. IX.97a–c. Male, 37 years old, with an epidermoid cyst of the terminal phalanx of the hallux. **a** Anteroposterior and lateral radiographs show a large osteolytic lesion, altered by secondary infection. **b** Photograph and **c** topographic photomicrograph showing destruction of the cortex where the cyst communicated with the surrounding soft tissue, giving rise to an inflammatory reaction. (Schajowicz et al. 1970) **c** ×10

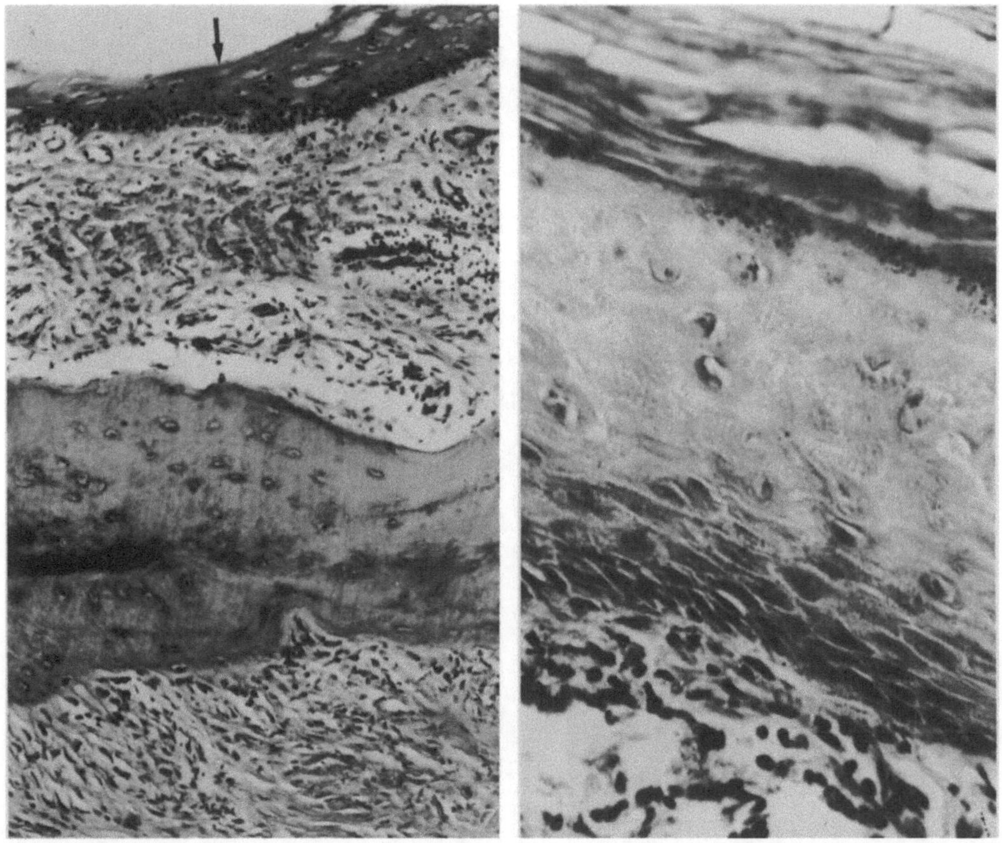

a b

Fig. IX.98a,b. Photomicrographs at lower and higher magnification demonstrating the typical pattern of a cyst, anuclear lamina of keratin, and a wall of flattened, stratified squamous epithelium with a granular layer. The newly formed, thinned cortex is seen in **a** (*bottom*). **a** ×100, **b** ×400

foreign-body giant-cell granulomas, occasionally containing cholesterol crystals surrounding keratin fragments.

The *treatment* consists of curettage or excision of the lesion. Amputation is indicated only in the few cases of advanced involvement.

Epidermoid or squamous cysts involving the *skull* (Fig. IX.99) (also classified as "cholesteatoma") were less frequent in our files (eight cases) and more often located in the frontoparietal region. Radiographically they showed a radiolucent appearance with sharply demarcated, generally slightly sclerotic margins. In this lesion the outer or inner cortex may be expanded, and it may displace adjacent soft tissues, producing neurologic symptoms or a palpable swelling of the cranium. The radiologic differential diagnosis with eosinophilic granuloma may be difficult. The pathologic features are identical to those described in the phalangeal cysts. Sometimes a larger number of cholesterol crystals may be found in the periphery of the epithelial wall, which explains the term "cholesteatoma" used by some authors. The etiology is probably a developmental defect, i.e., intraosseous inclusion of epidermoid cells during the embryonal period, rather than post-traumatic, which seems the most probable origin of the cysts involving the terminal phalanges. The treatment indicated in skull cysts is curettage or excision of the lesion.

10. Giant-Cell (Reparative) Granuloma (Giant-Cell Reaction)

Definition, WHO: "*An uncommon non-neoplastic lesion distinct from true giant-cell tumor, characterized histologically by a prominent spindle-celled fibrous stroma with areas of hemorrhage and nests of multinucleated giant cells, smaller than those of true giant-cell tumors. These lesions are histologically indistinguishable from the similar*

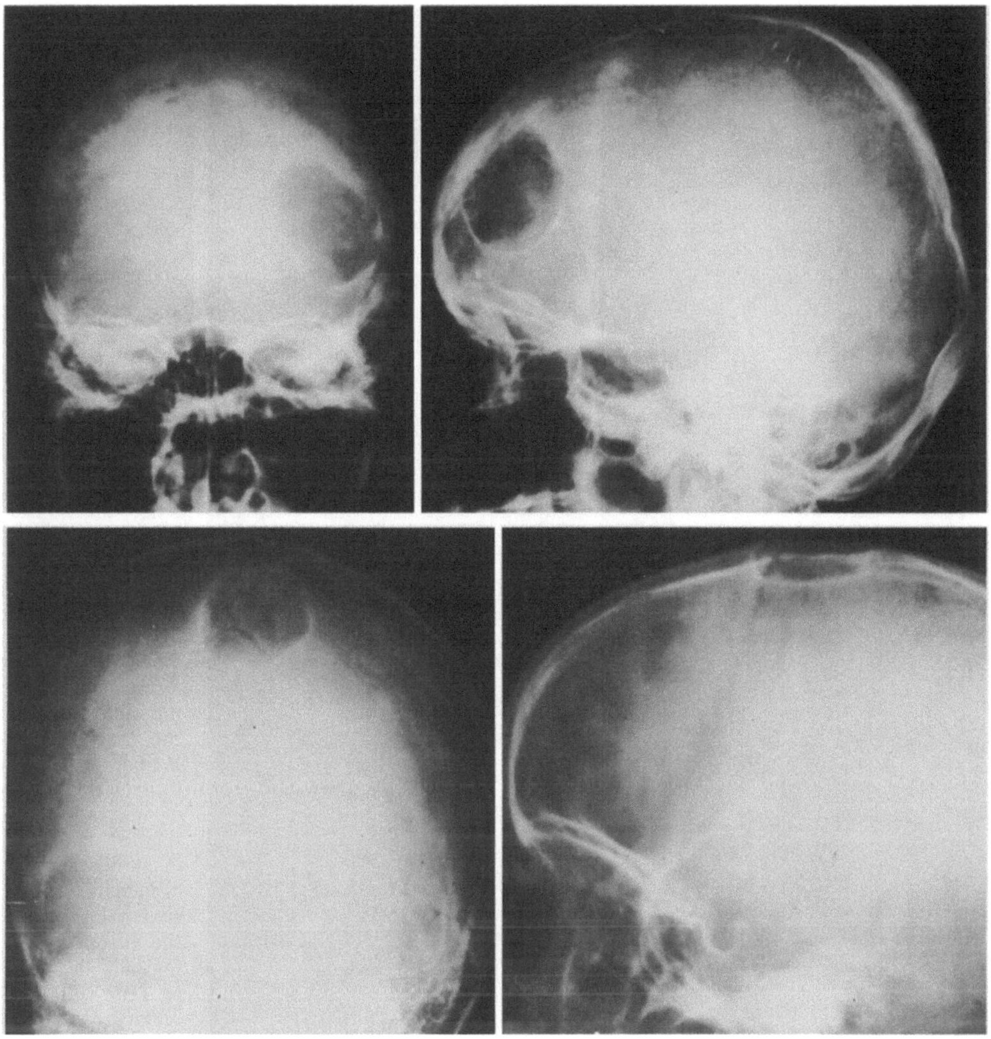

Fig. IX.99a,b. Two cases of epidermoid cyst in the skull. **a** Male, 54 years old, the anteroposterior and lateral radiographs showing a radiolucent roundish lesion, well delimited by a thin sclerotic border in the frontal bone. **b** Female, 28 years old, the radiographs illustrating a similar lesion in the parietal bone

lesions (brown tumors) in hyperparathyroidism. Conspicuous new bone formation is common."

Giant-cell (reparative) granuloma involves primarily the jaw bones (Jaffe 1953), but also the *tubular bones of hands and feet* and exceptionally the carpal, tarsal, and other bones. The adjective "reparative" has been dropped by many authors because a history of trauma is infrequent. Giant-cell granulomas of hands and feet have been previously reported under the term "giant-cell reaction of bone" in some publications (Ackerman and Spjut 1962; D'Alonzo et al. 1972; Jernstrom and Stark 1971; Schwinn 1976; Wold et al. 1990). Giant-cell granuloma of hands and feet is relatively infrequent; no more than 100 cases have been reported in the literature and only eight such lesions were found in our files. Giant-cell granulomas occur more commonly in males in some series (Ratner and Dorfman 1990) and in females in others (Campanacci 1990). The age range is from 6 to 53 years. Radiographically the lesions are osteolytic, slightly expanding the thinned cortex, and are often trabeculated; periosteal reaction is generally lacking (Fig. IX.100). Most lesions are metaphyseal, extending frequently into the diaphysis and more rarely into the epiphysis (Fig. IX.100). There have been several reports in the literature of recurrences after curettage, the incidence ranging from 30% to 50% of the cases (Lorenzo and Dorfman 1980; Picci et al. 1986; Wold et al. 1986).

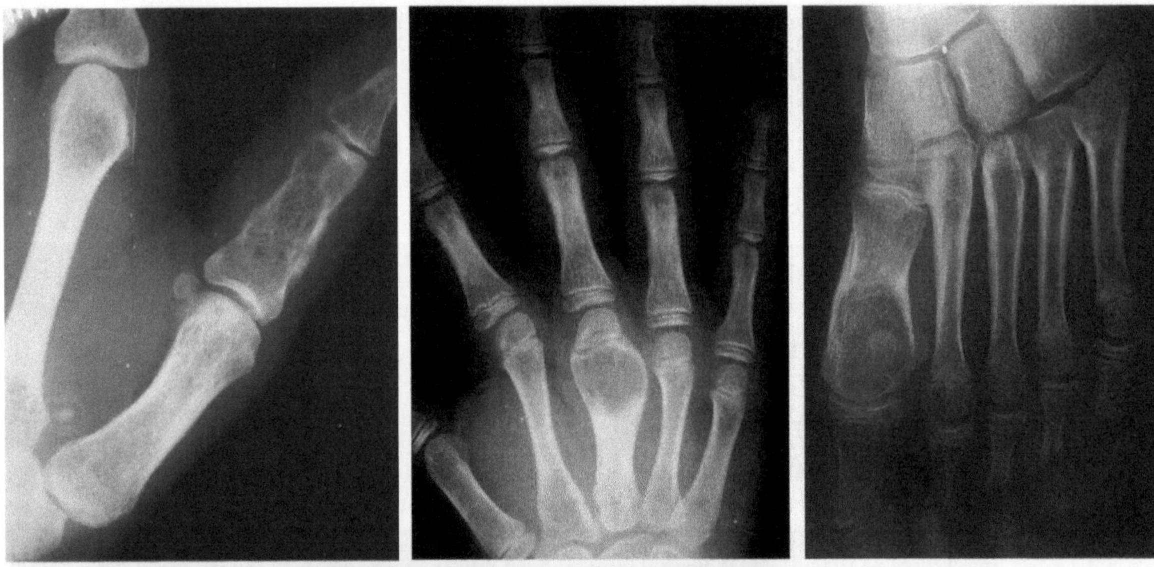

a b, c

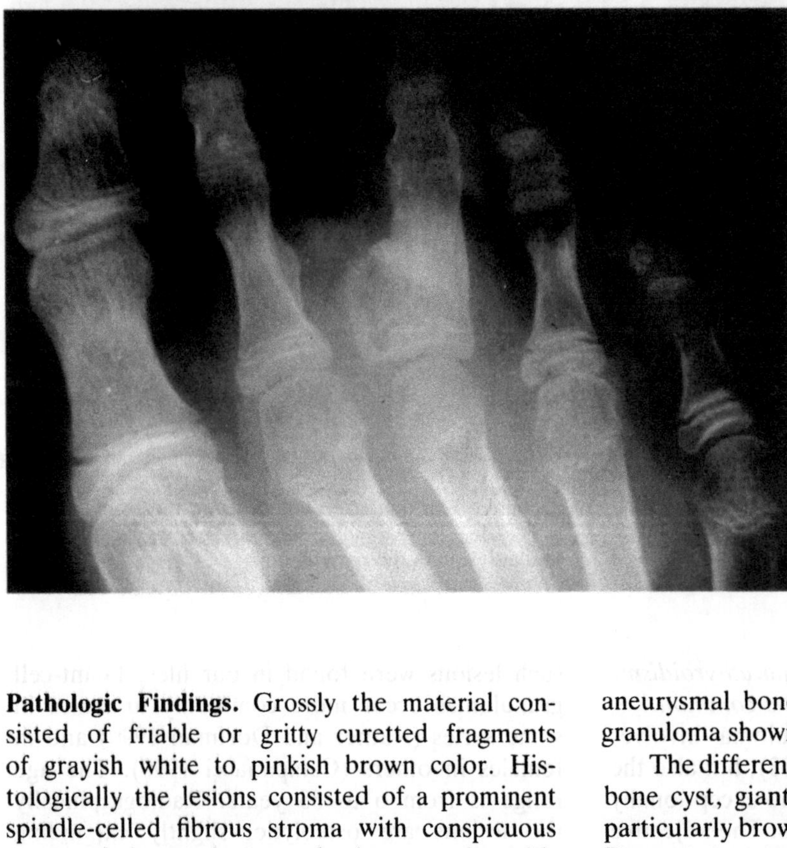

d

Fig. IX.100a–d. Radiographs of four cases of giant-cell granulomas of **a**,**b** hand and **c**,**d** foot bones. **a** Female, 22 years old, with radiolucent, trabeculated lesion, involving almost the entire diaphysis of the first phalanx of the thumb. **b** Male, 10 years old, with radiolucent lesion of the distal metaphysis of metacarpal bone, expanding the thinned cortex and suggesting a diagnosis of aneurysmal bone cyst. **c** Female, 10 years old, with a similar lesion in the distal end of the first metatarsal bone. Histologically the lesion was diagnosed as giant-cell granuloma with secondary aneurysmal bone cyst. **d** Twelve-year-old boy with an eccentric radiolucent lesion expanding the thinned cortex of the proximal end of the third phalanx of the right foot

Pathologic Findings. Grossly the material consisted of friable or gritty curetted fragments of grayish white to pinkish brown color. Histologically the lesions consisted of a prominent spindle-celled fibrous stroma with conspicuous areas of hemorrhage and clusters of multinucleated osteoclast giant cells, unevenly distributed and particularly evident in the areas of hemorrhage (Fig. IX.101). Reactive newly formed osteoid and bone formation is a frequent finding. Several reported cases contained focal areas with prominent cystic vascular spaces resembling an aneurysmal bone cyst. It is probable that some of the cases referred to as "solid aneurysmal bone cyst" correspond to giant-cell granuloma showing the above-described features.

The differential diagnosis includes aneurysmal bone cyst, giant-cell tumor, osteoblastoma, and particularly brown tumor of hyperparathyroidism. Brown tumor can be indistinguishable both radiographically and histologically from giant-cell granuloma, necessitating the study of the calcium metabolism to rule out hyperparathyroidism (see Chap. III on giant-cell tumors).

The correct diagnosis is essential for appropriate treatment. Curettage and bone grafting are effective; rarely, resection is indicated, most frequently in the recurrent lesions.

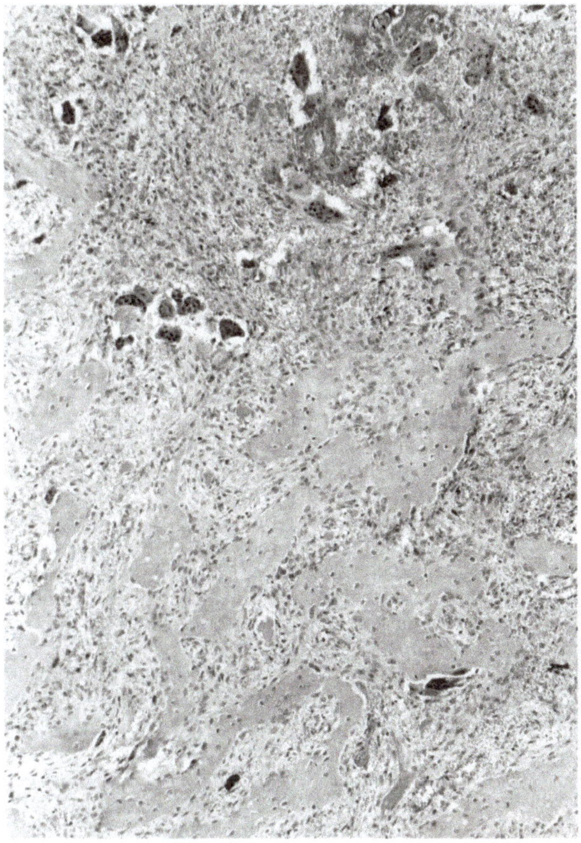
a

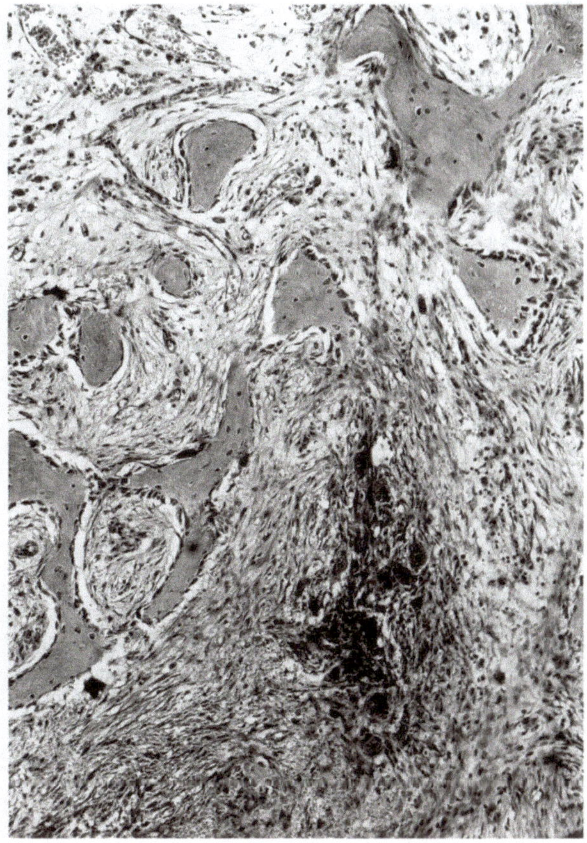
b

Fig. IX.101a–c. Photomicrographs show irregular distribution of multinucleated osteoclast giant cells, which are frequently clustered in areas of stromal hemorrhage. **a,b** The stroma is predominantly fibrous and shows evident reactive new-bone and osteoid formation. **c** These histologic features are indistinguishable from those seen in "brown tumor" of hyperparathyroidism. **a,b** ×100, **c** ×400

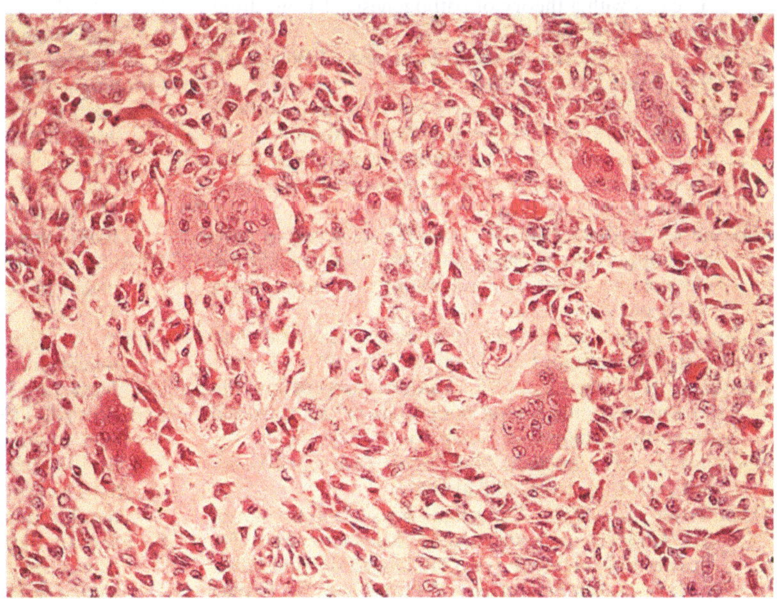
c

References

Solitary Bone Cyst (Simple or Unicameral Bone Cyst)

Adler CP (1985) Tumour-like lesions in the femur with cementum-like material. Does a "cementoma" of long bone exist? Skeletal Radiol 14:26–37
Boseker EH, Bickel WH, Dahlin DC (1968) A clinicopathologic study of simple unicameral bone cysts. Surg Gynecol Obstet 126:550–560
Campanacci M (1990) Bone and soft tissue tumors, Springer, Vienna New York
Campanacci M, DeSessa L, Bellando-Randone P (1976) Bone cysts: review of 275 cases. Results of surgical treatment and early results of treatment by methylprednisolone acetate injections. Chir Organi Mov 62:471–482
Campanacci M, DeSessa L, Trentani C (1977) Scaglietti's method for conservative treatment of simple bone cysts with local injections of methylprednisolone acetate. Ital J Orthop Traumatol 3:27–36
Campanacci M, Capanna R, Picci P (1986) Unicameral and aneurysmal bone cysts. Clin Orthop 204:25–36
Capanna R, Dal Monte A, Gitelis S, Campanacci M (1982) The natural history of unicameral bone cyst after steroid injection. Clin Orthop 166:204–211
Chigira M, Maehara S, Arita S et al. (1983) The aetiology and treatment of simple bone cysts. J Bone Joint Surg [Br] 65:633–637
Cohen J (1960) Simple bone cysts: studies of cysts fluid in six cases with a theory of pathogenesis. J Bone Joint Surg [Am] 42:609–616
Cohen J (1970) Etiology of simple bone cysts. J Bone Joint Surg [Am] 52:1493–1497
Cohen J (1977) Unicameral bone cysts: a current synthesis of reported cases. Orthop Clin North Am 8:4
Fahey JJ, O'Brien ET (1973) Subtotal resection and grafting in selected cases of solitary unicameral bone cysts. J Bone Joint Surg [Am] 55:59–68
Freund E, Moffert CB (1936) On different forms of nongeneralized fibrous osteodystrophy, localized, diffuse monostotic, unilateral and monostotic form. Surg Gynecol Obstet 62:541–563
Garceau GJ, Gregory CF (1954) Solitary unicameral bone cyst. J Bone Joint Surg [Am] 36:267–280
Gartland JJ, Cole FL (1975) Modern concepts in the treatment of unicameral bone cysts of the proximal humerus. Orthop Clin North Am 6:487–498
Geschickter CF, Copeland MM (1949) Tumors of bone, 3rd edn. Lippincott, Philadelphia
Haselhofer L (1937) Gutartige Riesenzellentumoren der Knochen und sogennante Knochenzysten. In: Lubarsch O, Henke F (eds) Handbuch der speziellen pathologischen Anatomie und Histologie, vol 9, part 3. Springer, Berlin Heidelberg New York, pp 477–555
Hutter RVP (1950) Unicameral bone cyst: report of unusual case. J Bone Joint Surg [Am] 32:430–432
Jaffe HL (1958) Tumors and tumorous conditions of the bones and joints. Lea & Febiger, Philadelphia
Jaffe HL, Lichtenstein L (1942) Solitary unicameral bone cyst. Arch Surg 44:1004–1025
Johnson LC, Kindred RG (1958) The anatomy of bone cysts. J Bone Joint Surg [Am] 40:1440
Johnson LC, Vetter H, Putschar WGJ (1962) Sarcomas arising in bone cysts. Virchows Arch [A] 335:428–451
Konjetzny GE (1922) Die sogenannte "lokalisierte Ostitis fibrosa." Arch Klin Chir 121–167
Lang FJ (1922) Beiträge zu den mikroskopischen Befunden bei Knochenzysten. Dtsch Z Chir 172–193
Lodwick GS (1958) Juvenile unicameral bone cysts: a roentgen reappraisal. Am J Roentgenol Radium Ther Nucl Med 80:495–506
Makley JT, Joyce MJ (1989) Unicameral bone cyst (simple bone cyst). Orthop Clin North Am 20:407–415
McGlynn FJ, Mickelson MR, El-Khoury G (1981) The fallen fragment sign in unicameral bone cyst. Clin Orthop 156:157–159
McKay LDW, Nason SS (1976) Surgical treatment of solitary unicameral bone cysts: a new concept. J Bone Joint Surg [Am] 58:734
Mikulicz I (1905) Über cystische Degeneration der Knochen. Verh Ges Dtsch Naturforsch Ärzte 76th meet, 2nd half, part II, p 107
Mirra JM, Bernard GW, Bullough PG et al. (1978) Cementum-like bone production in solitary bone cysts (so-called "cementoma" of long bones): report of three cases. Electron microscopic observations supporting a synovial origin to the simple bone cyst. Clin Orthop 135:295–307
Mönckeberg J (1904) Über Cystenbildung bei Ostitis fibrosa. Verh Dtsch Pathol Ges 7:232–234
Neer CS, Francis KC, Johnson AD, Kierman HA (1973) Current concepts on the treatment of solitary unicameral bone cyst. Clin Orthop 97:40–51
Nelson JP, Foster RJ (1976) Solitary bone cyst with epiphyseal involvement. Clin Orthop 118:147–150
Netherlands Committee on Bone Tumors (1973) Radiological atlas of bone tumors, vol 2. Williams & Wilkins, Baltimore, Maryland, pp 459–470
Ottolenghi CE, Schajowicz F, Raffa J (1969) Le kyste osseux essentiel uniloculaire. Etude clinique et anatomo-pathologique de 123 cas. Rev Chir Orthop 55:288–303
Pommer G (1919) Zur Kenntnis der progressiven Haematom und Phlegmasienveränderungen der Rohrenknochen. Arch Orthop Chir 17:17–34
Reynolds F (1969) The fallen fragment sign in the diagnosis of unicameral bone cysts. Radiology 92: 449–453
Sadler A, Rosenheim F (1964) Occurrence of two unicameral bone cysts in the same patient. J Bone Joint Surg [Am] 56:1557–1560
Sanerkin NG (1979) Old fibrin coagula and their ossification in simple bone cysts. J Bone Joint Surg [Br] 61:194–199
Scaglietti O (1974) L'azione osteogenetica dell'acetato di metilprednisolone. Bull Sci Med 146:159–160
Scaglietti O, Marchetti PG, Bertolozzi P (1976) Sull'azione topica dei corticoster steroide in microcristalli in alcune lesione delle schelet. Arch Putti Chir Organi Mov 27:9
Scaglietti O, Marchetti PG, Bertolozzi P (1979) The effects of methylprednisolone acetate in the treatment of bone cysts: results of three years follow-up. J Bone Joint Surg [Br] 61:200–204
Scaglietti O, Marchetti PG, Bertolozzi P (1982) Final results obtained in the treatment of bone cysts with methylprednisolone acetate (Depo-Medrol) and a discussion of results achieved in other bone lesions. Clin Orthop 165:33–42

Spence KF, Bright RW, Fitzgerland SP, Sell KW (1976) Solitary unicameral bone cyst: treatment with freeze-dried crushed cortical bone allograft. J Bone Joint Surg [Am] 58:636–641
Stelling CB, Martin W, Fechner RE et al. (1981) Case report 150. Diagnosis: solitary bone cyst with cementum-like bone production. Skeletal Radiol 6: 213–215
Virchow R (1876) Über die Bildung von Knochenzysten. Akad Wiss Berlin, pp 369–381
von Recklinghausen F (1891) Die fibröse oder deformierende Ostitis, die Osteomalacie und die osteoplastiche Carzinose in ihren gegenseitigen Beziehungen. Virchow Festschrift. G. Reimer, Berlin

Aneurysmal Bone Cyst (Multilocular Hematic Bone Cyst)

Aegerter E, Kirkpatrick JA Jr (1975) Orthopedic diseases: physiology, pathology, radiology, 4th edn. W.B. Saunders, Philadelphia
Aho HJ, Aho AJ, Einola S (1982) Aneurysmal bone cyst: a study of ultrastructure and malignant transformation. Virchows Arch [A] 395:169–179
Barnes R (1956) Aneurysmal bone cyst. J Bone Joint Surg [Br] 38:301–311
Bhaskar SN, Bernier JL, Godby F (1959) Aneurysmal bone cyst and other giant cell lesions of the jaws. Report of 104 cases. J Oral Surg 17:30–41
Biesecker JL, Marcove RC, Huvos AG, Mike V (1970) Aneurysmal bone cyst: a clinico-pathologic study of 66 cases. Cancer 26:615–625
Billings KJ, Werner LG (1972) Aneurysmal bone cyst of the first lumbar vertebra. Radiology 104:19–20
Bonakdarpour A, Levy WM, Aegerter E (1978) Primary and secondary aneurysmal bone cyst: a radiological study of 75 cases. Radiology 126:75–83
Buirski G, Watt I et al. (1984) The radiological features of "solid" aneurysmal bone cysts. Br J Radiol 57: 1057–1065
Buraczewski J, Dabska M (1971) Pathogenesis of aneurysmal bone cyst: relationship between the aneurysmal bone cyst and fibrous dysplasia of bone. Cancer 28:597–604
Campanacci M (1990) Bone and soft tissue tumors. Springer, Vienna New York
Capanna R, Albisinni U, Picci P et al. (1985) Aneurysmal bone cyst of the spine. J Bone Joint Surg [Am] 67:527–531
Capanna R, VanHorn JR, Biagini R et al. (1989) Aneurysmal bone cyst of the sacrum. Skeletal Radiol 18:109–113
Chuang VP, Soo CS, Wallace S et al. (1981) Arterial occlusion: management of giant cell tumor and aneurysmal bone cyst. AJR 136:1127–1130
Clough JR, Price CHG (1973) Aneurysmal bone cyst: pathogenesis and long-term results of treatment. Clin Orthop 97:52–63
Dabska M, Buraczewski J (1969) Aneurysmal bone cyst: pathology, clinical course and radiologic appearances. Cancer 23:371–389
Dahlin DC (1978) Bone tumors, 3rd edn. Charles C. Thomas, Springfield, IL
Dahlin DC, Besse BE, Pugh DG, Ghormley RK (1955) Aneurysmal bone cysts. Radiology 64:56–65
Dahlin DC, McLeod RA (1982) Aneurysmal bone cyst and other nonneoplastic conditions. Skeletal Radiol 8:243–250
Dahlin DC, Unni KK (1986) Bone tumors: general aspects and data on 8542 cases. Charles C. Thomas, Springfield, IL
Donaldson WF Jr (1962) Aneurysmal bone cyst. J Bone Joint Surg [Am] 44:25–39
Dos Santos R (1950) Arteriography in bone tumors. J Bone Joint Surg [Br] 32:17–29
Edling NPG (1965) Is the aneurysmal bone cyst a true pathologic entity? Cancer 18:1127–1130
Hadders HN, Oterdoom HJ (1956) The identification of aneurysmal bone cyst with hemangioma of skeleton. J Pathol Bacteriol 71:193–200
Hodgen JT, Frantz CH (1970) Subperiosteal giant cell tumor. J Bone Joint Surg [Br] 53:791
Hudson TM (1984) Fluid levels in aneurysmal bone cysts: a CT feature. AJR 142:1001–1004
Jaffe HL (1950) Aneurysmal bone cyst. Bull Hosp Joint Dis 11:3–13
Jaffe HL (1958) Tumors and tumorous conditions of the bones and joints. Lea & Febiger, Philadelphia
Jaffe HL (1962) Discussion following a paper by WF Donaldson Jr: aneurysmal bone cyst. J Bone Joint Surg [Am] 44:40
Jaffe HL, Lichtenstein L (1942) Benign chondroblastoma of bone: a reinterpretation of the so-called calcifying or chondromatous giant cell tumor. Am J Pathol 18:969–983
Levy WM, Miller AS, Bonakdarpour A, Aegerter E (1975) Aneurysmal bone cyst secondary to other osseous lesions: report of 57 cases. Am J Clin Pathol 63:1–8
Lichtenstein L (1950) Aneurysmal bone cyst: a pathological entity commonly mistaken for giant cell tumor and occasionally for hemangioma and osteogenic sarcoma. Cancer 3:279–289
Lichtenstein L (1953) Aneurysmal bone cysts, further observations. Cancer 6:1228–1237
Lichtenstein L (1957) Aneurysmal bone cyst: observations of fifty cases. J Bone Joint Surg [Am] 39:873–882
Lichtenstein L (1977) Bone tumors, 5th edn. C.V. Mosby, St. Louis
Lindbom A, Soderberg O, Spjut HJ, Sunnquist O (1961) Angiography of aneurysmal bone cyst. Acta Radiol 55:12–16
Martinez V, Sissons HA (1988) Aneurysmal bone cyst: a review of 123 cases including primary lesions and those secondary to other bone pathology. Cancer 61:2291–2304
Misasi N, Cigala F, Iaccarino V et al. (1982) Selective arterial embolisation in aneurysmal bone cysts. Int Orthop 6:123–128
Murphy WA, Strecker EB, Schoenecker PL (1982) Transcatheter embolisation therapy of an ischial aneurysmal bone cyst. J Bone Joint Surg [Br] 64: 166–168
Nobler MP, Higinbotham NL, Philips RF (1968) Irradiation superior to surgery in an analysis of 33 cases: the cure of aneurysmal bone cyst. Radiology 90: 1185–1192
Ruiter DJ, Lindeman J, Haverkate F, Hegt UN (1975) Fibrinolytic activity in aneurysmal bone cysts. Am J Clin Pathol 65:810–816

Ruiter DJ, Van Rijssel TG, Van der Velde EA (1977) Aneurysmal bone cysts: a clinicopathological study of 105 cases. Cancer 39:2231–2239
Sanerkin NG, Mott MG, Roylance J (1983) An unusual intraosseous lesion with fibroblastic, osteoclastic, osteoblastic, aneurysmal and fibromyxoid elements. "Solid" variant of aneurysmal bone cyst. Cancer 51:2278–2286
Schobinger R, Stoll HC (1957) The arteriographic picture of benign bone lesions containing giant cells. J Bone Joint Surg [Am] 39:953–960
Sherman RS, Soong KY (1957) Aneurysmal bone cyst: its roentgen diagnosis. Radiology 68:54–64
Steiner GC, Kantor EB (1978) Ultrastructure of aneurysmal bone cyst. Cancer 40:2967–2978
Tillman BP, Dahlin DC, Lipscomb PR, Steward JR (1968) Aneurysmal bone cyst: an analysis of 95 cases. Mayo Clin Proc 43:478–495
Wise DW, Bullough PG (1975) The natural history of aneurysmal bone cysts as shown in a review of 26 cases. J Hosp Spec Surg 1:1–23

Juxta-articular Bone Cyst (Intraosseous Ganglion)

Bugnion JP (1951) Lesions nouvelles du poignet. Acta Radiol [Suppl] (Stockh) 90:57–88
Campanacci M, Cervellati C (1971) Cisti mucose periostee e intraossee. Chir Organi Mov 60:221–232
Campanacci M, Gulino G (1974) Cisti mucose intraossee bilaterale. Chir Organi Mov 6:367–370
Catalano F (1969) Geodi sub-condrali non atrosici del ginocchio. Clin Orthop 21:499–506
Crabbé WA (1966) Intra-osseous ganglia of bone. Br J Surg 53:15–17
Crane AR, Scarano JJ (1967) Synovial cysts (ganglia) of bone. J Bone Joint Surg 49:355–361
Dominok GW, Crasselt C (1967) Das intraossäre Ganglion. Z Orthop 103:250–253
Eggers GW, Evans E, Blumel J, Nowlin D, Butler J (1963) Cystic change in iliac acetabulum. J Bone Joint Surg [Am] 45:669–686
Fairbanks HAT, Lloyd EI (1934) Cysts of the external cartilage of the knee with erosion of the head of the tibia. Br J Surg 22:115–118
Feldman F, Johnston A (1973) Intraosseous ganglion. Am J Roentgenol Radium Ther Nucl Med 118:328–343
Fisk GR (1949) Bone concavity caused by a ganglion. J Bone Joint Surg [Br] 31:220–221
Ghormley RK, Dockerty MB (1943) Cystic myxomatous tumors about the knee: their relation to cysts of menisci. J Bone Joint Surg [Am] 25:306–318
Golding C (1966) Radiology and orthopaedic surgery. J Bone Joint Surg [Br] 31:320–332
Goldman RL, Friedman NB (1969) Ganglia ("synovial cysts") arising in unusual locations: report of three cases, one primary in bone. Clin Orthop 63:184–189
Harrison MHM, Schajowicz F, Trueta J (1953) Osteoarthritis of the hip: a study of the nature and evolution of the disease. J Bone Joint Surg [Br] 35:598–626
Hicks JD (1956) Synovial cysts in bone. Aust NZ J Surg 26:138–143
Kambolis C, Bullough PG, Jaffe HL (1973) Ganglionic cystic defects of bone. J Bone Joint Surg [Am] 55: 596–605
Landells JW (1953) Bone cysts of osteoarthritis. J Bone Joint Surg [Br] 35:643–649
Lloyd-Roberts GC (1955) Osteoarthritis of hip: study of clinical pathology. J Bone Joint Surg [Br] 37:8–47
Magyar E, Talerman A, Fehér M, Wouters HW (1974) Giant bone cysts in rheumatoid arthritis. J Bone Joint Surg [Br] 56:121–129
Mainzer F, Minagi H (1970) Intraosseous ganglion: solitary subchondral lesion of bone. Radiology 94: 387–389
Menges V, Prager P, Cserhati MD, Becker WP, Griss P, Wurster K (1977) Das intraossäre Ganglion. Z Orthop 115:67–75
Nezelof C, Laurent M (1966) Inclusion capsulosynoviales intraosseuses. Rev Chir Orthop 52:225–240
Nigrisoli P, Beltrami P (1971) Subchondral cysts of bone. Scapello 1:65–75
Ondruch AS (1963) Cyst formation in osteoarthritis. J Bone Joint Surg [Br] 45:755–760
Pope TL, Fechner RE, Keats TE (1989) Intra-osseous ganglion: report of four cases and review of the literature. Skeletal Radiol 18:185–187
Prager PJ, Menges V, DiBiase M (1975) Das intraossäre Ganglion. Fortschr Roentgenstr 123:458
Rhaney K, Lamb DW (1955) The cysts of osteoarthritis of the hip: a radiologic and pathological study. J Bone Joint Surg [Br] 37:663–675
Salzer M, Salzer-Kuntschik M (1968) Ganglien mit Knochenbeteiligung. Arch Orthop Unfall-Chir 64: 87–99
Scaglietti O, Stringa G (1960) Geodi isolati sottocondrali. Arch Putti Chir Organi Mov 13:30–39
Schajowicz F, Blumenfeld I (1968) Pigmented villonodular synovitis of the wrist with penetration into bone. J Bone Joint Surg [Br] 50:312–317
Schajowicz, F, Clavel Sainz M, Slullitel JA (1979) Juxtaarticular bone cysts (intra-osseous ganglia): a clinicopathological study of 88 cases. J Bone Joint Surg [Br] 61:107–116
Seymour N (1968) Intraosseous ganglia. J Bone Joint Surg [Br] 50:134–137
Sim FH, Dahlin DC (1971) Ganglion cysts of bone. Proc Staff Meet Mayo Clin 46:484–488
Spjut HJ, Dorfman HD, Fechner RE, Ackerman LV (1977) Tumors of bone and cartilage. Atlas of tumor pathology, 2nd series, Fasc 5. Armed Forces Institute of Pathology, Washington, DC
Willems J, Mulier TC, Mortens M, Verhelts M (1973) Ganglion cyst of bone. Acta Orthop Scand 44:655
Woods CT (1961) Subchondral bone cysts. J Bone Joint Surg [Br] 43:758–766

Metaphyseal Fibrous Defect (Nonossifying Fibroma, Histiocytic Xanthogranuloma)

Bahls G (1936) Über ein solitares Xantom im Knochen. Zentralbl Chir 63:1041–1046
Bertoni F, Unni KK, McLeod RA et al. (1988) Xanthoma of bone. Am J Clin Pathol 90:377–384
Bhagwandeem SB (1966) Malignant transformation of a non-ossifying fibroma of bone. J Pathol Bacteriol 92:562–564

Blau RA, Zwick DL, Westphal RA (1988) Multiple non-ossifying fibromas. J Bone Joint Surg [Am] 70: 299–304
Burman MS, Sinberg SE (1938) Solitary xantohoma (lipoid granulomatosis). Arch Surg 37:1017–1032
Caffey J (1955) On fibrous defects in cortical walls of growing tubular bones. Adv Pediatr 7:13–51
Caffey J (1972) Pediatric X-ray diagnosis, 6th edn. Yearbook Medical, Chicago
Campanacci M, Laus M, Boriani S (1983) Multiple non-ossifying fibromata with extraskeletal anomalies: A new syndrome? J Bone Joint Surg [Br] 65:623–627
Campbell CJ, Harkess J (1957) Fibrous metaphyseal defect of bone. Surg Gynecol Obstet 104:329–336
Compere CL, Coleman SS (1957) Non-osteogenic fibroma of bone. Surg Gynecol Obstet 105:588
Cunningham BJ, Ackerman LV (1956) Metaphyseal fibrous defects. J Bone Joint Surg [Am] 38:797–808
Evans GA, Park WM (1978) Familial multiple non-osteogenic fibromata. J Bone Joint Surg [Br] 60: 416–419
Geschickter CF, Copeland MM (1949) Tumors of bone, 3rd edn. Lippincott, Philadelphia
Hastrup J, Jensen TS (1965) Osteogenic sarcoma arising in a non-osteogenic fibroma of bone. Acta Pathol Microbiol Scand 63:493–499
Hatcher CH (1945) The pathogenesis of localized fibrous lesion in the metaphyses of long bones. Ann Surg 122:1016–1030
Herrera GA, Reimann BEF, Scully TJ, Difiore RJ (1982) Nonossifying fibroma: electron microscopic examination of two cases supporting a histiocytic rather than a fibroblastic origin. Clin Orthop 167:269–276
Jaffe HL (1958) Tumors and tumorous conditions of the bones and joints. Lea & Febiger, Philadelphia
Jaffe HL, Lichtenstein L (1942) Non-osteogenic fibroma of bone. Am J Pathol 18:205–221
Kimmelstiel P, Rapp I (1951) Cortical defect due to periosteal desmoids. Bull Hosp Joint Dis 12:286–287
Kyriakos M, Murphy WA (1981) Concurrence of metaphyseal fibrous defect and osteosarcoma: report of a case and review of the literature. Skeletal Radiol 6:179–186
Llombart-Bosch A, Pedro-Olaya A, López-Fernández A (1974) Non-ossifying fibroma of bone: a histochemical and ultrastructural characterization. Virchows Arch [A] 362:13–21
Maudsley RH, Stanfsfeld AG (1956) Non-osteogenic fibroma of bone (fibrous metaphyseal defect). J Bone Joint Surg [Br] 38:714–733
Mirra JM, Gold RH, Rand F (1982) Disseminated non-ossifying fibromas in association with café-au-lait spots (Jaffe-Campanacci syndrome). Clin Orthop 168:192–205
Moser RP, Sweet DE, Haseman, Madewell J (1987) Multiple skeletal fibroxanthomas: radiologic-pathologic correlation of 72 cases. Skeletal Radiol 16:353–359
Murray RD, Jacobson HG (1971) The radiology of skeletal disorders. Williams & Wilkins, Baltimore, pp 356–360
Peuchmaur M, Forest M, Tomeno B et al. (1985) Multifocal nonosteogenic fibroma: report of a case with ultrastructural findings. Hum Pathol 16:751–753
Phelan JT (1964) Fibrous cortical defect and nonosseous fibroma of bone. Surg Gynecol Obstet 119:807–810
Phemister D (1929) Chronic fibrous osteomyelitis. Ann Surg 90:756–764
Ponseti IV, Friedman B (1949) Evolution of metaphyseal fibrous defect. J Bone Surg [Am] 31:582–585
Ritschl P, Karnel F, Hajek P (1988) Fibroma, metaphyseal defects: determinations of their origin and natural history using a radiomorphological study. Skeletal Radiol 17:8–15
Schroeder F (1932) Ein zentraler xanthomatöser Riesenzelltumor der Fibula. Arch Klin Chir 168:118
Schwartz AM, Ramos RM (1980) Neurofibromatosis and multiple nonossifying fibroma. AJR 135:617–619
Selby S (1961) Metaphyseal cortical defects in the tubular bones of growing children. J Bone Joint Surg [Am] 43:395–400
Sontag L, Pyle S (1941) The appearance and nature of cyst-like areas in the distal femoral metaphyses of children. Am J Roentgenol Radium Ther 46:185–188
Spjut HJ, Dorfman HD, Fechner RE, Ackerman LV (1971) Tumors of bone and cartilage. Atlas of tumor pathology, 2nd series, Fasc 5. Armed Forces Institute of Pathology, Washington, DC
Steiner GC (1974) Fibrous cortical defect and non-ossifying fibroma of bone: a study of the ultrastructure. Arch Pathol 97:205–210
Yagmai I (1978) Intra- and extraosseous xanthomata associated with hyperlipidemia. Radiology 128:49–54
Young JWR, Levine AM, Dorfman HD. Case report 293. Diagnosis: nonossifying fibroma (NOF) of the upper tibial diametaphysis with considerable increase in size over a three-year period. Skeletal Radiol 12:294–297

Eosinophilic Granuloma (Histiocytosis X, Langerhans Cell Granulomatosis)

Abt AF, Denenholz EJ (1936) Letterer-Siwe disease: splenohepatomegaly associated with widespread hyperplasia of non-lipoid-storing macrophages: discussion of the so-called reticuloendothelioses. Am J Dis Child 51:499–522
Aronson RP (1951) Streptomycin in Letterer-Siwe's disease. Lancet I:889
Avery ME, McAfee JG, Guild HG (1957) The course and prognosis of reticuloendotheliosis (eosinophilic granuloma, Schüller-Christian disease and Letterer-Siwe disease). Am J Med 22:636–652
Avioli LV, Lasersohn JT, Lopresti JM (1963) Histiocytosis X (Schüller-Christian disease): a clinico-pathological survey, review of ten patients and the results of prednisone therapy. Medicine (Baltimore) 42:119–147
Bass MH, Sapin SO, Hodes HL (1953) Use of cortisone and corticotropin (ACTH) in treatment of reticuloendotheliosis in children. Am J Dis Child 85:393
Basset F, Nezelof C, Turiaf J (1966) Présence en microscopie électronique de structures filamenteuses originales dans les lésiones pulmonaires et osseusses de l'histiocytose X. Mem Soc Med Hosp Paris 117:413
Batson R, Shaprio J, Christie A, Riley HD Jr (1955) Acute nonlipial disseminated reticuloendotheliosis. Am J Dis Child 90:323–343
Beier FR, Thatcher LG, Lahey ME (1963) The treatment of reticuloendotheliosis with vinblastine sulfate. J Pediatr 63:1087
Broadbent V, Pritchard J, Davies E et al. (1984) Spontaneous remission of multisystem histiocytosis X. Lancet I:253–254

Calvé JA (1925) Localized affection of the spine suggesting osteochondritis of vertebral body, with clinical aspects of Pott's disease. J Bone Joint Surg 7:41–46
Cancilla PA, Lahey ME, Carnes WH (1967) Cutaneous lesions of Letterer-Siwe disease. Cancer 20:1986
Capanna R, Springfield DS, Ruggieri P et al. (1985) Direct cortison injection in eosinophilic granuloma of bone: a preliminary report on 11 patients. J Pediatr Oncol 5:338–342
Cheyne C (1971) Histiocytosis X. J Bone Joint Surg [Br] 53:366–382
Christian HA (1920) Defects in membranous bones, exophthalmos and diabetes insipidus; an unusual syndrome of dyspituitarism: a clinical study. Med Clin North Am 3:849
Cohen M, Zornoza J, Cangir A et al. (1980) Direct injection of methylprednisolone sodium succinate in the treatment of solitary eosinophilic granuloma of bone. Radiology 136:289–293
Compere EL, Johnson WE, Coventry MB (1954) Vertebra plana (Calvé's disease) due to eosinophilic granuloma. J Bone Joint Surg [Am] 36:969–980
Dargeon HW (1967) Reticuloendothelioses in childhood. Charles C. Thomas, Springfield, IL
Doede KG, Rappaport H (1967) Long-term survival of patients with acute differentiated histiocytosis (Letterer-Siwe). Cancer 20:1782–1795
Elema JD, Atmosoerodjo-Briggs A (1984) Langerhans cells and macrophages in eosinophilic granuloma: an enzyme-histochemical, enzyme-cytochemical, and ultrastructural study. Cancer 54:2174–2181
Engelbreth-Holm J, Teilum G, Christensen E (1944) Eosinophilic granuloma of bone – Schüller-Christian's disease. Acta Med Scand 118:292–312
Enriquez P, Dahlin DC, Hayles AB, Henderson ED (1967) Histiocytosis X. Mayo Clin Proc 42:88–99
Farber S (1941) The nature of "solitary or eosinophilic granuloma" of bone. Am J Pathol 17:625–626
Finzi O (1929) Mieloma con prevalenza delle cellule eosinofile circoncritto all'osso frontale in un giovine di 15 anni. Minerva Med 9:239–241
Fisher RH (1953) Multiple lesions of bone in Letterer-Siwe disease. J Bone Joint Surg [Am] 35:445
Fowles JV, Bobechko WP (1970) Solitary eosinophilic granuloma in bone. J Bone Joint Surg [Br] 52:238–243
Friedman B, Hanaoka H (1969) Langerhans cell granules in eosinophilic granuloma of bone. J Bone Joint Surg [Am] 51:367–374
Galeotti-Flori A, Parenti GG (1937) Reticuloendoteliosi iperplasica infettiva ad evoluzione, granuloxantomatosa (tipo Hand-Schüller-Christian). Rev Clin Pediatr 35:193–263
Green WT, Farber S (1942) "Eosinophilic or solitary granuloma" of bone. J Bone Joint Surg [Am] 24:499–526
Gross P, Jacox HW (1942) Eosinophilic granuloma and certain other reticuloendothelial hyperplasias of bone. Am J Med Sci 203:673
Hajdu I, Zhang W, Gardon GB (1986) Peanut agglutinin binding as a histochemical tool for diagnosis of eosinophilic granuloma. Arch Pathol Lab Med 110:719–721
Hand A (1921) Defects of membranous bones, exophthalmos and polyuria in childhood: Is it dyspituitarism? Am J Med Sci 162:509
Hocking WG, Swanson M (1986) Multifocal eosinophilic granuloma: response of a patient to Etoposione. Cancer 58:840–842
Ide F, Iwase T, Saito I, Umemura S, Nakajima T (1984) Immunohistochemical and ultrastructural analysis of the proliferating cells of histiocytosis X. Cancer 53:917–921
Jaffe HL, Lichtenstein L (1944) Eosinophilic granuloma of bone. Arch Pathol 37:99–118
Jones B (1974) Chemotherapy of reticulo-endothelioses. Cancer 34:1011
Kondi ES, Deckers PJ, Gallitano AL, Khung CL (1972) Diffuse eosinophilic granuloma of bone: a dramatic response to Velban therapy. Cancer 30:1169
Kotz FL, Silva EG, DeSantos LA, Lukeman JM (1980) Diagnosis of eosinophilic granuloma of bone by cytology, histology and electron microscopy of transcutaneous bone-aspiration biopsy. J Bone Joint Surg [Am] 62:1284–1290
Letterer E (1924) Aleukanemische Retikulose (ein Beitrag zu den proliferativen Erkrankungen des Retikuloendothelialapparates). Frank Z Pathol 30:377–394
Lichtenstein L (1953) Histiocytosis X: integration of eosinophilic granuloma of bone, "Letterer-Siwe disease," and "Schüller-Christian disease" as related manifestations of a single nosologic entity. Arch Pathol 56:84–102
Lichtenstein L (1964) Histiocytosis X (eosinophilic granuloma of bone, Letterer-Siwe disease, and Schüller-Christian disease. J Bone Joint Surg [Am] 46:76–90
Lichtenstein L, Jaffe HL (1940) Eosinophilic granuloma of bone. Am J Pathol 16:595–604
Lieberman PH, Jones CR, Dargeon HWK, Begg CF (1969) A reappraisal of eosinophilic granuloma of bone, Hand-Schüller-Christian syndrome and Letterer-Siwe syndrome. Medicine (Baltimore) 48:375–400
McGavran HM, Spady HA (1960) Eosinophilic granuloma of bone. J Bone Joint Surg [Am] 42:979–992
Mercer W, Duthie RB (1956) Histiocytic granulomatosis. J Bone Joint Surg [Br] 38:279
Mickelson MR, Bonfiglio M (1977) Eosinophilic granuloma and its variation. Orthop Clin North Am 8:933–945
Morales AR, Fine G, Horn RC Jr, Watson JHL (1969) Langerhans cells in a localized lesion of the eosinophilic granuloma type. Lab Invest 20:412–423
Moseley JE (1968) Bone changes in hematologic disorders (roentgen aspects). Grune & Stratton, New York, pp 161–179
Murphy GI, Bhan AK, Sato S et al. (1981) A new immunologic marker from human Langerhans cells. N Engl J Med 304:791–792
Newton WA Jr, Hamoudi AB (1973) Histiocytosis: a histologic classification with clinical correlation. Perspect Pediatr Pathol 1:251–283
Nezelof C, Depres S, Barbey S et al. (1973) Histiocytosis X. Histogenic arguments for a Langerhans cell origin. Biomedicine 18:365
Nezelof C, Guibert C (1963) L'histiocytose X. Nosologie et prognostic. Arch Fr Pediatri 20:1063–1103
Oberman HA (1961) Idiopathic histiocytosis X: a clinicopathologic study of 40 cases. Pediatrics 28:301–327
Otani S (1957) Discussion of eosinophilic granuloma of bone, Letterer-Siwe disease and Schüller-Christian disease. J Mt Sinai Hosp NY 24:1079–1092

Otani S, Ehrlich JC (1940) Solitary granuloma of bone simulating primary neoplasm. Am J Pathol 16:479–490

Ponseti IV (1948) Bone lesions in eosinophilic granuloma, Hand-Schüller-Christian disease and Letterer-Siwe disease. J Bone Joint Surg [Am] 39:811

Ree HJ, Kadin ME (1987) Peanut agglutinin: a useful marker for histiocytosis X and interdigitating reticulum cells. Cancer 57:282–287

Rewald E (1960) Die Letterer-Christiansche Erkrankung. Ergeb Inn Med Kinderheilkd 3:143

Sbarbaro JL Jr, Francis KC (1961) Eosinophilic granuloma of bone. JAMA 178:706–740

Scaglietti O, Marchetti PG, Bartolozzi P (1976) Topical effect of corticosteroids in microcrystals in various diseases of the skeleton. Arch Putti Chir Organi Mov 27:9–31

Schairer E (1938) Ueber eine eigenartige Erkrankung des kindlichen Schädels. Zentralbl Allg Pathol Pathol Anat 71:113–117

Schajowicz F, Polak M (1947) Contribución al estudio del denominado "granuloma eosinofílico" y sus relaciones con la xantomatosis ósea. Rev Asoc Med Argent 61:218–226

Schajowicz F, Slullitel J (1973) Eosinophilic granuloma of bone and its relationship to Hand-Schüller-Christian and Letterer-Siwe syndromes. J Bone Joint Surg [Br] 55:545–565

Schajowicz F, Ackerman LV, Sissons HA (1972) Histological typing of bone tumours. World Health Organization, Geneva

Schüller A (1915–1916) Über eigenartige Schädeldefekte im Jugendalter. Fortschr Roentgenstr 23:12–18

Siegel S, Coltman CA (1966) Histiocytosis X: response to vinblastine sulfate. JAMA 197:403

Siwe SA (1933) Die Reticuloendotheliose, ein neues Krankheitsbild unter den Hepatosplenomegalien. Z Kinderheilkd 55:212–247

Stern MB, Cassidy R, Mirra J (1976) Eosinophilic granuloma of the proximal tibial epiphysis. Clin Orthop 118:153–156

Vogel JM, Vogel P (1972) Idiopathic histiocytosis. Semin Hematol 9:349–369

Wallgren A (1940) Systemic reticuloendothelial granuloma: nonlipoid reticuloendotheliosis and Schüller-Christian disease. Am J Dis Child 60:471–500

West WO (1973) Velban as treatment for diffuse eosinophilic granuloma of bone. J Bone Joint Surg [Am] 55:1755–1759

West WO (1984) Velban as a treatment for disseminated eosinophilic granuloma of bone: follow-up note after 17 years. J Bone Joint Surg [Am] 66:1128

Wester SM, Beabout JW, Unni KK et al. (1982) Langerhans' cell granulomatosis (histiocytosis X) of bone in adults. Am J Surg Pathol 6:413–426

Fibrous Dysplasia and Osteofibrous Dysplasia

Albright F, Reifenstein E (1948) The parathyroid glands and metabolic disease: selected studies. Williams & Wilkins, Baltimore

Albright F, Butler A, Hampton A, Smith P (1937) Syndrome characterized by osteitis fibrosa disseminata, areas of pigmentation and endocrine dysfunction, with precocious puberty in females: report of five cases. N Engl J Med 216:727

Benedict P, Szabo G, Fitzpatrick T, Sinesi S (1968) Melanotic macules in Albright's syndrome and in neurofibromatosis. JAMA 205:618

Benjamin D, McRoberts J (1973) Polyostotic fibrous dysplasia associated with Cushing's syndrome. Arch Pathol 96:175

Campanacci M (1976) Osteofibrous dysplasia of long bones, a new clinical entity. Ital J Orthop Traumatol 2:221–237

Campanacci M (1990) Bone and soft tissue tumors. Springer, Vienna New York

Campanacci M, Laus M (1981) Osteofibrous dysplasia of the tibia and fibula. J Bone Joint Surg [Am] 63:367–375

Campbell CJ, Hawk T (1982) A variant of fibrous dysplasia (osteofibrous dysplasia). J Bone Joint Surg [Am] 64:231–236

Castellote A, García-Peña P, Lucaya J, Lorenzo J (1988) Osteofibrous dysplasia: a report of two cases. Skeletal Radiol 17:483–486

Dabska M, Buraczewski J (1956) On malignant transformation in fibrous dysplasia of bone. Oncology 26:369

Danon M, Robboy S, Kim S et al. (1975) Cushing syndrome, sexual precocity and polyostotic fibrous dysplasia in infancy. J Pediatr 87:1019

DePalma A, Almad I (1973) Fibrous dysplasia associated with shepherd's crook deformity of the humerus. Clin Orthop 97:38

DeSmet AA, Travers H, Neff JR (1981) Chondrosrcoma occurring in a patient with polyostotic fibrous dysplasia. Skeletal Radiol 7:197–201

Ehrig V, Wilson D (1972) Fibrous dysplasia of bone and primary hyperparathyroidism. Ann Intern Med 77:234

Enneking WF, Gearen PF (1986) Fibrous dysplasia of the femoral neck: treatment by cortical bone grafting. J Bone Joint Surg [Am] 68:1415–1422

Freund E (1934) Osteodystrophia fibrosa unilateralis: report of a case. Arch Surg 28:849–869

Georgen TG, Dickman PS, Resnick D et al. (1977) Long bone ossifying fibromas. Cancer 39:2067–2072

Gibson MJ, Middlemiss JH (1971) Fibrous dysplasia of bone. Br J Radiol 44:1–13

Grabias SL, Campbell CJ (1977) Fibrous dysplasia. Orthop Clin North Am 8:771–783

Hall R, Warrick C (1972) Hypersecretion of hypothalamic releasing hormones: a possible explanation of the endocrine manifestations of polyostotic fibrous dysplasia (Albright's syndrome). Lancet I:1313

Harris WH, Dudley HR Jr, Barry RJ (1962) The natural history of fibrous dysplasia: an orthopaedic, pathological, and roentgenographic study. J Bone Joint Surg [Am] 44:207–233

Helawa M, Ahmad A (1984) Chondrosarcoma in fibrous dysplasia in the pelvis: a case report and review of the literature. J Bone Joint Surg [Br] 66:760–764

Henry A (1969) Monostotic fibrous dysplasia. J Bone Joint Surg [Br] 51:300–306

Huvos A, Higinbotham N, Miller T (1972) Bone sarcoma arising in fibrous dysplasia. J Bone Joint Surg [Am] 54:1042–1056

Jaffe HL (1958) Tumors and tumorous conditions of the bones and joints. Lea & Febiger, Philadelphia

Johnson LC (1972) Congenital pseudoarthrosis, adamantinoma of long bone and intracortical fibrous dysplasia of the tibia. J Bone Joint Surg [Am] 54:1355
Kempson RL (1966) Ossifying fibroma of the long bones: a light and microscopic study. Arch Pathol 82:218–233
Lichtenstein L (1938) Polyostotic fibrous dysplasia. Arch Surg 36:874
Lichtenstein L, Jaffe H (1942) Fibrous dysplasia of bone. Arch Pathol 33:777
MacMahna HE (1971) Albright's syndrome – 30 years later. Pathol Annu, p 81
Markel SF (1978) Ossifying fibroma of long bone: its distinction from fibrous dysplasia and its association with adamantinoma of long bone. Am J Clin Pathol 69:91–97
Mazabraud A, Semat P, Roze R (1967) Association of soft tissue fibromyxoma with fibrous bone dysplasia. Presse Med 75:2223–2228
Milgram JW (1975) Malignant degeneration of polyostotic fibrous dysplasia of bone. Bull Hosp Joint Dis 36:137–149
Nakashima Y, Yamamuro T, Fujiwara Y et al. (1983) Osteofibrous dysplasia (ossifying fibroma of long bones): a study of 12 cases. Cancer 52:909–914
Perkinson NG, Higinbotham NL (1955) Osteogenic sarcoma arising in polyostotic fibrous dysplasia: report of a case. Cancer 8:396–402
Pindborg JJ, Kramer IRH, Storloni HS (1971) Histological typing of odontogenic tumors, jaw cysts, and allied diseases. International Histological Classification of Tumours, No. 5. World Health Organization, Geneva
Reed RJ (1963) Fibrous dysplasia of bone: a review of 25 cases. Arch Pathol 75:480
Riddell, DM (1964) Malignant change in fibrous dysplasia: report of a case. J Bone Joint Surg [Br] 46:251–255
Rio Hortega P (1934) Anatomía microscópica de los tumores del sistema nervioso central y periférico. Madrid
Rio Hortega P (1943) Estudio citológico de los "neurofibromas" de Recklinghausen (lemocitomas). Arch Histol Normal Patol 1:373–419
Sanerkin NG, Watt I (1981) Enchondromata with annular calcification in association with fibrous dysplasia. Br J Radiol 54:1027–1033
Schajowicz F, Derqui JC (1968) Puncture biopsy in lesions of the locomotor system: review of results in 4050 cases, including 941 vertebral punctures. Cancer 21:531–548
Schajowicz F, Santini-Araujo E (1989) Adamantinoma of the tibia masked by fibrous dysplasia. Clin Orthop Rel Res 238:294–301
Schlumberger HF (1946a) Fibrous dysplasia (ossifying fibroma) of the maxilla and mandible. Am J Orthod Oral Surg 82:579–587
Schlumberger HF (1946b) Fibrous dysplasia of single bones. Milit Surg 99:504
Schoenecker PL, Swanson K, Sheridan JJ (1981) Ossifying fibroma of the tibia: report of a new case and review of the literature. J Bone Joint Surg [Am] 63:483–488
Schwartz DT, Alpert M (1964) The malignant transformation of fibrous dysplasia. Am J Med Sci 247:1–20
Sherman NH, Rao VM, Brennan RE et al. (1982) Fibrous dysplasia of the facial bones and mandible. Skeletal Radiol 8:141–143
Sissons H, Kancherla P, Wallace B (1983) Ossifying fibroma of bone: report of two cases. Bull Hosp Joint Dis 43:1–14
Slow IN, Stern D, Friedman EW (1971) Osteogenic sarcoma arising in pre-existing fibrous dysplasia: report of a case. J Oral Surg 29:126–129
Stewart M, Gilmer W, Edmonson A (1962) Fibrous dysplasia of bone. J Bone Joint Surg [Br] 44:302
Taconis WK (1988) Osteosarcoma in fibrous dysplasia. Skeletal Radiol 17:163–170
Thannhauser SJ (1944) Neurofibromatosis (von Recklinghausen) and osteitis fibrosa cystica localisata et disseminata (von Recklinghausen). Medicine 23:105–148
Valls J, Polak M, Schajowicz F (1950) Fibrous dysplasia of bone. J Bone Joint Surg [Am] 32:311–322
von Recklinghausen F (1882) Über die multiplen Fibrome der Haut und ihre Beziehung zu den multiplen Neuromen. Virchow Festschrift, Berlin
West R, Huvos AG, Lane JM (1983) Desmoplastic fibroma of bone arising in fibrous dysplasia. Am J Clin Pathol 79:630–633
Yabut SM, Kenan S, Sissons MA, Lewis MM (1988) Malignant transformation of fibrous dysplasia: a case report and review of the literature. Clin Orthop 228:281–289

Myositis Ossificans (Heterotopic Ossification)

Ackerman LV (1958) Extraosseous localized nonneoplastic bone and cartilage formation (so-called myositis ossificans). J Bone Joint Surg [Am] 40:279
Angervall L, Steiner L, Ahren CC (1969) Pseudomalignant osseous tumour of soft tissue. J Bone Joint Surg [Br] 51:654
Campanacci M (1990) Bone and soft tissue tumors. Springer, Vienna New York
Campanacci M, Gardini GF, Giunti A et al. (1980) Ossificazione muscolare e/o periostee pseutotumorali (studio di 57 casi). Ital J Orthop Traumatol 6:385–393
Chaplin DM, Harrison MHM (1972) Pseudomalignant osseous tumour of soft tissue: report of two cases. J Bone Joint Surg [Br] 54:334–340
Chung EB, Enzinger FM (1987) Extraskeletal osteosarcoma. Cancer 60:1132–1142
Dahlin DC (1978) Bone tumors, 3rd edn. Charles C. Thomas, Springfield, IL
Das Gupta TK, Hajdu SI, Foote FW Jr (1968) Extraosseous osteogenic sarcoma. Ann Surg 105:1011–1022
Dorfman HD, Norman A (1970) Juxtacortical circumscribed myositis ossificans: evolution and radiographic features. Radiology 96:301–306
Dupree WB, Enzinger FM (1986) Fibro-osseous pseudotumor of the digits. Cancer 58:2103
Fine G, Stout AP (1956) Osteogenic sarcoma of the extraskeletal soft tissues. Cancer 9:1027–1043
Huvos AG (1985) The spontaneous transformation of benign into malignant soft tissue tumors. Am J Surg Pathol 9[Suppl]:7–20
Jaffe HL (1958) Tumors and tumorous conditions of the bones and joints. Lea & Febiger, Philadelphia
Jeffreys T, Styles P (1966) Pseudomalignant osseous tumour of soft tissue. J Bone Joint Surg [Br] 48:488

Lagier R, Cox JN (1975) Pseudomalignant myositis ossificans: a pathological study of eight cases. Hum Pathol 6:653–665
Liefeld PA, Ferguson AB Jr, Fu FH (1982) Focal myositis: a benign lesion that mimics malignant disease. A case report. J Bone Joint Surg [Am] 64:1371–1373
Lorentzon R, Larsson SE, Boquist L (1979) Extraosseous osteosarcoma: a clinical and histopathological study of four cases. J Bone Joint Surg [Br] 61:205–208
Nora F, Dahlin DC, Beabout JW (1983) Bizarre parosteal osteochondromatous proliferations of the hands and feet. Am J Surg Pathol 7:245
Ogilvie-Harris HDJ, Hons CB, Fornasier VL (1980) Pseudomalignant myositis ossificans: heterotopic new-bone formation without a history of trauma. J Bone Joint Surg [Am] 62:1274–1283
Patel MR, Desai SS (1986) Pseudomalignant osseous tumor of soft tissue: a case report and review of the literature. J Hand Surg 11:66–70
Paterson DC (1970) Myositis ossificans circumscripta: report of four cases without history of injury. J Bone Joint Surg [Br] 52:296–301
Povysil C, Matejovsky Z (1979) Ultrastructural evidence of myofibroblasts in pseudomalignant myositis ossificans. Virchows Arch [A] 381:189–203
Rao U, Cheng A, Didolkar MS (1978) Extraosseous osteogenic sarcoma: clinicopathologic study of eight cases and review of literature. Cancer 41:1488–1496
Samuelson KM, Coleman SS (1976) Nontraumatic myositis ossificans in healthy individuals. JAMA 235:1132–1133
Shanoff LB, Spira M, Hardy SB (1967) Myositis ossificans: evolution to osteogenic sarcoma. Report of a histologically verified case. Am J Surg 113:537–541
Shea TE (1967) Calcified soft-tissue mass in the medial aspect of the thigh. JAMA 200:1050–1052
Sordillo PP, Hajdu SI, Magill GB et al. (1983) Extraosseous osteogenic sarcoma: a review of 48 patients. Cancer 51:727–733
Spencer JD, Missen GAK (1989) Pseudomalignant heterotopic ossification ("myositis ossificans"). J Bone Joint Surg (Br) 71:317–319
Spjut HJ, Dorfman HD (1981) Florid reactive periostitis of the tubular bones of the hands and feet. Am J Surg Pathol 5:423
Spjut HJ, Dorfman HD, Fechner RE, Ackerman LV (1971) Tumors of bone and cartilage. Atlas of tumor pathology, 2nd series, Fasc 5. Armed Forces Institute of Pathology, Washington, DC
Sumiyoshi K, Tsuneyoshi M, Enjoji M (1985) Myositis ossificans: a clinicopathologic study of 21 cases. Acta Pathol Jpn 35:1109–1122
Thickman D, Bonakdarpour A, Clancy M et al. (1982) Fibrodysplasia ossificans progressiva. AJR 139:935–941

"Brown Tumor" of Hyperparathyroidism

Albright FC, Reifenstein EC (1948) The parathyroid glands and metabolic bone disease. Williams & Wilkins, Baltimore
Black BM (1953) Hyperparathyroidism. Charles C. Thomas, Springfield, IL
Campanacci M (1990) Bone and soft tissue tumors. Springer, Vienna New York
Castleman B (1952) Tumors of the parathyroid glands. Atlas of tumor pathology, series IV, Fasc 15. Armed Forces Institute of Pathology, Washington, DC
Castleman B, Mallory TB (1935) Pathology of parathyroid gland in hyperparathyroidism. Study of 25 cases. Am J Pathol 11:1–72
Hellström J (1957) Experience from 105 cases of hyperparathyroidism. Acta Chir Scand 113:501–505
Pugh DG (1958) The roentgenographic diagnosis of hyperparathyroidism. Surg Clin North Am 32:1017–1030
Uehlinger E (1940) Osteofibrosis deformans juvenilis. Virchows Arch [A] 306:255
von Recklinghausen FD (1891) Die fibröse oder deformierende Ostitis, die Osteomalacie und die osteoplastische Carcinose in ihren gegenseitigen Beziehungen. Virchow Festschrift. G. Reimer, Berlin
Woolner LB, Keating FR, Black BM (1952) Tumors and hyperplasia of the parathyroid glands: review of pathological findings in 140 cases of primary hyperparathyroidism. Cancer 5:1069–1088

Intraosseous Epidermoid Cyst

Byers P, Mangle J, Salm R (1953) Epidermoid (epithelial) cyst of the skeleton. Am J Surg 85:327
Byers P, Mantel J, Salm R (1966) Epidermal cysts of phalanges. J Bone Joint Surg [Br] 48:577
Dahlin DC (1978) Bone tumors, 3rd edn. Charles C. Thomas, Springfield, IL
Goldsmith E (1966) Solitary bone cyst of the distal phalanx: a case report. J Am Podiatr Assoc 56:69
Lerner M, Southwick WO (1968) Keratin cyst in phalangeal bones. J Bone Joint Surg [Am] 50:365
Roth S (1964) Squamous cysts involving the skull and distal phalanges. J Bone Joint Surg [Am] 46:1442
Schajowicz F, Aiello C, Slullitel I (1970) Cystic and pseudocystic lesions of the terminal phalanx with special reference to epidermoid cysts. Clin Orthop 68:84–92

Giant-Cell (Reparative) Granuloma

Ackerman LV, Spjut HJ (1962) Tumors of bone and cartilage. Atlas of tumor pathology, Fasc 4. Armed Forces Institute of Pathology, Washington, Dc
Bertheussen KJ, Holch S, Schoidt T (1983) Giant cell lesion of bone of the hand with particular emphasis on giant cell reparative granuloma. J Hand Surg [Am] 8:46
Campanacci M (1990) Bone and soft tissue tumors. Springer, Vienna New York
Caskey PM, Wolf MD, Fechner RE (1985) Multicentric giant cell reparative granuloma of the small bones of the hand: a case report and review of the literature. Clin Orthop 193:199
D'Alonzo RT, Pitcock JA, Milford LW (1972) Giant-cell reaction of bone. J Bone Joint Surg [Am] 54:1267

Glass TA, Mills SE, Fechner RE et al. (1983) Giant cell reparative granuloma of the hands and feet. Radiology 149:65
Jaffe HL (1953) Giant cell reparative granuloma, traumatic bone cyst and fibrous (fibro-osseous) dysplasia of the jaw bones. Oral Surg 6:159
Jernstrom P, Stark HH (1971) Giant cell reaction of a metacarpal. Am J Clin Pathol 55:77–81
Lorenzo JC, Dorfman HD (1980) Giant-cell reparative granuloma of the short tubular bones of the hands and feet. Am J Surg Pathol 4:551
Merkow RL, Bansal M, Inglis AE (1985) Giant cell reparative granuloma in the hand: report of three cases and review of the literature. J Hand Surg [Am] 10:733
Picci, P, Baldini N, Sudanese A et al. (1986) Giant cell reparative granuloma and other giant cell lesions of the bones of the hands and feet. Skeletal Radiol 15:415
Ratner V, Dorfman HD (1990) Giant-cell reparative granuloma of the hand and foot bones. Clin Orthop Rel Res 260:251–258
Schwinn P (1976) Giant cell lesions of bone. In: Bones and Joints. IAP Monogr No 17. Williams & Wilkins, Baltimore, pp 236–299
Wold LE, Dobyns JH, Swee RG, Dahlin DC (1986) Giant cell reaction (giant cell reparative granuloma) of the small bones of the hands and feet. Am J Surg Pathol 10:491
Wold LE, McLeod RA, Sim FH, Unni KK (1990) Atlas of orthopedic pathology. W.B. Saunders, Philadelphia

CHAPTER X

Current Concepts of Treatment of Bone Tumors

1. Giant-Cell Tumor: Staging and Treatment

STEVEN GITELIS

Giant-cell tumor of bone is a locally aggressive neoplasm that presents a management dilemma. This tumor frequently occurs in proximity to major weight-bearing joints (see Chap. III). In most reported series of giant-cell tumor, almost half of the neoplasms involve the distal femur or proximal tibia. They frequently cause significant bone destruction, placing the joint at great risk for pathologic fracture. Because of the propensity of giant-cell tumors to involve subchondral bone, care must be taken to try to preserve the articular surface during surgical management (Fig. X.1).

Treatment historically has ranged from curettage to en bloc resection. The problem with curettage, especially through a limited cortical window, is the relatively high reported incidence of local recurrence (Fig. X.2). Recurrence rates have ranged from 27% to 54% with this type of management and have led to alternative forms of treatment (Dahlin et al. 1970; Goldenberg et al. 1970; Larsson et al. 1975; Sanerkin 1980; McDonald et al. 1986).

En bloc resection of giant-cell tumor is a better oncologic surgical procedure, with much lower local recurrence rate reported. In several published series, local recurrence after en bloc resection has ranged from 0% to 32%. The problem with en bloc resection is the need for extensive reconstruction with possible morbidity (Figs. X.3, X.6). When the tumor lies in proximity to the joint, en bloc resection necessitates sacrificing the joint and thus requires some form of arthroplasty or arthrodesis (Ottolenghi 1972; Larsson et al. 1975; Sung et al. 1982; Campanacci et al. 1987; Carrasco and Murray 1989) (Fig. X.4).

In summary, curettage alone is an inadequate oncologic procedure for giant-cell tumor, while en bloc resection is adequate oncologically but may be associated with disability.

Before discussing current concepts in the management of giant-cell tumor, some definitions regarding surgical margins and staging are necessary. The definitions should be credited to William Enneking, M.D., and associates. They allow us to be consistent in our surgical descriptions, and more importantly, conceptualize surgical margin as it relates to tumor management (Enneking 1983a,b).

Staging of Benign Bone Tumors

Three benign stages exist (Fig. X.5):

Stage 1: a latent benign tumor without the tendency for local progression

Stage 2: an active tumor that tends to progress locally but is limited by natural boundaries such as the articular cartilage or cortex

Stage 3: an aggressive lesion that is not limited by natural boundaries

A giant-cell tumor destroying the cortex with a soft tissue mass is stage 3. Of note is that most giant-cell tumors of bone are either stage 2 or stage 3. During the evaluation of benign giant-cell tumor of bone, it is important to examine the chest by plain x-ray and computed tomography. This is to detect pulmonary metastases. These lesions, when present, may be removed by thoracotomy or sternotomy. There have been cases of spontaneous regression of benign pulmonary metastases reported (Rock et al. 1984; Bertoni et al. 1985; Wray et al. 1990).

Surgical Margins (Fig. X.6)

Intralesional is defined as a removal of the neoplasm by entering the tumor. The old concept of curettage is actually an intralesional excision. If this is done through a limited cortical window,

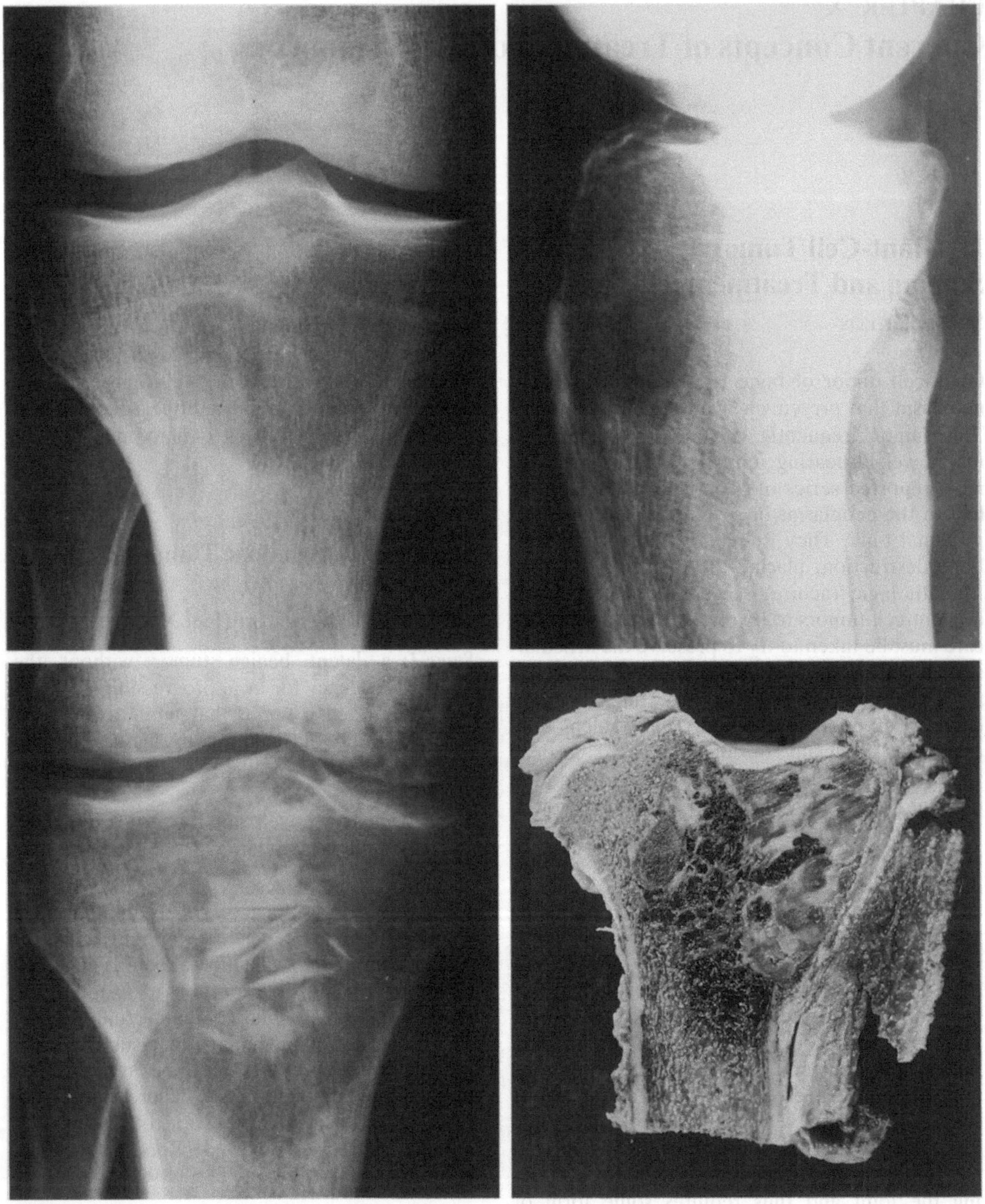
a
b
c

Fig. X.1. **a** Anteroposterior and lateral radiographs of giant-cell tumor of the proximal tibia. Note the extensive bone destruction in proximity to the articular surface. **b** Postoperative appearance after excision and autogenous bone graft; lytic area suggests local recurrence. **c** Specimen photograph after proximal tibial en bloc resection. A local recurrence is evident in the medial tibial plateau

Fig. X.2. Diagram of giant-cell tumor excision through a limited cortical window, "classic curettage"

Fig. X.3. Diagram of en bloc resection of giant-cell tumor of the distal femur. Depicted is an osteoarticular allograft reconstruction

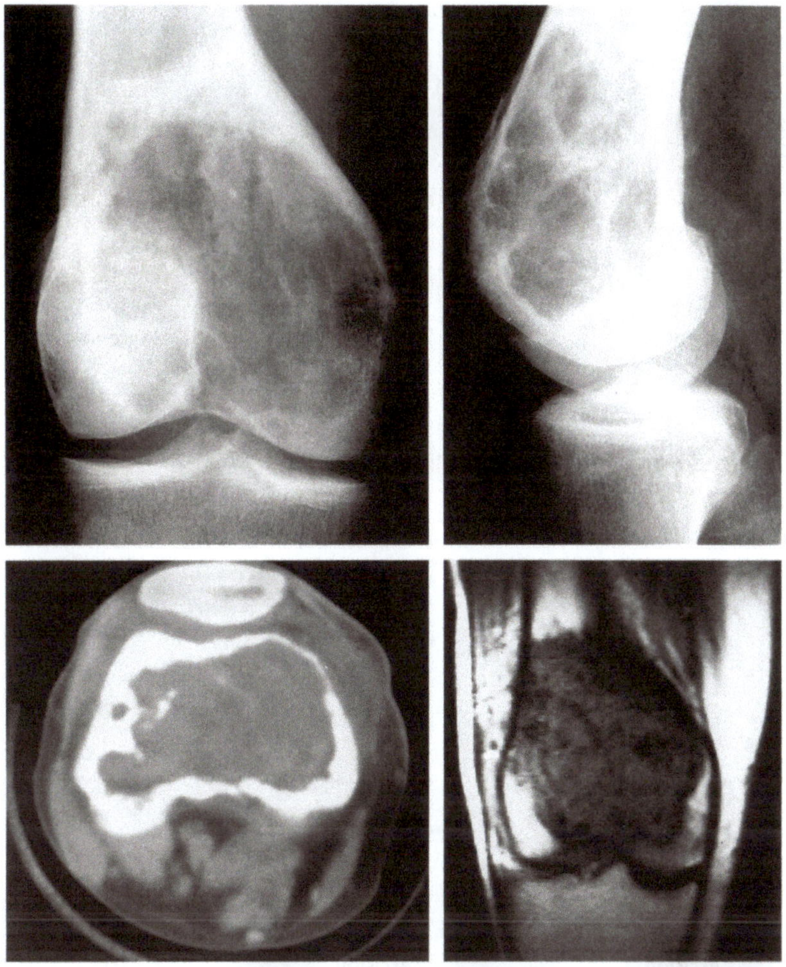

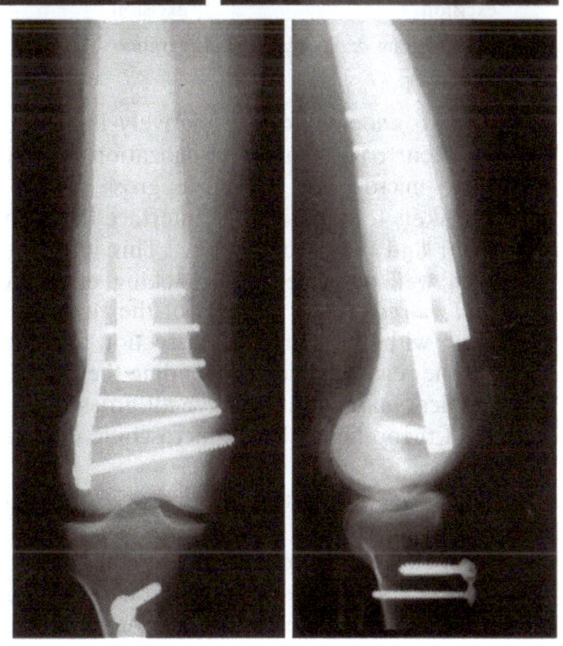

Fig. X.4. a Anteroposterior and lateral radiographs of distal femoral giant-cell tumor. **b** Computed tomogram of distal femoral giant-cell tumor. Note the marked bone destruction without soft tissue extension. **c** MR image (coronal) of distal femoral giant-cell tumor. T1-weighted coronal image shows the intraosseous extent of tumor. **d** Postoperative anteroposterior and lateral radiographs. Distal femoral giant-cell tumor treated by en bloc resection with osteoarticular allograft reconstruction. Note the preservation of the joint and excellent healing at the allograft–host junction

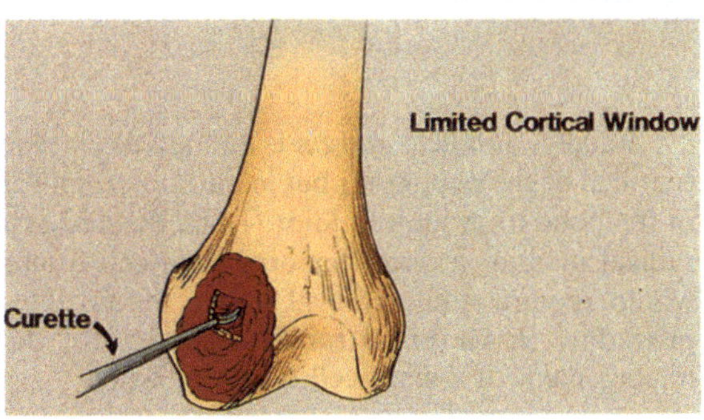

X.2

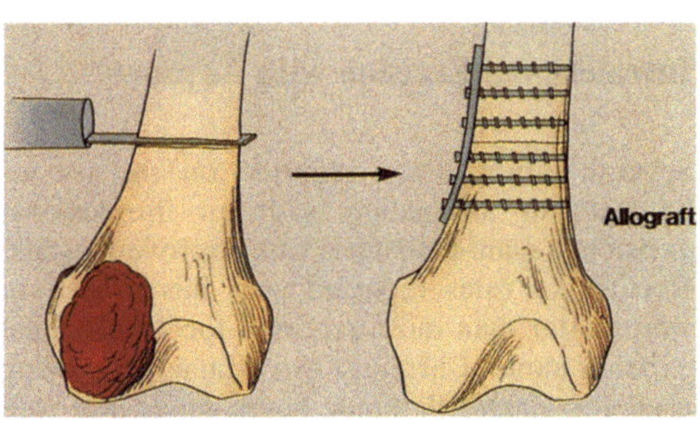

X.3

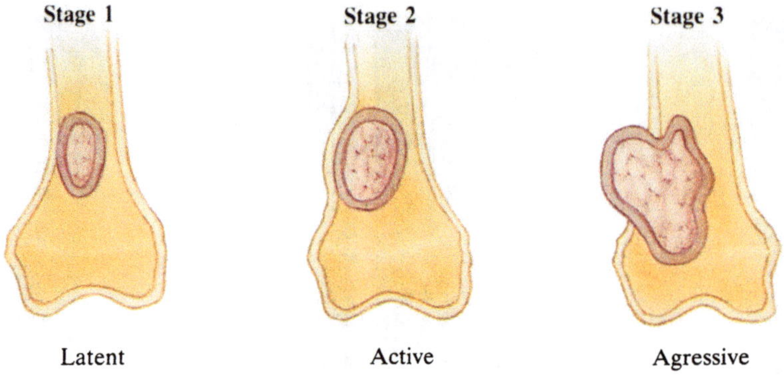

Fig. X.5. Diagram depicting the stages of benign bone tumors

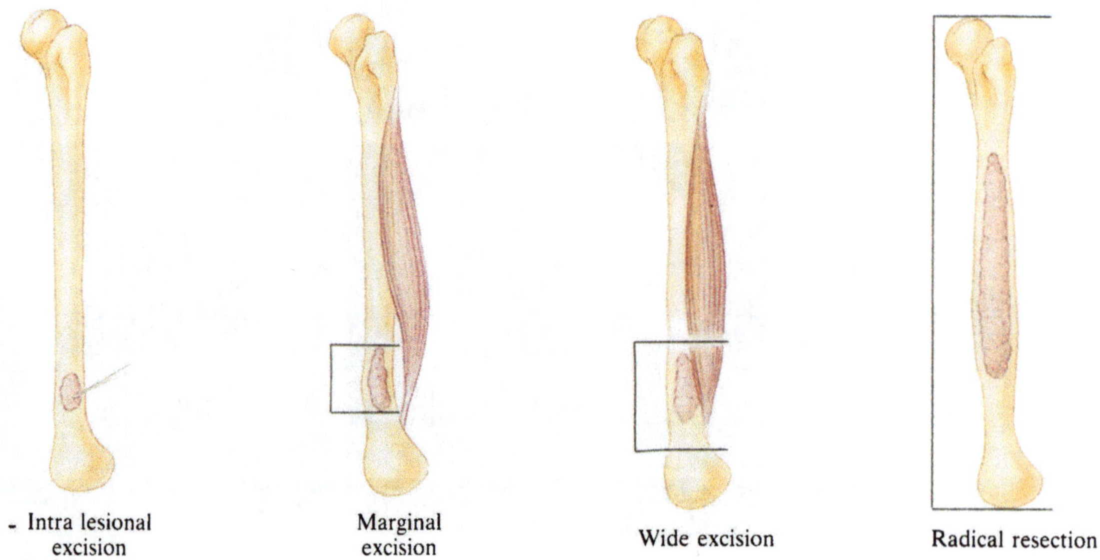

Fig. X.6. Diagram depicting surgical margins

it is easy to understand the relatively high rate of local recurrence. Tumor visualization is very poor, and microscopic as well as gross residual tumor is likely to remain at the interface between the tumor and the reactive bone. This interface has been well described by Enneking et al. A *marginal margin* is the removal of the tumor en bloc, but with the plane of dissection passing through the reactive zone surrounding the tumor. This surgical margin will remove all gross tumor but could theoretically leave microscopic disease in the tumor bed.

A *wide margin* is a surgical procedure that removes the tumor en bloc but takes a cuff of normal tissue completely encircling the tumor. The reactive zone and pseudocapsule are removed en bloc with the tumor. It must be emphasized that an en bloc procedure can be either marginal or wide, thus underlining the need for precise definitions when describing surgical margins.

Finally, a *radical margin* is defined as en bloc removal of the neoplasm, but in addition removal of the bone from joint to joint. To be defined as a radical margin, a distal femoral giant-cell tumor would require total removal of the femur. This procedure, however, is rarely necessary for the management of a giant-cell tumor of bone.

Intralesional Excision with Adjunct

Several authors have reported on the use of adjuncts in association with an intralesional excision of giant-cell tumor with improved results. Recurrence rates reported with this procedure were better than those reported for intralesional excision alone. Currently two adjuncts are being used for giant-cell tumor bone: liquid nitrogen and phenol. Liquid nitrogen causes thermal

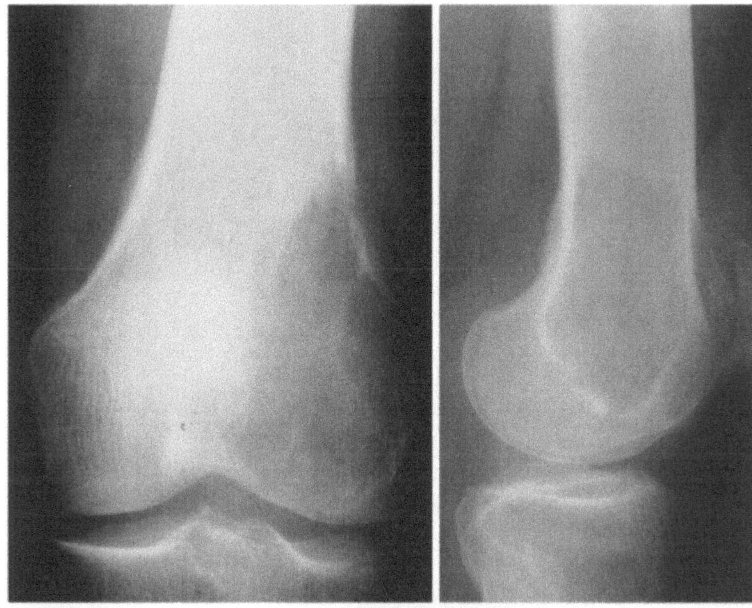

a

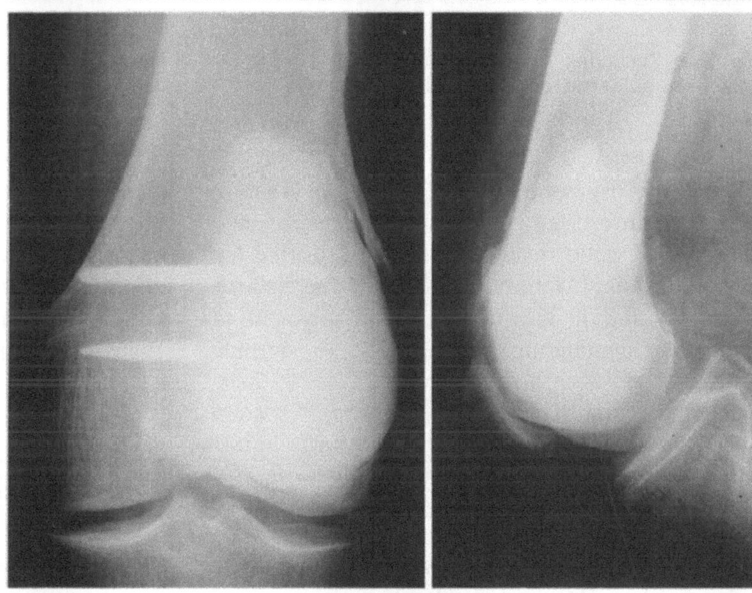

c

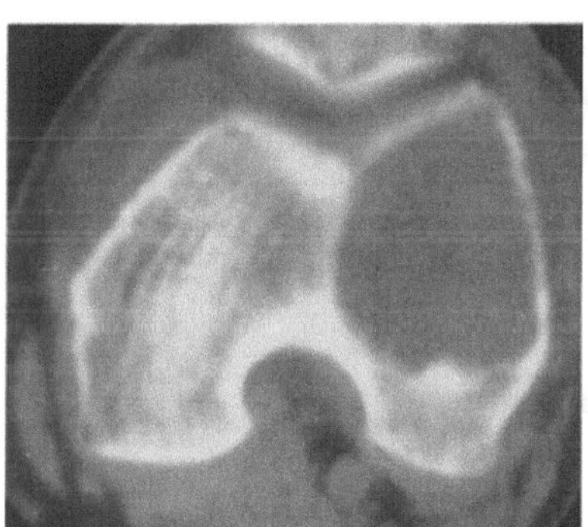

b

Fig. X.7. a Anteroposterior and lateral radiographs of distal femoral giant-cell tumor. **b** Computed tomogram of distal femoral giant-cell tumor. Note the bone destruction in the lateral femoral condyle. **c** Anteroposterior and lateral radiographs after intralesional excision. Note the internal fixation surrounded by methylmethacrylate. The acrylic supports the thin wafer of subchondral bone. **d** Anteroposterior radiograph of giant-cell tumor of the proximal tibia. **e** Cementations after intralesional excision

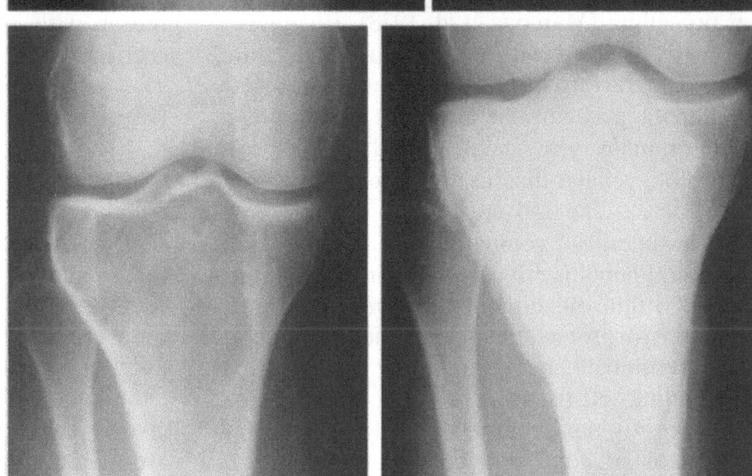

d e

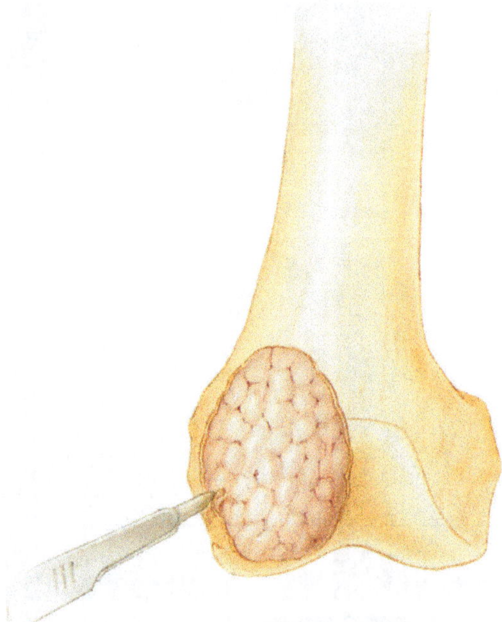

Fig. X.8. Rendering of the exteriorization process. A scalpel is used to excise the thinned cortical bone

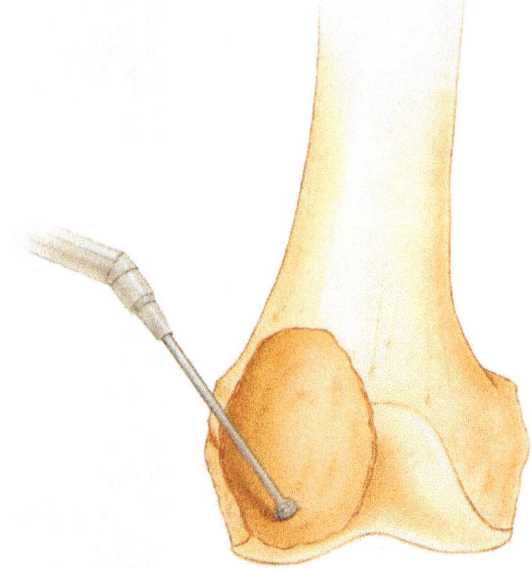

Fig. X.9. High-speed dental burr is used to clean the cavity after gross tumor debulking

necrosis by virtue of its freezing capacity. When it is used in an excised cavity after several freeze–thaw cycles, good results have been reported by several authors (Marcove et al. 1978; Jacobs and Clemency 1985). The use of liquid nitrogen is technically demanding (Lane 1989). A thermal couple is necessary to monitor the freeze–thaw cycle, and careful protection of the soft tissues is critical. One significant problem with liquid nitrogen is the amount of necrosis distal to the tumor cavity. The osseous necrosis extends centimeters beyond the cavity, leading to a relatively high incidence of pathologic fracture with this procedure (Marcove et al. 1978). Even when the cavity is filled with autogenous bone graft, pathologic fracture has been frequently reported.

Phenol is a cytotoxic substance that has been used for many years. When used in high concentration, cellular death can be seen (Lane 1989; Rock 1989). The kill created by phenol, however, is superficial compared with that of liquid nitrogen. Phenol is effective in killing any surface residue within the tumor bed. Great care must be taken to protect the soft tissues, as it does not discriminate between tumor and normal surrounding soft tissue.

Currently our preferred technique for giant-cell tumor of bone is a combination of intralesional excision, phenol cauterization, and methacrylation to reconstruct the bone defect. Methylmethacrylate acts as a bone filler and buttress, and may even have an adjunct oncologic effect by thermal necrosis and toxicity of the unpolymerized monomer (Persson and Wouters 1976; Mjöberg et al. 1984; Persson et al. 1984; Frassica et al. 1989; Rock 1989) (Fig. X.7).

Surgical Technique

The surgical procedure to remove a giant-cell tumor with an adjunct needs to be carefully carried out, in a very precise stepwise manner. The first part of the procedure is *exteriorization* (Fig. X.8).

The tumor is exposed and the thin cortical bone rim removed to expose the tumor completely. A useful technique is to excise the cortical shell with a scalpel until it no longer can cut the remaining bone. Once this cortical shell is removed, sponges are packed around the cavity to prevent spillage. The excision is performed initially with large instruments to perform a gross debulking of the tumor. Once the tumor has been grossly debulked, progressively smaller curettes are used until no visible tumor is seen. The cavity is further cleaned by using a high-speed dental

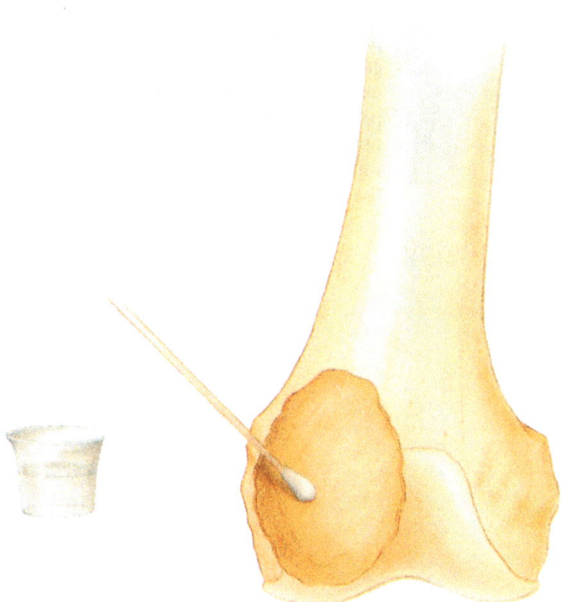

Fig. X.10. Phenol is applied to the cavity to chemically necrose any residual cells

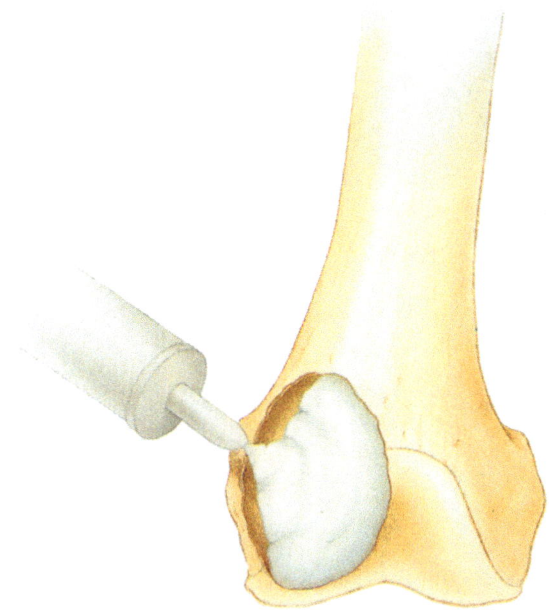

Fig. X.11. Methylmethacrylate is injected into the cavity. As the cement polymerizes, it is molded to the contour of the bone

burr on all bony surfaces (Fig. X.9). The exposed articular cartilage needs to be carefully cleaned but not traumatized.

Cauterization

Electrocautery is next used to cauterize the soft tissue margin around the tumor cavity where the dental burr cannot be used. Pulsatile lavage is used to clean the cavity, followed by careful drying. Phenol is dabbed into the bony cavity using a cotton-tipped applicator (Fig. X.10). After coating the cavity with the phenol solution, it is next removed by washing the surface with absolute alcohol, which brings the phenol into solution. The cavity is again cleaned with pulsatile lavage and, if necessary, the articular cartilage can be grafted with autogenous bone taken from the iliac crest (Frassica et al. 1989). After grafting has been completed, the cavity is packed with methylmethacrylate (Fig. X.11). Internal fixation is used when necessary. The methylmethacrylate needs to be molded while in its doughy form into the shape of the osseous defect.

Generally, early weight-bearing is allowed with joint rehabilitation. These patients are limited in their running and heavy lifting, but otherwise are allowed unrestricted use of their joint. At least conceptually, an intralesional excision with an adjunct will extend the margin from an intralesional margin to a wide margin.

In conclusion, an intralesional excision of giant-cell tumor alone does not appear to be an adequate oncologic procedure. An en bloc resection, while oncologically adequate, may be too aggressive and ultimately associated with morbidity and disability. An *intralesional excision* with adjunct may represent a solution to the surgical dilemma. It is oncologically adequate and allows joint preservation.

Just for completeness, there are giant-cell tumors that are not good candidates for an intralesional excision with adjunct. Expendable bones, such as the proximal fibula and ulna, are good candidates for en bloc resection (Fig. X.12). Since reconstruction is not necessary, morbidity is limited.

The radius is a common anatomic location for giant-cell tumor and needs special consideration. While some such tumors are amenable to intralesional excision, most require en bloc resection due to the large amount of bone destruction. If a decision is made to perform en bloc resection of the distal radius, various reconstructive options are available and need to be considered. If the patient is a candidate for an arthroplasty, this can be accomplished by either an autogenous bone and joint graft or an osteoarticular allograft. The

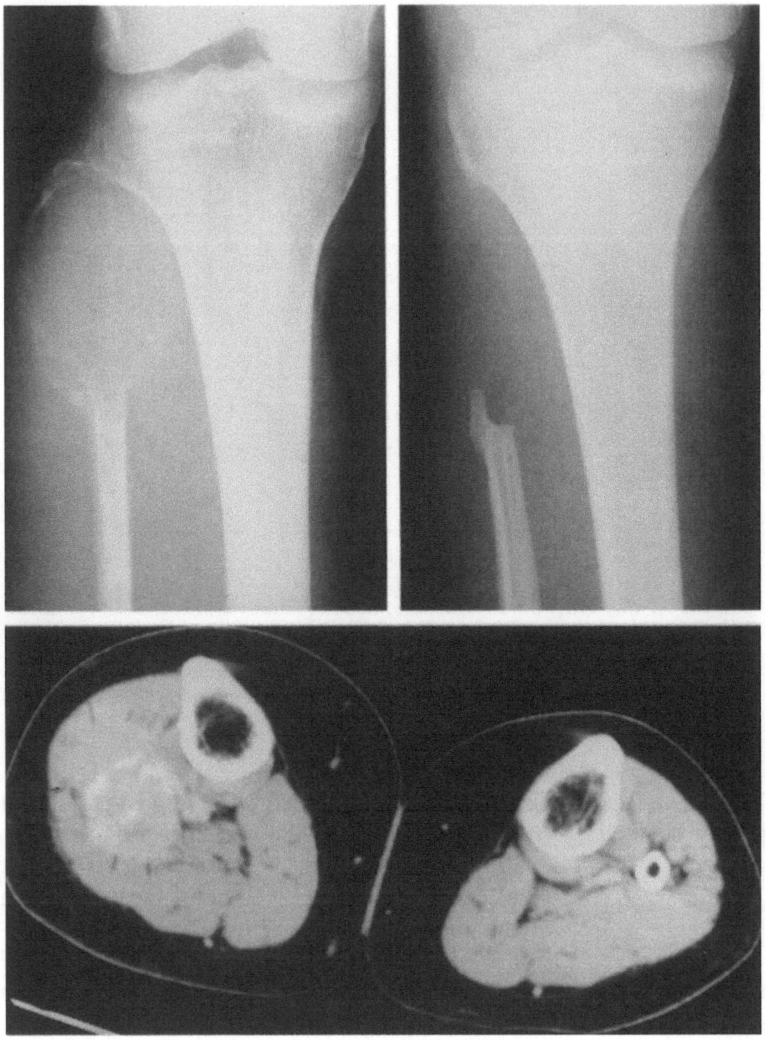

a c b

Fig. X.12. a Anteroposterior radiograph of giant-cell tumor of the proximal fibula. **b** Computed tomogram of right and left legs. Note the expansion and destruction of the right proximal fibula compared with the normal left fibula. **c** Anteroposterior radiograph after en bloc resection of the giant-cell tumor

proximal fibula has been successfully used as a replacement for the distal radius for many years (Lackman et al. 1987). The articular surface of the tibiofibular joint is similar to the distal radiocarpal articulation, and joint congruency can be obtained. The advantage of this form of arthroplasty is that the bone graft is autogenous, and as a result is rapidly incorporated. Its disadvantage is the disruption of the patient's tibiofibular joint with some inherent instability. An alternative to autogenous grafting is the use of a fresh-frozen osteoarticular allograft. This reconstruction will allow for a mobile wrist joint. Graft incorporation, fracture, and degeneration of the articulation are problems that are seen with this form of reconstruction. Centralization of the carpus over the ulna is a salvage type of reconstruction that can leave patients with a mobile wrist joint.

A second form of reconstruction after distal radius en bloc resection is an arthrodesis. An arthrodesed wrist is inherently stable and associated with fewer complications than an arthroplasty. It is particularly useful for heavy manual laborers. Arthrodesis can be achieved by either a fibular autograft or a fresh-frozen allograft.

Aggressive giant-cell tumor that destroys a large portion or a bone and joint that preclude joint preservation should be considered for an en bloc resection with reconstruction by either arthroplasty or arthrodesis. Reconstruction by autogenous grafting, allograft, or prosthesis should be individualized based on patient need, desire, and functional demand (Ottolenghi 1972; Campanacci and Costa 1979; Sim et al. 1987; Campanacci et al. 1987; Mankin et al. 1987; Hackbarth 1991) (Fig. X.13).

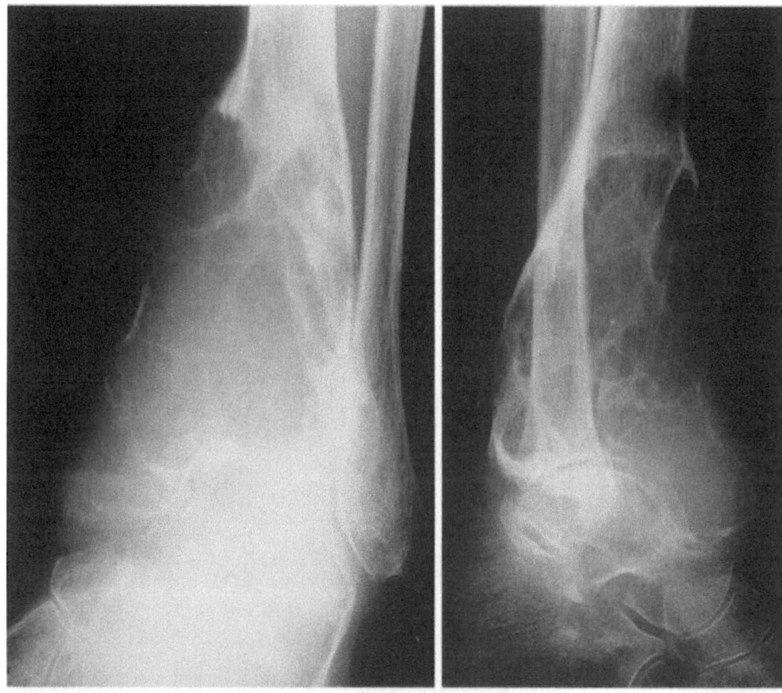
a

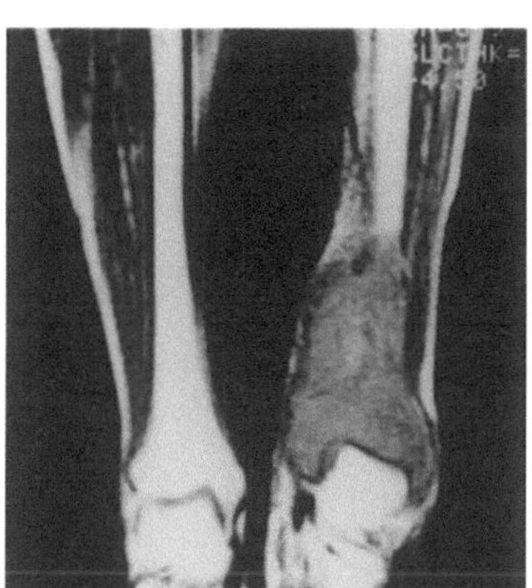
b

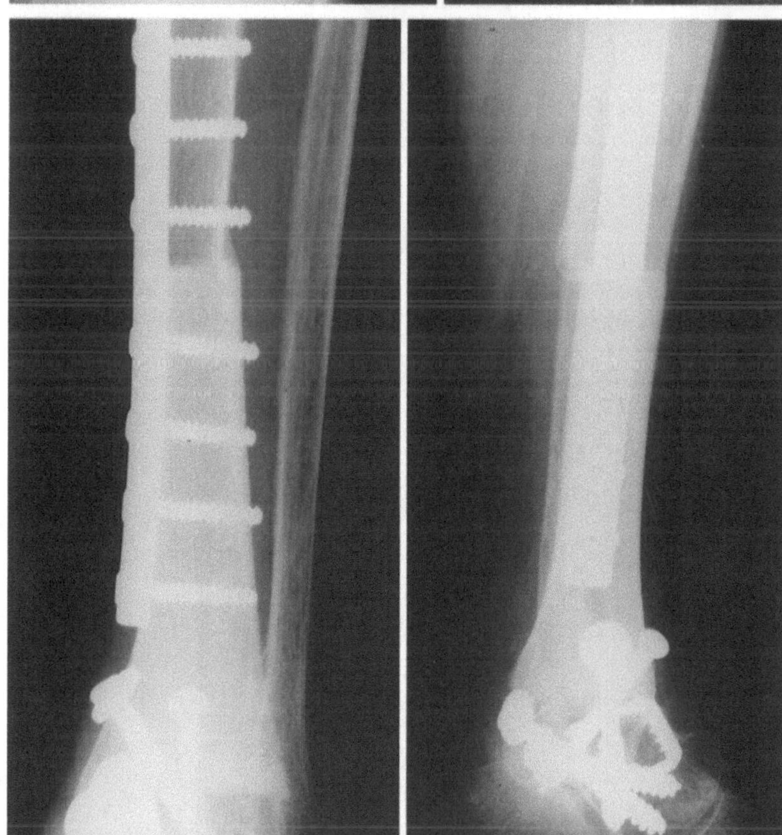
c

Fig. X.13. **a** Anteroposterior and lateral radiographs of large destructive giant-cell tumor of the distal tibia. **b** MR image (coronal) of distal tibial giant-cell tumor. **c** Anteroposterior and lateral radiographs after distal tibial en bloc resection. Intercalary allograft was used for ankle arthrodesis

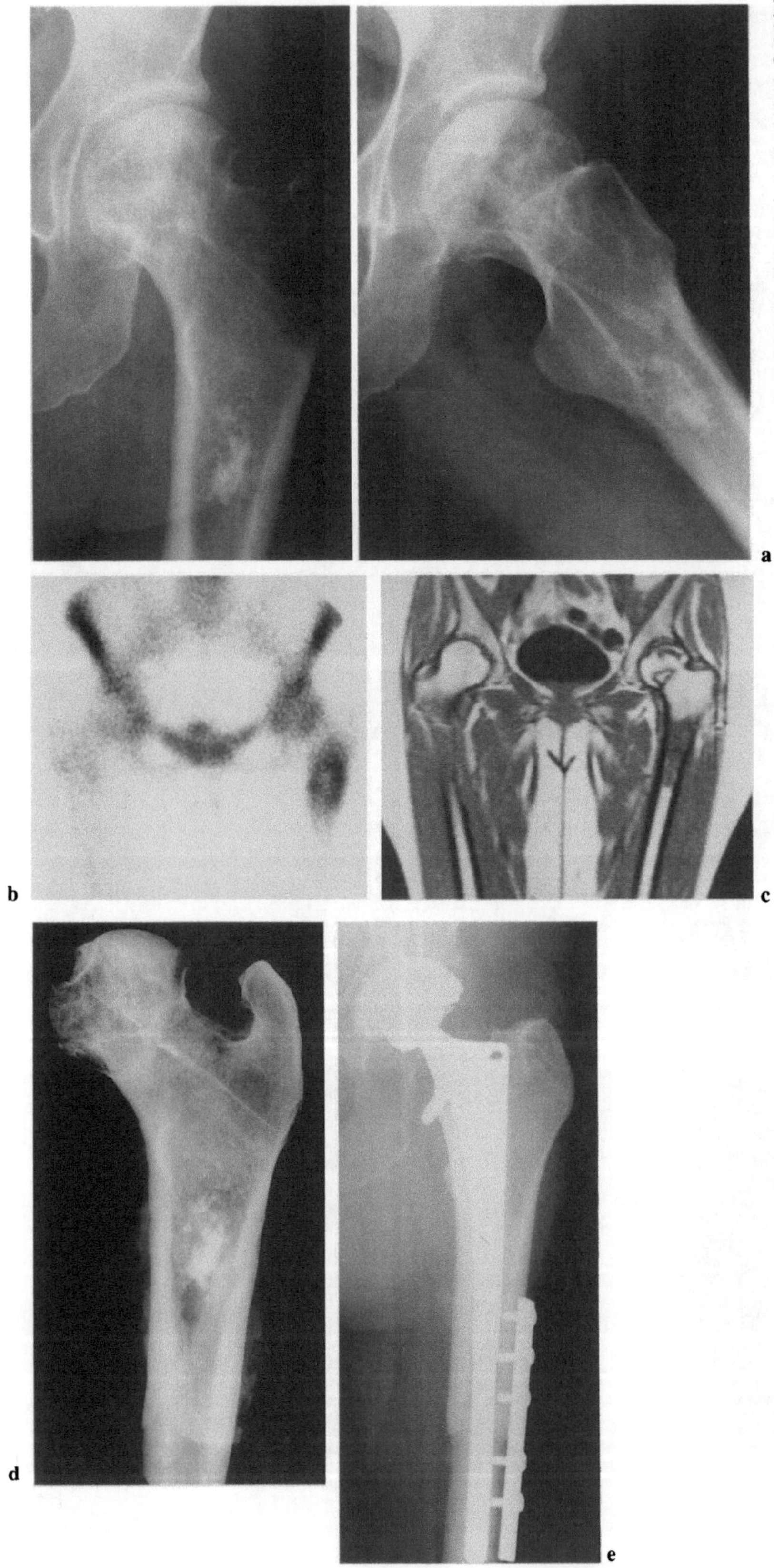

Fig. X.14. a Anteroposterior and lateral radiographs of dedifferentiated chondrosarcoma of hip and upper femur. Osteonecrosis of femoral head is evident. A calcified metadiaphyseal lesion is present, with surrounding lysis. **b** Technetium bone scan showing uptake by the tumor and secondary uptake by osteonecrosis of femoral head. **c** MR image of upper femur revealing both dedifferentiated chondrosarcoma and osteonecrosis of the femoral head. **d** Specimen radiograph. **e** Anteroposterior radiograph following wide en bloc resection of upper femur with allograft-prosthetic composite reconstruction

Giant-cell tumor located in a surgically inaccessible location such as the spine or sacrum poses an even greater problem (Turcotte et al. 1989). If it is felt that surgical excision is impossible, irradiation can be successfully used for local control. The risk of postradiation sarcoma is clearly present and needs to be strongly considered (Bell et al. 1983; Chen et al. 1986).

In a recent review of the management of giant-cell tumor of bone at Rush-Presbyterian-St. Luke's Medical Center, patients treated by en bloc resection (20) were compared with those treated with intralesional excision (20) along with phenol cauterization. The osseous defect in these cases was filled with methylmethacrylate. In this retrospective clinical review the local recurrence rate for both procedures was quite low, with only one (intralesional excision) of 40 patients suffering a local recurrence, 63 months following surgery. We found also that the complication rate for intralesional excision with adjunct was much lower than for en bloc resection, and functional results were far better for the former group.

We concluded that intralesional excision of giant-cell tumor of bone with adjunct is a successful oncologic procedure with excellent functional results and few complications. En bloc resection, while curative, is associated with significant morbidity, and should be reserved for expendable bones or large aggressive or recurrent giant-cell tumors.

2. Chondrosarcoma

Steven Gitelis

Chondrosarcoma of bone is a malignant neoplasm that can be both locally aggressive and potentially metastatic. Numerous studies have shown that survival is related to the stage of the tumor and the adequacy of its treatment (Evans et al. 1977; Sannerkin and Gallagher 1979; Gitelis et al. 1981).

For the most part, chondrosarcoma of bone is treated by surgery. The exceptions to this rule are two high-grade variants: dedifferentiated chondrosarcoma and mesenchymal chondrosarcoma. Both are associated with significant mortality and usually require a form of adjuvant or even neoadjuvant chemotherapy as part of their management (Harwood et al. 1980a; Bertoni et al. 1983; Huvos et al. 1983; Frassica et al. 1986; Capanna et al. 1988) (Fig. X.14). Conventional chondrosarcoma of bone, on the other hand, does not appear to be responsive to either radiation or chemotherapy, thus making surgery the mainstay of treatment.

Before biopsy, *staging of chondrosarcoma* must be performed. This is true not only for this neoplasm, but for all primary tumors of bone. The staging of bone tumors has been well described by Enneking (1983), and direct correlation between stage and prognosis has been reported. In order to stage a bone tumor, several facts need to be known, including the histologic grade of the tumor, its compartmental anatomy, and the presence or absence of metastatic disease (Fig. X.15).

The histologic grade is typically determined at the time of biopsy. The highest grade tissue from the biopsy determines the tumor grade. Even if the bulk of the tumor is low grade, as long as a small portion is high-grade sarcoma then the overall grade is considered high. This can be problematic because of sampling errors. It is not uncommon to see variable areas of malignancy within a chondrosarcoma.

Low-grade tumors such as grade I chondrosarcoma are considered stage I, whereas high-grade tumors such as dedifferentiated chondrosarcoma or mesenchymal chondrosarcoma are considered stage II. If metastatic disease is recognized, either regional lymphatic, bone, or pulmonary, then the tumor is regarded as stage III.

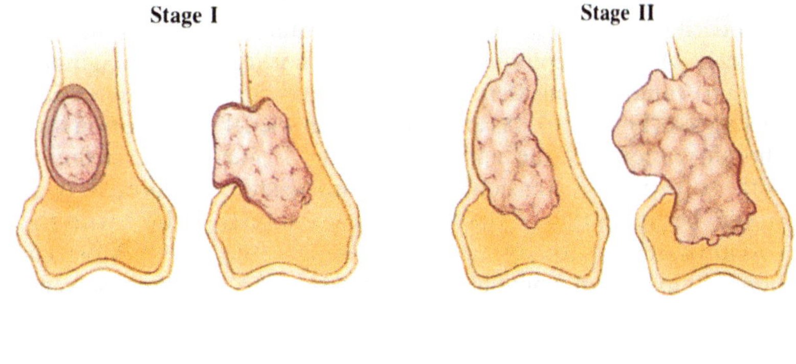

Fig. X.15. Diagram of staging of bone sarcomas. Low-grade lesions are stage I; high-grade lesions are stage II; metastatic lesions are stage III. Intraosseous lesions are "A" and extraosseous lesions are "B"

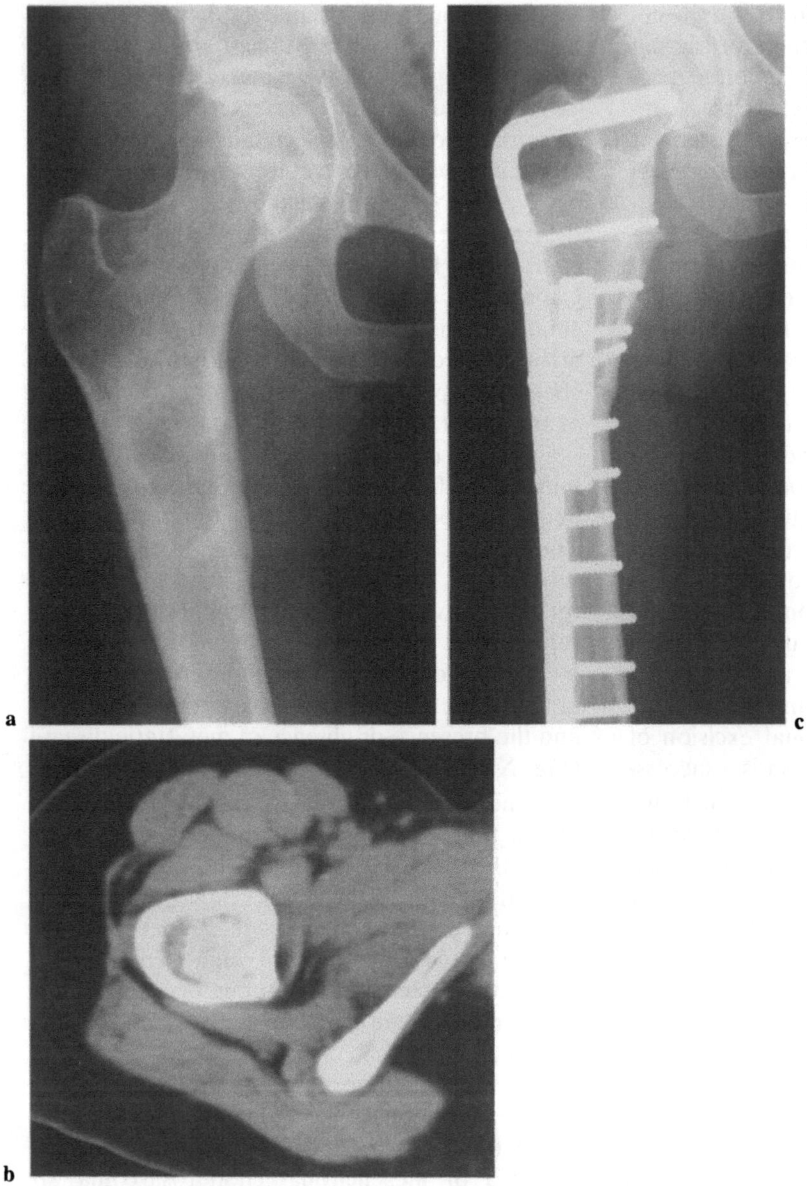

Fig. X.16. a Anteroposterior radiograph of low-grade (I) chondrosarcoma. Note the cortical thickening. **b** Computed tomogram of femur. Medullary calcification is evident but the lesion is contained within the bone (stage IA). **c** Anteroposterior radiograph after *wide* en bloc resection. Intercalary allograft was used to reconstruct the defect

Studies to specifically detect the presence of occult metastatic disease need to be performed prior to the completion of staging. Each stage is either stage A or B, based upon compartmental anatomy. For bone tumors, any lesion that destroys the cortex and extends to the soft tissues would be considered extracompartmental or stage B. A totally contained (within the cortical margin) tumor is considered intracompartmental or stage A (Fig. X.16). As an example, a grade III chondrosarcoma of the upper end of the femur with soft tissue extension, but nonmetastatic, would be stage IIB. A low-grade conventional chondrosarcoma totally contained within the bone compartment would be considered stage IA.

As stated earlier, conventional chondrosarcoma of bone, either central or peripheral, is best treated by surgery (Kaufman et al. 1977; Eriksson et al. 1980; Healy and Lane 1986). The goal of surgery is to achieve a wide margin at the time of en bloc resection (Gitelis et al. 1981). It is important to note that during biopsy of cartilaginous tumors, great care must be taken to minimize tumor spillage. These tumors are notorious for soft tissue implantation, and when the definitive surgical procedure is being performed, it is important to excise the biopsy site en bloc with the specimen.

Most chondrosarcomas can be managed by limb salvage (Smith and Simon 1975; Marcove

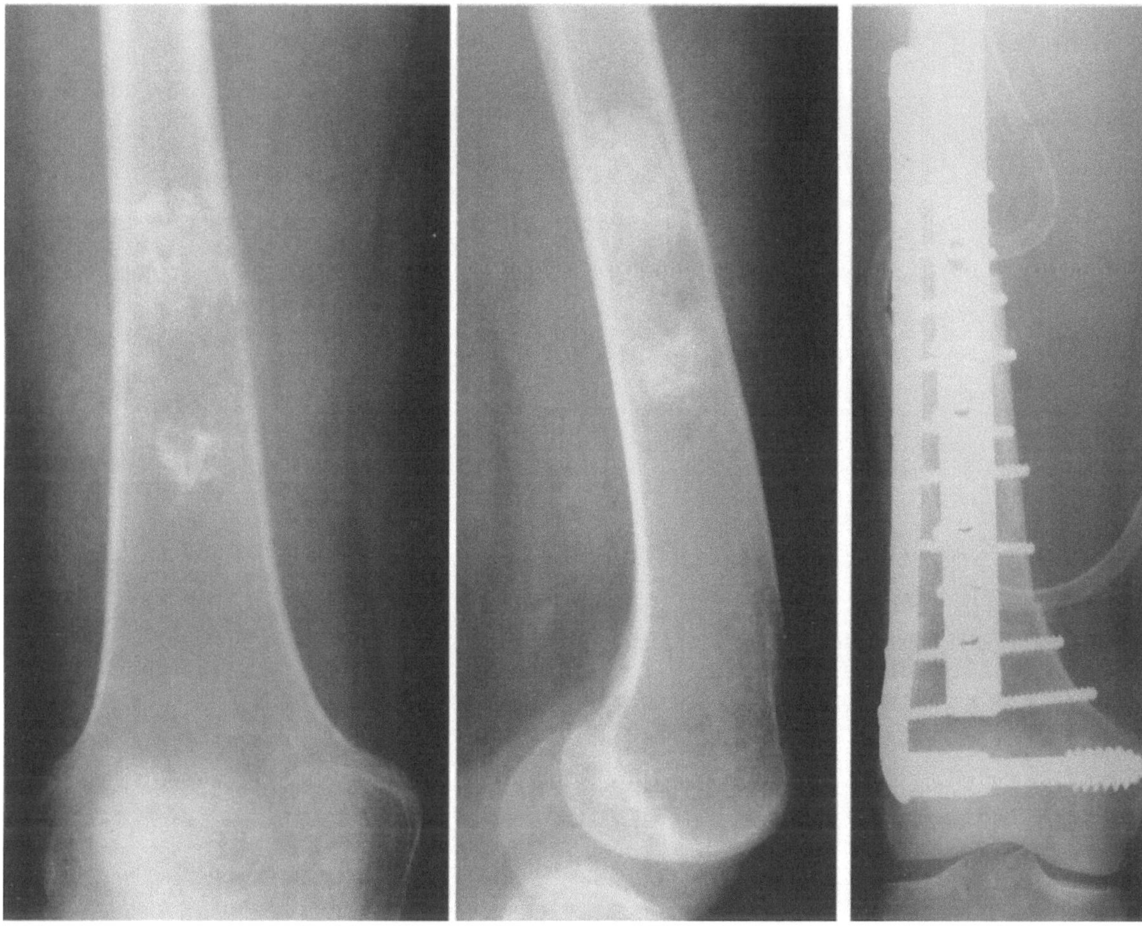

a b

Fig. X.17. **a** Anteroposterior and lateral radiographs of diaphyseal chondrosarcoma (low-grade, "I"). **b** Anteroposterior radiograph after *wide* en bloc resection with intercalary allograft reconstruction

1977; Malawer et al. 1985). The ideal surgical margin is *wide*. This implies en bloc removal of the tumor along with a cuff of normal tissue encircling the neoplasm (Fig. X.17). For intraosseous chondrosarcoma without soft tissue extension, a segment of bone needs to be removed extending well beyond the margins of the tumor. Imaging studies such as MRI and computed tomography are particularly useful in determining the extent of tumor, thus indicating where the surgical cuts in the bone need to be made (Hudson et al. 1984). Following wide en bloc resection, some form of reconstruction will be necessary. This can range from prosthetic replacement of bone and joint to fresh-frozen allograft reconstruction. The combination of these two techniques as an allograft prosthetic composite has also proven to be an effective means of reconstruction.

Intralesional excision with or without chemical cauterization has been used in some low-grade chondrosarcomas (Marcove et al. 1977b). This procedure should be reserved for very low grade lesions where en bloc resection cannot be performed. Peripheral chondrosarcomas require not only surgical excision of bone but also of surrounding muscle to achieve wide margins. MRI scans are particularly useful for this tumor to determine the relationship of the tumor to the neurovascular bundle. Reconstruction can be performed in a similar manner as described above.

The *pelvis* is a frequent location for chondrosarcoma. Various forms of wide en bloc resection of the pelvis have been described (Marcove et al. 1972; Guerra et al. 1985; Campanacci and Capanna 1991). There are three basic types of resection, each requiring a different form of reconstruction.

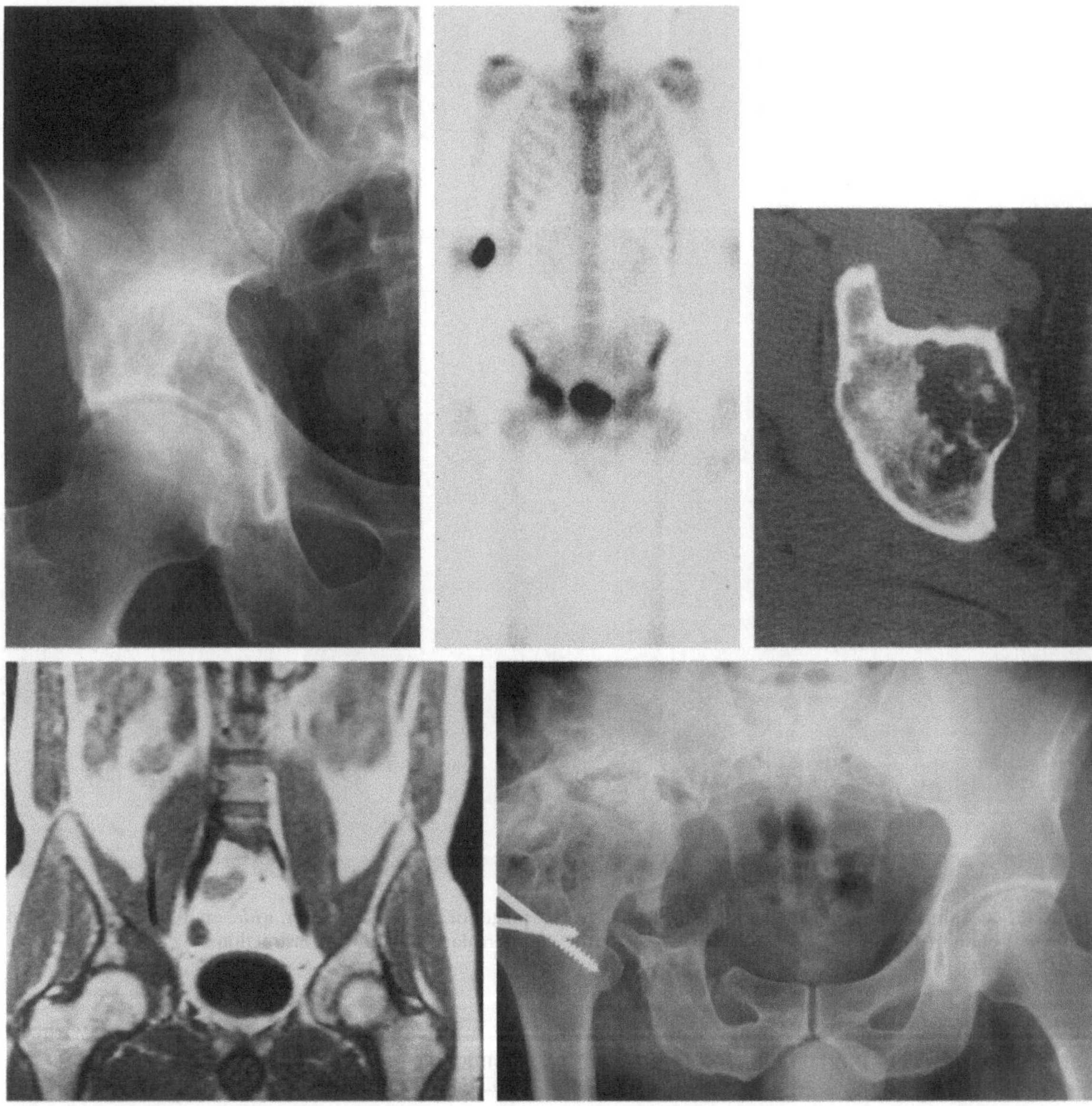

a b, c d e

Fig. X.18. **a** Anteroposterior radiograph of periacetabular chondrosarcoma (high-grade, "II"). **b** Technetium bone scan showing periacetabular uptake. **c** Computed tomogram of chondrosarcoma showing cortical destruction and soft tissue extension (stage IIB). **d** MR image of chondrosarcoma. Note the abnormal signal well visualized by the right acetabulum. **e** Postoperative anteroposterior radiograph. Periacetabular resection with pseudoarthrosis. Note the heterotopic bone present

Anterior arch resection below the level of the acetabulum and involving the superior and inferior pubic rami generally requires no reconstruction.

Chondrosarcoma that is located in a *periacetabular* location represents the most difficult reconstructive problem (Marcove et al. 1972) (Fig. X.18). Once a wide en bloc resection is performed, then the hip joint itself needs to be reconstructed. Options include: (a) allowing the femoral head to form a pseudoarthrosis up against the ilium or sacrum with inherent instability, (b) an osteoarticular pelvic allograft, (c) hip arthrodesis using a cobra plate fusing the femoral head to the ilium, and (d) a prosthetic replacement either in the form of a total hip arthroplasty or a custom pelvic prosthesis. A "saddle" prosthesis is available for this form of reconstruction.

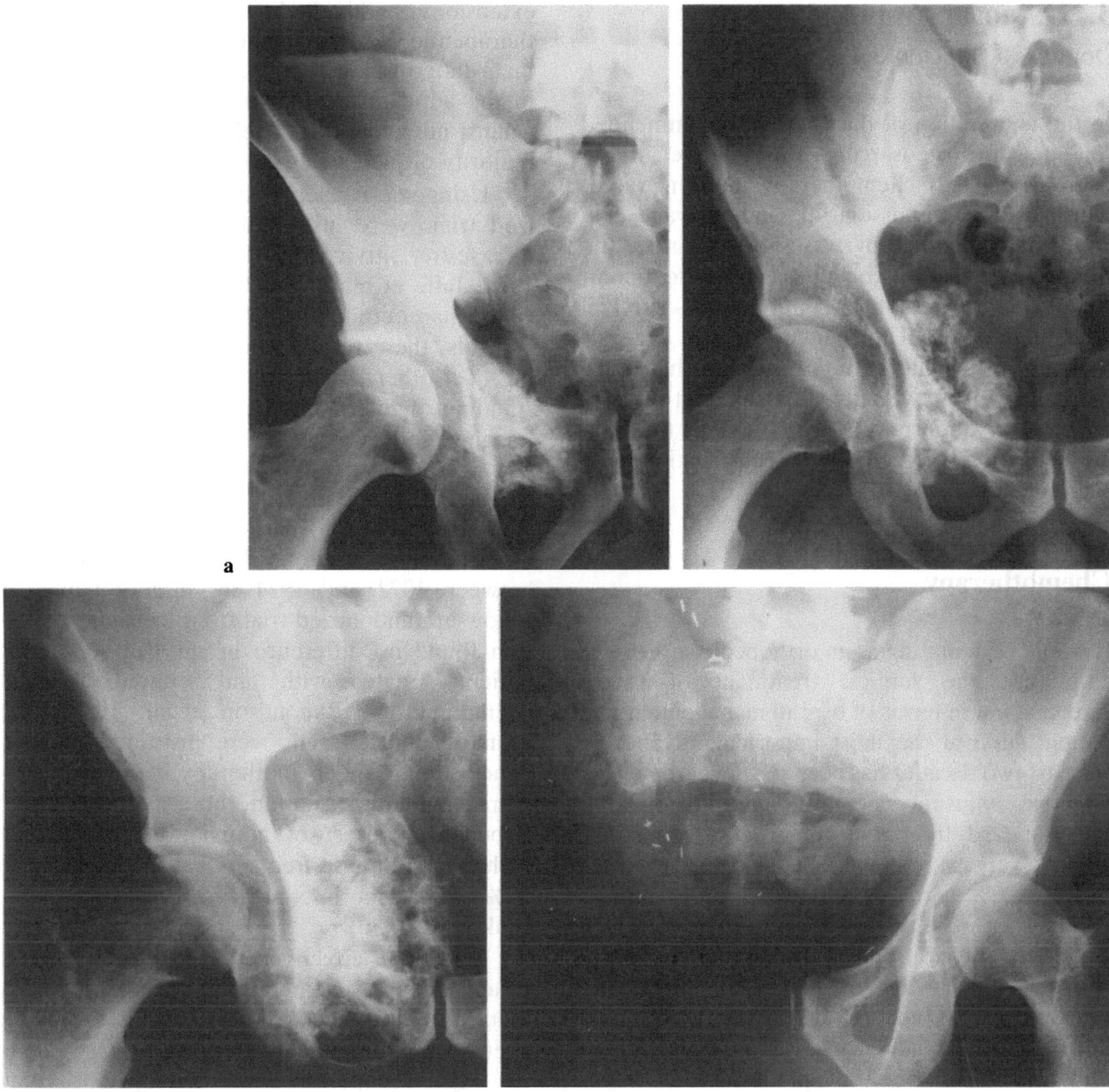

Fig. X.19. a Anteroposterior radiograph of peripheral chondrosarcoma. **b** Anteroposterior radiograph of chondrosarcoma showing progression despite conventional irradiation. **c** Anteroposterior radiograph showing further progression of the lesion. **d** Anteroposterior radiograph after hemipelvectomy

Finally, the third type of resection of the pelvis would be one of the *iliac wing*. This en bloc resection preserves the acetabulum, generally resecting bone above the sciatic notch. Reconstruction of the pelvic ring can be accomplished by autografts or allografts.

In conclusion, chondrosarcoma of bone should be treated by wide en bloc resection whenever possible, as this surgical margin will predictably achieve adequate local control. Chondrosarcoma located axially, such as in the spine, is more problematic from a surgical point of view. When it is felt that resection is impossible or wide en bloc margins cannot be achieved, the only reasonable alternative for local control is radiation (Fig. X.19). The only form of radiation that has proven to be effective for chondrosarcoma is neutron bombardment. If a linear accelerator is available, then this form of radiation should be considered for inoperable chondrosarcoma (Harwood et al. 1980b; Kim et al. 1983; Krochak et al. 1983; Cohen et al. 1984).

3. Osteosarcoma

DOUGLAS J. MCDONALD

In the first edition of this text the recommended treatment for osteosarcoma was ablative surgery with associated chemotherapy and/or radiotherapy. The discussion of limb salvage and adjuvant chemotherapy was short. Clearly, the treatment of osteosarcoma has evolved to a point where one can no longer simply discuss survival after amputation. The standard of care suggests that survival should be improved and that limbs be preserved. As we move into the next decade, limb preservation may not be enough; the limb must function better and the reconstruction must last longer.

Chemotherapy

It would be tempting as an orthopedic surgeon to emphasize the surgical treatment of osteosarcoma, yet in terms of overall management and patient survival the most important advance in the past two decades has been the development of effective adjuvant chemotherapy. Historically, the standard treatment for osteosarcoma was ablative surgical removal. Five-year survival rates of 15%–20% were reported by numerous authors and have become the historical controls by which current results are judged (Dahlin and Coventry 1967; Friedman and Carter 1972; Mike and Marcove 1978; Gehan et al. 1978). Clearly, with local recurrence after amputation occurring in only 2% of cases, most patients with osteosarcoma had metastatic disease at the time of their initial surgical treatment. With this observation it is reasonable to consider osteosarcoma a "systemic" disease at onset.

Crucial in the development of adjuvant treatment was the finding by Jaffe that intravenous methotrexate with citrovorum factor rescue could cause established metastatic disease to regress (Jaffe 1972; Jaffe et al. 1974). Further investigations found that the response was in part dose related, may potentiate the effects of radiotherapy, and overall gave a response rate of approximately 30% (Rosen et al. 1975; Jaffe et al. 1973, 1981). Other agents, particularly adriamycin and *cis*-platinum, were also found to have an effect on overt pulmonary disease (Bonnadonna et al. 1970; Gottlieb et al. 1975; Ochs et al. 1978; Pratte et al. 1985). The natural extension of this finding was that if chemotherapeutic agents could make measurable metastatic disease regress, then perhaps if used in the adjuvant setting they would be effective against micrometastases felt to be present in the majority of patients at presentation.

Using these agents, a number of randomized trials were instituted and reported 5-year disease-free survivals of 45%–60% (Cortes et al. 1974; Jaffe et al. 1978a; Rosenberg et al. 1979; Campanacci et al. 1981). Compared to historical controls, these results were obviously encouraging. Yet other factors, including a better understanding of tumor biology, improved diagnostic imaging, and an aggressive approach to diagnosis and treatment were also contributing to improved survival. Taylor et al. (1978), in a nonrandomized study, reported a 5-year survival of 62% with a disease-free survival of 43% in 41 patients treated between 1972 and 1974 by surgery alone. A follow-up randomized trial from the same institution found no difference in survival comparing patients treated with and without adjuvant chemotherapy (Edmondson et al. 1984). Yet as more clinical trials were instituted the evidence supporting chemotherapy became clearer. Almost without exception, these studies reported a beneficial effect of adjuvant chemotherapy, with 5-year disease-free survival in the range of 50%–70% (Goorin et al. 1985; Bacci et al. 1986; Link et al. 1986).

With the effectiveness of selected agents established in overt metastatic disease and micrometastatic disease, logic also suggested that the agents should be effective on the primary tumor as well. Preoperative or neoadjuvant treatment developed in conjunction with increased enthusiasm for limb salvage. Treatment was instituted immediately following diagnosis, during the period required to manufacture a custom prosthesis (Rosen et al. 1976; Jaffe et al. 1978b). With current modular prostheses and the availability of stored large fragment allografts, surgical resection does not have to be delayed for lack of a reconstruction, yet preoperative treatment does have a number of other potential advantages. Most importantly, it provides an in vitro test of the tumor's response to the agents used. High tumor necrosis measured at surgical resection has been correlated with improved patient prognosis (Rosen et al. 1982; Rosen 1985; Picci et al. 1985; Bacci et al. 1990). Poor response suggests that different chemotherapeutic agents should be used. The degree of necrosis which is considered "good" is controversial and subjective, but most authors suggest more than 90%. Another potential advantage of pretreatment is that it may allow for more limb salvage surgery. If the response to the treatment is good, the tumor stops growing and the soft tissue extension "matures" with an associated decrease in the local inflammatory response. This may create a margin between the tumor and uninvolved tissue which is more distinct, thus allowing for a safer limb-sparing resection. Many investigators have utilized preoperative chemotherapy as part of their treatment plan. Rosen (1985) reported the results of neoadjuvant treatment in four successive protocols over a 10-year period. Overall disease-free survival in 208 patients was 52%, with survival of 77% observed in 87 patients on the most recent (T-10) protocol. In general, survival with neoadjuvant treatment has been reported within the range of 60% to 75% with an associated increase in the use of limb salvage.

Whether neoadjuvant therapy is more effective than adjuvant treatment (using the same agents) in improving disease-free survival is unclear. Perhaps the "earlier" treatment of micrometastases may make a difference in a few patients, but the apparent increase in survival seen with some neoadjuvant trials may be secondary to the addition of more effective agents rather than the sequence of treatment. This is supported by the experience from the Rizzoli Institute, where patients treated with adjuvant therapy were compared with those patients who received the same drug in neoadjuvant form. No difference in disease-free survival was seen (Avella et al. 1988).

The major disadvantage of neoadjuvant treatment is the potential delay in definitive local treatment in the event that the patient does not respond. One study by Winkler et al. (1984) noted an increase in the incidence of pulmonary metastases in patients treated with preoperative chemotherapy and limb salvage surgery. A follow-up report, however, from the same authors concluded that preoperative chemotherapy was safe (Winkler et al. 1988). For the most part there is little to suggest an adverse effect of neoadjuvant treatment. A second potential disadvantage to preoperative treatment is that the complications of limb salvage, particularly wound healing and infection, may be more frequent. This could lead to a failure of the reconstruction, or at least a delay in resuming postoperative maintenance chemotherapy (McDonald et al. 1990). This effect from the chemotherapy itself, however, is probably small and in general complications are more related to tumor location, extent of resection, and type of reconstruction.

A challenge remains in the management of patients with established pulmonary metastasis. Telander et al. (1978) reported that with an aggressive surgical approach combined with chemotherapy approximately one-third of patients could be salvaged. Other studies have shown that time to metastasis of greater than 1 year and the completeness of resection are important prognostic variables associated with a better outcome (Han et al. 1981; Putman et al. 1983). Conversely, the appearance of more than three to five nodules has been associated with a poor outcome (Blasier et al. 1986; Meyer et al. 1987). Finally, Burk et al. (1991) found that although resection may improve the length of survival and the quality of survival, ultimate cure is probably not altered and most patients will eventually succumb to their disease.

Limb Salvage

Development of effective chemotherapy, along with improved imaging and reconstructive techniques, has contributed to the enthusiasm surrounding limb salvage surgery for osteosarcoma. Prior to 1980, limb salvage for osteosarcoma was reserved for small lesions, preferably stage IIA. If extraosseous involvement was present, it had to be small and away from important neurovascular structures before the patient was considered a candidate. With these guidelines, limb-sparing surgery was performed in approximately 6%–20% of patients (Campanacci et al. 1981; Sim et al. 1985). Recognizing that the primary goal of the orthopedic oncologist is to provide adequate control of the primary tumor, if a limb-sparing resection can ensure a local recurrence rate comparable to that achieved with amputation, yet provide a superior functional result, then resection represents a viable alternative. The ability to achieve a wide surgical margin is important in ensuring local control. In a large multi-institutional study, there was no significant difference in the local recurrence rate in 227 patients with osteosarcoma of the distal femur according to whether a wide surgical margin was achieved by amputation or by limb salvage (Simon et al. 1986). Only when a radical margin was achieved was there a noticeable improvement in local control. Other investigators have also noted a relatively low incidence (5%–10%) of local recurrence with limb salvage. Particularly low recurrence rates have been reported when a wide surgical margin was achieved in combination with adjuvant or neoadjuvant chemotherapy (Eckardt et al. 1987a; Kotz et al. 1989; Ueda et al. 1989). One may argue, however, that since local recurrence is associated with poor survival, any increase in local recurrence compared with the rate attained when a radical margin is achieved with ablative surgery is not justified. Fortunately the small increase in local recurrence with limb salvage does not seem to affect overall survival. There was no difference in survival in the multi-institutional study between patients treated with limb salvage and those treated with a radical surgical margin (Simon et al. 1986). Other series have also shown no adverse effect on survival provided a safe, wide surgical margin was achieved at resection (Sim et al. 1985; Gebhardt et al. 1989; Ueda et al. 1989; Tomita and Tsuchiya 1989).

As the functional results with limb salvage are generally superior to those with amputation, justification exists for considering most patients with high-grade osteosarcoma as potential candidates for limb salvage. In fact, most centers active in osteosarcoma treatment report that up to 80% of their patients are now being treated with limb-sparing surgery. Contraindications to limb salvage include extremely large lesions with obvious neurovascular involvement, lesions with pathologic fracture and subsequent contamination of multiple tissue compartments, distal lower extremity lesions, where the functional results of amputation and prosthetic fitting are generally good, and possibly local recurrences following a previous attempt at limb salvage. Another group of patients who may be best treated with amputation are the very young, in whom the anticipated leg length discrepancy at maturity becomes too great.

There is no universal optimum method of reconstruction after tumor resection and consideration must be given to location and extent of the lesion, the anticipated functional result, and functional demands of the patient, as well as the likelihood of associated complications. In principle, the reconstructive goal after removal of all or part of a major joint is to create a functional arthroplasty or stable arthrodesis. An arthroplasty can be biologic, utilizing an osteoarticular allograft segment, or nonbiologic by using an endoprosthesis. Composite arthroplasties can also be constructed where a large fragment allograft segment is used to reconstruct the skeletal defect together with a conventional prosthesis for the articulating portion of the joint. An arthrodesis, or for that matter an intercalary shaft reconstruction, can be achieved with autogenous bone, allogeneic bone, or a segmental replacement prosthesis.

Each option has advantages and disadvantages. From a functional standpoint patients prefer an arthroplasty, but a satisfactory arthroplasty generally requires preservation of intact musculotendinous units. In addition, an osteoarticular allograft arthroplasty requires at least partial preservation of ligament and capsular structures in order to maintain joint stability. While a successful arthrodesis is usually durable and can stabilize a joint after resection of important dynamic and static constraints, it does require prolonged healing time and may be difficult to achieve, and generally is functionally less satisfying to the patient. Furthermore, since osteosarcoma is an aggressive high-grade malignancy that in spite of extensive surgery and intensive chemotherapy may carry a 20%–40% 5-year mortality, the specific reconstruction should be selected with some short-term goals in mind, such as the early return of function and the avoidance of chemotherapy-delaying complications.

Reconstructive Techniques

In the upper extremity most lesions arise around the shoulder, usually in the proximal portion of the humerus. A classification of shoulder girdle resections developed by Malawar and associates (Malawar 1991) is useful in selecting appropriate reconstructive techniques depending on the amount of bone and soft tissue removed. For lesions requiring resection of the proximal humerus yet allowing preservation of the deltoid and scapula, an arthroplasty with potential functional abduction can be constructed with an endoprosthesis (Sim et al. 1980; Bos et al. 1987), an osteoarticular allograft (Gebhardt et al. 1990), or allograft–prosthesis composite (Rock 1987). Intra-articular resections of the proximal humerus, preserving the scapula, can also be treated with a glenohumeral arthrodesis. This can provide a good functional result with or without functioning abductors. Fusion techniques using

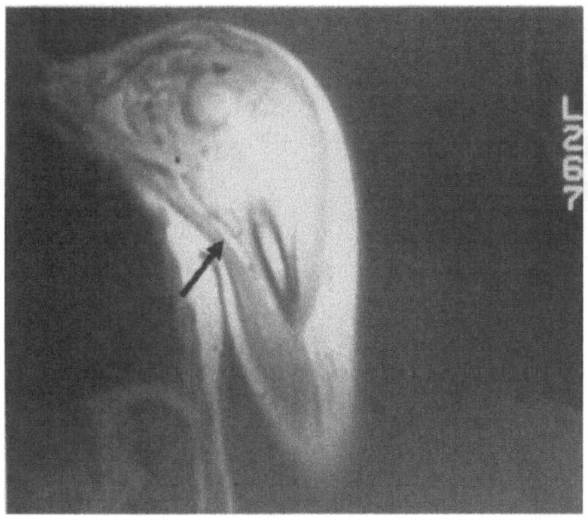

a

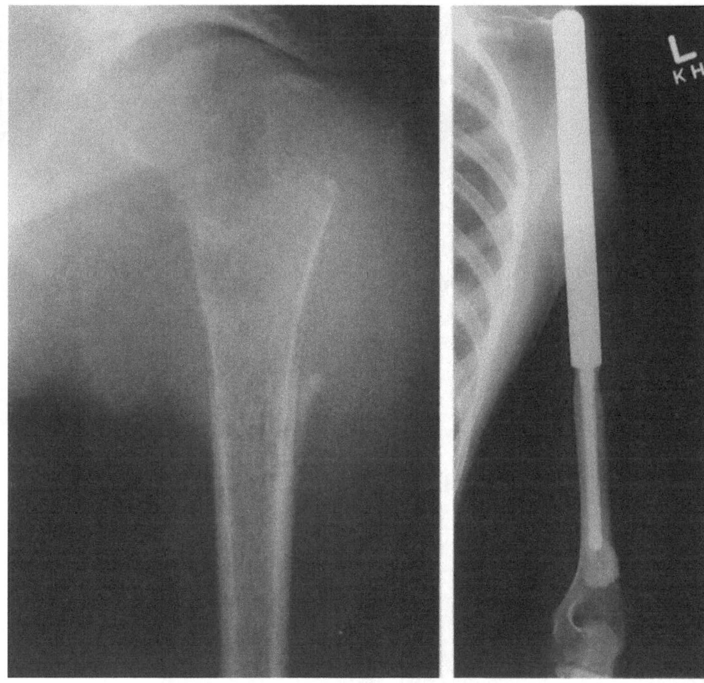

b, c

Fig. X.20. a T2-weighted coronal MR image which demonstrates the extent of the soft tissue mass, as well as proximity of the neurovascular bundle (*arrow*). **b** Anteroposterior radiograph of the proximal portion of the left humerus in a 16-year-old female. An obvious destructive lesion is present with soft tissue extension, as well as a Codman's reaction. **c** Postoperative radiograph after an extra-articular glenohumeral resection and proximal humeral spacer. This results in a flail shoulder but stabilizes the extremity for improved elbow and hand function

autogenous fibular grafts, as well as large fragment allografts, have been described (Gebhardt et al. 1987).

Extra-articular glenohumeral resection of the proximal humerus can also be reconstructed with an arthroplasty or arthrodesis provided the bony resection through the glenoid is minimal and allows adequate remaining bone stock. Glenohumeral resection necessitating significant scapular removal, as in the Tikhoff-Linberg procedure or its modifications, generally results in a flail shoulder (Linberg 1928; Marcove et al. 1977). If some degree of humeral stability can be achieved with a proximal humeral spacer or prosthesis secured to the remaining portion of the scapula, clavicle, or chest wall, then elbow, forearm, and hand function is generally improved (Capanna et al. 1989a; Frassica et al. 1991) (Fig. X.20). Preservation of neurovascular integrity in the distal extremity is a prerequisite to limb salvage in surgery around the shoulder. This usually implies adequate median and ulnar nerve function and preferably radial nerve function. The axillary nerve is generally sacrificed, and if need be the radial nerve can also be sacrificed with subsequent tendon transfers to restore its motor function.

In the lower extremity much attention has been given to limb-sparing procedures around the knee, for both distal femoral and proximal tibial lesions. The distal femur has no significant tendon attachments; therefore, satisfactory reconstruction after resection can be achieved by restoration of skeletal continuity and joint stability. If a functioning extensor mechanism, which spans the joint, can be preserved, an arthroplasty utilizing an endoprosthesis, osteoarticular allograft, or allograft-prosthesis composite can be achieved. The most predictable good results and early return to function follow endoprosthetic replacement (Sim and Chao 1987; Eckardt et al. 1987b) (Fig. X.21). Early complications with endoprosthetic replacements have been acceptable, and the functional result is dependent on the amount of quadriceps that can be spared (Capanna et al. 1991). Fortunately, for many intra-articular distal femoral resections the vastus medialis or vastus lateralis, as well as part of the rectus femoris, can be spared. Late problems with prosthetic loosening have been reported in up to 25% of cases at 5 years (Sim and Chao 1987). Newer modular designs with bone ingrowth potential as well as improved hinge design which allow rotation hold promise in reducing late failure. Capanna et al. (1989b) reported no cases of loosening in 63 distal femoral replacements using the uncemented KMFTR (Kotz modular femur and tibial reconstruction) prosthesis at a

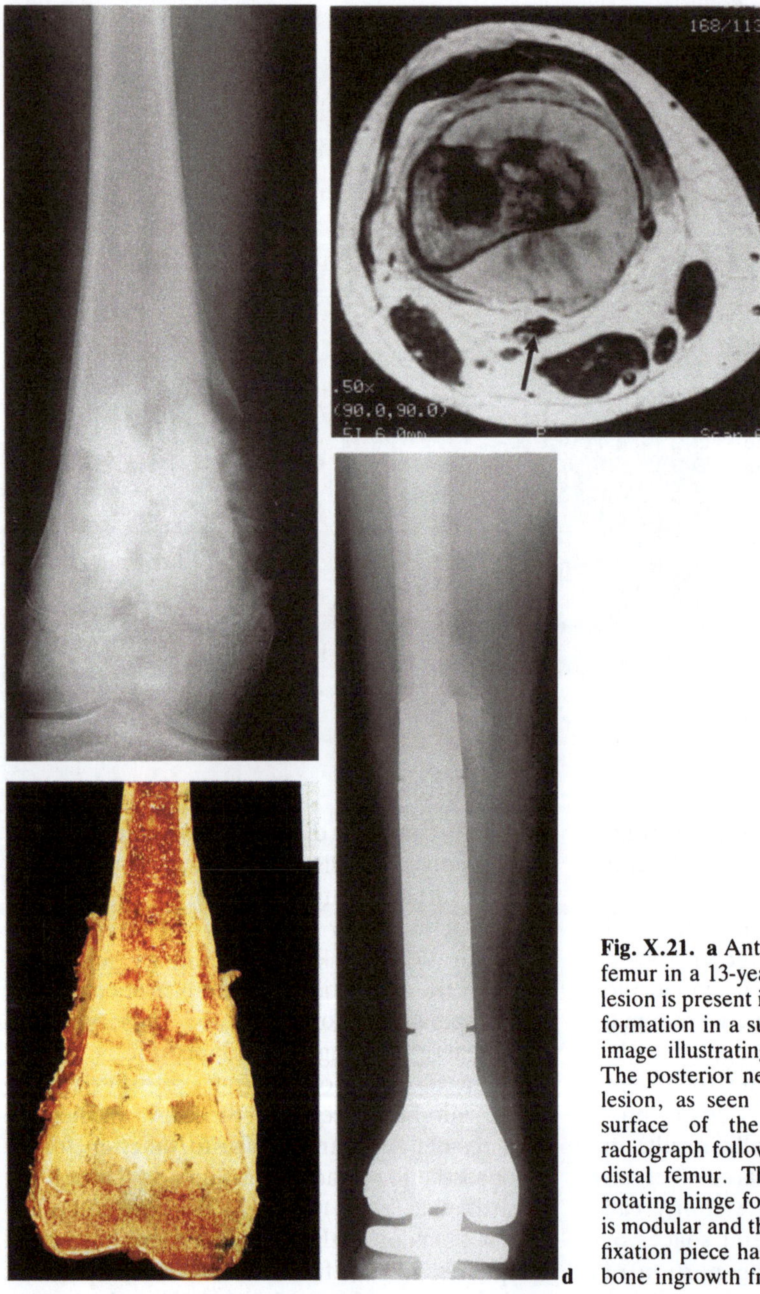

Fig. X.21. **a** Anteroposterior radiograph of the right distal femur in a 13-year-old female. A mixed lytic and sclerotic lesion is present in the metaphysis, with extraosseous bone formation in a sunburst pattern. **b** T1-weighted axial MR image illustrating the extraosseous extent of the lesion. The posterior neurovascular bundle is separate from the lesion, as seen at the *arrow*. **c** Photograph of the cut surface of the resected specimen. **d** Postoperative radiograph following endoprosthetic reconstruction of the distal femur. The prosthesis has an intrinsically stable rotating hinge for the articulating portion of the knee and is modular and therefore can be customized to length. The fixation piece has a porous surface which allows potential bone ingrowth from extracortical bone bridging

mean follow-up of 2 years, with good to excellent functional results in 75% of patients. Eckardt et al. (1991b) reported their large experience with cemented femoral replacements utilizing a rotating hinge. In 81 patients, good to excellent results were seen in 91%, with mechanical failure occurring in approximately 5% at a mean follow-up of more than 4 years.

Osteoarticular allografts create a pure biologic arthroplasty with the restoration of skeletal continuity, articular surface, and importantly, joint stability arising solely from the graft. Advantages include the ability to restore bone stock, provision of a site for soft tissue attachments, and intraoperative versatility. Mankin et al. (1982, 1987) have extensive experience with osteoarticular grafts about the knee and have reported overall satisfactory clinical and functional results in 76% of patients. Disadvantages of osteoarticular allografts include a long period of protected weight bearing, and therefore delayed functional return, and the tendency for com-

a, b
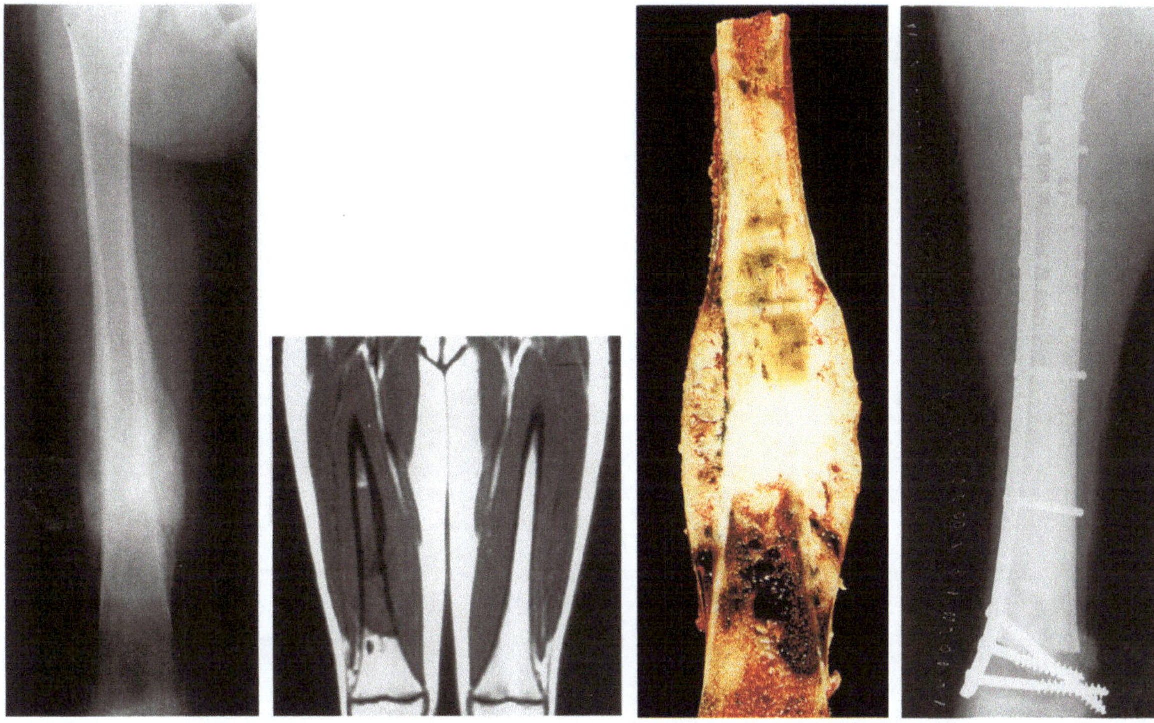
c, d

Fig. X.22. **a** Anteroposterior radiograph of the right femur in an 8-year-old female. A diaphyseal osteosarcoma is present. **b** T1-weighted coronal MRI illustrating the intraosseous extent of the tumor. The images suggest that it is almost a pure diaphyseal lesion with sparing of the metaphysis and growth plate. **c** Photograph of the cut surface of the resected specimen after preoperative chemotherapy. The proximal and distal margins appear grossly free of tumor. **d** Postoperative radiograph showing reconstruction of the defect with an intercalary allograft segment. The medullary portion of the graft was filled with methylmethacrylate to improve its strength and hopefully resist later fracture. The "composite" is secured to the host bone proximally and distally with plates and screws

plications, both early and late, in approximately 20%–30% of the patients. Early complications include infection and joint instability, while late complications include non-union, fracture, and articular collapse. If the knee joint can be spared, as is occasionally possible with a diaphyseal lesion, an intercalary allograft reconstruction can be done, which is associated with fewer complications and better functional results (Fig. X.22).

The allograft–prosthesis composite for distal femoral resection represents a compromise between an endoprosthesis and an allograft, and hopes to capitalize on the strengths of each. The allograft portion restores the skeletal defect and can be customized to length. A standard hinged prosthesis provides joint articulation and stability. Generally the prosthetic component is cemented into the allograft and the entire "composite" then fixed to the host bone (Fig. X.23). Hopefully, the restoration of bone stock will allow for better stress transfer through the composite.

Proximal tibia resections, although still "knee resections," differ from distal femoral resections by virtue of two further complicating features: the extensor mechanism attachment and minimal soft tissue coverage. When utilizing an endoprosthesis the patellar tendon is sutured to the prosthesis, with enhanced knee extension achieved by suturing the tendon to available muscle and fascial tissue, thus creating a functional soft tissue sleeve around the prosthesis (Eckardt et al. 1991a). An allograft, either osteoarticular or as a prosthetic composite, may provide a better potential site for extensor attachment (Fig. X.24). Soft tissue coverage of the reconstruction is critical in the proximal tibia, and almost universally requires a medial gastrocnemius muscle flap (Malawar and McHale 1989). The flap serves a dual purpose by also aiding reconstruction of the functional extensor sleeve.

For extra-articular resections of the knee or when a functioning extensor mechanism cannot be preserved, an arthrodesis may be done. The technique of resection arthrodesis of the knee

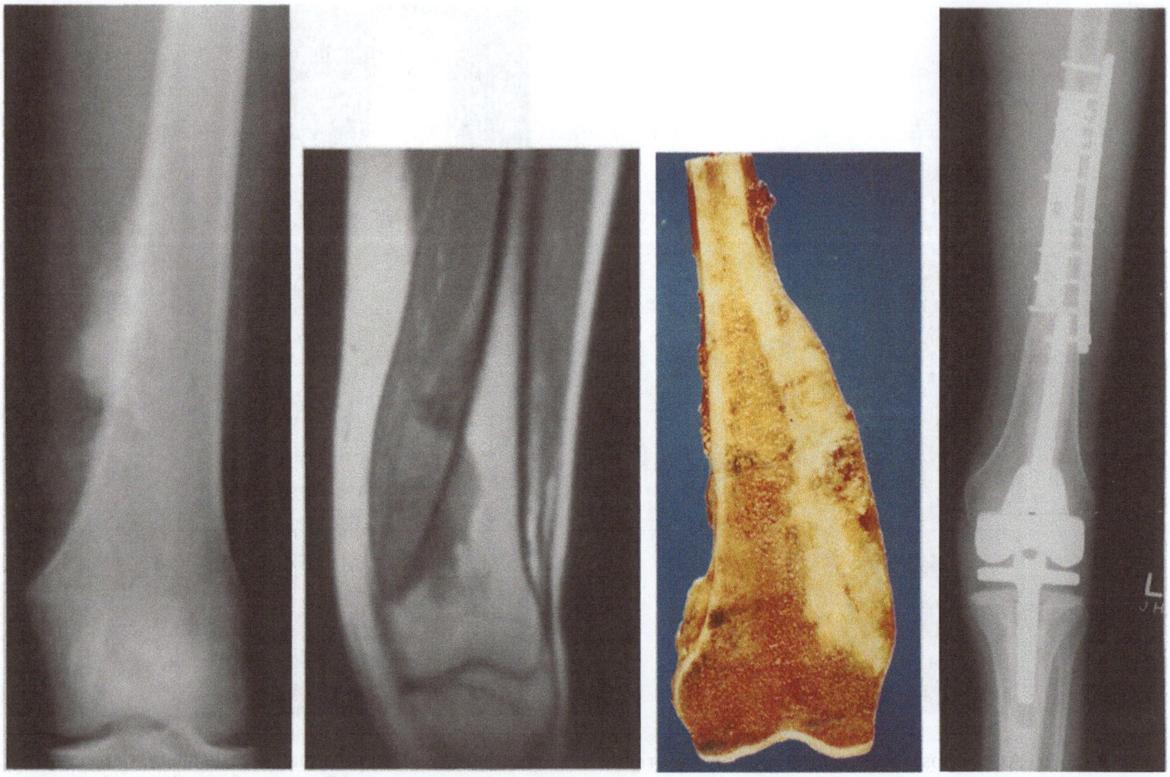

a, b c, d

Fig. X.23. **a** Anteroposterior radiograph of the left femur in a 16-year-old female. A lesion is present in the diaphyseal and metaphyseal portion of the bone, with both intraosseous and extraosseous bone formation. **b** T1-weighted coronal MRI illustrating the intraosseous, as well as the extraosseous, extent of the lesion. **c** Photograph of the cut surface of the resected specimen after preoperative chemotherapy. **d** Postoperative radiograph of the distal femur and knee illustrating an allograft–prosthesis composite reconstruction of the distal femur. A standard rotating hinge knee prosthesis is cemented into the distal femoral allograft and the entire composite then fixed to the host bone with double plates and screws

utilizing autogenous grafts is credited to Juvara (1921) with modifications by Merle D'Aubigné et al. (1958), Enneking and Shirley (1977), and Campanacci and co-workers (Campanacci and Costa 1979; Campanacci et al. 1987). Hemicylindrical grafts are harvested from the ipsilateral femur or tibia (depending on the site of tumor) and used to span the defect. Fibular grafts may also be used. A long intramedullary rod is generally used for internal fixation. An allograft arthrodesis, internally fixed with either a long intramedullary rod and short antirotation plates or plates and screws alone, is also effective. This has the advantage of being technically easier, requires less surgical exposure, and does not add potential donor site morbidity. Overall, satisfactory fusion with autogenous grafts occurs in more than 90% of patients, with complications of infection, delayed union, or fracture occurring in approximately 20% (Enneking and Shirley 1977; Campanacci and Costa 1979; Campanacci et al. 1987). Allograft fusions are also subject to complications, and overall lead to satisfactory results in approximately 60% of patients (Gebhardt et al. 1987; Makley 1985).

For lesions of the proximal femur the best results are obtained if an intra-articular resection can be done with either endoprosthetic or allograft–prosthesis composite reconstruction. Several authors have reported their experience with endoprosthetic replacement (Lewis and Chekofsky 1982; Katzner and Schwingt 1982; Khong et al. 1989; Capanna et al. 1989b). Good to excellent functional results are variably reported in approximately 50%–80% of patients, with better function observed when hip abductor strength is preserved or restored. Suturing the gluteal muscles to the fascia lata or vastus lateralis is the most common method of soft tissue reconstruction. Dislocation is the primary early postoperative problem, occurring in 5%–25% of patients. Late mechanical failure requiring

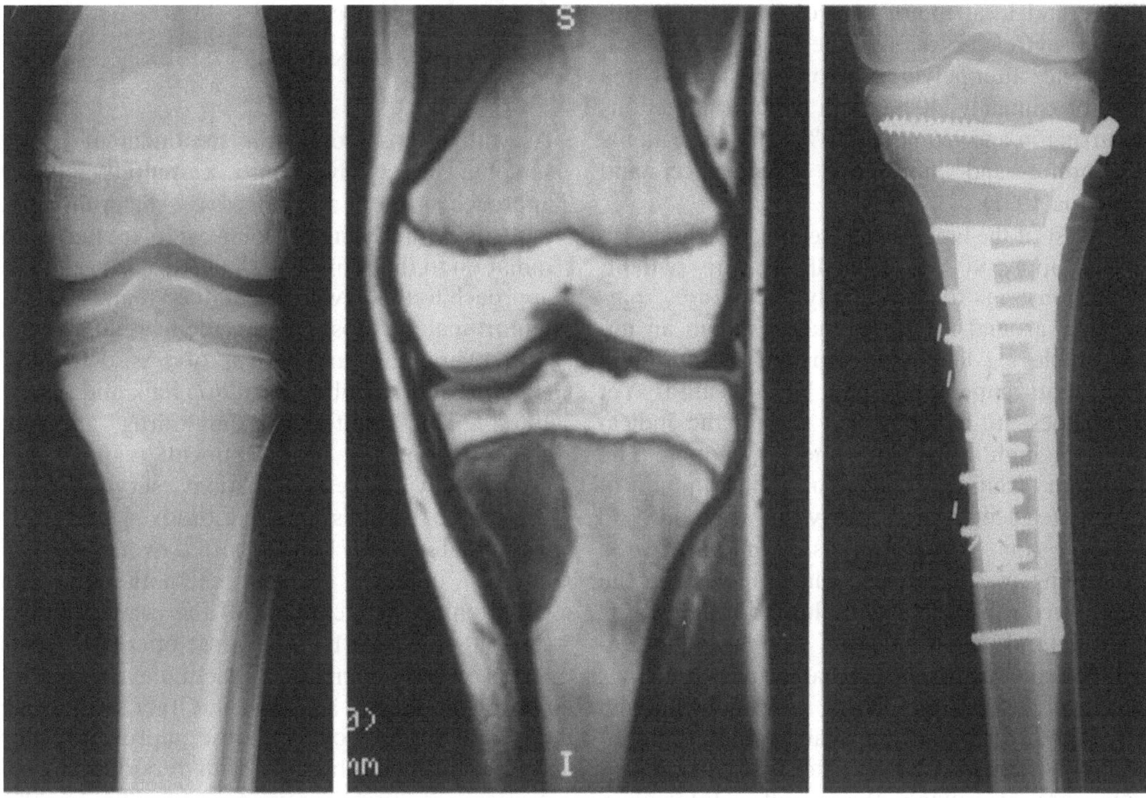

a b, c

Fig. X.24. **a** Anteroposterior radiograph of the left proximal tibia in a 13-year-old male. A sclerotic lesion is present in the proximal medial metaphysis of the tibia. No obvious extraosseous extension is noted. **b** Coronal T1-weighted MRI illustrating the intraosseous extent of the lesion. The lesion abuts the growth physis, but does not appear to cross it, and the extraosseous involvement is minimal. **c** Postoperative radiograph of the proximal tibia illustrating an osteoarticular allograft reconstruction of the defect. This allows preservation of distal femoral growth. At 6 months following surgery early healing of the graft–host junction is noted

revision was reported in only 4% by Khong et al. (1989). Allograft–prosthesis composite reconstruction holds promise in reducing instability and possibly enhancing function by allowing direct soft tissue reconstruction to the graft. Good to excellent results have been reported in 63%–88% of patients (Head et al. 1987; Gitelis and Piasecki 1991; Delepine and Delepine 1989). Osteoarticular allografts of the proximal femur have also been used as a primary reconstruction method for lesions of the proximal femur (Jofe et al. 1988). Used alone, however, they are subject to a higher rate of complications (infection, fracture, and non-union) and a delay in functional return.

The resection and reconstruction of pelvic osteosarcoma remains challenging. The classification system of Enneking and Dunham (1978) divides pelvic resections into three main types: type I includes all or part of the iliac wing, type II includes periacetabular resections, and type III consists of pubic rami resections. The most challenging reconstruction occurs in periacetabular resections, either from intra-articular pelvic lesions or following extra-articular proximal femoral resection. Unfortunately, most osteosarcomas of the pelvis will involve the periacetabular bone. From a functional standpoint, reconstructive techniques that allow restoration of the pelvic ring or at least stability between the femur and the sacrum are preferred. After type II resections an iliofemoral arthrodesis can be achieved primarily, or by using an intercalary allograft segment if more extensive resection of the ilium or proximal femur has been done. An ischiofemoral arthrodesis can also be done but fusion is more difficult and the functional result less predictable. The use of a saddle prosthesis as described by Nieder and co-workers (Nieder and Keller 1989; Nieder et al. 1990) creates a type of functional arthroplasty with reported good results. Complications after pelvic resections are higher and local tumor control is more difficult than in extremity lesions. The incidence of local recurrence after pelvic resection for osteosarcoma is approximately 40%, with wound infections occurring in approximately 20%–30% of patients (O'Connor and Sim 1989; Campanacci and Capanna 1991).

Most of the limb salvage techniques discussed so far apply to the skeletally mature patient. Resections in the skeletally immature, particularly around the knee, may result in an unacceptable leg length discrepancy at adulthood such that amputation may be indicated. Yet techniques are evolving that extend the indications for limb salvage into the very young. The optimum techniques depend upon the amount of anticipated length discrepancy and the ability to preserve the growth physis. For anticipated shortening of 2–3 cm, one can simply make the initial reconstruction slightly longer, followed by contralateral epiphysiodesis. For large discrepancies, the use of an expanding prosthesis has been advocated by Lewis (1986). Although associated with more complications than standard endoprosthesis, experience and design modifications are improving the results. Intercalary amputation and reimplantation of the distal extremity, as in the Van Nes (1950) rotation plasty, is also a reconstruction technique that can preserve growth. The functional result obtained is generally inferior to a below-knee amputation but preferable to an above-knee amputation, and when the technique is properly performed, it can provide satisfactory results (Kotz and Salzer 1982; Murray et al. 1985; Cammisa et al. 1990).

4. Ewing Sarcoma

Douglas J. McDonald

As with osteosarcoma, the treatment of Ewing sarcoma has evolved into a multidisciplinary approach. Prior to effective chemotherapy, patients with Ewing sarcoma were treated with radiation to the primary lesion and a wait-and-see approach to the development of systemic disease. Unfortunately, most patients died within 2 years, with overall 5-year survival of less than 20% (Phillips and Higinbotham 1967; Falk and Alpert 1967). The addition of multidrug adjuvant chemotherapy to the treatment regimen has dramatically increased patient survival. The Intergroup Ewing's Sarcoma Study – I (IESS-I) was initiated in 1971 and reported overall survival of 56% utilizing adjuvant chemotherapy with radiation as the treatment of the primary tumor (Nesbit et al. 1981). The most effective agents tested were vincristine, dactinomycin, cyclophosphamide, and adriamycin. Other series using the same agents confirmed the improved results seen with chemotherapy, with reported overall disease-free survival ranging from 39% to 79% (Rosen et al. 1981; Bacci et al. 1982; Jurgens et al. 1988; Sailer et al. 1988).

As survival improved it became apparent that radiation alone was inconsistent in controlling the primary lesion. Local recurrences in patients receiving radiation alone for local treatment were common, occurring in approximately 20%–50% of patients. Furthermore, autopsy studies by Telles et al. (1978) and Tepper et al. (1980)

Table X.1. Role of surgery in local control and disease-free survival for Ewing sarcoma

Series	Survival[a]		Local recurrence	
	Surgery or surgery/ radiation	Radiation	Surgery or surgery/ radiation	Radiation
Pritchard et al. (1975)	34.0%	10.5%	–	–
Rosen et al. (1981)	82.0%	76.0%	0%	21%
Bacci et al. (1982)	62.5%	23.0%	12.5%	35%
Bacci et al. (1985)	68.0%	31.0%	7.1%	31%
Wilkins et al. (1986)	74.0%	27.0%	3.7%	34.6%
Jurgens et al. (1988)	67.0%	44.0%	10%	47%
Sailer et al. (1988)	91.0%	46.0%	0%	31%
Bacci et al. (1989)	60.3%	28.0%	6.9%	36%

[a] Five-year continuous disease-free survival (real or projected)

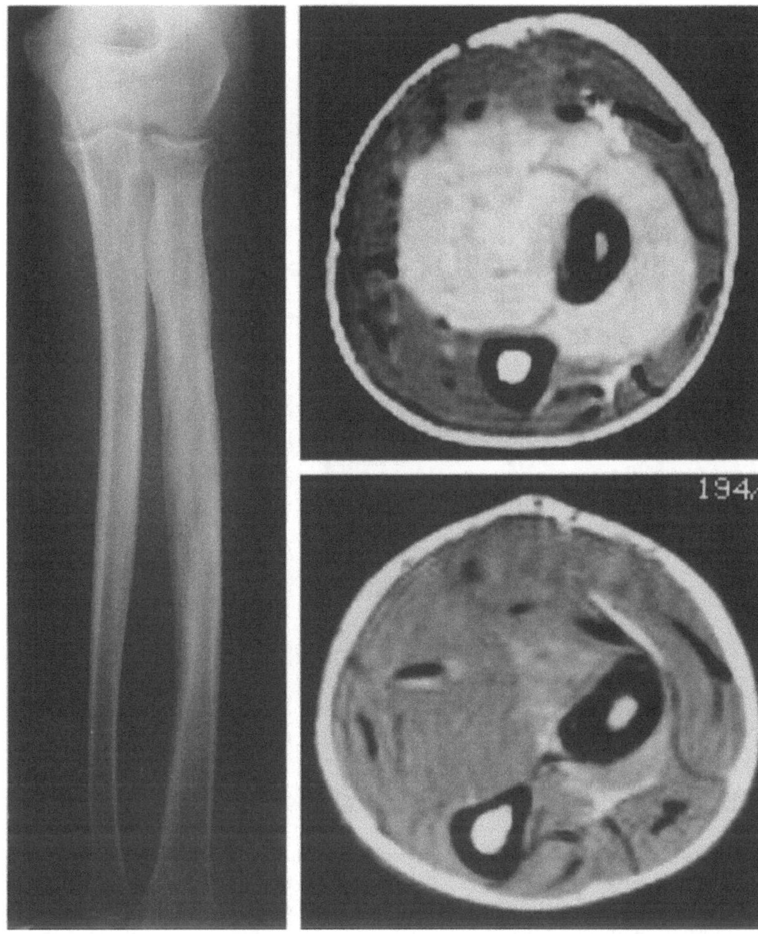

Fig. X.25. **a** Anteroposterior radiograph of the left forearm in a 16-year-old male. A long diaphyseal lesion is noted in the radius, with a permeative pattern of bone destruction consistent with a Ewing sarcoma. **b** Prechemotherapy T2-weighted axial MRI of the forearm. A large extraosseous component of the lesion is present, completely surrounding the radius. **c** Postchemotherapy T2-weighted axial MRI at the same level. Marked volumetric reduction of the soft tissue component of the lesion is seen

showed viable tumor in up to 65% of patients, suggesting potential local failure in the absence of clinical recurrence. With longer follow-up, radiation therapy also has been associated with severe functional deficits such as leg length discrepancy and joint ankylosis, as well as an increased potential for radiation-induced sarcoma.

The interest in the role of surgery grew when reports of increased survival and decreased local recurrence were seen after achievement of a wide surgical margin was added to the treatment regimen. In a retrospective view of the patients treated at the Mayo Clinic prior to 1969, Pritchard et al. (1975) noted 5-year survival of 45% in patients who had extremity lesions when a primary lesion was treated surgically, compared with 13% when nonsurgical methods were used. The IESS-I, although primarily designed to test different chemotherapy regimens with radiation as the usual treatment for the primary lesion, noted that in patients who did receive surgical resection, survival improved (Thomas et al. 1984; Evans et al. 1985). Additionally, surgical resection of the primary lesion also improved local control. In an updated report from the Mayo Clinic by Wilkins et al. (1986), both an increase in disease-free survival and a decrease in local recurrence were observed in patients who had surgical resections as part of the treatment protocol. Table X.1 summarizes the experience of multiple institutions worldwide who have specifically examined the role of surgery in patients with Ewing sarcoma.

Most current protocols contain provisions for surgical resection after preoperative induction chemotherapy. When surgical resection is done it is performed at approximately 9–12 weeks with the intent of achieving a wide margin. If wide margins are achieved, radiation can be avoided. If marginal or contaminated margins are achieved, local radiation is used at a lower dose (40 Gy) in the hope of diminishing the long-term effects of radiation. Unlike in the case of osteosarcoma, preoperative chemotherapy for Ewing sarcoma

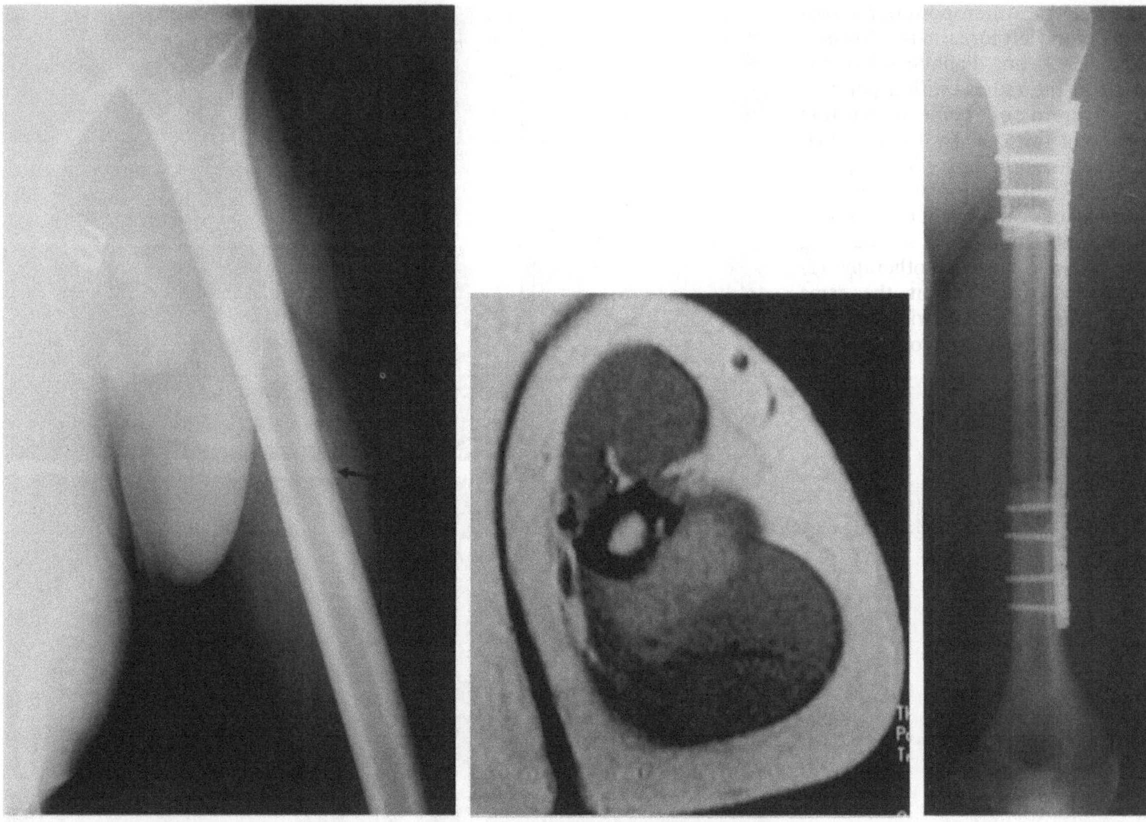

a b, c

Fig. X.26. **a** Anteroposterior radiograph of the left humerus in a 27-year-old female. There is a very subtle, permeative-type destruction of the lateral cortex near the midshaft with no obvious intramedullary extension (*arrow*). **b** T1-weighted axial MRI illustrating the cortical destruction, with an obvious soft tissue mass. **c** Following preoperative chemotherapy, an intercalary resection of the humerus was performed with reconstruction using a vascularized free fibula graft

will often result in a dramatic volumetric reduction in the soft tissue component (Fig. X.25). This may make resection technically easier and safer. Resection is most clearly indicated for small lesions in relatively expendable bones such as the proximal fibula, ribs, rays of hands or feet, body of the scapula, clavicle, or wing of the ilium, where no reconstruction is needed. For lesions around the knee, resection and reconstruction utilizing the same techniques used for osteosarcoma may be the only local treatment needed if wide margins can be achieved. The upper extremity lesions of the shoulder can also be resected and reconstructed as with osteosarcoma if the functional result is acceptable. Large lesions requiring sacrifice of the deltoid or extra-articular resection of the glenoid resulting in significant functional loss should be individualized and consideration given to radiotherapy. Lesions of the forearm in which one bone is involved can also be resected and the forearm reconstructed. Diaphyseal lesions, whether in the upper or lower extremity, should be considered for resection as the clinical and functional results with intercalary reconstructions are generally very good (Fig. X.26).

The optimal management for destructive lesions of the pelvis is less clear. Most large series have suggested that a pelvic or axial location is a poor prognostic variable (Rosen et al. 1981; Wilkins et al. 1986; Sauer et al. 1987; Bacci et al. 1989). Yet Li et al. (1983) suggested that resection could improve both local control and survival at short follow-up. They reported no local or distant relapses in ten patients treated with surgical resection, whereas five of eight patients treated without surgery developed either local recurrence or metastases. Evans et al. (1985), reporting on the IESS-I patients with pelvic primaries, noted a trend toward improved local control in patients with complete resection (18% recurrence) compared to those without surgical resection (28% recurrence), although this was not statistically significant. Capanna et al. (1990) noted no significant advantage in surgical resection for overall disease-free survival and only a slight trend toward improved local control when a wide margin was obtained. He suggested that resection of relatively expendable portions of the pelvis such as the wing of the ilium or the anteropubic arch may be worthwhile, but that for periacetabular resections and reconstruction, the increase in complications and poor functional result may not make surgery worthwhile. Lesions arising in the axial skeleton are rarely amenable to resection with wide margins as the only local treatment. Surgery is generally reserved for biopsy alone or, if needed, neurologic decompression and spinal stabilization.

Summary. The outlook for patients with osteosarcoma and Ewing sarcoma has improved dramatically over the last 20 years. An improved understanding of the biology and radiographic imaging of these tumors has led to more accurate and meaningful staging. Effective chemotherapy and techniques of reconstruction have improved survival and functional limb preservation. Importantly, with appropriate management limb salvage should be possible in a majority of these patients without compromise to their overall survival.

References

Giant-Cell Tumor

Bell RS, Harwood AR, Goodman SB et al. (1983) Supervoltage radiotherapy in the treatment of difficult giant cell tumors of bone. Clin Orthop Rel Res 174:208

Bertoni F, Present D, Enneking WF (1985) Giant cell tumor of bone with pulmonary metastases. J Bone Joint Surg [Am] 67:890

Campanacci M, Costa P (1979) Total resection of the distal femur or proximal tibia for bone tumors. J Bone Joint Surg [Br] 61:445

Campanacci M, Baldini N, Boriani S, Sudanese A (1987) Giant-cell tumor of bone. J Bone Joint Surg [Am] 69:106–114

Capanna R, Fabbri N, Bettelli G (1989) Curettage of giant cell tumor of bone: the effect of surgical technique and adjuvants on local recurrence rate. Chir Organi Movi 75:206–207

Carrasco CH, Murray JA (1989) Giant cell tumors. Orthop Clin North Am 20:395–405

Chen ZX, Gu DZ, Yu ZH et al. (1986) Radiation therapy of giant-cell tumor of bone: analysis of 35 patients. Int J Radiat Oncol Biol Phys 12:329

Dahlin DC, Cupps RE, Johnson EW Jr (1970) Giant cell tumor. A study of 195 cases. Cancer 25:1061–1070

Enneking WF (1983a) Staging musculoskeletal tumors. In: Enneking WF (ed) Musculoskeletal tumor surgery, vol 1. Churchill Livingstone, New York, pp 69–88

Enneking WF (1983b) Surgical margins. In: Enneking WF (ed) Musculoskeletal tumor surgery, vol 1. Churchill Livingstone, New York, pp 89–122

Frassica FJ, Sim FH, Pritchard DJ, Chao EYS (1989) Subchondral replacement: a comparative analysis of reconstruction with methylmethacrylate or autogenous bone graft. Chir Organi Movi 75:189–191

Goldenberg RR, Campbell CJ, Bonfiglio M (1970) Giant-cell tumor of bone. An analysis of two hundred and eighteen cases. J Bone Joint Surg [Am] 52:619–663

Hackbarth DA (1991) Resections and reconstructions for tumors of the distal radius. Orthop Clin North Am 22:49

Jacobs PA, Clemency RE (1985) The closed cryosurgical treatment of giant cell tumor. Clin Orthop Rel Res 192:149–158

Kreicbergs A, Lonnguist PA, Nilsson B (1985) Curettage of benign lesions of bone: factors related to recurrence. Int Orthop 8:287

Lackman RD, McDonald DJ, Beckenbaugh R, Sim FH (1987) Fibular reconstruction for giant cell tumor of the distal radius. Clin Orthop 218:232

Lane JM (1989) Liquid nitogren as an adjunct. Chir Organi Movi 75:198–203

Larsson SE, Lorentzon R, Boquist L (1975) Giant cell tumor of bone. J Bone Joint Surg [Am] 57:167–173

Mankin HJ, Gebhardt MC, Tomford WW (1987) The use of frozen cadaveric allografts in the management of patients with bone tumors of the extremities. Orthop Clin North Am 18:275

Marcove RC, Weis LD, Vaghaiwalla MR et al. (1978) Cryosurgery in the treatment of giant cell tumors of bone: a report of 52 consecutive cases. Cancer 41:957–969

McDonald DJ, Sim FH, McLeod RA, Dahlin DC (1986) Giant cell tumor of bone. J Bone Joint Surg [Am] 68:235–242

Mjöberg B, Petersson H, Rosenquist R, Rydholm A (1984) Bone cement, thermal injury and the radiolucent zone. Acta Orthop Scand 55:597–600

Ottolenghi CE (1972) Massive osteo and osteoarticular bone grafts. Clin Orthop Rel Res 87:156–164

Persson BM, Wouters HW (1976) Curettage and acrylic cementation in surgery of giant cell tumors of bone. Clin Orthop Rel Res 120:125–133

Persson BM, Ekelund L, Lövdahl R, Gunterberg B (1984) Favourable results of acrylic cementation for giant cell tumors. Acta Orthop Scand 55:209–214

Rock M (1989) Adjuvant management of benign tumors: basic concepts of phenol and cement use. Chir Organi Movi 75:195–198

Rock MG, Pritchard DJ, Unni KK (1984) Metastases from histologically benign giant cell tumor of bone. J Bone Joint Surg [Am] 66:269

Sanerkin NG (1980) Malignancy, aggressiveness and recurrence in giant cell tumor of bone. Cancer 46:1641–1649

Sim FH, Beauchamp CP, Chao EYS (1987) Reconstructions of musculoskeletal defects about the knee for tumor. Clin Orthop Rel Res 221:188

Sung HW, Kuo DP, Shu WP et al. (1982) Giant-cell tumor of bone: analysis of 208 cases in Chinese patients. J Bone Joint Surg [Am] 64:755–761
Turcotte RE, Biagini R, Sim FH, Unni KK (1989) Giant cell tumor of the spine and sacrum. Chir Organi Movi 75:104–108
Wray CC, MacDonald AW, Richardson RA (1990) Benign giant cell tumor with metastases to bone and lung. J Bone Joint Surg [Br] 72:486

Chondrosarcoma

Bertoni F, Picci P, Bacchini P et al. (1983) Mesenchymal chondrosarcoma of bone and soft tissue. Cancer 53:533
Campanacci M, Capanna R (1991) Pelvic resections: the Rizzoli Institute experience. In: Springfield DS (ed) The orthopedic clinics of North America, vol 1. W.B. Saunders, Philadelphia, pp 65–86
Capanna R, Bertoni F, Betelli G et al. (1988) Dedifferentiated chondrosarcoma. J Bone Joint Surg [Am] 70:60
Cohen L, Hendrickson F, Mansell J et al. (1984) Response of sarcomas of bone and of soft tissue to neutron beam therapy. Int J Radiat Oncol Biol Phys 10:821
Enneking WF (1983) Staging musculoskeletal tumors. In: Enneking WF (ed) Musculoskeletal tumor surgery, vol 1. Churchill Livingstone, New York, pp 69–88
Eriksson AI, Schiller A, Mankin HJ (1980) The management of chondrosarcoma of bone. Clin Orthop Rel Res 153:44
Evans HL, Ayala AG, Romsdahl MM (1977) Prognostic factors in chondrosarcoma of bone: a clinicopathologic analysis with emphasis on histologic grading. Cancer 40:818
Frassica FJ, Unni KK, Beabout JW et al. (1986) Dedifferentiated chondrosarcoma: a report of the clinicopathological features and treatment of 78 cases. J Bone Joint Surg [Am] 68:1197
Gitelis S, Bertoni F, Picci P, Campanacci M (1981) Chondrosarcoma of bone: the experience at the Istituto Ortopedico Rizzoli. J Bone Joint Surg [Am] 63:1249
Guerra A, Briccoli A, Capanna R et al. (1985) Resection with preservation of the lower limb in chondrosarcoma of the pelvis. Rev Chir Orthop 71:493
Harwood AR, Krajbich JI, Fornasier VL (1980a) Mesenchymal chondrosarcoma: a report of 17 cases. Clin Orthop 158:144
Harwood AR, Krajbich JI, Fornasier VL (1980b) Radiotherapy of chondrosarcoma of bone. Cancer 45:2769
Healy JH, Lane JM (1986) Chondrosarcoma. Clin Orthop Rel Res 204:119
Hudson TM, Springfield DS, Spanier SS et al. (1984) Benign exostoses and exostotic chondrosarcomas: evaluation of cartilage thickness by CT. Radiology 152:595
Huvos AG, Rosen G, Dabska M et al. (1983) Mesenchymal chondrosarcoma: a clinicopathologic analysis of 35 patients with emphasis on treatment. Cancer 51:1230
Kaufman JH, Douglass HO Jr, Blake W et al. (1977) The importance of initial presentation and treatment upon the survival of patients with chondrosarcoma. Surg Gynecol Obstet 145:357
Kim RY, Salter MM, Brascho DJ (1983) High-energy irradiation in the management of chondrosarcoma. South Med J 76:739
Krochak R, Harwood AR, Cummings BJ et al. (1983) Results of radical radiation for chondrosarcoma of bone. Radiother Oncol 1:109
Malawer MM, Sugerbaker PH, Lampert M et al. (1985) The Tikhoff-Linberg procedure: report of ten patients and presentation of a modified technique for tumors of the proximal humerus. Surgery 97:518
Marcove RC (1977) Chondrosarcoma: diagnosis and treatment. Orthop Clin North Am 8:811
Marcove RC, Miké V, Hutter RVP et al. (1972) Chondrosarcoma of the pelvis and upper end of the femur: an analysis of factors influencing survival time in 113 cases. J Bone Joint Surg [Am] 54:561
Marcove RC, Lewis MM, Huvos AG (1977a) En bloc upper humeral interscapulothoracic resection. The Tikhoff-Linberg procedure. Clin Orthop 124:219
Marcove RC, Stovell PB, Huvos AG et al. (1977b) The use of cryosurgery in the treatment of low and medium grade chondrosarcoma: a preliminary report. Clin Orthop 122:147
Nielsen HKL, Veth RPH, Oldhoff J et al. (1985) Resection of a peri-acetabular chondrosarcoma and reconstruction of the pelvis: a case report. J Bone Joint Surg [Br] 67:413
Sannerkin NG, Gallagher P (1979) A review of the behaviour of chondrosarcoma of bone. J Bone Joint Surg [Br] 61:395
Smith WS, Simon MA (1975) Segmental resection for chondrosarcoma. J Bone Joint Surg [Am] 57:1097

Osteosarcoma

Avella M, Bacci G, McDonald DJ et al. (1988) Adjuvant chemotherapy with six drugs (adriamycin, methotrexate, cisplatinum, bleomycin, cyclophosphamide and dactinomycin) for non-metastatic high-grade osteosarcoma of the extremities. Results of 32 patients and comparison to 127 patients concomitantly treated with the same drugs in a neoadjuvant form. Chemioterapia 9:133–137
Bacci G, Ghlerinzoni F, Picci P et al. (1986) Adriamycin-methotrexate high dose versus adriamycin-methotrexate moderate dose as adjuvant chemotherapy for osteosarcoma of the extremities: a randomized study. Eur J Cancer Clin Oncol 22:1337–1345
Bacci G, Picci P, Ruggieri P et al. (1990) Primary chemotherapy and delayed surgery (neoadjuvant chemotherapy) for osteosarcoma of the extremities: the Istituto Rizzoli experience in 127 patients treated preoperatively with intravenous methotrexate (high versus moderate doses) and intraarterial cisplatin. Cancer 65:2539–2553
Blasier D, Mayba T, Ferguson C et al. (1986) Metastatic osteosarcoma and multiple lung resection. J Bone Joint Surg [Br] 68:748
Bonnadonna G, Monfardi S, De Lena M et al. (1970) Phase I and preliminary phase II evaluation of adriamycin (NSC/123127). Cancer Res 30:2572–2582
Bos G, Sim FH, Pritchard DJ et al. (1987) Prosthetic proximal humerus replacement: the Mayo Clinic experience. In: Enneking WF (ed) Limb salvage in

musculoskeletal oncology. Churchill Livingstone, New York

Burk CD, Belasco JB, O'Neill JA Jr, Lange B (1991) Pulmonary metastasis and bone sarcomas. Clin Orthop 262:88–92

Cammisa FP, Glasser DB, Phil M et al. (1990) The Ven Nes tibial rotationplasty. J Bone Joint Surg [Am] 72:1541–1547

Campanacci M, Capanna R (1991) Pelvic resections: the Rizzoli Institute experience. Orthop Clin North Am 22:65–86

Campanacci M, Costa P (1979) Total resection of distal femur or proximal tibia for bone tumors. Autogenous bone grafts and arthrodesis in 26 cases. J Bone Joint Surg [Br] 61:455

Campanacci M, Bacci G, Bertoni F et al. (1981) The treatment of osteosarcoma of the extremities: twenty years' experience at the Istituto Ortopedico Rizzoli. Cancer 48:1569–1581

Campanacci M, Cervellati L, Guerra A et al. (1987) Knee resection-arthrodesis. In: Enneking WF (ed) Limb salvage in musculoskeletal oncology. Churchill Livingstone, New York

Capanna R, Giunti A, Biagini R et al. (1989a) Modular endoprosthesis for humerus and Tikhoff-Linberg resection. In: Yamamuro T (ed) New developments for limb salvage in musculoskeletal tumors. Springer, Tokyo

Capanna R, Leonessa C, Bettelli G et al. (1989b) Modular Kotz prosthesis: the Rizzoli experience. In: Yamamuro T (ed) New developments for limb salvage in musculoskeletal tumors. Springer, Tokyo

Capanna R, Ruggieri P, Biagini R et al. (1991) The effect of quadriceps excision on functional results after distal femoral resection and prosthetic replacement for bone tumors. Clin Orthop 267:186–196

Cortes EP, Holland JF, Wang JJ, Sinks LF (1972) Chemotherapy of advanced osteosarcoma. In: Price CHG, Ross FGM (eds) Bone – certain aspects of neoplasia. Butterworths, London

Cortes EP, Holland JF, Wang JJ et al. (1974) Amputation and adriamycin in primary osteosarcoma. N Engl J Med 291:998–1000

Dahlin DC, Coventry MB (1967) Osteogenic sarcoma: a study of six hundred cases. J Bone Joint Surg [Am] 49:101–110

Delepine G, Delepine N (1989) Titanium long-stem prosthesis combined with bone allografts in reconstructive surgery of high-grade bone sarcomas. In: Yamamuro T (ed) New developments for limb salvage in musculoskeletal tumors. Springer, Tokyo

Eckardt JJ, Eilber FR, Grant TT et al. (1987a) The UCLA experience in the management of stage IIB osteogenic sarcoma. In: Enneking WF (ed) Limb salvage in musculoskeletal oncology. Churchill Livingstone, New York

Eckardt JJ, Eilber FR, Kabo JM, Mirra JM (1987b) Kinematic rotating hinge knee-distal femoral replacement. In: Enneking WF (ed) Limb salvage in musculoskeletal oncology. Churchill Livingstone, New York

Eckardt JJ, Matthews JB, Eilber RF (1991a) Endoprosthetic reconstruction after bone tumor resection of the proximal tibia. Orthop Clin North Am 22:149–160

Eckardt JJ, Eilber FR, Rosen G et al. (1991b) Endoprosthetic replacement for stage IIB osteosarcoma. Clin Orthop 270:202–213

Edmonson JH, Green SJ, Ivins JC et al. (1984) A controlled pilot study of high-dose methotrexate as postsurgical adjuvant treatment for primary osteosarcoma. J Clin Oncol 2:152–156

Enneking WF, Dunham WK (1978) Resection and reconstruction for primary neoplasms involving the innominate bone. J Bone Joint Surg [Am] 60:731–746

Enneking WF, Shirley PD (1977) Resection-arthrodesis for malignant and potentially malignant lesions about the knee using an intramedullary rod and local bone grafts. J Bone Joint Surg [Am] 59:223

Frassica FJ, Chao EY, Shives TC, Sim FH (1991) Resection of malignant bone tumors about the shoulder. Clin Orthop 267:57–64

Friedman MA, Carter SK (1972) The therapy of osteogenic sarcoma: current status and thoughts for the future. J Surg Oncol 45:482–510

Gebhardt MC, McGuire MH, Mankin HJ (1987) Resection and allograft arthrodesis for malignant bone tumors of the extremity. In: Enneking WF (ed) Lung salvage in musculoskeletal oncology. Churchill Livingstone, New York

Gebhardt MC, Goorin AM, Traina J et al. (1989) Long-term results of limb salvage and amputation in extremity osteosarcoma: DFCI/TCH results in patients receiving postoperative weekly high-dose methotrexate and doxorubicin. In: Yamamuro T (ed) New developments for limb salvage in musculoskeletal tumors. Springer, Tokyo

Gebhardt MC, Roth YF, Mankin HJ (1990) Osteoarticular allografts for reconstruction in the proximal part of the humerus after excision of a musculoskeletal tumor. J Bone Joint Surg [Am] 72:334–345

Gehan EA, Sutow WW, Uribe-Botero G et al. (1978) Osteosarcoma: the MD Anderson experience, 1950–1974. Prog Cancer Res Ther 6:271–282

Gitelis S, Piasecki P (1991) Allograft prosthetic composite arthroplasty for osteosarcoma and other aggressive bone tumors. Clin Orthop 270:197–201

Goorin AM, Deloney M, Gelber R et al. (1985) Dana Farber Cancer Institute/The Children's Hospital adjuvant chemotherapy trials for osteosarcoma. Three sequential studies. Cancer Treat Symp 3:155–159

Gottlieb JA, Baker LH, O'Bryan RM et al. (1975) Adriamycin (NSC-123127) used alone and in combination with soft tissue and bone sarcoma. Cancer Chemother Rep 3:271–282

Han M, Telander R, Pairolero PC et al. (1981) Aggressive thoracotomy for pulmonary metastatic osteogenic sarcoma in children and young adolescents. J Pediatr Surg 16:928

Head WC, Berklacich FM, Malinin T, Emerson RH (1987) Proximal femoral allografts in revision total hip arthroplasty. Clin Orthop 225:22–36

Jaffe N (1972) Recent advances in the chemotherapy of metastatic osteogenic sarcoma. Cancer 30:1627–1631

Jaffe N, Farber S, Traggis D et al. (1973) Favorable response of metastatic osteogenic sarcoma to pulse high dose methotrexate with citrovorum rescue and radiation therapy. Cancer 31:1367–1373

Jaffe N, Frei E III, Traggis D et al. (1974) Adjuvant methotrexate and citrovorum factor treatment of osteogenic sarcoma. N Engl J Med 291:994–997

Jaffe N, Frei E III, Watts H, Traggis D (1978a) High-dose methotrexate in osteogenic sarcoma: a 5-year experience. Cancer Treat Rep 62:259–264

Jaffe N, Watts H, Fellows KE et al. (1978b) Local en bloc resection for limb preservation. Cancer Treat Rep 62:217–273
Jaffe N, Link M, Cohen D et al. (1981) High dose methotrexate in osteogenic sarcoma. In: Sarcomas of soft tissue and bone in childhood. NCI Monogr 56:201–206
Jofe MH, Gebhardt MC, Tomford WW, Mankin HJ (1988) Reconstruction for defects of the proximal part of the femur using allograft arthroplasty. J Bone Joint Surg [Am] 70:507–516
Juvara E (1921) Procédé de résection de la partie supérieure du tibia avec substitution, á la partie enlevée d'une grèffe prélevée sur le fémur. Presse Med 29:241
Katzner M, Schwingt E (1982) Etude de 100 arthroplasties totales de hanche avec mégaprothèse fémorale réalisées après reséction étendues de l'extrémité supérieure du fémur. Int Orthop 6:233–241
Khong KS, Chao EYS, Sim FH (1989) Long-term performance of custom prosthetic replacement for neoplastic disease of the proximal femur. In: Yamamuro T (ed) New developments for limb salvage in musculoskeletal oncology. Springer, Tokyo
Kotz R, Salzer M (1982) Rotation-plasty for childhood osteosarcoma of the distal part of the femur. J Bone Joint Surg [Am] 64:959–969
Kotz R, Winkler K, Salzer-Kuntschik M et al. (1989) Surgical margins influencing oncological results in osteosarcoma. In: Yamamuro T (ed) New developments for limb salvage in musculoskeletal tumors. Springer, Tokyo
Lewis MM (1986) The use of an expandable and adjustable prosthesis in the treatment of childhood malignant bone tumors of the extremity. Cancer 57:499–502
Lewis MM, Chekofsky KM (1982) Proximal femur replacement for neoplastic disease. Clin Orthop 171:72–79
Linberg BE (1928) Interscapulo-thoracic resection for malignant tumors of the shoulder region. J Bone Joint Surg 10:344
Link MP, Goorin AM, Miser AW et al. (1986) The effect of adjuvant chemotherapy on relapse-free survival in patients with osteosarcoma of the extremity. N Engl J Med 314:1600–1616
Makley JT (1985) The use of allograft to reconstruct intercalary defects of long bones. Clin Orthop 197:58–75
Malawar MM (1991) Tumors of the shoulder girdle: technique of resection and description of a surgical classification. In: Limb salvage in the treatment of musculoskeletal tumors. Orthop Clin North Am 22:7–35
Malawar MM, McHale KA (1989) Limb sparing surgery for high grade malignant tumors of the proximal tibia. Clin Orthop 239:231–248
Mankin HJ, Doppelt SH, Sullivan TR, Tomford WW (1982) Osteoarticular and intercalary allograft transplantation in the management of malignant tumors of bone. Cancer 50:613–630
Mankin HJ, Gebhardt MC, Tomford WW (1987) Use of frozen cadaveric osteoarticular allografts in the treatment of benign and malignant tumors about the knee. In: Enneking WF (ed) Limb salvage in musculoskeletal oncology. Churchill Livingstone, New York
Marcove RC, Lewis MM, Huvos AG (1977) En bloc upper humeral interscapulo-thoracic resection: the Tikhoff-Linberg Procedure. Clin Orthop 124:219–228
McDonald DJ, Capanna R, Gherlinzoni F, Campanacci M (1990) Complications of limb salvage surgery of the extremities. Cancer 65:1509–1516
Merle D'Aubigné R, Dejouany JP (1958) Diaphysoepiphysial resection for bone tumor at the knee. J Bone Joint Surg [Br] 40:385
Meyer WH, Schell MJ, Kumar APM et al. (1987) Thoracotomy for pulmonary metastatic osteosarcoma. Cancer 59:374
Mike V, Marcove RC (1978) Osteogenic sarcoma under the age of 21: experience at Memorial Sloan-Kettering Cancer Center. Prog Cancer Res Ther 6:283–292
Murray MP, Jacobs PA, Gore DR (1985) Functional performance after tibial rotationplasty. J Bone Joint Surg [Am] 67:392
Nieder E, Keller A (1989) The saddle prosthesis Mark II, Endo-Modell. In: Yamamuro T (ed) New developments for limb salvage in musculoskeletal tumors. Springer, Tokyo
Nieder E, Elson RA, Engelbrecht E et al. (1990) The saddle prosthesis for salvage of the destroyed acetabulum. J Bone Joint Surg [Br] 72:1014–1022
O'Connor MI, Sim FH (1989) Salvage of the limb in the treatment of malignant pelvic tumors. J Bone Joint Surg [Am] 71:481–494
Ochs JJ, Freeman AI, Douglass HO Jr et al. (1978) Cisdiammine-dichloroplatinum (II) in advanced osteogenic sarcoma. Cancer Treat Rep 62:239–245
Picci P, Bacci G, Campanacci M et al. (1985) Histologic evaluation of necrosis in osteosarcoma induced by chemotherapy. Cancer 56:1515–1521
Pratt CB, Champion JE, Senzer N et al. (1985) Treatment of unresectable or metastatic osteosarcoma with cisplatin or cisplatin doxorubicin. Cancer 56:1930–1933
Putnam JB Jr, Roth JA, Wesley NM et al. (1983) Survival following aggressive resection of pulmonary metastases from osteogenic sarcoma: analysis of prognostic factors. Ann Thorac Surg 36:516
Rock M (1987) Intercalary allograft and custom Neer prosthesis after en bloc resection of the proximal humerus. In: Enneking WF (ed) Limb salvage in musculoskeletal oncology. Churchill Livingstone, New York
Rosen G (1985) Preoperative (neoadjuvant) chemotherapy for osteogenic sarcoma: a ten year experience. Orthopedics 8:659–664
Rosen G, Tefft M, Martinez A et al. (1975) Combination chemotherapy and radiation therapy in the treatment of metastatic osteogenic sarcoma. Cancer 35:622–630
Rosen G, Murphy ML, Huvos A et al. (1976) Chemotherapy, en bloc resection and prosthesis bone replacement in the treatment of osteogenic sarcoma. Cancer 37:1–11
Rosen G, Caparros B, Huvos AG et al. (1982) Preoperative chemotherapy for osteogenic sarcoma: selection of postoperative adjuvant chemotherapy based on the response of the primary tumor to preoperative chemotherapy. Cancer 49:1221–1230
Rosenberg SA, Chabner BA, Young RC et al. (1979) Treatment of osteogenic sarcoma. I. Effect of adjuvant high-dose methotrexate after amputation. Cancer Treat Rep 63:739–751

Sim FH, Chao EYS (1987) Segmental prosthetic replacement of the knee after tumor resection. In: Enneking WF (ed) Limb salvage in musculoskeletal oncology. Churchill Livingstone, New York

Sim FH, Chao EYS, Pritchard DJ, Salzer M (1980) Replacement of the proximal humerus with a ceramic prosthesis: a preliminary report. Clin Orthop 146:161–174

Sim FH, Ivins JC, Taylor WF, Chao EYS (1985) Limb-sparing surgery for osteosarcoma: Mayo Clinic experience. Cancer Treat Symp 3:139–154

Simon MA, Aschliman MA, Thomas N, Mankin HJ (1986) Limb-salvage treatment versus amputation for osteosarcoma of the distal end of the femur. J Bone Joint Surg [Am] 68:1331–1337

Taylor WF, Ivins JC, Dahlin DC et al. (1978) Trends and variability in survival from osteosarcoma. Mayo Clin Proc 53:695–700

Telander RL, Pairolero PC, Pritchard DJ et al. (1978) Resection of pulmonary metastatic osteogenic sarcoma in children. Surgery 84:335

Tomita K, Tsuchiya H (1989) Intermediate results and functional evaluation of limb-salvage surgery for osteosarcoma: an intergroup study in Japan. J Surg Oncol 42:71–76

Ueda T, Uchida A, Yoshikawa H et al. (1989) Surgical management of osteosarcoma in extremities: survival between limb salvage and amputation. In: Yamamuro T (ed) New developments for limb salvage in musculoskeletal tumors. Springer, Tokyo

Van Nes CP (1950) Rotation-plasty for congenital defects of the femur. Making use of the ankle of the shortened limb to control the knee joint of a prosthesis. J Bone Joint Surg [Br] 32:1–16

Watts HG (1980) Introduction to resection of musculoskeletal sarcomas. Clin Orthop 153:31–38

Winkler K, Beron G, Kotz R et al. (1984) Neoadjuvant chemotherapy for osteogenic sarcoma: results of cooperative German-Austrian study. J Clin Oncol 2:318–325

Winkler K, Beron G, Dellinger G et al. (1988) Neoadjuvant chemotherapy of osteosarcoma: results of a randomized cooperative trial (COSS-82) with salvage chemotherapy based on histological tumor response. J Clin Oncol 6:329–337

Yasko AW, Lane JM (1991) Chemotherapy for bone and soft-tissue sarcomas of the extremities. Current concepts review. J Bone Joint Surg [Am] 73:1263–1271

Ewing Sarcoma

Bacci G, Picci P, Gitelis S et al. (1982) The treatment of localized Ewing's sarcoma: the experience at the Istituto Ortopedico Rizzoli in 163 cases treated with and without adjuvant chemotherapy. Cancer 49:1561–1570

Bacci G, Picci P, Gherlinzoni F et al. (1985) Localized Ewing's sarcoma of bone: ten years' experience at the Istituto Ortopedico Rizzoli in 124 cases treated with multimodal therapy. Eur J Cancer Clin Oncol 24:163–173

Bacci G, Toni A, Avella M et al. (1989) Long-term results in 144 localized Ewing's sarcoma patients treated with combined therapy. Cancer 63:1477–1486

Capanna R, Toni A, Sudanese A et al. (1990) Ewing's sarcoma of the pelvis. Int Orthop 14:57–61

Evans R, Nesbit M, Askin F et al. (1985) Local recurrence, rate and sites of metastases, and time to relapse as a function of treatment regimen, size of primary and surgical history in 62 patients presenting with non-metastatic Ewing's sarcoma of the pelvic bones. Int J Radiat Oncol Biol Phys 11:129–136

Falk S, Alpert M (1967) Five-year survival of patients with Ewing's sarcoma. Surg Gynecol Obstet 23:319–324

Jurgens H, Exner U, Gadner H et al. (1988) Multidisciplinary treatment of primary Ewing's sarcoma of bone: a 6-year experience of a European cooperative trial. Cancer 61:23–32

Li WK, Lane JM, Rosen G et al. (1983) Pelvic Ewing's sarcoma: advances in treatment. J Bone Joint Surg [Am] 65:738–747

Nesbit ME Jr, Perez CA, Tefft M et al. (1981) Multimodal therapy for the management of primary, nonmetastatic Ewing's sarcoma of bone: an intergroup study. NCI Monogr 56:255

Phillips RF, Higinbotham NL (1967) The curability of Ewing's endothelioma of bone in children. J Pediatr 70:391–397

Pritchard DJ, Dahlin DC, Dauphine RT et al. (1975) Ewing's sarcoma: a clinicopathological and statistical analysis of patients surviving five years or longer. J Bone Joint Surg [Am] 57:10–16

Rosen G, Caparros B, Nirenberg A et al. (1981) Ewing's sarcoma: ten-year experience with adjuvant chemotherapy. Cancer 47:2204–2213

Sailer SL, Harmon DC, Mankin HJ et al. (1988) Ewing's sarcoma: surgical resection as a prognostic factor. Int J Radiat Oncol Biol Phys 15:43–52

Sauer R, Jurgens J, Burgers JM et al. (1987) Prognostic factors in the treatment of Ewing's sarcoma. The Ewing's Sarcoma Study Group of the German Society of Paediatric Oncology CESS 81. Radiother Oncol 10:101–110

Telles NC, Rabson AS, Pomeroy TC (1978) Ewing's sarcoma: an autopsy study. Cancer 41:2321–2329

Tepper J, Glanbiger D, Lichter A et al. (1980) Local control of Ewing's sarcoma of bone with radiotherapy and combination chemotherapy. Cancer 46:1669–1673

Thomas PRM, Perez CA, Neff JR et al. (1984) The management of Ewing's sarcoma: role of radiotherapy in local tumor control. Cancer Treat Rep 68:703

Wilkins RM, Pritchard DJ, Burgert EO, Unni KK (1986) Ewing's sarcoma of bone: experience with 140 patients. Cancer 58:2551–2555

Subject Index

MIX
Papier aus verantwortungsvollen Quellen
Paper from responsible sources
FSC® C105338

If you have any concerns about our products,
you can contact us on
ProductSafety@springernature.com

In case Publisher is established outside the EU,
the EU authorized representative is:
Springer Nature Customer Service Center GmbH
Europaplatz 3, 69115 Heidelberg, Germany

Printed by Libri Plureos GmbH
in Hamburg, Germany